The
5-Minute
Urology
Consult

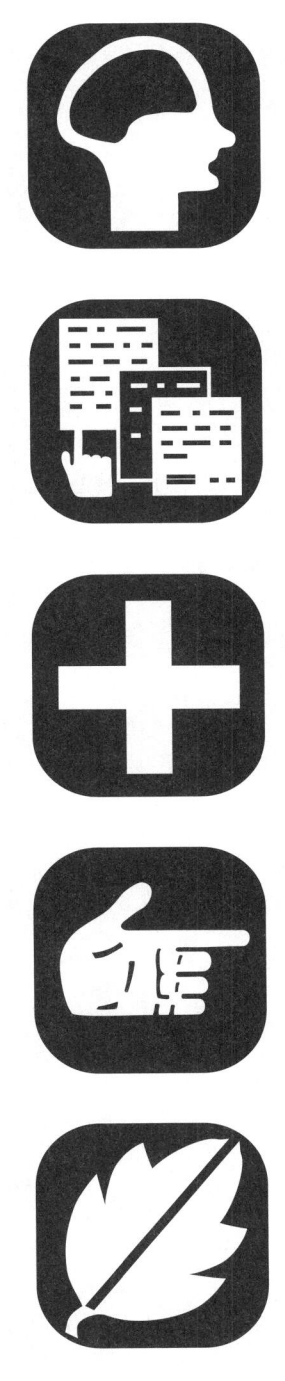
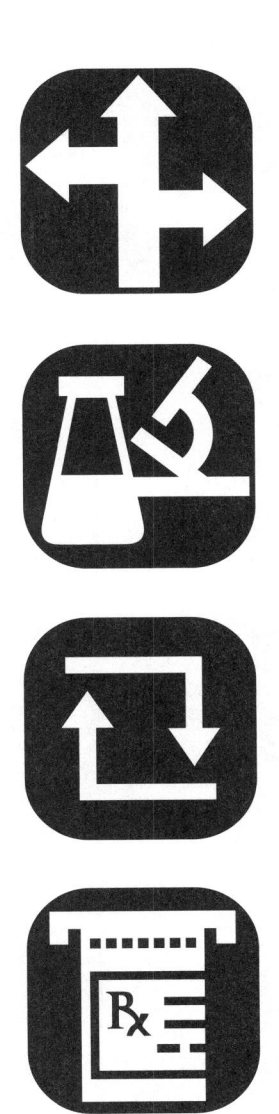

The
5-Minute
Urology
Consult

EDITOR

LEONARD G. GOMELLA, M.D., F.A.C.S

*THE BERNARD W. GODWIN, JR. ASSOCIATE
PROFESSOR OF PROSTATE CANCER*

DEPARTMENT OF UROLOGY

JEFFERSON MEDICAL COLLEGE

DIRECTOR OF UROLOGIC ONCOLOGY

KIMMEL CANCER CENTER

PHILADELPHIA, PENNSYLVANIA

CONSULTING EDITOR

MARK R. DAMBRO, M.D., F.A.A.F.P.

FORMERLY ASSISTANT PROFESSOR OF MEDICINE

DIRECTOR OF MEDICAL COMPUTING

UNIVERSITY OF ARIZONA

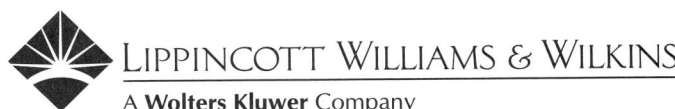
LIPPINCOTT WILLIAMS & WILKINS
A **Wolters Kluwer** Company
Philadelphia • Baltimore • New York • London
Buenos Aires • Hong Kong • Sydney • Tokyo

Associate Editor: Anne M. Sydor
Developmental Editors: Mildred G. Ramos and Andrea Allison-Williams
Manufacturing Manager: Kevin Watt
Supervising Editor: Mary Ann McLaughlin
Production Service: Colophon
Compositor: The PRD Group, Inc.
Printer: R.R. Donnelley Crawfordsville

© 2000 by LIPPINCOTT WILLIAMS & WILKINS
530 Walnut St.
Philadelphia, PA 19106
lww.com

Printed in the USA

Library of Congress Cataloging-in-Publication Data

The 5-minute urology consult / editor, Leonard G. Gomella.
        p. ; cm.
    Includes bibliographical references and index.
    ISBN 0-7817-2284-5 (alk. paper)
    1. Urology—Handbooks, manuals, etc.   2. Urinary organs—Diseases—Handbooks, manuals, etc.   I. Title: 5 minute urology consult.   II. Title: Five minute urology consult.
III. Gomella, Leonard G.
    [DNLM: 1. Urologic Diseases—Handbooks.   WJ 39 Z999 2000]
    RC872.9 .A14   2000
    616.6—dc21
                                                                    00-022180

Care has been taken to confirm the accuracy of the information presented and to describe generally accepted practices. However, the authors, editors, and publisher are not responsible for errors or omissions or for any consequences from application of the information in this book and make no warranty, expressed or implied, with respect to the currency, completeness, or accuracy of the contents of the publication. Application of this information in a particular situation remains the professional responsibility of the practitioner.

The authors, editors, and publisher have exerted every effort to ensure that drug selection and dosage set forth in this text are in accordance with current recommendations and practice at the time of publication. However, in view of ongoing research, changes in government regulations, and the constant flow of information relating to drug therapy and drug reactions, the reader is urged to check the package insert for each drug for any change in indications and dosage and for added warnings and precautions. This is particularly important when the recommended agent is a new or infrequently employed drug.

Some drugs and medical devices presented in this publication have Food and Drug Administration (FDA) clearance for limited use in restricted research settings. It is the responsibility of health care providers to ascertain the FDA status of each drug or device planned for use in their clinical practice.

10 9 8 7 6 5 4

TO

Tricia, Leonard, Patrick, Andrew, Michael, and my parents for their understanding and encouragement.

"El la tierra de los ciegos el tuerto es rey."

Preface

It is with great pride that I present the first edition of *The 5-Minute Urology Consult*. The goal of this book is to provide the reader with useful information in a quick reference format to help with the everyday care of patients with urologic problems. While written primarily for urologists, any health care practitioner who deals with urologic complaints and conditions should find the book useful. Students of urology and residents preparing for oral and written in-service and certification exams will find the book a useful study aid.

The topics addressed in this book are based on reviews of published literature, major textbooks, grand grounds case presentations, and actual patient consultations. Coverage includes adult and pediatric urology, as well as all subspecialty areas.

The organization of the book provides information on presenting problems, specific conditions, and new drug and lab reference data. Section I gives information on presenting urologic problems and a logical framework for initial management. Section II identifies specific urologic diseases and conditions in both adult and pediatric patients. Section III addresses brief topics of clinical importance. The remaining sections are references for diagnostic urine studies, common medications, alternative therapies, and other frequently needed reference data. The medication section is unique in that it presents additional urologic applications not often found on the package insert for "off label" indications commonly used in daily care. These "off label" applications are based on literature and the personal observations of the authors and editors.

In any project of this magnitude, there are many individuals responsible for its success. Carroll Cann provided the initial encouragement to proceed with a formal proposal for the book in 1996 and brought forth his extraordinary insight into what it takes to design a successful "5-Minute Clinical Consult" book. Dr. Mark Dambro, currently the masterful editor of the popular parent book known as *The 5-Minute Clinical Consult,* freely shared his secrets for success and serves as a consulting editor on this book. The general framework for his book design is followed with modifications that are more specific for a surgical discipline such as urology. Craig Percy, a long-time friend and colleague in the medical publishing arena, assumed the role of acquisitions editor after Lippincott Williams & Wilkins joined forces. His unique insight into what it takes to make the medical publisher-physician author interface a mutually beneficial activity is deeply appreciated.

Jennifer Wachter, Samantha Bruno, Denise Markham, and Melinda Lord provided administrative support to keep the project organized. My special thanks to the over 280 authors and editors who took the time to contribute to this effort. Anne Sydor, Peg Latham, Mary Ann McLaughlin, and the entire staff at Lippincott Williams & Wilkins went to extraordinary measures to move the publishing process along to meet certain critical deadlines, and for these efforts I am very grateful.

Lastly, I would like to thank my wife, Tricia, and my children, Leonard, Patrick, Andrew, and Michael, for allowing me to sacrifice my time with them at nights, weekends, and holidays to complete "the book."

Please contact me if you have suggestions for future editions of the book. I hope that *The 5-Minute Urology Consult* will provide useful information to allow all of us to care for our patients in the best way possible.

Leonard G. Gomella, M.D.
leonard.gomella@mail.tsu.edu

Contributing Authors

GREG ADEY, B.S.
Jefferson Medical College
Philadelphia, PA

HOWARD L. ADLER, M.D.
Assistant Professor
Department of Urology
State University of New York at Stony Brook
Stony Brook, NY

DAVID M. ALBALA, M.D.
Director of Endourology and Minimally Invasive Surgery
Professor, Department of Urology
Loyola Medical Center
Maywood, IL

RICHARD B. ALEXANDER, M.D.
Associate Professor
Department of Urology
University of Maryland
Baltimore, MD

MIHAI ALEXIANU, M.D.
Chief Resident
Department of Urology
Long Island Jewish Medical Center
New Hyde Park, NY

KEVIN R. ANDERSON, M.D.
Associate Professor
Department of Surgery
Yale University
New Haven, CT

GERALD ANDRIOLE, M.D.
Chief
Division of Urologic Surgery
Washington University
St. Louis, MO

CORLIS L. ARCHER, M.D.
Resident
Department of Urology
SUNY Health Science Center
Syracuse University Hospital
Syracuse, NY

ANTHONY ATALA, M.D.
Associate Professor
Department of Surgery
Harvard Medical School
Boston, MA

MARK S. AUSTENFELD, M.D.
Associate Clinical Professor
Department of Urology
Kansas University
Kansas City, KS

GOPAL H. BADLANI, M.D.
Professor of Urology
Department of Urology
Albert Einstein College of Medicine
New Hyde Park, NY

DEMETRIUS H. BAGLEY, M.D.
Professor of Urology and Radiology
Department of Urology
Thomas Jefferson Medical College
Philadelphia, PA

ROBERT R. BAHNSON, M.D.
Louis Levy Professor and Director
Division of Urology
Ohio State University
Columbus, OH

KEVIN BAN, M.D.
Medical Correspondent
ABC News
New York, NY

NATHALIE M. BARNES, M.D.
Resident
Department of Urology
University of California–San Francisco
San Francisco, CA

LAURENCE S. BASKIN, M.D.
Chief, Pediatric Urology
Department of Urology
University of California
San Francisco, CA

ASHOK K. BATRA, M.D., F.A.C.S.
Associate Professor
Department of Urology
SUNY Health Science Center
Syracuse, NY

STEPHEN D. W. BECK, M.D.
Resident
Department of Urology
Indiana University
Indianapolis, IN

JOHN A. BELIS, M.D.
Professor
Department of Urology
Penn State College of Medicine
Hershey, PA

ARIE S. BELLDEGRUN, M.D.
Professor
Department of Urology
UCLA School of Medicine
Los Angeles, CA

MICHAEL R. BERNSTEIN, M.D.
Division of Urology
West Jersey Health System
Voorhees, NJ

CHARLES D. BEST, M.D.
Resident
Department of Urology
Stanford University
Stanford, CA

JONATHAN D. BLOCK, M.D.
Chief Resident
Division of Urology
Albany Medical Center Hospital
Albany, NY

DAVID A. BLOOM, M.D.
Chief of Pediatric Urology
Department of Pediatric Urology
The University of Michigan Medical Center
Ann Arbor, MI

TIMOTHY B. BOONE, M.D., Ph.D.
Associate Professor
Scott Department of Urology
Baylor College of Medicine
Houston, TX

DARREN D. BRAY, B.S.
School of Medicine
Loma Linda University
Loma Linda, CA

ROBERT R. BYRNE, M.D.
Senior Urology Resident
Division of Urology
Duke University Medical Center
Durham, NC

DOUGLAS A. CANNING, M.D.
Associate Professor
Department of Urology
University of Pennsylvania School of Medicine
Philadelphia, PA

PETER R. CARROLL, M.D.
Professor and Chair
Department of Urology
University of California at San Francisco
San Francisco, CA

CULLEY C. CARSON III, M.D.
Professor and Chief
Department of Urology
University of North Carolina
Chapel Hill, NC

ANTHONY J. CASALE, M.D.
Associate Professor
Department of Urology
Indiana University
Indianapolis, IN

PASQUALE CASALE, M.D.
Resident
Department of Urology
Thomas Jefferson University
Philadelphia, PA

MICHAEL B. CHANCELLOR, M.D.
Associate Professor
Department of Urology
University of Pittsburgh School of Medicine
Pittsburgh, PA

MARK CHANG, B.S.
Thomas Jefferson University
Cherry Hill, NJ

SAM S. CHANG, M.D.
Resident
Department of Urology
Vanderbilt University Medical Center
Nashville, TN

GREGORY L. CHEN, M.D.
Fellow in Endourology
Thomas Jefferson University
Philadelphia, PA

ALLEN N. CHIURA, M.D.
Chief Resident in Urology
Thomas Jefferson University
Philadelphia, PA

BENJAMIN CHUNG, M.D.
Resident
Department of Urology
Lahey Clinic
Burlington, MA

TODD D. COHEN, M.D.
Assistant Professor
Department of Urology
Ohio State University
Columbus, OH

JOHN W. COLBERG, M.D.
Assistant Professor of Surgery
Section of Urology
Yale School of Medicine
New Haven, CT

MICHAEL J. CONLIN, M.D.
Assistant Professor
Department of Surgery/Urology
Oregon Health Sciences University
Portland, OR

MICHAEL SHAWN COOKSON, M.D.
Assistant Professor
Department of Urologic Surgery
Vanderbilt University
Nashville, TN

BENJAMIN N. CORN, M.D.
Former Vice Chairman
Department of Radiation Oncology
Thomas Jefferson University
Philadelphia, PA

MARLENE CORUJO, M.D.
Resident
Department of Urology
Long Island Jewish Medical Center
New Hyde Park, NY

MICHAEL CRAM, M.D.
Assistant Professor of Clinical Urology
Ohio State University
Columbus, OH

E. DAVID CRAWFORD, M.D.
Professor
Department of Surgery/Radiation Oncology
University of Colorado
Denver, CO

AKHIL DAS, M.D.
Assistant Professor
Department of Urology
New York Medical College
Valhalla, NY

SAKTI DAS, M.D., F.A.C.S., F.R.C.S.
Professor
Department of Urology
University of California
Davis Medical Center
Sacramento, CA ·

GREGORY E. DEAN, M.D.
Assistant Professor
Department of Surgery and Pediatrics
University of Medicine and Dentistry of New Jersey
Robert Wood Johnson Medical School at Camden
Camden, NJ

MICHAEL G. DESAUTEL, M.D.
Resident
Department of Urology
Long Island Jewish Medical Center
New Hyde Park, NY

CHRISTOPHER M. DIXON, M.D.
Assistant Professor of Urology
New York University Medical Center
New York, NY

CRAIG F. DONATUCCI, M.D.
Associate Professor
Department of Surgery
Duke University
Durham, NC

JAMES FRANCIS DONOVAN, JR., M.D.
Professor of Urology
Department of Urology
University of Oklahoma Health Sciences Center
Oklahoma City, OK

EHAB A. EL-GABRY, M.D.
Fellow, Urologic Oncology
Thomas Jefferson University
Philadelphia, PA

JOHN B. ELLSWORTH, M.D.
Chief Resident
Urology Service
Oregon Health Sciences Center
Portland, OR

PAMELA I. ELLSWORTH, M.D.
Assistant Professor
Department of Surgery/Urology and Pediatrics
Dartmouth–Hitchcock Medical Center
Lebanon, NH

MICHAEL J. ERHARD, M.D.
Pediatric Urologist
Assistant Professor, Mayo Medical School
Nemours Children's Hospital
Jacksonville, FL

DEBORAH R. ERICKSON, M.D.
Associate Professor of Surgery
Department of Surgery
Division of Urology
Pennsylvania State University College of Medicine
Hershey, PA

MARK S. ERNSTOFF, M.D.
Professor of Medicine
Chief of Medical Oncology
Dartmouth–Hitchcock Medical Center
Lebanon, NH

GARY J. FAERBER, M.D.
Associate Professor
Department of Surgery, Section of Urology
University of Michigan
Ann Arbor, MI

MARK L. FALLICK, M.D.
Director
Department of Male Infertility
Center for Urologic Care
Voorhees, NJ

SURENA FAZELI-MATIN, M.D.
Resident
Department of Urology
Cleveland Clinic Foundation
Cleveland, OH

MARK R. FENELEY, M.D.
Fellow
James Buchanan Brady Urological Institute
Johns Hopkins Institutes
Baltimore, MD

T. ERNESTO FIGUEROA, M.D.
Assistant Professor
Department of Urology
Thomas Jefferson University
Philadelphia, PA

ROBERT BRUCE FILMER, M.B., B.S.
Associate Professor
Department of Urology
Thomas Jefferson University
Philadelphia, PA

LEONARD H. FINKELSTEIN, D.O.
Professor
Department of Surgery, Division of Urology
Philadelphia College of Osteopathic Medicine
Philadelphia, PA

HUGH A. G. FISHER, M.D.
Associate Professor of Surgery
Division of Urology
Albany Medical College
Albany, NY

KENNETH J. FITZPATRICK, M.D.
Attending Urologist
Department of Urology
Paoli Memorial Hospital
Paoli, PA

ROBERT C. FLANIGAN, M.D.
Professor
Albert J., Jr. and Clair R. Speh Chair of Urology
Department of Urology
Loyola University Medical Center
Maywood, IL

MITCHELL C. FRAIMAN, M.D.
Senior Resident
Department of Urology
New York University Medical Center
New York, NY

ISRAEL FRANCO, M.D., F.A.C.S., F.A.A.P.
Assistant Professor
Department of Urology and Pediatrics
New York Medical College
Valhalla, NY

LEONARD A. FRANK, M.D.
Clinical Assistant Professor
Department of Urology
Thomas Jefferson University
Philadelphia, PA

STEPHEN J. FREEDLAND, M.D.
Resident
Department of Urology
University of California, Los Angeles
Los Angeles, CA

ELI A. FRIEDMAN, M.D.
Distinguished Teaching Professor
Chief
Renal Disease Division
SUNY Health Science Center at Brooklyn
Brooklyn, NY

MICHAEL P. GARDNER, M.D.
Resident
Department of Urology
University of Utah
Salt Lake City, UT

CHRISTOPHER GARLITZ, M.D.
Resident
Department of Urology
Thomas Jefferson University
Philadelphia, PA

JOHN P. GEARHART, M.D.
Professor and Chief
Department of Urology
Johns Hopkins School of Medicine
Baltimore, MD

K. SHANE GEIB, M.D.
Resident
Department of Urology
The George Washington University
Washington, DC

VALAL KORUTHU GEORGE, M.D.
Resident
Department of Urology
Wayne State University
Detroit, MI

GLENN S. GERBER, M.D.
Associate Professor
Department of Surgery
University of Chicago
Chicago, IL

MATTHEW T. GETTMAN, M.D.
Fellow
Department of Pediatric Urology
Nemours Children's Hospital
Jacksonville, FL

INDERBIR S. GILL, M.D.
Head
Section of Laparoscopic and Minimally Invasive Surgery
Cleveland Clinic Foundation
Cleveland, OH

PHILLIP C. GINSBERG, D.O., J.D.
Clinical Professor
Department of Urology
Philadelphia College of Osteopathic Medicine
Philadelphia, PA

DEBORAH T. GLASSMAN, M.D.
Resident
Division of Urology
University of Maryland Medical System
Baltimore, MD

GLADYS M. GLENN, M.D., Ph.D.
Clinical Investigator
Genetic Epidemiology Branch
National Cancer Institute
Rockville, MD

JOEL D. GLICKMAN, M.D.
Clinical Associate Professor
Department of Medicine
University of Pennsylvania
Philadelphia, PA

LEONARD G. GOMELLA, M.D., F.A.C.S.
The Bernard W. Godwin, Jr. Associate Professor of Prostate Cancer
Department of Urology
Thomas Jefferson University
Philadelphia, PA

BRIAN GRADY, M.D.
Chief Resident
Department of Urology
University of California at San Francisco
San Francisco, CA

MICHAEL GRASSO, III, M.D.
Professor of Urology
New York University School of Medicine
New York, NY

RICHARD E. GREENBERG, M.D.
Clinical Professor of Urology
Department of Surgery
Temple University
Philadelphia, PA

B. MAYER GROB, M.D.
Assistant Professor
Department of Urology
SUNY Downstate Medical Center
Brooklyn, NY

MARKO GUDZIAK, M.D.
Associate Professor of Urology
Director of Incontinence Center of Michigan
Michigan Institute of Urology
Pontiac, MI

MANTU GUPTA, M.D.
Assistant Professor
Department of Urology
Columbia University
New York, NY

GABRIEL P. HAAS, M.D.
Professor and Chairman
Department of Urology
Upstate Medical University
Syracuse, NY

SHAHANDEH HAGHIR, M.D.
Resident
Department of Pathology
State University of New York at Syracuse
Syracuse, NY

M. CRAIG HALL, M.D.
Associate Professor of Urology
Wake Forest University School of Medicine
Charlotte, NC

DAVID M. HALL, M.D.
Resident
Department of Urology
West Virginia University
Morgantown, WV

BLAKE D. HAMILTON, M.D.
Assistant Professor
Division of Urology
University of Utah
Salt Lake City, UT

RICHARD C. HARKAWAY, M.D.
Clinical Assistant Professor
Department of Urology
Temple University Hospital
Philadelphia, PA

JOSEPH F. HARRYHILL, M.D.
Assistant Clinical Professor
Division of Urology
University of Pennsylvania School of Medicine
Philadelphia, PA

JOHN A. HEANEY, M.D., B.Ch., F.R.C.S.I.
Professor
Department of Surgery/Urology
Dartmouth Medical School
Hanover, NH

JEREMY P. W. HEATON, M.D.
Professor
Department of Urology
Queen's University
Kingston, ON, Canada

WAYNE J. G. HELLSTROM, M.D., F.A.C.S.
Professor of Urology
Department of Urology
Tulane University School of Medicine
New Orleans, LA

IRVIN H. HIRSCH, M.D.
Clinical Professor
Department of Urology
Jefferson Medical College
Philadelphia, PA

MARK HOFFMAN, M.D.
Division of Hematology/Oncology
Department of Medicine
Long Island Jewish Medical Center
New Hyde Park, NY

JEFFREY M. HOLZBEIERLEIN, M.D.
Chief Resident
Department of Urologic Surgery
Vanderbilt University Medical Center
Nashville, TN

DAVID HOM, M.D.
Resident
Department of Urology
Long Island Jewish Medical Center
New Hyde Park, NY

ROBERT D. HONG, M.D.
Clinical Instructor
Section of Urology
Milton S. Hershey Medical School
Hershey, PA

MARK HOROWITZ, M.D.
Assistant Professor
Department of Urology
Downstate Medical Center
Brooklyn, NY

THOMAS H. S. HSU, M.D.
Resident
Department of Urology
Cleveland Clinic
Cleveland, OH

ROBERT P. HUBEN, M.D.
Chief
Department of Urologic Oncology
Roswell Park Cancer Institute
Buffalo, NY

SCOTT HUBOSKY, M.D.
Resident
Department of Urology
Thomas Jefferson University
Philadelphia, PA

TODD C. IGEL, M.D.
Assistant Professor of Urology
Department of Urology
Mayo Medical School
Jacksonville, FL

PIERCE B. IRBY
Assistant Professor of Urology
Uniformed Services University
Walter Reed Army Medical Center
Washington, DC

MOHAMMED T. ISMAIL, M.D.
Resident
Department of Urology
Thomas Jefferson University
Philadelphia, PA

MARK V. JAROWENKO, M.D.
Associate Professor of Surgery
Department of Surgery
Section of Urology
The Pennsylvania State University
The Milton S. Hershey Medical Center
Hershey, PA

JAVID JAVIDAN, M.D.
Resident
Department of Urology
Henry Ford Health System and Josephine Ford Cancer Center
Detroit, MI

V. KEITH JIMENEZ, M.D.
Resident
Division of Urology
Emory University
Atlanta, GA

GERALD H. JORDAN, M.D.
Professor of Urology
Department of Urology
Eastern Virginia Medical School
Norfolk, VA

BYRON D. JOYNER, M.D.
Chief
Department of Pediatric Urology
Madigan Army Medical Center
Tacoma, WA

SUK YOUNG JUNG, M.D.
Fellow
Department of Neuro-Urology and Female Urology
University of Pittsburgh School of Medicine
Pittsburgh, PA

ASHISH M. KAMAT, M.D.
Chief Resident
Department of Urology
West Virginia University
Morgantown, WV

RONALD P. KAUFMAN, JR., M.D.
Associate Professor of Surgery
Assistant Professor of Physiology and Cell Biology
Division of Urology
Albany Medical College
Albany, NY

SANKAR J. KAUSIK, M.D.
Resident
Department of Urology
Mayo Clinic Rochester
Rochester, MN

THOMAS E. KEANE, M.B., F.R.C.S.I., F.A.C.S.
Associate Professor
Department of Urology
Emory University
Atlanta, GA

MICHAEL C. KEARNEY, M.D.
Resident
Department of Urology
Columbia University College of Physicians and Surgeons
New York, NY

LOUIS L. KEELER III, M.D.
Director, Oncology Services
Department of Surgery (Urology)
Virtua-West Jersey Health System
Voorhees, NJ

FRANCIS XAVIER KEELEY, JR., M.D., F.R.C.S.
Consulting Urologist
Department of Urology
Bristol Urological Institute
Bristol, England

FERNANDO J. KIM, M.D.
Chief Resident
Department of Urology
Loyola University Medical Center
Stritch School of Medicine
Maywood, IL

ERIC A. KLEIN, M.D.
Head, Section of Urologic Oncology
Department of Urology
Cleveland Clinic Foundation
Cleveland, OH

LAURENCE KLOTZ, M.D.
Associate Professor
Department of Urology
University of Toronto
Toronto, ON, Canada

CARL G. KLUTKE, M.D.
Associate Professor
Department of Surgery, Division of Urology
Washington University School of Medicine
St. Louis, MO

MICHAEL O. KOCH, M.D.
Professor and Chairman
Department of Urology
Indiana University
Indianapolis, IN

FERNANDO C. KOLESKI, M.D.
Fellow
Department of Urology
Loyola University
Maywood, IL

MARK E. KOLLIGIAN, M.D.
Attending Pediatric Urologist
Clinical Assistant Professor of Urology
Department of Urology
Long Island Jewish Medical Center
Great Neck, NY

ARNON KONGRAD, M.D.
Director, South Florida Prostate Cancer Project
Investigator, The Stein Gerontological Institute
Geriatric Research Education and Clinical Center
Miami, FL

HARRY P. KOO, M.D.
Assistant Professor of Surgery
Department of Surgery, Section of Urology
University of Michigan Medical School
Ann Arbor, MI

EVAN B. KRISCH, M.D.
Assistant Professor of Surgery
Division of Urology
Robert Wood Johnson University Hospital System—Cooper Hospital
Camden, NJ

ELROY D. KURSH, M.D.
Urology Staff
Department of Urology
Cleveland Clinic Foundation
Cleveland, OH

ERIC A. KURZROCK, M.D.
Assistant Professor
Department of Urology
U. C. Davis School of Medicine
Sacramento, CA

YEGAPPAN LAKSHMANAN, M.D.
Resident
Department of Urology
University of Massachusetts Medical Center
Worcester, MA

RAYMOND S. LANCE, M.D.
Attending Urologist
Department of Surgery, Division of Urology
Madigan Army Medical Center
Tacoma, WA

JOHN P. LAVELLE, M.D.
Visiting Instructor/AFUD Scholar
Department of Urology
University of Pittsburgh
Pittsburgh, PA

MICHAEL A. LAWRENCE, M.D.
Chief Resident
Department of Urology
University of Southern California
Los Angeles, CA

GREGORY R. J. LEAL, M.D.
Resident
Department of Urology
Eastern VA Medical School
Norfolk, VA

DAVID LEE, M.D.
Resident
Department of Urology
Thomas Jefferson University
Philadelphia, PA

JAY LEE, M.D.
Resident
Department of Urology
Queen's University
Kingston General Hospital
Kingston, ON, Canada

W. MARSTON LINEHAN, M.D.
Chief
Urologic Oncology Branch
National Cancer Institute
Bethesda, MD

LOUIS S. LIOU, M.D.
Resident
Department of Urology
Cleveland Clinic Foundation
Cleveland Heights, OH

KEVIN R. LOUGHLIN, M.D.
Professor
Department of Surgery (Urology)
Harvard Medical School
Boston, MA

FRANKLIN C. LOWE, M.D.
Associate Professor of Clinical Urology
Department of Urology
Columbia University, College of Physicians and Surgeons
New York, NY

JEFFREY H. LUMERMAN, M.D.
Assistant Attending Physician
Department of Urology
Long Island Jewish Medical Center
New Hyde Park, NY

DONALD F. LYNCH, JR., M.D.
Professor
Department of Urology
Eastern Virginia School of Medicine
Norfolk, VA

JOHN H. LYNCH, M.D.
Professor and Interim Chairman
Department of Surgery
Division of Urology
Georgetown University School of Medicine
Washington, DC

RICHARD J. MACCHIA, M.D.
Professor and Chair
Department of Urology
State University of New York
Downstate Medical School
Brooklyn, NY

JOHN B. MAGGIONCALDA, M.D.
Resident
Department of Urology
University of Medicine and Dentistry of New Jersey
Camden, NJ

S. BRUCE MALKOWICZ, M.D.
Associate Professor
Department of Urology
University of Pennsylvania School of Medicine
Philadelphia, PA

MICHAEL J. MANYAK, M.D.
Professor of Urology
Acting Chairman
Department of Urology
The George Washington University Medical Center
Washington, DC

JOEL L. MARMAR, M.D.
Professor of Urology
Robert Wood Johnson Medical School at Camden
University of Medicine and Dentistry of New Jersey
Camden, NJ

JONATHAN F. MASOUDI, M.D.
Chief Resident
Department of Urology
University of Pennsylvania
Philadelphia, PA

WILLIAM M. McCORMACK, M.D.
Professor
Department of Medicine
Downstate Medical Center
Brooklyn, NY

DAVID E. McGINNIS, M.D.
Clinical Assistant Professor of Urology
Department of Urology
Thomas Jefferson University
Philadelphia, PA

MICHEL S. McGUIRE, M.D.
Assistant Professor of Urology
Northwestern University
Chicago, IL

DAVID G. McLEOD, M.D.
Professor
Department of Surgery
Uniformed Services University
Bethesda, MD

LEAH PEREZ McMANN, M.D.
Staff Physician
Department of Family Practice
Madigan Army Medical Center
Tacoma, WA

J. WILLIAM McROBERTS, M.D.
Professor and Chief
Department of Surgery (Pediatric Urology)
University of Kentucky
Lexington, KY

BRETT C. MELLINGER, M.D.
Associate Professor of Clinical Urology
Department of Urology
State University of New York at Stony Brook
Stony Brook, NY

MANI MENON, M.D.
Professor
Department of Urology
Case Western Reserve University
Cleveland, OH

PAUL A. MERGUERIAN, M.D.
Associate Professor
Division of Urology
Hospital for Sick Children
University of Toronto
Toronto, ON, Canada

EMILIO MERLINI, M.D.
Chief, Section of Pediatric Urology
Department of Pediatric Surgical Sciences
"C. Arrigo" Children's Hospital
Alessandria, Italy

EDWARD M. MESSING, M.D.
W. W. Scott Professor and Chairman
Department of Urology
University of Rochester School of Medicine
Rochester, NY

BADAR M. MIAN, M.D.
Resident
Department of Urology
Medical College of Virginia
Richmond, VA

DOUGLAS F. MILAM, M.D.
Assistant Professor
Urologic Surgery
Vanderbilt University
Nashville, TN

JAMES L. MOHLER, M.D.
Associate Professor
Division of Urology
University of North Carolina at Chapel Hill
Chapel Hill, NC

ROBERT M. MOLDWIN
Assistant Professor of Urology
Albert Einstein Medical College
New Hyde Park, NY

M. MONGA, M.D.
Resident
Department of Urology
Tulane University Medical School
New Orleans, LA

JOSE MORENO, M.D.
Clinical Assistant Professor
Department of Urology
Thomas Jefferson University
Philadelphia, PA

WILLIAM R. MORGAN, M.D.
Urologic Oncologist
Virginia Urology Center
Richmond, VA

JUDD W. MOUL, M.D.
Professor of Surgery
Department of Surgery
Uniformed Services University
Bethesda, MD

JOSEPH J. MOWAD, M.D., F.A.C.S.
Clinical Professor of Urology
Department of Urology
Jefferson Medical College
Philadelphia, PA

M. LOUIS MOY, M.D.
Resident
Department of Urology
Thomas Jefferson University
Philadelphia, PA

JOHN P. MULHALL, M.D.
Assistant Professor
Department of Urology
Loyola University Medical Center
Chicago, IL

S. GRANT MULHOLLAND, M.D.
The Nathan Lewis Hatfield Professor and Chairman
Department of Urology
Thomas Jefferson University
Philadelphia, PA

BRIAN P. MURRAY, M.D.
Resident
Division of Urology
Albany Medical Center
Albany, NY

JACK H. MYDLO, M.D.
Associate Professor of Urology
Department of Urology
SUNY Downstate Medical School
Brooklyn, NY

J. CURTIS NICKEL, M.D.
Professor
Department of Urology
Queen's University
Kingston General Hospital
Kingston, ON, Canada

PETER NIEMCZYK, M.D.
Mesa Urologists
Mesa, AZ

MARK J. NOBLE, M.D.
Staff Physician
Department of Urology
Cleveland Clinic, Gates Medical Center
Elyria, OH

UNYIME O. NSEYO, M.D.
Professor
Health Science Department of Urology
West Virginia University
Morgantown, WV

MICHAEL A. O'DONNELL, M.D.
Assistant Professor
Department of Surgery/Urology
Harvard Medical School
Boston, MA

KENNETH OGAN, M.D.
Resident
Department of Urology
The George Washington University
Washington, DC

JOHN OH, M.D.
Resident
Department of Urology
Thomas Jefferson University
Philadelphia, PA

GREGORY J. OLEYOURRYK, M.D.
Resident
Department of Urology
University of Rochester, Strong Memorial Hospital
Rochester, NY

MICHAEL G. PACKER, M.D.
Associate Professor of Surgery/Pediatrics
Section of Pediatric Urology
Robert Wood Johnson Medical School
Camden, NJ

JOHN J. PAHIRA, M.D.
Professor of Urology
Director, Georgetown University Medical Center
Center for Kidney Stone Disease and Lithotripsy Unit
Department of Surgery
Georgetown University
Washington, DC

BHALCHANDRA G. PARULKAR, M.D.
Clinical Assistant Professor
Division of Urology
Fallon Clinic
University of Massachusetts Medical Center
Worcester, MA

NICK PAVONA, M.D.
Associate Professor of Urology
Benjamin Franklin University
Chadds Ford, PA

DENNIS S. PEPPAS, M.D.
Assistant Professor
Departments of Surgery and Pediatrics
Uniformed Services University of the Health Services
Bethesda, MD

STEVEN P. PETROU, M.D.
Assistant Professor
Department of Urology
Mayo School of Medicine
Rochester, MN

PAUL KENNETH PIETROW, M.D.
Chief Resident
Department of Urologic Surgery
Vanderbilt University
Nashville, TN

PETER A. PINTO, M.D.
Resident
Department of Urology
Long Island Jewish Medical Center
New Hyde Park, NY

NATANIA Y. PIPER, M.D.
Resident
Department of Urology
San Antonio Uniformed Services Health Care Consortium
San Antonio, TX

MARC W. PLAWKER, M.D.
Assistant Professor
Department of Urology
State University of New York at Brooklyn
Brooklyn, NY

LOUIS F. PLZAK III, M.D.
Instructor
Department of Urology
University of Pennsylvania School of Medicine
Philadelphia, PA

DIX PHILLIP POPPAS, M.D.
Assistant Professor
Department of Urology
Cornell University
New York, NY

JOSEPH PRESTI, M.D.
Associate Professor
Department of Urology
University of California, San Francisco
San Francisco, CA

OWEN PROWSE, M.D.
Resident
Department of Urology
Montefiore Medical Center
New York, NY

SUNIL K. PUROHIT, M.D.
Resident
Department of Urology
Tulane University School of Medicine
New Orleans, LA

HYMAN H. RABINOVITCH, M.D.
Professor
Department of Surgery
MCP Hahnemann University
Philadelphia, PA

GANESH V. RAJ, M.D.
Resident in Urology
Department of Urology
Duke University Medical Center
Durham, NC

RAVI RAJAN, M.D.
Chief Resident
Department of Urology
Thomas Jefferson University
Philadelphia, PA

S. ADAM RAMIN, M.D.
Chief Resident
Department of Urology
Loma Linda University Medical Center
Loma Linda, CA

DAVID A. RIVAS, M.D.
Assistant Professor
Department of Urology
Jefferson Medical College
Philadelphia, PA

CARY N. ROBERTSON, M.D.
Associate Professor
Division of Urology
Duke University Medical Center
Durham, NC

JONATHAN H. ROSS, M.D.
Head, Section of Pediatric Urology
Department of Urology
Cleveland Clinic Foundation
Cleveland, OH

G. BINO RUCKER, M.D.
Resident
Department of Urology
New York Hospital–Cornell University
New York, NY

HERBERT C. RUCKLE, M.D.
Associate Professor of Surgery
Division of Urology
Loma Linda University School of Medicine
Loma Linda, CA

DANIEL RUKSTALIS, M.D.
Chief
Division of Urology
MCP Hahnemann University
Philadelphia, PA

RICARDO F. SANCHEZ-ORTIZ, M.D.
Instructor
Department of Urology
University of Pennsylvania School of Medicine
Philadelphia, PA

CHRISTOPHER G. SCHREPFERMAN, M.D.
Senior Resident
Department of Urology
University of Iowa Health Care
Iowa City, IA

BRADLEY F. SCHWARTZ, D.O.
Assistant Clinical Professor
Assistant Professor
Department of Urology
University of California at San Francisco
San Francisco, CA

WILLIAM A. SEE, M.D.
Professor and Chief
Division of Urology
Medical College of Wisconsin
Milwaukee, WI

E. JAMES SEIDMOND, M.D.
Professor of Urology and Diagnostic Imaging
Temple University
Philadelphia, PA

MATTHEW SHAHBANDI, M.D.
Resident
Department of Urology
University of Massachusetts Medical Center
Worcester, MA

ELLEN SHAPIRO, M.D.
Professor
Department of Urology
New York University School of Medicine
New York, NY

PATRICK J. SHENOT, M.D.
Instructor and Attending Physician
Department of Urology
Thomas Jefferson University
Philadelphia, PA

DAVID L. SHEPHERD, M.D.
Assistant Professor
Division of Urology
University of Texas
San Antonio, TX

W. BRUCE SHINGLETON, M.D.
Assistant Professor of Urology
Department of Surgery
University of Mississippi Medical Center
Jackson, MS

MARK SIGMAN, M.D.
Associate Professor of Surgery/Urology
Brown University School of Medicine
Rhode Island Hospital
Providence, RI

RICHARD I. SILVER, M.D.
Assistant Professor of Urology and Pediatrics
Jefferson Medical College
Thomas Jefferson University
Philadelphia, PA

JAMES A. SIMON, M.D.
Resident
Department of Urology
Washington University
St. Louis, MO

SATBIR SINGH, M.D.
Resident
Department of Urology
State University of New York Health Science Center at Syracuse
Syracuse, NY

STEVEN J. SKOOG, M.D., F.A.A.P., F.A.C.S.
Professor of Surgery and Pediatrics
Division of Urology and Renal Transplantation
Oregon Health Sciences University
Portland, OR

KEVIN M. SLAWIN, M.D.
Assistant Professor
Director, The Baylor Prostate Center
Scott Department of Urology
Baylor College of Medicine
Houston, TX

ARTHUR D. SMITH, M.D.
Professor
Department of Urology
Albert Einstein College of Medicine
Long Island, NY

MARK S. SOLOWAY, M.D.
Professor and Chairman
Department of Urology
University of Miami School of Medicine
Miami, FL

MEHRDAD SOROUSH, M.D.
Chief Resident
Department of Urology
Thomas Jefferson University
Philadelphia, PA

VICTORIA R. STAIMAN, M.D.
Urologic Surgery Associates
Elliot City, MD

BRADLEY W. STEELE, M.D.
Resident
Department of Urology
University of North Carolina
Chapel Hill, NC

JOHN P. STEIN, M.D.
Assistant Professor
Department of Urology
University of Southern California
Norris Comprehensive Cancer Center
Los Angeles, CA

GEORGE F. STEINHARDT, M.D.
Professor
Department of Surgery/Urology
St. Louis University School of Medicine
St. Louis, MO

ROBERT A. STEPHENSON, M.D.
Professor and Jon M. Huntsman Chair in Urological Oncology
Department of Surgery, Division of Urology
University of Utah
Salt Lake City, UT

MARSHALL L. STOLLER, M.D.
Professor
Department of Urology
University of California
San Francisco, CA

NELSON N. STONE, M.D.
Professor
Department of Urology and Radiation Oncology
Mount Sinai School of Medicine
New York, NY

STEVAN B. STREEM, M.D.
Head, Section of Stone Disease and Endocrinology
Department of Urology
Cleveland Clinic Foundation
Cleveland, OH

STEPHEN E. STRUP, M.D.
Assistant Professor
Department of Urology
Thomas Jefferson University
Philadelphia, PA

JOHN A. TAYLOR III, M.D.
Department of Urology
Columbia University
Columbia Presbyterian Medical Center
New York, NY

SEAMUS J. TEAHAN, M.D.
Fellow in Neuro-Urology and Female Urology
University of Pittsburgh School of Medicine
Pittsburgh, PA

MARTHA K. TERRIS, M.D.
Assistant Professor
Department of Urology
Stanford University
Stanford, CA

ASHUTOSH TEWARI, M.D.
Resident
Department of Urology
Henry Ford Health System and Josephine Ford Cancer Center
Detroit, MI

RAJU THOMAS, M.D., F.A.C.S., M.H.A.
Professor and Chairman
Department of Urology
Tulane University Medical Center
New Orleans, LA

MARK E. THOMPSON, M.D.
Resident
Department of Surgery
Loma Linda University
Loma Linda, CA

IAN MURCHIE THOMPSON, M.D.
Professor of Surgery
Chairman, Division of Urology
Department of Surgery
University of Texas Health Science Center at San Antonio
San Antonio, TX

J. BRANTLEY THRASHER, M.D.
William L. Valk Professor and Chairman
Section of Urology, Department of Surgery
University of Kansas Medical Center
Kansas City, KS

CHRIS B. THREATT, M.D.
Senior Resident
Department of Urology
Duke University Medical Center
Durham, NC

MATTHEW S. TOBIN, M.D.
Resident
Department of Urology
Harvard University
Boston, MA

EDOUARD J. TRABULSI, M.D.
Resident
Department of Urology
Thomas Jefferson University
Philadelphia, PA

J. C. TRUSSELL, M.D.
Chief Resident
Department of Urology
Upstate Medical University
Syracuse, NY

CHRISTOPHER K. TSAI, M.D.
Resident
Department of Urology
Loma Linda University Medical Center
Loma Linda, CA

RICHARD K. VALICENTI, M.D.
Assistant Professor
Department of Radiation Oncology
Thomas Jefferson University
Philadelphia, PA

KEITH VANARSDALEN, M.D.
Professor
Department of Urology
University of Pennsylvania Health Systems
Philadelphia, PA

JASON VARNER, M.D.
Jefferson Medical College
Philadelphia, PA

CHRISTOPHER L. VULIN, M.D., M.S.
Jefferson Medical College
Thomas Jefferson University
Philadelphia, PA

JOSEPH R. WAGNER, M.D.
Assistant Professor
Department of Urology
Albert Einstein College of Medicine
Bronx, NY

JONATHAN R. WALKER, M.D.
Resident
Department of Urology
Georgetown University Medical Center
Washington, DC

MARK J. WALTERSKIRCHEN, M.D.
Resident
Department of Urology
University of Kansas
Kansas City, KS

McCLELLAN M. WALTHER, M.D.
Staff Physician
Urologic Oncology Branch
National Institute of Health
Bethesda, MD

MICHAEL J. WEHLE, M.D.
Assistant Professor
Department of Urology
Mayo Clinic, Jacksonville
Jacksonville, FL

DAVID C. WEI, M.D.
Fellow
Department of Urology
Memorial Sloan-Kettering Cancer Center
New York, NY

GARY H. WEISS, M.D.
Assistant Professor
Department of Urology
Long Island Jewish Medical Center
New Hyde Park, NY

ROBERT M. WEISS, M.D.
Professor and Chief
Section of Urology
Yale University School of Medicine
New Haven, CT

HUNTER WESSELLS, M.D., F.A.C.S.
Assistant Professor
Section of Urology
University of Arizona
Tucson, AZ

JOHN S. WIENER, M.D.
Assistant Professor
Departments of Surgery and Pediatrics
Duke University
Durham, NC

JEFFREY F. WILLIAMS, M.D.
Resident
Department of Urology
University of Michigan Hospital
Ann Arbor, MI

HOWARD N. WINFIELD, M.D.
Associate Professor
Department of Urology
Stanford University
Stanford, CA

J. STUART WOLF, JR., M.D.
Assistant Professor
Department of Surgery/Urology
University of Michigan
Ann Arbor, MI

MARVIN J. YOUNG, M.D.
Resident
Department of Urology
University of Miami School of Medicine
Miami, FL

PAUL R. YOUNG, M.D.
Assistant Professor of Urology
Department of Urology
Mayo Medical School
Jacksonville, FL

J. PAUL YURKANIN, M.D.
Resident
Section of Urology
The University of Arizona
Tucson, AZ

MARK R. ZAONTZ, M.D.
Associate Professor
Department of Surgery and Pediatrics
University of Medicine and Dentistry of New Jersey
Robert Wood Johnson Medical School
Camden, NJ

MICHAEL K. ZENNI, M.D.
Resident
Department of Urology
University of Iowa
Iowa City, IA

ALI M. ZIADA, M.D.
Assistant Lecturer
Department of Urology
Cairo University
Cairo, Egypt

JEROME R. ZINK, M.D.
Resident
Department of Urology
Thomas Jefferson University Hospital
Philadelphia, PA

BURKHARDT H. ZORN, M.D.
Assistant Professor
Department of Surgery
Uniformed Services
University of the Health Sciences
Bethesda, MD

Contents

SECTION II: UROLOGIC DISEASES AND CONDITIONS / 185

SECTION III: SHORT TOPICS A TO Z / 617

SECTION IV: URINE STUDIES / 723

SECTION V: COMMONLY USED MEDICATIONS IN UROLOGY / 727

SECTION VI: ALTERNATE THERAPIES IN UROLOGY / 769

SECTION VII: APPENDIX/REFERENCE TABLES / 773

Presenting Problems

Abdominal Mass—Adult, Urologic Considerations

 Basics

DESCRIPTION

• Urologic abdominal masses are mostly retroperitoneal. They are generally

—Renal in origin
—Adrenal in origin

PATHOPHYSIOLOGY

Various urologic pathologic conditions may present with a mass:

• Primary renal neoplasms

—Malignant: RCC, renal sarcoma, adult Wilms' tumor, transitional cell carcinoma
—Benign: renal cortical adenoma, renal oncocytoma, and renal hamartoma (angiomyolipoma) fibroma

• Primary adrenal neoplasms

—Adrenal cortical carcinoma, pheochromocytoma, adrenal adenoma, paraganglioma

• Hydronephrosis
• Renal abscesses: usually follows insufficient treatment of lobar nephronia; needle aspiration may be needed to make a diagnosis. TB can cause cold abscess formation. Pus developing from a renal source may track alongside psoas muscle and appears in the groin, where it must be distinguished from hernia.
• Perinephric abscess: usually arises as a result of preexisting renal factors such as renal calculi, ureteral calculi, hydronephrotic changes, renal cystic disease, or infected carcinoma
• Hematomas: may be caused by a ruptured kidney or ureter avulsion. Blood in the retroperitoneal space may track to the corresponding iliac fossa.
• Renal cysts
• Bladder related: retention, tumor, and urachal abnormality

RISK FACTORS

• Infection: predisposing to abscess formation
• Trauma: may lead to hematoma
• Renal and adrenal cancer risk factors: See Section I, "Renal Masses."

 Differential Diagnosis

• GI tract tumors
• Metastatic tumors
• Hematoma (non-urologic): spine fracture, leaking abdominal aneurysm, acute pancreatitis
• Gynecologic causes: pregnancy, uterine fibroids, ovarian cysts and tumors
• Vascular: aneurysm
• Retroperitoneal cyst
• Primary retroperitoneal neoplasms arising from connective tissue: retroperitoneal lipoma, retroperitoneal sarcoma
• Retroperitoneal lymph nodes and nervous tissue tumors
• Hernia

 Database

HISTORY

• Weight loss, cachexia, nightsweats may be associated with chronic septic disease as TB, or malignancy.
• Spiking fever and throbbing pain are usually associated with abscess formation.
• Pain may be due to spontaneous renal hemorrhage, invasion by a tumor of neighboring tissues, clot colic with gross hematuria, or distant metastatic disease to bone or brain.
• Classic triad of hematuria, flank pain, and a flank mass is only seen in 10% of RCC cases.
• Medical history is significant for TB, lobar nephronia, upper tract stones, or infection.
• History of recent trauma

PHYSICAL EXAMINATION

• General examination may reveal lymphadenopathy or leg edema due to compression of lymphatics by the mass.
• Abdomino/pelvic examination

—Bimanual examination of the flank and upper abdomen may reveal a palpable mass.
—In the male patient, a varicocele may be present and seen more often on the right side when renal tumor clot forms and extends from the right renal vein into the vena cava.
—Scrotal examination for testicular masses is indicated since they may be associated with retroperitoneal lymphadenopathy.

Diagnostic Studies

LABORATORY TESTING

- Blood tests

—A full lab work-up for renal cancer should include CBC, blood calcium, urea and creatinine, and liver function tests to exclude metastasis.
—Adrenal metabolic work-up if adrenal mass is suspected
—Tumor markers: AFP and beta subunit of hCG if testicular neoplasm is suspected

- Urine tests

—U/A and culture if abscess is suspected
—Culture to exclude TB may be needed.

IMAGING

- Real-time ultrasound (US): probably best for detecting cystic lesions and should be used as an initial work-up
- Computerized tomography (CT) scan: best for solid abdominal masses
- Magnetic resonance imaging (MRI): may not offer any advantage over CT scan initially
- Intravenous urogram (IVU)
- Chest x-ray: to exclude metastatic disease

SPECIAL STUDIES

- Renal arteriography
- Venacavography

 Initial Management

- Urologic tumors: Early-stage renal and adrenal tumors are usually managed surgically. In the high stage, tumor radiation or chemotherapy may be used.
- Retroperitoneal lymphadenopathy associated with testicular cancer: RPLND and/or chemotherapy may be used, depending on the degree of node involvement.
- Cysts: Asymptomatic benign renal and adrenal cysts are usually left alone. Large symptomatic cysts may be treated by percutaneous aspiration under ultrasound guidance. Ethanol injection into an emptied renal cyst was shown to decrease cyst refill.

 Follow-Up

- Based on nature of diagnosed mass

 Miscellaneous

SYNONYMS: N/A

ASSOCIATED CONDITIONS

- RCC, renal cell carcinoma

NOTES

- See also Section I, "Renal Masses" and "Abdominal Mass—Newborn/Child"

ABBREVIATIONS

- RCC, renal cell carcinoma

REFERENCES

McDougal WS, Garnick M. Clinical signs and symptoms of renal cell carcinoma. In: Vogelzang NJ, Scardino PT, Shipley WV, et al., eds. *Comprehensive Textbook of Genitourinary Oncology*. Baltimore, Williams & Wilkins, 1996: 154–159.

Olsson CA, Sawczuk IS. Kidney tumors. *Urol Clin North Am* 1993;20(2):193–359.

Stenzl A, DeKernion JB. Pathology, biology, and clinical staging of renal cell carcinoma. *Semin Oncol* 1989;16[Suppl 1]:3–11.

Author: E. James Seidmond

Abdominal Mass—Newborn/Child

 Basics

DESCRIPTION

- Newborn abdominal mass in 1 in 1000 live births
- Most masses are nonsurgical; 87% of surgical lesions are benign; incidence of both surgical and malignant lesions increases with age.
- Two-thirds of abdominal masses in first month of life arise from the genitourinary tract.
- Prenatal ultrasound often detects lesions before delivery.

PATHOPHYSIOLOGY

- Normal abdominal examination in infant or child

—Rotund, soft, nontender abdomen
—The liver edge is palpable 1 to 2 cm below the right costal margin.
—The spleen is palpable until age 2.

- Any other masses detected need evaluation.

RISK FACTORS: N/A

 Differential Diagnosis

HYDRONEPHROSIS

- UPJ obstruction: most common cause of neonatal abdominal mass; typically presents as unilateral flank mass
- Less common causes of hydronephrosis: UVJ obstruction, PUV, VUR, megaureter and ureteroceles
- May present as mass in older child; often associated with intermittent hematuria after minor trauma
- 30% to 50% diagnosed prenatally; currently less than 15% of neonates with UPJ obstruction present with a mass.
- Two-thirds boys; 60% left side; 20% detected in first year are bilateral; after first year only 5%; contralateral unit often abnormal
- Older children present with abdominal/flank pain or UTI.
- Ultrasound, VCUG, and renal scan should be performed; may be needed to differentiate from MCDK

MULTICYSTIC DYSPLASTIC KIDNEY

- Second most common cause of neonatal mass; together with UPJ obstruction constitute 40% of all neonatal abdominal masses
- Usually presents as unilateral flank mass; more common on left; more frequent in boys; mass noted within first month of life
- Majority now detected prenatally
- Ultrasound diagnostic; seen as "cluster of grapes"; nuclear scan and IVP show nonvisualization on affected side
- Nephrectomy generally advised on elective basis (controversial); debate continues as to need for removal.

- Evaluation of contralateral side warranted, as 20% are abnormal; UPJ most common; 15% incidence of VUR, so VCUG necessary

NEUROBLASTOMA

- Most common solid neonatal abdominal mass; most common malignancy of newborn; almost 50% of all malignant tumors in children; 50% before age of 2 and 75% by age of 4
- A fixed, painful, irregular mass often crosses the midline; hepatic metastasis can be the cause of an abdominal mass in stage IV-S disease.
- Associated with fever, malaise, weight loss; child appears ill compared with patient with Wilms' tumor
- Ultrasound helpful but CT shows extrinsic renal displacement and calcification as well as metastases
- Diagnosis: 24 hour urine catecholamines, bone marrow aspiration, and tumor biopsy

MESOBLASTIC NEPHROMA

- Most common solid tumor of renal origin in neonate; benign; presents in first 3 months of life
- Solid appearance on ultrasound; nephrectomy curative

WILMS' TUMOR

- Rare in newborn, uncommon before age 3; 75% of cases detected between ages 1 and 5; peak age between 3 and 4; most common malignant neoplasm of urinary tract in children; most common childhood abdominal malignancy
- Abdominal mass and increasing girth most common signs; mass is firm, nontender, smooth and unilateral
- Ultrasound, CT, and MRI all help in confirming the kidney as the organ of origin, the patency of the renal vein and vena cava, metastases or bilateral disease.
- The combination of complete excision, chemotherapy, and radiotherapy yields success rates of 90% to 95% with favorable histology.

POLYCYSTIC KIDNEY DISEASE

- When diagnosed in neonatal period, most likely ARPKD; 50% of affected newborns die in first few hours or days of life; of the survivors, only 50% are alive at 10 years.
- Often detected prenatally; bilateral large, hard flank masses; do not transilluminate; associated oligohydramnios and Potter's facies common
- Usual age of presentation of ADPKD is third to fifth decade; neonatal cases occur, presenting with renomegaly; usually a family history is documented.

RENAL VEIN THROMBOSIS

- Most common cause of neonatal hematuria; 65% occur in neonatal period, 30% after age 1; male predominance
- Classic features include abdominal mass, hematuria, thrombocytopenia, leukocytosis, proteinuria, anemia, and coagulopathy.
- Occurs in conditions associated with dehydration, diabetic mothers, sepsis, diarrhea, congenital heart disease, or sickle cell disease

- Ultrasound shows renomegaly; IVP and renal scan show nonfunction.
- Conservative therapy indicated

INTESTINAL DUPLICATION

- GI lesions account for 12% of neonatal abdominal masses; duplication is most common GI cause; ileal most common
- A palpable abdominal mass with GI obstruction almost always originates in the GI tract.

HYDROCOLPOS

- Enlarged fluid-filled uterus due to obstruction from vaginal atresia, imperforate hymen, or cloacal anomaly
- Mass usually in pelvis in midline; ultrasound shows fluid-filled pelvic mass between bladder and rectum

OVARIAN CYST

- Incidence of ovarian mass is 1 in 3000 girls; most common cause of abdominal cystic tumor in female fetus; presents as large mobile mass in midabdomen
- Cysts and tumors occur throughout female life cycle; 17% in neonatal to age 4; 28% from 5 to 9 years; 55% from 9 to 18 years; prepuberty 50% are malignant, with teratoma most common

LIVER TUMOR

- Primary liver tumors are the third most common solid abdominal neoplasm in childhood, making up 15% of all abdominal masses in childhood.
- Benign lesions make up one-third; include hemangioendothelioma, mesenchymal hamartoma, adenoma, focal nodular hyperplasia, and congenital cysts
- Malignant lesions make up two-thirds; hepatoblastoma most common liver tumor in children under age 5; hepatocellular carcinoma presents in older children ages 12 to 15.

LYMPHOMA

- Most commonly occurs in abdomen; unusual in neonates; common in boys over 5 years of age
- Non-Hodgkin's lymphoma presents as an abdominal mass with ascites and bowel obstruction.
- Diagnosis confirmed by biopsy; treatment with chemotherapy

ORGANOMEGALY

- Hepatomegaly is the most common cause of liver mass; similarly splenomegaly is the cause of a splenic mass.
- More common in older child; need to rule out metastatic disease

POSTERIOR URETHRAL VALVES

- Most common cause of bladder outlet obstruction in newborn; caused by urethral fold extending from verumontanum
- 50% present within the first 6 months and 30% within a week of birth; a prenatal ultrasound can suggest diagnosis.
- 45% may present with an abdominal mass; an ultrasound shows bilateral hydroureteronephrosis with dilated bladder and posterior urethra.
- VCUG confirms diagnosis.

MISCELLANEOUS

• Gastric distension, urinary retention, fecal impaction

Database

HISTORY

• Age and sex of patient?

—Different conditions present at different times in a child's development.
—10% of all neonatal abdominal masses arise from the female genital system; sacrococcygeal teratomas and choledochal cysts are more common in girls.

• Maternal history?

—Maternal diabetes increases the risk for renal vein thrombosis.

• Family history?

—Parents of infants with ARPKD tend to be normal, unlike those with ADPKD.
—Urinary tract duplication is hereditary: An ectopic ureterocele or ureter should be sought.

• Was a prenatal ultrasound performed, and if so, was it normal?

—Reduced amniotic fluid volume (oligohydramnios) implies diminished renal function; anhydramnios may indicate urethral obstruction, bilateral renal agenesis, or bilateral multicystic kidneys; polyhydramnios may suggest impaired swallowing or a high GI obstruction.

• Concurrent symptoms and duration?

—Pain, tenderness, jaundice, weight loss, fever, melena, UTI, dysuria, and hematuria provide valuable diagnostic clues: fever: obstructive lesion; vomiting: GI disorder; weak stream: PUV.

PHYSICAL EXAMINATION

• Hypertension

—Neuroblastoma, polycystic kidney disease, pheochromocytoma, Wilms' tumor

• Aniridia

—Wilms' tumor as part of WAGR (Wilms' tumor, aniridia, genitourinary anomalies, and retardation) syndrome

• Subcutaneous nodules

—Neuroblastoma

• Abdomen mass

—Determine whether solid or soft, mobile or immobile, smooth or irregular, and tender or nontender. Determine size and location.

• Rectal mass

—Impaction, sacrococcygeal tumor, hydrocolpos in a girl

• Introital mass

—Bulging hydrocolpos or hematocolpos

Diagnostic Studies

LABORATORY TESTING

• CBC

—Neuroblastoma: anemia; leukemia/lymphoma: leukocytosis; infected hydronephrosis: leukocytosis with bandemia

• Electrolytes, BUN (blood urea nitrogen), creatinine

—Elevated BUN/creatinine: renal compromise, dehydration

• Urinalysis

—Hematuria seen in Wilms' tumor, renal vein thrombosis, UPJ obstruction after minor trauma

• 24-Hour urine

—Elevated catecholamine levels: neuroblastoma, pheochromocytoma

IMAGING

• Plain abdominal x-rays

—Bowel gas pattern can indicate obstruction or displacement.
—Calcification can suggest a neuroblastoma, teratoma, hepatoblastoma, or meconium peritonitis.

• Abdominal ultrasound

—Will establish location and size; more importantly, can determine cystic vs. solid; benign inexpensive test, can be performed at bedside without sedation

• VCUG

—Must be done to rule out reflux and assess for bladder outlet obstruction in boys when hydronephrosis or MCDK detected

• IVP

—Mostly supplanted by ultrasound; useful when duplication anomaly suspected

• CT scan

—Most versatile imaging modality for evaluation of abdominal masses; gives precise anatomic detail; more useful in older children

• Radionuclide scans

—Useful in certain abdominal mass evaluations; renal scans allow precise determination of renal function; biliary scans for evaluation of suspected choledochal cysts; liver–spleen scans in diagnosis of liver tumors or splenic enlargement

SPECIAL STUDIES: N/A

Initial Management

• Perform history and physical, then ultrasound; will often make diagnosis without any further imaging

• Eliminate these common diagnoses by using simple maneuvers—gastric dilatation: nasogastric tube; urinary retention: catheterization; and fecal impaction: enema.
• Categorize according to age, sex, and mass location; and whether cystic or solid; then proceed with further evaluation, if necessary.

Follow-Up

• Few entities require follow-up. Debate continues regarding when an MCDK needs to be removed. If observation is undertaken, routine ultrasound will show changes in size or solid components that may suggest the need for nephrectomy.
• UPJ obstruction is another entity still being debated. Previously, immediate surgery was the rule; now many are followed with serial ultrasound and scans.
• The remaining conditions are followed depending on the treatment undertaken.

Miscellaneous

SYNONYMS: N/A

ASSOCIATED CONDITIONS: N/A

NOTES: N/A

ABBREVIATIONS

• PUV, posterior urethral valves; VUR, vesicoureteric reflux; VCUG, voiding cystourethrogram; UVJ, ureterovesical junction; MCDK, multicystic dysplastic kidney; UPJ, ureteropelvic junction; ADPKD, autosomal dominant polycystic kidney disease; ARPKD, autosomal recessive polycystic kidney disease

REFERENCES

Caty MG, Shamberg RC. Abdominal tumors in infancy and childhood. *Pediatr Clin North Am* 1993;40(6):1253–1271.

Diamond DA, Gosalbez R. Neonatal urologic emergencies: In: Walsh PC, Retik AB, Vaughan ED, Wein AJ, eds. *Campbell's Urology,* 7th ed. Philadelphia: WB Saunders, 1998.

Grosfeld JL. Abdominal masses in infants and children. In: O'Donnell B, Koff SA, eds. *Pediatric Urology,* 3rd ed. London: Reed Educational and Professional Publishing LTD, 1997.

Taylor LA, Ross AJ III. Abdominal masses. In: Walker WA, Durie PR, Walker-Smith JA, Watkins JB, eds. *Pediatric Gastrointestinal Disease,* 2nd ed. St Louis: Mosby–Year Book, 1996.

Authors: Allen N. Chiura and Leonard G. Gomella

Adrenal Mass

 Basics

DESCRIPTION

• The adrenal glands are paired retroperitoneal organs that lie within the perinephric fat just anterior/superior/medial to the kidneys.
• The adrenal glands produce a number of steroid hormones and catecholamines that are essential for homeostasis.

PATHOPHYSIOLOGY

• The adrenal glands: two distinct regions, the adrenal cortex and the adrenal medulla

—Cortex has three zones: zona glomerulosa, zona fasciculata, and zona reticularis.
—Each region and zone produces specific, hormonally active products. Depending on the etiology of the adrenal mass, any of these regions or zones can overproduce or underproduce secretory products with resulting signs and symptoms.

• Adrenal cortex

—Zona glomerulosa: produces mineralocorticoid aldosterone (regulates sodium and fluid homeostasis; promotes exchange of potassium for sodium in the distal tubules)
—Zona fasciculata: produces glucocorticoid cortisol; regulates cellular metabolism, glucose metabolism, immune processes, and other regulatory functions
—Zona reticularis: produces adrenal androgens androstenedione, dehydroepiandrosterone (DHEA), and dehydroepiandrosterone sulfate (DHEAS).

• Adrenal medulla

—Produces catecholamines dopamine, norepinephrine, and epinephrine (act on alpha-adrenergic, beta-adrenergic, and dopaminergic receptors throughout the body)

• Masses may cause overproduction, underproduction, or no change in production of adrenal secretory products

—Cushing syndrome (CUS): excess cortisol production
—Conn syndrome (CON): excess aldosterone production; also known as primary hyperaldosteronism
—Pheochromocytoma (PHE): excess catecholamine production
—Sex steroid-secreting tumors (SEX): excess testosterone and/or estradiol, androstenedione, dehydroepiandrosterone (DHEA), and dehydroepiandrosterone sulfate (DHEAS); can be virilizing or feminizing
—Addison's disease (ADD): adrenal insufficiency
—Selective adrenal insufficiency: rare

RISK FACTORS

• Adrenal metastasis due to other malignancies, particularly breast, lung, and renal carcinomas
• Chronic steroid use may be associated with adrenal myelolipomas.
• Pheochromocytomas are associated with several syndromes, such as multiple endocrine neoplasias, Von Hippel-Lindau disease, Von Recklinghausen disease, tuberous sclerosis, and Sturge-Weber syndrome.

 Differential Diagnosis

• Adrenal adenoma
• Adrenal hyperplasia, unilateral or bilateral
• Adrenal metastasis
• Adrenocortical carcinoma
• Pheochromocytoma
• Adrenal myelolipoma
• Adrenal cyst
• Wolman's disease: rare congenital syndrome characterized by infiltration of multiple solid viscera with foam cells; may cause bilateral adrenal masses
• Adrenal varices: seen in portal hypertension, dilation of the adrenal vein may simulate a mass

 Database

HISTORY

• General: malaise (CUS, CON, PHE, ADD); weight loss (PHE, ADD); weight gain (CUS); anorexia (PHE, ADD)
• Gastrointestinal: abdominal pain (PHE, ADD); nausea/vomiting (PHE, ADD); diarrhea (ADD); constipation (PHE)
• Cardiovascular: orthostatic hypotension/syncope/dizziness (PHE, ADD); palpitations (PHE)
• Neurologic: headache (CON, PHE, ADD); muscle weakness (CUS, CON, PHE, ADD); paresthesias (CON); muscle cramps (CON); personality changes (CUS, PHE, ADD); tremor (CON, PHE)
• Skin: diaphoresis (PHE); purple striae (CUS); hirsutism (CUS, SEX); acne (CUS, SEX); gynecomastia (CUS, SEX)
• Menses: abnormal cycles (CUS, SEX)
• Genitourinary: frequency (CON); testes atrophy (SEX)
• Medical history: malignancies, syndromes
• Medications: exogenous steroids
• Family history: multiple endocrine neoplasias, Von Hippel-Lindau disease, Von Recklinghausen disease, tuberous sclerosis, and Sturge-Weber syndrome

PHYSICAL EXAMINATION

• Vital signs: hypertension (CUS, CON, PHE); hypotension (ADD); orthostasis (PHE, ADD); tachycardia (PHE, ADD)
• Skin: acne (CUS); purple striae (CUS); bruising (CUS)

• HEENT: moon facies (CUS); central obesity/ "buffalo hump" (CUS); retinopathy (RHE)
• Abdomen: mass (rare) (CUS, CON, PHE, ADD); obesity (CUS); cachectic (PHE, ADD)
• Heart: hyperdynamic (PHE, ADD)
• Chest: gynecomastia (CUS, SEX)
• Extremity: edema (CUS, ±CON)
• Genitourinary: testicular atrophy (SEX)
• Musculoskeletal: atrophy (CUS, PHE, ADD); osteoporosis (CUS)
• Neurologic: paresthesias (CON); weakness (CUS, CON, PHE, ADD); tremors (CON, PHE)

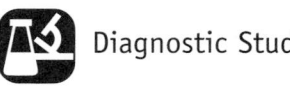 Diagnostic Studies

LABORATORY TESTING

• Cushing syndrome

—Serum electrolytes: hypernatremia, hyperglycemia
—AM and PM serum cortisol: Patients with Cushing syndrome show higher levels with less diurnal variation.
—24-hour urinary cortisol >100 μg
—Dexamethasone Suppression Test: 0.5 mg dexamethasone orally every 6 hours for 48 hours. Urinary cortisol should fall below 30 μg and serum cortisol below 5 μg/dL in normal subjects and those with Cushing disease (overproduction of ACTH). Patients with Cushing syndrome do not suppress.

• Conn syndrome

—Serum electrolytes: hypokalemia despite dietary supplementation
—Low plasma renin activity
—24-hour urine: potassium >40 mEq and aldosterone >15 μg
—Elevated plasma or urinary aldosterone level indexed against urinary sodium excretion after sodium loading with low plasma renin activity defines Conn syndrome.

• Pheochromocytoma

—24-hour urine for catecholamines. Numerous foods and drugs can affect levels.

• Sex steroid–secreting tumors

—Serum testosterone, estradiol, androstenedione, dehydroepiandrosterone (DHEA), and dehydroepiandrosterone sulfate (DHEAS)
—24-hour urine for 17-ketosteroids. Absence of increased 17-ketosteroid levels indicates a gonadal origin.

IMAGING

• Computerized tomography (CT)

—Hyperplasia: Diffuse thickening
—Adenoma: solitary with somewhat higher lipid content
—Myelolipoma: hematopoietic and fatty characteristics
—Carcinoma: large size, necrosis, and calcification

• Magnetic resonance imaging (MRI)

—Pheochromocytomas have a very high T2 signal.
—A high adrenal mass T2 signal compared with liver or spleen suggests the mass is not an adenoma.

• Metaiodobenzylguanidine (MIBG) scan

—MIBG is concentrated in APUD (amine precursor uptake and decarboxylation) cells like those in the adrenal medulla. Although MRI may soon largely replace MIBG scans, MIBG is a functional study that is highly sensitive and specific. It is also useful in identifying extra-adrenal pheochromocytomas.

SPECIAL STUDIES

• Adrenal vein sampling

—*Essential* for lateralizing hyperaldosteronomas
—10% incidence of adrenal adenomas at autopsy. Aldosterone-secreting tumors are often small and difficult to detect radiographically.
—To avoid removing a benign adenoma and leaving a contralateral functional hyperaldosteronoma, adrenal vein sampling must be performed.
—Occasionally useful for lateralizing cortisol-secreting tumors
—Given the excellent sensitivity and specificity rates for MRI and MIBG, there is little utility to use venous sampling to detect pheochromocytoma.

• Glucagon stimulation test

—Glucagon 1 mg IV stimulates catecholamine production in patients with pheochromocytoma. Blood pressure is carefully monitored, and serum catecholamine levels are drawn at 2 minutes. Regitine 5 mg IV should be available for hypertensive crises and does not affect serum catecholamine levels.

• Clonidine suppression test

—Clonidine 0.3 mg given orally causes a fall in serum catecholamines in patients with neurogenic hypertension. Patients with pheochromocytoma show no change in catecholamine levels.

• Iodocholesterol scan

—Can be used to demonstrate increased adrenal metabolic activity; rarely useful

 Initial Management

• All adrenal masses should be assessed with a biochemical evaluation.
• Pheochromocytoma: immediate alpha-adrenergic blockade

—Phenoxybenzamine 10 mg po bid
—Metyrosine 250 mg tid can be used to actually block catecholamine production.
—Calcium channel blockers or beta-blockers are added as needed.

• All biochemically active adrenal masses should be removed (79% of adrenal carcinomas are functional).
• Most adrenocortical carcinomas are >6 cm.

—Due to errors in measurement, masses >5 cm should be removed after biochemical evaluation.

• Laparoscopic management: option for adrenal masses <7 cm, including pheochromocytomas
• Biochemically inactive masses <5 cm are generally followed conservatively (unlikely to be carcinoma).

—There is evidence to support removing masses with a T2 signal twice that of the liver, as these lesions are less likely to be adenomas.
—Adrenal needle biopsies should *never* be performed without a biochemical evaluation.

—In the author's opinion, needle biopsy is rarely useful except in the setting of a known primary malignancy.

 Follow-Up

• Masses <5 cm: imaged every 6 months for 2 years

—If they become larger, the biochemical evaluation is repeated, and they are removed.

• Pheochromocytomas have malignant potential. They can also occur in the contralateral adrenal, particularly in the setting of a pheochromocytoma-associated syndrome. Patients should be monitored with periodic urinary catecholamine levels.
• Adrenal cortical carcinomas have a poor prognosis.

—If the tumor is biochemically active, it is not unreasonable to follow appropriate studies periodically. Chest and abdominal CT should be followed for chest, liver, or local recurrences. Bone involvement is also not uncommon. These tumors are radioresistant. Recurrences are generally treated with a chemotherapy regimen such as mitotane, with poor response rates.

• Biochemically active or inactive adenomas should not recur after removal. Patients are followed until metabolic studies become normal.

 Miscellaneous

SYNONYMS

• Adrenal incidentaloma

ASSOCIATED CONDITIONS: N/A

NOTES: N/A

ABBREVIATIONS

• CUS, Cushing syndrome; CON, Conn syndrome; PHE, pheochromocytoma; SEX, sex steroid–secreting tumors; DHEA, dehydroepiandrosterone; DHEAS, dehydroepiandrosterone sulfate; ADD, Addison disease; ACTH, adrenocorticotropic hormone; MIBG, metaiodobenzylguanidine scan; APUD, amine precursor uptake and decarboxylation

REFERENCES

Belldegrun A, et al. Incidentally discovered mass of the adrenal gland. *Surg Gynecol Obstet* 1986;163:203.

Luton JP, et al. Clinical features of adrenocortical carcinoma, prognostic factors, and the effect of mitotane therapy [see comments]. *N Engl J Med* 1990;322:1195.

Reinig JW, et al. Differentiation of adrenal masses with MR imaging: comparison of techniques [see comments]. *Radiology* 1994; 192:41.

Vargas HI, et al. Laparoscopic adrenalectomy: a new standard of care. *Urology* 1997;49:673.

Author: Joseph R. Wagner

Ambiguous Genitalia

 Basics

DESCRIPTION

• Ambiguous genitalia: genitalia that appear within the spectrum between male and female
• Gender identification allows for gender assignment and development of a gender role.
• Variable appearances of genitalia can make gender assignment difficult.

—Predominantly male but a small penis, hypospadias, bifid scrotum, and/or fewer than two palpable gonads
—Predominantly female but an enlarged clitoris or fusion of the labioscrotal folds

• Components of gender: Each must be evaluated before gender assignment.

—Genetic sex: XX or XY
—Gonadal sex: testes or ovaries
—Phenotypic sex: appearance of genitalia

• Ambiguous genitalia represents an emergency.

—Medical emergency: must exclude life-threatening condition (adrenal insufficiency)
—Psychological emergency: must make a gender assignment
—Social emergency: family needs support and guidance

PATHOPHYSIOLOGY

Normal Sexual Development

• SRY gene (Y chromosome) induces development of the testis (week 6 of gestation).
• MIF (Sertoli cells) causes regression of the mullerian ducts, except appendix testis and prostatic utricle (week 7).
• T (Leydig cells) causes development of the wolffian duct into male internal genitalia (week 8).
• Conversion of T to DHT by 5α-reductase results in development of the external genitalia.
• Development of an ovary, and the absence of male levels of T, DHT, and MIF, results in a female phenotype.

Causes

• Disturbed sexual development through an imbalance in fetal sex hormones.

—Insufficient androgen action in a genetic male; 80% due to androgen insensitivity, 20% due to T underproduction
   —Androgen insensitivity
   —Most common cause
   —Due to mutated AR (X chromosome)
   —Complete insensitivity: "testicular feminization syndrome"
   —Elevated LH and T; testosterone converted to estrogens by aromatase in peripheral tissues
   —Orchiectomy is delayed until after puberty to allow feminization (breast development).
   —Ectopic testes develop seminoma in 2% to 5%.
   —X-linked recessive inheritance
—Testicular insufficiency
   —Bilateral vanishing testes: due to intrauterine testicular torsion
   —Dysgenetic testes: high risk of malignancy
   —Absent testes: due to testicular agenesis; extremely rare; identified by presence of ipsilateral mullerian structures
   —Primary hypogonadism: inability to respond to gonadotropins (hypergonadotropic hypogonadism)
   —Secondary hypogonadism: understimulation by gonadotropins (hypogonadotropic hypogonadism)
—Adrenal/gonadal enzyme insufficiency: deficiency of five adrenal/gonadal enzymes can cause sexual ambiguity in the male.
   —20α-hydroxylase
   —3-β-ol-dehydrogenase: can also cause sexual ambiguity in the female
   —17α-hydroxylase
   —17,20-desmolase
   —17-ketosteroid reductase
   —Autosomal recessive inheritance
—5α-reductase deficiency: deficient conversion of T to DHT
   —DHT necessary for male external genital development
   —5α-reductase enzyme "type 2"
   —Autosomal recessive inheritance

• Excessive androgen action in a genetic female

—Adrenal enzyme insufficiency: Deficiency of three adrenal enzymes can cause sexual ambiguity in the female.
   —Most common cause of female pseudohermaphroditism
   —21-hydroxylase deficiency (95%)
   —11β-hydroxylase deficiency (rare)
   —3-β-ol-dehydrogenase deficiency: can also cause sexual ambiguity in the male
   —Autosomal recessive inheritance
—Excess androgen exposure (relatively rare)
   —External androgen exposure: drugs
   —Maternal virilizing tumors of the adrenal or ovary: arrhenoblastoma, corpus luteoma, adrenal neoplasms

• Deficient MIF in a genetic male: "Hernia uteri inguinale" indicates persistent mullerian duct syndrome

—External genitalia have male phenotype, but both male and female internal ducts are present.
—Usually identified during groin exploration for UDT or inguinal hernia

RISK FACTORS

• Exogenous factors
—Maternal drug exposure
• Endogenous factors
—Inherited genetic mutations
—Gonadal agenesis/maldevelopment
—Enzymatic insufficiency
—Target organ insensitivity

Differential Diagnosis

- Female pseudohermaphroditism: genetic female with two ovaries

—Most common cause of ambiguous genitalia
  —The most common diagnosis is congenital adrenal hyperplasia (CAH).
  —Adrenal overproduction of T due to adrenal enzyme deficiency at an intermediate step of cortisol synthesis
  —Ambiguous genitalia due to CAH is called the "adrenogenital syndrome."
  —95% due to deficiency of 21-hydroxylase

- Male pseudohermaphroditism: genetic male with two testes

—Due to insufficient androgen action at the cellular level; multiple causes

- True hermaphroditism: genetic male or female with both ovarian and testicular tissue present

—Karyotypes
  —46, XX with SRY gene present (70%)
  —Mosaicism, chimerism (20%)
  —46, XY (10%)
—Forms
  —Unilateral (40%): one ovotestis and one normal gonad
  —Lateral (40%): one testis and one ovary
  —Bilateral (20%): two ovotestes
—Gender assignment
  —Usually raised male; 80% have hypospadias; two-thirds of those raised female have clitoromegaly.

- Mixed gonadal dysgenesis: genetic mosaicism with one testis and one streak gonad

—Second most common cause of ambiguous genitalia
—Karyotype typically 45, XO/46, XY
—Unicornuate uterus and fallopian tube on side of streak gonad
—Gender assignment
  —60% are raised female, testes are dysgenetic, the streak gonad or testis develops seminoma, dysgerminoma, or gonadoblastoma in >30% of cases if not resected; risk of Wilms' tumor and Drash syndrome

- Pure gonadal dysgenesis

—Usually does not present with ambiguous genitalia
—Karyotype is 46, XX
—Autosomal recessive
—Bilateral streak gonads
—Gonadal tumors develop in the streaks if Y chromosome material is present.
—Gender assignment is female.

- Other rare anomalies in the differential diagnosis

—Penile agenesis: congenital absence of the penis; extremely rare
—Micropenis with or without an undescended testis

 ## Database

HISTORY

- Maternal and gestational history

—Pregnancy (illnesses and medications)
—Recent virilization (tumors)
—Previous children (neonatal death or genital abnormalities)
—Blood relatives with similar history

- Family history

—Unexplained neonatal death suggests CAH.
—Genital abnormalities (hypospadias, UDT) in male relatives suggest abnormal androgen physiology.
—Sterility, amenorrhea, hirsutism: suggests endocrine imbalance
—Consanguinity: increased risk of genetic transmission

- Patient history

—Primary amenorrhea (MGD or AIS) or masculinization at puberty (5αRD)
—Inguinal hernias
—Postpubertal testis tumors

PHYSICAL EXAMINATION

- General: vital signs, especially blood pressure; look for signs of dehydration

—CAH often associated with blood pressure abnormalities

- Specific: abdomen, gonads, phallus, scrotum, anus

—Areolae: Hyperpigmentation suggests CAH.
—Gonads: Finding a palpable gonad essentially excludes female pseudohermaphroditism and pure gonadal dysgenesis.
—Phallus: stretched length and configuration, position of urethral meatus
  —UDT and hypospadias: possible intersex
—Perineum: number of orifices
—Labia: Hyperpigmentation suggests CAH.
—Anus: digital rectal examination to feel for a uterus or prostate

 ## Diagnostic Studies

LABORATORY TESTING

- Biochemical evaluation

—Serum electrolytes: assess for mineralocorticoid deficiency
—Adrenal steroid hormones and precursors (accumulate with block in adrenal enzyme synthesis)
  —17-hydroxy-progesterone and -pregnenolone and urinary 17-ketosteroids and pregnanetriol
  —For rare enzyme deficiencies, measure precursor intermediate metabolites.
—Gonadotropins: LH (and FSH); elevated in gonadal failure, 5αRD, or AIS; decreased in pituitary failure
—T and DHT: Increased T:DHT ratio suggests 5αRD; use hCG stimulation to show between 3 months and puberty
—hCG stimulation test: stimulation of Leydig cells to produce T to demonstrate presence of testicular tissue
—Serum MIF: produced by Sertoli cells and can indicate presence of testicular tissue
—Note: Initial serum hormone levels may be normal and may need to be repeated.

- Karyotype analysis

—Determination of genetic sex
—Chromosome analysis to exclude mosaicism
—Buccal smears are unreliable; "Barr body" present in an XX karyotype (inactivated X, Lyon hypothesis)

- Genetic evaluation

—If a genetic defect is suspected, consider DNA sequence analysis.

(continued)

Ambiguous Genitalia (continued)

IMAGING

• Evaluation of internal anatomy: to look for Müllerian organs and gonads

—Ultrasound: advantage is that no sedation or ionizing radiation is required; often the first imaging study
—CT: requires both sedation and radiation, but may be more accurate than ultrasound
—MRI: may require sedation, but not radiation; most accurate imaging technique
—Radiographic imaging is less than 100% sensitive; exploration may be required for diagnosis.

• Evaluation of lower genitourinary tract

—Retrograde genitogram: the cervix may be seen as an impression in the opacified vagina
—Antegrade study (VCUG) is inadequate, since contrast may not fill the vagina.

SPECIAL STUDIES

• Exploration and gonadal biopsy may be necessary if internal genital anatomy and gonadal sex are unclear.

—Endoscopy in male pseudohermaphrodites is used to exclude female genital structures.
—Gonadal biopsies should be done longitudinally to exclude an ovotestis.

 Initial Management

• Exclude life-threatening emergency: e.g., CAH

—Close vital sign monitoring, intravenous fluids, frequent electrolyte evaluation

• Establish diagnosis by laboratory studies and radiographic imaging.
• Gender assignment: multidisciplinary approach

—Based on anatomy and potential for sexual function, not fertility
—Male gender assignment only if phallus can function as a penis
—Usual gender assignments
  —Female pseudohermaphrodite: female
  —Male pseudohermaphrodite: male or female
  —True hermaphrodite: male or female
  —Mixed gonadal dysgenesis: female
  —Pure gonadal dysgenesis: female

 Follow-Up

MEDICAL: HORMONAL SUPPLEMENTATION

• Replacement of inadequate adrenal steroids

—Mineralocorticoids: Florinef; monitor serum renin
—Glucocorticoids: hydrocortisone; monitor serum ACTH

• Estrogens: given to females at puberty if ovaries absent
• Testosterone: given to males at puberty if testes absent
• Growth hormone: mixed gonadal dysgenesis associated with short stature

SURGICAL

• Surgical reconstruction to allow for congruent sexual rearing

—Female: feminizing genitoplasty
  —Clitoroplasty: reduce size of the clitoris; glans and dorsal nerve preserved
  —Labioplasty: create labia minora and majora
  —Vaginoplasty: four types; choice based on severity of masculinization: (1) cutback; (2) flap vaginoplasty; (3) pull-through vaginoplasty; (4) vaginal reconstruction with skin grafts or bowel interposition
  —Gonadectomy: removal of gonads in phenotypic females with a Y chromosome to prevent malignancy
—Male: masculinizing genitoplasty
  —Phalloplasty: chordee release and/or hypospadias repair
  —Orchidopexy: for undescended testes
  —Scrotoplasty: repair of bifid scrotum
  —Mastectomy: for cases with gynecomastia
—Surgical removal of gonads predisposed to malignant degeneration
  —Streak gonads with a Y chromosome in the karyotype have a 15% to 25% incidence of malignancy (gonadoblastomas and dysgerminomas).
—Potential complications of surgical reconstruction
  —Adrenal insufficiency; Rx "stress doses" of steroids
  —Wound infection
  —Loss of sensation to phallus due to nerve injury
  —Urethral fistula or stricture
  —Vaginal stenosis or prolapse
  —Rectal injury during vaginal reconstruction

 Miscellaneous

SYNONYMS

• Intersex

ASSOCIATED CONDITIONS: N/A

NOTES

• See also Section II, "Intersex Disorders."

ABBREVIATIONS

• AIS, androgen insensitivity syndrome; AR, androgen receptor; CAH, congenital adrenal hyperplasia; DHEA, dehydroepiandrosterone; DHT, dihydrotestosterone; MGD, mixed gonadal dysgenesis; MIF, Müllerian inhibitory factor; T, testosterone; T Fem, testicular feminization; 5αRD, 5α-reductase deficiency; UDT, undescended testis; VCUG, voiding cystourethrogram.

REFERENCES

Allen TD. Disorders of sexual differentiation. *Urology* 1976;7(4)[Suppl]:1–32.

Blythe B, et al. Intersex. In: Gillenwater JY, Howards SS, Duckett JW, eds. *Adult and Pediatric Urology,* 2nd ed. St Louis: Mosby–Year Book, 1997:2141–2171.

Mandell J. Sexual differentiation: Normal and abnormal. In: Walsh PC, Retik AB, Vaughan ED, Wein AJ, eds. *Campbell's Urology,* 7th ed. Philadelphia: WB Saunders, 1998:2145–2154.

Raifer J, Walsh PC. The incidence of intersexuality in patients with hypospadias and cryptorchidism. *J Urol* 1976;116:769–770.

Silver RI, Gearhart JP. Ambiguous genitalia. In: *Glenn's Urologic Surgery,* 5th ed. Philadelphia: Lippincott-Raven, 1998:859–870.

Author: Richard I. Silver

Anuria and Oliguria

 Basics

DESCRIPTION

- Anuria: no urine output
- Oliguria: urine output <0.5 cc/kg/h

PATHOPHYSIOLOGY

- Decreased urine output is often the earliest sign of impaired renal or homeostatic function.
- The problem is usually a severe decrease in the glomerular filtration rate, which interferes with the kidneys' ability to eliminate nitrogenous wastes and maintain fluid, acid-base and electrolyte balances.
- Prompt evaluation and treatment may prevent protracted renal failure and its associated morbidity and mortality.

RISK FACTORS

- Preexisting renal disease (atherosclerotic, diabetic, intrinsic, etc.)
- Medications (aminoglycosides, etc.)

 Differential Diagnosis

- Prerenal
—Most common cause in hospitalized patients
—Absolute decrease in intravascular volume
  —Hemorrhage: postoperative, trauma
  —Dehydration: GI losses, inadequate fluid replacement
—Relative decrease in intravascular volume
  —Septic shock
  —Decreased venous tone
  —Spinal shock; autonomic neuropathy
—Myocardial failure
  —Ischemic heart disease
  —Cardiomyopathy
  —Valvular heart disease
  —Pericardial tamponade/constriction
—Renal/glomerular
  —Acute glomerulonephritis
  —Vasculitis
  —Goodpasture syndrome
  —Tubulointerstitial (acute interstitial nephritis, acute tubular necrosis, etc.)
—Vascular
  —Renal artery occlusion
  —Renal vein thrombosis
  —Vasculitis
- Postrenal
—Upper urinary tract obstruction
  —Nephrolithiasis
  —External compression of ureters: retroperitoneal fibrosis
—Lower urinary tract obstruction
  —Prostatic enlargement
  —Poorly functioning bladder
  —Urethral stricture

 Database

HISTORY

- Age and sex of patient
—Older males are more likely to have problems with bladder outlet obstruction.
- Duration of decreased urine output?
—Acute vs. chronic problem
- Associated symptoms?
—Flank pain may indicate stone disease of upper tract obstruction.
- History of renal problems?
—May predispose patient to renal failure
- Medical history?
—History of diabetes mellitus, hypertension, etc., may indicate underlying renal dysfunction.
- Previous surgeries?
—Solitary kidney
- Any recent dye administration?
—Potential cause of acute renal failure
- Medications?
—Many medications are nephrotoxic and may directly cause prerenal azotemia, renal failure, or may exacerbate an underlying condition.
—Medications such as antibiotics (aminoglycosides, amphotericin B), immunosuppressives (cycloserine), and chemotherapeutic agents (cisplatin, methotrexate) are often the offending agents.
- Hypotensive events?
- Weight gain or loss?
—Gives information regarding fluids status; daily weights are the best method to monitor acute gains or losses in overall body fluid.

PHYSICAL EXAMINATION

- Heart rate
—Bradycardia may be due to hypovolemia.
- Respiratory rate
—Tachypnea may compensate for a metabolic acidosis secondary to renal failure.
- Blood pressure
—Hypotension may be due to hypovolemia.
- Neurologic examination
—Lethargy may be a symptom of renal failure.
- Neck veins
—May estimate the central venous pressure. Jugular venous distension may indicate myocardial failure.
- Heart examination
—Murmurs may indicate endocarditis.
- Pulmonary examination
—Crackles may indicate fluid overload and heart failure.
- Abdominal or flank masses
—Can be found with abdominal aortic aneurysm or upper urinary tract obstruction
- Palpable bladder
—May indicate lower urinary tract obstruction or failure to empty
- Generalized edema (extremities, presacral area)
—Indicates overall fluid status
- Rectal examination
—May indicate enlarged prostate, which can cause bladder outlet obstruction

Diagnostic Studies

LABORATORY TESTING

- Serum electrolytes

—Blood urea nitrogen (BUN) to serum creatinine >20 suggests prerenal azotemia.
—There can be multiple electrolyte abnormalities associated with renal failure (hyperkalemia, hypocalcemia, hyperphosphatemia, and hypermagnesemia).

- Urinalysis

—Urine specific gravity >1.030 urine and/or urine osmolality >500 mOsmol/kg/h
—Urinary sediment
  —Prerenal failure may exhibit hyaline and fine granular casts.
  —Intrinsic renal failure: brown granular casts and tubular epithelial casts cells are present in 80% of patients.

- Urine electrolytes (spot urine sodium)

	Prerenal	Renal
Urinary sodium concentration (mmol/L)	<20	>40
Fractional excretion of sodium (%)	<1	>1
Ratio of urinary to plasma creatinine	>40	<20
Ratio of urinary to plasma osmolarity	>1.5	<1.1

IMAGING

- Renal/bladder ultrasound

—Hydronephrosis: may be able to visualize stone as cause of obstruction, and level may be noted secondary to level of ureteral dilation; can be used in all patients because there is no radiation exposure

- Nuclear renal scan may show blood flow and function of kidneys.
- IVP or contrast not generally indicated, as may exacerbate renal insufficiency

SPECIAL STUDIES: N/A

 ## Initial Management

- Diagnosing the cause of oliguria/anuria in a patient is the most important step, because this determines the proper treatment.
- All patients with oliguria/anuria should have a Foley catheter placed to accurately monitor urine output. Catheter placement also rules out lower urinary tract obstruction as a cause. If a catheter is already in place, check to ensure that it is functioning properly (i.e., not obstructed) and irrigates easily.
- Serum electrolytes should be checked and abnormalities corrected.
- If a prerenal cause has been diagnosed, this may be treated with crystalloid/colloids/blood products, vasoactive drugs, or cardiotropic drugs, depending on the exact cause.
- In the case of intrinsic renal failure secondary to acute tubular necrosis, two strategies may be employed:

—High-dose loop diuretics (1–3 g/d) may convert oliguric to nonoliguric ATN, which may have a more favorable prognosis.
—Low-dose dopamine (0.5–2.0 μg/kg/min) can be used to increase renal blood.
—These may facilitate management but have not been proven to reduce morbidity or mortality.

- If the cause is postrenal, then the obstruction must be relieved. This can be performed most quickly via percutaneous nephrostomy placement, ureteral stent placement, or Foley catheter insertion, depending on the level of obstruction and the overall condition of the patient.
- Treatment for patients in acute renal failure in which initial treatment is unsuccessful is hemodialysis.

—Indications for hemodialysis are
  —Severe hyperkalemia; symptomatic uremia
  —Severe volume overload resulting in pulmonary edema or severe hypertension
  —Refractory metabolic acidosis; uremic pericarditis

 ## Follow-Up

- Serial renal function testing for resolution

 ## Miscellaneous

SYNONYMS

- Decreased urine output

ASSOCIATED CONDITIONS: N/A

NOTES

- See Section I, "Renal Failure—Acute."

ABBREVIATIONS: N/A

REFERENCES

Klahr S, Miller SB. Acute oliguria. N Engl J Med 1998;338(10):671–675.

Walsh PC, Retik AB, Stamey TA, Vaughn ED, eds. Campbell's Urology, 6th ed. Philadelphia: WB Saunders, 1992:2045–2062.

Authors: Louis Moy and Leonard G. Gomella

Bacteriuria and Pyuria

 Basics

DESCRIPTION

• Bacteriuria: presence of bacteria in the urine

—Can be either symptomatic or asymptomatic
—Significant bacteriuria: quantitative count $>1 \times 10^5$ CFU/mL
—Majority of individuals with significant bacteria have significant pyuria
—Prevalence
  —Newborns: males: 1.5% to 3.6%; females: 0.4% to 1.0%
  —1 to 5 years: males: 0.0% to 0.4%; females: 0.7% to 2.7%
  —School age males: 0.04% to 0.2%; females 0.7% to 2.3%
  —Adult (middle-age): males $<-1\%$; females 4% to 6%
  —Older adults: males 11% to 13%; females 6% to 33%
—Usually one organism: a uropathogen
—More than one organism: either contamination or polymicrobic infection
—Polymicrobic infection: often associated with complicating medical or urologic factors

• Pyuria: presence of white blood cells in the urine

—Implies an inflammatory response
—Significant pyuria: >10 WBCs/HPF centrifuged
—96% of patients that are symptomatic and bacteriuric have >10 WBCs/HPF.
—Close association between pyuria and bacteriuria
—Abacteriuric: An asymptomatic patient rarely has >10 WBCs/μL.
—Sterile pyuria: associated with other disorders
  —Contamination: vaginal or prepuce
  —Infections: other than uropathogens (mycobacterial, tuberculosis, chlamydial, gonococcal, fungal [GU or systemic]), viral, hemophilus, bilharzia
  —Other organ infections: gastrointestinal (appendicitis, diverticulitis, prostatitis)
  —Noninfectious: nephritis, stones, foreign bodies, transplant rejection, trauma, malignancy, chemotherapy, nephrotoxic substance

PATHOPHYSIOLOGY

• Clean-catch midstream urine may contain contaminants of bacteria and WBCs.
• Contaminants: low-count non-uropathogens
• Pyuria: contaminant <5 WBCs/HPF
• Significant bacteriuria implies true infection.
• Bacteria have colonized urinary tract and are multiplying with an inflammatory response.
• Bacterial factors

—Bacteria successfully colonize the urinary tract in a retrograde manner.
—Bacteria originate from a fecal flora, traverse perineum, and colonize vagina, urethra, and bladder.

—Certain bacteria are more efficient at adhering to mucosal cells than are others due to fimbria.
—Virulence factors: hemolysis, adhesions, colicin, metabolic properties, etc.

• Host factor

—Cystitis prone: Certain patients are more prone to bacteriuria (transitional cell bacterial receptor sites).
—Menstrual cycle: bacteriuria; may be influenced by hormones
—Postmenopausal: increasing incidence of bacteriuria
—Vaginal pH: vagina normally acid pH with normal flora as pH increases; more conducive to colonization with uropathogens
—Competitive organisms: Normal vaginal flora discourage uropathogenic colonization.
—Buccal and vaginal cells: more receptive to uropathogens' adherence in cystitis-prone patients
—Local production of IgA, IgG: may play defense role
—Production of mucous protective layer as a local bladder defense
—Blood group antigen (secretors) saturate or block bacterial adherence

RISK FACTORS

• Bacteriuria/UTI

—With increasing age, increasing prevalence of bacteriuria
—Sexual intercourse
—Diaphragm
—Spermatocide
—Delayed postcoital micturition
—History of recent infection
—Previous antimicrobial infection
—Host and bacterial factors: favoring infection
—Newborn and early age highest incidence of pathology (congenital: vesicoureteral reflux, obstruction)
—Through childhood, incidence of pathology decreases.
—Postmenopausal: associated with sepsis, mortality, and morbidity
—Pregnancy: untreated bacteriuria; 30% incidence of subsequent pyelonephritis
—Complicating factors: obstruction, stones, foreign body, diabetes, neurologic disorders, and multiple medical problems
—Impaired host response

• Pyuria

—Lower tract: no risk factors unless ascension to upper tracts
—Upper tract: pyelonephritis
—Sterile pyuria: See associated disorders other than infection.

 Differential Diagnosis

• Cystitis: pyuria, positive culture, abrupt onset
• Urethritis: pyuria, negative urine culture, gradual onset
• Vaginitis: no pyuria, vaginal discharge, pruritus
• Pyelonephritis
• Noninfectious causes
• Interstitial cystitis
• Nonuropathogenic cause: as in sterile pyuria
• Contamination of specimen with vaginal organisms and/or cells

 Database

HISTORY

• Acute dysuria, frequency, urgency, malaise, rarely low-grade fever
• Occasionally hematuria (gross): especially in female patient; uncommon in children and men
• Fever and flank pain with upper tract origin: pyelonephritis
• Asymptomatic or atypical symptoms: young and old patients
• Young patients: abdominal discomfort, failure to thrive, fever, vomiting, jaundice
• Older patients: may be asymptomatic or have incontinence, fevers, frequency, urgency
• Varied symptoms with sterile pyuria associated with varied pathology
• History of childhood fevers: may imply UTIs and associated congenital abnormalities
• Problems with toilet training, urgency, incontinence
• Family history of UTIs: mothers, daughters, sisters
• History of a risk factor for bacteriuria

PHYSICAL EXAMINATION

• Suprapubic tenderness: cystitis
• Flank tenderness: pyelonephritis
• Fever: usually with upper tract infection
• Children may have abdominal discomfort, tenderness, distention.

Diagnostic Studies

LABORATORY TESTING

- Laboratory: culture technique

—Clean-catch midstream urine: most commonly used

- Catheterized urine: may be necessary to assure diagnosis or in special situations (i.e., children, patients unable to void, the debilitated, the obese)
- Segmented urine specimen, initial 10 mL, midstream, postexamination: for localization of bacteria or WBCs
- Quantitative counts in UTI are usually $>1 \times 10^5$ CFU/mL with a uropathogen

—Range 1×10^2 to 1×10^6
—$<10^5$ per milliliter in 47% of patients
—$<10^4$ per milliliter in 30% of patients
—$>10^2$ per milliliter: uropathogen; suspect UTI

- Conditions causing variation: hydration, bacterial growth rate, urinary pH, pyelonephritis, catheter specimen
- Usually single organism
- Multiple organisms: contamination or polymicrobic infection
- Uncomplicated infections: *E. coli,* other Enterobacteriaceae, *Staphylococcus saprophyticus,* enterococci
- Complicated infections: *E. coli,* other Enterobacteriaceae, *Pseudomonas, S. aureus,* coagulase negative staph, enterococci
- Contaminants: Lactobacilli, streptococci, diphtheroids, *Gardnerella, Mycoplasma,* coag.neg. staph
- In office, pad culture methods available
- Microscope

—Rapid in-office test: 80% accurate; usually fresh unspun
—Gram stain: may increase identification of bacteria
—Centrifugation: increases finding tenfold
—Difficult to see bacteria if $<1 \times 10^5$ CFU/mL
—Vaginal organisms may be misread as uropathogens: Lactobacilli and corynebacterium

- Dipstick: best for screening

—Leukocyte esterase (LE test)
  —Sensitivity 90%, specificity 95%
—Conversion of nitrate to nitrite (Greiss test): 70% to 80% sensitivity
—Catalase test: cannot differentiate infection from inflammation

IMAGING

- Bacteriuria

—Childhood: ultrasound, VCUG, radionuclide cystogram, intravenous pyelogram
—Adult: only indicated if suspicious of pathology or childhood history, obstruction, stone disease, hematuria
—Imaging in routine UTIs involving normal adult females: very low yield of pathology

- Pyuria

—Associated with infection and bacteriuria: same indications
—Sterile pyuria evaluation for other causes

SPECIAL STUDIES

- Localization of bacteria: segmented urine, ureteral catheterization, immunologic antibody studies
- Isotopic function studies and cystogram
- CT scans: localization of nidus or abnormality responsible for bacteriuria/pyuria (i.e., abscess)

 ## Initial Management

- Bacteriuria treated as a UTI in childhood and premenopausal men and women
- Persistent or recurrent bacteriuria: may need treatment for more prolonged periods followed by chronic low-dose medication
- High-risk patients (children with congenital abnormalities and adults with significant risk factors): may need chronic suppressive antimicrobial treatment
- Postmenopausal: treated only if symptomatic or associated with complicating factors

—Diabetes, obstruction, immunosuppression

 ## Follow-Up

- Repeat examination: 2 weeks posttreatment

—Microscopic: urinalysis
—Culture

- Periodic office visits to verify sterile urine

 ## Miscellaneous

SYNONYMS: N/A

ASSOCIATED CONDITIONS: N/A

NOTES

- See other sections on UTI in adults and children.

ABBREVIATIONS

- CFU, colony-forming units

REFERENCES

Hooten TM, Stamm WE. Diagnosis and treatment of uncomplicated urinary tract infections. *Infect Dis Clin North Am* 1997;11(3):551–582.

Kunin CM, ed. *Urinary Tract Infections: Detection, Prevention and Management,* 5th ed. Baltimore: Williams & Wilkins, 1997.

Mulholland SG. Bladder infections. In: Krane RJ, Siroky MB, Fitzpatrick JM, eds. *Clinical Urology.* Philadelphia: JB Lippincott, 1994.

Schaeffer AJ. Infection of the urinary tract. In: Walsh PC, Retik AB, Vaughan ED, Wein AJ, eds. *Campbell's Urology,* 7th ed. Philadelphia: WB Saunders, 1998.

Author: S. Grant Mulholland

Bladder Trauma

 Basics

DESCRIPTION

• There is a high incidence (>85%) of associated injuries with bladder rupture from external trauma.
• Treatment of most other injuries usually takes precedence, since there is a corresponding mortality rate of approximately 20% to 40%.

PATHOPHYSIOLOGY

• In the adult, the bladder is located extraperitoneally in the space of Retzius.
• In children, the majority are intraperitoneal.
• It is attached laterally and at the base to the bony pelvis.
• The body of the bladder is the most mobile portion.
• The shearing force of a pelvic fracture could tear the bladder.
• The weakest point is at the dome.
• Penetrating trauma to the pelvis can affect the bladder directly or indirectly.
• Contusion of the bladder can also be seen in blunt trauma.

RISK FACTORS

• 8% to 10% of all pelvic fractures have an associated bladder injury.

 Differential Diagnosis

• Extraperitoneal rupture

—More common than intraperitoneal rupture
—90% to 100% are associated with pelvic fractures.
—Usually associated with an empty bladder

• Intraperitoneal rupture

—Blunt force applied to a full bladder usually causes rupture at the dome.
—Associated with more seriously injured patients, with mortality rates of approximately 20% due to non-urologic injuries
—Also seen iatrogenically with bladder instrumentation

 Database

HISTORY

• History of blunt trauma involving the pelvis, or penetrating trauma to the pelvis
• The conscious patient usually complains of lower abdominal pain.
• A majority of patients cannot void if bladder rupture is present.
• Shoulder pain can be present if urine has reached to the diaphragm.

PHYSICAL EXAMINATION

• Bruising over the lower abdominal region
• Tenderness on palpation
• Blood at the meatus: *Urethral injury should first be ruled out with a urethrogram.*
• No blood at the meatus: A catheter should be placed.
• Late signs and symptoms

—Seen in patients with injuries in an acute alcoholic state, from domestic violence (reluctant to seek attention), or from physician misdiagnosis
—Abdominal pain
—Absence of voiding
—Elevated BUN/creatinine

Diagnostic Studies

LABORATORY TESTING

• U/A: macroscopic or microscopic hematuria; found in 95% to 100% of cases
• BUN and creatine elevation can be seen with extensive intraperitoneal bladder rupture; unusual with extraperitoneal rupture.

IMAGING

• Retrograde cystogram

—Passage of urethral catheter (after urethral injury excluded)
—At least 300 mL of water-soluble iodinated contrast instilled by gravity
—Anteroposterior, oblique, and post-drain films
—Postdrainage film essential to identify contrast outside bladder that may be obscured

• CT cystogram

SPECIAL STUDIES: N/A

 ## Initial Management

• If you are first to arrive at a trauma, verify that the ABCs (airway, breathing, circulation) have been secured.
• Blunt injuries

—Bladder wall contusions: catheter drainage
—Extravasating intraperitoneal bladder trauma: surgical exploration
—Minor extraperitoneal extravasation: catheter drainage

• Penetrating injuries: caused by gunshot, stab, or bony fragments

—Surgical exploration
—Cystoscopy plays no acute role.

 ## Follow-Up

• Bladder wall contusions require a few days of catheter drainage; then a trial of voiding should be instituted.
• Postoperative care is determined on an individual basis following surgical exploration.

 ## Miscellaneous

SYNONYMS: N/A

ASSOCIATED CONDITIONS: N/A

NOTES

• See also Section I, "Urethra—Trauma."

ABBREVIATIONS: N/A

REFERENCES

Cass AS. Diagnostic studies in bladder rupture. *Urol Clin North Am* 1989;16:267–273.

Corriere JN. Trauma to the lower urinary tract. In: Gillenwater J, et al., eds. *Adult and Pediatric Urology,* 2nd ed. St. Louis: Mosby–Year Book, 1991:400–513.

Peters PC. Intraperitoneal rupture of the bladder. *Urol Clin North Am* 1989;16:279–282.

Sagalowsky AI, Peters PC. Genitourinary trauma. In: Walsh PC, Ratik AB, Vaughan ED, Wein AJ, eds. *Campbell's Urology,* 7th ed. Philadelphia: WB Saunders, 1998:3104–3107.

Authors: Pasquale Casale and Leonard G. Gomella

Burns—External Genitalia and Perineum

 Basics

DESCRIPTION

• Burn can be caused by either thermal, electrical, or chemical injury.
• Characterization

—Partial thickness: first and second degree
—Full thickness: third degree

• Type

—Thermal: water scald or immersion; flame
—Electrical: passage of current
—Chemical: any caustic substance: lye (household cleansers), battery fluid, Clinitest tablets, acetic acid (used in evaluation of condyloma)

PATHOPHYSIOLOGY

• Burn may be isolated to the genitalia/perineum, but most often part of a larger burn
• Thermal: heat effects on tissues, resulting in various degrees of injury
• Electrical: Injury may be from electrothermal heat conduction, usually with extensive skin damage and minimal internal damage, although death may be caused by halting of cardiac and brain activity, leading to cardiac arrest.
• Chemical: alkaline or acidic effects on tissues

—Perineum and genitalia are fairly well protected secondary to their position and coverage by clothing.

RISK FACTORS

• Age: very young and old
• Type of employment (e.g., refrigeration technicians, firefighters, automotive repair)
• Sex: Female genitalia are less likely to be involved in burn injuries secondary to close proximity to the body.

 Differential Diagnosis

• Diagnosis is usually apparent.

 Database

HISTORY

• Children: scald and immersion injuries
• Type of burn: chemical, thermal, electrical
• Exact time and duration of contact
• Exact heat source: flame (often deep), hot water (often less thickness)
• Exact place: open vs. closed space; higher chance of pulmonary injury with closed space
• Presence of noxious substances: e.g., plastics, volatile chemicals
• Possibility of concomitant injuries: shrapnel, glass, fractures, motor vehicle accident (MVA)

PHYSICAL EXAMINATION

• Complete physical examination to include ATLS determination of

—Extent of burns: Rule of Nines, etc.
—Type: chemical, electrical, thermal
—Character of burn
  —First-degree burns involve only the dermis and are characterized by erythema.
  —Second-degree burns involve the epidermis and some of the dermis. Blistering and superficial denudation are prominent.
  —Third-degree burns are full thickness. All layers of the skin are destroyed; scarring is significant. The skin is tough, inelastic, and discolored (white or charred). It does not blanch and is anesthetic due to destroyed nerves and blood vessels.
—Neurologic examination: to include pulses of extremities to assess for compartment syndromes
—Genitourinary examination: involvement of phallus, meatus, glans, scrotum

 Diagnostic Studies

LABORATORY TESTING

• Electrical: CK levels and urine myoglobin to monitor for myoglobinuria secondary to extensive muscle injury
• *All* burns: Frequent electrolyte monitoring is needed secondary to extensive fluid resuscitation.
• Other lab studies based on medical treatment, patient's age, and associated medical problems

IMAGING

• None specific to urology

SPECIAL STUDIES: N/A

Initial Management

- Treat immediate, life-threatening conditions (ABCs).
- Estimation of burn extent: via Rule of Nines (estimation based on body surface area) or body surface nomogram (more accurate)
- Liberal pain management
- Tetanus prophylaxis
- Fluid resuscitation: started as soon as burn recognized

—Any burn >20% TBSA will need IV resuscitation; use the modified Brooke formula to estimate volume needed.
  —2 mL Ringer's lactate per kilogram of weight per percent of TBSA burned. One half this volume is given over the first 8 hours after the burn, and the balance is given the remaining 16 hours. The following days use 5% albumin or 5% dextrose at a rate to maintain urine output of 30 to 50 mL.

- Burn cleansing

—Initially with surgical detergent and water, bullae larger than 2 cm should be excised, as they are a nidus on infection.
—Chemical burns should be washed with copious amounts of fluids, and if chemical is known, neutralizing formulas should be used.
—Tar injuries are initially cooled with tap water and later with lipophilic solvent for removal.

- Electrical: Patients with burns caused by high voltage will need cardiac monitoring for 24 hours for latent arrhythmias.

—They will also need bladder catheterization to monitor for pigment. Delayed ocular injuries may present.

- Infection: There is no role for systemic prophylactic antibiotics; treat specific conditions as they arise.

—Funguria or candiduria: Treat with intravesical amphotericin B.

- Chemotherapy: topical application of chemotherapeutic agents to reduce infection

—Silver sulfadiazine: 1% suspension of silver sulfadiazine
  —Broad antimicrobial spectrum although without penetration of burn eschar
  —Ineffective against *Pseudomonas* and strains of *Enterobacter cloacae.*
  —Painless when applied
—Mafenide acetate (Sulfamylon) 11.1% suspension in a hydrophilic base, allowing penetration into burn eschar
  —Broad antimicrobial spectrum, including *Pseudomonas*
  —Inhibits carbonic anhydrase resulting in bicarbonate wasting with metabolic acidosis
  —Painful administration
  —Alternating application every 12 hours, with mafenide and sulfadiazine mostly used

—Silver nitrate: 0.5% solution
  —No penetration of burn eschar
  —Painless
  —Good antimicrobial spectrum
  —Electrolyte disturbances associated with use (losses of sodium, potassium, calcium, and chloride)

- Nonoperative management is the initial management for external genitalia burns.

—While full-thickness burns do not heal by re-epithelialization, perineal and genital burns of this depth often do. The loose and redundant skin of the penis and scrotum allow this.

- Operative intervention may be needed for extensive full-thickness burns: Epithelization should occur within 3 to 6 weeks.

—Split-thickness skin grafts, meshed/non-meshed depending on usage
—Frequent debridement of nonviable tissue, daily inspection until closure
—Electrical burns: more likelihood of surgical intervention secondary to contact points within the perineum, causing deep point of injury requiring debridement. These may require orchiectomy or penectomy.
—Testicular exposure: may be handled with temporary or permanent thigh implantation, creation of neoscrotum or free flaps
—Escharotomy: rare, but may be needed for the circumferential penile burn
—Female genital burn may result in vaginal stenosis secondary to contraction; repairs are best handled after 6 to 12 months with reconstruction.
—Male urethral meatal injury may require suprapubic catheter placement.

Follow-Up

- After 6 to 12 months most burns will have matured and the decision is made for any reconstruction.
- Long-term erectile dysfunction may be treated by release of any scar tissue bands or standard medical therapy or prosthesis placement.
- Other genital or perineal burn scar contractures: release of simple bands, split-thickness skin grafts, or Z-plasty

Miscellaneous

SYNONYMS: N/A

ASSOCIATED CONDITIONS: N/A

NOTES

- ATLS guidelines through the American College of Surgeons
- Rule of Nines (estimation of extent of burn): each arm, 9%; head, 9%; anterior and posterior body wall, 18%; each leg, 18%; and the genitalia/perineum, 1%

ABBREVIATIONS

- CK, creatinine kinase; ABC, airway, breathing, and circulation; ATLS, advanced trauma life support; TBSA, total body surface area

REFERENCES

Peck MD, et al. The management of burns to the perineum and genitals. *J Burn Care Rehabil* 1990; 11(1):54–56.

Sheridan R, Tompkins R. Burns. In: *Surgery, Scientific Principles, and Practice,* 2nd ed. 1997, Philadelphia: Lippincott-Raven, 422–438.

Waguespack RL, et al. Contemporary results of the management of burns of the genitalia and perineum. *J Urol* 1992;147(4):288A.

Waguespack RL, et al. *Genital and Perineal Burns.* AUA Update Series, 1995, Lesson 4; Volume XIV.

Authors: Natania Y. Piper and Ian M. Thompson

Contrast Allergy and Reactions

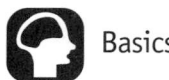 **Basics**

DESCRIPTION

• A complex of symptoms related to the intravenous administration of contrast agents. Reaction to topical/extravascular contrast is extremely rare.
• Iodinated contrast media are required for urography and imaging studies such as CT scan, venogram, etc.

—Currently, all commonly used radiographic materials have a basic chemical structure: a tri-iodinated benzene ring at the 2,4, and 6 positions.

• Three groups of contrast reactions: idiosyncratic, nonidiosyncratic, delayed

PATHOPHYSIOLOGY

• Idiosyncratic

—Typically begins within 20 minutes of administration
—Not in proportion to dose
—Urticaria, bronchospasm, upper airway edema, hypotension
—Not consistent with a true allergic reaction. No IgE anticontrast antibodies are found in patients; thus called *anaphylactoid*, not anaphylactic.
—Patients do not have to be previously exposed to contrast.
—Patients who do have a reaction are at increased risk for a second reaction. But not all patients will have a reaction.

• Nonidiosyncratic

—Dose-dependent reactions
—Sensation of warmth
—Metallic taste in mouth
—Nausea and vomiting
—Renal failure: 5% incidence in general population. Elevation of serum creatinine after 1 to 3 days is the first sign. Supportive measures are all that is needed, and function usually returns to baseline within 2 weeks.
—Patients are at increased risk if a reaction has occurred in the past.

• Delayed contrast reactions

—Typically after 30 minutes of injection
—Occur in up to 30% of patients
—Symptoms
  —Flu-like (malaise, upper respiratory infection, fever, chills, etc.)
  —Pain in injected extremity, rash, dizziness, headaches
  —Almost always resolve spontaneously

RISK FACTORS

• Previous adverse reaction

—7× for a mild reaction
—9× for a moderate reaction
—11× more likely for a severe reaction to recur

• Asthma: 5× the risk
• Allergies to substances other than contrast material: up to 2× the risk

—Shellfish allergy: however, no consistent data to support this theory

• Renal insufficiency/failure: up to 10× the risk
• No significant difference found between rapid or slow infusion of material, except

—Fast infusion is associated with higher incidence of warm feeling and headache.
—Slow infusion is associated with higher adverse reactions with use of Renografin.

• Diabetics are at increased risk of renal damage, especially if dehydrated.

 Differential Diagnosis

• The timing in relation to the contrast suggests the diagnosis.

 Database

HISTORY

• Current symptoms
• History of previous reactions to contrast
• Medical history, allergies, current medications

PHYSICAL EXAMINATION

• ABCs of resuscitation

—Current signs and objective symptoms

Diagnostic Studies

LABORATORY TESTING

- Usually not necessary in the acute setting
- Serum creatine must be known before administration of an agent.

IMAGING: N/A

SPECIAL STUDIES: N/A

 ## Initial Management

- Based on the severity of the reaction
- Support ABCs (airway, breathing, circulation) with appropriate resuscitative protocols as needed
- Idiosyncratic is most immediately life threatening
- Mild symptom: reassure
- Skin reactions (hives, pruritus)

—Benadryl 50 mg im/iv
—If severe (constructural edema, etc.)
   —Epinephrine 0.3–0.4 ml 1:1000 solution SQ

- Severe reactions

—IV fluids (i.e., saline)
—Pressors to support pressure if no response to fluids
—IV hydrocortisone 300–500 mg
—Epinephrine, as above

 ## Follow-Up

- Use of selective nonionic contrast media
- Premedication with corticosteroids (methyl-prednisolone 32 mg 12 hours and 2 hours before injection, or prednisone 50 mg 13, 7, and 1 hour prior to injection)
- Premedicate with antihistamines (diphenhydramine 50 mg 1 hour prior to study). An H2 blocker can be used in conjunction with H1, but never without H1 blockers.
- Adequate hydration 12 hours prior to until 2 hours after study for patients with history of renal failure/insufficiency. Furosemide and mannitol are controversial topics (never to be used without hydration).

 ## Miscellaneous

SYNONYMS: N/A

ASSOCIATED CONDITIONS

- Asthma
- Seafood/shellfish allergy

NOTES

- Non-ionic contrast agents may limit the reactions but cannot eliminate the possibility of a reaction.

ABBREVIATIONS: N/A

REFERENCES

Cohan RH, Ellis JH. Iodinated contrast material in uroradiology. *Urol Clin North Am* 1997;24(3): 471–490.

Shehadi WH. Contrast media adverse reactions: Occurrence, recurrence, and distribution patterns. *Radiology* 1982;143:11–17.

Authors: Pasquale Casale and Leonard G. Gomella

Costovertebral Angle Tenderness

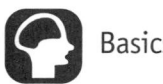 Basics

DESCRIPTION

- Pain arising in the kidney is referred to the ipsilateral flank, costovertebral angle, and upper anterior abdomen. Pain arising in the ureter may be referred to the ipsilateral lower abdomen, groin, and spermatic cord. Also, pain may be referred to the testicle and scrotum in the male and to the ovary or labia in the female.
- May be associated with anorexia, malaise, nausea, vomiting, fever, chills, gross hematuria, urinary frequency/urgency
- Colicky vs. noncolicky
- *Renal colic* is a misnomer; it does not wax and wane like gastrointestinal or biliary colic, but refers instead to pain involving the renal collecting system.

PATHOPHYSIOLOGY

- Urinary obstruction

—Local direct mechanical irritation of the collecting system or of the ureteral mucosa by stone(s) or other debris
—Interstitial edema and stretch of the renal capsule (especially when pyelonephritis is present)
—Obstruction may be intraluminal or extraluminal.

- The spinal reflex mechanism can cause muscle spasm or vascular responses in dermatomes and spinal nerve segments corresponding to the visceral origin of the pain.
- Gonadal pain: embryologic origin from the medial aspect of the most cephalic portion of the urogenital ridge, in close proximity to the nephrogenic ridge. Blood supply and innervation originate near the renal hilum; therefore, pain from the kidney and ureter can be referred along this pathway.
- Visceral pain

—Free nerve endings (stretch receptors) that tend to respond to changes in pressure or wall tension; most dense collections in renal capsule, renal pelvis (submucosal)
—Triggered by acute distension of the renal pelvis and upper ureter (rather than by ureteral hyperperistalsis or spasm); or by mucosal irritation

RISK FACTORS

- History of stones, family history of stones, hypercalcemia, chronic dehydration, warm arid climate, obstructive uropathy, excessive salt and protein intake
- Urinary risk factors: hypercalciuria, hyperuricosuria, hyperoxaluria, hypocitraturia

 Differential Diagnosis

- Renal colic

—Intraluminal causes: renal calculi, blood clots, fungal bezoar, tumor emboli, pedunculated fibroepithelial polyp, renal papillary necrosis, bullets and other penetrating foreign bodies, infundibular stenosis, calyceal diverticula, ureteropelvic junction obstruction, ureteral stricture
—Extraluminal causes: retroperitoneal fibrosis, ovarian vein syndrome, endometriosis, aortic dissection, abdominal aortic aneurysm, iliac artery aneurysm, retrocaval ureter, pregnancy, extrauterine pregnancy, mass lesions of the uterus or ovary, tubo-ovarian abscess, Crohn disease, diverticulitis, appendicitis, retroperitoneal mass, retroperitoneal hemorrhage, retroperitoneal lymphocele, pelvic lipomatosis

- Noncolicky pain

—Renal vascular events
    —Acute renal infarction, renal artery emboli associated with atrial fibrillation, acute myocardial infarction, endocarditis, artificial valve, ruptured atheroma from an aortic plaque
    —Polyarteritis nodosa or other inflammatory vascular disorders
    —Renal vein thrombosis
    —Nutcracker syndrome (compression of the left renal artery between the superior mesenteric artery and the aorta)
    —Arteriovenous fistula
—Infectious processes
    —Pyelonephritis
    —Renal cortical or corticomedullary abscess
    —Perinephric abscess

- Medical renal disease
    —Poststreptococcal glomerulonephritis
    —Rapidly progressive glomerulonephritis
    —IgA nephropathy (Berger disease)
    —Acute interstitial nephritis
    —Analgesic abuse nephropathy
—Renal trauma
—Loin pain/hematuria syndrome (related to oral contraceptive use)
—Polycystic kidney disease (autosomal dominant)
—Medullary sponge kidney (often accompanied by nephrocalcinosis, hyperparathyroidism, renal tubular acidosis)
—Renal tumors (angiomyolipoma especially prone to bleeding)
—Ptotic kidney (nephroptosis; usually on right side in thin women)

- Nonrenal causes of flank pain

—Muscular pain, skeletal/rib pain, herpes zoster, iliac osteomyelitis, pleural pain, aortic dissection or aneurysm, acute myocardial infarction, acute appendicitis, peptic ulcer disease, acute cholecystitis, acute diverticulitis, colon carcinoma, splenic infarction, splenic abscess, inflammatory bowel disease

Database

HISTORY

- Onset

—Acute vs. insidious
—Related temporally to large fluid intake? Suggestive of ureteropelvic junction obstruction

- Concurrent symptoms: low-grade fever, moderate leukocytosis common with uninfected obstruction; high fever suggestive of pyelonephritis/pyonephrosis
- Location of pain and tenderness? Flank, CVA pain suggestive of renal obstruction; lower abdominal pain, groin pain suggestive of ureteral pain. Nausea and vomiting are common, but peritoneal signs (rebound, guarding) are suggestive of intraperitoneal process.
- History of urolithiasis?
- Family history of urolithiasis?
- History of trauma?
- Symptoms of urinary tract infection? Gross hematuria? Dysuria?
- Other GU pathology (benign prostate hyperplasia, vesicoureteral reflux, etc.)
- History of upper respiratory infection? Associated with Berger disease and glomerulonephritis
- History of surgery (open or endoscopic, and laparoscopic)? Possible ureteral injury, fibrosis
- Medical history

—Diabetes mellitus, hemophilia, sickle cell disease or trait, analgesic abuse? Consider renal papillary necrosis.
—History of radiation therapy, inflammatory bowel disease, diverticulitis, appendicitis? Consider fibrosis, stricture.
—Endocarditis, atrial fibrillation, myocardial infarction, artificial cardiac valves? Consider emboli, infarction.
—Nephrotic syndrome, sickle cell? Consider renal vein thrombosis.
—Diabetes mellitus, long-term, broad-spectrum antibiotic use; steroids; transplantation; HIV; or cancer-related immunosuppression? Consider *Candida* or *Aspergillus* fungal bezoar.

- Menstrual history? Rule out pregnancy-related causes (e.g., ovarian vein thrombosis). Cyclic pain can be associated with endometriosis.

PHYSICAL EXAMINATION

- Vital signs

—Fever, especially with tachycardia, can be indicative of pyelonephritis (with chills, nausea, vomiting, and dull, aching pain); obstructing renal calculi without superimposed infection are rarely present with fever.
—Hypotension: urosepsis; hypertension. Consider vascular emergency such as dissection.

- Palpation

—Palpable flank or abdominal mass?
—Severe, intense pain suggestive of abscess
—Pain with flexion of back, thigh. Consider perinephric/psoas abscess?

- Pelvic examination: Distal ureteral stones may be palpable transvaginally.
- Decreased breath sounds on affected side, rales, splinting, dullness to percussion, hiccups are all suggestive of renal caruncle.
- Inability to find a comfortable position is suggestive of renal colic (obstruction).
- Flank ecchymoses is suggestive of trauma; flank blistering is suggestive of severe perinephric infection.
- Flank fistula tracts: associated with long-standing obstructive uropathy, especially with urolithiasis
- Right-sided varicocele is suggestive of vascular occlusive process in retroperitoneum.

 Diagnostic Studies

LABORATORY TESTING

- Urinalysis: hematuria, WBC (infection, tuberculosis), proteinuria (glomerulonephritis, IgA nephropathy, nephrotic syndrome), casts (leukocyte: pyelonephritis; RBC: sickle cell), pH (<5.5 suggestive of uric acid or cystine lithiasis; >7.2 suggestive of infection calculi associated with urease-producing organisms resulting in magnesium ammonium phosphate calculi [normal urine pH 5.8–6.0]), crystalluria (helpful with unique crystals such as cystine; calcium oxalate crystals normal finding)
- Urine culture for bacteria; consider fungal cultures in diabetics, other immunocompromised states
- Complete blood count: mild-to-moderate leukocytosis, even in uninfected obstruction, anemia associated with long-standing infectious process
- Blood cultures for pyelonephritis, abscess
- Electrolytes, urea nitrogen, creatinine, calcium, phosphorus, uric acid, parathyroid hormone

(continued)

Costovertebral Angle Tenderness (continued)

IMAGING

- KUB: to look for extraosseous calcifications, nephrocalcinosis, renal contours, bowel gas pattern, prior surgery (missing rib, clips), intrarenal air

—Radiopaque stones: calcium oxalate, calcium phosphate, magnesium ammonium phosphate (rarely a primary ureteral stone, more commonly staghorn configuration), cystine (ground-glass appearance with smooth edges)
—Radiolucent stones: uric acid, matrix, xanthine, protease inhibitor–associated stones

- IVP: to assess renal position, shape, orientation, axis and size, renal contours/uptake and excretion of contrast; caliber of collecting system (renal and ureteral), masses, calculi, filling defects
- Ultrasound: cannot assess ureter well. Posterior acoustic shadowing helps confirm presence of calculi. Identification of small ureterovesical junction stones may be enhanced through the acoustic window of a full bladder. Can exclude hydronephrosis. Helpful in determining solid vs. cystic masses. Doppler to assess vascular structures, flow. Useful when renal failure precludes contrast administration
- CT: to assess renal mass (solid vs. cystic), intraabdominal pathology; can give limited information on vascular system

—Noncontrast study to identify renal and ureteral calculi (all stones irrespective of appearance on KUB will give appearance of bonelike density, with the exception of pure protease inhibitor–associated calculi). It may become the first-choice imaging modality for calculi.

- MRI: to assess renal veins, vena cava; stones poorly visualized
- Nuclear medicine: to assess renal function, rule out UPJO; bisphosphates bind to calculi

SPECIAL STUDIES

- Cystoscopy, retrograde pyelography: if ureteral pathology suspected, excretory urography suboptimal, or renal failure present
- Ureteroscopy
- Renal biopsy to diagnose nephropathy, interstitial nephritis
- Antegrade nephrostogram, ureterogram

 Initial Management

- Initial work-up should include imaging studies; first line dependent on equipment availability, operator experience, and cost
- Additional studies as indicated to confirm or rule out other pathology
- "Medical" renal causes of pain: Tailor the work-up to preliminary findings (e.g., consider renal biopsy with proteinuria).
- Volume: intravenous fluids to achieve a euvolemic state; excessive intravenous fluid will *not* promote stone clearance; effective ureteral peristalsis requires coaptation of the ureteral walls.
- Analgesia

—NSAIDs (half-life, hours)
  —Ibuprofen: 400 mg q4–6h [2]
  —Naproxen: 550-mg loading dose, 275 mg q6–8h [13]
  —Fenoprofen: 400 mg q4–6h [3]
  —Diflunisal: 500 to 1000 mg q6–8h [12]
  —Ketorolac: 30 mg IV/IM loading, 15 mg IV/IM q6h (use with caution in the elderly and in those with renal failure)
—Aspirin: 650 to 1000 mg q4–6h
—Acetaminophen: 800 to 1000 mg q4h (not to exceed 4000 mg/24 h)
—Narcotics
  —Morphine sulfate: 0.1 mg/kg IM/IV q4h
  —MS Contin (long-acting oral morphine): 30 mg po q12h
  —Meperidine: 1 mg/kg IM q3–4h
  —Hydromorphone: 1 to 2 mg IM q4–6h, 2 to 4 mg po q4–6h
  —Oxycodone: 5 mg po q6h
  —Methadone: 2.5 to 10.0 mg po q3–4h
  —Codeine: 15 to 60 mg po q3–4h
  —Propoxyphene (Darvon)
  —Pentazocine (Talwin)
—Adjuvants
  —Tricyclic antidepressants: amitriptyline: 25 to 75 mg po qhs
  —Antihistamines: hydroxyzine: 25 mg IM/po q4–6h
—Acupuncture: works via beta-endorphins, met-enkephalin

- Chronic pain management
—Same medications as with acute pain
—Sedatives: dangerous, habit-forming (barbiturates, benzodiazepines)
—Carbamazepine can be helpful in pain of CNS origin
—Tricyclic and SRI antidepressants helpful with psychological component of chronic pain
—Nerve blockade: can be both diagnostic and therapeutic
—Nephropexy to exclude ptotic kidney (when all other measures fail)

- Intravenous antibiotics for pyelonephritis
- Surgical intervention after failed conservative observation (awaiting spontaneous stone passage)

—Acute obstruction: retrograde ureteral stent placement or percutaneous nephrostomy
—To remove calculi: ureterorenoscopy with or without intracorporeal lithotripsy, ESWL, percutaneous nephrolithotomy, open lithotomy, laparoscopic lithotomy
—Drainage of abscess, cysts: now safely performed percutaneously, laparoscopically, or in an open fashion

Follow-Up

• Outpatient metabolic evaluation and treatment for calculi

—Evaluation with 24-hour urine collection (volume, calcium, uric acid, oxalate, citrate, phosphorus, creatinine, sodium) and blood chemistries obtained under routine diet intake and activities

—Treatments based on 24-hour urine parameters

—Hypercalciuria: absorptive Type I (dietary independent, treat with binders such as cellulose phosphate or with hydrochlorothiazide), absorptive Type II (dietary dependent, reduce calcium intake by 50% to 400–500 mg/24 h), absorptive Type III (phosphate renal leak, treat with bioavailable phosphate), resorptive (primary hyperparathyroidism, surgery only effective treatment), renal (hydrochlorothiazide therapy effective over long term)

—Hyperuricosuria: dietary modification; if unsuccessful, treat with allopurinol

—Hyperoxaluria: Treat underlying diarrheal state; provide calcium intake with meals.

—Hypocitraturia: Treat underlying metabolic acidosis; use potassium citrate or lemonade.

—Specific therapy for unusual stone types/ 24-hour urine parameters

• KUB and renal ultrasound to rule out silent hydronephrosis and calculi

• Office visit to check compliance with medications; emphasis on optimizing diet (decreased sodium and protein intake, aim for voided volume of 1.6 L per day; calcium restriction *only* if indicated based on 24-hour urine finding of absorptive Type I hypercalciuria), reevaluation of 24-hour urine parameters, and patient reassurance

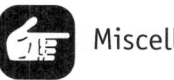 Miscellaneous

SYNONYMS: *N/A*

ASSOCIATED CONDITIONS: *N/A*

NOTES: *N/A*

ABBREVIATIONS

• IgAN, immunoglobulin A nephropathy; UPJO, ureteropelvic junction obstruction; DM, diabetes mellitus; SRI, serotonin reuptake inhibitor antidepressant; EHL, electrohydraulic lithotripsy; ESWL, extracorporeal shock wave lithotripsy; NSAIDs, nonsteroidal antiinflammatory drugs

REFERENCES

Gupta M. Acute and chronic renal pain. In: Coe FL, et al., eds. *Kidney Stones: Medical and Surgical Management.* Philadelphia: Lippincott–Raven, 1996.

Tanagho EA, et al., eds. *Smith's General Urology,* 14th ed. Norwalk, CT: Appleton & Lange, 1995.

Walsh PC, AB, Vaughan ED, Wein AJ, eds. *Campbell's Urology,* 7th ed. Philadelphia: WB Saunders, 1998.

Authors: Brian P. Grady, Bradley F. Schwartz, and Marshall L. Stoller

Dyspareunia

 Basics

DESCRIPTION

- Pain during or resulting from sexual intercourse
- May be anatomic, psychological, or mixed
- Described in *Diagnostic and Statistical Manual of Mental Disorders* (DSM-IV) as a subclassification of sexual dysfunction

PATHOPHYSIOLOGY

- The anatomic site of pain during intercourse may be subdivided into three areas.

—Entrance dyspareunia: pain concentrated at the vaginal opening
—Vaginal dyspareunia: pain along the entire length of the vagina
—Deep-thrust dyspareunia: pelvic pain during partner's thrust

RISK FACTORS

- Traumatic deliveries
- Vaginal infections
- Menopause

 Differential Diagnosis

- Congenital: rigid hymen, hymenal tags, imperforate hymen, vaginal deviations, vaginal agenesis, uterine retroversion
- Vaginal masses: cystocele, rectocele, uterine prolapse, neoplasm
- Vaginal stenosis: narrowing of the introitus or vaginal canal due to surgery or radiation
- Senile atrophy of the vagina: loss of lubrication due to hormonal influences
- Childbirth trauma: episiotomies or rectal tears
- Infections of the vulva or vagina: HPV, herpes simplex, STDs, fungal (*Candida*), PID
- Vulvar dystrophies: hyperplasia, lichen sclerosis (white plaque)
- Inflammatory lesion of the urethra: urethral caruncle, urethral diverticulum, urethritis, neoplasm
- Lesions within the pelvis: endometriosis, fibroids, ectopic pregnancy, adnexal cysts, adnexal prolapse, pelvic adhesions, neoplasm, pelvic floor muscle spasm
- Allergic reactions of the vagina: contraceptives or douching materials, latex
- Rectal causes: constipation, proctitis, hemorrhoids
- Psychological causes

—Lack of arousal: due to hormonal influences and decreased lubrication
—Guilt, shame, tension: due to new or unusual sexual situations
—Fear, anxiety: history of sexual abuse

 Database

HISTORY

- Is pain at vaginal opening, entire vagina, or associated with deep thrusts?

—Localized anatomic site of pain

- Has pain always been present with sexual intercourse?

—Primary dyspareunia. Consider congenital causes or pelvic floor spasm.

- Is pain a recent occurrence with sexual intercourse?

—Secondary dyspareunia. Decreased lubrication, vulvar dystrophies, infection/inflammation, fibrosis, neoplasm

- Have you had prior pelvic or vaginal surgery or radiation?

—May cause vaginal stenosis or pelvic adhesions

- Any childbirth trauma?

—Episiotomy, rectal tears

- Are you postmenopausal?

—If not on hormonal replacement, may have decreased lubrication

- Is pain related to your menstrual cycle?

—Endometriosis

- Any recent use of new deodorants or feminine hygiene (douches)?

—Consider allergic reactions.

- Is there a history of sexual abuse?

—May point toward psychological causes

PHYSICAL EXAMINATION

• Erythema of vulva

—Allergic reaction or infection

• Ulcers and lesions surrounding vulva and introitus

—Infectious causes, STDs, clear cell carcinoma of the vagina

• Decreased lubrication with thinning of the vaginal mucosa

—Vaginal atrophy

• Tenderness at vestibule and hymenal area

—Vulvovaginitis or vulvovestibulitis

• Pain with vaginal palpation of the pelvic floor muscles

—Pelvic floor muscle spasm

• Palpable mass on anterior vaginal wall that may exude discharge per urethra when compressed

—Urethral diverticulum

• Tenderness with palpation of the cul-de-sac, if uterus is not retroverted

—May be endometriosis or pelvic adhesions

• Tenderness with gentle manipulation of the cervix

—Suggestive of PID/cervicitis

 Diagnostic Studies

LABORATORY TESTING

• Urine culture to evaluate for infection

IMAGING

• Endovaginal ultrasound may identify ovarian, uterine, or other pelvic masses.

SPECIAL STUDIES

• PAP smear to rule out malignancy
• KOH test of cervical secretions to differentiate between *Gardnerella* and *Trichomonas*
• Endocervical culture to rule out infection with *Chlamydia* or *Gonorrhea*
• Colposcopy of the vulva and cervix to identify HPV, malignant changes
• Vaginal mucosal biopsy to identify vulvar dystropies
• Diagnostic laparoscopy to differentiate endometriosis from adhesions
• VCUG "double balloon urethrogram" to identify a urethral diverticulum

 Initial Management

• Vulvovaginitis: Avoid vaginal deodorants, douches, or constant use of a panty liner.
• Vaginal atrophy: estrogen replacement (oral, transdermal, intramuscular)
• Vulvar dystrophy

—Hyperplastic dystrophy: topical corticosteroid applied 2 to 3× daily
—Lichen sclerosis: testosterone propionate 2% ointment applied 2 to 3× daily for 3 to 6 months

• Vaginal stenosis or shortening: passive dilation with vaginal dilators used daily
• Endometriosis: laparoscopic laser, fulguration, or excision or with GnRH analogues (e.g., Lupron)
• Pelvic adhesions: laparoscopic lysis of adhesions
• Retroverted uterus: Change sexual position to allow a more anterior entry.

—Pessary to antevert uterus out of cul-de-sac.
—Surgical treatment with uterine suspension

 Follow-Up

• Recommendations: Close follow-up is recommended when behavior or medical therapy is instituted to treat dyspareunia. When patient satisfaction is increased, time to follow up is gradually lengthened to a routine annual check-up.

 Miscellaneous

SYNONYMS: N/A

ASSOCIATED CONDITIONS: N/A

NOTES: N/A

ABBREVIATIONS

• STD, sexually transmitted disease; HPV, human papilloma virus; PID, pelvic inflammatory disease

REFERENCES

Leventhral JL, et al. Treatment of dyspareunia following medical illness. *West J Med* 1992;156: 196.

Meana M, et al. Dyspareunia: Sexual dysfunction or pain syndrome? *J Nerv Ment Dis* 1997; 185:561.

Sandberg G, et al. Dyspareunia: An integrated approach to assessment and diagnosis. 1987; 24:66.

Sarazin SK, et al. Causes and treatment options for women with dyspareunia. *Nurse Pract* 1991; 16:30.

Steege JF, et al. Dyspareunia: A special type of chronic pelvic pain. 1993;20:779.

Authors: Marlene Corujo and Gopal H. Badlani

Dysuria

 Basics

DESCRIPTION

- Painful urination that is usually caused by inflammation
- Sensation of pain or burning may be felt at start of, during, or at the end of micturition
- Usually not indicative of serious disorder; infection or inflammation is most common cause.

—Unexplained persistent dysuria should never be ignored, as this subgroup may have occult carcinoma.

- Dysuria is frequently accompanied by urinary frequency and urgency.
- Dysuria work-up is often guided by the presence of other symptoms or findings (e.g., hematuria).

PATHOPHYSIOLOGY

- Painful urination is usually related to irritation of nerve endings in the bladder, urethra, or prostate.
- Sensation may be interpreted as pain or "burning" on urination.
- Pain originating in the bladder is commonly referred to the urethral meatus or the distal urethra in men.

RISK FACTORS

- Female sex, recent trauma, urinary tract surgery or instrumentation, immunosuppression, indiscreet sexual activity, family history of renal calculi, pelvic radiation, recent febrile illness, history of similar complaint in partner

 Differential Diagnosis

- Inflammatory causes

—Bladder: cystitis (bacterial, viral, parasitic, specific, e.g., tuberculosis), interstitial cystitis, radiation cystitis
—Urethra: urethral caruncle, urethritis (specific and nonspecific), foreign body induced, postinstrumentation, radiation induced
—Prostate: prostatitis (bacterial, nonbacterial [chemical])
—Adjacent organs: e.g., appendix, uterus and vagina, small bowel, colon, rectum

- Tumors

—Primary urologic tumors: bladder cancer, prostate cancer, urethral carcinoma
—Secondary urologic tumors: e.g., invasion of the bladder by tumors of the bowel or gynecologic organs

- Foreign bodies

—Stones in bladder, distal ureter, urethra; postinstrumentation

- Obstructive

—Bladder neck contracture, posterior urethral valves, BPH, stones, urethral stricture, meatal stenosis

 Database

HISTORY

- Age and sex?

—Urinary tract infection (UTI) common in females. Likelihood of cancer increases with increasing age.

- Timing and location of pain?

—Pain at the start of urination indicates urethral pathology (e.g., urethral caruncle).
—Pain present in urethra during micturition indicates urethral stricture or inflammation. Look for urethral discharge.
—Pain at the end of urination is usually of bladder origin (strangury). Sometimes felt as a tingling or pricking sensation in the glans penis. Indicates an inflammatory or irritative process at the trigonal region of the bladder such as calculus, cystitis. Transitional cell carcinoma (TCC) at the base.
—Note that sometimes a calculus in the distal intramural portion of the ureter may give severe pain at the end of micturition.

- History of urethral discharge?

—Implicates the urethra or prostate as site of inflammation

- Any vaginal symptoms?

—Vulvar irritation, vaginal discharge, itching, odor indicate probable vaginitis.

- Any associated bleeding?

—Hematuria without documented UTI or persistent hematuria after treatment of UTI must be worked up as outlined in the section on Hematuria. Finding hematuria takes precedence over the symptom of dysuria.

- Recent trauma or instrumentation to urinary tract?

—Can cause inflammatory response or introduce infection

- Lower urinary tract symptoms?

—Frequency, nocturia, slowing of stream, etc., may indicate benign prostatic hypertrophy (BPH) in men or urethral stricture in women. Incomplete bladder emptying predisposes to infection and to stones.

- Significant medical or surgical history?

—Renal or urologic disease or surgery. Sexually transmitted disease or urethral instrumentation can cause strictures. History of pelvic radiation; history of tuberculosis; malignancies; diabetes

- Current medications?

—Topical podophyllins for penile condyloma, allergic reaction to intravaginal douches, substances that can cause phosphaturia and/or crystalluria

- Sexual history?

—Recent onset or initiation of sexual intercourse
—Young men with dysuria, frequency, and urethral discharge following sexual intercourse most likely have urethritis.

- History of tobacco use?

—Associated with TCC and recurrent UTIs

- Family history?

—History of urinary calculi, diabetes, urologic cancer, reflux

- Other accompanying symptoms?

—Suprapubic pain and/or pressure is suggestive of cystitis.
—Fever implicates tissue invasion by infectious agents and necessitates urgent treatment.
—Male children may have a meatal ulcer from ammoniacal dermatitis.
—Symptoms suggestive of primary pathology in other organ systems

PHYSICAL EXAMINATION

- Vital signs

—Fever, tachycardia, or other indications of systemic inflammatory response

- Abdominal examination

—Flank tenderness suggests pyelonephritis or urolithiasis.
—Suprapubic tenderness suggests inflammation of bladder.
—Abdominal mass may be felt arising from other organ systems.

- Genital examination

—Associated inflammation such as orchitis or epididymitis
—Examine urethra for presence of meatal stenosis, meatitis, urethral caruncle, urethral prolapse.
—Evaluate for urethral discharge, especially after prostate massage.

- Digital rectal examination

—Tender, boggy prostate with acute prostatitis; nodularity suggests cancer
—Prostate massage can be used to diagnose prostatitis.
—Evaluate rectum for inflammation.
—Hemoccult testing to screen for gastrointestinal pathology

- Pelvic examination

—Adnexal masses or tenderness, bimanual examination for bladder cancer, vaginal inflammation, vaginoscopy
—Evidence of chlamydial or gonococcal infection (e.g., mucopurulent discharge and organisms seen on smear)

 Diagnostic Studies

LABORATORY TESTING

- Urinalysis/dipstick

—Note nitrates, leukocyte esterase, pH, blood, and glucose.

—Test strips that detect nitrites (bacteria) and leukocyte esterase (WBCs) are accurate predictors of bacteruria.

—Nitrite test: A positive nitrite suggests the presence of greater than 10^5 organisms/mL. Being positive for only the coagulase-splitting bacteria, this test is accurate only in 50% to 60% cases when used alone. A false-negative nitrite test can result if the bacteria do not contain nitrate reductase, urine is not present in the bladder for >4 hours, absence of dietary nitrite, or ingestion of ascorbic acid.

—Leukocyte esterase test: identifies WBCs and a positive result indicates 10 to 12 WBCs/HPF. Used together, the two tests are as predictive of UTI as microscopic analysis. Glucosuria, vitamin C, nitrofurantoin, Pyridium, or rifampin can produce a false-negative leukocyte esterase reaction.

—pH: If greater than 7.0, this suggests the presence of urea-splitting organisms such as *Proteus, Klebsiella, Pseudomonas, Providentia,* and *Staphylococcus.*

—Hematuria: may coexist with UTI or indicate other underlying pathology

—Glucose: could indicate diabetes mellitus, which predisposes patients to UTIs

• Microscopic analysis

—In the sediment from a clean-catch specimen from men or a catheterized specimen from women, 5 to 8 WBCs/hpf is considered as abnormal and indicates pyuria. Also more than 3 RBCs/hpf is significant and warrants work-up as outlined in the section on Hematuria

—Sterile pyuria, the presence of pyuria without bacteria, may indicate renal tuberculosis and, if persistent, should prompt acid-fast staining to detect the organism.

—A careful study of the urine can often reveal "old" leukocytes (small, wrinkled cells) which are present in the vagina of women and thus indicate contamination. "Fresh" leukocytes indicate acute urinary tract injury.

—The identification of bacteria or yeast in an uncontaminated specimen is pathognomic for UTI. Five bacteria per high power field are equivalent to a colony count of 100,000 organisms/mL.

—Preliminary identification of the type of bacteria or yeast on the basis of Gram stain or acid-fast stain gives a clue to the appropriate choice of antibiotic.

• Urine culture

—Formal culture and sensitivities will further direct the choice of antibiotics. For routine UTIs, identification of the offending microorganism and its sensitivity may not be necessary.

—It is a standard that 10^5 organisms per milliliter of midstream urine are needed to diagnose a UTI. Several authors have challenged this. Note that the concentration of urine can alter the colony count and that in a dilute specimen, fewer bacteria may be significant.

—If urinary tuberculosis is suspected, special methods for growth of *Mycobacteria* should be used. These organisms grow slowly, taking 6 to 8 weeks or longer.

—In men, use Stamey collection method (see Section III)

• Urinary cytology

—Perform if indicated by other findings. Detects high-grade TCC; may miss low-grade TCC

• Renal function tests

—Serum creatinine may be needed prior to intravenous urogram (IVU)

• Complete blood count

—An elevated white count may be seen with systemic inflammatory response.

—Anemia may be present from chronic disease.

• Other laboratory tests

—Tuberculous skin testing to rule out TB

IMAGING

• Based on history and physical, may obtain KUB (plain film of kidney ureter bladder) or IVP (intravenous pyelogram)

• KUB

—Look for stones along ureters, in bladder, or in prostatic tissue.

—Look for foreign bodies in urinary tract.

• Intravenous urogram (IVU)

—IVU in cases of recurrent UTIs

—May detect stones, masses; collecting-system filling defects may signify tumors, fungal balls, or stones; useful to look at anatomy and rule out tumors, stones, foreign objects in upper urinary tract

• Abdominal ultrasound

—Perform if indicated by other findings. Useful in children in place of IVU

• Abdominal CT scan or MRI

—Perform if indicated by other findings. Useful in imaging tumors

SPECIAL STUDIES

• Cystoscopy

—Identifies lower urinary tract pathology

—Retrograde pyelograms or ureteroscopy as indicated

—Evaluate urethra, prostatic channel, bladder

—Look for inflammation, especially at trigone, and evidence of old inflammation such as trigonitis and squamous metaplasia.

• Bladder washings

—Obtain cytology if indicated in history or if suspicious findings are seen on cystoscopy or IVU.

• Urethral calibration

—Important especially in women

—Calibration done with Olive-tip sounds after liberal use of local anesthesia

—If urethral opening is small (<24 French), dilate with graded sounds to at least 28 French.

• Other studies

—Perform as indicated by other findings (e.g., uroflow to evaluate coexisting poor stream or straining).

 ## Initial Management

• "Standard" urologic evaluation as outlined above

• Work-up often modified or tailored by associated symptoms or findings (e.g., hematuria takes precedence)

• Treatment directed toward causative etiology

• Symptomatic relief (only for temporary relief or concurrent with definitive therapy)

—Phenazopyridine hydrochloride
    —An azo dye with local anesthetic and analgesic effects on the urinary tract
    —Contraindicated in renal insufficiency and children less than 12 years of age
    —Side effects include renal and hepatic toxicity, methemoglobinemia, hemolytic anemia, stain undergarments.

 ## Follow-Up

• Persistent dysuria with no apparent cause must be evaluated again to rule out early carcinoma in situ of the bladder.

• Follow-up dictated by associated finding or etiology of dysuria

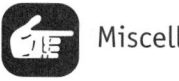 ## Miscellaneous

SYNONYMS: N/A

ASSOCIATED CONDITIONS: N/A

NOTES

• See also Section I, "Bacteruria and Pyuria," and Section II, "Urethral Syndrome."

ABBREVIATIONS

• IVU, intravenous urogram; TCC, transitional cell carcinoma; US, ultrasound

REFERENCES

Gillenwater JY, Grayhack JT, Howards SS, Duckett JW, eds. *Adult and Pediatric Urology,* 3rd ed. St Louis: Mosby, 1996.

Tanagho, McAninch, eds. *Smith's General Urology,* 14th ed. Norwalk, CT: Appleton & Lange, 1996.

Walsh PC, Retik AB, Vaughan ED, Wein AJ, eds. *Campbell's Urology,* 7th ed. Philadelphia: WB Saunders, 1998.

Authors: Ashish M. Kamat and Unyime O. Nseyo

Edema—External Genitalia

 Basics

DESCRIPTION

- Part of generalized edema or localized to the scrotum with or without involvement of penis
- If localized to the scrotum, may be unilateral or bilateral
- Must rule out any underlying testicular pathology

PATHOPHYSIOLOGY

- Extreme laxity of scrotum aided by gravity predisposes to accumulation of fluid.
- May indicate increased fluid inflow (as in volume overload) or decreased outflow (as in lymphatic obstruction).

RISK FACTORS

- If part of generalized edema

—Cardiac conditions resulting in fluid overload
—Renal disorders leading to fluid overload and protein loss
—Malnutrition with hypoproteinemia

- If localized edema

—Infection
—Recent surgery
—Trauma

 Differential Diagnosis

- First exclude testicular problems with secondary edema of the scrotum (see Section I, "Testicular Mass—Adult and Pediatric").
- In adults, congestive heart failure and volume overload after recent surgery are major causes.
- In children, testicular pathology and infections are common causes.

—Congenital
  —Neonatal torsion (especially in the premature infant)
  —Neonatal incarcerated/strangulated hernia

- Hypoproteinemic states
- Traumatic

—Direct injury to scrotum: may be unilateral
—Pelvic trauma with urethral rupture and violation of Buck's fascia, causing superficial extravasation of urine, limited by Colles' fascia

- Iatrogenic

—Fluid overload after any major surgery
—Decreased pelvic venous return after pelvic surgery
—Altered lymphatic drainage, e.g., after inguinal lymph node surgery or radiation therapy
—Peritoneal dialysis (usually associated with a hernia)

- Inflammatory

—Spreading cellulitis from abdominal wall infections or from periurethral abscesses
  —Associated with pain and erythema
—Early Fournier's gangrene

- Tropical elephantiasis

—Lymphatic obstruction by *Wuchereria bancrofti* infestation
—Transmitted by mosquito bites
—Associated with penile swelling and hydroceles

- Neoplastic

—Metastatic deposits to inguinal nodes

- Idiopathic cyclical scrotal edema in boys

—Self limited: usually resolves in 72 hours
  —Usually unilateral, may be recurrent in 20% of cases

 Database

HISTORY

- Age

—Cardiac problems predominate in older men, while infections are more common in younger ages.

- Onset

—Usually gradual; sudden onset may indicate rapidly spreading cellulitis, e.g., Fournier's

- Associated symptoms

—Shortness of breath or swelling of extremities indicates CHF.

- History of trauma

—Local injury
—Inability to urinate after pelvic trauma may indicate urethral injury.

- History of recent surgery

—Volume overload
—Pelvic surgery affecting venous return
—Procedures interrupting lymphatic drainage

- Significant PMH

—Renal or cardiac diseases
—Nutritional disorders

PHYSICAL EXAMINATION

- Generalized edema

—Cardiac or renal etiology

- Abdominal or inguinal scars

—Recent surgery or trauma

- Testicular pathology

—Tenderness may indicate infection or torsion.

Diagnostic Studies

LABORATORY TESTING

- Urinalysis and urine culture

—Proteinuria may be associated with systemic edema.

- Renal function tests

—May suggest renal failure

- Peripheral smear for larva of *W. bancrofti*

IMAGING

- Ultrasonography

—Define testicular pathology if clinically not clear.

- In trauma: Pelvic fractures may indicate associated soft-tissue injuries.
- Urethrogram

—To assess urethral injuries

SPECIAL STUDIES

- Doppler ultrasonography

—To assess testicular viability

- Renal biopsy

—To confirm diagnosis of renal disease

 ## Initial Management

- Every male patient with the acute onset of pain and swelling of the scrotum requires an immediate evaluation to have testicular torsion diagnosed or excluded.
- Treat underlying cause.
- Infection

—Appropriate antibiotics and local debridement as needed

- Urinary drainage

—Suprapubic diversion may be needed in urethral ruptures.

- Elevation of scrotum

—May relieve edema
—Treat skin breakdown.

 ## Follow-Up

- Depending on etiology
- To assess efficacy of initial therapy

 ## Miscellaneous

SYNONYMS: N/A

ASSOCIATED CONDITIONS: N/A

NOTES

- See also Section I, "Edema—Lower Extremity" and "Testicular Mass."

ABBREVIATIONS: N/A

REFERENCES: N/A

Authors: Yegappan Lakshmanan and Bhalchandra G. Parulkar

Edema—Lower Extremity

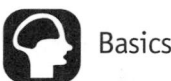 ## Basics

DESCRIPTION

- Retention of fluids in extravascular space, leading to swelling and stretching of skin
- Initially the problem may be indolent, evidenced by increase in weight only.
- May be caused by cardiac, hepatic, or renal disease; IVC compression from tumors; RT; etc.
- When pain is present, it is usually associated with an acute process.
- Edema associated with renal disease may be seen first as facial puffiness.
- Later swelling in dependent parts of the body, lower extremities, "pitting" edema evident
- Anasarca develops, if fluid retention continues.

PATHOPHYSIOLOGY

- Usually represents excessive water and Na+ in the extracellular space due to abnormal renal excretion
- Usually an indication of another disease process, rather than a primary disease
- May be acute or chronic, and may be aggravated by existing venous insufficiency
- Increased peripheral venous pressure causes movement of fluids into extracellular space.
- Postoperative usually associated with lymphatic occlusion

—Often unilateral
—Pelvic lymphocele can occlude venous/lymphatic return.

RISK FACTORS

- Cardiovascular failure, liver insufficiency, renal failure, malnutrition, and thyroid disorders
- Inactivity, excessive dependent position, bedridden
- IV fluid overhydration
- Inferior vena cava obstruction, due to urinary bladder distention, bladder cancer, prostate cancer, uterine or cervical cancer that compresses the veins and/or invades the lymphatic channels
- Treatment with interleukin-2 (IL-2) and alpha-interferon (IFN-α) can cause protein leakage from plasma to the interstitium.
- Renal cell carcinoma presenting as nephrotic syndrome secondary to tumor extension into vein
- Endocrine therapy, brachytherapy, or external beam therapy

—Prostate, bladder, cervical, ovarian, etc.

- Inferior vena cava obstruction from retroperitoneal fibrosis
- Protein calorie malnutrition
- Deep venous thrombosis: malignancy related or postoperatively
- Pelvic node dissection, inguinal node dissection, etc.
- Leg edema due to a medication
- Penile edema after BCG instillation
- Streptococcal venereal edema of the penis

 ## Differential Diagnosis

- For acute scrotal swelling

—Rule out torsion of testis or appendages, hydrocele, varicocele, trauma, tumor, idiopathic scrotal edema, cellulitis, and Henoch-Schönlein purpura.

- For penile swelling

—Rule out cellulitis, penile fracture, urethral abscess, priapism.

- For lower extremity edema

—Rule out deep vein thrombosis, cellulitis, obesity, CHF, renal disease, venous compression from distended bladder, tumors of the pelvis, anatomic or vascular malformations, fibrosis/scar.

 ## Database

HISTORY

- Age and sex of patient?

—Usually occurs in older males and females with numerous medical problems, but can occur in younger bedridden patients or those with malignancy

- History of trauma?

—Crush injury to pelvis can lead to vascular, lymphatic malformations.

- Any associated pain?

—Pain is usually associated with acute process; chronic process is usually painless.

- Symptoms of urinary tract infection, bladder outlet obstruction?

—Suggests BPH or CAP, which may compress IVC

- Significant medical or surgical history?

—Cardiac history, renal history; surgical, radiation, or endocrine therapy for malignancy

- Current medications?

—Calcium channel blockers, nonsteroidals, clonidine, minoxidil, hydralazine, methyldopa, diazoxide, guanethidine, steroids, estrogen, progesterone, and testosterone are common medications causing edema. Hx of alcoholism is associated with malnutrition, leading to edema.

- Occupational risk factors?

—Sedentary position

PHYSICAL EXAMINATION

- Hypertension

—May indicate cardiac disease, renal disease, or renal failure

- Heart murmurs

—May indicate underlying heart disease

- Palpable abdominal or pelvic masses

—May indicate bladder distension, BPH or CAP, or pelvic malignancy

- Pelvic examination

—Uterine prolapse, cystocele, may compress pelvic vasculature.

- Digital rectal examination

—BPH, CAP, rectal mass

- Must categorize leg edema as local or systemic, acute or chronic, unilateral or bilateral, painful or painless

Diagnostic Studies

LABORATORY TESTING

- Urine analysis

—May reveal RBCs suggestive of bladder or prostate neoplasm
—If specific gravity low, suggests poor concentrating ability due to renal disease
—RBC casts suggest glomerulonephritis.

- Urine cytology

—May reveal TCC of bladder, which may infiltrate or compress vascular/lymph channels

- Renal function tests, serum Na+

—May indicate prerenal, renal, or postrenal impairment

- Complete blood count

—May reveal anemia in intrinsic renal disease

IMAGING

- Chest x-ray to rule out cardiac failure
- Ultrasound

—May reveal renal mass (with tumor extension into vein) or hydronephrosis

- IVP

—May reveal hydronephrosis from tumors, retroperitoneal hydronephrosis, etc.

- Nuclear medicine renal scan

—If unable to obtain contrast study, may indicate etiology of renal condition

- Abdominal CT

—May distinguish between renal masses, hydronephrosis, pelvic mass, retroperitoneal fibrosis, or other possible sources of compression of IVC

- Duplex Doppler ultrasound lower extremity

—Generally replaces venography
—Useful to evaluate for deep venous thrombosis

SPECIAL STUDIES

- Cystoscopy

—May reveal bladder cancer

- Renal biopsy

—Used in suspected glomerulonephritis

 ## Initial Management

- Treatment of CHF if confirmed
- Treatment of renal failure (if by hydronephrosis, stents, or percutaneous nephrostomy)
- To exclude deep vein thrombosis, can utilize venography or duplex ultrasonography

—Anticoagulant therapy if DVT confirmed

- A thorough pelvic examination may obviate the need for pelvic ultrasound or CT as screening test.

—CT may be necessary in obese patients to rule out venous compression from tumors.
—Elective surgery to remove pelvic masses causing compression

- Elevation of lower extremities, scrotal support
- Lymphedema compression device for leg
- Dietary counseling, if due to malnutrition, alcoholic history
- If cellulitis, treat with antibiotics (i.e., cephalosporin)

 ## Follow-Up

- Edema may be multifactorial: After treatment of cardiac or renal disease, the patient may still have an undiagnosed condition causing compression of IVC and/or edema.
- Excision of abdominal/pelvic masses requires F/U CT to rule out recurrences, scar tissue, etc.

 ## Miscellaneous

SYNONYMS: N/A

ASSOCIATED CONDITIONS: N/A

NOTES

- See also Section I, "Edema—External Genitalia," and Section II, "Deep Venous Thrombosis and Pulmonary Embolism."

ABBREVIATIONS

- IVC, inferior vena cava; RT, radiotherapy; DVT, deep venous thrombosis; CAP, cancer of prostate; TCC, transitional cell carcinoma

REFERENCES

Benderev TV, et al. Inferior vena cava obstruction secondary to adenocarcinoma of the prostate. Role of orchiectomy in treatment. *Arch Intern Med* 1986;146:598.

Ciocon JO, et al. Leg edema in the elderly: A practical diagnostic approach. *Compr Ther* 1994;20:586.

Palma L, Peterson MC, Ingebretsen R. Iliac vein compression syndrome from urinary bladder distension due to prostatism. *South Med J* 1995; 88:959.

Pilepich MV, et al. Complications of definitive radiotherapy for carcinoma of the prostate. *Int J Radiat Oncol Biol Phys* 1981;7:1341.

Rabinowitz R, Hulbert WC Jr. Acute scrotal swelling. *Urol Clin North Am* 1995;22:101.

Author: Jack Mydlo

Enuresis—Adult

 ## Basics

DESCRIPTION

- Enuresis is the involuntary loss of urine.
- Nocturnal enuresis (NE) is nighttime incontinence.
- Adult nocturnal enuresis occurs as two separate entities.

—Persistent primary NE (1% of adult population)
  —May have subtle diurnal symptoms: mild urgency, frequency, and urge incontinence (UI)
  —More UDS findings than children: 28% to 70%; usually detrusor instability
  —Incidence of organic disease in adults with NE similar to that in children with NE
—Adult onset or secondary NE: is not uncommon, particularly in the elderly
  —Usually associated with diurnal symptoms, voiding dysfunction and UI
  —UDS needed to assess for lower urinary tract dysfunction (anatomic or neurologic)
  —The majority of adults with secondary NE have organic disease.

PATHOPHYSIOLOGY

- Primary persistent NE

—As in children, the exact cause is unknown, but there are several theories:
—Subtle neurologic maturational arrest
  —Disturbance in sensory function, cortical arousal, or sphincter function
—Alteration in vasopressin secretion or atrial natriuretic factor release
—Obstructive sleep apneas: associated with NE

- Secondary NE: multiple etiologies (refer to Section I, "Urinary Incontinence—Adult Male" and "Urinary Incontinence—Adult Female")

RISK FACTORS

- Primary persistent NE

—Family history of NE

- Secondary NE

—Increased age: increased incidence of concomitant medical and urologic disease
—Altered mental status
—Impaired mobility

 ## Differential Diagnosis

- Persistent nocturnal enuresis
—Emotional disturbances/psychological diseases
—Spina bifida occulta
—Obstructive sleep apnea
—Idiopathic detrusor instability
—Previously unrecognized myelopathy or neuropathy (multiple sclerosis, tethered cord, epilepsy)
—Rule out causes of secondary NE.

 ## Database

HISTORY

- Primary persistent NE (for secondary NE, see Section I, "Urinary Incontinence—Adult Female" and "Urinary Incontinence—Adult Male")

—Never achieved total nocturnal urinary continence or achieved nighttime dryness for less than 1 year
—Minimal or no daytime symptoms: frequency, urgency, urge UI occasionally reported
—No clearly identifiable medical or neurologic conditions

PHYSICAL EXAMINATION

- Neurologic examination: Abnormalities may be subtle.
- Careful urologic examination (DRE)
- Findings are usually all normal.

Diagnostic Studies

LABORATORY TESTING

- Urinalysis and urine culture
—UTI
—Rule out proteinuria, glycosuria, and poor concentrating ability.
—Rule out hematuria and pyuria.
- BUN and creatinine: suspected renal insufficiency
- Urine cytology if carcinoma/CIS suspected

IMAGING

- IVP, renal ultrasound, voiding cystourethrogram, or retrograde pyelogram
—Rule out anatomic abnormalities
  —Duplication and ureteral ectopia
  —Urethral strictures or diverticula
- Spine x-rays: spina bifida occulta

SPECIAL STUDIES

- Urodynamics are recommended in adults, particularly with diurnal symptoms.
—Identify: anatomic abnormalities, neurogenic vesical dysfunction
—Abnormalities found in up to 70%
  —Bladder instability most common
  —Reduced cystometric capacity

 ## Initial Management

- If no anatomic or neurologic abnormalities are found, treatment is the same as in children (see Section I, "Enuresis—Pediatric").
- Reduce caffeine intake: reduces bedwetting in adult enuretics
- DDAVP should be used judiciously or avoided in patient at risk for electrolyte changes or fluid retention (congestive heart failure, renal insufficiency, and cystic fibrosis).

 ## Follow-Up

- Long-term follow-up until NE resolves
- Worsening of symptoms: reevaluation
- Patients on DDAVP need monitoring for fluid retention and hyponatremia

 ## Miscellaneous

SYNONYMS: N/A

ASSOCIATED CONDITIONS: N/A

NOTES

- See also Section I, "Enuresis—Pediatric," "Urinary Incontinence—Adult Male," and "Urinary Incontinence—Adult Female."

ABBREVIATIONS

- NE, nocturnal enuresis; UDS, urodynamic studies; LUT, lower urinary tract; UI, urge incontinence

REFERENCES

Karaman MI, et al. Rationale of urodynamic assessment in adult enuresis. *Eur Urol* 1992; 21:138–140.

Torrens MJ, Collin CD. The urodynamic assessment of adult enuresis. *Br J Urol* 1975;47:118–121.

Authors: Marko Gudziak and Valal K. George

Enuresis—Pediatric

Basics

DESCRIPTION

- Enuresis is the involuntary loss of urine.
- Nocturnal enuresis is wetting that occurs at night during sleep.
- Five to 7 million enuretic children in the United States
- 10% to 20% of normal children have nocturnal enuresis at age 5.
- After age 5, 15% of enuretics per year resolve spontaneously.
- Diagnosis of nocturnal enuresis is made in a child of 5 and older who has nocturnal enuresis at least twice per week for more than 3 months (DSM-IV, American Psychiatric Association, 1994).

—Primary enuresis: urinary incontinence/wetting that has never completely resolved or recurs after a dry period of less than 1 year
—Secondary enuresis: recurrent wetting after at least 1 year of continence

PATHOPHYSIOLOGY

- Both functional and organic causes

—Organic urologic causes: 1% to 4% enuresis in children
  —UTI, occult spina bifida, ectopic ureters, lazy bladder syndrome, irritable bladder with wide bladder neck
—Organic non-urologic causes
  —Epilepsy, diabetes mellitus, sleep apnea, food allergies
  —Sleep apnea: There is an increased release of atrial natriuretic factor, which may increase urine output and contribute to enuresis.

- Deficiency of nocturnal production of arginine vasopressin, antidiuretic hormone, by the anterior pituitary is seen in the majority of enuretic patients.
- Certain food, such as milk and its products and drinks containing caffeine, may increase the incidence of enuresis.
- Central nervous system maturational delay is implicated as a cause.

—These children have been found to have a delay in other developmental milestones.

- Emotional and psychological problems have been identified in children with primary enuresis.
- An increased incidence of family and social problems has been seen.

—Death in the family, temporary separation of mother, moving, accidents, or surgery

- Sleep disorders or alteration in sleep pattern: no evidence

—Nocturnal enuresis occurs in all stages of sleep.
—Sleep patterns in enuretics are no different than those in normal children.

RISK FACTORS

- Enuresis tends to be familial.

—In 70% of families with an enuretic child, enuresis occurred in more than one member of the family.
—If both parents were enuretics: 77% chance of enuresis in their offspring; with one parent, 44% chance

Differential Diagnosis

- See "Pathophysiology"

Database

HISTORY

- A general detailed medical history needs to be taken in regard to symptoms.
- Presenting symptoms

—Type of enuresis primary/secondary
—Duration and frequency of night wetting, day-time voiding, and diurnal continence
—Quality of urinary stream and voiding pattern
—History of urinary tract infection
—Degree of success with toilet training

- Further history

—Uropathology such as obstruction, reflux, duplication, or ectopic ureter
—History of hospitalization
—History of previous surgeries
—Allergies to foods and medicines
—Past and present medications
—Family history of enuresis (see above)

PHYSICAL EXAMINATION

- Examination carried out with child completely undressed
- Abdominal examination to assess for distention

—Rule out distended bladder and distended bowels due to constipation.

- Genital examination for congenital anomalies
- Evaluate rectal sphincter tone and perenial sensation: Assess for stool impaction.
- Lower extremity reflexes
- Examination of lower spine for deformities
- Determine any gait abnormalities.

Diagnostic Studies

LABORATORY TESTING

- Urine analysis to rule out UTI, hematuria, proteinuria, glycosuria, and fixed low specific gravity
- Urine culture

IMAGING

- Ultrasonography of kidneys and bladder

—Rule out anatomic abnormalities of kidneys.
—Bladder: bladder wall thickening, size, post-void residual urine

- Voiding cystourethrography (VCUG): history of UTI to rule out reflux

SPECIAL STUDIES

- Urodynamic evaluation to rule out significant voiding dysfunction

—Indications: recurrent UTI, daytime incontinence, abnormal neurologic examination, failure of conservative measures

 ## Initial Management

- Treatments: pharmacotherapy, psychotherapy, and behavioral modifications
- Pharmacotherapy: anticholinergic/antispasmodic agents

—Improved success: Combine with behavioral modification and bladder training.

- Oxybutynin (Ditropan) (see Section V, "Commonly Used Medications in Urology")

—Anticholinergic: increases functional bladder capacity and helps in time voiding
—Ditropan 5 mg single nighttime dose: success rate of 30% to 50%; 50% relapse with stopping drug
—Best in children with frequency, urgency, concomitant daytime wetting, and urodynamic evidence of uninhibited detrusor contractions (success rate: 85% to 91%)

- Imipramine

—Tricyclic antidepressant with anticholinergic effects; success rate of 25% to 30% when used >3 months
—0.9 to 1.5 mg/kg/d (maximum 2–5 mg/kg/d) (see Section V, "Dosing")

- DDAVP (Desmopressin): decreases nocturnal urine output

—Intranasally at a dose of 10 to 40 μg (see Section V, "Dosing")
—Success rate: 10% to 60%
—Safe even when used for more than 12 months
—Caution in patients with cystic fibrosis (hyponatremia)

- Psychotherapy

—Requires participation of child along with the entire family

- Behavioral modifications: These include

—Self-monitoring/record keeping: primary technique to improve enuresis
—Motivation and responsibility training: child made responsible for changing/laundering bed linen
—Efficacy: 25%; 5% relapse rate

- Bladder training

—Exercises to increase bladder capacity; may include biofeedback
—Effectiveness in nocturnal enuresis: variable
—Enuresis alarms: 70% success; 30% relapse

- Diet

—Reduce fluid intake after 6 PM; restrict caffeine consumption

 ## Follow-Up

- Follow until spontaneous resolution
- Nocturnal enuresis is generally a self-limiting condition
- 1% will persist as adult nocturnal enuresis; require detailed evaluation for organic causes
- Self-concept and self-esteem are adversely effected by enuresis, therefore early successful treatment is advocated.

 ## Miscellaneous

SYNONYMS

- Bed wetting

ASSOCIATED CONDITIONS: N/A

NOTES

- See also Section I, "Enuresis—Adult."

ABBREVIATIONS

- UDS, urodynamic study

REFERENCES

Bond T, et al. Overview and management of sleep enuresis in children. *AUA Update Series* 1996;16.

Kaplan WE. Office management of nocturnal enuresis. *AUA Update Series* 1989;19.

Authors: Marko Gudziak and Valal K. George

Epididymis—Mass

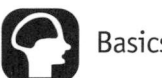 Basics

DESCRIPTION

- Small solid paratesticular mass located in any portion of the epididymis
- Frequently asymptomatic, usually discovered on routine urologic physical examination
- Occasionally, pain is the presenting complaint.
- Enlarging masses are more indicative of possible tumor.

PATHOPHYSIOLOGY

- Benign epididymal cysts are extremely common with aging.
- Most solid lesions are benign tumors.
—Malignant tumors are less common.
- Metastasis is rare but reported.

RISK FACTORS

- Cyst adenomas are frequently seen in association with Von Hippel-Lindau disease.
- DES exposure in utero causes increased incidence of epididymal cyst.

 Differential Diagnosis

- Epididymal cyst (spermatocele)
—Most common mass of epididymis
- Epididymitis
—Thickened inflamed epididymis, positive UA
—Bacterial epididymitis usually in males over age 40
—Chlamydial epididymitis in males less than age 40
- Benign solid tumors
—Adenomatoid tumor is most common; 80% are in globus minor
—Cystadenoma: frequency with VHL syndrome
—Leiomyomas
—Lipomas, teratomas, adrenal cortical, fibromas are all uncommon.
- Primary malignant tumor in adults
—Mesenchymal tumors (sarcomas) are most common.
—Rhabdomyosarcomas are more frequent than leiomyomas, fibrosarcomas, or liposarcomas.
—Seen in older men
—Adenocarcinomas are much less common.
—When diagnosis is adenocarcinoma, always consider metastatic disease from other sources (i.e., GU or gastrointestinal).
- Metastatic tumors
—Prostate metastatic are most common.
—Also GI and breast reported
—Not infrequently, metastatic tumor is the initial presentation of an occult carcinoma.
- Pediatric tumors
—Paratesticular rhabdomyosarcomas are uncommon.
—MNTI: melanotic neuroectodermal tumor of infancy
- Lymphomas
—Isolated epididymal lymphomas are rare; usually testicular involvement is seen as well.
- Primary mesenchymal tumors are more common than epithelial tumors.

 Database

HISTORY

- Age of patient: Solid tumor is more frequent in males under 40.
- History of pain: Inflammatory benign conditions are more likely.
- Stable or enlarging mass
—A painless enlarging mass suggests a malignant tumor.
- Symptoms of associated urinary tract infection
—Frequency, urgency, dysuria, slow stream, fever, chills
- History of cancer or infection
—Metastatic adenocarcinoma or tuberculosis is not uncommon.
- Travel history
—Foreign travel or immigrants: increased incidence of tuberculosis

PHYSICAL EXAMINATION

- Location in scrotum
—Relationship to testicle: upper, middle, or lower pole of epididymis
- Rule out hernia.
- Hydrocele/spermatocele
—Hydroceles can mask benign malignant epididymal tumors.
- Fixed or mobile lesion of epididymis
- Digital rectal examination
—Tender prostate: Consider epididymal orchitis as well as prostatitis.
- Findings in contralateral testicle and scrotum
- Rule out testicular tumor.
—Check groin, neck nodes, and abdominal examination.

Diagnostic Studies

LABORATORY TESTING

• Urinalysis

—Pyuria, nitrate, or leukocyte esterase positive or bacteruria suggests infection.

• Chest x-ray PPD testing: when examination and history suggest tuberculosis
• WBC: shift to left, increased WBCs suggest infection.
• Testes tumor markers

—AFP, beta-hCG, LDH

IMAGING

• Scrotal ultrasound

—Cyst vs. solid
—Testicular vs. paratesticular epididymal lesion
—Ultrasound of solid lesion cannot differentiate benign vs. malignant tumor.
—Scrotal MRI may be useful in select cases to avoid exploration.

SPECIAL STUDIES

• Transcrotal biopsy contraindicated if tumor is suspected

 Initial Management

• Observation for asymptomatic cyst/spermatocele
• Inguinal exploration and radical orchiectomy for malignant tumors
• Transcrotal excision of epididymal structures for cyst or clearly benign tumor
• Quinolone or sulfa antibiotics for bacterial epididymitis

—May use tetracycline or quinolones for presumed chlamydial epididymitis

• Tubercular epididymitis frequently requires orchiectomy as well as tuberculosis antibiotics.

 Follow-Up

• Solid benign tumors: routine postoperative care
• Malignant primary tumors

—Depends on cell types: Outlook is frequently poor.
—Rhabdomyosarcomas of childhood do well with multimodal therapy.

 Miscellaneous

SYNONYMS: N/A

ASSOCIATED CONDITIONS: N/A

NOTES

• See also Section II, "Von Hippel-Lindau Disease/Syndrome."

ABBREVIATIONS: N/A

REFERENCES

Gill WB, Schumacher GFB, Bibbo M, et al. Association diethylstilbestrol exposure in utero with cryptorchidism, testicular hypoplasia and semen abnormalities. *J Urol* 1979:122:36.

Rowland RG. Scrotum and testis. In: Gillenwater JY, Grayhack JT, Howards SS, Duckett JW, et al., eds. *Adult and Pediatric Urology*. St Louis: Mosby–Year Book, 1991.

Author: Louis Keeler III

Erectile Dysfunction

 Basics

DESCRIPTION

- The consistent inability to obtain and/or maintain an erection sufficient for satisfactory sexual relations
- Estimated to affect 2 to 30 million men in the United States
- 52% of men 40- to 70-years-old have some degree of ED.
- Complete ED affects 5% of men at 40 years and 25% of men at 65 years of age.

PATHOPHYSIOLOGY

- 90% of ED is primarily organic in nature.
- ED may be the harbinger of diabetes, occult neurologic diseases, AAA, or subclinical coronary artery disease.
- 10% of patients have a primary psychogenic etiology.
- Etiologies of organic ED include vascular disease (70%), medications (10%), surgical procedures (10%), neurologic diseases (5%), endocrine disorders (3%), and trauma (2%).

RISK FACTORS

- Diabetes mellitus
- Cardiovascular diseases: hypertension, myocardial infarction, CABG surgery, peripheral vascular disease, stroke
- Hypercholerolemia
- Cigarette smoking
- Radical pelvic surgery: radical prostatectomy, pelvic colorectal surgery
- AAA surgery
- Transurethral surgery
- Pelvic fracture
- Long-distance cycling
- Hypogonadism, hyperprolactinemia
- Multiple sclerosis, Parkinson disease
- Lumbar disk disease
- Depression, psychotic states
- Medications: digoxin, antiandrogens, psychotropics, antihypertensives, H-2 blockers, others

 Differential Diagnosis

- Neurologic
- Endocrine
- Vascular

—Arteriogenic
—Venogenic

- Psychogenic
- Medication induced
- Aging
- Systemic diseases

 Database

HISTORY

- Medical history
- Surgical history
- Medication history
- Social history: cycling, cigarettes, recreational drugs
- Sexual history: partner age, masturbation activity, sexual practices
- ED history: onset (sudden vs. gradual), duration (number of months), rigidity level (0%–100%), penetration ability, maintaining capability, early morning/nocturnal erection presence, ejaculation/orgasm, penile curvature presence

PHYSICAL EXAMINATION

- Visual fields: Check for bitemporal hemianopsia.
- Breasts: Check for gynecomastia.
- Abdomen: Check for cirrhosis, AAA.
- Femoral pulses: Check for large vessel disease (Leriche syndrome: buttock pain, buttock wasting, erectile dysfunction secondary to internal iliac artery occlusion).
- Penis: circumcision status, penile compliance (stretch capability of the penis), Peyronie disease plaques
- Digital rectal examination
- Neurologic assessment: In cases where neurogenic ED is suspected, check for perianal sensation and lower limb neurologic integrity (bulbocavernosus reflex is only of significance if present, as it is absent in 30% of normal men).

 Diagnostic Studies

LABORATORY TESTING

- NIH Consensus Conference Panel (1993) recommends (if not previously done)

—CBC, chemistry panel, random glucose level
—Early-morning total serum testosterone (sT) level
—If sT is abnormal, repeat in combination with a free testosterone, LH, and prolactin levels.

- Consideration may be given to withholding testosterone estimation in older men (>60 years of age) and men with overt causes for their ED (multiple vascular risk factors, radical prostatectomy).
- Thyroid function tests should be performed in patients with symptoms of hypo- or hyperthyroidism.

IMAGING

- See below.

SPECIAL STUDIES

- The vast majority of men with ED require no further testing.
- Further testing should be considered in young men (<40 years of age), men with no risk factors for ED, men with penile deformity and ED, and in medicolegal situations.
- Testing should be aimed at defining whether the patient is curable/treatable or educating the patient regarding potential response to therapy.
- Vascular testing: aimed at defining whether the patient has arterial occlusion (synonyms: cavernosal artery insufficiency, arteriogenic ED), corporo-venocclusive dysfunction (synonyms: venous leak, venogenic ED)
- All vascular testing must be performed in the presence of an erection induced by administration of vasoactive agents by penile injection.
- Historical tests: Tests that no longer have any significant role in the evaluation of the man with ED include penile-brachial index evaluation and plethysmography.
- Vascular studies: Two tests have replaced all others: duplex Doppler penile ultrasonography and dynamic infusion cavernosometry/cavernosography (DICC).

- Neurologic testing: No single test yields information concerning the entire neural pathway. The reliability and reproducibility of such tests in the impotent male is unclear.
- Neurologic tests include biothesiometry, pudendal nerve EMG, somatosensory evoked potential analysis, and corpus cavernosal EMG.
- Nocturnal erection analysis: Historical forms of such testing include postage stamp application and snap-gauges.
- Nocturnal penile tumescence and rigidity (NPTR) analysis (RigiScan): simple ambulatory test that measures the nocturnal erection frequency, rigidity, and duration

—NPTR is useful in defining two specific etiologies: psychogenic (when the tracing is completely normal) and neurogenic (when the tracing is completely flat).

- Selective internal pudendal arteriography: reserved for men with vascular test-proven pure arteriogenic (no venous leak) ED with normal hormonal assay and normal neurologic evaluation who are candidates for and have expressed interest in penile artery bypass (revascularization) surgery

 ## Initial Management

- Patients should be counseled regarding the available options that include oral therapy (Viagra), penile injection therapy, transurethral prostaglandin therapy (MUSE), vacuum erection device therapy, penile revascularization, and penile implant surgery.
- Historical oral therapies include yohimbine, trazodone, isoxsuprine, and pentoxifylline.
- Viagra

—Advantages: simplicity, efficacy (60%)
—Disadvantages: lack of spontaneity (usually needs to be taken 60 minutes prior to onset of relations), cost, systemic side effects (headache 15%, facial flushing 10%, GI upset 7%, nasal congestion 4%, visual disturbances)
—Contraindications: concomitant nitrate use, documented retinopathy, patients prone to priapism

- Penile injection therapy

—Advantages: efficacy (60%–90% depending on agents used), consistency of response, spontaneity (erection occurs within 5–10 minutes)
—Disadvantages: concept of needle use, local complications (occur in approximately 3% of men and include ecchymosis, hematoma, penile nodules, scarring, priapism)
—Contraindications: concomitant use of monoamine oxidase medications, poor patient manual dexterity

- MUSE

—Advantage: simplicity
—Disadvantages: efficacy 30% to 40%, lack of spontaneity (15–30 minutes for erection to occur and patient must remain standing until rigid erection develops), lack of consistency (in responders, approximately 60% of administrations will induce an erection sufficiently rigid for intercourse), cost
—Contraindications to use: pregnant partner, patients prone to priapism

- Vacuum device therapy

—Advantages: simplicity, good insurance coverage
—Disadvantages: poor cosmesis, difficulty integrating therapy into sexual relations, adverse effects (pain, sensory changes in penis, ecchymosis, hematoma formation). Consider withholding such therapy in men on anticoagulant therapy or with penile curvature.

- Penile implant surgery is an excellent management strategy in the carefully selected patient with ED.

—Advantages: spontaneity, rigidity/girth profile
—Disadvantages: cost, lack of reversibility, postoperative morbidity (most men will lose 1 week from work), complications (infection 2%, mechanical malfunction 2%, reoperation 15% at 10 years)

- Penile revascularization is the only curative treatment modality that exists.

—Advantages: cures approximately 60% of men who have this procedure performed following careful investigation and selection
—Disadvantages: cost, postoperative morbidity

- Testosterone skin patches: In hypogonadal men, daily application of testosterone patches produces hormone levels that parallel the endogenous pattern of serum testosterone characteristic of normal men.

—Advantages: improvements in mood, energy, libido, and sexual function
—Disadvantages: skin irritation, transient local itching, and discomfort related to the patch

 ## Follow-Up

- Based on etiology
- Often may be the first manifestation of a systemic disease

 ## Miscellaneous

SYNONYMS

- Impotence, ED

ASSOCIATED CONDITIONS: N/A

NOTES: N/A

ABBREVIATIONS

- ED, erectile dysfunction; sT, total serum testosterone; DICC, cavernosometry/cavernosography; NPTR, nocturnal penile tumescence and rigidity

REFERENCES

Feldman HA, Goldstein I, Hatzchristou G, et al. Impotence and its medical and psychosocial correlates: Results of the Massachusetts male aging study. *J Urol* 1994;151:54–61.

Garcia-Reboll L, Mulhall JP, Goldstein I. Drugs for the treatment of impotence. *Drugs Aging* 1997;11(2):140–151.

Krane RJ, Goldstein I, Saenz de Tejada I. Impotence. *N Engl J Med* 1989;321:1648–1659.

NIH Consensus Conference. Impotence. NIH Consensus Development Panel on Impotence. *JAMA* 1993;270:83–87.

Author: John P. Mulhall

Filling Defect—Upper Urinary Tract

 Basics

DESCRIPTION

• Radiolucency identified on excretory urogram, retrograde ureteropyelography, or contrast CT scan

PATHOPHYSIOLOGY

• Any radiolucent mass within the upper urinary tract will appear as a filling defect.

RISK FACTORS

• Prior history of stones or transitional cell carcinoma
• Urinary tract infection (bacterial, fungal)
• Diabetes, sickle cell, analgesic abuse
• Bleeding disorder

 Differential Diagnosis

• Malignant
—Transitional cell carcinoma
　—The most common malignant cause of upper urinary tract filling defects
—Renal cell carcinoma
　—Usually found in conjunction with renal mass on ultrasound or CT scan; has been reported without associated renal mass
• Benign
—Renal papilla
　—Ectopic or "end on" renal papilla can be misidentified as a filling defect.
—Fibroepithelial polyp
—Inverted papilloma
—Sloughed papilla
—Blood clot
—Fungus ball
—Air
　—May be iatrogenic during retrograde pyelography, or due to ureteroenteric fistula, or emphysematous pyelonephritis
—Vascular impression
—Protein matrix
—Mucus
　—Urinary diversion patients

 Database

HISTORY

• History of urinary calculi?

—Especially uric acid and cysteine stones

• History of transitional cell carcinoma of the bladder?

—15% to 30% incidence of upper tract tumor development

• History of diabetes, analgesic abuse, or sickle cell disease?

—Potential causes of sloughed papilla

• History of gross hematuria?

—May indicate malignancy or blood clot as cause of filling defect

• History of inflammatory bowel disease, or long-term *E. coli* urinary tract infection?

—Potential causes of air in the upper urinary tract

• History of urinary diversion?

—Urinary diversion can be associated with urolithiasis, protein matrix production, and mucus within the upper urinary tract.

• History of fungal UTI?

PHYSICAL EXAMINATION

• Evidence of CVA tenderness

Diagnostic Studies

LABORATORY TESTING

• Urinalysis and culture

—If the urine pH is greater than 6.5, uric acid stones are unlikely.
—Hematuria can indicate either malignancy or clot.
—Fungal elements on urinalysis raises the possibility of a fungus ball.
—Mixed aerobic and anaerobic bacteria may indicate ureteroenteric fistula.

• Urine cytology

—Positive cytology would indicate possible transitional cell carcinoma.
—Negative cytology does not rule out transitional cell carcinoma.
   —False negatives are common (up to 60%).

IMAGING

• Ultrasonography

—Ultrasound can usually distinguish stones from soft-tissue masses within the upper urinary tract. However, it is not as sensitive or specific as a CT scan.

• CT scan

—A CT scan with and without contrast will differentiate stones, tissue densities, and air. It will also rule out any parenchymal mass.

SPECIAL STUDIES

• Ureteroscopy

—Diagnosis can often be made by direct inspection alone.
—Ureteroscopic biopsy can also provide histologic confirmation.

 Initial Management

• Establish the diagnosis. Once the initial laboratory studies are completed, a CT scan is recommended.

—Calculus: Appropriate treatment is initiated.
   —Uric acid calculus: initially consists of urinary alkalinization
   —If this is unsuccessful, the stone can be treated with ESWL, ureteroscopy, or percutaneous nephrostolithotomy.
—Soft-tissue density is found within the collecting system; further evaluation with ureteroscopy and biopsy is recommended.

• Because ureteroscopy is now so safe, and the differential diagnosis of upper urinary tract filling defects so broad, any doubt about the cause of the filling defect should be confirmed ureteroscopically.

—Ureteroscopy, when needed, should consist of direct inspection of the lesion, lavage for cytology, and biopsy with 3-French biopsy forceps or a flat wire basket.

• Nephroureterectomy is the treatment of choice for upper urinary tract transitional cell carcinoma. However, ureteroscopic treatment and surveillance may be indicated in patients who cannot undergo nephroureterectomy because of comorbidities or renal insufficiency. Other benign tumors of the upper urinary tract, such as fibroepithelial polyps and inverted papillomas, can also be treated successfully ureteroscopically.

• Holmium laser is a useful tool for ureteroscopic treatment of soft-tissue lesions of the collecting system. It is very effective in ablating tissue, and its limited tissue penetration (0.4 mm) makes it very safe.

• Fungal UTIs should be treated prior to any endoscopic manipulation.

• Fungus balls, sloughed papilla, blood clot, mucus, and protein matrix can also be treated endoscopically during the initial ureteroscopic evaluation. Further endoscopic treatment from a percutaneous route may be necessary if the volume of these lesions is large.

• Endoluminal ultrasound during ureteroscopy can confirm the presence of an extrinsic vessel causing compression of the upper urinary tract.

• A ureteroenteric fistula usually requires open repair.

• Emphysematous pyelonephritis requires aggressive antibiotic treatment, and often nephrectomy.

 Follow-Up

• Patients with upper urinary tract transitional cell carcinoma are treated endoscopically.

—Ureteroscopy has been shown to be more accurate than retrograde ureteropyelography, and should be performed every 6 months once the patient is tumor-free.
—Cystoscopic inspection of the bladder must also be included in the surveillance protocol, because of the relatively high frequency (39%) of asynchronous transitional cell carcinoma of the bladder in these patients.

• Patients with radiolucent stones are the same as other urolithiasis patients. Metabolic evaluation is recommended.

• Patients with confirmed successful treatment of benign upper urinary tract tumors should not need any further imaging unless signs or symptoms return.

 Miscellaneous

SYNONYMS

• Filling defect, ureter; filling defect, kidney

ASSOCIATED CONDITIONS: N/A

NOTES: N/A

ABBREVIATIONS: N/A

REFERENCES

Bagley DH. Treatment of upper urinary tract neoplasms. In: Smith AD, et al., eds. *Smith's Textbook of Endourology.* St Louis: Quality Medical Publishing, 1996.

Clayman RV, et al. Endourology of the upper urinary tract: Noncalculous applications. In: Gillenwater JY, Grayhack JT, Howards SS, Duckett JW, et al., eds. *Adult and Pediatric Urology.* St Louis: Mosby-Year Book, 1996.

Author: Michael J. Conlin

Fistula—Enterovesical

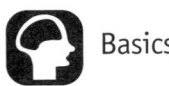 Basics

DESCRIPTION

- Abnormal connection between bladder and any portion of the GI tract
- Symptoms of suprapubic pain, recurrent UTIs, cystitis
- May have pneumaturia or fecaluria
- Incidence estimated to be 1 to 3 patients per 100,000 hospital admissions
- Most commonly results from diverticulitis (50%), Crohn disease, or bowel neoplasms
- Can also be caused by penetrating injuries or spontaneous drainage of abscess

PATHOPHYSIOLOGY

- By definition, a *fistula* is an extraanatomic, epithelialized channel between two hollow organs or a hollow organ and the body surface.
- Can organize when proliferative processes, trauma, or inflammation go beyond organ borders
- Colovesical fistula is the most common. Ileovesical fistulas are more prevalent in cancer and Crohn disease.
- Colovesical is usually seen in diverticular disease, and rectovesical is seen in cancer or trauma.
- A fistula on the left part of the dome suggests diverticulitis; on the right side, it suggests Crohn disease.
- Less common in females than in males; thought to be due to position of uterus between colon and bladder

RISK FACTORS

- Recent bowel or bladder surgery, external beam radiotherapy, recent GU manipulation, trauma, inflammatory bowel disease, bladder/prostate/bowel neoplasm, ovarian abscess, small bowel lymphoma with or without AIDS, Meckel's diverticulum, pelvic actinomycosis, foreign bodies or stones in bowel or bladder, and congenital fistulas associated with an imperforate anus

 Differential Diagnosis

- UTI, stones, prostatitis, cystitis, and tumors may all simulate the symptoms of fistula.
- Pneumaturia may be caused by recent GU instrumentation, or gas-forming infection.
- Iatrogenic injury
- Foreign body
- Radiation cystitis/enteritis
- Endometriosis
- Interstitial cystitis (both male and female)
- Fecaluria is pathognomonic, as is an oral charcoal test.

 Database

HISTORY

- Age and sex of the patient?
—More frequently in males (uterus "protects" females), most common above age 50
- History of trauma?
—Penetrating trauma may be the etiology for fistula.
- History of surgery, radiation?
—Seen after surgery or RT for tumors (cervix, bladder, prostate, etc.)
- History of inflammatory bowel disease or bowel surgery, GU manipulation, venereal disease?
—Inflammatory bowel disease is seen in a majority of patients. Ulcerative colitis: rule out colon CA.
—Urethral stricture disease may lead to abscess, fistula formation, repeated GU instrumentation.
- Pneumaturia
—May be seen in 60% of cases, but may also be seen in *Clostridium* infections, diabetic urine, and GU instrumentation.
- Fecaluria
—Occurs in 40% of cases and is also pathognomonic for fistula
- Any associated pain?
—Could be acute or chronic suprapubic pain, generalized abdominal ache, or back pain; may be associated with chills, fever, or diarrhea
- Current medications?
—A history of diabetes may lead to poor wound healing after bowel/bladder surgery.
—Steroid use may indicate bowel disease, or may even cause spontaneous bowel perforation.
- Occupational risk factors?
—Construction, military may expose to penetrating injuries, foreign-body "missiles."

PHYSICAL EXAMINATION

- Hypertension, elevated pulse
—May suggest type "A" personality with inflammatory bowel disease
- Suprapubic or abdominal mass
—Could suggest abscess, tumor
- Lacerations or healed scars
—May be due to penetrating injury, previous bowel or bladder surgery
- Rectal examination
—May be tender or boggy, suggestive of abscess, fistula formation

Diagnostic Studies

LABORATORY TESTING

• Urine analysis: must include the standard urine dipstick and microscopic evaluation

—Color: may be red, suggestive of tumor, erosion, and/or breakdown of tissue; brown suggests old clots

—Particulate matter, especially food particles, stool, mucus, suggests fistula.

• Urine culture

—Usually have WBCs in urine but may have negative cultures

• Urine cytology

—May detect aggressive or infiltrative TCC; less sensitive for well-differentiated tumors

—"Atypical" cytology may indicate tumor, stone, foreign body, inflammation, or erosion.

• Complete blood count

—Anemia may be present in chronic fistula with loss of blood, but not usual.

—Elevated WBC suggests infection, abscess, etc.

IMAGING

• Excretory urography (IVP)

—May demonstrate filling defect in bladder, suggestive of tumor, foreign body, or stone.

—Contrast may be seen in bowel or rectum.

• Cystogram

—May demonstrate filling defect, suggestive of tumor, fistula; may see contrast in bowel

—May detect fistulas in 20% to 60% of cases

• Barium enema

—May demonstrate colon carcinoma; may reveal contrast in bladder

—May detect fistulas in 10% to 40% of cases

• CT scan

—May identify abscess, bowel/bladder/prostate tumor, bowel disease

—May reveal intravenous contrast in bowel or oral contrast in bladder

—More than 96% diagnostic in confirmation of fistula, and usually its etiology

SPECIAL STUDIES

• Cystoscopy

—Identifies bladder, prostate, urethral pathology (tumors, fistula, stricture)

—The exact site of fistula may be visualized.

—Biopsy of bladder tissue may reveal TCC, colon adenocarcinoma, or just inflammation.

• Colonoscopy

—May identify bowel disease, neoplasm

• Oral charcoal test

—Oral ingestion resulting in subsequent dark or gray urine is pathognomonic for fistula. It can also strain urine on a filter to detect charcoal.

• Bourne test

—Plain film of urine after barium enema

 ## Initial Management

• Standard work-up for fistula includes IVP, urine cytology, and cystoscopy. CT scan is currently considered the most cost-effective approach in making diagnosis.

• Spontaneous closure of fistula occurs in about 2% of cases, usually with trauma etiology.

• If fistula due to neoplasm, must determine if bladder, prostate, bowel, or other

—Must treat primary tumor first; deal with fistula as described below

• If fistula is due to inflammatory bowel disease

—Surgical repair is usually directed at bowel first; repair of bladder is secondary.

—Usually a segment of bowel is resected after thorough bowel prep and antibiotics.

—Usually a portion of bladder wall is resected and closed in layers.

—Interposition of omentum is suggested when possible.

—One-stage procedure recommended if colon is unobstructed and the fistulous tract is matured with no infection

• Staged repair and colostomy may be necessary in the presence of infections or abscess, large resections, or poorly healing tissues.

• A Foley catheter is left in place for 7 to 10 days and removed after a negative cystogram.

 ## Follow-Up

• After corrective surgery, may repeat CT with IV and/or oral contrast for baseline image

—May also repeat IVP, cystogram, barium enema, or cystoscopy, depending on original etiology

• Periodic UAs and cytology

• Recurrence is more likely in cases of infection, and radiation requires more compulsive follow-up.

 ## Miscellaneous

SYNONYMS: N/A

ASSOCIATED CONDITIONS: N/A

NOTES

• See also Section I, "Pneumaturia," and Section II, "Inflammatory Bowel Disease—Urologic Considerations."

ABBREVIATIONS

• TCC, transitional cell carcinoma

REFERENCES

Carson CC, Malek RS, Remine WH. Urologic aspects of vesicoenteric fistulas. *J Urol* 1978;1 19:744.

Goldman SM, Fishman EK, Gatewood OMB, Jones B, Siegelman SS. CT in the diagnosis of enterovesical fistulae. *AJR* 1985;144:1229.

Karamchandani MC, West CF Jr. Vesicoenteric fistulas. *Am J Surg* 1984;147:681.

Larsen A, Johansen TEB, Solheim BM, Urnes T. Diagnosis and treatment of enterovesical fistula. *Eur Urol* 1996;29:318.

Author: Jack Mydlo

Fistula—Vesicovaginal, Ureterovaginal

 Basics

DESCRIPTION

- Communication from the bladder, urethra and/or ureter to the vagina

PATHOPHYSIOLOGY

- Urine leaks into vagina, then out through the vaginal introitus.

RISK FACTORS

- Most common cause in developing countries: obstetric trauma
- Most common cause in developed countries: pelvic surgery
- Other causes: radiation, malignancy, trauma, foreign body, inflammation (e.g., tuberculosis)

 Differential Diagnosis

- Leak of peritoneal fluid into vagina
- Drainage of pus into vagina (e.g., cervicitis, pelvic abscess)
- If leak is truly urine, differential diagnosis includes

—Incontinence through urethra
—Reflux of urine into vagina while voiding, and urine leaks out of the vagina later
—Leaking urine from urethral diverticulum
—Ectopic ureter (congenital anomaly, so leak is present from birth)

 Database

HISTORY

- Time of symptom onset (leak may begin days to weeks after pelvic surgery)
- History of predisposing factors: pelvic surgery, childbirth, trauma, radiation, pelvic inflammation, malignancy
- When does urine leak occur?

—Classic history for fistula: continual leak of urine, even at night
—With severe stress incontinence, urine leak may be continual when upright but usually stops at night.
—With small fistula, urine leak may be intermittent.
—Leaking soon after voiding suggests vaginal reflux.
—Stress or urge incontinence may be present in addition to fistula, or may be mistaken for fistula by the patient.

PHYSICAL EXAMINATION

- Appearance of vaginal skin

—Healthy, inflamed, irradiated?

- Urine pooled in vagina is classic.
- Appearance of fistula

—Location: anterior vaginal wall or vaginal cuff
—Size
—Is bladder neck or urethra involved?
—If inflamed, delay surgical repair.
—May need special tests to identify fistula (see "Special Studies" below)

- Concomitant pathology: urethral mobility, stress incontinence, urethral diverticulum, cystocele, pelvic prolapse
- Caliber and flexibility of vagina (adequate exposure for vaginal surgery?)

Diagnostic Studies

LABORATORY TESTING

- Urinalysis, urine culture
- Appropriate preoperative tests for age and medical condition

IMAGING

- Cystogram

—Confirms fistula; not essential if fistula is evident on physical examination

- Excretory urogram or retrograde pyelogram

—Essential: Up to 10% of vesicovaginal fistulas have ureteral involvement.

SPECIAL STUDIES

- Cystoscopy

—Evaluate fistula position and proximity to ureteral orifices.
—Does fistula appear inflamed? If so, defer repair until inflammation resolves.
—Look for multiple fistulas.
—Look for other intravesical pathology.
—If history of pelvic malignancy, biopsy fistula site.

- Red/white/blue test

—Useful if fistula is suspected, but not seen on examination
—Vaginal tampon, oral phenazopyridine, intravesical methylene blue solution
—Remove tampon: wet but no color: peritoneal fluid leak; blue: vesicovaginal fistula (with or without ureteral involvement); orange: ureterovaginal fistula

 ## Initial Management

- A small fistula may close with conservative treatment.

—Indwelling catheter drainage
—Anticholinergics (control bladder spasms)
—Consider cauterizing fistula tract.
  —Only if tract is small, mature, epithelialized
  —Pediatric Bugbee electrode, minimal current
  —Avoid enlarging the tract.
—Endoscopic treatment: a few cases reported

- Timing of surgical repair

—Automatic 3- to 6-month delay is not needed.
—Repair when inflammation has resolved and tissue is healthy and pliable.

- Surgical approach: vaginal or abdominal?

—Most important factor: surgeon's training and expertise. "The best repair is the first repair."
—Vaginal approach contraindicated if
  —Concomitant abdominal pathology
  —Fistula involving or adjacent to ureter (reimplant will be needed)
  —Vagina too small or scarred for adequate exposure

- Key surgical principles

—Sterilize urine; use perioperative broad-spectrum antibiotics (include anaerobe coverage).
—Close without tension.
—Close in multiple layers; avoid overlapping suture lines.
—Interpose a vascularized graft between bladder and vagina if repair is at all tenuous.
  —Omentum
  —Peritoneal flap
  —Martius labial fat pad
  —Gracilis muscle or rectus abdominis myocutaneous flap (large or radiated fistulas)
—If bladder neck or urethra is involved, special reconstructive techniques are needed.
—Stent if the fistula is close to the ureter.

- Key principles for postoperative care

—Uninterrupted bladder drainage
—Aggressive anticholinergics (e.g., belladonna and opium suppositories) to prevent bladder spasms
—No coitus or tampons for at least 2 months

 ## Follow-Up

- Cystogram to confirm closure before removing catheter (at least 10 to 14 days)
- Renal imaging if ureter(s) were involved
- Late recurrence of fistula is rare.

Miscellaneous

SYNONYMS: N/A

ASSOCIATED CONDITIONS: N/A

NOTES

- See also Section I, "Urinary Incontinence: Adult Female."

ABBREVIATIONS: N/A

REFERENCES

Blaivas JG, et al. Early versus late repair of vesicovaginal fistulas: Vaginal and abdominal approaches. *J Urol* 1995;153:1110.

Davits RJ, et al. Conservative treatment of vesicovaginal fistulas by bladder drainage alone. *Br J Urol* 1991;68:155.

Leach GE, et al. Surgery for vesicovaginal and urethrovaginal fistula and urethral diverticulum. In: Walsh PC, Retik AB, Vaughan ED, Wein AJ, eds. *Campbell's Urology*, 7th ed. Philadelphia: WB Saunders, 1998.

Raz S, et al. Transvaginal repair of vesicovaginal fistula using a peritoneal flap. *J Urol* 1993;150:56.

Stovsky MD, et al. Use of electrocoagulation in the treatment of vesicovaginal fistulas. *J Urol* 1994;152:1443.

Author: Deborah R. Erickson

Flank Pain

 Basics

DESCRIPTION

- Pain arising in the area below the rib cage and above the ilium

—May be local or referred
—Renal pain typically a dull constant ache in the costovertebral angle. Pain may radiate along subcostal border towards the umbilicus or lower abdominal quadrant.

PATHOPHYSIOLOGY

- Flank pain: stretching of an organ capsule or by peritoneal irritation

—Renal pain: sudden distention of the renal capsule by edema (acute pyelonephritis) or back pressure (acute obstruction/hydronephrosis)
  —Some renal diseases painless due to slow progression (cancer, staghorn calculus, chronic obstruction)
—Ureteral pain produced by acute obstruction (calculi, clot)
  —Pain: due to renal pelvic and ureteral muscle spasm, and renal capsular distention. Pain follows the course of the ureter, radiating to low abdominal quadrants and the groin.
  —Proximal ureter radiates pain to the testicle or round ligament.
  —Mid-ureter radiates to the low anterior abdominal wall (mimicking appendicitis on the right and diverticulitis on the left).
  —Stones in the distal ureter: urinary urgency and frequency

RISK FACTORS

- Urinary tract infection, pregnancy, history of urinary calculi, history of prior urologic surgery, trauma, family history of urologic neoplasm, congenital anomaly, polycystic kidney disease, tuberous sclerosis

 Differential Diagnosis

- Inflammatory
—Acute pyelonephritis
  —Usually ascending UTI; females more common
  —Typical organisms are *E. coli, Proteus* (predispose to struvite calculi), and *Klebsiella*.
  —Emphysematous pyelonephritis: kidney infection with gas-forming bacteria; typically seen in diabetics, immunocompromised
—Xanthogranulomatous pyelonephritis (XGP), or pyonephrosis
  —Chronic bacterial infection with parenchymal damage; usually a nonfunctioning, obstructed renal unit.
—Papillary necrosis: ischemic necrosis of the renal papilla or entire pyramid (diabetics, sickle cell disease, analgesic abuse)

—Renal abscess: indolent fever, chills, flank mass and tenderness, occasionally weight loss or malaise, gram-negative septicemia

- Obstructive
—Urinary lithiasis (2%–3% prevalence)
  —Obstruction causes renal/ureteral colic.
  —Pain begins in flank, may gain intensity, coursing laterally around abdomen, then radiating to groin/testicles or labia majora/round ligament.
—Congenital
  —Ureteropelvic junction (UPJ) obstruction: pain, hematuria, or urinary infection in older children; palpable abdominal mass in infants; pain may be associated with increased fluid intake
  —Ureterocele: Occasionally, flank pain is the presenting symptom.
  —Autosomal dominant polycystic kidney disease
—Stricture: may result from ureteral devascularization and/or scarring (radiation therapy or surgery)
—Extrinsic compression: AAA, iliac aneurysm, fibroids, ovarian cysts, diverticulosis, tumors

- Pregnancy-related
—"Physiologic" hydronephrosis of pregnancy: mechanical and humoral factors
  —Dilated collecting system predisposes to urinary stasis and infection (90%–95% of pregnant women have asymptomatic hydronephrosis).
  —Spontaneous forniceal rupture (rare)
—Renal calculi occur in 1 of 1500 pregnancies, usually diagnosed in second or third trimesters.
—Bacteriuria is present in 4% to 7%. Twenty percent to 40% of untreated bacteriuria will subsequently develop pyelonephritis.

- Neoplastic
—Renal cell carcinoma (RCC)
—Transitional cell carcinoma (TCC): pain from obstruction (tumor or clot, rarely, locally invasive or metastatic disease)
—Angiomyolipoma (benign): tumors >4 cm more likely symptomatic (pain, hemorrhage)

- Traumatic
—Renal/ureteral injury caused by penetrating or blunt trauma, surgical injury, radiation damage, or urinary calculi

- Miscellaneous
—Radiculitis
  —Irritation to costal nerves produces costovertebral pain that may radiate to ipsilateral lower abdominal quadrant.
  —Unlike true renal pain, pain is positional and related to physical activity.
—Retroperitoneal hemorrhage (ruptured AAA)
—Subdiaphragmatic abscess
—Gynecologic: cervical cancer, endometriosis
—Biliary disease
—Factitious/drug seeking
  —Typically give history of multiple narcotic allergies, allergies to contrast, multiple prior stones

 Database

HISTORY

- Age, sex of the patient?
- Characterize the pain?

—Dull or sharp?
—Constant or intermittent?
—Sudden or gradual onset?
  —Stones tend to have a sudden onset.
—Alleviating, aggravating factors?
  —UPJ obstruction is aggravated with increased fluid uptake.
—Similar prior episodes?
  —Possible stone recurrence
—Location? Does the pain radiate?

- Associated symptoms?

—Fever, chills, dysuria?
  —Suggest inflammatory/infectious etiology
—Weight loss?
  —Suggest chronic infection, malignancy
—Hematuria?
  —Painless hematuria suggests malignancy (see Section I, "Hematuria—Adult" and "Hematuria—Pediatric")

- Medical history?

—History of diabetes?
  —Diabetics have higher incidence of infection and are predisposed to more severe infections, such as emphysematous pyelonephritis, XGP, and renal abscess.
—Previous urinary tract calculi?
  —History of stone disease has 10% one-year, 35% five-year, and 50% ten-year recurrence rate.
—History of radiation therapy?
  —Causes for flank pain following radiotherapy include recurrent tumor and obstruction of the ureter.
—History of blunt or penetrating trauma?
—History of intravenous drug abuse?
  —Gram-positive bacteria predispose to renal abscess, particularly if patient is immunocompromised.
—Pregnancy?

- Surgical history?

—Many procedures, including hysterectomy, salpingo-oophorectomy, vesicourethral suspension, femoral-popliteal or AAA bypass, and ureteroscopy, can damage the ureter, causing immediate or delayed obstruction.

- Family history of urologic cancer or polycystic kidney disease?
- Habits? Smoking is a risk factor for renal and transitional cell carcinoma.

PHYSICAL EXAMINATION

- Vital signs

—Fever
—Tachycardia may be a result of pain response.

—Hypertension can be seen in renal parenchymal disease, renal cystic disease, renal vascular disease, or renal neoplasia. It may also be a response to pain stimuli.
—Hypotension may reflect sepsis or hemorrhage and requires immediate treatment.

• Inspect abdomen: ecchymosis, purpura, penetrating injury, surgical scars
• Palpation of flank: Note size, location of masses, and tenderness.

—Costovertebral angle tenderness with fist percussion suggests acute pyelonephritis or other inflammatory process.
—Abdominal/flank mass: tumor (RCC), hydronephrosis, renal cystic disease (see also Section I, "Abdominal Mass—Newborn/Child")
—Tenderness: Tumors are usually minimally tender to palpation. Significant flank tenderness on palpation usually represents inflammatory response.

• Renal colic

—Patients can rarely find a comfortable position.
—Fever is not present unless there is concomitant infection.
—Pulse rate and blood pressure can be elevated due to pain.

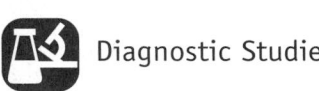 ## Diagnostic Studies

LABORATORY TESTING

• Urinalysis

—Rule out UTI and screen for hematuria.
—Hematuria: Confirm dipstick-positive hematuria with microscopic analysis for RBCs.
 —Degree of hematuria does not correlate with the seriousness of its etiology.
 —Dipsticks are sensitive to 5 RBCs per HPF.
 —False positives: myoglobinuria, oxidizing agents
 —5% to 15% of patients with urolithiasis will not have hematuria.
—Nitrite or leukocyte esterase positive; pyuria: suggests infection
 —Nitrite test depends on bacterial conversion of nitrate to nitrite; directly dependent on bacterial counts. Enterococci do not convert nitrate and are not detected by this test.
 —Leukocyte esterase identifies leukocyte concentrations >5 cells per HPF.

• Cultures and sensitivities to document infection and ensure appropriate antibiotic coverage

—Blood cultures: if septicemia is suspected

• Urine cytology

—Performed routinely in work-up of hematuria (in addition to IVP and cystoscopy)
 —Other urine tests for malignancy include assays for NMP-22 and BTA-stat.
—The first morning's voided specimen has the highest yield.

• Complete blood count (CBC)

—Evaluate leukocytosis and anemia.
—Leukocytosis suggests inflammatory response.

• Renal function tests

—Electrolytes, BUN, CR to evaluate renal function. (CR <2.0 for IV contrast)

• Chemistry profile

—In malignant process, elevated LFTs may suggest liver metastasis.
—Elevated alkaline phosphatase is suspicious for bony metastasis.
—Hypercalcemia is present in some malignancies.

IMAGING

• Intravenous pyelography (IVP)

—Study of choice for complete visualization of the urinary tract; may be replaced by spiral CT
—Indications: flank pain, hematuria, known symptomatic lithiasis, abnormal urine cytology
—Contraindicated: renal insufficiency (CR >2.0), allergy to iodine, multiple myeloma
—Delay in appearance of contrast confirms decreased renal function or obstruction.
 —80% of urinary calculi are radiopaque.
 —Excretion of contrast through the affected kidney helps delineate renal masses and location and degree of obstruction.
 —Delayed films (up to 24 hours) may be needed to delineate the entire ureter.

• Ultrasonography

—Evaluates the renal collecting system, parenchyma, and retroperitoneum for hydronephrosis, calculi, and abscesses
—Differentiates solid and cystic masses
—Usual initial examination in pregnant patients
—Advantages: easy to perform, noninvasive, no ionizing radiation, widely available, visualizes radiolucent calculi
—Disadvantages: tissue nonspecificity, lack of contrast media, small field of view, dependence on operator skill and patient physique

• Computed tomography (CT)

—Images renal parenchyma, urinary tract, and surrounding tissue; ideal for neoplasms, trauma, and abscess. Spiral CT may replace IVP for evaluation of urolithiasis.
—Advantages: wide field of view, detailed visualization of anatomy, urinary system imaged with administration of IV contrast, readily available
—Disadvantages: need for contrast media, cost, low soft-tissue contrast resolution
—Examination for malignancy *must* have pre- and postcontrast images.
—A solid enhancing mass is renal cell carcinoma until proven otherwise.

SPECIAL STUDIES

• Lasix washout renogram

—Estimates relative renal function and evaluates obstruction

• Whittaker test (see Section III)

 ## Initial Management

• Evaluation and baseline lab and imaging studies should help narrow the differential diagnosis.
• Hypotension should be treated immediately with fluid resuscitation and investigation into underlying cause (sepsis, hemorrhage).
• Infectious: appropriate antibiotics

—Infection with high-grade obstruction requires immediate attention: drainage of abscess.

• Pain management: Once diagnosis is made, use appropriately effective analgesics (rapid relief obtained by IV administration).
• Patients with calculi generally can be seen as outpatients if pain and nausea are controlled and there is no infection.
• Malignancy: may need admission for pain control, dehydration, or hemorrhage. Stable patients may be evaluated as outpatients.

 ## Follow-Up

• Follow-up is dictated by the diagnosis.
• If no urologic cause is identified, non-urologic etiologies should be investigated.

 ## Miscellaneous

SYNONYMS: N/A

ASSOCIATED CONDITIONS: N/A

NOTES

• See also Section I, "Costovertebral Angle Tenderness."

ABBREVIATIONS

• XGP, xanthogranulomatous pyelonephritis; UPJ, ureteropelvic junction; AAA, abdominal aortic aneurysm; RCC, renal cell carcinoma; TCC, transitional cell carcinoma

REFERENCES

AUA Update Series, Vol XII, Lesson 30, Houston, 1993.

Gillenwater JY, Grayhack JT, Howards SS, Duckett JW, eds. *Adult and Pediatric Urology*, 3rd ed. St Louis: Mosby, 1996.

Walsh PC, Retik AB, Vaughan ED, Wein AJ, eds. *Campbell's Urology*, 7th ed. Philadelphia: WB Saunders, 1998.

Authors: Christopher K. Tsai and Herbert C. Ruckle

Foley Catheter Problems

 Basics

DESCRIPTION

• Foley catheter problems generally fall into two categories: inability to insert or inability to remove.

PATHOPHYSIOLOGY

• Indications for catheterization include monitoring fluid balance, overcoming outflow obstruction, urinary incontinence, and diagnostic purposes.

 Differential Diagnosis

• Common causes of difficult Foley placement

—Strictures: primarily male patients (history of prior instrumentation, surgery, trauma, or STD)
—BPH: primarily elderly men
—Cancer of the prostate: primarily elderly men (obstructive symptoms usually present late in the disease)
—Bladder neck contracture; late complication of prostate surgery
—Meatal stenosis: congenital or acquired (meatal instrumentation, balanitis xerotica obliterans, postcircumcision, STD)
—Tight phimosis: primarily diabetics, children, and elderly men
—Buried penis: short shaft length and/or a large suprapubic fat pad
—Posterior urethral valves: primarily male infants/children
—Hypospadias: smaller meatal opening with associated duplex urethras or false passages
—Tumors: prostate cancers and, rarely, bladder, penile, and urethral cancers can cause distortion of normal anatomy. Also, local spread of cancers of nearby structures (i.e., vaginal, cervical, uterine, rectal)
—Trauma: Intrinsic from instrumentation or extrinsic to the urethra and/or bladder can cause false passages, stricture, or complete transection of the urethra (i.e., pelvic fracture).
—Miscellaneous: A foreign body/stone in urethra/bladder or, rarely , a prolapsing ureterocele can cause obstruction.

• Difficult Foley removal

—Catheter malfunction (most common): To prevent this problem, test the catheter balloon prior to placement.
—Obstruction of the balloon channel or balloon port from debris or crystals; sometimes caused by placement of solutions, other than the recommended sterile water, to inflate the balloon (i.e., saline, sorbitol, contrast, etc.)
—Long-term indwelling catheters can become encrusted by calcium.

 Database

HISTORY

• Age and sex of patient
• Onset/duration of symptoms
• Associated symptoms (frequency, nocturia, urgency, dysuria)
• History of trauma, prior surgery, or instrumentation. Discuss previous attempts at catheter passage.

PHYSICAL EXAMINATION

• Abdomen: palpable bladder, pain
• GU: blood at meatus, phimosis, meatal stenosis, hypospadias
• Rectal: floating prostate with urethral trauma; nodularity with cancer
• Bimanual examination: abnormal anatomy, tumor

 Diagnostic Studies

LABORATORY TESTING

Urinalysis: Hematuria can suggest tumor, BPH, stone, or other foreign body. Pyuria can occur with stones, foreign bodies, and infectious processes.

IMAGING

• Rarely needed acutely
• Urethrography: Retrograde, antegrade, and combined urethrograms can help diagnose the presence and extent of strictures, valves, false passages, and urethral trauma.

SPECIAL STUDIES

• Cystourethroscopy: Direct visualization of urethra and bladder can help in both diagnosis and placement of catheter.

 Initial Management

• Catheterization problems

—External sphincter spasm: reassurance patient, local anesthesia, distraction of patient, and patience
—Suspected or known stricture: Retrograde urethrography can be carried out to assess the urethra. Filiform and followers to dilate stricture. Cystoscopic placement of guidewire can be done at bedside with local anesthesia. In an impassible stricture, a suprapubic tube is indicated.
—Bladder neck obstruction: The coudé tip catheter or catheter stylette is useful and avoids risk of trauma.
—Trauma: confirm via radiologic modalities. Percutaneous cystostomy is always a safe, reliable option. Direct visualization with flexible cystoscopy is also a viable option.

• Catheter placement

—If necessary, use 2% lidocaine jelly (URO-JET/ASTRA) for anesthesia.
—In females, with difficult anatomy, the hand may be placed into the vagina with gentle downward traction to allow better determination of the urethral meatus.
—In males, fill the urethra with lubricant jelly and maintain stretch on the penis to keep the urethra straight.
—If the catheter does not enter the bladder easily, the most likely causes are spasm of the external sphincter, stricture, or bladder neck obstruction. BPH rarely prevents the passage of a catheter.
—If urine is not obtained or if there is doubt regarding position of the catheter balloon, do not inflate the balloon (this may cause severe urethral trauma or rupture). Hand irrigation with normal saline and catheter tip syringe can help check catheter position. If one can irrigate in and withdraw easily, the catheter is most likely within the bladder and the balloon can be inflated safely. If not, continue to instill water and then withdraw. If again not successful, withdraw the catheter and reintroduce or try other options.
—The coudé catheter with a curved hard tip is designed to guide the catheter over the prostate/bladder neck.
—Catheter stylettes: malleable metal guides that, when placed into a Foley or other type of catheter, can be used to provide stiffness and a particular contour. Can be used following TURP to avoid undermining the bladder neck; should only be used by experienced operators

—If stricture prevents placement
—Van Buren sounds: solid metal sounds curved in the shape of the male urethra (sizes 16Fr–30Fr), used for dilation
—Filiforms and followers: thin, pliable, solid catheters for dilating urethral stricture (sizes 1Fr–6Fr). The tip may be straight, pigtailed, or coudé type. They have a female screw tip on the proximal end to allow attachment of the follower (sizes 12Fr–30Fr), which may be solid or hollow.
—Laforte sounds: similar to Van Buren sounds except for the presence of a male screw fitting on the end, permitting attachment to a filiform
—Coaxial dilators: dilators that can be passed into the bladder over a flexible wire
—Perform flexible/rigid cystoscopy to pass a guidewire under direct vision
—Council catheters: similar to a Foley catheter except for a small perforation at its tip, which can engage a filiform or guidewire. Safest to place after difficult dilation

• Percutaneous cystostomy trocars: used when the bladder cannot be entered through the urethra; bladder must be distended

—Stamey trocar: Malecot catheter into the bladder
—Argyle trocar: Foley-type can be used to irrigate.
—Cystocath: 8Fr or 12Fr simple tube retained in the bladder by skin glue and/or skin suture
—Contraindications: prior lower abdominal surgery and the presence of surgical scars in the suprapubic area (because small bowel may be interposed in the retropubic space)
—If the bladder is not distended sufficiently to permit blind cystostomy, a long spinal needle may be used to determine location of the bladder, and the bladder can be filled with saline through this needle (or distend the bladder by putting the catheter into the distal aspect of the urethra and introduce saline retrograde to fill the bladder). The trocar can then be passed into the bladder safely.
—Occasionally, ultrasound guidance can be used to help with percutaneous cystostomy.

• Bladder irrigation for clots

—Whistle-tip catheter: a straight catheter with a beveled opening at the tip and another opening in the side; provides better irrigation and drainage
—A large catheter will irrigate clots better than a three-way catheter due to the larger lumen.
—A resectoscope sheath can be used to irrigate clots.

• Children

—Female children: Catheterization is similar to that for adult women, but smaller catheters are used (size 8Fr–12Fr).
—Male children: Some prefer to use an 8Fr feeding tube rather than a Foley because the Foley balloon is somewhat larger than the catheter itself and can be difficult to pass.

• Techniques for catheter removal

—Deflate the balloon and test the balloon channel before proceeding with any other procedure. The problem may be as simple as incomplete balloon deflation.
—Cut the distal port of the balloon channel. This aspect of the catheter may be the sole area which is blocked in the balloon channel, and cutting it may allow the fluid from the balloon to drain without obstruction.
—Balloon perforation: A stiff guidewire may be passed into the channel to try to perforate the balloon. Also a suprapubic technique for balloon perforation under ultrasound guidance can be utilized using a suprapubic needle. Blind needle placement is not recommended.
—Hyperinflation is not recommended (bladder injury and balloon segments within the bladder); remove these segments because they can become focuses for stone formation and infection.
—External crystal formation: Bladder instillations of Renacidin or diluted vinegar (for struvite stones), or alkaline solutions (i.e., k-citrate, $NaHCO_3$) (for uric acid stones), have been used. ESWL may be required to disrupt stones.
—Finally, flexible or rigid cystoscopy may be necessary to remove the catheter.

 Follow-Up

• Bleeding/hematuria: common following instrumentation; usually clears spontaneously within 24 hours. Maintain a high fluid intake to promote diuresis and prevent clot formation. Irrigation may sometimes be indicated.
• Perforation of the urethra: can occur when excessive force is used. Diagnosis is made by retrograde urethrography. If minimal extravasation is present, antibiotic coverage and urinary drainage for 1 to 2 days is a reliable treatment. If major extravasation into the perineum or extraperitoneal extravasation occurs, drainage of fluid or surgery may be necessary.
• Infections: range from simple bacteriuria to sepsis. Antibiotic prophylaxis and coverage is sometimes indicated.

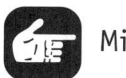 Miscellaneous

SYNONYMS: N/A

ASSOCIATED CONDITIONS

• BPH, stricture, prostate cancer

NOTES

• Catheters are made of various materials (latex, rubber, silicone, polymers, plastic, metals), calibrated according to the French (Fr) scale, in which each unit equals 0.33 mm in diameter (i.e., a 30Fr catheter has a 10-mm outer diameter) (see appendix).

ABBREVIATIONS

• STD, sexually transmitted diseases; BPH, benign prostatic hypertrophy; ESWL, extracorporeal shock wave lithotripsy; TURP, transurethral resection of prostate; EHL, electrohydraulic lithotripsy

REFERENCES

Gomella LG, ed. Bladder procedures. In: *Clinician's Pocket Reference*, 8th ed. Norwalk, CT: Appleton & Lange, 1997.

Authors: Matthew Shahbandi and Bhalchandra G. Parulkar

Foreign Body—Bladder and Urethra

 ## Basics

DESCRIPTION

• Nonphysiologic solid material within the bladder or urethra

—Generally nontherapeutic, or beyond its therapeutic usefulness

• May or may not be symptomatic

—Often found on plain radiograph when the object is metallic or calcified

PATHOPHYSIOLOGY

• Any solid object within the bladder or urethra that does not belong there

—Most foreign bodies with the urinary tract used for therapeutic reasons are temporary

• May be placed directly into the bladder or urethra or migrate from another location

—Iatrogenic, purposely or inadvertently left by a surgeon or clinician
—Inserted transurethrally by the patient or another person

• Medical devices

—Suture, catheters, stents, calculi admixed with foreign body, IUDs, wires, prosthetic devices, staples, clips

• Nonmedical objects

—Pencils, safety pins, nails, glue, electrical wire, etc.

RISK FACTORS

• Previous surgery in or near the urinary tract where nonabsorbable material is left within the body
• Psychiatric disorder

—Schizophrenia
—Self-mutilation

• Sexual experimentation
• Torture

 ## Differential Diagnosis

• Stones
• Infection
• Tumor
• Interstitial cystitis
• Bladder outlet obstruction
• Urethral stricture
• Urethral diverticulum
• Endometriosis
• Ectopic ureter

 ## Database

HISTORY

• May be asymptomatic
• Common complaints: dysuria, gross hematuria, stranguria, pneumaturia, urgency, frequency, slow stream, foul odor, abdominal pain, dyspareunia, spasm
• Onset of symptoms, history of placing any object within the urethra, is incontinence present?

—Incontinence might represent a fistula.
—Obstructive symptoms may be intermittent or constant.

• Prior surgery or instrumentation

—Were any implants or devices placed within the urinary tract?
—What type of suture, clips, or staples were used near the bladder or urethra?

• Sexual history?

—Experimentation with insertion of objects for sexual pleasure

• Psychiatric history?

—Schizophrenia or depression/self-mutilation

PHYSICAL EXAMINATION

• Fever
• Suprapubic tenderness; palpable mass in urethra (males), in bladder (females)
• Abdominal

—Pain, peritoneal signs, surgical scar

• Genitourinary

—Urethral bleeding, discharge, trauma
—Palpable mass within the urethra

• Vaginal

—IUD, discharge, tenderness, mass, pessary

Diagnostic Studies

LABORATORY TESTING

Urinalysis

—Hematuria, pyuria, bacteriuria

- Microbiology

—Multiple organisms could indicate vesico-enteric fistula.

IMAGING

- Plain abdominal radiograph

—May be the initial method of diagnosis
—Often can diagnose the foreign body simply by its shape

- Computed tomography/ultrasound

—May be performed to rule out differential diagnosis and discover the foreign body

SPECIAL STUDIES

- Cystourethroscopy

—Direct visualization of the object

- Retrograde urethrogram

—May indicate the degree of urethral trauma and extravasation

 ## Initial Management

- Foreign body removal: type specific

—Endourologic: for small objects that can be through the urethra with minimal trauma, clips, staples, fragmented pieces of catheters and stents, some small metallic objects such as nails and pins
—Open cystotomy: for larger objects, such as pencils, open safety pins, etc.
—Urethrotomy: for objects lodged within the urethra

- Repair of concomitant injuries

—Strictures, perforations, fistulas, and diverticula

 ## Follow-Up

- Cystourethroscopy

—Assure complete healing and complete removal

- Psychiatric evaluation and treatment where indicated

 ## Miscellaneous

SYNONYMS: N/A

ASSOCIATED CONDITIONS: N/A

NOTES: N/A

ABBREVIATIONS

- IUD, intrauterine device

REFERENCES

Blasco Hernandez P, Camacho Martinez E, Quintero Rodriguez R, et al. Migration of an intrauterine device. An unusual cause of bladder foreign. *Actas Urol Esp* 1995;19(10):798–801.

Chitale SV, Burgess NA. Endoscopic removal of a complex foreign body from the bladder. *Br J Urol* 1998;81(5):756–757.

Derevianko IM, Derevianko TI, Ryzhkov VV. The urological complications of contraception using intrauterine. *Urol Nefrol* 1997;(5):27–30.

Author: Kevin R. Anderson

Frequency and Urgency

 Basics

DESCRIPTION

- *Frequency* is voiding more often than normal (typically 5 to 6 times per day, 0 to 2 times per night).
- *Urgency* is the sudden impulse to void. Uncontrollable voiding after this impulse is termed *urge incontinence*.

PATHOPHYSIOLOGY

- Frequency can be caused by
—Increased urine output (polyuria)
—Direct bladder abnormalities (e.g., decreased capacity, outlet obstruction, etc.)
—Adjacent pathology (e.g., pelvic masses, neurologic disease, etc.)
- Urgency is usually a severe form of frequency.

RISK FACTORS

- Depends on etiology (see "Differential Diagnosis," below)

 Differential Diagnosis

- Congenital/inherited
—Spina bifida and other neurologic malformations
—Posterior urethral valves and other urologic malformations
- Traumatic
—Pelvic trauma: bladder or urethral injury
—Neurologic trauma: brain or spinal cord
—Iatrogenic trauma: surgical injury to brain, spinal cord, pelvic nerves, bladder, or urethra
—Foreign body: Foley catheter, ureteral stents, etc.
- Inflammatory
—UTI: most common cause of frequency/urgency; also causes dysuria, fever, bacteriuria, pyuria
—Specific infections: tuberculosis, schistosomiasis
—Radiation cystitis: pelvic irradiation for malignancy (cervical, prostate, etc.)
—Urethritis: STD usually from chlamydia, gonorrhea, etc.; also causes dysuria, urethral discharge
—Interstitial cystitis
- Metabolic
—Polyuria
　—Excessive fluid intake
　—Diabetes mellitus, usually with glucosuria and poorly controlled or undiagnosed
　—Diabetes insipidus
　—Urinary calculi: bladder or intramural ureter
- Neoplastic
—BPH: Bladder outlet obstruction can induce urgency, frequency, nocturia, and obstructive symptoms.
—Prostate cancer: also by the mechanism of bladder outlet obstruction
—Bladder cancer and CIS
—Urethral cancer
—Non-urologic cancers, by local extension: cervical, rectal, etc.
—Metastatic cancer: rare

- Miscellaneous
—Drugs
　—Diuretics: induce polyuria
　—Caffeine: medication or coffee, tea, sodas, chocolate, etc.
　—Alcohol: induces polyuria
—Neurologic
　—Cerebral or brainstem: CVA, dementia, brain tumor, Parkinson disease, cerebral palsy, etc.
　—Spinal cord: trauma, spina bifida, polio, multiple sclerosis, disk disease etc.
　—Peripheral neuropathies: radical pelvic surgery, diabetes mellitus, etc.
—Gastrointestinal: obstipation/impaction, irritable bowel, etc.
—Gynecologic: gynecologic cancers, fibroids, pelvic floor relaxation, pelvic pain syndromes, etc.

 Database

HISTORY

- Irritative voiding symptoms?
—Urgency, frequency, urge incontinence, nocturia
- Obstructive voiding symptoms?
—Hesitancy, slow stream, post-void dribbling, straining to void, retention
—Consider causes of outlet obstruction: BPH, strictures, cancer.
- Incontinence (stress, urge, total, etc.)?
—Female stress incontinence may be related to pelvic prolapse
- Symptoms of UTI or prostatitis?
—These are easily treated with antibiotics.
- Hematuria?
—Will need careful evaluation for UTI, cancer, stones with upper tract study and cystoscopy
- History of stone disease?
- Fluid intake?
- Change in bowel habits or sexual function?
—May imply neurologic etiology
- History of gynecologic or gastrointestinal problems?
- Significant medical or surgical history?
—Neurologic, diabetes, radiation, trauma, pelvic surgery, etc.
- Current medications?
—Drugs as noted above
- History of tobacco use?
—Associated with bladder cancer
- History of caffeine use?
—Causes diuresis, stimulates bladder directly
- Family history?
—Particularly bladder and prostate cancers, urolithiasis

PHYSICAL EXAMINATION

- Neurologic

—Mental status, cognitive deficits
—Motor deficits
—Sensory deficits
—Reflexes: particularly bulbocavernosus, cremasteric, and anal

- Palpable abdominal masses

—Retention, fibroids, or uterine masses

- Pelvic examination for masses, pelvic floor support

—Fibroids, gynecologic cancers, pelvic floor relaxation, urethral lesions, urethral diverticula
—Valsalva maneuver to detect SUI, pelvic floor descensus

- Genital examination in men

—Phimosis, meatal stenosis, urethral scarring

- Digital rectal examination

—Prostate size, nodules, estimate of PVR
—Rectal masses, fecal impaction
—Perineal sensation, anal sphincter tone (passive and active), bulbocavernosus reflex

- General examination for edema

—May contribute to nocturia

 ## Diagnostic Studies

LABORATORY TESTING

- Urinalysis (UA)

—Specific gravity: Poorly concentrated urine suggests polydipsia.
—Leukocyte esterase, nitrate, pyuria: suggests UTI
—RBCs: suggest need for hematuria work-up (rule out stone, tumor, etc.)
—Glucosuria: rule out diabetes mellitus
—Proteinuria: suggests nephritis or nephrotic syndrome

- Urine culture: if UA suggests UTI
- BUN and creatinine

—If neurogenic bladder suspected, severe bladder obstruction, or retention

IMAGING

- Renal ultrasound

—If neurogenic bladder suspected, severe bladder outlet obstruction, or retention
—If renal insufficiency found

- Pelvic ultrasound

—If adnexal mass or uterine enlargement noted on pelvic examination
—Estimate of PVR

SPECIAL STUDIES

- Voiding diary

—Documents voiding pattern and incontinence

- Cystoscopy

—If hematuria, pyuria, or persistent/worsening symptoms
—May detect stones, bladder tumors, BOO (strictures, BPH)

- Urodynamics (CMG, EMG, uroflow, PVR, pressure/flow)

—PVR very important to r/o retention
—Evaluate for neurogenic causes.
—Evaluate for incontinence, BOO.
—Define treatment options.

 ## Initial Management

- Standard evaluation is history, physical examination and UA.

—Additional evaluation based on clinical findings
—Opinion divided on indications for cystoscopy, urodynamics, or imaging in the setting of symptoms without other significant findings

- Treatment based on underlying disorder

—Treatment types include behavioral, pharmacologic, and surgical

- Behavioral treatment

—Bladder training involves suppressing urges to void and delaying voiding.
—Timed voiding or prompted voiding involves scheduled voiding to preempt urgency.

- Kegel's exercises to strengthen the pelvic floor musculature may improve SUI and inhibit urgency.
- Biofeedback involves using electronic measurements to assist patients in changing or inhibiting bladder behavior.
- Pharmacologic treatment (see Section VII)

—Anticholinergics to inhibit detrusor overactivity: oxybutynin, hyoscyamine, Propantheline, or tolterodine
—Alpha blockers to decrease outflow obstruction due to BPH: terazosin, doxazosin, or tamsulosin
—Other agents are occasionally used: imipramine, topical estrogens (in postmenopausal women), etc.

- Surgical treatment

—Correction of pelvic floor prolapse (e.g., bladder neck suspension, sling, cystocele repair, etc.)
—Correction of bladder outlet obstruction due to BPH (e.g., TURP, etc.)
—If disabling and associated with incontinence: bladder augmentation or urinary diversion

 ## Follow-Up

- Periodic follow-up depending on etiology, treatment, and response

 ## Miscellaneous

SYNONYMS

- Urethral syndrome (refers to urgency, frequency, etc., in women)

ASSOCIATED CONDITIONS: N/A

NOTES

- See also Section II, "Urethral Syndrome."

ABBREVIATIONS

- BOO, bladder outlet obstruction; CMG, cystometrogram; EMG, electromyogram (of urinary sphincter); SUI, stress urinary incontinence

REFERENCES

Steers WD, et al. Voiding dysfunction: Diagnosis, classification, and management. In: Gillenwater JY, Grayhack JT, Howards SS, Duckett JW, eds. *Adult and Pediatric Urology*, 3rd ed. St Louis: Mosby, 1996.

Urinary Incontinence Guideline Panel. Urinary incontinence in adults: Clinical practice guideline. AHCPR Pub. No 92-0038, Dept. of HHS, 1992.

Author: David E. McGinnis

Groin Mass

 Basics

DESCRIPTION

- Palpable abnormality generally located in the inguinal region. Most commonly due to

—Hernia: presents with bulge (sometimes sudden onset), often after period of crying/cough/strain
—Cryptorchid testis: usually present at birth; may be retractile
—Lymphadenopathy: infectious, inflammatory of malignant conditions

PATHOPHYSIOLOGY

- Cryptorchidism

—Improper gubernaculum shortening with (?) associated diminished androgen levels during first 3 months' gestation
—Histologic changes of testicle at 18 months (if not in scrotum)
—Diminished fertility and increased risk for testicular cancer
—90% of cryptorchids have hernia sacs.

- Hernia

—Congenital (majority): processus vaginalis is not obliterated (increases with low birth weight and prematurity).
    —Congenital abnormalities (such as pelvic deformities and bladder extrophy) can cause abnormal inguinal canal formation.
    —Collagen deficiency increases risk for direct hernia formation.
—Acquired: Wear-and-tear stresses such as straining (urine/stool), coughing, heavy lifting
    —Cigarette smoking is associated with increased risk (increased serum elastolytic activity).
—Incarcerated bowel (rare in children): acute abdomen and bowel necrosis

- Lymphadenopathy

—Lymphadenitis with STD and HPV infections; skin infections of lower extremity
—Malignant adenopathy (decreasing frequency): melanoma, squamous cell carcinoma of penis/urethra, lymphoma

RISK FACTORS

- Cryptorchidism

—Incidence based on birth weight (inversely proportional): Full-term (>2500 g), 3.4%; premature, 30.3%; <900 g, 100%; adult, <1%
—No geographic or racial predisposition
—Persistent Müllerian duct syndrome (PMDS): form of pseudohermaphroditism
    —Failure of Müllerian duct regression in a phenotypically normal male with normal testosterone

- Hernia: 3.5% to 5.0% full-term newborns; higher if premature; 60% bilateral; 9:1 male:female ratio

 Differential Diagnosis

- Inguinal or femoral hernia
- GU: cryptorchid/ectopic testes, varicocele, hydrocele, epididymitis, testicular torsion
- Infectious: lymphadenitis, tuberculosis
- Malignant: lymphoma, metastatic
- Lipoma
- Hematoma
- Femoral aneurysm/pseudoaneurysm
- Sebaceous cyst
- Hidradenitis of inguinal apocrine glands
- PMDS

 Database

HISTORY

- Family history of malignancy such as lymphoma?
- Medical history

—Birth history: premature or low birth weight: hernia/cryptorchidism
—Mass present at birth or recently developed?
—Both testes present in scrotum?
    —"Vanishing" testes with hyperactive cremasterics
    —Increasing size of mass with abdominal straining suggests hernia.
    —Is bulge absent in AM and gets larger in PM? Suggests hernia
    —Fever or recurrent illness suggests lymphadenitis.

- Surgical history

—Previous herniorrhaphy (60% of hernia defects in children are bilateral)

PHYSICAL EXAMINATION

- Examine scrotum and contents: epididymitis, absent testicle.
- External genitalia for evidence of malignancy, lesion of STD
- Extremity for infectious lesions
- Inguinal mass

—If tender, likely infectious etiology; if nontender, likely malignancy

- Cryptorchidism: testis locations

—Abdominal: inside internal ring; diagnostic study for conformation of location
—Canalicular: between internal and external rings
—Ectopic: away from normal path of descent
    —"Wayward gubernaculum": most common location is superficial inguinal pouch

—Retractile: "vanishing"; examine patient in warm, comfortable environment.

- Hernia

—Examine with patient in standing position; visually inspect for a discrete bulge in the inguinal region.
—Place fingertip in canal and have patient Valsalva.
    —Indirect: bulges lateral to medial
    —Direct: from deep onto tip of finger
    —Femoral: from below inguinal ligament
—Synchronous palpation of both spermatic cords; roll finger over pubic tubercles
    —"Bulky" cord is consistent with hernia sac.
—Palpate for testes (6% congenital inguinal hernias have incomplete testicular descent).
—If incarcerated, may attempt manual reduction; gangrenous bowel must be repaired surgically.

Diagnostic Studies

LABORATORY TESTING

- Urinalysis
- Gonadotropin/androgen levels for cryptorchid testicle

IMAGING

- Note: most diagnosed by physical findings
- Ultrasound: helps with testes in canal; not reliable for: intraabdominal testis/hiding under external oblique
- CT scan: location of bilateral impalpable testes; identify/characterize suspicious inguinal masses.
- MRI: not commonly used
- Angiography of testicular vessels: *Avoid!* Invasive—femoral artery thrombosis is disastrous.

SPECIAL STUDIES

- Fine-needle aspiration: undetermined lymphadenopathy
- Laparoscopy: Evaluate possible abdominal testes.

 ## Initial Management

- Cryptorchidism: usually will not descend after 3 months

—See Section I, "Undescended Testicle (Cryptorchidism)."

- Retractile testis: gonadotropins
- Infectious lymphadenopathy: specific antibiotics for pathogen
- Metastatic lymphadenopathy: Consider inguinal lymph node dissection.
- Persistent Müllerian duct structure: Remove Müllerian structures (uterus, fallopian tubes), taking care to preserve the distal end of the vas, then orchiopexy.
- Hernia

—Attempt reduction (especially if incarcerated).
—Preemie hernias: observed for resolution (with increasing age, have increased bowel diameter relative to inguinal ring size). Otherwise, hernias do not improve with time.
—Unless incarcerated/strangulated, elective surgical repair is recommended: Bassini/McVay (Cooper ligament repair)/Shouldice.

 ## Follow-Up

- Metastatic lymphadenopathy: surveillance for recurrence and lymphedema of distal extremities
- Cryptorchidism

—Increased risk for malignancy or torsion with undescended testes
—Decreased fertility damage to seminal tubules
—Patient *must* perform monthly testicular self-examinations.

- Hernia

—Watch for recurrence, or occurrence, on the contralateral side.

 ## Miscellaneous

SYNONYMS: N/A

ASSOCIATED CONDITIONS: N/A

NOTES: N/A

ABBREVIATIONS: N/A

REFERENCES

Lima M, et al. Persistent mullerian duct syndrome associated with transverse testicular ectopia: A case report. *Eur J Pediatr Surg* 1997;60.

Sabiston D, ed. *Textbook of Surgery*, 15th ed. Philadelphia: WB Saunders, 1997;32:1218.

Walsh PC, Retik AB, Vaughan ED, Wein AJ, eds. *Campbell's Urology*, 7th ed. Philadelphia: WB Saunders, 1998:1543.

Authors: J.C. Trussell and Gabriel P. Haas

Gynecomastia

 Basics

DESCRIPTION

- The mammary gland contains both glandular ductal epithelium and periductal connective tissue.
- Gynecomastia in males is a proliferation of the ductal epithelium of the breast with hyperplasia and edema of the surrounding stroma and connective tissue.

PATHOPHYSIOLOGY

- In males, due to an alteration in the estrogen-to-testosterone ratio
—Due to an elevation of estrogens (estradiol/estrone)
—Due to a decrease in synthesis or recognition of androgens (testosterone/androstenedione)
- Due to abnormal tissue response to circulating hormones

RISK FACTORS

- Endocrinopathies
- Intersex
- Alcoholism
- Prostate cancer (side effect of therapy)
- Renal failure
- Obesity

 Differential Diagnosis

- Congenital

—Androgen insensitivity: Genetic males with testosterone receptor defects have normal female genitalia and breast development.
—Male pseudohermaphrodism: frequently have enzymatic defect in the production of testosterone, allowing an unopposed action of estrogen on the breast
—Partial testicular feminization: ambiguous genitalia with variable gynecomastia
- Developmental
—Neonatal
  —Due to high estrogen levels in the fetal/placental unit and resolves spontaneously
—Prepubertal (>2 years old, <12 years old)
  —Rare; predominantly benign
  —Need to differentiate from other breast masses: abscess, carcinoma, fatty necrosis, hemangiomas, lipomas, lymphangiomas, metastatic disease
  —Must evaluate for Leydig cell tumor of the testis
—Pubertal
  —Normal part of development; highest incidence at 14 years of age
  —Occurs in 70% of boys during puberty
  —Occurs in early puberty because estrogens derived from adrenal androgens rise during the 24-hour period, while testosterone from the testis is secreted only at night, thus causing an imbalance in the estrogen:testos-

terone ratio during the daytime and subsequent gynecomastia
  —Time limited and benign: enlarges approximately 1 year after the onset of puberty and subsides within 2 years
—Aging
  —Mild primary testicular failure, causing a high estrogen:androgen ratio and ultimately gynecomastia
  —Increased percentage of body fat, allowing aromatization of androgens to estrogen
- Testicular failure
—Primary: chronic stimulation of Leydig cells by LH with decreased testosterone and elevation of circulating estrogen
  —Chromosomal defects: i.e., Klinefelter (XXY karyotype)
  —Congenital defects in androgen production
  —Iatrogenic injury, trauma, torsion
  —Cryptorchidism that was not corrected
—Secondary
  —Kallmann syndrome: defect in gonadotropin-releasing hormone (anosmia, infertility, gynecomastia)
  —Pituitary failure: infarction, neoplasm
  —Pituitary adenoma: increased prolactin, visual field defects, gynecomastia, and galactorrhea
- Medications/drugs
—Diethylstilbestrol (DES): used for treatment of prostate carcinoma; very high incidence of gynecomastia
—Nonsteroidal antiandrogens (flutamide, bicalutamide)
  —Competitively binds to androgen receptor, thereby blocking conversion of testosterone to dihydrotestosterone (DHT)
  —Circulating testosterone is increased and is converted by aromatase to estradiol, which stimulates ductal proliferation of the breast.
  —Breast and nipple tenderness is reported in 42% to 53% of patients, and gynecomastia in 14% to 51%.
—Finasteride
  —Blocks conversion of testosterone to DHT by inhibiting the enzyme 5-alpha reductase
  —Breast tenderness reported in 10% to 62%, and gynecomastia in 30% to 54%
—Growth hormone (GH): given for GH deficiency
  —Proposed that GH receptors in breast tissue are directly stimulated by GH, or indirectly stimulate breast tissue by inducing production of insulin-like growth factor (IGF)
  —Causes bilateral gynecomastia; time limited and benign
—Anabolic steroids
—Antipsychotics
  —Influence secretion of hormones in pituitary by dopaminergic (D2) receptor blockade
  —Elevation of prolactin, hypogonadism, gynecomastia, and galactorrhea
—Tricyclic antidepressants
—Dilantin
  —Enhances the conversion of testosterone to estradiol

—Cimetidine (blocks binding of testosterone to its receptor)/omeprazole/metoclopramide
—Nifedipine, digitalis, isoniazid
—Ketoconazole/spironolactone
  —Inhibits androgen production and prevents binding of androgens to their receptors; induces sex hormone–binding globulin (SHBG), which binds testosterone more readily than estrogen
—Chemotherapy
  —Platinum-based, for testicular tumors
  —Toxic effect on Leydig cells; increased gonadotropins cause an increased secretion of testicular estrogens
—Marijuana/heroin/alcohol
- Neoplasia
—Testicular
  —Choriocarcinoma: 10% found to have gynecomastia; increased B-hCG causes Leydig cell stimulation, leading to increased release of estradiol over testosterone by the interstitial cells
  —Leydig cell: occurs at all ages; 90% unilateral and benign; adults present with gynecomastia, loss of libido, feminine hair patterns, and genital underdevelopment; testosterone decreased 30% to 50% with normal or elevated FSH; 50% secrete estrogen; 20% present with gynecomastia, which may appear months or years before tumor becomes evident
  —Sertoli cell: Approximately 20% will present with gynecomastia; tumor cells stimulate neighboring Leydig cells to secrete androgens, which are aromatized to estrogens, ultimately causing bilateral gynecomastia.
—Breast
  —Male breast cancer accounts for 1% of all breast cancer; unilateral; often associated with bloody nipple discharge, skin fixation, ulcer, and axillary adenopathy
—Adrenal (carcinoma): androstenedione production is increased, which is peripherally converted to estrone by aromatase
—Lung (giant cell carcinoma): secretes B-hCG, which stimulates Leydig cells to increase testosterone and estradiol production
—Hepatic: increased aromatase, inducing breast tissue proliferation
—Others: sarcomas, gastric, pancreatic, pituitary
—Metastatic disease
- Systemic/medical illnesses
—Cirrhosis
  —Prevalence of gynecomastia noted to be approximately 50%
—Hyperthyroidism
  —Increased production of androstenedione, providing a substrate for increased formation of estrogens through aromatization of androgens at extraglandular sites
—End-stage renal failure
  —Elevated FSH/LH, low testosterone, and normal-to-high estrogens
—HIV/AIDS
  —Testicular atrophy, hypogonadotropic hypogonadism

Database

HISTORY

- Age
—Infant (<2 years old): congenital
—Prepubertal (>2 years old, <12 years old): usually benign, must differentiate between other types of breast masses as noted
—Pubertal: normal development; if does not resolve, consider other causes
—Adult (>25 years old): Consider medication and drug use, medical conditions, hypogonadism, or testicular carcinoma.
- Medications
—Drugs as noted
- Medical conditions
—Symptoms of pulmonary disease, hepatic dysfunction, and hyperthyroidism
- Length of time and progression of gynecomastia
—Greater than 12 months leads to fibrosis and is often not reversible.
- Painful breasts, nipple discharge
- Associated fevers
—Consider breast abscess.
- History of cryptorchidism
—Consider testicular tumor, primary hypogonadism.
- History of testicular trauma
- Sexual maturation (children)
- Change in libido, erectile dysfunction and infertility (adults): associated with hypogonadism

PHYSICAL EXAMINATION

- Weight of patient
—Aromatase, which converts testosterone to estradiol and subsequently causes breast tissue proliferation, is found in adipose tissue.
- Body hair patterns
—More dense and extensive, and earlier completion of body hair development in 18- to 26-year-old males with gynecomastia as compared with those without gynecomastia
- Breast
—Firm, mobile disk arising from underneath the nipple/areolar region
—Unilateral vs. bilateral gynecomastia
—Measurements (baseline and posttherapy)
  —Sternal notch to nipple, midclavicular line to nipple, nipple to nipple
- Lymph nodes
- Testicular
—Palpable lesion/atrophy

 ## Diagnostic Studies

LABORATORY TESTING

- Liver function tests, thyroid function tests
- FSH, LH, testosterone, estradiol, estrone, B-hCG, AFP, prolactin

IMAGING

- Testicular ultrasonography
- CT scan of the abdomen and pelvis/chest

—To aid in diagnosis of tumors of the adrenals, liver/lungs
- Mammography
—Can distinguish fat from mammary tissue and recognize cancer

SPECIAL STUDIES

- Needle biopsy/biopsy for suspicious masses of the breast
- Exclude systemic medical illnesses as a cause of gynecomastia.
- Review medications and adjust accordingly.
- Testicular lesions (palpable)
—Check serum B-hCG: If the level is low, confirm the lesion on ultrasonography and perform a radical orchiectomy.
—Check serum testosterone: If markedly elevated, confirm the lesion on ultrasonography and perform a radical orchiectomy.
- No testicular lesion palpable
—Check serum testosterone, estradiol, B-hCG, LH/FSH, and testicular sonography.
  —All normal: idiopathic gynecomastia
  —Low testosterone with elevated LH/FSH: primary hypogonadism, enzymatic defect, or testicular defect
  —Low testosterone with low LH/FSH: secondary hypogonadism, possible prolactin-secreting pituitary tumor if prolactin elevated
  —Elevated testosterone and elevated LH: androgen resistance, possible hyperthyroidism if T4 high and TSH low
  —Elevated B-hCG and normal testicular sonography requires CXR and/or abdominal and pelvis CT scan to rule out extragonadal germ cell tumors, bronchial carcinoma, pancreatic carcinoma, or gastric carcinoma
  —Elevated estradiol and a normal testicular sonogram requires an abdominal and pelvis CT scan to rule out adrenal tumors or hyperplasia
  —For elevated B-hCG and an abnormal testicular sonogram: testicular germ cell tumor (choriocarcinoma, embryonal, mixed)
  —For elevated estradiol and abnormal testicular sonogram: non–germ cell tumor (Leydig cell, Sertoli cell, mixed)

 ## Initial Management

- Testicular tumors: radical orchiectomy
—For Leydig cell tumors: gynecomastia likely to resolve; therefore, no mastoplasty/mastectomy until 1 year after orchiectomy performed
- Discontinuation of medication or treatment of underlying condition causing gynecomastia
—Often causes resolution of gynecomastia
—If gynecomastia is prolonged (usually greater than 12 months), periductal fibrosis and hyalinization occurs, and the gynecomastia is usually not reversible.
- Neoadjuvant irradiation of the breasts
—Can prevent the development of gynecomastia in 76% to 89% of patients treated with estrogen

- Tamoxifen citrate
—A synthetic drug that acts by blocking estrogen receptors in the breast
—Circulating estrogens are increased but can no longer exert their effect on the breast, leading to normalization of gynecomastia and resolution of pain.
—Reported to have 66% to 100% resolution of mastodynia in patients with idiopathic gynecomastia; however, breast size reduction was marginal
—The dosage of 10 mg/d controlled breast size and resolved breast tenderness in patients taking flutamide—finasteride combination therapy for prostate cancer.
—Side effects: mild nausea and abdominal discomfort; rarely, elevated liver function tests
- Liposuction
—Only effective in removing excess fat, not mammary tissue
- For nonresolving gynecomastia after initial treatment
—Subcutaneous mastectomy
  —Anatomic parameters for proper breast position in adult males are found to be sternal notch to nipple, 20 cm; midclavicular line to nipple, 18 cm; nipple to nipple, 21 cm; and areolar diameter, 28 mm.

 ## Follow-Up

- Depends on etiology
—If malignancy, routine cancer follow-up
—If endocrinopathy, biannual evaluation

Miscellaneous

SYNONYMS: N/A

ASSOCIATED CONDITIONS: N/A

NOTES: N/A

ABBREVIATIONS

- B-hCG, beta-human chorionic gonadotropin; AFP, alpha-fetoprotein

REFERENCES

Braunstein GD. Gynecomastia. *N Engl J Med* 1993;328:490–495.

Glass AR. Gynecomastia. *Endocrinol Metab Clin North Am* 1994;23:825–837.

Lemack GE, Poppas DP, Vaughan ED. Urologic causes of gynecomastia: Approach to diagnosis and management. *Urology* 1995;45:313–319.

Mahoney CP. Adolescent gynecomastia: Differential diagnosis and management. *Pediatr Clin North Am* 1990;37:1389–1404.

Authors: Victoria R. Staiman and Franklin C. Lowe

Hematospermia

 Basics

DESCRIPTION

- Defined as gross (visible) blood in the ejaculate
- Semen can be reported as "rust colored" or "darkened."
- May be a single episode or repeated, lasting up to several months
- Usually younger men, mean age 37

PATHOPHYSIOLOGY

- Normal ejaculate does not contain RBCs.
- Almost always resolves spontaneously, usually in a number of weeks
- Rarely associated with malignancy

RISK FACTORS

- Infection, inflammation, stone, trauma, bleeding dyscrasias, prior prostate biopsy, or malignancy (about 2%)

 Differential Diagnosis

- Prostate: polyps, vascular lesions (telangiectasia or varices), calculi, inflammatory disorders (prostatitis), malignancy
- Bladder and urethra: urethritis, condyloma, stricture, polyps, utricular cyst, malignancy (urethral)
- Seminal vesicals: congenital seminal vesicle cyst, associated with either ipsilateral renal agenesis or ipsilateral absence of the vas deferens, malignancy (primary carcinoma of the SV: associated with hematospermia in 6 of 39 cases reviewed), seminal vesiculitis, lymphoma or papillary tubular adenocarcinoma, SV calculi, SV amyloidosis
- Infections: tuberculosis, cytomegalovirus, schistosomiasis, hydatid disease (caused by the *Echinococcus* worm)
- Trauma: perineum, postprostatic biopsy or prostate surgery, self-instrumentation, local nerve block, testicular, posthemorrhoidal injection
- Systemic disorders: hypertension, chronic liver disease, lymphoma
- Bleeding disorders: hemophilia, Von Willebrand disease, others

 Database

HISTORY

- Recent trauma, surgery, or infection?

—Hematospermia common after TRUS prostate biopsy; microwave hyperthermia and laser prostate procedures as well

- Medical conditions?

—Hypertension, liver diseases, bleeding disorders

- Are there urinary symptoms?

—Obstructive or irritative voiding symptoms

- Hematuria or other evidence of bleeding?

PHYSICAL EXAMINATION

- Hypertension can be associated.
- Penis

—Urethral lesion, discharge, masses, condylomata

- Scrotum and vas deferens

—Evaluate for the presence or absence of the vas, testicular lesion or tenderness
—Induration of the vas deferens may indicate tuberculosis.

- Prostate

—Nodularity, tenderness, masses

- Seminal vesicles

—Palpate for stones or fullness; fullness associated with schistosomiasis correlates with egg burden.
—Note: A normal SV should not be palpable.

Hematospermia

 Diagnostic Studies

LABORATORY TESTING

- Urinalysis and culture

—Incidence of infection is low (from 6%–29%)
—Urine culture for acid-fast bacilli

- Urethral swab: Evaluate for nonspecific and gonococcal urethritis.
- Semen analysis: Confirm diagnosis with RBCs in the ejaculate; may see *Schistosoma haematobium* eggs

—Semen culture sometimes helps.

- PT/PTT, platelet count and function
- PSA: Evaluate for the possible presence of malignancy.
- Urinary cytology: possible transitional cell carcinoma of the prostate/bladder

IMAGING

- Transrectal ultrasound

—To evaluate the prostate, seminal vesicles, and possible Müllerian remnants
—Most common findings of dilated seminal vesicles (30%), ejaculatory duct cysts, or seminal vesicle stones
—Evaluate for the presence or absence of vas deferens, often associated with seminal vesicle cysts and ipsilateral renal agenesis.
—Recommend for all patients being evaluated for hematospermia.

- Magnetic resonance imaging

—Normal seminal vesicles are depicted on T-2–weighted images as a mixture of high and low signal granules or as a convolution of tubules with a diameter of less than 0.5 cm.
—Dilatation or cyst formation was seen in 13 of 15 patients evaluated.
—Abnormal signal intensity may represent subacute hemorrhage.
—Recommended study if the patient is unable to undergo a transrectal ultrasound or if further clarification of the ultrasound is desired.

SPECIAL STUDIES

- Cystourethroscopy

—Evaluate for the presence of polyps, tumors, or stones.
—Should evaluate the bladder for coexistent pathology as well

 Initial Management

- Infections: appropriate antibiotic treatment (empiric quinolone for suspected prostate/SV infection); other based on C&S or clinical setting
- Bleeding disorders: Treat the underlying systemic disorder.
- Urethral or prostatic varices: fulguration
- Palpable mass or abnormality: Assess with imaging and biopsy.
- Cystoscopic lesion: resection/biopsy if a tumor or polyp
- Stones: excision transurethrally; historically patients have undergone open bilateral seminal vesiculectomy
- Abnormal PSA: transrectal biopsy

 Follow-Up

- Reevaluate semen analysis.

 Miscellaneous

SYNONYMS

- Hemospermia, hematospermia, bloody ejaculate

ASSOCIATED CONDITIONS: N/A

NOTES: N/A

ABBREVIATIONS

- PSA, prostate-specific antigen

REFERENCES

Maeda H. Magnetic resonance images of hematospermia. *Urology* 1993;41:5.

Mulhall JP. Hemospermia: Diagnosis and management. *Urology* 1995;46:4.

Worischeck JH. Chronic hematospermia: Assessment by transrectal ultrasound. *Urology* 1994;43:4.

Authors: James A. Simon and Gerald L. Andriole

Hematuria—Adult

 Basics

DESCRIPTION

- Hematuria can either be gross (visible) or microscopic.
- Serious urologic disease is present in 5% to 20% of adults with microscopic hematuria.
- Gross hematuria has a high incidence of serious urologic disorders.
- Confirm a positive dipstick with microscopic examination.

PATHOPHYSIOLOGY

- Normal urine contains a small number of RBCs (normal less than 3 RBCs/HPF on an unspun urine).
- False-positive dipsticks for blood: oxidizing agents (hypochlorite, povidone, bacterial peroxidases), myoglobinuria
- False-negative dipsticks for blood: reducing agents (high-dose vitamin C), urine pH <5.1

RISK FACTORS

- Recent trauma, urinary tract surgery or instrumentation, some medications, family history of renal disease, calculi, pelvic radiation, recent febrile illness and others

 Differential Diagnosis

- In adults neoplasms, UTI, stones, and benign prostatic hypertrophy are major causes of hematuria. In children, glomerulonephritis and UTI are common causes (see Section I, "Hematuria—Pediatric").
- Pseudohematuria: Other causes of discolored urine are drugs (e.g., Pyridium); vegetables, dyes, or pigments; myoglobin and free hemoglobin (microscopic analysis should be negative); menstrual periods; and dysfunctional uterine bleeding.
- Congenital/inherited

—Cystic renal disease: polycystic kidney disease, medullary sponge kidney, medullary cystic disease, and solitary renal cysts
—Benign familial hematuria or thin basement membrane nephropathy (TMN): common benign condition (incidence 2.5%–9.2%) in general population, diagnosed on renal biopsy
—Alport syndrome: micro- and/or gross hematuria, proteinuria, progressive renal insufficiency, and high-frequency hearing loss. X-linked dominant with incomplete penetrance
—Inherited renal tubular disorders: Renal tubular acidosis type I, cystinuria, and oxalosis can cause stones.
—Hematologic abnormalities: bleeding dyscrasias and sickling disorders (4% and 12%, respectively); cases of hematuria; sickle hemoglobinopathies (Blacks and Mediterranean Caucasians)
—Anatomic: phimosis, posterior urethral valves, diverticula, UPJ obstruction, and vesicoureteric reflux
—Vascular malformations: hemangiomas and others (rare)

- Traumatic

—Trauma: Degree of hematuria is a poor indicator of the severity of the injury.
  —Abdominal trauma: renal or ureteral injury
  —Pelvic fracture: bladder or urethral injury
  —Iatrogenic trauma (fistula, etc.) after abdominal or pelvic surgery
—Exercise-induced hematuria ("athletic hematuria"): gross or microscopic, follows exercise, resolves with rest; no underlying abnormality
—Foreign bodies: Foley catheter, stents, etc.

- Inflammatory

—UTI: pyuria: bacteruria and voiding symptoms
—Specific infections: schistosomiasis, tuberculosis, toxoplasmosis, and malaria (most outside United States)
—Glomerulonephritis: mostly children/young adults; IgA nephropathy most common (4%)
—Radiation: radiation nephritis (renal dose >23 Gy); radiation cystitis (pelvic irradiation)

- Metabolic

—Urinary calculi: Up to 85% have hematuria. If there are calculi without hematuria, obstruction may prevent passage of urine. Even with a calculus, evaluate to rule out neoplasm.
—Hypercalciuria: hematuria due to microcalculi or nephrocalcinosis; most common cause in children without UTI or proteinuria

- Neoplastic

—Any GU benign or malignant lesion (prostate, bladder, renal, ureteral, urethral) can present with hematuria. Hematuria is often the only sign of GU cancer. Cancer is found in 20% to 40 % with gross hematuria and in 5.1% of microscopic hematuria.

- Miscellaneous
- —Drugs
    - —Nephrotoxic (aminoglycosides, cyclosporine, cytotoxic cancer drugs); cause tubular necrosis and altered membrane permeability
    - —Drug-induced interstitial nephritis (penicillin, sulfas, nonsteroidal antiinflammatory agents, analgesics, cephalosporins, furosemide)
    - —Analgesic abuse: analgesic nephropathy, and/or papillary necrosis
    - —Hemorrhagic cystitis: cyclophosphamide, mitotane, methicillin
    - —Indirect hematuria: either urolithiasis (triamterene and carbonic anhydrase inhibitors) or induction of urothelial malignancy (cyclophosphamide, phenacetin)
    - —Anticoagulation: at recommended levels, does not cause hematuria unless pathology present. If gross hematuria, underlying disease is likely; incidence of microscopic hematuria in anticoagulated is similar to that of the general population. Most anticoagulated patients with microscopic hematuria are found to have GU disease.
- —Nutcracker syndrome: compression of the left renal vein between aorta and superior mesenteric artery, with venous stasis, parenchymal congestion
- —Loin pain hematuria syndrome: young woman on oral contraceptives; rarely, in men. Characterized by renal colic, low-grade fever, with isolated dysmorphic hematuria, occasionally gross hematuria
- —Benign prostatic hypertrophy (BPH): exclude other pathology; common cause in males over 65 years
- —Renal vessel disease: C3 arteriolar deposition, arterial emboli or thrombosis, or renal vein thrombosis
- —Obstructive uropathy: hydronephrosis from any cause
- —Idiopathic urethrorrhagia: prepubertal boys with dysuria and blood spotting on their underwear; microscopic hematuria in 57%
- —Endometriosis of the urinary tract: rare; suspect in a female with cyclic hematuria
- —Postoperative: Microhematuria can persist for several months after urinary tract surgery.
- —Benign essential hematuria: an older term for an identifiable cause of hematuria (most probably have thin membrane nephropathy)

 Database

HISTORY

- Age and sex of the patient?

—Cancer most commonly seen in men >50 years of age; in children, GN is most common cause. GU cancer is greater in males than in females; females may have vaginal bleeding.

- History of trauma?

—A large crush injury or burn may result in myoglobinuria; abdominal or pelvic trama may cause urinary tract injury.

- Timing of blood during urinary stream?

—Initial hematuria: prostatic or urethral pathology
—Terminal hematuria: vesical calculus
—Hematuria throughout the stream: vesical or upper tract origin

- Any associated pain?

—Painless gross hematuria is the hallmark of bladder cancer. Flank pain with gross hematuria and an abdominal mass is pathognomonic of renal cell carcinoma. Ureteral colic is usually caused by calculi, but can also be due to a tumor or blood clot.

- Symptoms of urinary tract infection or prostatitis?

—Infection can cause hematuria.

- Lower urinary tract symptoms present (frequency, urgency, nocturia, etc.)?

—BPH may cause hematuria. Incomplete bladder emptying predisposes to infection and/or stones.

- Hematuria associated with any activity?

—Exercise-induced or trauma should be sought.

- History of recent upper respiratory tract infections?

—Associated with GN or IgA nephropathy

- Significant medical or surgical history?

—A history of renal or urologic disease or surgery must be sought. Sexually transmitted diseases or urethral instrumentation (including catheterization) can cause stricture; a history of tuberculosis; pelvic irradiation; and bleeding diatheses.

- Current medications?

—Drugs, as noted, can cause hematuria.

- History of tobacco use?

—Associated with TCC

- Menstrual history?

—Vaginal bleeding (normal or dysfunctional) can be mistaken for hematuria.

- Family history?

—Conditions such as benign familial hematuria, Alport syndrome, sickle cell disease or trait, polycystic kidney disease, coagulation abnormalities, familial hypertension, nephrolithiasis, cancer (prostate, renal), or chronic renal failure may be relevant.

- Occupational risk factors?

—Exposure to naphthylamine, benzidine, and 4-aminobiphenyl, often in rubber, dye petroleum, industries, predisposes to TCC.

PHYSICAL EXAMINATION

- Hypertension

—Renal parenchymal disease, renal failure, renal cystic disease, or renal vascular disease

- Pallor

—Anemia is associated with several abnormalities: hemolytic anemia, SLE, and renal failure.

- Rashes

—Henoch-Shönlein purpura and SLE

- Generalized edema

—Nephrotic syndrome or renal failure

- Hearing loss

—Alport syndrome

- Heart murmurs

—Subacute bacterial endocarditis

- Palpable abdominal or flank masses

—Hydronephrosis, renal cystic disease, renal tumors, renal vein thrombosis, and distended bladder

- Flank tenderness

—Pyelonephritis or urolithiasis

- Flank lacerations, contusions, or rib fractures

—Underlying renal injury

- Urethral prolapse, meatitis, or meatal stenosis

—May cause hematuria in children

- Digital rectal examination

—Boggy, tender, warm prostate with acute prostatitis; nodularity suggests cancer; floating prostate suggests urethral disruption in the presence of pelvic fracture

- Pelvic examination findings

—Urethral caruncle or vaginal prolapse, vaginal bleeding

(continued)

Diagnostic Studies

LABORATORY TESTING

• Urine analysis: must include the standard urine dipstick and microscopic evaluation

—Color: bright red with urologic/anatomic causes; brown or tea-colored urine suggests GN or old clots
—Specific gravity: Poorly concentrated urine (low specific gravity) suggests hydronephrosis with renal impairment or intrinsic renal disease.
—Proteinuria: if heavy (3–4+), suggests GN
—Leukocyte esterase or nitrite positive; pyuria: suggests infection
—Red cell casts: pathognomonic of a glomerular source of bleeding
—Crystalluria: suggests urolithiasis

• Urine culture: if UA suggestive of infection
• Urinary cytology

—Detects high-grade TCC; less effective with well-differentiated TCC (renal or prostate cancer are not diagnosed by cytology). "Atypical cells" can be seen with calculi or inflammation. (Note: Newer rapid urine tests [BTA-Stat, NMP-23] are undergoing study in TCC.)

• Renal function tests (creatinine and blood urea nitrogen)

—Renal impairment associated with underlying pathology

• Complete blood count

—Anemia is rarely caused directly by microhematuria, more likely with gross hematuria. Chronic renal disease may result in anemia. Elevated white counts with a left shift suggest infection.

• Other laboratory tests

—Streptozyme (antistreptolysin-O titer), serum complement and ANA, total serum proteins, and albumin : globulin ratios in the diagnosis of GN

—Urinary calcium : creatinine ratio: A ratio of > 0.18 is significant and suggests hypercalciuria.
—Peripheral smear: Sickle cell disease or trait is suspected.
—Coagulation profile/bleeding studies: coagulopathy
—TB skin test and urinary mycobacterial cultures: Rule out tuberculosis.

IMAGING

• Excretory urography (ExU; intravenous pyelogram)

—May detect renal masses; collecting system filling defects may signify tumors or stones. Rough estimation of kidney function and bladder emptying (contraindicated if creatine is >2 mg/dL)

• Abdominal ultrasonography

—More sensitive for renal masses than ExU. Poor in diagnosing filling defects in upper tract unless due to stones. Useful in children and when contrast is contraindicated.

• Abdominal CT or MRI: usually if US or ExU suggests mass. Spiral CT in rapid evaluation of suspected urolithiasis.
• Nuclear renal scans, arteriography, retrograde urethrogram, cystogram as clinically indicated

SPECIAL STUDIES

• Cystoscopy: identifies lower urinary pathology (i.e., neoplasms, stricture)

—Bleeding site often visualized (i.e., bladder tumor, etc); not recommended in children
—Retrograde pyelograms used in cases of contrast allergy
—Ureteroscopy as needed to evaluate upper tracts

• Renal biopsy: US guided; used in suspected GN
• Phase contrast microscopy of urinary sediment: differentiates glomerular and nonglomerular bleeding based on the presence of distorted RBCs in glomerular bleeding; sensitivity of 95% and specificity 100%
• Urinary RBC acanthocytosis: ring-formed cells with one or more protrusions. If >5% of total RBC, glomerular disease likely

Initial Management

- The "standard" urologic evaluation of hematuria (gross and microscopic) has been ExU, cystoscopy, and cytology. Currently, work-up is undergoing refinement to determine the most cost-effective approach.
- Additional testing based on clinical findings (i.e., urine culture with pyuria)
- Always consider "medical" causes of hematuria (e.g., GN, IgAN) based on presentation, lab data, or if evaluation for anatomic lesion is negative.
- Gross hematuria

—Usually requires urgent evaluation to prevent/treat clot retention
—Patients with clots and retention
   —Place three-way Foley catheter (24Fr–26Fr) and continuous bladder irrigation.
   —Irrigate clots from the bladder; a large-bore, two-way Foley catheter is sometimes more effective than a three-way to clear clots (larger lumen). For difficult clots, a cystoscope sheath may help.
—Renal biopsy may be urgently needed in gross hematuria and renal failure; crescentic nephritis may necessitate immediate immunosuppressive therapy.

- Microscopic hematuria

—Work-up is usually elective unless associated with traumatic injury.
—In trauma, the degree of hematuria may have no relation to the degree of injury.

 ## Follow-Up

- After evaluation, the cause of hematuria is undiagnosed in up to 35% of patients. Opinion is divided on follow-up.
- 19% with pathology may have at least one negative UA within 6 months of diagnosis. Neoplasms are found in 9% with initial negative work-up and persistent microhematuria.
- Frequency of repeat standard urologic evaluation is unclear. Some recommend periodic UA and cytology. One study suggests that only the symptomatic patient should be reinvestigated.

 ## Miscellaneous

SYNONYMS: N/A

ASSOCIATED CONDITIONS: N/A

NOTES

- See also Section I, "Hematuria—Pediatric."

ABBREVIATIONS

- ExU, excretory urography; GN, glomerulonephritis; IgAN, immunoglobulin A nephropathy

REFERENCES

Bagley DH. Hematuria in the adult. In: Coe FL, et al., eds. *Kidney Stones: Medical and Surgical Management.* Philadelphia: Lippincott-Raven, 1996.

Clarkson AR. Microscopic hematuria: Whom to investigate. *Aust N Z J Med* 1996;26:7.

Sultana SR, et al. Microscopic hematuria using a standard protocol. *Br J Urol* 1996;78:691.

Authors: Mohammed Ismail and Leonard G. Gomella

Hematuria—Pediatric

 ## Basics

DESCRIPTION

- Hematuria can be gross (visible) or microscopic.
—Normal excretion of red blood cells: <50,000 RBCs/h in a 24-hour urine
—Microscopic hematuria: >5 RBCs/HPF. Occurs in 0.5% to 5% of urine specimens
—Prevalence: 1% to 2% for two or more positive samples in children 6 to 15 years of age
—Gross hematuria uncommon (1 in 1000 pediatric visits)
—Acute bacterial urinary tract infection: most common cause of gross hematuria in the pediatric age group; especially in boys
—Rare to find significant pathologic conditions in children for whom microscopic hematuria is the only significant finding on history and physical examination
—The cause of microscopic hematuria is usually a medical, not a surgical, problem.
- Most causes are benign and self-limiting in duration.
—Serious disorders such as progressive renal disease or cancer must be ruled out.

PATHOPHYSIOLOGY

- The color of the urine depends on the source of blood, urine pH, and briskness of bleeding.
- Substances can mimic hematuria and positive dipsticks but reveal no red blood cells on microscopic urinalysis: hemoglobin, myoglobin, antibiotics, infected urine with high levels of bacterial peroxidase, food coloring, laxatives, salicylates.

—In newborns, normal physiologic clearance of urate leads to urate crystals precipitating in the urine, which can lead to a pink/red discoloration of the urine.

RISK FACTORS

- Urinary tract infection, calculi, glomerular bleeding, glomerulonephritis, recent upper respiratory illness, sickle cell anemia or trait, hemophilia, renal papillary necrosis, Alport syndrome, benign familial hematuria, cystinuria, anaphylactoid purpura, systemic lupus erythematous, Henoch-Schönlein purpura

 ## Differential Diagnosis

- Divided into categories, depending on the source of bleeding: renal parenchyma, renal vessel diseases, urinary tract diseases, and systemic coagulation disorders
- Postinfectious glomerulonephritis (GN): edema, hypertension, and oliguria. Usually follows a group A beta-hemolytic streptococcal sore throat or pyoderma. Positive ASO titers and decreased serum complement (C3) are usually present.
- Renal vessel diseases: C3 arteriolar deposition, renal vein thrombosis (approximately 20% of gross hematuria occurring in the first months of life), AV malformations, AV fistulas, nutcracker syndrome, renal artery emboli/thrombosis
- Renal parenchymal

—Neoplasm
—IgA nephropathy or Berger disease (recurrent, gross, painless hematuria, often following a mild fever, viral respiratory infection, or exercise)
—Membranoproliferative glomerulonephritis, lupus nephritis
—Hemolytic uremic syndrome (hemolytic anemia, renal failure, and thrombocytopenia)
—Henoch-Schönlein purpura (rash on the dependent parts of the body that is heralded by a prodrome of malaise, arthralgia, and/or abdominal pain)
—Goodpasture syndrome (pulmonary hemorrhage associated with severe and progressive GN)
—Familial benign hematuria (hematuria in patient and first-degree relatives without hearing loss or renal insufficiency)
—Nail-patella syndrome (dystropic fingernails and toenails, absence of one or both patellae, iliac crest horns, and renal disease)
—Alport syndrome (microhematuria, proteinuria, progressive renal insufficiency, high-frequency hearing loss)
—Renal vasculitis, interstitial nephritis, analgesics, pyelonephritis, sickle cell nephropathy, polycystic kidneys, trauma/surgery/biopsy, exercise

- Urinary tract diseases: idiopathic hypercalciuria, Munchausen syndrome, neoplasia, obstructive uropathy, cysts, papillary necrosis, infections (e.g., tuberculosis), infestations (e.g., schistosomiasis), radiation nephritis, hepatitis, HIV, drug induced cystitis, sickle cell disease, urethral prolapse, caruncle, meatal stenosis, ureterocele, urethritis, menstruation, catheters, foreign bodies, exercise
- Systemic coagulation disorders: platelet defects, coagulation protein deficiency, scurvy, anticoagulant therapy

 ## Database

HISTORY

- Age and timing of onset
—Poststreptococcal GN occurs 7 to 14 days after the onset of the sore throat.
—IgA nephropathy hematuria develops at the time of or shortly after the respiratory infection.
—Hematuria secondary to Henoch-Schönlein purpura develops 1 to 3 months after the rash.
- Determine the duration of hematuria and whether episodes of gross hematuria are followed by periods of microscopic hematuria or resolve completely.
- Characterize the pattern of hematuria: gross (suggests a urologic cause) or microscopic (suggests a nephrologic cause), initial or terminal.
—Indicates a lower tract source versus total hematuria, which is typical of upper tract bleeding
- Blood clots or blood that is not persistent throughout voiding is suggestive of nonglomerular bleeding.
- Any precipitating events? Onset of hematuria after an upper respiratory illness, skin infection, or viral illness directs the evaluation toward postinfectious GN.
- Any urinary symptoms associated with the hematuria, such as frequency, urgency, dysuria, flank pain, orabdominal pain, are suggestive of nonglomerular hematuria.
- Oliguria, symptomatic hypertension, and symptoms of systemic disease (e.g., arthritis, arthralgias, rash, or respiratory problems) are more suggestive of glomerular disease.
- Obstructive symptoms suggest posterior urethral valves, urethral strictures, or polyps.
- Trauma, strenuous exercise, foreign bodies, and sexual or physical abuse
- Family history of specific renal diseases, stones, end-stage renal disease, neurosensory hearing loss, and urinary tract infections may focus laboratory and radiologic evaluation.
- Any other bleeding suggestive of coagulation disorder
- Current medications

PHYSICAL EXAMINATION

- What is the blood pressure?

—Make sure to use an age-appropriate blood pressure cuff.
—High BP is highly suggestive of glomerular disease, as is presence of edema.

- Look for evidence of SLE, Wegener granulomatosis, Goodpasture syndrome, etc.
- Hearing loss suggests Alport's disease.
- Presence of palpable abdominal or flank mass, bruit, or tenderness
- Eyes should be examined for evidence of acute or long-standing hypertension.
- Rashes and arthritis can occur in Henoch-Schönlein purpura and SLE.
- Examine the genitalia for meatal stenosis, urethral prolapse, ureterocele, trauma, or sexual abuse.

 ## Diagnostic Studies

LABORATORY TESTING

- Persistent hematuria is defined as three positive urinalyses, based on a test strip and microscopic examination, over a 2- to 3-week period.

—False-negative results occur in samples with high specific gravity or with high ascorbic acid concentrations.
—False-positive results occur in the presence of myoglobin, free hemoglobin, and oxidizing agent's (i.e., household bleach).

- Urinalysis

—Is the patient able to acidify and concentrate urine?
—Is proteinuria present?
—Does the microscopic analysis show casts, crystals, or WBCs?
—Are the RBCs eumorphic or dysmorphic? Dysmorphic red cells predict glomerular bleeding with a sensitivity of 93% to 95% and a specificity of 95% to 100%.

- Concomitant proteinuria, cellular casts, and brown, tea-, or cola-colored urine suggest glomerular causes of bleeding.
- Urine culture

—If infected, repeat the urinalysis after treating the infection.

- Other laboratory tests: serum creatinine, blood urea nitrogen, CBC with differential, C3/C4 levels (may be lowered in case of SLE, mesangiocapillary GN, or acute GN), CH50, ANA, plasma IgA levels (may be increased with IgA nephritis or Henoch-Schönlein purpura), antistreptolysin-O titer, calcium:creatinine ratio (requires urine specimen)
- Urine calcium:creatinine ratio should be less than 0.18. If more than 0.18, usually indicates that the 24-hour excretion of calcium is more than 4 mg/kg/d.

IMAGING

- Renal and bladder sonography

—Evaluating for renal parenchymal disease, stones, tumors, or anatomic abnormalities

- Voiding cystourethrogram

—Evaluate for vesicoureteral reflux, posterior urethral valves, other anomalies.

SPECIAL STUDIES

- Renal biopsy: Open or closed, heavy proteinuria, or worsening renal function are the main indications for biopsy. It should only be done if the results will alter therapy.
- Cystoscopy: rarely indicated
- Hearing tests

 ## Initial Management

- Based on clinical diagnosis

 ## Follow-Up

- The current recommendation of the American Academy of Pediatrics is to perform a screening urinalysis at school entry (ages 4 or 5 years) and once during adolescence. More important are recommendations for annual measurements of height and weight and annual blood pressure measurement after age 3 years.

 ## Miscellaneous

SYNONYMS: N/A

ASSOCIATED CONDITIONS: N/A

NOTES

- See also Section I, "Hematuria—Adult."

ABBREVIATIONS

- GN, glomerulonephritis; SLE, systemic lupus erythematous

REFERENCES

Cilento BG, et al. Hematuria in children: A practical approach. *Urol Clin North Am* 1995;22:43.

Feld LG, et al. Hematuria: An integrated medical and surgical approach. *Pediatr Clin North Am* 1997;44:1191.

Fogazzi GB, et al. Microscopic hematuria diagnosis and management. *Nephron* 1996;72:125.

Yadin O. Hematuria in children. *Pediatr Ann* 1994;23:474.

Author: Mark Horowitz

Hesitancy and Intermittency

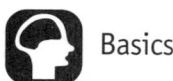 Basics

DESCRIPTION

• Urinary hesitancy and intermittency are commonly encountered symptoms in a urologic evaluation.

—*Hesitancy* is defined as the delay in initiating micturition.
—*Intermittency* is defined as the stopping and starting of the urinary stream during voiding.
—Commonly seen as part of the symptom complex referred to as obstructive voiding pattern
—Population at risk are elderly men with enlarged prostates; 40% to 60% of men may have obstructive symptoms by the age of 70.
—Less commonly seen in women

PATHOPHYSIOLOGY

• Bladder outlet obstruction: Increased resistance requires more time to generate adequate detrusor pressures.
• May also be seen with inability to initiate or maintain adequate detrusor contraction (detrusor hypocontractility)

RISK FACTORS

• Bladder outlet obstruction

—Usually secondary to mechanical obstruction from BPH, prostate cancer, bladder neck contracture, bladder stones, urethral valves, urethral strictures, or large cystocele

• Detrusor hypocontractility

—Multiple causes: can be idiopathic, neurogenic in origin (i.e., secondary to diabetes, Parkinson's) or nonneurogenic (dysfunctional voider)

 Differential Diagnosis

• In adult males, mechanical obstruction is the major cause of hesitancy and intermittency. In females, neurogenic obstruction or previous pelvic surgery are more common causes.
• Benign prostate hyperplasia

—Most common cause in men
—Degree of symptoms may not correlate with severity of bladder outlet obstruction.

• Bladder neck contracture

—Seen in patients who have undergone previous urologic surgery (either TURP or radical prostatectomy)

• Bladder stone/foreign body
• Prostate cancer

—Locally advanced prostate cancer can present with obstructive symptoms.

• Urethral stricture

—Formation of scar that reduces caliber of urethra; may be termed *urethral stenosis* in females

• Urethral cancer
• Meatal stenosis
• Neurogenic obstruction

—Bladder neck dyssynergia: failure of the bladder neck to relax appropriately
—Detrusor–sphincter dyssynergia: seen in patients with multiple sclerosis or spinal cord lesions

• Previous pelvic surgery

—Can result in injury to pelvic nerves with secondary detrusor hypocontractility
—Antiincontinence surgery in women can cause voiding dysfunction secondary to iatrogenic obstruction.

 Database

HISTORY

• Age and sex of patient

—BPH and prostate cancer are common causes in older men. In younger men, urethral stricture is more likely. Women rarely have anatomic bladder outlet obstruction.

• Associated lower urinary tract symptoms

—Other obstructive symptoms (poor urinary stream, incomplete emptying often present)
—Symptoms of bladder irritability (i.e., frequency, urgency) may alter differential diagnosis and work-up.

• Symptoms of UTI or prostatitis

—Prostatitis can present with acute, severe obstructive symptoms.

• History of hematuria

—Seen in patients with BPH, prostate cancer, and bladder neck pathology
—Mandates full evaluation of urinary tract, including cystoscopy and upper tract imaging

• History of urologic surgery

—Can predispose to bladder neck contracture and urethral strictures

• Significant medical and surgical history

—Prior pelvic surgery can result in detrusor hypocontractility.
—History of sexually transmitted disease: Gonorrhea is a leading cause of urethral strictures.
—Prior pelvic irradiation can affect bladder contractility.
—A history of neurologic disease (spinal cord injury, multiple sclerosis, Parkinson disease) can cause neurogenic functional bladder obstruction.
—History of pelvic carcinoma: may cause secondary symptomatology

• Family history

—Important in assessing risk of prostate cancer, colon/rectal cancer

• Medication

—Over-the-counter medications for colds frequently contain alpha-sympathomimetics (e.g., Ornade, phenylephrine) or anticholinergics and may exacerbate voiding symptoms.

PHYSICAL EXAMINATION

• Should be systematic and meticulous
• Abdominal examination

—Palpable kidney if hydronephrosis is present.
—Percussion and palpation are important in assessing bladder size and elevated residual urine.

• Urethral meatal stenosis

—Can cause obstruction in boys

- Digital rectal examination

—Enlargement is graded from normal to 4+; a normal gland is approximately 20 g in size.
—Nodularity and induration suggest prostate cancer.
—Boggy, tender prostate seen in acute prostatitis

- Pelvic examination

—A large cystocele may be a cause of obstruction in women.
—Urethral abnormality may indicate carcinoma, infection, or diverticulum.

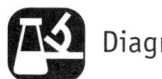 ## Diagnostic Studies

LABORATORY TESTING

- Several additional tests may aid in formulating a final clinical impression and treatment plan.
- Urine analysis

—Standard urine dipstick for glucose, protein, pH level, and blood
—Microscopic analysis for RBCs
—Positive leukocyte esterase, nitrites, and pyuria are suggestive of infection.

- Urine culture

—If UA is suggestive of infection

- Renal function tests (serum creatinine and BUN)

—Rule out renal impairment.

- Serum PSA

—Evaluate for prostate cancer.

Imaging

- Evaluation of upper tracts by IVP/ultrasound are not routinely performed unless warranted by history, examination, or laboratory evaluation.
- If impaired renal function is present, ultrasound of the kidneys is indicated to rule out obstruction.
- If urethral stricture disease is suspected, retrograde urethrography should be performed.
- Transrectal ultrasound and biopsy are performed only if clinical suspicion of prostate cancer is high.
- CT and MRI are rarely indicated.

SPECIAL STUDIES

- Catheterized or scanned post-void residual: may indicate outlet obstruction or voiding dysfunction
- Cystoscopy if post-void residual is high
- Urodynamic evaluation indicated only in select patients

 ## Initial Management

- Patients with mild symptoms can be managed by watchful waiting.
- Patients with bothersome symptoms secondary to BPH may benefit from medical therapy.

—Finasteride (5 mg/d), a 5-alpha reductase inhibitor, results in a decrease of prostatic volume, which may improve symptoms by reducing the level of outlet obstruction. Be aware that finasteride might drop PSA levels by 50%.
—Adrenergic antagonists (Hytrin, Cardura, Flomax) can reduce resistance from bladder outlet and provide symptomatic relief. Be aware that blood pressure may be iatrogenically lowered. In addition, patients may have nasal congestion or retrograde ejaculation with side effects.

- Surgical therapy is indicated in patients with BPH who fail medical therapy or develop complications (i.e., stones, recurrent UTIs, hydroureteronephrosis).

—TURP is a commonly performed operation and remains the gold standard of surgical therapy for outlet obstruction.

- Minimally invasive therapies such as microwave therapy, laser therapy, balloon dilation, and urethral stents are alternatives to the standard TURP.

 ## Follow-Up

- Outcome of bladder outlet obstruction depends on the cause, site, and degree of specific etiology.
- Patients on watchful waiting or medical management for BPH may remain stable over a number of years.
- Development of complications, including worsening symptoms, warrants surgical intervention.
- It is difficult to predict which patients may progress and develop complications.
- Physical examination, UA, and PVR assessment are cornerstones of evaluation.
- Prevention: N/A

 ## Miscellaneous

SYNONYMS: N/A

ASSOCIATED CONDITIONS: N/A

NOTES: N/A

ABBREVIATIONS

- BPH, benign prostatic hypertrophy; TURP, transurethral resection of prostate

REFERENCES

Gillenwater JY, Grayhack JT, Howards SS, Duckett JW, eds. *Adult and Pediatric Urology,* 3rd ed. St Louis: Mosby, 1996.

Resnick, Older, eds. *Diagnosis of Genitourinary Disease,* 2nd ed. New York: Thieme Medical Publishers, 1997.

Authors: Sankar J. Kausik and Steven P. Petrou

Hydrocolpos and Hydrometrocolpos

 Basics

DESCRIPTION

- Congenital anomalies of the female reproductive tract
- Hydrocolpos (HC) is gross distension of the vagina due to an imperforated hymen.
- Hydrometrocolpos (HMC) is gross distension of the vagina and uterus.

PATHOPHYSIOLOGY

- Congenital: HC or HMC occurs due to incomplete canalization of the vagina by the twentieth week of gestation.
- Results in accumulation of excess mucus secretions proximal to the site of obstruction

RISK FACTORS

- Imperforated hymen: Accumulated secretions avert membrane.
- High transverse vaginal septum
- Partial agenesis of the anterior of the vagina

 Differential Diagnosis

- Hematometrocolpos: accumulation of menstrual blood due to obstruction at menarche
- Interlabial masses

—Prolapsed urethra: donut-shaped urethral meatus in center of normal vaginal introitus
—Periurethral cyst: eccentric smooth mass displacing urethral meatus

- Ovarian cysts
- Dermoid cysts
- Anterior meningocele
- Bladder outlet obstruction secondary to ureterocele
- Rhabdomyosarcoma: cluster of grapelike masses protruding from vaginal introitus

 Database

HISTORY

- Newborn may have history of a sonolucent mass on prenatal ultrasound.
- Newborn may present with difficulty voiding due to bladder outlet obstruction.
- Amenorrhea is seen in pubertal females.

PHYSICAL EXAMINATION

- Lower abdominal midline
- Bulging cystic vaginal introital mass due to imperforate hymen
- Palpable suprapubic mass due to distended bladder when bladder outlet obstruction is associated with this problem
- Lower extremity lymphedema due to decreased venous return

Diagnostic Studies

LABORATORY TESTING

• Not usually helpful

IMAGING

• Abdominal ultrasound shows large sonolucent midline mass displacing bladder anteriorly and rectum posteriorly.

—Layering of debris can sometimes be seen.

• IVP may show hydroureteronephrosis and a distended bladder.
• VCUG may demonstrate an anteriorly displaced bladder.
• CT and MRI

SPECIAL STUDIES: N/A

 ## Initial Management

• Surgical: depends on level of anatomic obstruction

—Imperforated hymen: simple incision

 ## Follow-Up

• Abdominal ultrasound to test decompression of the urinary tract and HC/HMC

 ## Miscellaneous

SYNONYMS: N/A

ASSOCIATED CONDITIONS: N/A

NOTES: N/A

ABBREVIATIONS

• HC, hydrocolpos; HMC, hydrometrocolpos

REFERENCES

Brown MR. Common office problems in pediatric urology and gynecology. *Pediatr Clin North Am* 1997;44(5):1091–1115.

Zaontz MR. Abnormalities of the external genitalia. *Pediatr Clin North Am* 1997;44(5):1267–1297.

Author: Ellen Shapiro

Hydronephrosis—Adult

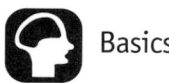 Basics

DESCRIPTION

- Hydronephrosis is usually caused by obstructive uropathy or vesicoureteral reflux.
- Obstruction of ureters, bladder, or urethra may be involved.
- Progressive renal damage occurs.
- Symptoms vary from acute flank pain to chronic vague flank discomfort or fullness.
- Urinary infection and sepsis may be superimposed.

PATHOPHYSIOLOGY

- Elevated ureteral pressure and decreased renal blood flow
- Impairment of most renal functions
- Gradual destruction of renal parenchyma
- Oliguria or anuria may occur with acute obstruction.

RISK FACTORS

- Congenital anomalies, calculi, urothelial cancer, retroperitoneal process, BPH, prostate cancer, neurogenic bladder

 Differential Diagnosis

- In adults, calculi, urinary neoplasms, extrinsic retroperitoneal process, BPH, prostate cancer, and voiding dysfunction are major causes. In children, vesicoureteral reflux, congenital ureteropelvic obstruction, neurogenic bladder, and posterior urethral valves are common causes.
- Congenital/inherited

—Most common cause of a neonatal abdominal mass
—Ureteropelvic junction obstruction (most common site of obstruction in neonate, often detected on fetal ultrasonography)
—Renal cystic dysplasia (most common is multicystic dysplastic kidney)
—Duplication anomalies of the upper urinary tract (usually associated with ureterocele or reflux)
—Prune-belly syndrome (renal and collecting system abnormalities, undescended testis, and deficient abdominal wall musculature)
—Autosomal recessive polycystic kidney disease
—Neurogenic bladder (often with myelodysplasia with or without vesicoureteral reflux)
—Vesicoureteral reflux
—Posterior urethral valves (thick-walled bladder, incomplete bladder emptying, dilated posterior urethra)
—Ureterovesical junction obstruction (congenital megaureter)
—Sepsis (can produce hydronephrosis in neonate, complete reversal with antibiotic treatment)
—Retrocaval ureter

- Adult/intrinsic
—Urinary calculi (usually present with flank pain and hematuria)
—Malignant tumors of the uroepithelium (transitional cell carcinoma in the majority)
—Renal cell carcinoma with invasion of the urinary collecting system
—Fibroepithelial polyp of the ureter
—Trauma (injuries to the renal pelvis and ureter)
—Neurogenic bladder (from any cause, with or without reflux)
—Benign prostatic hyperplasia (bladder outlet obstruction)
—Carcinoma of prostate (may produce bladder outlet obstruction or obstruct ureters by direct extension)
—Urethral stricture

- Adult/extrinsic

—Vascular lesions (abdominal aortic aneurysm, iliac artery aneurysm, aberrant arterial anomalies), obstruction of the ureter after arterial repair or replacement, venous obstruction (ovarian vein syndrome, postpartum ovarian vein thrombophlebitis)
—Benign pelvic masses (pregnancy, extrauterine pregnancy, mass lesions of the uterus and ovary, ovarian remnants, Gartner's duct cyst)
—Pelvic conditions (tubo-ovarian abscess, endometriosis, periureteral inflammation associated with contraceptives, uterine prolapse)
—Trauma (ureteral ligation and intraoperative ureteral injury)
—Gastrointestinal diseases (granulomatous ileitis, granulomatous colitis, appendicitis, diverticulitis, carcinoma of the pancreas, pancreatic pseudocyst, acute pancreatitis)
—Retroperitoneal processes (retroperitoneal fibrosis, radiation fibrosis, chronic urinary tract infection and urinary extravasation, tuberculosis, lymphangitis, extravasation of medical materials such barium, retroperitoneal hemorrhage/abscess/inflammation)
—Retroperitoneal masses (primary retroperitoneal tumors; metastases to the retroperitoneum, usually from prostate, bladder, or cervix; lymphocele; pelvic lipomatosis)

 Database

HISTORY

- Age and sex of the patient?

—Diagnosis by prenatal ultrasonography, association with posterior urethral valves in male neonates
—Calculi most common in middle aged men

- Blood in urine?

—Usually noted with urinary tract malignancies and may be painless; may be associated with flank pain when caused by calculi or blood clots in ureter

- Any associated pain?

—Acute ureteral obstruction produces severe flank pain, but chronic obstruction may be asymptomatic.

- History of voiding difficulty?

—Benign prostatic hyperplasia, prostate cancer, and urethral strictures in older men; neurogenic bladders in children with myelodysplasia and in adults with diabetes or neurologic disorders

- Symptoms of urinary tract voiding obstruction?

—BPH, prostate cancer, and urethral strictures in men

- History of gastrointestinal disorders?

—History of regional enteritis, granulomatous colitis, intestinal malignancy, pancreatic tumors, or pancreatic pseudocysts

- Significant medical or surgical history?

—Pelvic surgical history with potential ureteral injury

- Gynecologic history?

—Association with endometriosis, benign and malignant pelvic masses, uterine prolapse

- Family history?

—History of urinary calculus disease, BPH, prostate cancer

- Occupational risk factors?

—Association of smoking with urothelial malignancies

PHYSICAL EXAMINATION

- Hypertension

—Frequent association of hydronephrosis with hypertension

- Pallor

—Anemia associated with chronic renal failure from hydronephrosis

- Abdominal or flank mass

—Hydronephrosis is the most common abdominal mass in neonates. Hydronephrosis associated with ureteropelvic junction obstruction may produce a palpable flank mass.

- Flank tenderness

—Calculi, pyelonephritis, pyonephrosis, retroperitoneal abscess, tubo-ovarian abscess

- Pelvic mass

—Benign and malignant gynecologic masses

- Vaginal examination

—Uterine prolapse, urethral prolapse, prolapse of ureterocele through urethra

- Digital rectal examination

—Enlarged prostate associated with BPH, nodule of prostate suggestive of prostate cancer

Diagnostic Studies

LABORATORY TESTING

- Urine analysis

—Evidence for urinary tract infection or hematuria

- Urine culture: if UA suggestive of infection
- Renal function tests (BUN and creatinine)

—Assessment of severity of obstruction

- CBC

—Assessment of overall status of patient. Anemia is associated with chronic renal insufficiency, and elevated white blood cell count with infection.

- Other laboratory tests

—Serum chemistries (especially hyperkalemia)
—Serum PSA

- Urinary cytology

—May detect high-grade transitional cell carcinoma

IMAGING

- Intravenous urography

—If serum creatinine is not significantly elevated (should be <2 ng/dL), used for identification of obstructive uropathy and in determining location of obstruction

- Ultrasonography

—Useful first study, noninvasive
—Differentiates ureteropelvic junction obstruction from multicystic dysplastic kidney in neonates and children
—Hydroureters may be detected.
—Find extrinsic retroperitoneal and pelvic mass, abscess.
—Aid placement of nephrostomy tube when indicated.

- Computed tomography (CT) (adults)

—Often delineates point of obstruction
—Assess extrinsic retroperitoneal and abdominal disorders.
—CT-guided percutaneous procedures and biopsies when indicated

- Magnetic resonance imaging (MRI) (adults)

—May provide additional information to CT when a vascular anomaly is involved

- Radionuclide imaging (diuretic renogram)

—Useful in determining renal function and recovery after relief of obstruction; assessment of significance of UPJ obstruction

- Angiography

—When vascular lesion requires further evaluation

- Barium enema/upper GI series

—When gastrointestinal disease is suspected cause of hydronephrosis

SPECIAL STUDIES

- Cystoscopy: to identify lower urinary tract pathology
- Ureteroscopy: to identify upper urinary tract pathology
- Retrograde pyelography: when noninvasive imaging fails to identify location or extent of obstruction

 ## Initial Management

- Neonates and infants

—See Section I, "Hydronephrosis—Prenatal" and "Hydronephrosis—Pediatric."

- Adults

—Initial management depends on clinical circumstances.
—A unilaterally obstructed, infected kidney in a septic patient requires drainage.
—Placement of ureteral stent and percutaneous nephrostomy are the most common methods for drainage.
—Calculi in a noninfected patient may be initially managed therapeutically with ESWL or ureteroscopy.
—Vascular lesions (aortic aneurysm) may require urgent initial management.
—Renal failure and electrolyte abnormalities should be corrected in conjunction with drainage.
—Renal dialysis may be necessary in the acutely ill patient.
—Treatment may be limited. (An obstructed kidney in a terminally ill patient with a normal opposite kidney and satisfactory serum creatinine and electrolytes may require no intervention.)

 ## Follow-Up

- After initial drainage and stabilization, the location and cause of obstruction should be determined.
- Effective treatment of *causes* should be addressed.
- A permanent form of urinary drainage may be necessary in some patients.

 ## Miscellaneous

SYNONYMS

- Hydroureteronephrosis

ASSOCIATED CONDITIONS: N/A

NOTES

- See also Section I, "Hydronephrosis—Prenatal" and "Hydronephrosis—Pediatric."

ABBREVIATIONS: N/A

REFERENCES

Docimo SG, Silver RI. Renal ultrasonography in newborns with prenatally detected hydronephrosis. *J Urol* 1997;157:1387.

Koelliker SL, Cronan JJ. Acute urinary tract obstruction: Imaging update. *Urol Clin North Am* 1997;24:571.

Liu JS, Hrebinko RL. The use of two ipsilateral ureteral stents for relief of ureteral obstruction from extrinsic compression. *J Urol* 1998;159:179.

Author: John A. Belis

Hydronephrosis—Pediatric

 Basics

DESCRIPTION

- Hydronephrosis is the condition where the collecting system of the kidney is dilated with urine.
- May be diagnosed antenatally on maternal ultrasound or at any age throughout childhood
- Complete evaluation is always required to determine cause and severity.
- May present with UTI, abdominal pain, hematuria, an abdominal mass, or on an imaging study in an asymptomatic patient

PATHOPHYSIOLOGY

- May be physiologic or pathologic in nature
- Physiologic hydronephrosis
—Function and drainage of the kidney may be within normal limits.
—Dilation of the urinary tract may be due to maldevelopment.
- Pathologic hydronephrosis may be due to obstruction.
—Ureteropelvic junction (UPJ) obstruction: most common in children
  —Most diagnosed on antenatal ultrasound
  —Intrinsic and extrinsic types occur.
  —Intrinsic obstruction involves a narrow segment of ureter at the UPJ.
  —Extrinsic obstruction is due to pressure on or kinking of the UPJ (usually by a lower pole renal artery).
—Ureterovesical junction obstruction may be primary or secondary.
  —Primary UVJ obstruction: due to disorganized muscle and fibrosis of the distal ureter
  —Secondary UVJ obstruction: due to neuropathic bladder, posterior urethral valves, or urethral stricture
  —UVJ obstruction may be due to a distal ureter that is either stenotic or aperistaltic.
  —More common in males; more common on the left side
—Neuropathic bladder dysfunction
  —Causes hydronephrosis because of increased bladder pressures
  —Uninhibited detrusor contraction or detrusor sphincter dyssynergia
- Hydronephrosis due to vesicoureteral reflux
—Little correlation of the degree of reflux and the severity of hydronephrosis
—Degree of hydronephrosis varies with the cycle of bladder filling and voiding.
- Hydronephrosis due to excessive urine output
—Diabetes insipidus; psychogenic polydipsia
- Hydronephrosis due to UTI
—Bacterial toxins may inhibit smooth muscle peristalsis in the urinary tract.
- Behavioral disorders
—Dysfunctional voiding and holding urine
—If extreme, hydronephrosis can result (Hinman syndrome).

- Consequences of hydronephrosis
—Renal tubular damage
  —Unable to concentrate urine or adequately conserve sodium
  —Decreased hydrogen ion excretion leading to acidosis
—Renal glomerular damage: decreased glomerular filtration rate
—Increased risk of infection and stones due to stasis of urine

RISK FACTORS

- Neurologic conditions: myelomeningocele and spinal cord injury
- Congenital conditions: anorectal anomalies and congenital heart disease
- History of multiple family members with hydronephrosis
- Trisomies 13 and 18 (20% have hydronephrosis)
- Trisomy 21 and Turner syndrome (4% are affected)

 Differential Diagnosis

- Multicystic dysplastic kidney (MCDK)
—MCDK: often confused with hydronephrosis on antenatal and infant ultrasound
—Ultrasound image of MCDK
  —Multiple cysts of various size without a central dominant cyst
  —Reniform shape is lost; no identifiable parenchyma
—Nuclear renogram: no function of the MCDK
- Solid renal tumors
—May present as flank masses
—Wilms' tumor, neuroblastoma, mesoblastic nephroma, and renal cell carcinoma
—Ultrasound can easily differentiate hydronephrosis from solid tumor.
- Swollen kidneys
—May be palpable in the flank or abdomen
—This can be due to renal vein thrombosis or pyelonephritis.
—Ultrasound, nuclear scans, and CT can distinguish from hydronephrosis.
- Hyperechoic pyramids
—In infants, can appear on ultrasound as dilated calyces to inexperienced observers
—Collecting tubules are dilated very early in life.
—Pyramids are distinctly more lucent than the remainder of the parenchyma.
—On ultrasound
  —The lucent areas are arranged in a radial pattern around the medulla.
  —The central complex (renal pelvis) is not dilated.

 Database

HISTORY

- A family history of renal abnormalities may uncover familial conditions.
- Children may have a history suggestive of renal colic.
—Intermittent flank or abdominal pain
—Intermittent nausea and vomiting
—Flank or abdominal pain associated with minor abdominal trauma
—Parents may notice infants exhibiting a pattern of intermittent crying and pulling up their legs.
- A history of UTI at any age is important.
—Urinary stasis increases the risk of infection.
—A history of unexplained febrile illnesses may indicate an undiagnosed UTI.
- A history of other urologic problems deserves evaluation (i.e., gross hematuria, incontinence, etc.).
- Some systemic complaints may indicate renal disease.
—Vomiting, dehydration, infants with failure to thrive, hypertension

PHYSICAL EXAMINATION

- Most common finding: flank or abdominal mass
- Costovertebral angle or abdominal tenderness
- Auscultation of the abdomen may reveal a lack of bowel sounds on the hydronephrotic side.

 Diagnostic Studies

LABORATORY TESTING

- There is no urine or blood test to screen for hydronephrosis.
—Urinalysis: hematuria and signs of UTI
—Serum electrolytes, BUN, and creatinine: to determine total renal function

IMAGING

- Initial diagnosis is usually made by ultrasound.
—Ultrasound reveals urine within the collecting system.
—Dilation of the renal pelvis without dilation of the interrenal collecting system is often insignificant clinically.
—Dilatation within the kidney is more likely to be a pathologic process.
—Most pediatric hydronephrosis today is diagnosed on antenatal ultrasound.
—Fetal hydronephrosis is the most common abnormality found on antenatal ultrasound (1 in 500).
—Most antenatal hydronephrosis is physiologic and does not require surgery.

- Diuretic renography is the most helpful test in determining function and obstruction.

—Technetium-99m-Mag 3 is the isotope of choice for diagnosing obstruction.

—Obstruction demonstrated by
  —Decreased and delayed uptake of isotope by the obstructed kidney
  —Prolonged renal transit time
  —Delayed drainage of isotope from the collecting system

- Excretory urography is useful detecting obstruction in older children.

—Delayed concentration of contrast

—Prolonged nephrogram phase of the study

—Dilated collecting system drains slowly

—Difficult to interpret in infants due to poor visualization of kidneys

—Infants are unable to concentrate contrast medium

- CT scan may be helpful in evaluating complex cases.

SPECIAL STUDIES

- If other studies do not define obstruction, a Whitaker Perfusion test

—Percutaneous nephrostomy and Foley catheter placed; kidney infused with saline or contrast at up to 10 mL/min

—Interrenal pressure is measured during infusion.

—Normal: at this rate of infusion with pressures <15 cm of H_2O

—Pressures >20 cm of H_2O indicate obstruction.

—Pressures 15 to 18: intermediate and must be correlated with other factors to determine significance

—If contrast is used, anatomy can be imaged during the test and correlated with pressures.

- Cystoscopy may be necessary to evaluate the bladder and urethra.
- Ureteroscopy or retrograde pyelography can define upper tract anatomy.

 ## Initial Management

- Based on etiology

—Obstruction always requires intervention.
  —Temporary drainage of obstruction: percutaneous nephrostomy or suprapubic tube
  —Protect from infection with suppressive antibiotics until definitive repair is performed.
  —UPJ obstruction: pyeloplasty (or endopyelotomy in older children in some centers)
  —UVJ obstruction: ureteral reimplant (and tapering of the ureter in most cases)
  —Posterior urethral valves: catheter drainage initially, followed by ablation of the valves endoscopically, or vesicostomy in very small infants
  —Neuropathic bladder: anticholinergic medication and intermittent catheterization initially or with vesicostomy; occasionally bladder augmentation is necessary to reduce bladder pressures and to increase urine storage capacity

—Vesicoureteral reflux: treated medically or surgically, depending on its severity

—Hydronephrosis without obstruction or reflux: observation to ensure that it does not progress to obstruction

 ## Follow-Up

- Ultrasound is the most helpful study to evaluate the degree of hydronephrosis.
- Diuretic renography is necessary to evaluate function and drainage.

 ## Miscellaneous

SYNONYMS: N/A

ASSOCIATED CONDITIONS: N/A

NOTES

- See also Section I, "Hydronephrosis—Antenatal."

ABBREVIATIONS

- UPJ, ureteropelvic junction; UVJ, ureterovesical junction

REFERENCES

Kass EJ, et al. Radioisotopic evaluation of the dilated urinary tract. *Urol Clin North Am* 1990;17:273.

King LR. Hydronephrosis. When is obstruction not obstruction? *Urol Clin North Am* 1995;22:31.

Peters, CA. Urinary tract obstruction in children. *J Urol* 1995;154:1874.

Tripp BM, et al. Neonatal hydronephrosis—The controversy and the management. *Pediatr Nephrol* 1995;9:503.

Author: Anthony J. Casale

Hydronephrosis—Prenatal

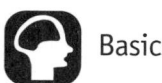 Basics

DESCRIPTION

- In utero sonographic detection of fetal renal dilatation, pelviectasis, or hydronephrosis
- May represent a normal developmental variant or severe obstructive uropathy
- Hydronephrosis may be evident from the fifteenth week of gestation onward, but the diagnosis cannot be made with certainty until 18 to 20 weeks of gestation.
- One of 100 to 500 pregnancies is found to have fetal hydronephrosis.
- Assessment should also offer information regarding contralateral kidney, amniotic fluid volume, renal parenchymal appearance, ureteral dilatation, and bladder distention.

PATHOPHYSIOLOGY

- Ureteropelvic junction obstruction
- Transitional hydronephrosis (recanalization of ureter)
- Ureterovesical obstruction (megaureter, obstructed and nonobstructed)
- Vesicoureteral reflux
- Bladder outlet obstruction (posterior urethral valves, urethral atresia)

RISK FACTORS

- Family history of renal abnormalities
- Previous fetal loss secondary to urinary tract anomalies
- Family history of vesicoureteral reflux

 Differential Diagnosis

- Renal: UPJ obstruction, duplication anomalies, transitional hydronephrosis
- Vesicoureteral: reflux, UVJ obstruction

—Prune-belly syndrome
—Megacystis–megaureter microcolon syndrome

- Multicystic dysplastic kidney
- Autosomal recessive polycystic kidney disease
- Intestinal disorders

—Intestinal duplication
—Mesenteric cysts
—Imperforate anus
—Persistent cloaca
—Cloacal exstrophy

- Ovarian cysts
- Tumors

—Neuroblastoma
—Congenital mesoblastic nephroma

 Database

HISTORY

- Timing of detection

—Earlier detection implies more severe condition

- Renal pelvic dilatation and severity of hydronephrosis (ureteropelvic junction obstruction)

—Correlation between renal pelvic AP diameter and age of fetus
  —8 mm by 25 weeks
  —10 mm by 32 weeks
  —15 mm at term
  —Presence of calyectasis
  —Renal cortical thinning or cysts

- Unilateral vs. bilateral
- Bladder distention: Suspect valves.
- Change in dilation in relation to bladder filling and emptying: vesicoureteral reflux
- Presence of oligohydramnios

—Suggests compromised renal function
—Associated with severe obstructive uropathy, usually posterior urethral valves, urethral atresia
—May lead to pulmonary hypoplasia, and fetal or postnatal demise
—Prenatal intervention for relief of hydronephrosis to restore amniotic fluid and prevent pulmonary hypoplasia

- Unilateral hydronephrosis may produce polyhydramnios by compressing the fetal intestinal tract.

PHYSICAL EXAMINATION

- Prenatal maternal physical examination for fundal height: oligohydramnios
- Postnatal physical examination

—Palpable kidney or mass; tense kidney
—Distended bladder
—Genital anomalies
—Urinary stream

Diagnostic Studies

LABORATORY TESTING

- Maternal α-feto protein may be elevated in some cases of fetal renal anomalies.
- Amniotic fluid level

—Composed mostly (90%) of fetal urine after the sixteenth week of gestation
—Correlates with fetal renal function

- Fetal karyotype
- Assessment of fetal urinary electrolytes

—"Good outcome": sodium <100 mg/dL; osmolarity <210 mOsmol/dL; chloride <90 mg/dL; urine output >2 mL/h

- Postnatal serum electrolyte assessment

—Nadir creatinine
—CO_2: acidosis
—Urinalysis and urine culture

IMAGING

- Prenatal: serial fetal sonography
- Postnatal assessment

—Unilateral hydronephrosis
—Delay initial renal/bladder ultrasound 2 to 7 days postbirth to avoid false readings secondary to perinatal oliguria.
—Repeat (second) renal/bladder ultrasound at 30 days.
—Voiding cystourethrogram (VCUG) at 7 to 10 days
—Diuretic nuclear renal scan (MAG-3) at 30 days
—Bilateral hydronephrosis
　—Male
　—Early postnatal assessment with sonography, VCUG to exclude posterior urethral valves
—An intravenous urogram may be of value in cases of UVJ obstruction or renal duplication anomalies.

SPECIAL STUDIES

- Fetal urinary electrolyte assessment in cases of severe bilateral hydronephrosis

—Controversial: one vs. multiple examinations

- Assessment of pulmonary maturity (lecithin : sphingomyelin ratio)
- Whitaker test: may be used in cases of postnatal uncertain status of hydronephrosis (historical interest)

 Initial Management

PRENATAL MANAGEMENT

- Assessment of hydronephrosis, oligohydramnios
- For unilateral cases

—Serial fetal sonography every 4 weeks; deliver at term
—Severe progressive hydronephrosis: Consider intrauterine drainage for dystocia.

- For bilateral cases, oligohydramnios

—Observation
—Termination
—Early delivery: steroid treatment for pulmonary immaturity
—Fetal intervention
　—Tapping of fetal bladder
　—Percutaneous urinary (bladder) to amniotic space shunting
　—Fetoscopy and intrauterine ablation of urethral valves (limited experience and results)

POSTNATAL MANAGEMENT

- Pulmonary support if respiratory compromise
- Antibiotic prophylaxis

—Amoxicillin at one-third of therapeutic dose for weight of infant (50 mg/kg/d divided in 3)

- Imaging based on unilateral vs. bilateral involvement

—Suspected posterior urethral valves: Place "feeding tube" urinary catheter.
—For tense hydronephrosis, consider percutaneous nephrostomy tube placement.
—Early vs. late pyeloplasty for UPJ obstruction
　—Differential function less than 35%
　—Grade IV hydronephrosis or solitary kidney

 Follow-Up

- Prenatal: sonographic evaluation every 4 weeks
- Postnatal: Based on initial evaluation, subsequent imaging may be necessary.

 Miscellaneous

SYNONYMS

- Antenatal hydronephrosis, fetal hydronephrosis

ASSOCIATED CONDITIONS: N/A

NOTES: N/A

ABBREVIATIONS

- VCUG, voiding cystourethrogram; PUV, posterior urethral valves

REFERENCES

Mandell J, et al. The natural history of structural genitourinary anomalies defects detected in utero. *Radiology* 1991;178:193.

Mandell J, et al. Diagnosis and management of congenital anomalies. In: Walsh PC, Retik AB, Stamey TA, Vaughn ED, eds. *Campbell's Urology*, 6th ed. Philadelphia: WB Saunders, 1992.

Author: T. Ernesto Figueroa

Hypertension—Urologic Considerations

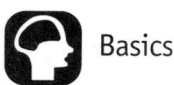 **Basics**

DESCRIPTION

- Sustained elevation of blood pressure above 140/90 mm Hg

—For children, sustained pressures above the 90th percentile are considered hypertensive.

- Uncontrolled hypertension causes small vessel disease.

—Organ failure may result: heart, kidneys, CNS.

PATHOPHYSIOLOGY

- Hypertension is sustained by structural renal and systemic vascular changes.

—Renin-angiotensin-aldosterone system: big role in hypertension and sodium/volume regulation
—Renin-angiotensin system activity may only be subtly elevated in chronic hypertension.
—Small structural changes will greatly alter resistance.
—Resistance changes with the fourth power of the radius (Poiseuille's law)

- The kidney is almost wholly responsible for control of blood pressure.

—Renovascular hypertension (RVH) is the cause in 5% to 10%.
—Atherosclerosis and fibromuscular disease account for most RVH.

RISK FACTORS

- RVH is mostly sporadic.

—Young adults, abrupt onset, Whites

- Smoking is associated with fibromuscular RVH, but less so than in atherosclerotic disease.

 Differential Diagnosis

ESSENTIAL HYPERTENSION

- Atherosclerotic hypertension
- Fibromuscular hyperplasia
- Intimal fibroplasia
- Medial fibroplasia (most common)
- Perimedial fibroplasia

 Database

HISTORY

- Any family history?
- Onset <25 or >45 years?
- Abrupt onset and severity?
- Headaches?
- Cigarette usage?
- White race?
- Good response to angiotensin converting enzyme inhibitors?

PHYSICAL EXAMINATION

- Blood pressure measurement technique is critical.

—Three separate occasions, correct blood pressure cuff size

- The "white coat effect" is of uncertain significance.
- Secondary changes

—Retinopathy
—Bruits

Hypertension—Urologic Considerations

 ## Diagnostic Studies

LABORATORY TESTING

- Hypokalemia may be seen.

—Due to high aldosterone or as excessive response to hydrochlorothiazide

- Plasma renins

—High false negative makes this alone a poor screening test.

- Single-dose captopril test

—Good screening test
—No antihypertensives, normal salt
—Increase in indices of plasma renin activity distinguish RVH from essential.

IMAGING

- Angiography

—Medial fibroplasia: string of beads, mainly women
—Intimal fibroplasia: focal stenosis in mid-artery
—Perimedial fibroplasia: tight stenosis with collaterals

- Ultrasound

—Visible size differences and scars (infarcts)
—Doppler studies for flow asymmetries

SPECIAL STUDIES

- Hypertensive renogram

—Isotope test showing decreased perfusion of affected kidney after dose of captopril

- Renal vein renin sampling

—Plasma renins may be elevated.
—High renal vein:arterial renin ratios

 ## Initial Management

- Medical management

—Antihypertensives to control hypertension
—Angiotensin converting enzyme inhibitors or angiotensin receptor blockers
—Less morbidity, threat to renal function

- Angioplasty

—Easy to do, 5% to 10% restenosis
—Most successful in fibromuscular dysplasias, with up to 88% improved

- Vascular stents

—Rapidly developing technique
—Long-term results not available

- Surgery

—Renal artery bypass or nephrectomy
—Patient selection is the key issue.
—Many different techniques, up to 93% improvement

 ## Follow-Up

- Blood pressure

—Watch for secondary changes.

- Renal function

—Primary need to preserve long-term renal function
—Ultrasound follow-up of changes in renal size

 ## Miscellaneous

SYNONYMS: N/A

ASSOCIATED CONDITIONS: N/A

NOTES: N/A

ABBREVIATIONS: N/A

REFERENCES

Dustan HP. Renal arterial disease and hypertension. *Med Clin North Am* 1997;81(5):1199–1212.

Greco BA, Breyer JA. The natural history of renal artery stenosis: Who should be evaluated for suspected ischemic nephropathy? *Semin Nephrol* 1996;16(1):2–11.

Ploth DW, Fitzgibbon W. Pathophysiology of altered renal function in renal vascular hypertension. *Am J Kidney Dis* 1994;24(4):652–659.

Author: Jeremy P.W. Heaton

Infertility

Basics

DESCRIPTION

- 10% to 15% of couples are unable to conceive within 1 year.

—20% due to pure male factor
—30% due to combined male and female factors

- Begin basic evaluation when the couple presents with infertility. Do not wait for 1 year of attempted conception.

PATHOPHYSIOLOGY

- Male fertility requires

—Potency
—Spermatogenesis
 —A full spermatogenic cycle lasts 74 days.
 —Any insult to spermatogenesis may have an effect for at least one spermatogenic cycle.
 —Any treatment to improve spermatogenesis will not have an effect for at least one spermatogenic cycle.
 —Requires testosterone and FSH
—Ejaculation
—Intercourse in periovulatory period

RISK FACTORS

- Cryptorchidism, testicular infection, trauma, or torsion
- Use of hot tub, Jacuzzi, steamroom
- Radiation or chemotherapy, alcohol abuse, possibly cigarettes

Differential Diagnosis

- Endocrine or pretesticular causes

—Pituitary disease
 —Hypogonadotropic hypogonadism (decreased FSH, LH, testosterone; normal prolactin)
 —Kallmann syndrome (with anosmia)
 —Fertile eunuch syndrome deficiency
 —Isolated FSH deficiency
—Congenital syndromes: Prader-Willi syndrome, Laurence-Moon-Bardet-Biedl syndrome
—Androgen excess: exogenous anabolic steroids, endogenous (metabolic abnormality or androgen-secreting tumor)
 —Decreased FSH, LH; elevated testosterone
—Estrogen excess: estrogen-secreting tumors, hepatic dysfunction, morbid obesity
 —Decreased FSH, LH, testosterone; elevated estrogen
—Prolactin excess: pituitary tumor, idiopathic
 —Elevated prolactin, decreased FSH, LH, testosterone
—Hyperthyroidism
 —Patients usually present with clinical symptoms of hyperthyroidism, not infertility
—Glucocorticoid excess
 —May suppress LH secretion, resulting in androgen insufficiency

- Testicular causes

—Genetic/karyotype abnormalities
 —10% to 15% of azoospermic patients
 —4% of oligospermic patients
 —1% of normospermic patients
 —Klinefelter syndrome: elevated gonadotropins; azoospermic, mosaic patients may have oligospermia
 —XYY syndrome: tall and azoospermic or severely oligospermic
 —XX male: small firm testes, gynecomastia, azoospermia
 —Androgen abnormalities: defects in androgen synthesis or conversion of testosterone to dihydrotestosterone, androgen receptor abnormalities
 —47, XY, phenotypes range from pseudohermaphroditism to a normal male phenotype with infertility
 —Noonan syndrome: cryptorchidism, testicular atrophy, elevated gonadotropins, azoospermia
 —Azoospermia factor deletions: Spermatogenesis genes are located on the short arm of the Y chromosome.
 —Deletions of DAZ (deleted in azoospermia), and RBM genes: azoospermia/oligospermia
 —Diagnosed by sequence tagged site analysis of Y chromosome; not widely available
—Nongenetic abnormalities
 —Bilateral anorchia (vanishing testes syndrome): XY males with nonpalpable testes
 —Cryptorchidism
 —Bilateral: 50% have low sperm counts
 —Unilateral: 30% have low sperm counts
—Varicocele
 —Found in 30% to 40% of infertile men
 —Decreased motility found in 90% of patients, low sperm counts in 65%
 —Low percentage of normal morphologic forms with stress pattern (increased number of amorphous cells and immature germ cells, >15% tapered forms)
 —Diagnosed by physical examination; utility of diagnosing and treating subclinical varicoceles unproved
—Sertoli-cell only syndrome
 —Small- to normal-sized testes, azoospermia
 —Testis biopsy reveals seminiferous tubules lined by Sertoli cells.
 —FSH is elevated or normal; testosterone and LH are normal.
—Myotonic dystrophy
 —Myotonia, premature frontal baldness, posterior subcapsular cataracts, cardiac conduction defects
 —Testicular atrophy develops during adulthood with normal Leydig cells, testosterone, and LH.
—Gonadotoxins
 —Chemotherapy, radiation
 —Alcohol abuse, cigarettes (controversial), marijuana (decreased testosterone, gynecomastia, low sperm counts), nitrofurantoin (high doses), lead, arsenic, sulfa drugs
—Ultrastructural defects
 —Immotile cilia syndrome (Kartagener syndrome if associated with situs inversus)

—Immotile viable sperm and immotile respiratory cilia
—Orchitis
 —Postpubertal mumps involves testis in 30% of patients, 70% to 90% are unilateral, 10% to 30% are bilateral.
 —Usually results in scarring and atrophy of involved testis
 —Other causes: bacterial epididymoorchitis, syphilis, gonorrhea, and leprosy.
—Antisperm antibodies
 —Ductal obstruction is a clear risk factor; possible risk factors include epididymal or testicular infection, torsion, cryptorchidism, genital trauma, and varicoceles.
 —Occur in 60% of men following vasectomy, and in 10% of infertile men
—Testicular cancer: oligospermia present in 60% of patients
—Idiopathic: abnormal SA in 25% of infertile patients with no clear cause

- Posttesticular causes

—Ductal obstruction (see Section II)
 —Congenital bilateral absence of vas (CBAVD)
 —Ejaculatory duct obstruction
 —Other causes of epididymal or vasal obstruction: vasectomy, infection, scarring.
—Ejaculatory dysfunction
 —Retrograde ejaculation: TURP, bladder neck surgery, retroperitoneal lymph node dissections, pelvic surgery, spinal cord injury, diabetes, multiple sclerosis, drugs that block sympathetics
 —Absent or low-volume ejaculate associated with sperm in postejaculate urine specimen
 —Anejaculation: Causes are the same as for retrograde ejaculation; orgasm occurs without antegrade or retrograde ejaculation; postejaculate urine is negative.

Database

HISTORY

- Sexual history

—Duration of sexual relations with and without birth control, methods of birth control, sexual technique, potency, use of lubricants (most harm sperm), frequency and timing of intercourse

- History

—Developmental history
 —Cryptorchidism, age of puberty, gynecomastia, congenital abnormalities of urinary tract or central nervous system
—Surgical history
 —Orchidopexy, retroperitoneal or pelvic surgery, sympathectomy, hernia, vasectomy, injury to scrotum, spinal cord injury
—Medical history
 —UTI, STD, mumps orchitis, renal disease, diabetes mellitus, recent fever, epididymitis, radiotherapy, tuberculosis, other chronic diseases

—Drugs, habits, and occupation
—Exposure to heat and chemicals, hot baths, steamrooms, cigarettes, alcohol, radiation
—Marital history of both partners
Family history
—Intersex disorders, testicular atrophy, cystic fibrosis

• Female reproductive history and results of female evaluation

PHYSICAL EXAMINATION

• Female habitus suggests karyotype abnormality.
• Under androgenization: low testosterone
• Gynecomastia: elevated estrogens or low testosterone
• Situs inversus: Kartagener syndrome (immotile cilia syndrome)
• Respiratory wheezes: immotile cilia syndrome
• Liver abnormalities: abnormal steroid hormone metabolism, elevated estrogens
• Hypospadias: abnormal deposition of semen
• Chordee: interferes with intercourse if severe
• Presence or absence of testes, epididymides, and vas deferens
• Testicular atrophy: primary or secondary hypogonadism
• Epididymal induration: may indicate obstruction
• Varicocele
• Prostatic tenderness

 ## Diagnostic Studies

LABORATORY TESTING

• Semen analysis (see also Section III)

—Volume: normal, >1.5 mL
—Low volume associated with incomplete collection, retrograde ejaculation, ejaculatory duct obstruction
—Count: normal, at least 20 million sperm/mL
—Azoospermia suggests CBAVD, vasal or epididymal obstruction, germ cell or testicular failure, hypogonadotropic hypogonadism
—Oligospermia: usually associated with other seminal defects, deficiency of FSH, LH, prolactinoma, idiopathic
—Motility: normal, at least 60%
—Low motility associated with antisperm antibodies, partial ejaculatory duct obstruction, infection if associated with pyospermia, immotile cilia syndrome (motility <10%), idiopathic
—Sperm agglutination suggests antisperm antibodies.

• Second-level tests

—Antisperm antibodies: obtain if history of obstruction, testicular infection or trauma, cryptorchidism, low sperm motility, sperm agglutination, abnormal postcoital test, unexplained infertility
—WBC staining of semen: if excess numbers of round cells are consistently found in semen

—Cultures
—Semen or urethra: *Mycoplasma* and *Chlamydia* if evidence of genital tract infection, bacterial semen cultures usually contaminated by distal urethral organisms
—Urine culture with cystitis or urethritis
—Hormone studies
—FSH and testosterone with sperm counts 10 million/mL or under androgenization on physical
—LH and prolactin if testosterone low or evidence of prolactinoma

IMAGING

• Transrectal ultrasonography

—To identify ejaculatory duct obstruction: dilatation of seminal vesicles or ejaculatory ducts
—Complete obstruction: azoospermic patients with acidic, small seminal volumes
—Partial obstruction: low volume, very low motility semen sample

SPECIAL STUDIES

• Testicular biopsy

—Azoospermic patients to differentiate between obstructive and nonobstructive azoospermia
—May be combined with sperm retrieval for in vitro fertilization
—Not needed for diagnosis in patients with bilateral testicular atrophy and FSH >2 to 3 times normal

• Functional assays

—SPA, acrosome reaction assay, hemizona assay; evaluate fertilizing capacity of sperm prior to ART.

• Vasography

—Indicated in azoospermic patient with normal-sized testes, normal FSH levels, and spermatogenesis present on testis biopsy

 ## Initial Management

• Basic evaluation consists of history, physical examination, and two to three semen analyses
• Second-level testing based on basic evaluation
• Determine if male factor infertility is present; determine the cause of infertility: Initially, fix the underlying problem; the goal is conception through intercourse. Treatments are not available for all etiologies.

—Hormone deficiency: Treat the cause (i.e., prolactinoma) or replace deficient hormones.
—Varicocele: Repair if SA is abnormal.
—Gonadotoxins, drugs: Remove exposure.
—Antisperm antibodies: steroids minimally effective, ART most often employed
—Idiopathic oligospermia: empiric clomiphene 25–50 mg/d for 6 months
—Ductal obstruction: microsurgical repair for vasal or epididymal obstruction, TURED for ejaculatory duct obstruction

—Ejaculatory dysfunction: medical therapy
—Phenylpropanolamine 75 mg bid
—Ephedrine sulfate 25 to 50 mg qid
—Pseudoephedrine hydrochloride 60 mg qid
—Imipramine hydrochloride 25 mg bid
—Sperm retrieval: Alkalinize urine to pH >7.0; adjust fluid intake to achieve isotonic urine in patients with retrograde ejaculation that cannot be converted to antegrade: sodium bicarbonate 650 mg qid for 12 to 48 hours; baking soda 1 to 3 tsp with glass of water night before and morning of collection.
—Vibratory stimulation for patients with spinal cord injury, electroejaculation for all neurologic causes of anejaculation
—Assisted reproductive techniques (ART)
—Goal: conception through IUI or IVF
—Male: not treated, although sperm retrieval may be necessary

 ## Follow-Up

• SA 3 months after treatment
• If no conception after treatment of male fertility, consider ART
• Options of donor insemination and adoptions should be considered if the above fail.

Miscellaneous

SYNONYMS: N/A

ASSOCIATED CONDITIONS: N/A

NOTES

• See also Section III, "Semen Analysis—Abnormal."

ABBREVIATIONS

• CBAVD, congenital bilateral absence of vas deferens; IUI, intrauterine insemination; IVF, in vitro fertilization; ART, assisted reproductive techniques; DAZ, deleted in azoospermia; RBM, RNA binding motif; SPA, sperm penetration assay; SA, semen analysis; TURED, transurethral resection of ejaculatory ducts

REFERENCES

Goldstein M. Surgical management of male infertility and other scrotal disorders. In: Walsh PC, et al., eds. *Campbell's Urology*. Philadelphia: WB Saunders, 1998.

Lipshultz LI, et al. *Infertility in the Male*. Baltimore: Mosby, 1997.

Sigman M, et al. Male infertility. In: Walsh PC, et al., eds. *Campbell's Urology*. Philadelphia: WB Saunders, 1998.

Author: Mark Sigman

Inguinal Lymphadenopathy

 Basics

DESCRIPTION

• Palpable inguinal nodes secondary to infectious, inflammatory, or neoplastic processes
• Determination of nodal size, consistency, mobility, and tenderness is critical to aid in diagnosis.

PATHOPHYSIOLOGY

• Inguinal nodes act as drainage sites for the penis, urethra, lower extremities, lower abdominal wall (extending to the umbilicus), gluteal region, and parts of the anal canal.
• Preputial, penile, and scrotal skin drain into superficial inguinal nodes bilaterally.
• Glans penis and corporal drainage are via the superficial and deep inguinal lymphatics.
• Superficial inguinal nodes lie in the superficial fascia, 1 cm inferior to the inguinal ligament and along the saphenous vein.
• Deep inguinal nodes lie deep to the roof of the femoral triangle.

RISK FACTORS

• Trauma, lower extremity infection, perianal infection or inflammation, perirectal inflammation, STDs, urethritis, perineal neoplasia, fixed drug reactions, systemic neoplasia (lymphoma), HIV

 Differential Diagnosis

• Infectious and inflammatory causes remain the most common in both adults and children.
• Infectious

—Superficial lower extremity infections, i.e., phlebitis, cellulitis, usually staph
—STDs
  —Herpes, both herpes viruses 1 and 2
  —Chancroid, caused by *Haemophilus ducreyi*
  —Lymphogranuloma venereum, caused by *Chlamydia trachomatis*
  —Syphilis, caused by *T. pallidum tremponema*
  —HIV infections with generalized lymphadenopathy

• Neoplasia

—Penile, scrotal, and distal urethral neoplasia may give palpable nodes.
  —50% of patients with penile cancer have palpable nodes.
  —These nodes may be secondary to metastasis, infection, or inflammation.
  —Only half of those who present with enlarged nodes will have metastasis.
  —Vaginal or labial alignancies
  —Lymphoma

 Database

HISTORY

• Age

—Infections are more common in the 20 to 40 age group but may be present in all ages. They are rarer in children, except for systemic infections. Neoplastic processes are more common in older age groups.

• Sex

—Infectious processes affect sexes nearly equally.

• History of trauma, perineal or lower extremity
• Medications and allergies?
• Sexual practices?

—History of STDs
—Prior genital lesions

• Occupational history

—Scrotal cancer has a high association with exposure to soot and hydrocarbon (i.e., those who work as chimney sweeps).

• Recent weight loss

—Associated with neoplastic process

• Ethnicity

—Penile cancer is almost never found in cultures that perform neonatal circumcisions (i.e., Jews).

PHYSICAL EXAMINATION

• Vitals

—Fever especially important

• General appearance

—Cachexia of neoplasia or HIV
—Presence of Kaposi's sarcoma associated with HIV infection

• Node survey

—Neck, axillary, inguinal, maxillary for generalized process

• Abdomen

—Palpable abdominal mass suggestive of enlarged abdominal or pelvic nodes

• Inguinal nodes: careful characterization of nodes

—Extent, size, tenderness, firmness, overlying erythema, purulence, fluctuance
—Painful adenopathy suggestive of herpes, chancroid, LGV
—Painless lesions more suggestive of inflammatory or neoplastic process
—Fluctuant nodes more suggestive of chancroid or LGV
—Firm nodes suggest herpes or syphilis.
—Chancroid with characteristic overlying erythema
—Neoplastic and strictly inflammatory nodes often large and matted or adherent to adjacent structures
—Femoral artery pulse to assess involvement of surrounding structures

• Genitalia

—Presence of foreskin almost always seen with penile cancer. Prepubertal circumcision is usually protective.
—Circumcision later in life is not protective.
—Penile or scrotal lesions, ulcers, phimosis, erythema, fluctuance, purulence
—Painful ulcers seen with herpes, chancroid
—Painless ulcers associated with granuloma inguinale, syphilis, neoplasia
—Neoplastic lesions may be large or subtle, often papillary or erosive.
—HIV associated with Kaposi's sarcoma

• Digital rectal examination

—Attention to perianal area for abscess, infection, erythema, tenderness, purulence. Anal sphincter stenosis may suggest inflammatory process.

• Lower extremities

—Inspect for lesions, phlebitis, erythema, purulence, scaling of skin

Diagnostic Studies

LABORATORY TESTING

• If associated with penile or scrotal lesions: The lesion must be biopsied to identify possible cancer.
• If associated with genital ulcer
• A culture of the ulcer should be performed to diagnose the infective organism.

—If syphilis is suspected, then dark-field microscopy of the ulcer bed scrapings will show characteristic organisms.

• Preferred tests for specific organisms

—Herpes viral culture
—Chancroid-selective media culture
—LGV-complement fixation or immunofluorescence
—Syphilis dark-field microscopy

• When no associated lesions exist and no historical evidence is suggestive of a diagnosis, then nodal biopsy is indicated either by needle or open procedure.

IMAGING

• Inguinal ultrasound

—May help identify surrounding structures, i.e., invasion into femoral vessels

• Computerized tomography of the abdomen and pelvis

—May show involvement of other nodal beds, i.e., iliac nodes in higher stages of penile or scrotal cancers, or with lymphoma

• Lymphangiogram

—Old test that may help differentiate neoplastic from inflammatory nodes. Inflammatory nodes will not usually show filling defects, while neoplastic nodes or metastatic nodes will more likely appear irregular and display filling defects.

SPECIAL STUDIES: N/A

 Initial Management

• Diagnosis essential for management
• Infections

—Herpes: acyclovir 200 mg po qid for approximately 10 days
—Chancroid: erythromycin 500 mg po qid for 10 days
—LGV: tetracycline or doxycycline 500 mg po qid/100 mg bid for 14 days or until healed
—Syphilis: penicillin G 2.4 million U IM × 1 dose
—Lower extremity infection (i.e., phlebitis or cellulitis): cephalexin 500 mg po tid or qid until resolved
—Perianal infections/abscess: drainage of abscess, broad-spectrum antibiotic coverage, i.e., quinolone
—Scrotal/penile infection/abscess: drainage of abscess, cephalexin 500 mg po tid or qid

• Penile or scrotal cancer

—Nodes may be neoplastic or inflammatory
—Treat initially with cephalexin 500 mg po tid or qid for 4 to 6 weeks. See Section II, "Penis Cancer—General" for further management

 Follow-Up

• If diagnosis remains unclear and/or nodes remain enlarged after antibiotic therapy, biopsy is indicated.

—Recommend a return visit about 6 weeks after initiating therapy.

 Miscellaneous

SYNONYMS: N/A

ASSOCIATED CONDITIONS: N/A

NOTES

• See Section II, "Penis Cancer—General," and specific infectious agent.

ABBREVIATIONS

• LGV, lymphogranuloma venereum

REFERENCES

Crawford ED, Das S, eds. Penile, urethral and scrotal cancer. *Urol Clin North Am* 1992;19(2)211–415.

Mellinger BC, Smith AD, eds. Sexually transmitted diseases and other lesions of the external genitalia. *Urol Clin North Am* 1992;19(1)35–46.

Authors: Todd D. Cohen and Robert R. Bahnson

Libido—Diminished

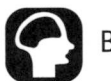 **Basics**

DESCRIPTION

- Libido (sexual desire) is mediated by the cerebral cortex and limbic system.
- Diminished libido: lack of desire to engage in a sexual experience

PATHOPHYSIOLOGY

- Psychological

—Psychological disturbances of all degrees, from anxiety to major psychiatric disorder
—May be secondary to other medical conditions (i.e., congenital anomalies, disfiguring injuries, etc.)

- Hormonal

—Hypogonadism: androgen deficiency, particularly testosterone, whether primary (testicular defect) or secondary to hypothalamic–pituitary dysfunction
—Hyperprolactinemia with or without pituitary lesion
—Thyroid: Both hyper- and hypothyroidism can lead to diminished sexual desire.

- Drugs: beta-blockers, clonidine, diuretics, lithium, major tranquilizers, methyl-dopa, sedatives, ketoconazole, alpha-blockers, DHT-inhibitors, cimetidine, antiandrogens, LHRH analogues

RISK FACTORS

- Therapy for prostate cancer (decreased testosterone)
- Congenital, inflammatory, or surgical causes of testicular dysfunction

 Differential Diagnosis

- Psychiatric disturbances
- Hormonal disturbances
- Drug induced

 Database

HISTORY

- Sexual history

—Frequency and level of sexual desire?
—Difficulty in achieving or maintaining an erection?
—Evidence of ejaculation disorder, overall satisfaction with sexual life?

- History of psychiatric illness?
- Previous/current medications?
- History of endocrine problems?
- Therapy for prostate cancer?

PHYSICAL EXAMINATION

- Assessment of secondary sexual characteristics

—Absence of secondary sexual characters suggests hormonal etiology.

Diagnostic Studies

LABORATORY TESTING

- Serum testosterone
- Serum prolactin
- If any abnormality in the above, then serum FSH and LH measurements

IMAGING

- MRI of brain: if prolactin is elevated

SPECIAL STUDIES: N/A

 ## Initial Management

- Determine if obvious cause exists, and correct if possible.

—Decreased testosterone, etc., hormonal supplementation

- Psychiatric consultation/sex function therapist
- Endocrinologic consultation

 ## Follow-Up

- With appropriate practitioner

 ## Miscellaneous

SYNONYMS: N/A

ASSOCIATED CONDITIONS: N/A

NOTES

- See also Section I, "Erectile Dysfunction."

ABBREVIATIONS: N/A

REFERENCES

Brendler CB. Evaluation of urologic patient. In: Walsh PC, Retik AB, Vaughan ED, Wein AJ, eds. *Campbell's Urology*, 7th ed. Philadelphia: WB Saunders, 1998:131–157.

Wilson B. The effect of drugs on male sexual function and fertility. *Nurse Pract* 1991;16:12.

Authors: Ehab El-Gabry and Irvin H. Hirsch

Neurogenic Bladder

 **Basics**

DESCRIPTION

• Multiple reversible and irreversible etiologies that lead to malfunction of one or both normal bladder functions (storage/emptying)
• Definitions

—Detrusor hyperreflexia: insuppressible involuntary bladder contractions during filling (spontaneous or provoked)
    —Unstable detrusor: similar syndrome but without definable neurologic disorder
—Detrusor–sphincter dyssynergia: detrusor contraction with an involuntary contraction of the urethral/periurethral striated sphincter

PATHOPHYSIOLOGY

• Normal bladder function

—Low-pressure filling and storage with continence
    —Sympathetic α-adrenergic stimulation of bladder neck and posterior urethra increases tone (T_{10}-L_2 via hypogastric nerve).
    —Sympathetic (β-adrenergic stimulation of bladder fundus decreases tone (T_{10}–L_2 via hypogastric nerve).
    —Somatic innervation of external urethral sphincter increases tone (S_2–S_4 via pudendal nerve).
—Voluntary low-pressure micturition with complete bladder emptying
    —Decrease in somatic output to external urethral sphincter decreases tone.
    —Inhibition of sympathetic output and/or receptors in bladder neck
    —Parasympathetic cholinergic stimulation of bladder causing contraction (S_2–S_4 via pelvic nerve)

• Lapides classification (with specific neurologic insult): historically important; frequent overlapping categories

—Sensory neurogenic bladder (peripheral or central sensory fibers): diabetes mellitus, tabes dorsalis
    —Impaired sensation, bladder overdistension and decompensation, residual urine
—Motor paralytic bladder (parasympathetic detrusor motor supply): pelvic surgery, trauma, zoster, polio
    —Inability to initiate voiding, painful distension, bladder overdistension and decompensation, residual urine
—Uninhibited neurogenic bladder ("corticoregulatory tract": inhibitory system on sacral reflexes): CVA, tumor, Parkinson's, demyelinating disease
    —Frequency/urgency/urge incontinence, detrusor hyperreflexia
—Reflex neurogenic bladder (sensory and motor suprasacral spinal cord pathways): trauma, transverse myelitis
    —Initial spinal shock (acontractile and areflexic bladder with baseline outlet tone), urinary retention
    —Absent sensation, inability to initiate voiding, detrusor hyperreflexia, striated sphincter dyssynergia
—Autonomous neurogenic bladder (sacral cord, sacral roots, pelvic nerves): trauma, surgery, tumor
    —Absent sensation, inability to initiate voiding, absent reflex activity, bladder overdistension and decompensation, residual urine, possible late decrease in compliance

• Anatomic classification (of the neurologic lesion): "Classic" findings do not always correlate with urodynamic findings.

—Supraspinal (above the brainstem)
    —Involuntary bladder contractions, smooth and striated sphincter synergy, sensation intact
—Spinal (above cord level S2; after initial spinal shock)
    —Involuntary bladder contractions, smooth sphincter synergy, striated sphincter dyssynergia, sensation absent
—Sacral spinal
    —Detrusor areflexia $\pm$ decreased compliance, open smooth sphincter, residual striated sphincter tone, sensation absent
—Peripheral (motor and/or sensory)
    —Detrusor areflexia $\pm$ decreased compliance, open smooth sphincter, residual striated sphincter tone
    —Nerve root irritation may lead to detrusor hyperreflexia.

• Functional classification (Wein): logically associates with treatment modalities; frequent overlapping categories

—Failure to store
    —Because of bladder (detrusor hyperactivity, detrusor hypersensitivity)
    —Because of outlet incompetence
—Failure to empty
    —Because of bladder (neurologic, myogenic, psychogenic, idiopathic)
    —Because of outlet obstruction (anatomic, functional)

RISK FACTORS

• Myelodysplasia, trauma (intracranial, spinal, pelvic), vascular (intracranial, spinal cord), surgery (intracranial, spinal, pelvic), neurologic disorder (CNS, spinal cord, peripheral)

Differential Diagnosis

- Supraspinal processes

—Cerebrovascular disease
  —Rare initial detrusor areflexia (initial urinary retention); detrusor hyperreflexia (chronic incontinence, frequency, and urgency)
—Dementia
  —Loss of awareness vs. detrusor hyperreflexia (incontinence)
—Concussion (uncommon urinary sequela)
  —Initial detrusor areflexia (initial urinary retention); chronic detrusor hyperreflexia (incontinence, frequency, and urgency)
—Brain tumor (especially tumors in superior frontal lobes)
  —Detrusor hyperreflexia with smooth and striated sphincter synergy, loss of awareness (incontinence)
—Normal pressure hydrocephalus (dementia/ataxia/incontinence)
  —Detrusor hyperreflexia with smooth and striated sphincter synergy (incontinence)
—Cerebral palsy
  —Detrusor hyperreflexia with smooth and striated sphincter synergy (incontinence)
—Parkinson disease (voiding symptoms in 35%–70%)
—Detrusor hyperreflexia with smooth and striated sphincter synergy, normal compliance (incontinence)
—Involuntary striated sphincter contractions (not obstructive); poor voluntary striated sphincter control
—Shy-Drager syndrome (urinary symptoms frequently predate diagnosis)
  —Detrusor hyperreflexia with smooth and striated sphincter synergy (initial incontinence, frequency, and urgency)
  —Decreased compliance (distal spinal involvement); striated sphincter denervation (late)

- Spinal processes
—Myelodysplasia (depends on type and level of lesion; may evolve over time)
  —Most commonly detrusor areflexia with baseline striated sphincter tone (overflow incontinence)
  —May have detrusor hyperreflexia with detrusor–sphincter dyssynergia
—Multiple sclerosis (demyelination most commonly in cervical spinal cord, but can be throughout; exacerbation/remission)
  —Detrusor hyperreflexia $\pm$ striated sphincter dyssynergia $\pm$ impaired contractility; sensation intact
—Spinal cord injury (sacral cord begins at T12-L1)
  —Initial spinal shock (acontractile, areflexic bladder with resting sphincter tone); overflow incontinence
  —C1 to T7-8: detrusor hyperreflexia, asensate, smooth and striated sphincter dyssynergia; autonomic hyperreflexia
  —T9 to S2: detrusor hyperreflexia, asensate, smooth sphincter synergia, striated sphincter dyssynergia
  —Below S2: detrusor areflexia with initial high/normal compliance and chronic decreased compliance; chronically open smooth sphincter with baseline striated sphincter tone
  —Autonomic hyperreflexia: headache, hypertension, bradycardia, flushing above the lesion; massive sympathetic response to specific stimuli (primarily bladder/rectal dilatation or manipulation) in patients with cord levels above T6-8 (sympathetic outflow)
—Tabes dorsalis, pernicious anemia "sensory neurogenic bladder"
  —Classically, loss of sensation with large residual urine volumes

- Peripheral processes
—Spinal disc disease (1%–18% incidence of voiding dysfunction after herniated disc; not always reversed by laminectomy)
  —Areflexic bladder with normal compliance (residual urine, difficulty voiding)
—Pelvic surgery (pelvic plexus injury): 10% to 60% acutely and 15% to 20% permanently (often transient/avoid early definitive TX)
  —Impaired bladder contractility, decreased compliance, baseline striated sphincter tone (retention/overflow incontinence)
—Herpes zoster (sacral nerve root viral invasion; usually with painful dermatomal eruptions)
  —Areflexic bladder (retention/overflow incontinence) with resolution in 1 to 2 months
—Diabetes mellitus (sensory $\pm$ motor neuropathy)
  —Insidious onset of impaired sensation, increased capacity, decreased contractility, decreased flow
—Guillain-Barré syndrome
  —Retention in 10% to 30% (usually transient)

- Hinman-Allen syndrome (nonneurogenic neurogenic bladder/dysfunctional voiding)

—Urodynamic/clinical evidence of involuntary obstruction at the striated sphincter without evidence of neurologic disease

(continued)

Neurogenic Bladder (continued)

 Database

HISTORY

- Duration and quantity of bladder symptoms (voiding diary)?

—Acute or chronic, stable or progressive, primary or subsequent to a period of normal bladder function

- Bladder sensation?

—Filling, fullness, need to void, voiding

- Quality of micturition?

—Spontaneous or only after stimulation, Valsalva or Credé

- Incontinence?

—Primary or secondary, continuous dribbling or intermittent leakage, stress or urge incontinence, pre-void or post-void, nocturnal or diurnal (or both), quantity (number of pads, etc.)

- Additional symptoms?

—Changes in bowel habit, gait, or erectile function; back or leg pains; seizures

- Prior management of urinary symptoms?

—Medical and surgical therapies

- Social history?

—Stress, family dynamics, parent–child relationships

PHYSICAL EXAMINATION

- Neurologic examination (gait, balance, muscular symmetry, reflexes)

—CNS disease, neuropathy/radiculopathy

- Back examination (skin tags, tufts of hair, dimples, scars)

—Occult myelodysplasia, previous surgery

- Abdominal examination (kidney size, bladder distention, colon distention, scars)

—Ability to stimulate micturition by suprapubic massage or to express urine by suprapubic compression

- Genital examination (excoriation, hypospadias or meatal stenosis, urogenital anomalies, scars)

—Evidence of incontinence, previous surgery

- Rectal examination (perianal sensation, anal tone, prostate size, stool quality)

—Bulbocavernosus reflex (external sphincter contraction elicited by squeezing the glans penis or clitoris due to an intact sacral reflex arc)

 Diagnostic Studies

LABORATORY TESTING

- Urinalysis

—Collection: infants (bag technique or midstream collection after stimulated void); adults (clean catch if possible; otherwise catheter or suprapubic specimen)
—Signs of infection (pyuria, leukocyte esterase), with culture if indicated

- Serum creatinine, electrolytes

—If elevated or there is evidence of renal scarring, measure creatinine clearance.

IMAGING

- Plain abdominal film

—Bony abnormalities, severe constipation, stones

- Upper tract evaluation (ultrasound, intravenous pyelogram, radionucleotide scan)
- Voiding cystourethrogram (can be performed in conjunction with urodynamics)

—Especially in children to rule out vesicoureteral reflux in setting of voiding dysfunction

SPECIAL STUDIES

- Urodynamic studies

—Noninvasive: uroflow (not specific)
—Simultaneous pressure–flow videocystourethrography
  —Quality and quantity of storage/emptying dysfunction
  —Difficult in children

 Initial Management

- Complete neurologic and urodynamic evaluation to identify likely cause
- Upper-tract damage risk factors related to intravesical pressure and leak point pressure
- Goal: low-pressure storage with periodic emptying
- Numerous medical and surgical therapies available; must be tailored to the degree and functional type of dysfunction
- Watchful waiting occasionally reasonable as long as upper tracts not threatened and incontinence tolerated (infants and neurologically devastated)
- Failure to store (because of bladder; because of outlet)

—Detrusor hyperactivity
  —Anticholinergics: propantheline 15 to 30 mg q4–6h, hyoscyamine (Cystospaz); anticholinergic side effects, unproved efficacy
  —Anticholinergic/smooth muscle relaxants: oxybutynin (Ditropan) 5 mg tid/qid; dicyclomine (Bentyl) 10 to 20 mg tid/qid; tolterodine (Detrol) 1 to 2 mg bid; side effects (less with tolterodine, reportedly due to bladder specificity)
  —Tricyclics: imipramine 25 mg tid/qid (anticholinergic, smooth muscle relaxant, increased outlet resistance); anticholinergic side effects
—Decreased compliance
  —Anticholinergic/smooth muscle relaxants
  —Advanced: dorsal rhizotomy (abolish detrusor motor input); augmentation cystoplasty
—Decreased outlet resistance
  —α-Adrenergic agonists: pseudoephedrine 30 to 60 mg qid; ephedrine, phenylpropanolamine; adrenergic side effects (BP)
  —Tricyclics: imipramine 25 mg tid/qid
  —Surgery: periurethral bulking agents, urethral sling procedures, artificial urethral sphincter

- Failure to empty (because of bladder; because of outlet)

—Decreased detrusor contractility
  —Mechanical: clean intermittent catheterization (CIC), external compression (Credé), Valsalva; reflex contractions
  —Cholinergic agonists: bethanechol (Urecholine) 10 to 50 mg bid/qid; cholinergic side effects, little contractile effect
  —Advanced: electric stimulation
—Outlet obstruction (essential to treat specific location of outlet obstruction)
  —Mechanical: CIC, external compression (Credé), Valsalva
  —α-Adrenergic blockade: terazosin (Hytrin) and doxazosin (Cardura) 1 to 10 mg qhs; tamsulosin (Flomax) 0.4 to 0.48 mg qhs (GU selective); bladder neck and smooth sphincter relaxation, best effects seen in BPH (prostatic capsule relaxation), some cardiovascular side effects, first-dose phenomenon
  —Surgical: bladder neck incision, striated sphincterotomy (for unresponsive sphincter dyssynergia), urinary diversion

- Catheterization

—Clean intermittent catheterization: in emptying failure and in combined failure (after storage failure attenuated surgically or pharmacologically); unsterile, but low risk of infection unless VUR; some recommend suppressive antibiotics
—Continuous catheterization: initial management; long-term complications (urethral complications avoided with suprapubic tube); SP tube does not eliminate urethral leakage; suppressive antibiotics indicated

 Follow-Up

- Periodic lifelong reevaluation essential, especially in children
- Evaluation for upper tract damage and side effects/complications of therapy

—Periodic KUB if on CIC for stones

 Miscellaneous

SYNONYMS

- Neurogenic voiding dysfunction, neuropathic bladder, atonic bladder, spinal bladder

ASSOCIATED CONDITIONS: N/A

NOTES: N/A

ABBREVIATIONS

- CIC, clean intermittent catheterization

REFERENCES

Bellinger MF. Myelomeningocele and neuropathic bladder. In: Gillenwater JY, Grayhack JT, Howards SS, Duckett JW, eds. *Adult and Pediatric Urology*. St Louis: Mosby, 1996:2489–2528.

Staskin DR. Classification of voiding dysfunction. In: Krane RJ, Siroky MB, eds. *Clinical Neuro-Urology*. Boston: Little, Brown, 1991: 411–424.

Wein AJ. Neuromuscular dysfunction of the lower urinary tract and its treatment. In: Walsh PC, Retik AB, Vaughan ED, Wein AJ, eds. *Campbell's Urology*. Philadelphia: WB Saunders, 1997:953–1005.

Wein AJ. Pathophysiology and categorization of voiding dysfunction. In: Walsh PC, Retik AB, Vaughan ED, Wein AJ, eds. *Campbell's Urology*. Philadelphia: WB Saunders, 1997:917–926.

Authors: Robert R. Byrne and Craig F. Donatucci

Nocturia

 Basics

DESCRIPTION

• Nocturia is a manifestation of one or a combination of voiding dysfunction, medical condition, or sleep disorder.

• As a completely isolated symptom, it may more often represent a non-urologic problem or medical condition.

• Elucidating its etiology requires a careful history and assessment of associated voiding symptoms.

• Nocturia is usually the most "bothersome" symptom of prostatic outlet obstruction.

• It should be distinguished from nocturnal enuresis in children, which is currently thought to represent one or a combination of developmental delay, concentrating defect, or sleep disorder.

PATHOPHYSIOLOGY

• While voiding one to seven times per day may be in the range of normal, awakening even one time per evening may be considered abnormal.

—If sleep hours do not significantly exceed usual daytime voiding intervals, the patient should theoretically not have to awaken to void.
—Volumes consistently in excess of or substantially less than average daytime volumes suggest an abnormality.

• See specific diseases under "Differential Diagnosis."

RISK FACTORS

• Elderly, sleep disorders, volume-related disorders, lower urinary tract dysfunction (physiologic or anatomic)

 Differential Diagnosis

• Elderly

—May have reversed circadian voiding patterns in which two-thirds of 24-hour volume is excreted in the night hours and only one-third in the daytime, as opposed to the converse seen in younger controls
—Higher incidence of associated medical conditions
—Multiple medications that alter volume or voiding dynamics
—Possible age-related changes in voiding
  —Detrusor instability, detrusor hyperactivity with impaired contractility (DHIC), increased incidence of outflow obstruction and overflow

• Sleep disorders

—Sleep apnea, mood disturbances such as depression or anxiety, chronic pain syndromes, unspecified insomnia

• Volume-related disorders: Once supine, dependent peripheral edema is mobilized, filtered, and excreted.

—Congestive heart failure
—Liver disease/hypoalbuminemia
—Peripheral vascular disease (chronic venous insufficiency or lymphedema)
—Excessive fluid intake, especially in evening hours
  —True psychogenic polydipsia typically does not manifest as nocturia but rather daytime frequency.

• Pharmacologic

—Diuretics, alcohol, caffeine (may act as a diuretic or cause sleep disturbance), theophylline (can promote diuresis), calcium channel blockers (causing peripheral edema), lithium (impairs vasopressin response), steroids (may reverse normal circadian voiding patterns or cause osmotic diuresis via hyperglycemia)
—Has patient been started on any other medications that may alter normal voiding physiology?
  —Tricyclics (i.e., imipramine), psychiatric or cold remedies (anticholinergic properties), alpha-blockers (terazosin, doxazosin, tamsulosin), anticholinergics (hyoscyamine, tolterodine, propantheline), musculotropic relaxants (oxybutynin)

• Lower urinary tract dysfunction

—Anatomic
  —Diminished capacity (previous surgery, radiation), outflow obstruction (overflow or obstruction-induced instability), impaired compliance (previous radiation, long-standing outflow obstruction), stress incontinence (stress-induced instability), atrophic vaginitis (menopause)
—Physiologic
  —Detrusor instability, detrusor hyperreflexia (presence of neurologic etiology), sensory urgency, impaired sensation or hypocontractility (diabetic cystopathy) with resultant overflow
  —Nocturia may often be the only remaining bothersome symptom following medical or surgical relief of outflow obstruction.

• Metabolic or endocrine disorder

—Hypercalcemia or hypokalemia may result in osmotic diuresis.
—Diabetes insipidus (nephrogenic or central)
  —Nocturia almost uniformly accompanied by daytime frequency
  —Also marked by high-volume output
—Diabetes mellitus: daytime frequency and/or nocturia associated with polydipsia, osmotic diuresis
—Hyperaldosteronism: nocturia often present but unlikely as an isolated symptom

• Tubulointerstitial disease

—Analgesics abuse, specific antibiotics, etc.

 Database

HISTORY

• Age and gender
• Duration of problem
• Change of overall well-being?

—Depression, stresses, anxieties, menstrual cycle abnormalities or menopause, chronic pain

• Details of nocturia

—Does patient awaken and *subsequently* void or awaken *because* of an urge to void?
—Times per night, volume per void, associated incontinence

• Associated daytime symptoms?

—Frequency, urgency, dysuria, hesitancy, straining, diminished force of stream, sensation of incomplete emptying

• Other new complaints

—Dyspnea, lower extremity swelling, weight loss, fatigue, change in bowel habits

• Other medical problems
• Surgical history, prior radiation
• Medications

—Time of dosing, especially diuretics

• Drinking habits

—Types, volume, timing

PHYSICAL EXAMINATION

• Overall disposition

—Anxious, depressed, obvious shortness of breath
—Other signs of systemic illness (fatigue, cachexia)

• Signs of volume overload

—Auscultation of lungs for crackles, rales, wheezes
—Dependent edema or signs of chronic venous insufficiency

• Palpable abdominal mass or suprapubic distention consistent with retention
• Digital rectal examination of the prostate, fecal impaction
• Pelvic examination

—Cystocele, urethral hypermobility, atrophy

• Global or focal neurologic deficits

Diagnostic Studies

LABORATORY TESTING

• Urine

—Dilute or concentrated (examine color and specific gravity)
—Microscopic urinalysis and culture, cytology only if clinically indicated
—Calculation of osmolality if necessary
  —Persistently low values (normal range: 50–1200 mOsmol/kg) suggest inappropriate water excretion.

• Hematologic

—Serum chemistries (electrolyte levels)
—Complete blood count (anemia may be secondary to volume overload or chronic disease process)
—Prostate specific antigen (PSA) if indicated

• Other specific tests

—Fractional excretion of sodium (in the azotemic patient)
—Urinary calcium:creatinine ratio

IMAGING

• Limited role in the evaluation of isolated nocturia
• A renal sonogram may demonstrate hydronephrosis in the obstructed patient or medical renal disease.
• Bladder sonogram with post-void volume determination for suspected retention
• Urethrogram if history suggests stricture

SPECIAL STUDIES

• Voiding diary

—Patient should record actual sleep hours, time of nocturia, volume, and any associated voiding symptoms associated with each episode (urgency, incontinence, quality of stream).
—The nighttime diary should be compared with a similar daytime diary to see if voiding patterns differ.
—May consider a log of fluid intake (type and quantity)

• Urodynamics

—With or without video (fluoroscopy), depending on working diagnosis
—Look for instability, measure capacity, check for residual, rule out obstruction (prostatic, bladder neck dysfunction or contracture, stricture), sensory urgency, stress incontinence.
—Prior to the study, the clinician must be aware of all of the patient's medications that may alter voiding dynamics.

• Cystoscopy

—Unlikely to add much information to diagnosis of isolated nocturia unless other pathology is suspected or found by laboratory or radiographic analysis

 ## Initial Management

• Management will depend on the assignment of the diagnosis to one of the three categories: sleep disorder, medical condition, or lower urinary tract dysfunction.

—Rarely will nocturia be the only symptom of lower urinary tract dysfunction, but it may be the only bothersome symptom.

• In the absence of any of these conditions, the patient may need no other treatment than reducing nighttime fluid intake, avoiding alcohol or caffeine in the evening, and voiding just prior to bedtime.

• Sleep disorder

—May need counseling regarding stress management or evaluation of mood disturbance
—Elderly patients may need to reduce daytime napping to improve nighttime sleep patterns.
  —Early-morning awakening and deprivation of stage IV of the sleep cycle is characteristic of aging.
—Medications that cause insomnia may need to be withdrawn or taken at alternative times.
—May need evaluation of sleep apnea
  —Partial: such as plain snoring, which can be minimized by avoiding alcohol, sedatives/hypnotics, or antihistamines in the evening hours, or by changing sleep positioning
  —Severe (pickwickian): requires weight reduction and possible otolaryngologic evaluation

• Medical condition

—Evaluation by internist, nephrologist, or cardiologist, etc., depending on the etiology of volume overload disorder or other medical condition
—Vascular referral for lymphedema or chronic venous insufficiency
—Change certain medications or alter the timing of administration (especially medications with a diuretic effect).

• Lower urinary tract dysfunction

—Consider all medications that may alter physiology.
—Outflow obstruction or retention with overflow (in the presence of adequate detrusor function) may be treated with the appropriate pharmacologic or surgical intervention.
  —Caution the patient that nocturia is often the last or only symptom to persist.
  —Relief of fecal impaction may be therapeutic.

—For instability, hyperreflexia, or diminished capacity, antimuscarinic or musculotropic agents are the mainstay primary treatment.
  —Although a trial is warranted, sensory urgency and impaired compliance respond less favorably.
—Stress-induced instability might respond to correction of the incontinence.
  —Conversely, exacerbation or de novo instability may result from correction of stress urinary incontinence.
—Postmenopausal women with atrophic vaginitis (poor urethral coaptation) may respond to topical or oral estrogen replacement therapy.
—Retention/overflow secondary to detrusor hypo- or areflexia may respond best to clean intermittent catheterization or an indwelling catheter in patients who are not eligible for CIC.

 ## Follow-Up

• There are no standard recommendations for the interval of follow-up.

—Will depend on the etiology of nocturia
—Urologic follow-up is not always warranted if the evaluation demonstrates no dangerous urologic pathology, an untreatable condition, a non-urologic condition that is best treated by another specialist, or treatment options to which the patient is not amenable.

 ## Miscellaneous

SYNONYMS: N/A

ASSOCIATED CONDITIONS: N/A

NOTES: N/A

ABBREVIATIONS: N/A

REFERENCES

Kirkland JL, Lye M, Levy DW, Banerjee AK. Patterns of urine flow and electrolyte excretion in healthy elderly people. *BMJ* 1983;287:1665.

Author: Marc W. Plawker

Pelvic Pain—Chronic Female

 Basics

DESCRIPTION

- Any type of pelvic pain that has lasted 6 months or longer
- Lacks apparent physical cause sufficient to explain the pain (laparoscopy disclosed minimal, if any, pathology)
- Accompanied by significantly altered physical activity, including work, recreation, sexual life, as well as disturbance of mood

PATHOPHYSIOLOGY

- The exact pathogenesis of pelvic pain is unclear; however, combined psychosocial alterations and nociceptive stimuli from tissue damage have led to a biopsychosocial model.
- Biologic events sufficient to initiate nociception

—Sexually transmitted diseases
—Endometriosis
—Recurrent bladder and vaginal infections
—Primary or secondary dyspareunia
—Alterations of bowel habits

- Alterations of lifestyles and relationships over time
- Anxiety and affective disorders

—Depression may accompany chronic pain.

- A circular interaction of these elements, creating a "vicious cycle"

RISK FACTORS

- Depression
- Prior sexual or physical abuse
- Previous diagnosis of PID; fourfold increased risk
- Chronic pain experience among first-degree family members

 Differential Diagnosis

- Irritable bowel syndrome, inflammatory bowel disease, diverticulitis
- Urethral syndrome, interstitial cystitis
- Endometriosis, PID, cervical stenosis
- Pelvic floor tension myalgia (constant painful contraction of levator musculature)

 Database

HISTORY

- A complete history must include a family history; a social background, including family and professional responsibilities; and a medical, gynecologic, and obstetric history; including the patient's sexual life.
- Any childhood or adult sexual and physical abuse
- Any emotional stressors present

—Effect on personal and professional functions
—Psychological consultation is helpful.
—Up to 70% of patients have sleep disorders.
—Up to 50% of patients have depression.

- Lifetime substance abuse

—Should include patient's visits to other physicians and use of pain medications

- Previous low-back trauma

—Rule out possible nerve or musculoskeletal damage.

- Previous abdominal or pelvic surgeries

—May suggest pelvic adhesive disease or abdominal wall trigger points from scars

- Site and radiation of pain

—Relation to posture, movement, menses, micturition, and defecation
—Presence of associated symptoms

- Onset, duration, and severity

—Need for analgesics

PHYSICAL EXAMINATION

- Abdominal examination

—Search for trigger points
—Gently pinching the abdominal wall or light touch with a cotton tip in the dermatomes T10-S5 may elicit a hyperesthetic dermatome.
—Deeper palpation in usual fashion; suprapubic tenderness should be differentiated from right and lower quadrant tenderness

- Back and musculoskeletal system

—Posture and gait may reveal scoliosis or lordosis as a cause of both back and subsequent pelvic pain.
—Low-back pain may be musculoskeletal in nature or referred from a pelvic condition.

- Pelvic examination should be performed in a stepwise fashion, proceeding from external to internal.

—Inspect vulva for lesions, irritation, trauma, or significant pelvic relaxation.
—Speculum examination with a Pederson (narrow) speculum
—Finger or one-handed pelvic palpation to identify muscular pain, tenderness of the urethra, base of bladder, vaginal fornix, and cervix
—Bimanual examination: Assess shape, direction, and mobility of uterus and adnexa and presence of associated masses or tenderness.
—Rectovaginal examination: Evaluate presence of induration or nodularity of rectovaginal septum, cul-de-sac, or uterosacral ligaments.

Diagnostic Studies

LABORATORY TESTING

- CBC

—Elevated white counts with shift suggest infection.

- ESR

—Elevated in subacute or chronic inflammation

- CA-125 level

—Elevated in endometriosis, PID, and malignant neoplasms

- Urine analysis

—Urine culture if urinalysis suggestive of infection
—Urine cytology if hematuria present and urine culture is negative

- Cervical cultures
- PAP smear

IMAGING

- Ultrasonography

—Transvaginal sonography permits evaluation of the uterus and adnexa.
—Renal and pelvic sonography in combination are useful in detecting pyeloureteral diseases and mullerian anomalies.

- Plain x-ray

—KUB can identify ureteral calculi or dermoid cyst.
—Spine and bony films are indicated when osteoarticular disease is suspected.

- Hysterosalpingography

—Useful in assessment of uterus and fallopian tubes

- Pelvic phlebography

—May document pelvic venous congestion

- Contrast radiography of the gastrointestinal tract, MRI, or CT may be useful in selected instances.

SPECIAL STUDIES

- Laparoscopy

—Sources differ on percentage and type of pathology seen on diagnostic laparoscopy.
—Published data indicate a disease entity in over 60% of patients with CPP, while various studies have found up to a 66% negative laparoscopy rate.
—The most common disease entities appear to be endometriosis (3%–47% prevalence) and pelvic adhesions.

 Initial Management

- Evaluation for CPP includes a detailed history and physical examination; in the absence of clinical signs and a normal pelvic examination, diagnostic imaging is rarely helpful.
- Ultrasonography may be helpful if the pelvic examination is not satisfactory.
- Additional testing is based on clinical findings.
- Laparoscopy is traditionally used for evaluation of pelvic pain.

—Negative findings do not exclude a somatic cause.
—And positive findings do not necessarily correspond to the cause of the pain.

- Multidisciplinary evaluation, including psychological and environmental factors

 Follow-Up

- Variable, dependent on findings of a somatic cause for pain

 Miscellaneous

SYNONYMS: N/A

ASSOCIATED CONDITIONS: N/A

NOTES

- Trigger points are superficial local areas of hyperesthesia that cause pain that may be referred, due to neurologic innervation of the pelvis and lower abdomen.

ABBREVIATIONS

- CA, cancer antigen; CPP, chronic pelvic pain; ESR, erythrocyte sedimentation rate; PID, pelvic inflammatory disease

REFERENCES

Milburn A, et al. Multidisciplinary approach to chronic pelvic pain. *Obstet Gynecol Clin North Am* 1993;20:643.

Porpora MG. The role of laparoscopy in the management of pelvic pain in women of reproductive age. *Fertil Steril* 1997;68:765.

Ryder RM. Chronic pelvic pain. *Am Fam Physician* 1996;54:2225.

Steege JF. Office assessment of chronic pelvic pain. *Clin Obstet Gynecol* 1997;40:554.

Steege JF. Chronic pelvic pain in women: Toward an integrative model. *Obstet Gynecol Surv* 1993;48:95.

Authors: Corlis L. Archer and Ashok K. Batra

Penis—Curvature and/or Pain

 Basics

DESCRIPTION

- Congenital curvature is known as *chordee*.
- Acquired curvature and pain most commonly due to Peyronie disease
- Peyronie disease prevalence approximately 1%; typically in men ages 40 to 60

—Curvature in 50% to 100% of patients
—Pain in 30% to 70%
—Palpable plaque present in 78% to 100%

PATHOPHYSIOLOGY

- Chordee is secondary to abnormal development of urethra, corporal tissue, Buck's fascia, or penile skin.
- Peyronie disease is secondary to inflammatory process in tunica albuginea; a tear leads to bleeding, fibrosis, collagen deposition, and scarring.

—Microtrauma to tunica during intercourse results in tears, especially at the junction of the tunica and corporal septum.
—25% of scars calcify.

RISK FACTORS

- Penile trauma, chronic irritation
- Injection therapy and vacuum devices for erectile dysfunction
- Dupuytren's contracture (fibrosis in hand): 3% to 10%
- Other connective tissue diseases: Ledderhose disease of plantar fascia, scleroderma, Paget bone disease
- Curvature due to scarring in corpora can result, with trauma, infection, and priapism.

 Differential Diagnosis

- Congenital curvature: ventral

—Hypospadias: One-third of cases have curvature, usually ventral.
—Chordee without hypospadias: 0.6% of boys have curvature with normal urethra.
—May also be due to short urethra

- Congenital curvature: dorsal or lateral

—Epispadias are often associated with dorsal curvature.
—Lateral curvature is due to skin asymmetry or disproportion of the corpora cavernosum.

- Acquired curvature secondary to trauma/scarring in skin, urethra, Buck's fascia, or tunica albuginea
- Peyronie disease: curvature, pain, tunical plaques, and sometimes erectile dysfunction
- Penile pain

—With Peyronie disease
—Nonbacterial prostatitis/prostatodynia
—Psychogenic

 Database

HISTORY

- Age of patient
- Onset of symptoms: related to traumatic incident?
- Duration of symptoms: important for determining appropriate therapy and timing of any surgical intervention

—Assess for degree of angulation.
—Dorsal/ventral/lateral
—Does curvature interfere with sexual activity?

- Presence of palpable plaque
- Presence and duration of pain

—Pain may resolve prior to other symptoms.
—Avoid surgery during a painful period.

- Erectile function: important for determining successful treatment
- Other medical diseases: especially connective tissue diseases as above.
- Previous genital/pelvic surgery
- Medications or illegal drugs

—At one time, beta-blockers were felt to be causative, but currently are not implicated.

PHYSICAL EXAMINATION

- Circumcised or uncircumcised penis
- General assessment of penile length

—Plication/Nesbit procedures associated with loss of penile length
—Plaque incisions/excision with grafting better for preserving penile length

- Palpation for plaques

—Glans penis held on stretch
—Shaft palpated with other hand
—Assess location; often dorsal midline
—Assess for size/extent/multifocal plaques.
—Hourglass deformities

- Check for associated diseases such as Dupuytren's contracture of hands.

Diagnostic Studies

LABORATORY TESTING: N/A

IMAGING

- Plain films

—Can perform ventral/dorsal and lateral views to assess position and size of plaques
—Low kilovoltage recommended

- Duplex ultrasound

—Can measure plaque size and location
—Used with Doppler and pharmacologic injection, can determine penile blood flow and response to medication
—Assess degree of curvature with erection.

- Cavernosography/cavernosometry can be used to further assess erectile function when history and ultrasound are inconclusive.

SPECIAL STUDIES

- Patient photos

—Polaroid photos documenting curvature from dorsal, lateral, and frontal views are very helpful.

- Nocturnal penile tumescence studies.

—May be helpful in assessing erectile function and determining if there is a psychological component of problem

 Initial Management

- Conservative treatment of Peyronie disease is the best initial step.

—Disease should be stable for 12 months prior to surgical intervention.
—Pain may decrease/resolve after the initial period.

- Medical treatment

—Vitamin E 400 IU bid is the most favored initial treatment.
  —Low cost
  —No significant toxicity
  —Up to two-thirds of patients will have improvement or resolution.
—Potassium aminobenzoate (POTABA) is also used but is expensive and requires large doses.
—Colchicine and tamoxifen are also reported as effective but not proven in placebo-controlled studies.

- Intralesional injections have been advocated by some, but it is unclear whether plaque resolution is due to a mechanical or pharmacologic effect.
- Pain has been controlled with nonsteroidal antiinflammatories and antihistamines.
- Psychological counseling/couples therapy has been beneficial.
- Treatment of chordee requires surgery.

—Best performed prior to age 2 for psychological reasons
—May require release of chordee/urethra, one-stage urethroplasty, or plication of tunica albuginea

 Follow-Up

- Surgical treatment is indicated for curvature interfering with sexual activity.

—Plication/Nesbit procedures straighten penis and do not interfere with erectile function, but result in loss of penile length.
—Plaque incision or excision with graft placement is also very successful.

- Higher risk of erectile dysfunction than plication, but preserves length and is therefore best for shorter penises
- Graft materials include dermal patch, vein, tunica vaginalis, Gore-Tex and Dacron.
- Can be combined with venous ligation surgery or placement of penile prosthesis.

—Placement of prosthesis with or without plaque incision/grafting has been used to straighten the penis.

- Penile modeling can be used to crack plaques and straighten the penis with the prosthesis inflated.
- The patient should be reminded that the goal of therapy is to restore sexual function and to avoid expectations of a perfect penis postoperatively.
- Pain unresponsive to medical management has been relieved with ultrasound or low-dose radiation. However, radiation has resulted in penile fibrosis/scarring.

 Miscellaneous

SYNONYMS

- Chordee

ASSOCIATED CONDITIONS

- Dupuytren contracture

NOTES

- See also Section II, "Chordee" and "Peyronie Disease."

ABBREVIATIONS: N/A

REFERENCES

Ehrich, Alter, eds. *Reconstructive and Plastic Surgery of External Genitalia.* Philadelphia: WB Saunders, 1998.

Jordon GH, Schlossberg SM, Devine CJ Jr. Peyronie's disease. In: Lytton B, et al., eds. *Advances in Urology,* vol. 8. St Louis: Mosby-Year Book, 1995.

Levine LA, Eterman L. Peyronie's disease and its medical management. In: Hellstrom W, ed. *Male Infertility and Sexual Dysfunction.* New York: Springer, 1997.

Author: Mark L. Fallick

Penis—Lesion

 Basics

DESCRIPTION

- Can occur in either adult or pediatric population
- Oftentimes occurs in conjunction with cutaneous lesions elsewhere
- May be a manifestation of systemic, sexually transmitted, or metastatic disease

PATHOPHYSIOLOGY

- Many lesions resemble each other. Therefore, a careful history and physical are essential.
- A correct diagnosis may require biopsy and/or laboratory evaluations.
- Descriptive terms for the lesions include *erythema, patch, nodule, papule, bulla, erosion, vesicle, scale, crust,* and others.

RISK FACTORS

- Recent trauma, sexual contact (heterosexual and homosexual), change in laundry/bath soaps or lotions, recurrent infections, use of medications, contact with animal or plant life, family history, degree of personal hygiene, and others

 Differential Diagnosis

- In adults, lesions can occur in either circumcised or uncircumcised males. In children, the vast majority of penile lesions are found in uncircumcised males.
- Papulosquamous disorders. A scaly lesion on an erythematous base

—Psoriasis: affects about 1% of the population; is a hyperproliferation of the epidermis, begins generally in the third decade and can be lifelong. Genital involvement rarely occurs without nongenital disease.
—Seborrheic dermatitis: most often found on hair-bearing regions, can cause a lifetime of exacerbation and remission
—Lichen planus: a pruritic inflammatory disease. When present on the genitalia, it most often affects the glans penis.
—Lichen nitidus: very small, flat-topped papules. They can be flesh-colored, pink, or yellow-red. Cause is unknown.
—Reiter syndrome: most commonly affecting immunocompromised individuals. It is a systemic illness as a result of *Gonococcus, Chlamydia, Yersinia, Shigella, Campylobacter, Neisseria,* or *Ureaplasma.*
—Lichen sclerosis: In later stages, it becomes balanitis xerotica obliterans. Patients with this tend to have a high prevalence of autoimmune diseases.
—Fixed drug eruption: a reaction to parenterally administered medication. A lesion tends to occur in the same location with each challenge.

- Eczematous (allergic) dermatitis. usually involving the outer layer of skin, appearing red and weepy, with or without crusting

—Eczema: a set of cutaneous illnesses that lead to epidermal damage. The cause is unknown. The lesions are red and scaly and tend to weep and form yellow crusts.
—Contact dermatitis: the response by the skin to an externally applied allergen. The response may take several days to manifest itself, but is most often immediate in nature. The lesions are a result of a localized inflammation that produces scales and crust formation.
—Erythema multiforme: can be minor or major variants. The major variant is Stevens-Johnson syndrome, and is manifested by targetoid lesions, blisters, and mucosal membrane involvement.

- Vestibulobullous disorders

—Bullous pemphigoid: an immune-mediated blistering, most commonly found in the elderly
—Pemphigus vulgaris: an IgG-mediated blistering of the skin, directed at keratinocytes
—Dermatitis herpetiformis: an IgA-mediated blistering of the skin, directed at the basement membrane

- Ulcers: These are lesions that extend into the dermis, and are most commonly related to sexually transmitted diseases.

—Pyoderma gangrenosum: a chronic, painful ulcer associated with the cutaneous manifestations of Crohn disease, ulcerative colitis, or collagen vascular disease
—Traumatic ulcers: may be secondary to sexual activity, body ornamentation, or cleansing techniques
—Sexually transmitted diseases: includes herpes simplex, primary syphilis, chancroid, lymphogranuloma venereum, and granuloma inguinale. The diagnosis is based on specific tests that will appear later in this section.
—Behçet disease: a syndrome comprised of oral and genital ulceration, uveitis, and nonmucous membrane skin lesions. Lesions are painful, and one must rule out other forms of ulcerative lesions, as the treatment is more supportive in nature than the sexually transmitted ulcerative lesions.

- Malignancy: local and metastatic

—Bowen disease (squamous cell carcinoma in situ/erythroplasia of Queyrat): sharply demarcated erythematous plaques. The lesions may be present for months to years prior to the patient seeking medical attention.
—Squamous cell carcinoma: can be a fungating lesion, most often seen in uncircumcised individuals. Poor hygiene and recurrent infections may be predisposing factors.
—Bowenoid papulosis: resembles squamous cell carcinoma in situ, occurring usually in the third and fourth decades of life and associated with human papillomavirus infections.
—Kaposi's sarcoma: associated with herpes virus and AIDS (3% of males with HIV present with this lesion).

—Melanoma: commonly found on the glans penis. Lesions may be blue, red, black, brown, or nonpigmented and have an irregular border.
—Basal cell carcinoma: the most common cutaneous malignancy, but the penis is an uncommon location
—Verrucous carcinoma: also known as Buschke-Lowenstein tumor; a variant of squamous cell carcinoma; incidence of 20% to 25% of all penile tumors
—Extramammary Paget disease: if on the genitalia, can be associated with malignancies of the urethra, bladder, rectum, and sweat glands

- Infections/infestations

—Erythrasma: may appear like tinea cruris ("jock itch"), but is due to a member of the Corynebacteriaceae
—Balanoposthitis: inflammation of the glans and foreskin, occurring exclusively in uncircumcised males of any age. Recurrent episodes may lead to phimosis.
—Folliculitis: an infection of the follicles in hair-bearing areas
—Furunculosis: otherwise known as a "boil," is a red, tender, fluctuant pustule or abscess
—Genital warts: most commonly associated with HPV types 6 and 11. Passage of this lesion to a female may lead to cervical carcinoma.
—Pediculosis pubis: infestation with the crab louse
—Scabies: infestation with the mite *Sarcoptes scabiei.* The pruritus resulting from this infestation is so severe, excoriation may be what is initially identified on examination.
—Molluscum contagiosum: results from a virus related to the pox family; requires skin-to-skin contact

- Common benign lesions

—Pearly penile papules: commonly seen in uncircumcised males, are the small, raised papules that encircle the corona
—Angiokeratoma of Fordyce: small ectasias of the dermal blood vessels; may cause concern due to periodic bleeding
—Cysts: most commonly are epidermal inclusion cysts, and can be postsurgical in nature, following circumcision or hypospadias repair.
—Phimosis: the inability to retract the foreskin; may be a manifestation of a systemic illness, such as diabetes
—Penile melanosis: pigmented papule of the penis, difficult to distinguish from melanoma
—Sclerosing lymphangitis: commonly associated with sexual activity and is a translucent, cordlike lesion
—Zoon's balanitis: a patchlike lesion seen only in uncircumcised men, and must be differentiated from squamous cell carcinoma in situ
—Balanitis xerotica obliterans: contraction and fixation of the foreskin to the glans
—Vitiligo: sharp depigmentation of the skin, which results in patches of varying size

Database

HISTORY

• Age of the patient?

—Children most commonly will have balanoposthitis or phimosis.
—Adults will require a thorough history and physical.

• History of trauma?
• Sexual practices: homosexual, heterosexual, promiscuity (greater than one partner), sexual contact with any cutaneous or mucosal lesions?
• Family history of dermatologic disorders?
• History of similar lesions?
• History of systemic illness?
• History of change in laundry/bath soaps or lotion?
• History of sharing of clothing with another who demonstrates symptoms consistent with dermatologic disease?
• Any friends or social contacts with similar symptoms? (infestation among children)
• History of contact with strange plants, strange animals or insects?
• Associated with a urethral discharge?
• Associated with pruritus?
• Associated with pain?
• Length of time of symptoms?
• History of blood transfusion?
• Types of self-treatments attempted?
• History of cancer?
• History of medication use?
• Occupational risk factors: chemical/industrial exposure?
• Recent travel?

PHYSICAL EXAMINATION

• Thorough dermatologic examination of the body

—Like lesions elsewhere on the body (eczema, seborrheic dermatitis)?
—Are the skin folds/pubic region involved as well (fungal infection, infestation)?

• Circumcised/uncircumcised
• Can the foreskin be retracted?
• Is the foreskin fixed to the glans?
• Urethral discharge

—Sexually transmitted disease

• Character of the lesion

—Macular, papular
—Raised, smooth
—Erythematous, patchy, scaly, weepy, bullous
—Nodular, plaque, vesicle, pustule, ulcerative
—Fungating, painful, color of lesion(s)

• Adenopathy

 Diagnostic Studies

LABORATORY TESTING

• Urinalysis
• Urethral swab for Gram stain and culture
• Serum chemistry profile

—Diabetes is occasionally diagnosed in phimosis

• HIV

—Kaposi's sarcoma

IMAGING: N/A

SPECIAL STUDIES

• Aspiration

—Pap smears can identify intranuclear inclusions.
—Cytologic examination

• Incisional/excisional biopsy (to include punch biopsy)

—Viral culture (HSV, etc.)
—Special stains (IgG, IgA, immunofluorescent, etc.)
—Level of depth of lesion
—Tzanck preps (molluscum contagiosum, herpes, varicella)
—Pathologic examination of specimen

• Tzanck preps
• Immunofluorescence
• Potassium hydroxide preps
• Antibody stains

 Initial Management

• Diagnosis can be made in the majority of cases by history and physical examination.
• If infectious, choose an antibiotic based on the differential.
• Change medications, if implicated.
• Change soaps/lotions.
• Consider circumcision, if indicated.
• Aspirate/biopsy
• Consider topical steroids/tar-based medication.
• Acetic acid prep

 Follow-Up

• Examination should be followed up, depending on initial therapy.
• If oncologic, follow-up should be individualized, based on diagnosis.
• If associated with HIV, follow-up should also be based on level of disease.

 Miscellaneous

SYNONYMS: N/A

ASSOCIATED CONDITIONS: N/A

NOTES

• See also Section II, "Balanitis Xerotica Obliterans" and "Balanitis and Balanoposthitis," and specific sexually transmitted diseases.

ABBREVIATIONS: N/A

REFERENCES

Berger RE. Sexually transmitted diseases: The classic triad. In: Walsh PC, et al., eds. *Campbell's Urology,* 7th ed. Philadelphia: WB Saunders, 1998.

Krieger JN. Acquired immunodeficiency syndrome and related conditions. In: Walsh PC, et al., eds. *Campbell's Urology,* 7th ed. Philadelphia: WB Saunders, 1998.

Margolis DJ. Cutaneous diseases of the male external genitalia. In: Walsh PC, et al., eds. *Campbell's Urology,* 7th ed. Philadelphia: WB Saunders, 1998.

Authors: Dennis S. Peppas and Judd Moul

Penis—Trauma and Fracture

 Basics

DESCRIPTION

• Classified into five categories (Culp):

—Nonpenetrating: blunt trauma, contusions, and fracture of the corpora/urethra
—Penetrating: punctures, lacerations, gunshot wounds, and amputations (self or traumatic)
—Avulsions: traumatic emasculations, degloving injuries of the penis, etc.
—Burns: thermal, electrical, and chemical
—Radiation: direct vs. indirect

PATHOPHYSIOLOGY

• The position and mobility of the penis is a natural defense against traumatic injury.
• Penile layers: skin; dartos fascia; Buck's fascia; tunica albuginea
• Tunica albuginea: barrier against intrusion

RISK FACTORS

• Frequent vigorous sexual intercourse (penile corporal/urethral disruption)
• Proximity to rotating machinery (industrial, garden, or farming equipment): avulsion injury, amputation, etc.
• Athletes (football, hockey, basketball, etc.): blunt trauma

 Differential Diagnosis

• Penile fracture: disruption of tunica albuginea and corpora cavernosum

—Most commonly: result of vigorous intercourse or patient rolling over on erect penis during sleep
—Often feeling and hearing snap followed by penile swelling and pain
—Buck's fascia is often disrupted; with hematoma confined by dartos fascia.
—20% associated urethral disruption; retrograde urethrogram for confirmation
—Early diagnosis and treatment: minimize scarring and penile deviation

• Penile contusion
• Penile laceration: clean vs. contaminated
• Avulsion (e.g., degloving injury): clothes get entangled in rotating machinery or use of suction device for sexual arousal

—Skin and dartos layer are often the only layers involved.
—Urethra: should be evaluated with retrograde urethrogram

• Amputation of penis: ultimate penile injury

—Immediate microvascular reimplant (i.e., Wayne Bobbitt)
—Consider time elapsed since injury, the care given to the amputated penis, and severity of injury.

• Burns: similar to that for any burn
• Radiation injury

—Direct radiation therapy for a penile lesion
—Radiation to pelvis or pelvic lymph node dissection with chronic lymphedema
—Involves dartos fascia and the dermis layer of the skin

 Database

HISTORY

• Careful, detailed history regarding events pre- and postinjury

—Penile fracture
—Recent vigorous intercourse?
—Distinct pop or snap heard before onset of swelling/pain?
—Difficulty voiding or blood at urethral meatus?
—Penile laceration/avulsion/amputation
—Clean or contaminated?
—Time elapsed since injury?
—Difficulty voiding or any urethral bleeding?
—For amputation injury: Documented care of the amputated penis is important (storage, proper cooling, etc.).

PHYSICAL EXAMINATION

• GU examination (including abdomen, penile, scrotal, and rectal)

—Is the skin intact, or is there any discoloration?
—Presence of hematoma?
—Blood at the urethral meatus suggests urethral injury.

• Burns: classified by burn depth (body surface area)

—Genitalia represent approximately 1% of total body surface area (BSA)
—First-degree burns primarily involve the epidermis.
—Appear pink to red (no blisters)
—Second-degree burns involve the epidermis and dermis.
—Superficial dermal burns: characteristic bullae; hypersensitive; skin remains elastic; heal within 2 weeks
—Deep dermal burns: more severe; skin less elastic and is hyposensitive; may result in hypertrophic scar; usually heal by 3 weeks
—Third-degree burns: involve full-thickness dermis; pearly white or charred appearance; sensation absent

Diagnostic Studies

LABORATORY TESTING

• Not usually needed, unless extensive blood loss; check CBC

IMAGING

• Retrograde urethrogram if suspicious of urethral injury

—Evaluates anterior urethra (penile, bulbar, membranous)
—Foley catheter into distal urethra until balloon disappears; fill balloon with 1 to 2 cc of water
—Plain film in right posterior oblique position while injecting 30 to 40 cc of half-strength contrast

SPECIAL STUDIES: N/A

Initial Management

• Penile contusion: bedrest, ice pack, elevation of penis, analgesia
• Penile laceration: primary suture repair if wound is clean

—If contaminated, open dressing; delayed primary closure

• Penile fracture: immediate exploration; repair corpus cavernosum

—Deglove penis; evacuate hematoma; repair tunica albuginea with 2-0 absorbable suture, inverted knots
—Urethral injury: 4-0 or 5-0 absorbable suture; Foley catheter 7 to 14 days
—Close all layers of the penis.

• Avulsion injury: skin usually removed on an avascular plane; limits blood loss

—Small: primary closure (clean) or delayed (contaminated)
—Large: cool saline packs; keep tissue moist
  —Debride distal skin; excise to level of coronal sulcus; distal penile skin prone to chronic lymphedema
  —If unable to mobilize tissue for coverage, apply split-thickness skin graft (0.15 cm).

• Penile amputation: Cold ischemia allows for reimplantation up to 18 to 24 hours.

—Tourniquet base of penis to control bleeding; reimplant as soon as possible
—Amputated piece: clean, sterile bag with saline solution; bag placed on ice for transport
—Microsurgical technique
  —Two-layer urethral reanastomosis (urethral mucosa and spongiosa fascia)
  —Repair corpora cavernosa with 2-0 absorbable suture (Dexon).
  —Reanastomosis: two dorsal penile arteries, the vein, and as many nerves as possible; 8-0 to 11-0 nonabsorbable suture
  —If skin contaminated: excise and split-thickness skin graft
—Unable to find the amputated penis: partial penectomy

• Penile burns: initial management by burn team (BSA, fluid requirements, etc.)

—Limit debridement: The penis is highly vascular and heals well.
—Topical antibiotic cream using sterile technique
—Chemical burns: usually superficial
  —Flush with sterile water and treat as a thermal burn.
—Electric burn: can be serious injury
  —Injury to deep penile structures despite appearance of minimal skin injury ("tip of the iceberg")
  —Conservative treatment for the first 18 to 24 hours; divert urine with suprapubic catheter
  —After, debride to the point of viable tissue; often needs reconstruction

• Radiation injury

—Chronic suppurative gangrene: partial penectomy and reconstruction
—Chronic lymphedema
  —Excise the edematous tissue (skin and dartos fascia) to Buck's fascia; excise distally to the coronal sulcus.
  —Apply a split-thickness skin graft.

Follow-Up

• Penile fracture: wound check, 7 to 10 days

—If urethral injury: periurethrogram to exclude extravasation before Foley removal
—Follow for possible chordee from the fibrosis.

• Avulsions/severe lacerations/amputation: check viability of tissue; debridement, grafting, dressing changes, as needed
• Burns: follow for skin contractures; may need release or skin graft

—Reconstruction, if required, after healing complete

Miscellaneous

SYNONYMS: N/A

ASSOCIATED CONDITIONS: N/A

NOTES: N/A

ABBREVIATIONS

• BSA, body surface area; RUG, retrograde urethrogram

REFERENCES

Dixon CM. Genitourinary trauma. *Spec Rev Urol* 1997;292–294.

Jordan GH, et al. Surgery of the penis and urethra. In: Walsh PC, Retik AB, Stamey TA, Vaughn ED Jr, eds. *Campbell's Urology*, 7th ed. Philadelphia: WB Saunders, 1997:3338.

Jordan GH, et al. Male genital trauma. AUA Updates Series, Vol 4, Lesson 20, 1985.

McAnich JW. Management of genital skin loss. *Urol Clin North Am* 11989;6:369.

Sagalowsky AI, et al. Genitourinary trauma. In: Walsh PC, Retik AB, Stamey TA, Vaughn ED Jr, eds. *Campbell's Urology*, 7th ed. Philadelphia: WB Saunders, 1997:3114.

Authors: Sunil K. Purohit and Wayne J.G. Hellstrom

Perineal Pain

 Basics

DESCRIPTION

- Perineal pain encompasses symptomatology related to a multitude of pathologies.
- Perineal symptoms could point to major underlying pathology.
- Vague, nonspecific, and chronic symptoms may be attributed to nondescript diagnoses, such as prostatodynia.
- Usually found in male patients

PATHOPHYSIOLOGY

- Since the perineal innervation is cross-linked from L5 to S4 nerve roots, a variety of pathologies could present as perineal pain.
- Important to distinguish patients who are at risk for a major pathology

RISK FACTORS

- Diabetes mellitus: Patients are prone to infective processes, such as Fournier's gangrene.
- Urethral stricture disease: Patient's are prone to perineal abscesses and urethrocutaneous fistula.
- Rectal pathology: Associated problems, such as rectal fissure, can masquerade as prostatic pathology.

 Differential Diagnosis

- Congenital
—Persistent prostatic utricle
- Traumatic
—Rectal fissures
—Urethral stricture disease (USD), urethral diverticulum, urethrocutaneous fistula
- Inflammatory
—Prostatitis
—Urethritis
—Abscess (Fournier's gangrene, especially in diabetics)
—Skin rash, abscesses, etc.
—Urinary tract infection
- Neoplastic
—Perineal skin cancer
—Malignant lesions, such as carcinoma of the prostate (rare)
- Other
—Bladder stones
—Rarely, lower ureteral stones may present with referred pain in the external genitalia.
—Post operative (radical prostatectomy, etc.)

 Database

HISTORY

- Age and sex of patients
—Usually present in male patients
—Of the above-mentioned traumatic and inflammatory causes, the patients are usually young, in their 20s, 30s, or 40s.
—Females with perineal pain usually initially present to a gynecologist.

- Diagnostic criteria: Clinical presentation could vary from an acute process, such as an abscess formation, to chronic perineal pain secondary to long-standing chronic prostatitis. Clinical correlation is essential to rule out an acute and potentially life-threatening presentation.
- Fever and chills may be associated with acute prostatitis and/or abscess formation in the perineum. Close monitoring of these patients is essential.
- If infection is left undrained or untreated, the patient could present with impending sepsis or progression of his abscess.

PHYSICAL EXAMINATION

- If the perineum and scrotum are normal, then transrectal evaluation of the prostate is recommended. If acute prostatitis is suspected and the perineum is normal on inspection, rectal examination should be judicious, since it might aggravate the acute prostatitis episode.
- If perineal examination reveals an inflammation or an abscess, prompt management, such as drainage and/or debridement is recommended.

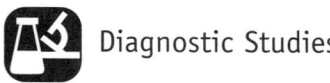 Diagnostic Studies

LABORATORY TESTING

- Urine analysis may be suggestive of pyuria and/or urinary tract infection.
- If a patient is diagnosed as having chronic prostatitis, further evaluations, such as urine cultures using the VB1, VB2, and VB3 specimens, are recommended (pre- and postprostatic massage).
- A blood sugar evaluation should diagnose diabetes.
- An elevated white blood cell count can point toward an infective process.

IMAGING

- Plain x-ray of the abdomen and pelvis should reveal presence of bladder or lower ureteral calculi.
- Contrast studies, such as retrograde urethrogram, will diagnose conditions such as urethral stricture disease, fistula, or other associated perineal pathology.
- Bladder ultrasound can diagnose conditions such as calculi, presence of enlarged prostate, etc.

SPECIAL STUDIES

- Cystoscopy to evaluate any urethral, prostatic, or bladder pathology may be indicated.
- Anoscopy can evaluate for any associated rectal pathology, such as fissures or internal hemorrhoids.
- Transrectal ultrasound of the prostate: Caution is advised in the presence of acute prostatitis.
- Expressed prostatic secretions (EPS) are normal with negative urine analysis in patients with nonbacterial prostatitis and prostatodynia.
- Specialized cultures for mycoplasma and ureaplasma may be indicated.
- Video-urodynamic studies: Most patients with prostatodynia may have "spastic" dysfunction of the bladder neck, depressed urinary flow rates, incomplete relaxation of the bladder neck and prostatic urethra, and abnormally high maximal urethral closure pressures at rest.

 Initial Management

- Prostatitis, appropriate urinary cultures as described above, followed by a course of antibiotics is recommended. Fluoroquinolones are considered the initial treatment of choice.
- If an infective process is found (abscess, etc.), this must be drained. Any necrotic tissue must be excised and appropriate systemic antibiotic usage initiated.
- Any rectal pathology should be treated appropriately.
- Any other pathology, such as calculus disease, suspected to be the cause of the perineal pain should be managed.
- If the patient has chronic prostatitis requiring frequent office visits with negative urine cultures, secondary modalities, such as use of alpha-blockers, dietary restrictions (discontinue stimulants such as caffeine, alcohol, etc.), or judicious use of transurethral microwave thermotherapy (TUMT), is recommended.
- Inadequately treated conditions will tend to recur.

 Follow-Up

- Acute prostatitis is followed up to rule out any additional pathology, such as urethral stricture disease, UTI, etc.
- Infective processes, such as Fournier's gangrene, should be carefully monitored for adequate healing and for control of any other factors, such as diabetes mellitus, urethral stricture disease, etc.

 Miscellaneous

SYNONYMS: N/A

ASSOCIATED CONDITIONS

- USD, diabetes mellitus, Fournier's gangrene

NOTES

- Initial history and physical examination are critical.
- Minor complaints of perineal pain or discomfort may be a precursor to a major underlying problem.
- Careful follow-up is important.

ABBREVIATIONS

- USD, urethral stricture disease; EPS, expressed prostatic secretions

REFERENCES

Barbalias GE, Meares EM Jr, Sant GR. Prostatodynia: Clinical and urodynamic characteristics. *J Urol* 1983;130:514–517.

Clayton MD, Fowler JE Jr, Sharifi R. Causes, presentation, and survival of 57 patients with necrotizing fasciitis of the male genitalia. *Surg Gynecol Obstet* 1990;170:49–55.

McCallum RW. The adult male urethra: normal anatomy, pathology, and method of urethrography. *Radiol Clin North Am* 1979;17:227–244.

Meares EM Jr. Acute and chronic prostatitis: Diagnosis and treatment. *Infect Dis Clin North Am* 1987;1:855–1873.

Neal DE Jr, Moon TD. Use of terazosin in prostatodynia and validation of a symptom score questionnaire. *Urology* 1994;43:460–465.

Paty R, Smith AD. Gangrene and Fournier's gangrene. *Urol Clin North Am* 1992;1(19):149–162.

Author: Raju Thomas

Pneumaturia

 Basics

DESCRIPTION

- Defined as the passage of gas per urethra
- Uncommon symptom, which usually prompts thorough investigation
- Evaluation aims to distinguish between a gas-forming UTI and a fistula between the GI and urinary tracts.

PATHOPHYSIOLOGY

- Pneumaturia may be simply the result of instrumentation but is associated with pathology in vast majority of cases.

—The most common source of gas is a fistula from the GI tract.
—Urinary stasis and glucosuria may promote growth of gas-forming organisms.
—Trauma, instrumentation may introduce gas into the bladder.

RISK FACTORS

- Diverticulitis

—Fistula from sigmoid colon to bladder typical

- Inflammatory bowel disease

—Crohn disease typically causes fistula from ileum to bladder; ulcerative colitis less likely to cause fistula

- Gas-forming UTI often associated with diabetes mellitus (DM)
- Pelvic malignancy, prior irradiation

 Differential Diagnosis

- Inflammatory/infectious: diverticulitis; Crohn disease; UTI (emphysematous cystitis)
- Neoplastic: carcinoma of the bladder, colon, cervix, or ovaries; role of BPH less clear
- Iatrogenic: postoperative; catheterization
- Trauma

 Database

HISTORY

- Fever, chills are nonspecific.
- Fecaluria, GI symptoms suggest enterovesical fistula.
- Hematuria suggests malignancy.
- Abdominal pain most consistent with Crohn
- Any recent instrumentation, surgery?
- History of bowel disease, especially Crohn, diverticulitis?
- History of pelvic malignancy?
- Prior radiation therapy?
- History of DM?

—Associated peripheral/autonomic neuropathy?

PHYSICAL EXAMINATION

- Fever with diverticulitis, cancer, UTI
- Abdominal tenderness with diverticulitis, Crohn
- Pelvic mass may be distended bladder
- Flank tenderness with pyelonephritis
- Digital rectal examination: tender prostate with acute prostatitis; mass may be palpable in rectal or bladder CA

Diagnostic Studies

• Note: Gas-forming UTI is a diagnosis of exclusion.

LABORATORY TESTING

• Urinalysis: Particulate matter or rhabdomyocytes suggests fistula.
• Urine culture nonspecific: positive in 100% of UTIs, 88% of fistulas

—*E. coli, Enterobacter aerogenes* found in >80% of gas-forming UTIs

• WBC elevated in half of patients with fistulas; variable in gas-forming UTIs
• Electrolytes, BUN, creatinine usually normal in fistula patients

—Serum glucose, creatinine may be elevated in patients with DM.

IMAGING

• CT of abdomen/pelvis best first test (diagnostic in 60%–90%)

—Can detect gas in bladder, pelvic mass, inflammation

• Cystography, barium enema used selectively depending on history and CT findings
• IVU generally not helpful

SPECIAL STUDIES (TO DETECT FISTULA)

• Cystoscopy typically demonstrates edema, erythema around the fistula tract.
• Colonoscopy generally nondiagnostic
• Bourne test

—Plain film of urine after barium enema

• Charcoal test

—Ingested orally; urine examined 12 to 48 hours later; paper stone filter useful to identify charcoal residue
—Diagnostic in 50% to 100% of cases

• Neither the Bourne test nor the charcoal test identifies the site of fistula.

 ## Initial Management

• Enterovesical fistula: Identify site and underlying etiology.

—Modern antibiotics, bowel prep, and nutritional support allow for one-stage repair in most cases.

• Gas-forming UTI

—Organism-specific antibiotic treatment; treat underlying obstruction if present; UDS may be indicated if bladder dysfunction secondary to DM suspected

 ## Follow-Up

• Urine cultures, urinalysis, symptom assessment for gas-forming UTIs
• Repeat studies following definitive treatment in enterovesical fistula patients generally unnecessary

 ## Miscellaneous

SYNONYMS: N/A

ASSOCIATED CONDITIONS: N/A

NOTES

• See also Section I, "Fistula—Enterovesical," and Section II, "Cystitis—Emphysematous," "Inflammatory Bowel Disease—Urologic Considerations."

ABBREVIATIONS: N/A

REFERENCES

Glick SH, Low RK, Fishman JR. Evaluation of pneumaturia. *Infect Urol* 1994;Jan/Feb:7–10.

Goldman SM, Fishman EK, Gatewood OMB. CT in the diagnosis of enterovesical fistulae. *Am J Radiol* 1985;144:1229–1233.

Kirsch GM, Hampel N, Shuck JM, Resnick MI. Diagnosis and management of vesicoenteric fistulas. *Surg Gynecol Obstet* 1991;173:91–97.

McNamara MJ, Fazio VW, Lavery IC, Weakley FL, Farmer RG. Surgical treatment of enterovesical fistulas in Crohn's disease. *Dis Colon Rectum* 1990;33:271–276.

Pontari MA, McMillen MA, Garvey RH, Ballantyne GH. Diagnosis and treatment of enterovesical fistula. *Am Surg* 1992;58:258–263.

Author: Francis X. Keeley, Jr.

Polyhydramnios/Oligohydramnios

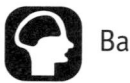 ## Basics

DESCRIPTION

- Abnormal amniotic fluid volume (AFV)

—Increased incidence of fetal and neonatal morbidity and mortality

- AFV historically determined by uterine fundal height for fetal age
- Currently, ultrasound and other methods are used to determine AFV.
- Brace and Wolf plotted the AFV change and gestational age using dilution and direct measurement.

—2.5% of pregnancies are at the end of the spectrum (i.e., polyhydramnios or oligohydramnios).

- Polyhydramnios: excessive amniotic fluid relative to gestational age, or >2000 mL at 30 weeks of gestation

—Associated with fetal gastrointestinal or CNS anomalies
—Incidence: 0.4% (clinical assessment), 1% (ultrasound)
—Usually found in second trimester; as rapid accumulation of fluid (acute polyhydramnios)
—Chronic polyhydramnios (more common) usually evident in the third trimester
—40% of polyhydramnios have normal AFV at term; no increased fetal or maternal morbidity
—With persistent polyhydramnios, 35% show fetal malformation; 10% show a karyotypic anomaly.

- Oligohydramnios: reduced AVF; <300 mL at 30 weeks

—Associated with fetal renal anomalies and severe obstructive uropathy
—Associated with pulmonary hypoplasia and fetal compression anomalies
—Incidence: 0.5 to 5.5%
—Acute oligohydramnios: usually PROM
—Chronic oligohydramnios: fetal anomalies or placental insufficiency

PATHOPHYSIOLOGY

- AF provides a supportive environment for fetal development.

—Allows for fetal movement, musculoskeletal and pulmonary development
—Protects the fetus and umbilical cord

- After the sixteenth week of gestation, AF production reflects fetal urine production.

—The fetus swallows AF, and fetal urine becomes amniotic fluid.
—At term, fetus produces 500 to 700 mL urine; fetus swallows 1000 mL of fluid/d; balance returned to mother via placenta

- AFV increases through pregnancy and plateaus at 33 weeks.
- At term, the AVF averages 700 to 800 mL; at postterm, it decreases to 500 to 550 mL.
- Polyhydramnios: abnormal swallowing mechanism, faulty fetal formation or release of antidiuretic hormone in fetuses with CNS anomalies

—Causes: maternal (15%), fetal (13%), or idiopathic (67%)
—Maternal causes: glucose intolerance (causes fetal polyuria), infections (syphilis, rubella, cytomegalovirus, toxoplasmosis, and parvovirus), isoimmunization, fetomaternal hemorrhage
—Fetal causes: abnormalities of CNS, GI, respiratory, cardiovascular systems, fetal renal hamartoma, twin–twin transfusion

- Oligohydramnios: inadequate fetal urine production or fluid loss

—Prerenal: placental insufficiency, fetal demise, maternal hypovolemia, maternal hypertension, autoimmune disorders, maternal drugs (NSAIDs, ACE inhibitors)
—Renal: renal agenesis, polycystic or multicystic dysplastic kidneys
—Postrenal (obstructive uropathy): bilateral UPJ obstructions, posterior urethral valves, urethral atresia
—Other: PROM, chronic amniotic leak

RISK FACTORS

- Polyhydramnios

—Maternal glucose intolerance, infections
    —Polyhydramnios may cause PROM, premature labor, and can complicate labor and produce postpartum hemorrhage (uterine atony).

- Oligohydramnios: placental insufficiency

 ## Differential Diagnosis

- Polyhydramnios

—CNS: anencephaly, encephalocele, spina bifida, microcephaly
—GI: esophageal or duodenal atresia, pyloric stenosis
—Klippel-Feil syndrome
—Cleft palate
—Achondroplasia
—Diaphragmatic hernia
—Cystic adenomatoid malformation of the lung

- Oligohydramnios

—Renal agenesis
—Obstructive uropathy: posterior urethral valves, bilateral UPJ obstructions, urethral atresia
—Chronic amniotic leak, PROM

 ## Database

HISTORY

- Polyhydramnios: rapid (acute) or chronic accumulation of fluid

—Increased maternal weight, and growth of fundal height

- Oligohydramnios: poor weight gain, or fetal growth

—Assess for PROM.

PHYSICAL EXAMINATION

- Polyhydramnios: large fundal height; fetus may show evidence of hydrops fetalis; exclude multiple gestations
- Oligohydramnios: diminished fundal height for gestational age

—Fetal compression anomalies (Potter's appearance, compression of lateral aspect of knees)

Diagnostic Studies

LABORATORY TESTING

• Polyhydramnios: maternal testing for glucose intolerance, viral agent

—Consider karyotype; maternal antibody screen; glucose screen; TORCH titers; parvovirus titer.

• Oligohydramnios

—Suspected fetal renal anomaly, consider amniocentesis for fetal karyotype and analysis of fetal urinary electrolytes. Assess fetal pulmonary maturity; maternal antinuclear antibody, anticardiolipin antibody, lupus anticoagulant.

IMAGING

• Sonographic assessment: noninvasive, safe, reproducible, and cost effective. Downside: the ability of ultrasound measurements to represent actual AFV is unproved. There is no accurate model to determine exact volume. Ultrasound measurements are operator dependent.

—Maximum vertical pocket (MVP): deepest amniotic fluid pocket
  —2 to 8 cm being normal
  —Polyhydramnios: pockets >8 cm
  —Oligohydramnios: pockets <1 cm in vertical length
—Amniotic fluid index (AFI): the sum of the sonographic measurements obtained by dividing the maternal abdomen into four quadrants. Each quadrant is scanned to measure the largest AF pocket.
  —Favored technique for noninvasive measurement of AFV
  —Near term: average 12 cm
  —Oligohydramnios AFI <5 cm
  —Polyhydramnios AFI >25 cm

SPECIAL STUDIES

• Direct quantitative measurement of AFV: invasive, only done at delivery or termination of pregnancy; cannot be used to obtain prenatal information
• Indicator dilution technique: A known amount of a specific substance (indicator, i.e., sodium aminohippurate [PAH]) is instilled into the amniotic space. The indicator mixes in the AF, a sample is withdrawn, and indicator concentration is inversely proportional to the AFV.

—Risk of infection, induction of labor, PROM, and fetal injury

 ## Initial Management

• Polyhydramnios: serial sonographic observation, accurate fetal assessment. Karyotype. Discuss with family the possibility of fetal malformation. Diuretics are not indicated. AF aspiration for maternal respiratory distress.
• Oligohydramnios: serial measurement; assess for fetal renal anomaly. Karyotype. Discuss with family the possibility of fetal malformation. Consider amnioinfusion with saline for severe cases. Early delivery if pulmonary maturity can be determined.

 ## Follow-Up

• Polyhydramnios: serial ultrasound every 3 to 4 weeks. Maintain pregnancy until week 38. Aspirate fluid at the time of delivery (controlled amniotomy). Observe for possible uterine hemorrhage after delivery.
• Oligohydramnios: serial measurements and assessment for fetal viability using biophysical profiles. Consider steroids to induce pulmonary maturity and allow for early delivery. Transfer the newborn to the intensive care nursery.

 ## Miscellaneous

SYNONYMS

• Hydramnios

ASSOCIATED CONDITIONS: N/A

NOTES

• Polyhydramnios, if severe, may compromise maternal respiration.

ABBREVIATIONS

• AVF, amniotic fluid volume; AF, amniotic fluid; AFI, amniotic fluid index; MVP, maximum vertical pocket; PROM, premature rupture of membranes; UPJ, ureteropelvic junction

REFERENCES

Brace RA, Wolf EJ. Normal amniotic fluid volume changes throughout pregnancy. *Am J Obstet Gynecol* 1989;161:282.

Ergun A, et al. Predictive value of amniotic fluid volume measurements on perinatal outcome. *Gynecol Obstet Invest* 1998;45:19.

Larmon JE, Ross BS. Clinical utility of amniotic fluid volume assessment. *Obstet Gynecol Clin North Am* 1998;25:639.

Piazze JJ, et al. The effect of polyhydramnios and oligohydramnios on fetal lung maturity index. *Am J Perinatol* 1998;15:249.

Author: T. Ernesto Figueroa

Premature Ejaculation

 Basics

DESCRIPTION

- Recurrent or persistent ejaculation with minimal stimulation before, during, and shortly after vaginal penetration
- Causes distress or relationship difficulty
- Not due to direct effects of a substance
- Primary PE vs. secondary PE
- Life-long vs. acquired
- Psychological vs. mixed factors
- Specific vs. generalized situations

PATHOPHYSIOLOGY

- Psychological

—Traditional assumption, easily treated with sex-therapy behavioral techniques

- Physiologic

—Decreased vibratory threshold at glans penis measured by biothesiometry
—Greater mean amplitudes of dorsal nerve and glans penis somatosensory evoked potentials
—Rarely, hypothalamic pituitary dysfunction

RISK FACTORS

- Presence of erectile, libidinal, or arousal difficulties
- Psychological factors

—Beginning sexual activity; relationship difficulties, interpersonal conflicts

 Differential Diagnosis

- Concomitant erectile dysfunction

 Database

HISTORY

- Complaint and duration

—Acquired vs. lifelong
—Precipitating event
—Temporal relationship to some life event
—Does patient have voluntary control?
—Treatments or solutions tried
—Other sexual dysfunction in patient or partner
—Quality of couple's relationship

- Assessment of mean latency with coitus, masturbation, other sexual activity

PHYSICAL EXAMINATION

- Signs of hypogonadism

—Extent of virilization, male-pattern baldness, gynecomastia

- Genital examination

—Penile deformity, plaques; testicular volume; DRE; sphincter tone and reflexes

Diagnostic Studies

LABORATORY TESTING

- Not always indicated except with signs of hypogonadism; libidinal or arousal difficulties

—Testosterone: FSH, LH, prolactin

IMAGING

- When erectile dysfunction present
- Duplex Doppler with intracavernous injection of vasoactive drug

—Elevated prolactin, obtain MRI of pituitary

SPECIAL STUDIES

- Usually not indicated
- Penile biothesiometry, glans penis somatosensory evoked potentials
- Rigiscan-NPTR when erectile dysfunction present

 ## Initial Management

- Psychotherapeutic behavioral techniques, usually initiated by psychotherapist/sex therapist

—Stop–start or squeeze techniques

- Topical anesthetics

—Lidocaine–prilocaine cream (EMLA) 2.5 g, applied with condom, 30 minutes before sexual activity

- Pharmacotherapy, selective serotonin reuptake inhibitors (SSRI)

—Clomipramine 25 mg qid, qod, or the day of anticipated coitus
—Sertraline 25 to 50 mg qid or 6 hours before
—Paroxetine 20 mg qid or prn
—Fluoxetine 20 mg qid or prn

 ## Follow-Up

- Assessment of therapeutic efficacy; need for referral to psychotherapist/sex therapist
- Assessment of treatment for other sexual dysfunction (erectile dysfunction, hypogonadism); referral to other specialist (endocrinologist)

 ## Miscellaneous

SYNONYMS: N/A

ASSOCIATED CONDITIONS: N/A

NOTES: N/A

ABBREVIATIONS

- PE, premature ejaculation; SSRI, selective serotonin reuptake inhibitors

REFERENCES

Berkovitch M, et al. Efficacy of prilocaine-lidocaine cream in the treatment of premature ejaculation. *J Urol* 1995;154:1360.

Haensel SM, et al. Clomipramine and sexual function in men with premature ejaculation and controls. *J Urol* 1996;156:1310.

Kara H, et al. The efficacy of fluoxetine in the treatment of premature ejaculation: A double-blind placebo controlled study. *J Urol* 1996;156:1631.

Xin ZC, et al. Penile sensitivity in patients with primary premature ejaculation. *J Urol* 1996;156:979.

Author: Brett C. Mellinger

Priapism

 Basics

DEFINITION

• A prolonged erection developing in the absence of sexual stimulation and unrelieved by ejaculation
• The duration of the erection must be >6 hours.
• Named after the Greek god of fertility and lust: Priapus.
• Categorized into veno-occlusive (synonymous with ischemic, low-flow) and arterial (high-flow, nonischemic)
• Proper categorization is essential, as the management of the two conditions is very different.

PATHOPHYSIOLOGY

• *Venocclusive* priapism: continuous veno-occlusion and a failure of blood to drain from the erectile chamber

—May result from paralysis (persistent relaxation) of the erectile smooth muscle (pharmacologic) or from sludging of blood (hematologic) with subsequent prevention of venous outflow

• *Arterial* priapism: unregulated inflow of arterial blood into the corpora cavernosa secondary to a fistula between the cavernous artery and the corpus cavernosum

—This results from blunt or penetrating trauma to the perineum or penis.

RISK FACTORS

• Erectile dysfunction
• Sickle cell
• Perineal/penile trauma
• Psychiatric disturbances

 Differential Diagnosis

• Venocclusive

—Intracavernosal injection therapy
—Psychotropics
—Ganglion-blocking drugs
—Recreational drugs
—Toxins (spider venom, rabies)
—Total parenteral nutrition (especially utilizing high lipid content)
—The incidence of priapism in penile self-injection programs ranges between 0.5% and 6.0%.
—Most of the literature implicating drugs and priapism is case report–based.
—Sickle cell disease, thalassemia, leukemia
  —Sickle cell disease is the most common cause of priapism in the pediatric population.
  —40% of sickle cell disease patients have at least one episode of priapism in their lives.
  —Sickle cell disease is the most common cause of stuttering priapism.
  —Stuttering priapism is a form of veno-occlusive priapism whereby the patient experiences frequent episodes of prolonged erection short of formal priapism. This condition usually precedes an episode of true priapism.
—Idiopathic priapism

• Arterial

—Any form of trauma (blunt or penetrating) to the penis or perineum may cause arterial priapism.

 Database

HISTORY

• History and physical examination are aimed primarily at differentiating between the two forms of this condition.
• Veno-occlusive

—Painful erection, which is typically fully rigid
—Careful questioning is necessary regarding the above-listed etiologic conditions.
—Defining the amount of time that has passed is essential, as the longer the episode of priapism, the more likely that permanent ischemic damage to the erectile tissue is to have occurred.
—It is estimated that priapism of 24 hours' duration is associated with a 50% incidence of permanent erectile dysfunction.

• Arterial

—Erection that is usually less than fully rigid and painless
—Usually some form of penile or perineal trauma

PHYSICAL EXAMINATION

• Attention to the degree of rigidity and tenderness may allow differentiation between the two forms.

Diagnostic Studies

LABORATORY TESTING

• Definition of the nature of the condition is based on the oxygen content of the corporal blood.
• A corporal blood gas analysis can define the oxygen content.

—Veno-occlusive priapism: oxygen content that is venous in nature (≤40 mm Hg)
—Arterial priapism: oxygen content of that is arterial in nature (≥70 mm Hg)

IMAGING

• Venocclusive priapism: none
• Arterial priapism: Confirmation of the location of the arteriocavernous fistula by duplex Doppler ultrasonography is necessary.

—Ultrasonography should be performed both on the penis and through the perineum.
—Pudendal arteriography may be both diagnostic and therapeutic options.

SPECIAL STUDIES: N/A

 Initial Management

• Veno-occlusive priapism is a true urologic emergency, and rapid detumescence is required.
• Arterial priapism is not a medical emergency, as the corporal tissue is fully oxygenated.
• Veno-occlusive: Institute pharmacologic detumescence.

—Primary detumescence: intracavernosal injection with an alpha-adrenergic agonist (most frequently used in United States is phenylephrine [Neo-Synephrine, not available in Europe])
—Other agents: epinephrine and metaraminol
—Administration requires strict blood pressure and pulse monitoring (occasional hypertension and bradycardia).
—No safe maximum dose of this agent has been defined.
—In patients with a significant cardiac history, consultation with a cardiologist is advised.
—Using a 10 mg (10,000 μg)/mL stock solution, dilution with 9 mL of normal saline creates a 1000 μg/mL solution.
—Intracavernosal injection of 500 μg (0.5 mL) should be administered slowly.
—Repeat at 5- to 10-minute intervals; if erection is ≤8 hours in duration, 2 to 4 injections are generally successful.
—When detumescence does not result, corporal aspiration is necessary.
—Place a 19-gauge butterfly needle into the corporal body and aspirate the sludged blood.
—Follow this by irrigation with normal saline and further phenylephrine injection.
—This will result in detumescence in the vast majority of cases.
—Failure to achieve detumescence warrants surgical intervention to create a shunt between the corpus cavernosum and corpus spongiosum.
—In hematologic veno-occlusive priapism, correction of the underlying condition is the primary therapy.
—This requires oxygenation, hydration, and alkalinization.
—In some recalcitrant cases, plasmapheresis may be required.
—These patients should also have intracorporal phenylephrine injection contemporaneously.
—This maneuver is aimed at reversing any corporal smooth muscle paralysis resulting from the intracorporal acidosis.

• Arterial

—This condition is not a true medical emergency.
—The patient must be informed that expectant management is an option.
—Closure of the fistula may be attempted using angioembolization.
—If expectant management is instituted, serial follow-up of the fistula with ultrasonography is indicated.

 Follow-Up

• Determine recovery of erectile function.

 Miscellaneous

SYNONYMS: N/A

ASSOCIATED CONDITIONS: N/A

NOTES

• See also Section II, "Sickle Cell Disease—Urologic Considerations."
• Neonatal priapism associated with polycythemia

ABBREVIATIONS: N/A

REFERENCES

Bastuba MD, Saenz de Tejada I, Dinclenc CZ, Sarazen A, Krane RJ, Goldstein I. Arterial priapism: Diagnosis, treatment and long-term follow-up. *J Urol* 1994;151:1231–1237.

Forsberg L, Mattiasson A, Olsson AM. Priapism: Conservative treatment versus surgical procedures. *Br J Urol* 1981;53:374.

Fowler JE, Koshy M, Strub M, Chinn SK. Priapism associated with sickle cell hemoglobinopathies: Prevalence, natural history and sequelae. *J Urol* 1991;145:65.

Lee M, Cannon B, Sharifi R. Chart for preparation of dilutions of alpha-adrenergic agonists for use in the treatment of priapism. *J Urol* 1995;153:1182–1183.

Mulhall JP, Honig S. Emergency management of priapism. *Acad Emerg Med* 1996;3(8):810.

Author: John P. Mulhall

Prostate Nodule

 Basics

DESCRIPTION

- Usually no presenting complaints
- Detected by physician by digital rectal examination
- Consistency of nodule can denote underlying pathology.
- Rapidity of appearance and changes in size and consistency can infer malignant potential.
- Size can vary from 1 to 2 mm to involve the entire prostate.

PATHOPHYSIOLOGY

- Normal prostate has soft, uniform consistency
- Prostate enlarges with aging
- Becomes rubbery in consistency and has feel of "hypothenar eminence"
- Nodule often graded as to degree of "hardness"

—Grade 1: slightly firm
—Grade 2: moderately firm
—Grade 3: hard

- The nodule can be well circumscribed or irregular and diffuse.

RISK FACTORS

- Prostate cancer

—Family history increases likelihood of cancer by 2.5 times.
—High prostate-specific antigen (PSA) level above 4.0 ng/mL increases likelihood
—Rapidly growing nodule

- Benign nodule

—"Softer" nodule
—No change in size over 1 year
—History of prostate infection

- Prior therapy with intravesical BCG
- Prior prostate surgery (i.e., turp)
- Prior episodes of prostatitis

 Differential Diagnosis

- Neoplasm: malignant

—Adenocarcinoma: commonly called *prostate cancer*
—Transitional cell carcinoma: commonly called *bladder cancer*
—Lymphoma: primary and secondary
—Sarcoma, other rare tumors

- Neoplasm: benign

—Calculus/calcifications
—Scarring from previous surgery or infection
—Benign prostatic hyperplasia
—Cyst-ejaculatory duct
—Granulomatous prostatitis

- Rectal wall lesions (thrombosed hemorrhoid, etc.)

 Database

HISTORY

- Age

—Age >50 years, increased likelihood of malignancy
—Men >70 years, high likelihood of prostate cancer

- Symptoms

—Usually no complaints
—Patients with infection may have irritative voiding symptoms and fever.
—Patients with transitional cell carcinoma may have hematuria and irritative symptoms.
—Younger patients with lymphoma may have obstructive symptoms.

- History of prior prostatitis

—Abscess
—Chronic prostatitis can make the prostate firm.
—Usually gram-negative organisms
—Patients with exposure to tuberculosis may develop granulomatous prostatitis.

- Prior surgery

—Biopsy
—Benign prostatectomy (TURP or open)

- Prior treatment

—External beam irradiation
—Brachytherapy

PHYSICAL EXAMINATION

- Digital rectal examination

—Prostate cancer (adenocarcinoma and transitional cell carcinoma): grade 2 or 3 nodule; can be 5 mm in size or involve entire prostate. Extensive lesion extends outside of gland. Advanced cancer patients may also complain of hip or back pain.
—Lymphoma: diffusely firm gland
—Prostatitis: warm, boggy, tender, poorly circumscribed nodule
—BPH: grade 1 to 2 nodule, rubbery, involves both lateral lobes
—Calculus: stony, hard, small nodule

Diagnostic Studies

LABORATORY TESTING

- Urine analysis

—Prostate cancer: usually normal; locally advanced cases may have microscopic or gross hematuria

—Transitional cell carcinoma: microscopic or gross hematuria almost always present

—Lymphoma: same as above

—Prostatitis: few to many white blood cells, microhematuria usually present

—BPH: usually normal

—Calculus: usually normal

 —Urine culture: usually positive for gram-negative organisms in acute and chronic bacterial prostatitis

—Urine cytology: positive about two-thirds of the time in transitional cell carcinoma, rarely positive in locally advanced adenocarcinoma

- Prostate-specific antigen

—Prostate cancer: elevated above 4.0 ng/mL in 80% to 90% of cases. Above 10 ng/mL with nodule denotes cancer more than 80% of the time. About 20% of prostate cancer cases will have a nodule and PSA <4.0 ng/mL.

—Transitional cell carcinoma: PSA <4.0 ng/mL

—BPH: PSA usually between 4.0 and 10 ng/mL, makes distinguishing from prostate cancer difficult. Free PSA, which measures the percent PSA not bound to serum proteins, is usually less than 15% to 25% in cancer cases.

—Prostatitis can elevate PSA many-fold: need to wait until infection cleared and repeat PSA

- Other laboratory tests

—Prostate cancer: in advanced cases, can have elevations of acid phosphatase and if bone metastases are present, elevations of alkaline phosphatase and calcium

IMAGING

- Prostate ultrasonography

—Prostate cancer: Lesions can be hypo-, iso-, or hyperechoic. Large lesions can extend outside of the prostate, involving the capsule, seminal vesicles, or base of the bladder. Often, a prostate ultrasound is normal.

—Transitional cell carcinoma: centrally located lesion, often invading base of bladder

—Lymphoma: diffuse enlargement of prostate

—BPH: enlargement of lateral lobes and central zone

—Prostatitis: very hyperechoic, asymmetric enlargement

- Excretory urography

—Advanced lesions (prostate cancer, TCC, lymphoma, BPH): lesion extending into bladder, large post-void residual, lateral displacement of ureters, hydroureteronephrosis

- Abdominal CT or MRI

—Malignant lesions: enlargement of pelvic (obturator, hypogastric, and iliac) lymph nodes; extension of cancer outside of prostate

SPECIAL STUDIES

- Cystoscopy: identifies outlet obstruction; used to evaluate bladder when hematuria is present with nodule
- Prostate biopsy: All prostate nodules should be biopsied using transrectal ultrasound guidance.

Initial Management

- Standard work-up includes measurement of serum PSA followed by prostate biopsy.
- Ultrasound imaging and biopsy represents the gold standard for prostate nodules.
- Cystoscopy is only necessary if obstructive symptoms or hematuria is present.
- CT or MRI is reserved for diagnosis of malignancy.

Follow-Up

- Negative biopsy with abnormal PSA may require repeat biopsy. Biopsy is positive about 20% of time with PSA <4.0 ng/mL and >50% of time with PSA >10 ng/mL.
- Biopsy positive for malignancy will require treatment depending on type of malignancy and stage of cancer.

Miscellaneous

SYNONYMS

- Prostate lesion

ASSOCIATED CONDITIONS: N/A

NOTES

- See Section II, "Prostate Cancer—General" and "Prostatitis—Granulomatous"

ABBREVIATIONS

- PSA, prostate-specific antigen; DRE, digital rectal examination

REFERENCE

Morton RA, Lepor H. Prostate disorders: Benign and malignant. In: Noble J, ed. *Textbook of Primary Care Medicine*. St Louis: Mosby, 1996:1782–1792.

Author: Nelson N. Stone

Proteinuria

 Basics

DESCRIPTION

- The normal kidney excretes 80 to 150 mg of protein daily in urine; excess is consistent with proteinuria.
- Proteinuria may be a first indication of renal parenchymal disease.
- Must confirm dipstick proteinuria with quantitative 24-hour urine protein measurement
- False-negative dipstick proteinuria is due to alkaline urine, dilute urine, or urinary protein other than albumin.

PATHOPHYSIOLOGY

- Proteinuria is classified into glomerular, tubular, overflow, or tissue etiologies.

—Glomerular proteinuria most commonly results from increased glomerular capillary permeability primarily to albumin.
  —Nephrotic syndrome is >3 g/d glomerular proteinuria, with hypoalbuminemia, lipiduria, and edema due to severe renal disease. Associated with ascites, edema etc.

—Tubular proteinuria results from failure to reabsorb low-molecular-weight proteins such as immunoglobulins, and seldom exceeds 2 to 3 g/24 h.
—Overflow proteinuria occurs in the absence of renal disease caused by abnormal accumulation or overproduction of immunoglobulins and low-molecular-weight proteins.
—Tissue proteinuria is associated with inflammatory, benign prostatic hyperplasia, or bladder cancer.

RISK FACTORS

- Glomerular renal diseases with nephrotic syndrome
- Multiple myeloma
- Glomerulonephritis
- Tumor necrosis syndrome/glomerular toxin exposure (cadmium, iodinated contrast)
- Myeloproliferative states
- Fanconi syndrome

 Differential Diagnosis

- Glomerular proteinuria

—IgA nephropathy
—Diabetic nephropathy
—Medication induced: mercurials, heroin, penicillamine, probenecid, captopril, lithium, and NSAIDs
—Minimal-change disease
—Primary glomerulonephritides
—Autoimmune: SLE, Henoch-Schönlein purpura, and amyloidosis
—Infusion of norepinephrine
—Congestive heart failure
—Other: exercise-induced, orthostatic, and febrile proteinuria

- Tubular proteinuria

—Obstructive uropathy
—Toxins and drugs
—Aminoaciduria
—Glucosuria
—Phosphaturia
—Fanconi syndrome

- Overflow proteinuria

—Multiple myeloma
—Hemoglobinuria and myoglobinuria
—Leukemia

- Tissue proteinuria

—Acute inflammation of urinary tract: cystitis, acute prostatitis, and uroepithelial tumors

 Database

HISTORY

- Timing is very important: transient, intermittent, or persistent.

—Transient proteinuria is most common in pediatric patients and usually resolves spontaneously within days to weeks. It may be caused by fever, exercise, emotional stress, and renal venous hypertension in CHF.
—Intermittent proteinuria is frequently related to orthostasis and may be due to excessive pressure on the renal vein while the patient is standing. No further treatment is needed if renal function is normal.
—Persistent proteinuria requires complete evaluation and is often of glomerular etiology.

PHYSICAL EXAMINATION

- Focus on signs of nephrotic syndrome and azotemia, such as peripheral edema and papilledema, and also skin rash signs or arteritis, flank bruit, abdominal mass, and pericardial rub.

Diagnostic Studies

LABORATORY TESTING

- Dipstick sensitive to determine albuminuria 20 to 30 mg/dL
- 3% sulfosalicylic acid demonstrates proteinuria as low as 15 mg/dL, and more sensitive to reveal non-albumin protein.
- Quantitative protein measurement with 24-hour urinalysis for all qualitative proteinuria findings

—Protein electrophoresis for proteinuria of 300 to 2000 mg/24 h
  —Normal proteins consistent with tubular proteinuria
  —Light-chain immunoglobulins (Bence-Jones protein) due to multiple myeloma

- Fasting glucose for patients with evidence of renal insufficiency and proteinuria to rule out diabetes mellitus

IMAGING

- Renal ultrasound for any patient with evidence of significant proteinuria and/or renal insufficiency
- Nuclear renal scan for differential function in patients with renal insufficiency
- Proceed with IVP if renal function adequate and associated hematuria

SPECIAL STUDIES

- Renal biopsy: nephrotic syndrome, acute renal failure of unknown etiology, transplanted kidney

 ## Initial Management

- Management depends on etiology. Hydration and repeated studies for patients suspected of exercise-induced or transient proteinuria
- Nephrology consultation for all patients with persistent proteinuria
- Oncology evaluation for patients found to have Bence-Jones proteinuria due to multiple myeloma

 ## Follow-Up

- Based on underlying condition

 ## Miscellaneous

SYNONYMS: NA

ASSOCIATED CONDITIONS: N/A

NOTES

- See also Section II, "Nephrotic Syndrome."

ABBREVIATIONS

- IgA, immunoglobulin A; SLE, systemic lupus erythematosus

REFERENCES

Brendler CB. Evaluation of the urologic patient. In: Walsh PC, Retik AB, Vaughan Ed, Wein AJ, eds. *Campbell's Urology,* 7th ed. Philadelphia: WB Saunders, 1998.

Glassrock RJ. Proteinuria. In: Bennett JC, Plum F, eds. *Massry and Glassrock's Textbook of Nephrology,* 3rd ed. Baltimore: Williams & Wilkins, 1995.

Authors: Raymond S. Lance and J. Brantley Thrasher

PSA Elevation

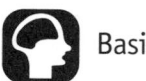 Basics

DESCRIPTION

• PSA >4.0 ng/mL based on the Baltimore Longitudinal Study of Aging and adopted in initial studies

—Age-specific and race-specific guidelines have been proposed (see Section III).
—PSA >2.5 ng/mL: may be used in African-American men >40 or if there is a family history of CaP >40

PATHOPHYSIOLOGY

• Prostate-specific antigen (PSA) is a member of the kallikrein gene family (gene on chromosome 19).
• Serine protease: produced by the prostatic epithelium and periurethral glands
• Responsible for liquefying the seminal coagulum
• Secreted into the seminal fluid in high concentrations (mg/mL)
• Found in the serum in low concentrations (ng/mL)
• Complexed to antiproteases alpha1-antichymotrypsin (ACT) and alpha2-macroglobulin (MG), yet a small proportion remains free, or otherwise termed *free PSA* (FPSA)
• PSA bound to ACT and that which is free are detected by assay, while that bound to MG is not detected by assay.
• Complexed PSA hepatic clearance (half-life of 2–3 days); FPSA is cleared by glomerular filtration (half-life of 2–3 hours)
• Serum PSA elevation occurs due to disrupted prostatic architecture.
• Physiologic variation in serum PSA from 15% to 30% in the short term. BPH can vary up to 30%.
• Infection, infarction, trauma, or prostatic manipulation can produce transient serum elevations (not routine DRE).
• Androgens strongly influence PSA levels with treatment of prostatic diseases (BPH, CaP, infection) will lower PSA
• Finasteride, a 5-alpha-reductase inhibitor, lowers serum PSA by approximately 50% over 6 to 12 months

RISK FACTORS

• Malignancy, infection, prostatic infarction, recent manipulation (e.g., trauma, biopsy, or vigorous massage)

 Differential Diagnosis

• Adenocarcinoma of the prostate
• Benign prostatic hyperplasia
• Prostatitis (usually bacterial infection)
• Prostatic infarction: may occur after shock, sepsis, or recent cardiac bypass surgery
• Urethral manipulation, recent cystourethroscopy, Foley catheter placement
• Prostatic massage (not routine DRE)
• Ejaculation within 24 hours of PSA blood draw; only in the setting of a marginally elevated PSA

 Database

HISTORY

• Difficulty with urination, such as hesitancy, straining, weak stream, or intermittency?
• Urinary retention?
• Dysuria, frequency, or urgency?
• Any previous PSA levels?
• Any previous prostate biopsies?
• Known history of prostate cancer?
• Family history of prostate carcinoma?

PHYSICAL EXAMINATION

• Digital rectal examination

—Evaluate for the presence of nodules, induration, asymmetry, tenderness

 Diagnostic Studies

LABORATORY TESTING

• FPSA: helpful to differentiate if serum PSA elevation is due to benign or malignant disease (see below)

IMAGING

• Transrectal ultrasound of the prostate

—Determine prostatic size used: to calculate PSA density
—Most hypoechoic lesions are not cancer, but hypoechoic areas are twice as likely to contain cancers as are isoechoic areas (25%–50% of cancers missed if only hypoechoic areas biopsied).
—Evaluate for extraprostatic extension in advanced disease.
—Most useful to guide systematic needle biopsy of the prostate

SPECIAL STUDIES

- PSA derivatives

—PSA density (PSAD): PSA divided by volume of prostate in grams

    —Correlates serum PSA to TRUS determined prostatic size in order to attempt to distinguish BPH versus CaP

    —Useful with PSA levels 4.0 to 10.0 ng/mL and a previous negative biopsy

    —The cut-off point of 0.15 ng/mL/cm^3 improves specificity by 50% but misses 27% to 48% of cancers.

    —A cut-off point of 0.1 avoids 31% of biopsies, yet misses 10% of cancers.

    —A cut-off point of 0.8 avoids 12% of biopsies, yet misses 5% of cancers.

- PSA slope (velocity)

—Rate of PSA increase per year, based on the theory that PSA rises more rapidly if clinically significant CaP present

—In the Baltimore Longitudinal Study, 72% of men with CaP had a PSA rise >0.75 ng/mL/yr vs. 10% of men with BPH.

—In prospective trials, 47% of men with a velocity >0.75 ng/mL/yr had CaP vs. 11% of men with velocities <0.75.

—Note: A minimum testing interval of 18 months with three repeated PSA measurements is necessary for accurate velocity determination.

- Free PSA

—Men with CaP have a lower amount of FPSA; it is postulated that CaP cells produce more ACT.

—Measured as the percent of FPSA/total assayed PSA

—TPSA levels 4.0 to 10.0 ng/mL: if <10% FPSA, 90% chance of cancer; if FPSA >25%, <10% chance of cancer (Hybritech assay)

—FPSA is more specific in men with prostates less than 50 g; not valid if TPSA >10

—Verify parameters specific to each commercial assay

- AGE/RACE corrected PSA (see Section III)

 Initial Management

- If there is clinical evidence of acute prostatitis, treat with antibiotics and repeat PSA after 3 to 4 weeks.
- Total PSA 2.5 to 10.0 ng/mL

—Obtain FPSA

    —F/T PSA >25%: Repeat PSA and DRE in 6 months.

    —F/T PSA <25%: 6 to 12 core biopsy

- Total PSA >10.0 ng/mL

—Sextant biopsy

 Follow-Up

- Biopsy

—Positive biopsy for CaP: Evaluate for staging and discuss treatment options.

—Negative biopsy: Repeat PSA and DRE in 6 months.

- Total PSA <2.5 ng/mL

—Repeat PSA and DRE in 1 year.

- Total PSA 2.5 to 10.0 ng/mL: Discuss options.

—Repeat PSA and DRE in 6 months.

—Or 6 to 12 peripheral zone biopsy and 4 transitional zone biopsy

—Or biopsy only if PSA density >0.1, PSA slope >0.75 ng/mL/yr, or F/T PSA <30%

- Total PSA >10.0 ng/mL

—6 to 12 peripheral zone biopsy and 4 transition zone biopsy

 Miscellaneous

SYNONYMS: N/A

ASSOCIATED CONDITIONS: N/A

NOTES

- See also Section I, "PSA Elevation Following Definitive Therapy for Localized Prostate Cancer."

ABBREVIATIONS

- CaP, adenocarcinoma of the prostate; TPSA, total PSA; FPSA, free PSA; F/T, free total

REFERENCES

Babaian RJ, et al. Comparative analysis of prostate specific antigen and its indexes in the detection of prostate cancer. *J Urol* 1996;156: 432–437.

Catalona WJ, et al. Comparison of digital rectal examination and serum prostate specific antigen in the early detection of prostate cancer: Results of a multicenter trial of 6630 men. *J Urol* 1994;151:1283–1290.

Catalona WJ, et al. Serum free prostate specific antigen and prostate specific antigen density measurements for predicting cancer in men with prior negative biopsies. *J Urol* 1997; 158:2162–2167.

Partin AW, Oesterling JE. The clinical usefulness of prostate specific antigen: Update 1994. *J Urol* 1994;152:1358–1368.

Woodrum DL, et al. Interpretation of free prostate specific antigen clinical research studies for the detection of prostate cancer. *J Urol* 1998;159:5–12.

Authors: James A. Simon and Gerald L. Andriole

PSA Elevation Following Definitive Therapy

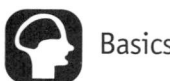 Basics

DESCRIPTION

- Prostate-specific antigen (PSA) is a single-chain glycoprotein produced almost exclusively by prostatic epithelial cells or prostatic malignancy.
- Destruction or removal of malignant prostate tissue reduces PSA, making it a useful marker to monitor patients after treatment.
- Characteristics of rising PSA after initial therapy may direct next treatment.

PATHOPHYSIOLOGY

- Assays report total serum level; standard sensitivity, 0.1 ng/mL; ultrasensitive assays, 0.01 ng/mL.

—Fractionated PSA (free:total ratio) is under study in this setting.

- Time to PSA nadir after treatment depends on therapy.

—Radical prostatectomy (RP) should reduce PSA to <0.1 ng/mL within 3 to 4 weeks.
—External beam radiotherapy (EBRT) reduces PSA to nadir 12 to 18 months after treatment and depends on the definition of *PSA nadir* (most use <0.5).
—Brachytherapy may require 2 to 3 years before PSA nadir; transient elevation is common before nadir.
—Cryoablation will cause PSA decline for 6 to 12 months.

RISK FACTORS (FOR PSA [BIOCHEMICAL] FAILURE)

- RP 5-year failure is 20% to 30%, and 10-year the failure rate is 30% to 50% and can be estimated based on both pretreatment and posttreatment parameters.

—Risk of high-stage malignancy and PSA failure have a direct relationship to pretreatment total serum PSA; 5-year risk is 29% if PSA >10 ng/mL, and 5% if <10 ng/mL.
—Preoperative Gleason score and recurrence: 5-year failure rates—Gleason ≥7: 45%; Gleason score ≤6: 8%
—Bulky peripheral zone tumors are at higher risk of PSA failure than are smaller nonpalpable ones.

- Pathologic staging after RP is predictive of failure.

—Risk of PSA failure when tumor is organ confined: 10%
—Risk when margins are positive or seminal vesicals involved: 26% and 60%, respectively
—Risk of lymph node spread is now <5%, but when present indicates systemic disease (>90% PSA failure rate).

- The characteristics of falling and rising PSA are also useful to predict PSA recurrence and direct second-line treatment.

—If PSA never reaches "0.0" immediately after RP, distant is likely.
—If PSA failure occurs >2 years following surgery and the doubling time is over 6 months, then local failure is likely.

- PSA recurrence following EBRT or brachytherapy can also be estimated using PSA, Gleason score, and clinical stage.

—There is no accepted definition of "normal" PSA after radiation, but "lower is better"; 5-year failure is 10% when PSA <0.5 ng/mL, but nearly 60% if it does not.
—Pretherapy PSA is predictive; failure at 4 years for PSA 0 to 4 ng/mL is 9%, for 4 to 10 ng/mL is 57%, and for over 10 ng/mL is 60%.

- Pretreatment PSA more important in predicting biochemical failure than stage

—T1/T2 staged groups with PSA greater than 15 ng/mL outcomes were the same as stage T3 groups.
—Increasing Gleason sums also appear to have an increasing chance of biochemical failure.

- Using combination androgen ablation and EBRT, 5-year PSA recurrence rates have been reported as low as 15%.

 Differential Diagnosis

- PSA rise after definitive treatment: Only rarely could anything other than cancer be the cause.
- Stable elevations can be problematic.

—After prostatectomy, benign tissue at the bladder neck or urethra
—Following radiotherapy, EBR, brachytherapy, persistence of viable benign prostatic tissue
—Salivary glands and periurethral glands can produce minor amounts of PSA, but they rarely reach the bloodstream.

- More important differential may be between local cancer recurrence vs. distant disease as sources of PSA

—High pretreatment Gleason's grade (7 or above) and PSA >20 associated with distant sources of PSA failure
—After prostatectomy, cancer spread to seminal vesicals, PSA failing to reach 0, and early PSA rises are all predictive of distant recurrences.
—Pretreatment Gleason's score <6, cancer at the urethral margin, greater than 2 years before, and slow PSA doubling times are most consistent with local recurrences.
—Isolated local recurrences after prostatectomy are present in 30% to 50% of cases.
—After EBRT or brachytherapy, PSA nadir >0.5 ng/mL to 1.0 ng/mL and then short (<6-month) PSA doubling rates suggest distant failure.

 Database

HISTORY

- Type of treatment and dates performed

—Any androgen ablation or adjuvant therapy

- Pretreatment: PSA, Gleason sum, tumor stage (ploidy, RT-PCR, microvessel density, if available)
- Posttreatment: PSA nadir, time to PSA failure, rate of PSA rise (doubling time)
- Review pathology of prostatectomy specimen, if available.

—Final Gleason sum, estimated tumor volume, ploidy, microvessel density
—Involvement of lymph nodes, seminal vesicals, margins, capsule, apical urethra, and bladder neck

PHYSICAL EXAMINATION

- Rectal examination

—For prostatectomy patients, check for locally palpable nodules along neurovascular bundles or posterior pubic ramus.
—For radiation patients, check for nodularity, side-wall extension, and character or texture of the prostate.

- General physical examination to check for cutaneous nodular metastasis, presence of testes, or atrophy of genitalia
- Palpate for spinal or other bony tenderness.

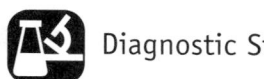 Diagnostic Studies

LABORATORY TESTING

- Total serum PSA (fractionated assay currently under investigation in this setting)
- Serial serum PSA to establish rate of increase or doubling time
- Prostatic acid phosphatase (PAP) of limited value
- Serum chemistry, particularly alkaline phosphatase, liver function studies, and serum creatinine level

IMAGING

- Bone scan still useful to evaluate for osteoblastic lesions
- CT and MRI may reveal intraabdominal pelvic soft-tissue spread, although it is only present in 10% to 12% of patients with early metastatic recurrences.
- A ProstaScint scan may be useful to identify the source of PSA recurrence (local vs. distant) to direct secondary therapy.
- Transrectal ultrasound after RP: to detect hypoechoic lesions around vesicourethral (VU) anastomosis and/or direct anastomotic biopsies; color Doppler flow signal usually associated with positive biopsy

SPECIAL STUDIES

- Prostatic or prostatic bed biopsies

—US-guided biopsy of VU anastomosis is positive in about 40% to 50% of patients with PSA failure after radical prostatectomy.
—After radiotherapy, may direct biopsies of prostate to restage and grade local recurrences
—Positive biopsy rate after radiotherapy is variable and depends on pretreatment stage, Gleason score, and PSA level.

- Bone marrow biopsy and RT-PCR are investigational, and their role has not yet been determined.

 Initial Management

- Observation or delayed androgen ablation

—Option for all patients with PSA failure because of prolonged period before clinically evident recurrences
—Benefits include no side effects or expense of secondary treatment
—Risks include anxiety of "doing nothing," progression to symptomatic recurrences or progression from local to metastatic disease, possible shortened interval of suppression when androgens are used late, and less curable local disease when radiotherapy is postponed.
—The best candidates are those with a Gleason score of 6 or below, slow PSA doubling rates, diploid tumors, low anxiety, and active sex lives.

- Radiotherapy

—Option for patients who fail after RP; best outcome if PSA <2.0, RT dose at least 64 Gy
—Additional RT not beneficial in men failing primary RT; brachytherapy salvage under study
—Benefits include potential for cure and delay in use of long-term androgen deprivation.
—Risks include complications of radiotherapy, such as radiation cystitis, hematuria, bladder neck contracture, incontinence, and impotence.
—Combination with temporary (6–12 months) androgen deprivation may improve long-term outcomes.
—Best outcome in isolated local recurrence; low preoperative PSA (<10 ng/mL), low Gleason's score (<6), positive apical or bladder neck margins, negative seminal vesicals, negative lymph nodes
—Biopsy-proven local recurrence may be helpful but not necessary, since 40% to 50% still have PSA nadir to 0.

- Early androgen deprivation

—Option for all patients with PSA failure
—Benefits: treats subclinical metastasis, may offer prolonged clinical disease-free interval over delayed treatment
—Best candidates: high risk of distant failure; high preoperative PSA (>10 ng/mL), Gleason score >7, high-stage disease, positive lymph nodes or seminal vesicals involved
—Options of androgen deprivation include GnRH analogs, orchiectomy, or combinations with antiandrogens. Administration of oral antiandrogens alone or combined with finasteride is under study and an option in potent patients.
—Intermittent therapy under study; benefit of reduced long-term side effects and cost. Efficacy is unknown. A minimum period of deprivation is usually 6 to 9 months.

 Follow-Up

- Usually PSA and rectal examination every 3 to 6 months
- Bone scan every year; for PSA doubling, 6 months or less; and every 2 years for slower PSA increases

 Miscellaneous

SYNONYMS

- Biochemical failure

ASSOCIATED CONDITIONS: N/A

NOTES: N/A

ABBREVIATIONS

- RP, radical prostatectomy; EBRT, external beam radiation therapy; RT, radiation therapy; VU, vesicourethral

REFERENCES

Critz FA, et al. The PSA that indicates potential cure after radiotherapy for prostate cancer. *Urology* 1997;49:322.

Nasseri KK, et al. PSA recurrence after definitive treatment of clinically localized prostate cancer. AUA Update, Lesson 11, Volume XVI.

Partin AW, et al. Evaluation of serum prostate-specific antigen velocity after radical prostatectomy to distinguish local recurrence from distant metastases. *Urology* 1994;43:649.

Ragde H, et al. Interstitial iodine-125 radiation without adjuvant therapy in the treatment of clinically localized prostate cancer. *Cancer* 1997;80:442.

Shinohara K, et al. Cryosurgical ablation of prostate cancer: Patterns of cancer recurrence. *J Urol* 1997;158:2206.

Authors: Mark S. Austenfeld and Mark J. Walterskirchen

Renal Failure—Acute

 Basics

DESCRIPTION

• Acute renal failure (ARF) is a relatively abrupt decline in renal function, over a period of hours to days, sufficient to raise the level of nitrogenous waste products in the blood and, usually, a decline in the urine output.
• Occurs in up to 5% of all hospitalized patients and in up to 20% of all ICU patients. 50% of hospital ARF can be considered iatrogenic in origin.
• Reduced renal perfusion (prerenal disease) and acute tubular necrosis (ATN) account for approximately 75% of all cases.
• Acute renal failure can be oliguric (urinary output <400 mL/d) or nonoliguric (≥400 mL/d).
• There is confusion in terminology and wide disparity in the definition of terms.

PATHOPHYSIOLOGY

• The degree of renal dysfunction is directly proportional to the decrease in the glomerular filtration rate (GFR) measured in mL/min.
• Prerenal: decreased amount of blood delivered to the kidney

—Systemic hypotension stimulates the renin-angiotensin–aldosterone axis, antidiuretic hormone release, and sympathetic nervous system: redistribution of blood flow away from the renal cortex, avid reabsorption of sodium, water, and urea. Urine and sodium output declines and osmolality increases. Blood urea nitrogen increases. Reduction in renal blood flow decreases GFR. Acute tubular necrosis can happen if hypoperfusion is sustained.

• Renal: malfunction of the kidney parenchyma. Several mechanisms explain pathophysiology:

—Tubular destruction: after major traumatic injury, with release of myoglobin from skeletal muscle cells. Myoglobin can precipitate in the tubule with subsequent obstruction. This leads to increased intratubular pressure and decreased glomerular filtration.
—Vasomotor therapy: ARF can occur after an initial insult that results in an increased renin-angiotensin level. Afferent arteriolar vasoconstriction results, with subsequent redistribution of blood away form cortical nephrons, resulting in a decrease in glomerular function.
—Decreased permeability in glomerular membrane

• Postrenal: obstruction to the flow of urine

—Renal blood flow is significantly decreased, as is GFR.
—The renin–angiotensin system is probably responsible for decreased delivery of filtrate to the proximal convoluted tubule.
—Decreased concentrating ability and impaired acid excretion are lost with postrenal failure.
—With correction of the obstruction, large volumes of urine containing sodium, potassium, and solutes are excreted.
—Concentrating ability may be lost for days or weeks.

RISK FACTORS

• Surgery (especially if patients are elderly or have previous elevated levels of creatinine)
• Volume depletion
• Aminoglycoside therapy, congestive heart failure, contrast exposure, septic shock, nephrotoxic drugs

 Differential Diagnosis

• Prerenal

—Intravascular volume depletion
—Hemorrhage
—Gastrointestinal losses (vomiting, diarrhea, fistulas)
—Renal losses (nephritis, glycosuria, diuretics)
—Skin losses
—Respiratory losses
—Sequestration in third spaces (pancreatitis, peritonitis, intestinal obstruction)
—Inadequate fluid replacement
—Burns
—Reduced cardiac output (cardiogenic shock, congestive heart failure, pericardial tamponade, massive pulmonary embolism, sepsis, cirrhosis with ascites)
—Systemic vasodilatation
  —Anaphylaxis, antihypertensive drugs, sepsis: drug overdose
—Systemic or renal vasoconstriction
  —Anesthesia, surgery, alpha-adrenergic agonists or high-dose dopamine
  —Hepatorenal syndrome
—Hyperviscosity syndromes: multiple myeloma or macroglobulinemia

• Renal (70% of the patients will have concurrent causes)
• Renal hypoperfusion (50%)
• Toxic causes: exogenous (25%)

—Antibiotics (aminoglycosides, cephalosporins, penicillins, tetracyclines, sulfa derivatives, rifampicin, acyclovir, amphotericin)
—Nonsteroidal antiinflammatory agents
—Diuretics (furosemide, thiazides, triamterene)
—Antihypertensives (captopril, alpha-methyldopa)
—Anticonvulsants (carbamazepine, phenytoin, phenobarbital, valproic acid)
—Chemotherapeutic agents (cisplatin, methotrexate, mitomycin)
—Immunosuppressive agents (cyclosporine)
—Cimetidine, allopurinol, azathioprine, penicillamine
—Heavy metals (mercury, lead, arsenic)
—Radiographic contrast media
—Organic solvents (ethylene glycol)

• Toxic causes: endogenous (25%)

—Myoglobin, Hemoglobin, Calcium phosphate precipitation, Uric acid

• Postrenal

—Pediatric patients
  —Posterior urethral valves
  —Bilateral ureteral obstruction
  —Meatal stenosis

• Adults
—Pregnancy
—Bilateral renal calculi
—Retroperitoneal disorders
—Neurogenic bladder dysfunction
—Iatrogenic (ureteral ligation)

• Elderly
—Benign prostatic hypertrophy
—Carcinoma (prostate, bladder, cervix, colon)
—Papillary necrosis
—Coagulated blood
—Fungus

 Database

HISTORY

• Evaluation of the patient's history usually will reveal the source of ARF.
• Which drugs have been given, how frequently, in what doses, duration of drug usage?
• Presence of irritative or obstructive symptoms, hematuria, history of stones, trauma or previous episodes of ARF
• History of cardiac disease or other disorders that cause extracellular fluid volume loss
• Previous surgery on the urinary tract or abdominal vasculature
• History of fevers or rashes suggesting allergy
• History of cancer or previous chemotherapy or radiotherapy
• Bone pain in an elderly patient should suggest multiple myeloma.

PHYSICAL EXAMINATION

• Volume depletion suggests prerenal causes.
• Cardiac dysfunction with signs and symptoms of congestive heart failure (pulmonary edema, peripheral edema, ventricular gallop, jugular venous distension)
• Flank pain, suprapubic distension, and incontinence suggest obstructive causes.
• Harsh abdominal bruits or a palpable aortic aneurysm suggests vascular causes.
• Palpable purpura, pulmonary hemorrhage, and sinusitis suggest systemic vasculitis, with glomerulonephritis as a cause.

 Diagnostic Studies

LABORATORY TESTING

• Urinalysis
—Proteinuria
—Hematuria
—Brown granular urinary casts
—Urinary renal tubular epithelial cells
—Urine sediment
  —Coarse granular sediments
  —Renal tubular epithelial cells
  —Eosinophils (AIN)
  —Red cell or hemoglobin casts (RPGN)
  —Crystals (lithiasis, obstruction)

- Urine electrolytes/osmolality

—Increased urine sodium (>20 mEq/L), increased fractional excretion of sodium (>3%)
  —Calculation: Fractional excretion of sodium = [(urine Na/serum Na)/Urine creatinine/serum creatinine)] × 100
—Urine isotonic to plasma
  —Low urine sodium (<10 mEq/L), low fractional excretion of sodium (<1%), concentrate urine osmolality (>500 mOsmol/L)

- Other

—Azotemia
—Decreased creatinine clearance
—Hyperosmolarity
—Hyperphosphatemia
—Hyperkalemia
—Decreased serum bicarbonate
—Increased plasma volume
—Decreased hemoglobin, hematocrit
—Hypocapnia
—Increased serum magnesium
—Acidemia
—Increased serum amylase/lipase
—Hyponatremia
—Hypocalcemia
—Increased serum uric acid
—Increased bleeding time
—Impaired phagocytic function

Differential Diagnosis between ATN and Prerenal Azotemia

	ATN	*Prerenal Azotemia*
Urine/plasma creatinine	<20	>40
Urine/plasma BUN	<3	>8
Urine/plasma osmolality	<1.2	>1.2
Urine sodium (mEq/L)	>40	<20
Urinalysis	Casts or cells	No casts

IMAGING

- Kidney ultrasound; considered by most as standard approach

—IV contrast studies are generally contraindicated in ARF.

- Findings

—Medical renal disease: normal-size kidneys
—Ischemia: kidney size disparity
—Postrenal causes: hydronephrosis
  —If suspicion of obstruction remains, proceed with antegrade or retrograde contrast studies.
  —A nondilated collecting system does not necessarily exclude the possibility of obstruction, especially when the condition is acute.

SPECIAL STUDIES

- Angiogram (renal vascular disease)
- Cystoscopy (bladder outlet obstruction)
- Retrograde ureterogram/ureteroscopy (ureteral obstruction)

- Renal biopsy is indicated when prerenal and postrenal causes have been excluded and a primary renal disease other than ischemic or toxin-related ARF is suggested.
- Bleeding time

 ## Initial Management

- The aim of treatment: maintain the patient while assessing the cause of the ARF
- The key to effective treatment is making the correct diagnosis.
- General measures
—Placement of a urethral catheter may be useful to monitor urine output, but is not essential.
—Restriction of fluid intake to 500 mL every 24 hours, plus the daily urine volume
—Fluids are best given orally, but may need to be administered intravenously.
—Dopamine (2–5 mg/kg/min) and furosemide (10–15 mg/kg/h) in order to improve urine output. Higher doses of furosemide should not be used. This measure will convert the patient from an oliguric state to a nonoliguric one.
—Overexpansion of plasma volume should be avoided because it may result in water intoxication. Accurate fluid balance is usually done by daily weighing.
—Restrict sodium intake (20–30 mmol/d).
—Hyperkalemia can be lowered by intravenous infusion of glucose (50 g) and insulin (10 U) and maintenance at safe levels by ion-exchange resins.
—Help of a clinical nutrition team for maintenance of nutritional status. Ideally, patients should receive 100 g of carbohydrate and 3000 to 3500 kcal daily, with 60 to 80 g of nitrogen.
—There is no place for prophylactic antibiotics, but careful monitoring for infections must be done. If confirmed, an infection should be treated vigorously. If possible, avoid foreign bodies (catheters, intravenous cannula).
—Use H2-receptor antagonists and antacids, since gastrointestinal bleeding is a major contributing factor in a patient's death.
—Always be aware of potential problems with toxicity due to impaired renal excretion when prescribing drugs in ARF. Modify dosages of drugs excreted by the kidneys.
—If drug induced, discontinue offending agent.
—Dialysis is indicated if conservative measures fail to control the situation. Peritoneal dialysis is the simplest form of treatment, but hemodialysis may be necessary.
—Persistent anuria may be an indication of renal biopsy to exclude vascular occlusion, which has a very poor prognosis and is normally irreversible.

 ## Follow-Up

- Clinical course
—Oliguric phase: It usually starts early, although it may be delayed for a week or so, and may last up to 60 days.

—Diuretic phase: It can be quite abrupt; sometimes it is a signal that recovering is occurring.
  —Take great care with fluid and electrolyte intake, since the kidneys are unable to deal with a solute load.
  —50% of the deaths occur during this phase.
—Postdiuretic phase
  —Renal function gradually improves over 3 to 12 months, but GFR returns to a normal level only in young patients.
  —Distal tubular function remains permanently impaired, although usually undetectable.
—Prognosis
  —Nonoliguric ARF has a better prognosis than oliguric renal failure.
  —Gastrointestinal bleeding, anemia, coagulopathies, and poor wound healing contribute significantly to morbidity.
  —Mortality rates in ARF range from 7% among patients admitted to a hospital with prerenal azotemia to more than 80% among patients with postoperative ARF.
  —Mortality among patients with severe ARF requiring dialysis has not decreased appreciably over the past 50 years. Of the patients who survive, 30% require dialysis and 20% to 40% have a decrease in glomerular filtration for a year or more.
  —Multiorgan failure, especially in patients with severe hypotension or the acute respiratory distress syndrome: Mortality: 50% to 80%.

 ## Miscellaneous

SYNONYMS: N/A

ASSOCIATED CONDITIONS: N/A

NOTES

- See also Section I, "Renal Failure—Chronic" and "Anuria and Oliguria."

ABBREVIATIONS

- ATN, acute tubular necrosis; ARF, acute renal failure; AIN, acute interstitial nephritis; GFR, glomerular filtration rate; RPGN, rapidly progressive glomerulonephritis

REFERENCES

Bullock N, et al. Renal failure, dialysis and transplantation. In: *Essential Urology*, 2nd ed. Churchill Livinsgstone, 1994:179–195.

Guzman NJ, et al. Acute renal failure. In: *Nephrology*, 2nd ed. Baltimore: Williams & Wilkins, 1993:60–74.

Thadani R, et al. Medical progress: Acute renal failure. *N Engl J Med* 1996;334(22):1448–1460.

Authors: David M. Albala and Fernando C. Koleski

Renal Failure—Chronic

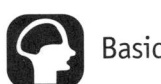 Basics

DESCRIPTION

- Irreversible uremia may follow unresolved acute renal failure (shock kidneys, eclampsia, abruptio placenta, nephrotoxic drugs, hemolytic-uremic syndrome).
- Typically, predictable outcome of gradual loss of renal function (glomerular filtration rate) over months to years
- Plotting reciprocal of serum creatinine concentration (1/CR) against time yields straight line indicating estimate of onset of end-stage renal disease (ESRD).
- Elevated serum creatinine level (>8 mg/dL), normochromic normocytic anemia, acidosis
- Serum creatinine may be lower (<5 mg/dL) in advanced ESRD in children, elderly, and cachectic patients.
- Proteinuria of 1 g/d usual; if greater than 3.5 g/d, suggests nephrotic syndrome
- Persistent urinary obstruction (prostatism, calculi, neoplasm) may culminate in irreversible ESRD.
- Consequence of neurogenic bladder in paraplegia or postspinal surgery
- Radiation "nephritis" following tumor therapy
- Systemic disease involving kidneys (systemic lupus erythematosus, amyloidosis, systemic sclerosis)
- Exclude urethral (prostate, uterine) and ureteric (calculi, tumor, retroperitoneal fibrosis) urinary obstruction.
- ESRD has greater incidence (3×) in African Americans and Native Americans than in Caucasians.

—Hispanics have 2× greater incidence.
—Mean age of incident ESRD patients is now 65 years.

PATHOPHYSIOLOGY

- Reduced clearance of nitrogen-containing compounds (urea, creatinine, and uric acid) and some cations (potassium, magnesium). The most popular laboratory indicators of progressive renal insufficiency are blood levels of urea and creatinine.
- Azotemia, acidosis, from retained solutes and unexcreted organic acids
- Anemia resulting from deficient renal secretion of erythropoietin
- Metabolic bone disease (osteofibrosis, osteosclerosis, osteoporosis) from deficient synthesis of active vitamin D (1,25-dihydroxycholecalciferol)
- Extracellular volume overload leading to edema, ascites, pleural effusions, pericardial effusion
- Muscle wasting, loss of fat due to metabolic toxicity of retained nitrogenous wastes, plus hyperphosphatemia
- Urochrome (orange-green) skin discoloration
- Neuropathy with loss of neurolemmal cells in alpha-myelinated nerves more severe in lower than upper extremities

- Suspected uremic toxins: urea, creatinine, guanidines (methylguanidine, guanidinoacetic acid, guanidinosuccinic acid), indoles, furans, amines, parathyroid hormone, pyrimidines, uric acid

RISK FACTORS

- Hypertension, family history of renal disease (autosomal polycystic kidney disease) and deafness (Alport syndrome), medullary cystic disease, nephrocalcinosis, bilateral renal calculi, instrumentation of atheromatous arteries (atheroembolic renal disease), pelvic surgery (ureteral ligation), plasma cell dyscrasia, hepatitis C, hepatitis B
- Analgesics abuse, nonsteroidal antiinflammatory drugs, aminonucleoside antibiotics, lithium, lead nephropathy
- Systemic lupus erythematosus
- Gout, Fabry disease (alpha-galactosidase A deficiency), hyperoxaluria
- Sickle cell disease
- Glomerulonephritis: mainly children and young adults, focal segmental glomerulonephritis (African Americans) and IgA nephropathy (Asians), Wegener granulomatosis, Goodpasture syndrome
- Vascular disease: malignant hypertension, nephrosclerosis, dissecting aneurysm
- Thrombotic microangiopathies (thrombotic thrombocytopenic purpura)
- Diabetes accounts for 40% of all ESRD in adults.

—Diabetic retinopathy is clinically present in more than 90% of individuals whose ESRD is due to diabetic nephropathy.

 Differential Diagnosis

- Distinguish between primary renal disorder (polycystic kidneys) and systemic disease afflicting kidneys (diabetes). In hypoproteinemic states, identify the relative contribution of deficient albumin synthesis (liver) and protein loss (bowel).
- Renal malfunction in HIV-associated nephropathy and heroin nephropathy
- Interstitial nephritis: Balkan nephropathy, heavy metal poisoning, analgesic abuse
- Inherited renal tubular disorders: Cystinosis, cystinuria, oxalosis, and Fanconi syndrome may cause calculi and obstructive uropathy.
- Congenital malformations: posterior urethral valves, horseshoe kidney, ureteric reflux
- Urosepsis: ESRD though emphysematous pyelonephritis (air discernible on pyelogram) and cystitis are rare, often fatal complications of urinary infection in diabetes.
- Hepatic insufficiency (anemia, hypoalbuminemia, hepatorenal syndrome)
- Advanced malignancy
- Anemia
- Hypothyroidism
- Miscellaneous

—Diuretic toxicity (prerenal azotemia BUN: creatinine level >15:1)
—Profound hypoalbuminemia with intravascular volume contraction (nephrosis, burns)

—Nephrotoxic chemotherapeutic agents: alkylating agents (cisplatin, cyclophosphamide, streptozotocin), antimetabolites (methotrexate, 5-fluorouracil, cytosine arabinoside, 6-thioguanine), antitumor antibiotics (mitomycin, mithramycin, Adriamycin), biologic agents (interferons, interleukins)
—Rhabdomyolysis-induced kidney injury: CRACK toxicity, familial paralysis, porphyria

 Database

HISTORY

- Age, race, gender?

—Glomerulonephritis in young adults, membranous nephritis in middle age, systemic disease, diabetic nephropathy, malignancy in elderly
—Family history of kidney disease or diabetes

- Exposure to nephrotoxins?
- Duration of known hypertension?
- Obtain prior lab test results and/or report of renal biopsy?
- Occupational exposure (lead, mercury, solvents)?
- Substance abuse, drugs, chemotherapy, and antibiotics?

PHYSICAL EXAMINATION

- Hypertension

—85% of ESRD patients: may be primary (malignant hypertension) or secondary to renal insufficiency

- Edema

—Pitting in nephrosis and diabetic nephropathy, associated with pleural and pericardial effusions

- Ecchymosis, oral, anal, renal bleeding

—Defective platelets

- Pallor

—Anemia associated with diminished erythropoietin, bleeding tendency

- Hearing loss

—Alport syndrome

- Rashes

—SLE, Henoch-Schönlein purpura

- Pulsus paradoxus

—Pericardial tamponade

- Abdominal (flank) masses

—Autosomal polycystic kidney disease

- Flank "punch" tenderness (Murphy's sign)

—Active pyelonephritis

- Suprapubic mass, rectal mass

—Obstructed bladder, prostatic hypertrophy malignancy

- Funduscopic abnormalities

—Hypertensive, diabetic, sickle cell retinopathy

- Tophi

—Gouty nephropathy

- Vascular access for hemodialysis, intraperitoneal dialysis catheter

—Established ESRD under treatment by dialysis

- Palpable suprafemoral mass under healed incision scar

—Renal transplant in situ indicating prior ESRD

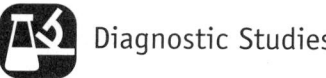 ## Diagnostic Studies

LABORATORY TESTING

- Urine analysis: dipstick and microscopic

—Color: Red indicates current hematuria; brown indicates rhabdomyolysis, chronic renal disease.
—Proteinuria: if 3 to 4+, suggests diabetic nephropathy or nephrotic syndrome
—Red cell casts: active glomerular inflammation (glomerulonephritis)
—Doubly refractile fat bodies under polarized light: nephrotic syndrome

- 24-hour urine collection

—Daily protein excretion: >3.5 g defines nephrotic syndrome.
—Daily creatinine excretion: computation of endogenous creatinine clearance

- Freshly collected urine culture

—Detects active urinary infection if colony count >100,000/mL in women, >10,000/mL in men

- Blood chemistry

—Elevated serum creatinine defines renal failure, low serum albumin in nephrosis, and hyperuricemia in gout.

- Blood antibodies

—ANA in SLE, hepatitis B, C antibody titer, anti-GBM in Goodpasture disease, and rapidly progressive glomerulonephritis

IMAGING

- Abdominal sonography

—Hydronephrosis, enlarged bladder, renal size, opaque calculi

- Abdominal CT or MRI

—Defines renal masses and renal size

- Nuclear renal scans, arteriography, retrograde urethrogram, cystogram as clinically indicated
- Excretory urography

—Defines collecting system filling defects and radiolucent calculi. Contraindicated if serum creatinine >2.0 mg/dL

SPECIAL STUDIES

- Percutaneous kidney biopsy guided by ultrasound

—Indicates need for immunosuppressive therapy in amyloidosis, membranous glomerulonephritis, renal allograft rejection

- Cystoscopy

—Identifies reversible obstruction. Obtain tumor biopsy.

- Renal artery catheterization and angioplasty in bilateral stenosis
- Urodynamics

—Detects adynamic bladder presenting as obstruction with overflow

 ## Initial Management

- Imminent decompensation: seizures, excessive bleeding, hyperkalemia, pericardial tamponade

—Urgent peritoneal or hemodialysis
—Sodium bicarbonate for hyperkalemia in electrocardiogram

- Educate patient and family.

—Options in uremia therapy include peritoneal dialysis, hemodialysis, renal transplantation, and no further intervention.

- Establish access for dialytic regimen.

—Cimino fistula in wrist for hemodialysis or Tenckhoff catheter in abdomen for peritoneal dialysis

- Refer for kidney transplant consideration.

—ACE tissue-typing screening for anti-HLA antibodies

- Control hypertension.

—Inhibitor, calcium channel blocker, diuretics if persistent urine formation

- Administer erythropoietin.

—Raise hematocrit to 35%.
—Measure transferrin and ferritin to determine need for supplemental intravenous iron.

- Reduce hyperphosphatemia.

—Administer calcium carbonate for intestinal binding of dietary phosphorous.
—Limit dietary protein to 0.6 to 0.8 g/kg body weight.
—Synthetic vitamin D to increase dietary calcium absorption, thereby reducing parathormone bone resorption

 ## Follow-Up

- Continue patient education, including reinforcement of social support system.

—Inventory intrafamilial transplant donors, and consider home hemodialysis or continuous ambulatory peritoneal dialysis.

- Monitor blood pressure regulation.

—Adjust doses of antihypertensive drugs (ACE inhibitors may cause hyperkalemia and worsening azotemia).

 ## Miscellaneous

SYNONYMS

- Chronic renal failure, uremia, end-stage renal disease (ESRD)

ASSOCIATED CONDITIONS: N/A

NOTES

- See also Section I, "Renal Failure—Acute."

ABBREVIATIONS

- ESRD, end-stage renal disease; SLE, systemic lupus erythematosus

REFERENCES

Andreoli SP. Renal manifestations of systemic diseases. *Semin Nephrol* 1998;18:270–279.

Brand DA. Perfect timing, no remorse, and kidney transplantation. *Med Decis Making* 1998;18:249–255.

Ifudu O, Dawood M, Homel P, Friedman EA. Timing of initiation of uremia therapy and survival in patients with progressive renal disease. *Am J Nephrol* 1998;18:193–198.

Obrador GT, Pereira BJ. Early referral to the nephrologist and timely initiation of renal replacement therapy: A paradigm shift in the management of patients with chronic renal failure. *Am J Kidney Dis* 1998;31:398–417.

U.S. Renal Data System, USRDS 1998 Annual Data Report, The National Institutes of Health, National Institute of Diabetes and Digestive and Kidney Diseases, Bethesda, MD, April 1998.

Weigert AL, Schafer AI. Uremic bleeding: Pathogenesis and therapy. *Am J Med Sci* 1998;316:94–104.

Author: Eli A. Friedman

Renal Masses—Benign and Malignant

 Basics

DESCRIPTION

- Renal masses are common and are incidentally identified with radiographic imaging with increased frequency.
- These masses are benign or malignant, cystic or solid, unilateral or bilateral, single or multiple, and primary or metastatic.
- Most common: simple renal cyst
- Most common solid tumor 85%: is renal cell carcinoma (RCC)
- 0.33% of adults undergoing screening renal ultrasonography (US) are found to have a malignant renal mass.
- Most common renal mass in newborns: hydronephrosis

PATHOPHYSIOLOGY

- RCC arises from the proximal convoluted tubule cell. A pseudocapsule forms around the tumor. Hemorrhage and necrosis are common. May extend locally and may spread into renal vein and inferior vena cava (IVC) as a tumor thrombus (10%). Metastasizes by both hematogenous and lymphatic routes (regional lymph node, lungs, liver, bone)

RISK FACTORS

- Simple renal cysts: advancing age (rare up to 18 years; 20% incidence age 40; 33% age 60)
- Renal cortical adenoma: adult polycystic kidney disease (APCKD), chronic renal failure (hemodialysis and/or peritoneal dialysis)
- Renal abscess: immunocompromised state, intravenous drug use, diabetes mellitus (DM)
- Xanthogranulomatous pyelonephritis (XGP): middle-aged women (thrice common), DM, chronic obstructing urinary calculi
- Renal cell carcinoma (RCC): male sex (twice common), advancing age, chronic renal failure (hemodialysis and/or peritoneal dialysis), pipe/cigar smoking, family history of von Hippel-Lindau (VHL) or tuberous sclerosis (TS)
- Transitional cell carcinoma (TCC) of renal pelvis: tobacco use, chronic analgesic use (phenacetin), Balkan nephropathy, exposure to aniline dyes, bladder cancer, cyclophosphamide

 Differential Diagnosis

- Cystic renal masses

—Solitary simple cyst: usually an incidental radiographic finding; US diagnosis with 98% accuracy when strict radiographic criteria satisfied (smooth-walled, cystic mass without internal echoes [homogeneous] and increased through transmission)

—Complex renal cyst: cystic mass that does not meet all strict criteria of a simple cyst (solid components, septations, hyperdense, heterogenous, non-through transmission, calcifications); occasionally associated with malignancy; minimally complicated complex cysts have low association with cancer but radiographic follow-up imaging required; complex cysts with solid and cystic components may have a 50% association with malignancy and require further evaluation (radiographic or surgical exploration with possible partial or radical nephrectomy)

—Malignant cysts: Radiographic features are consistent with cancer (e.g., tumor nodules on cyst wall) and are treated surgically with partial or radical nephrectomy.

—Pyogenic cyst: rare complication of renal cystic disease. Infected cyst that responds to drainage and antibiotic therapy

—Multilocular cystic nephroma: benign dysplastic renal mass comprised of multiple cysts with intervening thick, fibrous septations; oftentimes difficult to distinguish from malignant masses; found most commonly in young boys or middle-aged women; requires surgical resection

—Adult polycystic kidney disease: autosomal dominant with 100% penetrance; causes 10% of renal failure; most patients identified between ages of 30 to 50 years; associated findings (bilateral, large, multicystic kidneys; hypertension [HTN]; hepatic, pancreatic, and pulmonary cysts; cerebral berry aneurysms of the circle of Willis; colon diverticula; mitral valve prolapse)

—Acquired renal cystic disease: cystic degeneration of end-stage kidneys: Extent of cystic disease is dependent on duration of renal failure (most commonly develops in patients undergoing hemodialysis or peritoneal dialysis) and is associated with RCC.

- Benign solid renal masses

—True oncocytoma: male > female, median size 6 cm, 6% bilateral, well-circumscribed tumor that is difficult to distinguish from malignant tumors by radiographs alone (spoke-wheel appearance angiography), oftentimes coexists with renal malignancies; preferred therapy is radical or partial nephrectomy

—Renal cortical adenoma: most commonly found incidentally, usually less than 3 cm in diameter, considered benign, but may represent earliest stage of RCC (controversial); radiographic characteristics indistinguishable from RCC; most treated surgically

—Hemangioma: congenital tumor derived from endothelium of blood and lymphatic vessels. Patients present with intermittent hematuria. Renal angiography may localize lesion.

—Angiomyolipoma (AML) (renal hamartoma): <0.5% of renal tumors, right side involved 80% of time for unknown reasons; develops in >50% of patients with tuberous sclerosis (hereditary, mental retardation, epilepsy, adenoma sebaceum, multiorgan hamartomas); however, majority of patients with AML (most commonly middle-aged women) do not have TS; TS (small, multiple, bilateral tumors), non-TS (larger, unilateral tumors); AML histologically composed of blood vessels, adipose, and smooth muscle elements; CT scan makes diagnosis secondary to intratumoral fat; may be cause of spontaneous perirenal hemorrhage

—Renal pelvis papilloma: benign transitional cell tumor; multiple papillomas associated with future development of malignant TCC

—Hemangiopericytoma: renin-secreting tumor arising from capillary pericytes in juxtaglomerular apparatus. Patients present with HTN and elevated renal vein renin levels.

—Pseudotumor: normal variant, appears as questionable mass on IVP or US (dDx fetal lobulation, hypertrophied column of Bertin, dromedary hump, nodular compensatory hypertrophy). DMSA renal scan confirms diagnosis (95% sensitivity).

—Other less common benign solid renal masses include fibroma, lipoma, leiomyoma, renal capsule tumor, and arteriovenous malformation.

- Inflammatory renal masses

—Renal abscess (carbuncle): renal collection of purulent material; arises from pyelonephritis (gram-negative organisms) or from distant sites from hematogenous spread (*Staphylococcus aureus*). Patients usually present with greater than 5-day history of fever, flank pain and tenderness, and urinary tract infection. It is treated with intravenous antibiotics and percutaneous or open surgical drainage.

—Xanthogranulomatous pyelonephritis: Chronic renal parenchymal infection is usually secondary to high-grade obstruction (usually ureteropelvic junction), which gives rise to a renal mass lesion that often mimics RCC. Patients present with recurrent urinary tract infection, renal calculi, and constitutional symptoms commonly; they may present with anemia and reversible hepatic dysfunction (hypoalbuminemia and elevated liver function tests [LFTs]). Histology reveals lipid-laden macrophages, termed *foam cells*.

—Genitourinary tuberculosis: follows prior pulmonary infection (may be asymptomatic). Renal infection is slow and usually asymptomatic. Mass lesions are secondary to renal abscesses or urinary tract obstruction.

- Malignant renal masses

—Renal cell carcinoma (hypernephroma, internist's tumor): represents 90% of malignant renal tumors. Patients present in myriad ways. Incidence increases with advancing age, 2:1 male sex predominance, 2% are bilateral (synchronous or asynchronous). The most common distant metastasis site is the lung, followed by liver, bone, adrenal, and contralateral kidney. Clear cell is most common histological type. The sarcomatoid type carries the worst prognosis. Treatment is radical or partial nephrectomy. Overall survival is dependent on pathologic stage. Occasionally it is predominantly cystic in appearance and is known as renal papillary cystadenocarcinoma.

—TCC of renal pelvis: 4% of urinary tract TCC; 30% of patients with upper tract TCC will develop lower urinary tract TCC; 50% present with superficial disease. Radical nephroureterectomy with excision of a cuff of bladder is the treatment of choice. Patients with a solitary kidney may sometimes be treated with conservative measures (endoscopic resection, partial nephrectomy).

—Squamous cell carcinoma of kidney: arises from renal pelvis epithelium secondary to chronic urinary tract infection and irritation from nephrolithiasis. Patients present with advanced disease and respond poorly to treatment.

—Renal sarcomas: represent 3% of malignant renal tumors; difficult to distinguish from RCC radiographically. Radical nephrectomy with adjuvant therapy is the current treatment. Pathology reveals leiomyosarcoma (most common), liposarcoma, rhabdomyosarcoma, and malignant fibrous histiocytoma.

—Renal lymphoma: Primary renal lymphoma is rare, and renal involvement usually follows systemic disease. Treatment is directed toward the primary tumor. Nephrectomy is indicated only for severe symptoms, a solitary lesion, or severe bleeding.

- Metastatic renal masses

—Metastases to the kidney from nonrenal cancers (breast most common, followed by lung, intestine, and contralateral kidney) are usually multiple and silent clinically. Prognosis depends on treatment of the primary tumor.

- Special pediatric renal masses

—Hydronephrosis: most common cause of pediatric abdominal mass
   —Ureteropelvic junction (UPJ) obstruction: most common etiology of prenatal hydronephrosis
—Multicystic dysplastic kidney: most common cause of renal cystic disease in infants, characterized by small, benign, dysplastic, nonfunctioning fetal kidney; high incidence of contralateral upper urinary tract abnormalities; nephrectomy if patient symptomatic or has associated hypertension
—Mesoblastic nephroma: most common solid renal benign tumor in newborns. Treatment is nephrectomy.
—Wilms' tumor (nephroblastoma): most common childhood renal malignancy, with median age of diagnosis at 3 years

 Database

HISTORY

- General characteristics of the patient?

—Most renal masses today are incidentally discovered radiographically.
—Both simple renal cysts and malignant renal tumors rarely present prior to the age of 20.

- Fever?

—May signify inflammatory renal mass. 20% of patients with RCC have intermittent fever of unknown origin.

- Hematuria?

—60% of patients with RCC have either gross or microscopic hematuria. Painless hematuria should be considered a genitourinary malignancy until proven otherwise.

- Flank pain?

—Inflammatory process (e.g., XGP).
—Symptom secondary to renal capsule tumor invasion or urinary obstruction. 41% of patients with RCC have flank pain.
—The classic triad of flank pain, hematuria, and flank mass is present in only 10% of RCC patients and usually suggests advanced disease.

- Weight loss, nightsweats?

—Common in RCC, but may be presenting symptoms of renal tuberculosis or lymphoma

- Renal failure/hemodialysis?

—Duration of end-stage renal disease is directly related to the incidence of acquired renal cystic disease and concomitant RCC.

(continued)

Renal Masses—Benign and Malignant (continued)

- Family history?

—VHL: hereditary disease characterized by multiple tumors (bilateral renal cell carcinoma and renal cysts, cerebellar hemangioblastomas, retinal hemangiomas, pheochromocytomas, pancreatic islet cell tumors, and epididymal cystadenomas). RCC occurs in up to 38% of affected individuals, and nearly 45% die of kidney cancer.

—TS: patients at risk for AML (see above); 2% develop RCC

—APCKD: Patients oftentimes develop renal cortical adenomas.

—RCC: Familial RCC has been described (less common).

- Tobacco use?

—Evidence suggests tobacco use is related to TCC of the renal pelvis.

—Cigar/pipe smoking may be related to RCC.

- Occupational risk factors?

—Exposure to aniline dyes predisposes to TCC of the renal pelvis.

PHYSICAL EXAMINATION

- General

—Cachexia may suggest metastatic disease.

- Fever

—Suggests UTI, inflammatory or malignant renal mass

- Hypertension

—APCKD, hemangiopericytoma. 22% of patients with RCC have HTN.

- Hypotension

—Spontaneous perirenal hemorrhage secondary to RCC or AML

- Varicocele

—A left-sided varicocele (most common) suggests left renal tumor extension into the left renal vein, and a right-sided varicocele suggests right renal tumor extension into the inferior vena cava with obstruction.

 Diagnostic Studies

LABORATORY TESTING

- Urinalysis

—Gross or microscopic hematuria suggests genitourinary disease and requires further evaluation.

—Nitrite or leukocyte esterase positive. Pyuria suggests infection or an inflammatory renal mass.

- Urine culture

—Performed when clinical findings suggest renal or urinary tract infection

—Sterile pyuria may suggest genitourinary tuberculosis.

- Voided urine cytology

—May detect TCC of urinary tract (good specificity)

—Positive in only 7% of patients with RCC

- Complete blood count (CBC)

—Anemia is most common laboratory abnormality with RCC; occasionally erythrocytosis (3%) secondary to increased erythropoietin secretion

- Renal function tests (BUN and creatinine)

—Evaluate baseline renal function.

- Liver function tests (LFTs)

—Up to 20% of patients with RCC may have abnormal LFTs (most commonly elevated serum alkaline phosphatase) secondary to Stauffer syndrome (nonmetastatic reversible hepatic dysfunction); LFTs may also be abnormal in the setting of tumor metastases.

—Oftentimes abnormal in XGP

- Serum calcium

—May be elevated in RCC secondary to paraneoplastic syndrome; tumor secretes parathormone related protein. Elevation may also occasionally signify bony metastases.

IMAGING

- Chest x-ray

—Useful for preoperative clinical staging when malignant renal mass diagnosis made

—May also evaluate for primary tuberculosis

- KUB

—Detects enlarged or malpositioned renal shadow and identifies 90% of renal calculi; occasionally detects perirenal gas, which is a urologic emergency

—Loss of psoas margin signifies a retroperitoneal process (ipsilateral).

- Intravenous pyelogram (IVP; excretory urogram) with renal tomography

—Imaging method of choice for hematuria; evaluates upper urinary tract and kidney (not ideal for bladder)

—Detects renal masses; however, sensitivity for those <3 cm is only 67%

—Identifies urinary obstruction; defines contralateral renal function

—Filling defects in the collecting system may signify tumor.

- Renal ultrasonography (US)

—More sensitive in detecting renal masses than IVP

—Cost-effective follow-up radiographic imaging study to suspicious IVP

—Characterizes solid and/or cystic nature of renal mass

—Upper urinary tract imaging study of choice in children

- Abdominal CT scan (CT)

—"Gold standard" for evaluating renal masses

—Small tumors and complex renal cysts best evaluated with 5-mm "thin-cut" slices before and after IV contrast administration

—Useful in cancer staging (identifies tumor local extension, renal vein or IVC involvement, intraabdominal metastases), defining surgical anatomy, and evaluating contralateral kidney

- Abdominal MRI

—Generally not preferred to CT; may define local extension of tumor

—Best to evaluate vascular structures with RCC (extent of venous tumor involvement)

- Renal arteriography

—Largely replaced by CT/digital subtraction angiography

—Used primarily for planning partial nephrectomy surgery

- Retrograde pyelography, nuclear medicine DMSA scan as clinically indicated

SPECIAL STUDIES

- Cystoscopy and/or retrograde pyelography

—Should be performed on patients with hematuria to exclude lower urinary tract (bladder) pathology

- Percutaneous renal mass aspiration or biopsy

—Not recommended for patients except when there is high suspicion of lymphoma, nonrenal cancer metastatic to the kidney, or abscess; associated with tumor seeding of the needle tract and false-negative biopsies

 Initial Management

- Patients presenting with urologic symptoms, especially hematuria or flank pain, should undergo urinalysis (urine culture and/or urine cytology based on clinical findings) and appropriate radiographic imaging when indicated.
- Patients with hematuria should undergo IVP.
- Suspicious renal mass abnormalities detected on IVP should be further investigated with renal US.
- Solid masses or complex cysts detected by US should be further studied by CT scan.
- Inflammatory renal masses (renal abscess, XGP, emphysematous pyelonephritis [gas in affected kidney]) need urgent urologic evaluation and appropriate treatment.
- Solid renal masses usually need surgical treatment with radical or partial nephrectomy (tumor <4 cm and contralateral kidney normal, bilateral renal tumors, systemic disease [e.g., DM, HTN] predisposing to chronic renal failure).
- AML diagnosed by CT may be observed if small (<4 cm), stable in size, and asymptomatic. Larger tumors have an increased tendency to spontaneously bleed and are therefore best treated with radical or partial nephrectomy. Angioembolization has a role in selected cases.
- Once the diagnosis of a malignant renal mass is made, clinical staging continues with CXR and also with a bone scan in patients with either bone pain or elevated serum alkaline phosphatase.

 Follow-Up

- Simple renal cysts defined by US need no further follow-up unless the patient becomes symptomatic or other signs develop.

—Symptomatic simple cysts can be treated with aspiration and sclerosis with alcohol with high success rates.

- Complex renal cysts warrant periodic radiographic surveillance or surgical exploration with radical or partial nephrectomy, because a proportion of these will eventually prove to be malignant

 Miscellaneous

SYNONYMS: N/A

ASSOCIATED CONDITIONS: N/A

NOTES
- See Section II for specific tumor types.

ABBREVIATIONS
- AML, angiomyolipoma; APCKD, adult polycystic kidney disease; dDx, differential diagnosis; DM, diabetes mellitus; HTN, hypertension; RCC, renal cell carcinoma; TCC, transitional cell carcinoma; TS, tuberous sclerosis; VHL, von Hippel-Lindau; XGP, xanthogranulomatous pyelonephritis

REFERENCES

Belldegrun A. Renal tumors. In: Walsh PC, Retik AB, Vaughan ED, Wein AJ, eds. *Campbell's Urology,* 7th ed. Philadelphia: WB Saunders, 1998: 2283–2326.

Pritchett TR. Clinical manifestations and treatment of renal parenchymal tumors. In: Skinner DG, Lieskovsky G, eds. *Diagnosis and Management of Genitourinary Cancer.* Philadelphia: WB Saunders, 1988:337–361.

Stein JP, Skinner DG. Radical nephrectomy. In: Petrovich Z, et al., eds. *Carcinoma of the Kidney, Testis, and Uncommon Tumors of the Genitourinary Tract.* Berlin: Springer-Verlag, (*in press*)

Wolf JS. Evaluation and management of solid and cystic renal masses. *J Urol* 1998;159:1120.

Authors: Michael A. Lawrence and John P. Stein

Renal Trauma

 Basics

DESCRIPTION

• Renal injuries occur from a blunt or penetrating injury and are not always obvious.

PATHOPHYSIOLOGY

• Blunt trauma

—80% to 90% of renal injuries from blunt injury
—Direct blow to the flank or abdomen

• Laceration from lower rib fractures or transverse processes of L1-L3 vertebral bodies
• Main vessel stretching/avulsion from a deceleration injury or direct contusion
   —Intimal tearing, arterial thrombosis, and renal ischemia

• Penetrating trauma: stab or gunshot wounds

—Many factors involved: bullet yaw, fragmentation, velocity, and tissue characteristics
—High risk for major renal injury. Accurate staging is essential for expectant management.
—The blast effect may cause contusion in proximity of the bullet path.

• Vascular injuries can occur from blunt or penetrating injury.

RISK FACTORS

• Adult: blunt trauma

—Deceleration injury, direct blow to flank, flank pain/contusions, and lower rib or lumbar transverse processes fractures
—Major laceration(s) with >one-third to one-half of devascularized tissue have an increased risk of complications.

• Adult: penetrating trauma

—Major injury occurs in 40% to 67% of penetrating renal injuries.

• Pediatric: blunt or penetrating

—Pediatric kidney relatively larger and less protected
—Preexisting abnormalities more likely; approximately 10% of pediatric hydronephrosis/tumor present with trauma.

 Differential Diagnosis

• Diagnosis usually straightforward
• Do not confuse with a congenital anomaly, e.g., congenitally absent kidney.

 Database

HISTORY

• Information sometimes limited in trauma setting

• Pediatric history is less reliable, i.e., a minimal history of trauma may be associated with a major renal injury.
• Key elements for initial decision making

—Mechanism of injury: stratifies high (penetrating) vs. lower (blunt) risk
—Initial BP: <90 mm Hg in adult
—Gross hematuria indicates a need for imaging studies.
—Triage associated injuries for overall management strategy.
—Hypotension: late sign of severe injury in children, therefore unreliable

• Medical history

—Inquire about medical conditions affecting renal function: hypertension, diabetes, etc.
—Previous renal surgery for stones, cancer, trauma
—Iodine, contrast allergy
—General health, cardiac, pulmonary history

PHYSICAL EXAMINATION

• Vital signs: in particular, systolic blood pressure
• General examination for any signs of acute injury
• Note previous surgical scars
• Specific signs of genitourinary injury

—Flank contusions/tenderness
—Abdominal tenderness/distension
—Pelvic fractures
—GU: meatal or urinary bleeding, rectal examination

 Diagnostic Studies

LABORATORY TESTING

• Urinalysis

—Hematuria >90% of renal injuries
—Best indicator of renal trauma, but, 19% to 36% of pedicle injuries have normal urinalysis.
   —Check first (preferably voided) urine
   —Significant hematuria is >5 RBCs/HPF (arbitrary definition).
   —Dipstick excellent: sensitivity and specificity of 98%

IMAGING

• Defines injury severity to direct management
• Clinical staging determines the need for radiographic staging.
• Adults sustaining blunt trauma with microscopic hematuria and stable blood pressure rarely have a major renal injury (0.5%). If there is no clinical indicator, it is extremely unlikely that a major renal injury is present. Imaging is not required.
• Indications for radiographic staging

—Adult: blunt trauma
   —Hypotension (systolic <90 mm Hg) and any hematuria
   —Presence of gross hematuria

—Clinical indicators of renal injury from history and physical examination
—Pediatric (≤16 years old): blunt trauma
   —In children, imaging is recommended with any degree of hematuria after trauma.
   —Parameters determining the need for radiographic imaging in children are not well established.
   —Probably higher risk group
—Adult or pediatric: penetrating trauma
—Imaging should be performed after any penetrating injury with any degree of hematuria.

• Intravenous urography: intraoperative

—Confirms contralateral renal function; may localize injury but not define it
—2 cc/kg IV contrast bolus, maximum 150 cc. Check the IV site during infusion.
—Intraoperative "one-shot" IVP: Expose film at 10 minutes, repeat if necessary.
—33% to 60% of IVPs may not be adequate to exclude a major injury.

• Ultrasound

—Not for initial work-up: does not determine function; difficult to distinguish hematoma from extravasation

• CT scan

—Best single study for staging renal injuries
—Most sensitive study for urinary extravasation
—Identifies associated organ injury(s)
—Renal artery thrombosis has a characteristic image and can be reliably diagnosed.
—Scanning can be too rapid; i.e., image after contrast has entered the collecting system.

SPECIAL STUDIES

• Arteriography: largely replaced by CT; useful if embolization necessary (rare)

 Initial Management

• Accurate injury detection and classification

—Staging is the process of determining the extent of renal injury. It consists of three parts.
   —Clinical, radiographic, and surgical

—Some patients only require clinical staging and others more extensive evaluation.
—Accurate staging leads to selective surgery.
—Renal injury classification: severity of parenchymal damage by the Organ Injury Scaling Committee of the American Association for the Surgery of Trauma. Minor Injury: I to II; major injury: III to V
   —Grade I: microscopic or gross hematuria, normal radiographic study(s), contusion/contained subcapsular hematoma, no parenchymal laceration
   —Grade II: nonexpanding perirenal hematoma or cortical laceration <1 cm deep
   —Grade III: laceration >1 cm into the parenchyma without extravasation

—Grade IV: laceration >1 cm (beyond corti-comedullary junction) with extravasation or segmental arterial thrombosis.
—Grade V: multiple major lacerations, or thrombosis/avulsion of the main renal vessels

- Selecting a radiographic study: examples

—Coordinate with the trauma team and tailor to the clinical situation.
—Renal imaging required, CT planned to assess possible splenic rupture: Kidneys will be evaluated.
—Aortogram planned to evaluate vessels: Additional "IVP" films should be taken. If injury is suspected, selective renal artery injection is possible.
—Stab wound to the flank, laparotomy not required: CT scan to evaluate the kidneys
—Intraoperative consult: A "one-shot" IVP is the only practical study to confirm contralateral function.

- Definitive management

—General rule: In the case of blunt injury, there should be compelling reasons *to* operate, whereas in the case of penetrating injury, there should be compelling reasons *not* to operate.
—Blunt trauma: general principles
  —Degree of hematuria does *not* correlate to injury severity.
  —Minor injuries are safely and properly managed expectantly.
  —Most renal injuries are due to blunt trauma; only 2% to 3% require surgery.
—Blunt trauma: major lacerations
  —Course unpredictable; early complications: bleeding (most common), urinoma, abscess
  —Management controversial; most observed
  —Completely transected or shattered kidneys are uncommon but require surgery.
  —Large segments of devitalized tissue and major laceration higher risk; surgery considered
  —If laparotomy planned for associated injury, repair kidney
—Penetrating injuries
  —Most penetrating injuries are major; surgery is required.
  —Laparotomy is usually required after gunshot wounds. Adequate preoperative staging often is not possible. Renal exploration (surgical staging) is necessary in this situation.
  —Selected patients that do not require laparotomy, e.g., flank stab wound, can be observed if accurately staged by CT scan.
—Vascular injuries
  —Segmental arterial thrombosis leads to parenchymal infarct and is diagnosed by CT.
  —Observation is recommended if there is no major laceration.

—Main renal vessel injury
—Artery 70%, vein 20%, both 10% (blunt trauma)
—Bilateral arterial injury: 5%
—Poorest renal salvage rates with arterial injury; slightly better if only vein injured
—Usually occur in a multiply injured patient, preventing time-consuming, complicated vascular repair
—Early diagnosis and repair is the only hope for salvage. The literature is not clear on time intervals. Return of function is rare.
—Some injuries may be partial and allow delayed reconstruction and salvage.
—Absolute indications for renal exploration
  —Renal bleeding with hemodynamic instability
  —Expanding or pulsatile retroperitoneal hematoma found during laparotomy
  —Main artery injury bilaterally or in a solitary kidney
—Relative indications for renal exploration
  —Nonviable tissue and major laceration
  —Urinary extravasation
  —Renal artery thrombosis
  —Incomplete injury staging
  —Concomitant laparotomy for associated injury(s)
—Renal surgery: general considerations
  —Constant awareness of patient's condition (i.e., save the patient)
  —Confirm contralateral function by contrast study. Palpation is not sufficient!
  —Injuries addressed in order of severity, e.g., pedicle injury
—Renal surgery: vascular control
  —Midline incision: always
  —First step: control artery and vein in the midline over aorta
  —12% need temporary arterial occlusion; no predictor of the need for occlusion (hematoma size, etc.)
  —Prolonged artery occlusion (>20–30 minutes) requires surface cooling with slush.
—Renal surgery: principles of renal repair
  —Complete mobilization of the injured kidney
  —Debridement of nonviable tissue
  —Suturing of bleeding vessels: chromic
  —Collecting system closure: chromic
  —Closed drainage of perirenal area
  —Stents or nephrostomy tubes rarely necessary
—Renal surgery: types of repair
  —Suture of parenchymal laceration
  —Renorrhaphy with Gelfoam bolster
  —Renorrhaphy with omental coverage
  —Partial nephrectomy
  —Nephrectomy
  —Main vessel repair
    —Suture repair: Prolene
    —Excision with or without vascular grafting
    —Autotransplantation: rarely necessary

Follow-up

- Postoperative care

—Ambulate when urine clears; early drain removal to prevent infection
—Follow-up imaging based on clinical course (i.e., fever, ileus, etc.). Consider a CT scan.

- Postoperative complications: early

—Delayed bleeding, urinoma, perinephric abscess

- Postoperative complications: late

—Hypertension: about 5%. Responds best to surgical treatment during the first year
—Arteriovenous fistula: usually closes spontaneously; otherwise embolize

- Follow-up

—Observed major lacerations reimaged before hospital discharge or sooner if needed
—Frequent blood pressure and UAs during first year

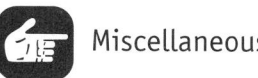

Miscellaneous

SYNONYMS: *N/A*

ASSOCIATED CONDITIONS: *N/A*

NOTES: *N/A*

ABBREVIATIONS: *N/A*

REFERENCES

Carroll PR, McAninch JW. Staging of renal trauma. *Urol Clin North Am* 1989;16:193–202.

Dixon CM, McAninch JW. Traumatic renal injuries, Part I. Patient assessment and management. AUA Update Series, Vol X, Lesson 35, 1991.

Dixon CM, McAninch JW. Traumatic renal injuries, Part II. Operative management. AUA Update Series, Vol X, Lesson 36, 1991.

McAninch JW, Carroll PR. Renal exploration after trauma: Indications and reconstructive techniques. *Urol Clin North Am* 1989;16:203–212.

Mee SL, McAninch JW, Robinson AL, Auerback PS, Carroll PR. Radiographic assessment of renal trauma: 10 year prospective study of patient selection. *J Urol* 1989;141:1095–1098.

Author: Christopher M. Dixon

Retrograde Ejaculation

 Basics

DESCRIPTION

• Ejaculation is the expulsion of semen from the urethra and has three distinct phases: emission, closure of the bladder neck, and propulsion.
• Retrograde ejaculation is the backward propulsion of semen into the bladder.

—Complete retrograde ejaculation presents as lack of ejaculation.

• Retrograde ejaculation can occur with varying degrees of antegrade ejaculation.

—Combination antegrade and retrograde ejaculation presents as low-volume ejaculation.

PATHOPHYSIOLOGY

• Antegrade ejaculation requires coordination between the ejaculatory ducts, bladder neck, bulbo/ischiocavernosus muscles, and external sphincter.

—Processes that interfere with the anatomy, innervation, or function of the ejaculatory ducts, bladder neck, bulbo/ischiocavernosus muscles, and external sphincter can cause abnormal ejaculation. Ejaculatory innervation is primarily T10-L3; somatic efferents arising in S2-S4 innervate the bulbo/ischiocavernosus muscles.

RISK FACTORS

• Surgical procedures

—Bladder neck surgery, retroperitoneal lymph node dissection, extensive pelvic surgery, and prostate surgery

• Neurologic abnormalities

—Diabetes mellitus, multiple sclerosis, and spinal cord abnormalities

• BPU

—Use of alpha blockers (i.e., terazosin, etc.)

 Differential Diagnosis

• Lack of ejaculation: complete retrograde ejaculation
• Lack of ejaculation: lack of emission; semen is not expulsed into the posterior urethra.

—Agenesis of seminal vesicles, ejaculatory duct obstruction, neurologic abnormalities, and psychological disturbances
—Hypogonadism

• Low-volume ejaculation: combination of antegrade and retrograde ejaculation
• Low-volume ejaculation: can occur without retrograde ejaculation

—Unilateral agenesis of seminal vesicle, partial ejaculatory duct obstruction, and neurologic abnormalities
—Hypogonadism

• Collection artifacts

—Incomplete collection, short abstinence period, and low volumes with masturbation

 Database

HISTORY

• Ejaculatory symptoms

—Amount of ejaculation and relation to duration of abstinence; ?painful ejaculation (can be sign of obstruction); ?cloudy postejaculate urine (due to semen in urine)

• Medical history

—Surgical procedures (bladder neck, prostate, retroperitoneal, pelvic); neurologic abnormalities (including diabetes, multiple sclerosis, spinal cord injury, transverse myelitis, myelodysplasia); prior children/pregnancies; personal or family history of cystic fibrosis; posterior urethral valves

• Medications

—α-Blockers, antidepressants, antipsychotics, narcotics, and benzodiazepines are the most common pharmaceutical causes of retrograde ejaculation.

PHYSICAL EXAMINATION

• General

—Habitus; secondary sex characteristics; back (dimpling or signs of occult spinal dysraphism)

• Genitourinary

—Epididymis: A firm or enlarged epididymis may indicate obstruction.
—Vas deferens: Palpate from the convoluted portion to the external ring. An absent vas is associated with an absent unilateral seminal vesicle and kidney.
—Testes: size and consistency. Small, soft testes can be a sign of hypogonadism.
—Digital rectal examination: enlarged (obstructed) or absent seminal vesicle (can be difficult to palpate)

• Neurologic

—Complete motor/sensory examination
—Reflexes: abdominal (T6-L2), cremasteric (L1-L2), anal/bulbocavernosus (S2-S5), quadriceps (L3-L4) DTR, and ankle (L5-S2) DTR

Diagnostic Studies

LABORATORY TESTING

- Semen analysis

—Particular attention to volume, sperm concentration, and total sperm count

- Postejaculate urine specimen

—Centrifuge specimen for 10 minutes at >300 g. More than 5 to 10 sperm per high power field indicates retrograde ejaculation.

—Determine sperm concentration and total sperm count of postejaculate urine. To determine the degree of retrograde ejaculation, compare the sperm counts of the postejaculate urine specimen with those of the antegrade specimen.

- Serum testosterone level

IMAGING

- TRUS

—Absence of sperm in the postejaculate urine with absent or low-volume ejaculate may indicate ejaculatory duct obstruction or seminal vesicle agenesis. TRUS is an excellent modality to image the ejaculatory ducts and seminal vesicles.

- MRI

—Can be useful to delineate spinal cord abnormalities or unclear findings on TRUS

SPECIAL STUDIES

- Evoked neurologic potentials

 ## Initial Management

- α-Sympathomimetic agents and antihistamines: Success depends on etiology (higher success rates for neurologic abnormalities).

—Phenylpropanolamine 75 mg bid; pseudoephedrine 60 mg qid; ephedrine 25 to 50 mg qid; imipramine 50 mg qhs

- Assisted reproduction

—Fluid intake is adjusted to ensure the urine is isotonic, and the urine is alkalized with sodium bicarbonate 650 mg qid. Ham's F-10 culture medium can be instilled into the bladder prior to ejaculation. Sperm are recovered from the bladder and washed with Ham's F-10 medium. Intrauterine insemination, in vitro fertilization, or intracytoplasmic sperm injection is performed as indicated.

 ## Follow-Up

- Retrograde ejaculation is a benign condition. Follow-up should be performed as indicated for associated medical problems or to achieve pregnancy.

 ## Miscellaneous

SYNONYMS: N/A

ASSOCIATED CONDITIONS: N/A

NOTES: N/A

ABBREVIATIONS

- DTR, deep-tendon reflex

REFERENCES

Gilja I, et al. Retrograde ejaculation and loss of emission: Possibilities of conservative treatment. *Eur Urol* 1994;25:226.

Meacham RB, et al. Male infertility. In: Gillenwater JY, Grayhack JT, Howards SS, Duckett JW, eds. *Adult and Pediatric Urology*, 3rd ed. St Louis: Mosby–Year Book, 1996:1747–1802.

Okada H, et al. Treatment of patients with retrograde ejaculation in the era of modern assisted reproduction technology. *J Urol* 1998;159:848.

Yavetz H, et al. Retrograde ejaculation. *Hum Reprod* 1994;9:381.

Author: Joseph R. Wagner

Retroperitoneal Mass

 Basics

DESCRIPTION

- A mass in the retroperitoneal space may be solid, cystic, inflammatory, or infectious.

—Solid: tumor arising from/in retroperitoneal tissue, excluding tumors of solid organs (kidney, adrenal, ureter, pancreas)
—Cystic mass: congenital or acquired
—Inflammatory: retroperitoneal fibrosis (see Section II, "Retroperitoneal Fibrosis")
—Infectious: retroperitoneal abscess (see Section II, "Retroperitoneal Abscess")

PATHOPHYSIOLOGY

- Incidental or present with vague abdominal, GI, or GU complaints and palpable mass

—The retroperitoneum has no significant anatomic barriers.
—Retroperitoneal masses here can grow to a large size before symptoms occur.

- Solid mass

—Metastases with or without lymphadenopathy
  —Testicular, breast, colon, kidney, and gastric cancer (common)
—Primary retroperitoneal sarcoma (1000 cases/yr)
  —Arise from any connective tissue element
  —Peaks at sixth decade of life; can occur anytime
  —Equal incidence in men and women
  —Slow-growing, locally aggressive; rare lymphatic metastases
  —Metastases late primarily via hematogenous route (lung, liver, bone)
—Primary benign tumors: slow growth; encroachment of adjacent organs
—Cystic masses
  —Congenital: may represent urogenital remnant; in females, wolffian duct remnants
  —Acquired: conditions predisposing to accumulation of fluid in the retroperitoneum
—Retroperitoneal fibrosis
  —Insidious onset, usually idiopathic
  —Progressive pain and renal impairment secondary to obstruction

- Retroperitoneal abscess
  —GU causes: stone, infected urinoma, perirenal hematoma
  —GI cause: infected appendiceal, duodenal, or colonic process

RISK FACTORS

- History of malignancy
- Cryptorchidism (testicular cancer)
- Increased incidence of sarcoma in

—Genetic diseases: Gardner syndrome, neurofibromatosis (von Recklinghausen disease), tuberous sclerosis, Li-Fraumeni syndrome
—Patients treated for retinoblastoma in childhood or previous exposure to ionizing radiation

- Spontaneous retroperitoneal or perirenal hematoma should raise suspicion for underlying neoplasm.
- Teratomas and dermoid cysts most common in children

 Differential Diagnosis

- Most common cause of solid retroperitoneal mass is metastatic disease: testicular, breast, gastric, colon, kidney
- Primary retroperitoneal tumors

—Malignant (85%)
  —Primarily sarcoma (50%; liposarcoma most common)
  —Lymphoma (25%)
  —Primary retroperitoneal germ cell tumor (rare)
—Benign (15%)
  —Neural origin (30%), cystic (22%), lipoma (16%)

- Cystic mass

—Congenital: most common in females, usually located posterior to gonadal vessels
—Acquired
  —Urinary: recent history of stone passage (forniceal rupture with urinoma formation)
  —Lymphatic: history of lymphadenectomy, abdominal or vascular surgery
  —Hematoma: in presence of neoplasm, may be caused even by minimal trauma
  —Teratoma: may have both cystic and solid elements; most common in children

- Inflammatory

—Primary (idiopathic) retroperitoneal fibrosis
—Secondary to known agent (methysergide, methyldopa, LSD, radiation therapy)
—Secondary to vascular disease (abdominal aortic aneurysm, periaortitis) or malignancy with desmoplastic reaction

- Infectious: retroperitoneal abscess (GI or GU pathology)

 Database

HISTORY

- Age and sex of the patient?

—Breast cancer: common cancer in women
—Testicular cancer: most common malignancy in 15- to 35-year-old men
—Malignant fibrous histiocytoma: older patients

- Low-grade fever?

—Infection or tumor necrosis (sarcoma)

- Abdominal pain?

—Stretching of peritoneum

- Back pain?
- Enlarging abdominal girth?
- Constitutional symptoms

—Unintentional weight loss, anorexia, malaise?

- Obstructive GI symptoms

—Early satiety, bloating, nausea/vomiting, new-onset constipation?

- GU symptoms

—Flank pain, urgency/frequency?
  —Mass effect and decreased bladder capacity
—History of UTIs or stones?

- Neurologic symptoms?

—Nerve root impingement or peripheral nerve (genitofemoral, ilioinguinal) invasion

- Medical and surgical history

—History of malignancy and treatment?
—Previous abdominal or pelvic surgery?
—History of childhood diseases or surgeries?

- Medications?
- Family history?

PHYSICAL EXAMINATION

- Palpable abdominal mass

—Most common physical finding; often painless; hard or ballotable

- Cachexia: underlying malignancy or chronic disease
- Lymphadenopathy: metastatic disease, lymphoma
- Breast examination: breast cancer
- Testicular examination: mass or varicocele that does not decompress with reclining
- Lower extremity edema: venous compression by retroperitoneal mass

Diagnostic Studies

LABORATORY TESTING

• Complete blood count

—Leukocytosis with infection
—Anemia: hemorrhage, chronic disease, azotemia, or malignancy

• Creatine/BUN: possible obstruction
• Urinalysis: hematuria with renal tumors or stones
• Serum markers

—Alpha-feto protein and beta-hCG in males (testicular cancer)
—ESR often elevated in retroperitoneal fibrosis/abscess

• Complete chemistry panel

—Elevated liver function tests suggest hepatic invasion or biliary obstruction.
—Elevated alkaline phosphatase should raise suspicion of bony metastases.

IMAGING

• Abdominal CT: most important modality

—Nodal enlargement separate from great vessels suggests malignancy (metastases, lymphoma).
—A dense mass surrounding great vessels and ureters without lymphadenopathy suggests retroperitoneal fibrosis.

• IVP: diagnosis of retroperitoneal fibrosis (medial deviation of ureters)
• MRI: additional information on relationship of mass to adjacent organs and vessels
• Testicular US: to rule out testicular cancer
• Mammogram: breast cancer screening

SPECIAL STUDIES

• Biopsy

—Percutaneous with US or CT guidance
—Open biopsy/laparoscopic provides the best chance of diagnosis (larger specimen).

• Angiogram

—Provides important information for planning surgical resection of large vascular mass
—Possible preoperative arterial embolization

• Assessment of bilateral renal function

—The kidney is the most frequent adjacent organ removed during resection of sarcoma.
—Function is estimated by contrast CT, but a renal scan is better.

• Metastatic evaluation

—Bone scan
—Chest CT: Metastatic sarcoma is often peripheral and may not be seen on CXR.

 ## Initial Management

• Clinical suspicion is confirmed with CT scan, additional imaging (e.g., testicular ultrasound), and laboratory studies.
• Testicular cancer with retroperitoneal metastasis

—Orchiectomy for staging and histologic diagnosis; treat based on primary

• Sarcoma

—Biopsy for diagnosis of surgery: only chance of cure; chemotherapy and radiation no advantage

• Lymphoma

—Surgery not indicated; percutaneous biopsy/FNA followed by chemotherapy

• Benign primary retroperitoneal masses may require removal.

—Malignancy cannot be ruled out; local symptoms/enlarging mass

• Cystic mass: open or percutaneous drainage, especially if infected or symptomatic
• Retroperitoneal fibrosis (see Section II, "Retroperitoneal Fibrosis")
• Abscess (see Section II, "Retroperitoneal Abscess")

 ## Follow-Up

• Testicular cancer: based on specific tumor type
• Sarcoma

—Examination every 3 months; CXR and CT scan every 6 months for 2 years
—Recurrence: 90% after 5 years (less for completely resected tumors)
—Recurrence usually associated with grade progression

• Benign primary retroperitoneal tumors

—Can recur if incompletely resected; follow-up recommended

• Retroperitoneal hematoma: when stabilized, follow-up imaging after resorption of hematoma to rule out neoplasm
• Cystic masses and retroperitoneal abscesses: repeat imaging
• Retroperitoneal fibrosis: Long-term follow-up is warranted, with imaging (IVP) and renal function studies.

 ## Miscellaneous

SYNONYMS: N/A

ASSOCIATED CONDITIONS: N/A

NOTES

• See also Section II, "Retroperitoneal Abscess" and "Retroperitoneal Sarcomas."

ABBREVIATIONS

• FNA, fine-needle aspiration

REFERENCES

Baker LR, et al. Idiopathic retroperitoneal fibrosis: A retrospective analysis of 60 cases. *Br J Urol* 1988;60:497.

Hall MC, et al. Diseases of the retroperitoneum. In: Gillenwater JY, Grayhack JT, Howards SS, Duckett JW, eds. *Adult and Pediatric Urology*, 3rd ed. St. Louis: Mosby, 1996.

Richie JP. Neoplasms of the testis. In: Walsh PC, Retik AB, Vaughan ED, Wein AJ, eds. *Campbell's Urology*, 7th ed. Philadelphia: WB Saunders, 1998.

Storm FK, Mahvi DM. Diagnosis and management of retroperitoneal soft-tissue sarcoma. *Ann Surg* 1991;214:2.

Authors: Surena Fazeli-Matin and Inderbir S. Gill

Scrotal and Testicular Trauma

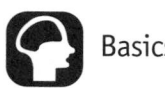 Basics

DESCRIPTION

- Injuries are classified by mechanism as blunt, penetrating, avulsion, or burn.
- Initial concern is for testicular injury and genital skin loss.

—Associated structures that can be injured include the corpora cavernosa, urethra, and spermatic cord.

PATHOPHYSIOLOGY

- Blunt injuries: direct blow, fall, straddle injury, motorcycle accident, or sport-related injury
- Penetrating injuries: gunshot and stab wounds, human or animal bites
- Avulsion injuries: machinery accidents, bizarre sexual practices, or high-speed MVAs
- Burn injuries: flame, electrical, or chemical related

RISK FACTORS

- Underlying neoplasms may cause testicular rupture when associated with trivial injury.
- Spermatic cord injury puts testicular viability at risk.

 Differential Diagnosis

- Torsion of the testicle or one of its appendages (i.e., epididymis, appendix epididymis, appendix testis), causing swelling and tenderness
- Pelvic hematoma secondary to pelvic FX extending into the scrotum, causing discoloration, a mass, and tenderness
- Testicular neoplasm causing a mass with or without tenderness

—Tenderness is due to acute bleeding within the tumor.

- Infectious epididymo-orchitis with or without reactive hydrocele, causing tenderness with or without a mass
- Ruptured varicocele, causing discoloration or tenderness
- Hematoma of the scrotal wall, epididymis, or spermatic cord, causing tenderness

 Database

HISTORY

- History of traumatic event to the genitalia

—Detail the type of injury and the magnitude of the force causing the injury.
—Determine the caliber and velocity of the bullet for GSWs.
—Investigate contamination of objects used in stab injuries.
—Determine the species of the animal in biting injuries.
—Include questions about recent sexual activity.
—Torsion may be falsely attributed to minor trauma.

- Ask about scrotal discoloration, pain, swelling, and tenderness.

—Focus on timing of symptoms in relation to the traumatic event.
  —Minor degrees of trauma are associated with a delayed onset of pain, swelling, and discoloration.
  —Testicular rupture is usually immediately painful, with a rapid onset of swelling.
  —Tumors are associated with more chronic symptoms.
—Ambulation increases scrotal pain.

- Associated symptoms: nausea with or without emesis and syncope

PHYSICAL EXAMINATION

- Assess scrotal swelling, ecchymosis, tenderness, disfigurement, and masses

—Transillumination of scrotal masses may provide information on mass content; hydroceles are clear and will transmit light; hematoceles and tumors are solid and will not transmit light.
—Usually with testicular rupture, the epididymis cannot be palpated separate from the testis or a hematoma.

- Testicular displacement into the inguinal canal may occur due to scrotal hematoma formation.
- Blood at the urethral meatus may indicate urethral or other GU tract injury.
- Entrance and exit wounds should be assessed in cases of penetrating injuries.
- Ecchymosis, disfigurement, and tenderness along the penis or spermatic cord are indicative of traumatic injury and should prompt thorough scrotal, penile, and urethral examination.

Diagnostic Studies

LABORATORY TESTING

• Urine analysis: Perform both urine dipstick and microscopic evaluations.

—Gross or microscopic hematuria may indicate other urinary tract injuries.
—Pyuria suggests infectious epididymo-orchitis.

• Urine culture if UA suggests infection
• Complete blood count with differential if the wound appears infected

IMAGING

• High-resolution scrotal ultrasound

—Look for normal homogeneity of testicular parenchyma; loss of continuity of the tunica albuginea, intraparenchymal hematoma, and parenchymal heterogeneity are the hallmarks of rupture.
  —Disruption of the tunica albuginea may not be apparent.
—Color Doppler flow aids in differentiating torsion.

• Retrograde urethrogram if urethral injury suspected

—Urethral injury is most common in straddle injuries or penetrating injuries.

SPECIAL STUDIES: N/A

 Initial Management

• Blunt injuries with scrotal skin intact and a nonruptured, viable testicle

—Ice pack, analgesics, elevation, and bed rest

• Scrotal skin laceration, but underlying layers intact with a nonruptured, viable testicle

—Debride devitalized scrotal skin and obtain meticulous hemostasis.
—Primarily close noninfected wounds with absorbable suture (i.e., 4-0 Vicryl or 4-0 Chromic Gut), with simple interrupted sutures.
  —Do not close infected wounds; leave open and begin twice-daily wet to dry dressings with normal saline; consider a 3- to 7-day course of cephalexin or dicloxacillin, depending on the severity of infection (i.e., bite wounds) and amount of skin debrided.
—Ice pack, analgesics, elevation, and bed rest
—Debridement and wound closure can be performed in the emergency department.

• Deep scrotal laceration through the tunica vaginalis with a nonruptured, viable testicle

—Immediate surgical exploration with debridement of devitalized tissue
—If gross contamination is absent, close the wound in layers.
—Consider leaving a drain in the wound bed.

• Ruptured testicle with or without scrotal skin injury

—Immediate surgical exploration, with testicular preservation being the goal
—Excise extruded seminiferous tubules.
—Orchiectomy if testicle not salvageable
—Close the tunica albuginea in a running fashion with 3-0 Vicryl suture.

• Flame, electrical, and chemical burn injuries

—Expectant management to allow for demarcation of nonviable tissue
—After demarcation, debride necrotic tissue.
—Testicles are usually spared.

• Evaluate the need for tetanus and/or rabies immunization.

 Follow-Up

• Testicular preservation is the goal for endocrine purposes and cosmesis; normal sperm production and sperm transport are not expected after repair of testicular rupture.

—Fertility studies may be indicated.

• Monitor wounds for appropriate healing.

—Healing is reliable in the well-vascularized scrotum.
—Remove drains after 24 or 48 hours.
—Burn injuries may need grafting after debridement.

• Fournier's gangrene may occur after local trauma.

—It is a rapidly progressive, fulminating, gangrenous infection of the genitalia due to aerobic and anaerobic organisms.
—Observe patients for malaise, fever, chills, sweats, and increasing genital discomfort.
—Monitor wounds for erythema, tenderness, induration, and black discoloration.

 Miscellaneous

SYNONYMS: N/A

ASSOCIATED CONDITIONS: N/A

NOTES

• See also Section I, "Penis—Trauma and Fracture" and "Burns—External Genitalia and Perineum."

ABBREVIATIONS

• MVA, motor vehicle accident; FX, fracture; GSW, gunshot wound

REFERENCES

Fournier GR, et al. Scrotal ultrasonography and the management of testicular trauma. *Urol Clin North Am* 1989;16:377.

Cline KJ, et al. Penetrating trauma to the male external genitalia. *J Trauma* 1998;44:492.

Wessells H, McAninch JW. Testicular trauma. *Urology* 1996;47:750.

Wessells H, McAninch JW. Injuries to the urogenital tract. *Sci Am: Surgery* 1997;IV:10.

Wolf JS, et al. Dog bites to the male genitalia: Characteristics, management, and comparison with human bites. *J Urol* 1993;149:286.

Authors: J. Paul Yurkanin and Hunter Wessells

Scrotum—Mass and/or Pain (Acute Scrotum)

 Basics

DESCRIPTION

- A "lump" in the scrotal sac; can be painful or painless
- May be benign or malignant
- May be associated with structures in the scrotum or independent of them

—For example, testicular mass vs. scrotal wall lipoma

PATHOPHYSIOLOGY

- The mass can result from abnormal growth of tissue or inflammatory causes.
- Etiology varies with age of patient.

RISK FACTORS

- Recent trauma, infection, or instrumentation of urinary tract; congenital anomaly; prior neoplasm of testis, hematopoietic malignancy, vasculitis

 Differential Diagnosis

- Differs between adults and children (i.e., torsion more likely in child/adolescent than in adult)
- Congenital

—In utero testicular torsion
—Testicular torsion: due to "bell-clapper" deformity; most common in pediatric population
—Hydrocele: due to patent processus vaginalis; may also be acquired
—Inguinal hernia: abdominal wall defect with migration of abdominal contents into scrotum
—Unilateral/bilateral testicular enlargement: associated with Beckwith–Wiedemann syndrome
—Supernumerary testis
—Pachyvaginalitis: thickening of the tunica vaginalis around the testicle
—Epidermal cyst: usually in midline raphe

- Traumatic

—Hematoma
—Fractured testis: more common in penetrating trauma

- Inflammatory

—Epididymitis/epididymo-orchitis: associated with UTI or instrumentation of urethra
—Scrotal cellulitis
—Testicular torsion, torsion of testicular appendages can lead to necrosis.

- Neoplastic

—Scrotal wall lesions
  —Squamous cell carcinoma of scrotum: "chimney sweep's disease," ulcerative pruritic lesion, often painless; seen in middle-aged men
  —Sarcomas: fibrosarcoma, Kaposi's, histiocytic, rhabdomyosarcoma
  —Sclerosing lipogranuloma
  —Hemangioma: aggravated by venous stasis in scrotum, may cause "bleeding" in undergarment
  —Lymphangioma: capillary, cavernous, cystic

—Intrascrotal paratesticular lesions
  —Adenomatoid tumor: most common paratesticular tumor, usually in epididymis, 30- to 40-year-old men, benign
  —Sarcomas: rhabdomyosarcoma (most common), fibrosarcoma, leiomyosarcoma, liposarcoma
  —Papillary cystadenoma: epididymal, associated with VHL (in 40% of VHL patients), benign; one-third are bilateral.
  —Leiomyoma: second most common epididymal tumor, associated with hydrocele
  —Carcinoma of rete testis: rare; may present with draining sinus or skin nodule in addition to scrotal mass
  —Epidermoid cyst; fibrous pseudotumor of testicular tunic, ectopic adrenal rests; mesothelioma (<20 reported)
—Spermatic cord tumors
  —Lipoma: most common, two-thirds of all spermatic cord tumors, benign
  —Sarcomas: see above; aggressive rhabdomyosarcoma more often in children
—Testicular tumors
  —Germ cell neoplasm: seminoma, embryonal cell teratoma, choriocarcinoma, yolk sac tumor
  —Non-germ cell neoplasm: Leydig cell tumor, gonadal stromal tumors (sex-cord tumors), gonadoblastoma, Sertoli cell tumor
  —Benign tumors (adenomatoid etc.)
  —Metastases or hematopoietic (lymphoma, etc.) neoplastic infiltration
  —Carcinoid: primary or metastatic (extremely rare)

- Miscellaneous

—Varicocele: " bag of worms," engorged pampiniform plexus, in 20% of males, associated with infertility; if on right, may be associated with retroperitoneal mass
—Spermatocele: collection of sperm/fluid in epididymis
—Henoch-Schönlein purpura: in up to 15% of patients with the disease
—Idiopathic fat necrosis of scrotum

Database

HISTORY

- Age of patient?
—Torsion more likely in children
- Onset of symptoms?
—Associated with trauma or antecedent infection or instrumentation?
—Acute or insidious onset?
  —Differentiate acute torsion from mass or infection.
- Associated with any pain?
—In the absence of trauma, pain suggests infection or torsion. Malignancy is often painless.
- Medical history of neoplasm, vasculitis, scrotal surgery, or intranatal trauma?

PHYSICAL EXAMINATION

- Vital signs: fever or tachycardia as sign of infection
- Skin: signs of Henoch-Schönlein purpura or petechiae
- Abdomen: palpating for hernia defects or inguinal masses
- Penis: chancre or plaques to indicate infection
- Scrotum

—Inspect for lesions, cellulitis, sinus tracts. "Blue dot" sign with torsion of testicular appendage
—Palpate testes: normal adult size approximately 3.5 cm, smooth, nontender, nonboggy, firm but not hard, able to separate epididymis from testis
—Palpate for mass: intratesticular vs. extratesticular, epididymal or spermatic cord involvement
—Transilluminate to evaluate for hydrocele.
—Valsalva maneuver to evaluate for varicocele in supine and upright positions. Varix should disappear when supine.

- Lymph nodes: Palpate the inguinal area for enlarged nodes associated with infection.

—Note: testicular tumor metastasizes to pelvic and retroperitoneal nodes, not inguinal nodes
—Rectal examination: Evaluate the prostate for evidence of prostatitis, and seminal vesicles for fullness.

 Diagnostic Studies

LABORATORY TESTING

- Urine analysis: signs of infection suggesting epididymitis
- Urine culture: if UA suggestive of infection
- Urethral swab to rule out gonorrhea/chlamydia
- Complete blood count
—WBC count to evaluate for infection or leukemia/lymphoma
—HCT to evaluate for anemia associated with malignancy
- Tumor markers: β-hCG, AFP, LDH for testicular malignancy
- RPR or FTA to evaluate for syphilis

IMAGING

- Do not unduly delay operative evaluation of suspected torsion to obtain radiologic imaging studies!!
- The gold standard is transcrotal ultrasound.
—Used to determine location and size of a mass (intra- vs. extratesticular), rule out simple hydrocele
—Echo texture used to differentiate types of masses
—Duplex/Doppler used to evaluate for blood flow
  —Torsion of testicle: decreased or absent blood flow compared with contralateral side
  —Increased flow to testis/epididymis associated with infection
  —May help evaluate a varicocele
- Nuclear testicular blood flow scans are sometimes used to rule out torsion.
- Magnetic resonance imaging of the testis may be used to evaluate masses not clearly seen by ultrasound.

SPECIAL STUDIES: N/A

 Initial Management

- Depending on the suspected cause of the scrotal mass, the first-line treatment may be surgical.

—Testicular torsion is a urologic emergency! It is a diagnosis usually made based on history and physical examination and requires immediate scrotal exploration.
—Testicular tumors require urgent removal to limit metastasis. This is done through an inguinal approach.

- Many scrotal masses can be followed over time without treatment.
- Treatment of systemic diseases as appropriate

 Follow-Up

- Advise patients to do monthly testicular self-examinations, particularly those ages 20 to 40.
- For benign diseases, periodic surveillance is sufficient.
- For cancer, postoperatively, there are several protocols.
- For torsion, contralateral orchiopexy at time of surgery

 Miscellaneous

SYNONYMS

- Acute scrotum, acute orchalgia

ASSOCIATED CONDITIONS: N/A

NOTES: N/A

ABBREVIATIONS

- VHL, Von-Hippel Lindau disease; hCG, human chorionic gonadotropin; AFP, alpha-feto protein; HCT, hematocrit; UA, urinalysis

REFERENCES

Aragona F. Painless scrotal masses in the pediatric population: Prevalence and age distribution of different pathologic conditions—A 10-year retrospective multicenter study. *J Urol* 1996;155:1424.

Chin JL. Paratesticular tumors. *Specialty Review in Urology*. CME Video Programs, 1997.

Rabinowitz R, Hulbert WC. Acute scrotal swelling. *Urol Clin North Am* 1995;22(1):155.

Rowland RG, Foster RS, Donohue JP. Scrotum and testis. In: Gillenwater JY, Grayhack JT, Howards SS, Duckett JW, eds. *Adult and Pediatric Urology*, 3rd ed. St Louis: Mosby, 1996.

Authors: Deborah Glassman and Richard B. Alexander

Shock—Septic (Urosepsis)

 Basics

DESCRIPTION

- Sepsis syndrome: bacteremia resulting in clinical instability

—Clinical evidence of infection
—Tachypnea, tachycardia, hyperthermia or hypothermia
—Evidence of inadequate organ perfusion (hypoxemia or elevated plasma lactate or oliguria)

- Septic shock: sepsis syndrome with hypotension (sustained decrease in systolic blood pressure <90 mm Hg in the face of adequate hydration)
- Urosepsis: as above, with evidence of GU source; roughly 25% of all cases of sepsis
- Multisystem organ failure: end-point along the spectrum of sepsis syndrome; often terminal

—Pulmonary: adult respiratory distress syndrome (ARDS)
—Renal: acute renal failure due to prerenal state, ATN
—Heme: disseminated intravascular coagulopathy (DIC), pancytopenia
—Hepatic: elevated LFTs, synthetic failure
—Neuro: mental status changes, obtundation, coma

- Mortality 20% to 95% (median probably 50%–60%), thirteenth leading cause of death, approximately 150,000 deaths per year
- Estimated treatment costs of $5 billion to $10 billion per year

PATHOPHYSIOLOGY

- Most frequently triggered by gram-negative pathogens (*E. coli* > *Klebsiella, Enterobacter, Serratia, Proteus, Pseudomonas*), although gram-positive bacteria (*Enterococcus, Staphylococcus, Streptococcus* sp.), viral, fungal, and parasitic sources are possible
- Powerful cascade of inflammatory mediators released in response to insult, especially triggered by endotoxin (lipopolysaccharide) from gram-negative bacterial cell wall

—Interleukins (IL-1, 2, 4, 6, 8), tumor necrosis factor
—Eicosanoids: prostaglandins, leukotrienes, thromboxane
—Bradykinins
—Complement cascade

RISK FACTORS

- GU related: urinary tract instrumentation, urolithiasis, indwelling catheter or foreign body (e.g., ureteral or urethral stent, artificial sphincter, penile prosthesis), urinary diversion (all types), obstructive uropathy (BPH, stone, stricture, valve, UPJO), neurogenic bladder
- Non-GU related: diabetes, hospitalization, immunocompromised state, malnourishment, debilitated state

 Differential Diagnosis

- Shock from any other cause

—Hypovolemic
—Cardiogenic
—Anaphylactic

 Database

HISTORY

- Fevers, chills, hematuria, cloudy urine, foul-smelling urine, stone passage, history of stone formation, renal colic, indwelling catheter, back pain, obstructive voiding symptoms, mental status changes
- Review risk factors as noted above.
- Surgical history

—GU instrumentation
—Stents/foreign body
—Urinary diversion or GU reconstruction
—Abdominal procedure: risk of inadvertent ureteral/bladder injury during abdominal or pelvic procedure

PHYSICAL EXAMINATION (with emphasis on GU source)

- Review vital signs.

—Need to see evidence of systemic illness/response

- Assessment of hydration

—Skin turgor, mucous membranes
—Urine output

- Abdominal examination

—Point tenderness, peritoneal signs
—Abdominal masses
—Presence of stoma
—Presence of fistula
—Postoperative wounds
—Rule out incarcerated hernia: include inguinal, femoral, parastomal.

- Costovertebral angle (CVA) tenderness: pyelonephritis, stone, acute obstruction
- GU examination: must be thorough

—Scrotal contents: including testes, epididymes, cord contents
—Perineum: fistulas, abscess, Fournier gangrene
—Rectal: enlarged prostate (BPH), nodular (PCa), boggy (acute prostatitis)
—Catheters, nephrostomy tubes

Diagnostic Studies

LABORATORY TESTING

• Culture all potential sources (urine, blood, sputum, lines, abscess).

—Aerobic
—Anaerobic
—Fungal: especially if nosocomial, recent or chronic antibiotic therapy, chronic bacteriuria
—Collect before the first dose of antibiotic if possible, but do not delay antibiotics for the sake of collection.

• Serum chemistries (assess renal function, electrolytes, LFTs)
• Complete blood count with differential
• Arterial blood gas: Assess oxygenation, assess adequacy of ventilation, rule out acidosis.

IMAGING

• CXR: infiltrates, volume status, free air under diaphragm
• KUB if stone suspected; possible IVP to evaluate for obstruction, stricture, urolithiasis
• US: new hydronephrosis significant but not specific for GU source of sepsis
• CT: can visualize radiolucent stones (during noncontrasted portion of scan), abscess/emphysematous process, anatomic variants, edema, parenchymal thickening, hydronephrosis. CT-guided drainage
• Renogram: can demonstrate parenchymal defects due to pyelonephritis
• Retrograde pyelogram: if obstruction suspected but contrast allergy present; not first-line test

SPECIAL STUDIES: N/A

 ## Initial Management

• Fluid resuscitation is *crucial;* must overcome increased capillary permeability, support BP. Inadequate volume loading can predispose to ARF and further tissue hypoxia.
• IV antibiotics (broad spectrum): Knowledge of local bacterial flora/sensitivities is helpful.

—Empiric
—Ampicillin 1 g q6h + gentamicin 4 to 5 mg/kg q24h (check trough): most appropriate for community-acquired infections and those patients unlikely to harbor resistant organisms
—Penicillinase-resistant penicillin (e.g., piperacillin 3–4 g q4–6h) + gentamicin: if resistance is likely
—Vancomycin 1 g q12h + gentamicin (if MRSA prevalent)
—Amphotericin B 1 mg/kg/d: used in known fungal sepsis; multiple potential side effects
—Adjust doses in the face of renal impairment.
—Tailor antibiotics as cultures and sensitivities return.

• Intensive care unit as clinically indicated
• Supplemental oxygen: nasal cannula; increase as needed to keep oxygen saturation elevated. Consider intubation/mechanical ventilation for pulmonary collapse or patient fatigue.
• Invasive lines as clinically indicated

—Foley catheter: relieves infravesical obstruction, monitors urine output (and response to resuscitation)
—Central venous catheter: allows for easier blood draws, provides access for parenteral nutrition, delivers multiple medications simultaneously, is the preferred route for vasoactive medications
—Arterial catheter: patients with persistently labile blood pressures, intubated, with need for frequent blood gas checks

• Swan-Ganz catheter: assess cardiovascular parameters when suspect major aberration (decreased SVR, decreased BP, increased CO with early sepsis, decreased CO with circulatory collapse, CVP/PCWP/EDV as estimates of volume status); monitor response to vasoactive medications
• Vasoactive medications: patients unresponsive to volume resuscitation, need predicts >80% mortality

—Dopamine: 2 to 20 μg/kg/min
—Norepinephrine: 0.05 to >0.30 μg/kg/min
—Dobutamine: 2 to 20 μg/kg/min
—Epinephrine: 2 to 4 μg/kg/min

• Relieve obstruction

—Foley catheter: relieves infravesical obstruction (stricture, prostatic enlargement)
—Suprapubic tube: bypasses urethra
—Percutaneous nephrostomy: drains renal unit, bypasses ureter
—Ureteral stent: requires visit to operating room, allows retrograde study

• Monoclonal antibodies: no efficacy despite multiple studies of many targets in inflammatory cascade
• Corticosteroids: no proven efficacy, likely detrimental

 ## Follow-Up

• Repeat cultures to determine response to therapy

 ## Miscellaneous

SYNONYMS

• Systemic inflammatory response syndrome (SIRS)

ASSOCIATED CONDITIONS: N/A

NOTES: N/A

ABBREVIATIONS

• ATN, acute tubular necrosis; PCa, prostate cancer; SVR, systemic vascular resistance; CO, cardiac output; CVP, central venous pressure; PCWP, pulmonary capillary wedge pressure; EDV, end diastolic volume; MRSA, methacillin resistant staph aureus

REFERENCES

Ackermann RJ. Bacteremic urinary tract infection in older people. *J Am Geriatr Soc* 1996;44(8):927.

Bone RC. The sepsis syndrome: Definition and general approach to management. *Clin Chest Med* 1996;17(2):175.

Wiessner WH, et al. Treatment of sepsis and septic shock: A review. *Heart Lung* 1995;24(5):380.

Authors: Paul K. Pietrow and Douglas Milam

Spermatic Cord Mass

 Basics

DESCRIPTION

• The spermatic cord extends from the internal inguinal ring to the testicle, passing through the inguinal canal.
• A mass or swelling in the spermatic cord can be cystic or solid (uncommon), asymptomatic or painful.
• Most solid masses are benign.

PATHOPHYSIOLOGY

• Spermatic cord contains vas deferens, internal and external spermatic arteries, artery to the vas, pampiniform (venous) plexus, lymphatics, nerves, investing layers of fascia, and cremaster muscle.
• A cord mass can arise from cord contents or from structures above or below the cord.
• A cord mass can be palpated in the inguinal region or the upper scrotum.

—Varicocele
  —Dilatation of pampiniform plexus
  —Present in 10% to 15% of adults, usually unilateral in 80% to 90%
  —More common on left
  —A right-sided varicocele requires further work-up (renal or retroperitoneal tumor with compression of the spermatic vein).
  —Grade I: palpable with Valsalva; grade II: palpable without Valsalva; grade III: visible
  —May cause infertility, presumably by increasing scrotal temperature and inhibiting spermatogenesis
—Hydrocele of the cord
  —Incomplete obliteration of the processus vaginalis can result in cystic fluid collection confined to the cord.
—Communicating hydrocele with hernia
  —Patent processus vaginalis results in a hydrocele with an inguinal hernia if communication with the peritoneal cavity is large.
  —A narrow communicating channel results in a hydrocele only.
  —More common in children
—Inguinal hernia in adults
  —Direct (through the floor of inguinal canal) or indirect (through the internal ring)
  —Can present as a mass in the inguinal region or extend through the external ring into scrotum
—Spermatocele
  —Arises from epididymal tubules, usually in the area of the head of the epididymis
  —Contains cloudy fluid with sperm
  —Common finding at scrotal sonography, usually asymptomatic
—Lipoma of the cord
  —Benign and the most common tumor of the cord
  —Arises from adipose tissue of the cord
  —Clinically rare, but not an uncommon finding during inguinal hernia repair
—Adenomatoid tumor
  —Uncommon, benign, and of uncertain histologic origin

—Most common epididymal tumor
—Usually seen in second to fourth decade
—More common on the left
—40% to 50% will arise from the head of the epididymis.
—Sarcomas
  —Rare lesions of spermatic cord, epididymis, and paratesticular soft tissue
  —May arise from muscle, adipose, or connective tissue (mesenchymal origin)
  —Leiomyosarcoma and rhabdomyosarcoma are the most common, followed by fibrosarcoma and liposarcoma.
  —May involve the cord in the inguinal region or in the scrotum
  —Incidence has two peaks: 15 to 25 years and 50 to 80 years.
—Funiculitis: inflammation of the spermatic cord either secondary to severe epididymitis or due to trauma. Severe inflammation can result in granulomatous and sclerosing endophlebitis of the spermatic cord due to parasites (e.g., *Schistosoma hematobium, Wucheria bancrofti* filariasis).

RISK FACTORS: N/A

 Differential Diagnosis

• Most spermatic cord masses are cystic (70%–75%).
• Most of the solid masses are benign (75%–80%) and usually asymptomatic.
• Cystic

—Varicocele
—Patent processus vaginalis with communicating hydrocele: may have associated inguinal hernia, more common in children
—Hydrocele of the cord: can mimic solid mass when tense
—Inguinal hernia containing bowel or omentum
—Spermatocele: when large, may be misdiagnosed as a scrotal hydrocele

• Solid

—Lipoma of the cord: can be mistaken for hernia
—Adenomatoid tumor: usually found on routine examination
—Sarcomas: often misdiagnosed as inflammatory lesions when pain is a presenting feature

Database

HISTORY

• Most patients will present with pain or a mass.
• Pain

—Most masses (cystic or solid) are painless from the onset.
—Pain may be associated with a malignant or inflammatory lesion or an expanding cystic lesion.

—Presence or absence of pain does not distinguish between a benign or a malignant mass.
—For cystic masses, size usually determines the degree of discomfort or pain.

• Onset and duration

—Sudden onset is a nonspecific finding.
—Most masses will have a history of several years.
—Acute onset of a right varicocele may herald the presence of a renal tumor invading the renal vein or a retroperitoneal mass compressing the gonadal vein.
—Sudden appearance of a mass associated with pain and strenuous activity may occur with acute inguinal hernia.

• Change in size

—Any rapid increase in size can result in worsening pain.
—A slow increase in size over years can result in a heavy, dragging sensation or a dull ache in the groin or abdomen.
—Spermatoceles, hernias, and varicoceles generally grow slowly over many years and present due to large size and discomfort.

• Alleviating factors

—Recumbent position may result in disappearance of the mass and the pain.
  —Varicocele
  —Communicating hydrocele with or without hernia

• Scrotal elevation may provide relief of groin or abdominal dragging pain if the mass is large.

PHYSICAL EXAMINATION

• The patient should be examined in upright and supine positions.
• The mass should be palpated between the thumb and first two fingers of both hands.
• Transillumination of the mass by placing a light on its posterior surface signifies a cystic mass.

—Some cystic masses will not transilluminate due to a thick wall, chronic inflammation, or blood.

• A varicocele is best palpated in a standing position as a painless or tender mass of veins ("bag of worms").

—Usually palpable posterior to and above the testicle
—A small varicocele may become more obvious in an upright position with the Valsalva maneuver.
—The ipsilateral testis may be atrophic.

• Spermatoceles: usually palpable superior and posterior to the upper pole of testis and head of epididymis

—Usually small, these are palpable separate from the testis.
—A large spermatocele may surround the testis and mimic a hydrocele (these will transilluminate).
—Aspiration (rarely indicated) will yield a cloudy fluid containing sperm.

- The hydrocele of the cord is palpated as a round or fusiform cystic mass in the upper scrotum or inguinal region.

—Occasionally firm, can mimic a solid mass
—Palpation can determine the superior and inferior extent of the mass (unlike inguinal hernia).
—A testicular hydrocele usually does not co-exist.

- A communicating hydrocele may have an associated indirect inguinal hernia.

—Supine position results in drainage of fluid into peritoneal cavity; becomes smaller
—If a hydrocele is present, it will transilluminate.
—Bowel sounds may be present over the mass when associated with a hernia.
—With a hernia, the proximal limit is not palpable since contents extend through the internal ring.

- An adult hernia may be direct or indirect, reducible or incarcerated.

—It is not possible to palpate the superior extent of the mass.
—Bowel sounds may be audible over the mass.
—In the supine or Trendelenburg position, an attempt is made to reduce the hernia with gentle pressure.
—After reduction, a finger is inserted through the external ring, into the inguinal canal.
—A cough or Valsalva will produce an impulse, caused by abdominal contents, felt at the fingertip.

- A lipoma of the cord is palpated as a smooth, firm mass in the inguinal canal or upper scrotum.

—Nontender, does not transilluminate or change with position
—More often found incidentally during inguinal procedures

- Adenomatoid tumors are painless, well circumscribed, and hard.

—Do not transilluminate
—The testis can be easily separated from the epididymis and the mass.
—Nearly half are present in the head of the epididymis.

- Sarcomas present as a hard mass that is occasionally tender.

—Depending on local extent, they may be well circumscribed or invade surrounding tissues.

- There are no specific symptoms or signs to differentiate between a benign or a malignant solid mass.

 Diagnostic Studies

LABORATORY TESTING

- No specific tests
- Microscopic analysis of a spermatocele will reveal sperm and confirm the diagnosis (rarely indicated).

IMAGING

- Ultrasound

—Most useful study to distinguish between solid and cystic mass
—Cannot differentiate between a benign or malignant solid mass
—Bowel can be easily identified in a hernia sac.

- Duplex Doppler can aid in the diagnosis of a low-grade varicocele.

SPECIAL STUDIES: N/A

 Initial Management

- Most cystic lesions do not need treatment.
- Decision to treat cystic masses often depends on symptoms

—Spermatocele: excise through scrotal incision
—Hydrocele of the cord: inguinal incision and excise
—Varicocelectomy may be performed to relieve pain or to improve fertility (see Section II, "Varicocele—Adult" and "Varicocele—Pediatric").
—A communicating hydrocele will resolve spontaneously in most children in the first year.
   —An inguinal incision is made to expose the cord. High ligation of the processus vaginalis is performed
   —The testicular artery and the vas deferens must be preserved.

- All solid masses should be explored to rule out malignancy.

—Inguinal incision; testis is delivered
—Early control of the cord at internal ring (reduce risk of tumor dissemination)
—After excluding the operative field with towels, a biopsy to confirm the diagnosis
—Adenomatoid tumors: simple excision
—Sarcomas: radical orchiectomy with high ligation of cord

 Follow-Up

- For benign lesions, no follow-up is needed.
- After radical orchiectomy for a malignant tumor, further work-up is needed to rule out metastasis.

—Lymphatic metastases are to the retroperitoneum.
—Hematogenous spread is common.
—Retroperitoneal lymphadenectomy with adjuvant radiotherapy and/or chemotherapy is indicated in many patients.

 Miscellaneous

SYNONYMS: N/A

ASSOCIATED CONDITIONS: N/A

NOTES

- See also Section II, "Spermatic Cord Tumors."

ABBREVIATIONS: N/A

REFERENCES

Lemack GE, Uzzo RG, Schlegel PN, Goldstein M. Microsurgical repair of adolescent varicocele. *J Urol* 1998;160(1):179.

Lioe TF, Biggert JD. Tumors of the spermatic cord and paratesticular tissue. A clinicopathological study. *Br J Urol* 71993;1(5):600.

Martin LC, Share JC, Peters C, Atala A. Hydrocele of the spermatic cord: Embryology and ultrasonographic appearance. *Pediatr Radiol* 1996;26(8):528.

Authors: Badar M. Mian and William R. Morgan

Suprapubic Pain

 Basics

DESCRIPTION

• Pain in midline of lower abdomen, most often due to genitourinary (GU) disease, occasionally GI or gynecologic causes

PATHOPHYSIOLOGY

• GU tract pain is usually associated with inflammation or obstruction.

—Inflammatory pain is typically more severe if it involves the parenchyma of the organ.

• Constant suprapubic pain unrelated to urinary retention is rarely of genitourinary origin.

• Tumors from GU tract malignancies generally do not produce pain unless they cause obstruction or extend into adjacent nerves. Pain is usually a late manifestation.

• Prostate

—Usually secondary to inflammation with secondary edema and distention of the prostatic capsule
—Symptoms are localized primarily in the perineum, but frequently pain is referred to the suprapubic area.
—Severe edema may produce acute urinary retention.

• Vesical

—Usually produced by overdistention of the bladder secondary to acute urinary obstruction or inflammation
—Chronic, slowly progressing urinary retention is usually asymptomatic despite large residual volumes.
—Inflammation of the bladder usually produces intermittent suprapubic discomfort.
　—Bacterial and interstitial cystitis is most severe when the bladder is full, and symptoms improve when the bladder is empty.
　—Sharp and stabbing pain at the end of micturition
　—Pain can be referred to the distal urethra and is associated with irritative voiding symptoms (urgency, frequency).

• Urethra

—Urethral strictures
　—Infection, trauma
　—Can cause acute urinary retention
—Urethral syndrome
　—Dysuria, frequency, and suprapubic discomfort in women without objective findings of urologic abnormality
　—Etiology unclear

RISK FACTORS

• Recurrent infections
• Benign prostatic hypertrophy

—May cause acute urinary retention

• Urolithiasis
• Immunocompromised patients

—Increased susceptibility to infections

• Radiation treatment for malignancy

 Differential Diagnosis

• Urologic causes

—Urethra
　—Urethral syndrome
　—Urethral stenosis
—Prostate
　—Nonbacterial prostatitis
　—Acute and chronic bacterial prostatitis
　—Prostatodynia
　—Acute nonspecific granulomatous prostatitis
—Vesical
　—Interstitial cystitis
　—Bladder calculi, foreign body
　—Acute bacterial cystitis
　—Cancer
　—Urinary retention
—Distal ureter
　—Calculi
　—Ascending infection
　—Foreign body
　—Urachal abnormalities

• Pain in midline of lower abdomen due to alternate conditions

—Large or small bowel
　—Appendicitis
　—Inflammatory bowel disease
　—Diverticulitis, fecal impaction, malignancy
—Gynecologic
　—Pelvic inflammatory disease, uterine fibroids, ectopic pregnancy, endometriosis

 Database

HISTORY

• Constant suprapubic pain that is unrelated to urinary retention is seldom of urologic origin.
• Acute urinary retention

—Marked edema and distention of prostatic capsule (prostatitis, cancer)
—Urethral stricture
—Benign prostatic hyperplasia
—Distal ureteral calculi
—Neurogenic bladder

• Irritative urinary symptoms (frequency, dysuria, nocturia, and urgency)

—Infection urinary tract or soft tissue
—Interstitial cystitis
—Urethral syndrome
—Prostatodynia
—Urolithiasis
—Foreign body
　—Stents, catheters, etc.
—Hematospermia

• Painful ejaculation
• Trauma
• Radiation treatment for cancer

PHYSICAL EXAMINATION

• Rectal examination

—Tender, swollen, and/or boggy prostate during palpation
　—Bacterial, nonbacterial, and granulomatous prostatitis
—Firm and indurated prostate; warm to the touch
　—Bacterial prostatitis

• Abdominal examination

—Abdominal distention
　—Acute retention due to dilated bladder
—Rebound tenderness
—Suprapubic tenderness to palpation
　—Urinary obstruction
　—Inflammation and infection

Diagnostic Studies

LABORATORY TESTING

- CBC

—Leukocytosis with left shift
  —Infection and inflammation

- Urine analysis and culture

—Pyuria, nitrite, and bacteria with infection
—pH, crystals/calcium, uric acid, oxalate, citrate, 24-hour exertion
  —Urolithiasis

- Urine cytology

—Malignancy

IMAGING

- Plain films

—Little value in inflammatory disease
—Important in evaluation of urolithiasis, tumors, and foreign bodies

- Retrograde urethrogram

—Evaluation of urethral strictures

- CT scan

—Staging for GU tumors
—Evaluation of calculi
—No role in uncomplicated infections of GU tract

- Ultrasound bladder (residual urine, stone, etc.)

SPECIAL STUDIES

- Cystoscopy

—Contraindicated during acute bacterial prostatitis
—Interstitial cystitis
  —Perform under anesthesia to allow sufficient distention of the bladder.
  —First therapeutic modality
—Observe calculi
—Assess mucosa for lesions and areas of inflammation.

- Urodynamics

—Assess bladder capacity in interstitial cystitis.
—Evaluate neurogenic bladder.

- Ureteroscopy

—Visualize upper tract, remove calculi.

 ## Initial Management

- Retention: urethral catheterization
- Prostatitis, acute

—Transurethral catheterization is contraindicated.
—A suprapubic catheter may be placed until spontaneous voiding resumes.
—Antibiotics
  —Fluoroquinolones or trimethoprim-sulfamethoxazole until culture and sensitivities available

- Benign prostatic hyperplasia

—Transurethral catheterization to relieve acute obstruction; if unable to perform, then suprapubic catheter should be placed
—Transurethral resection of prostate or other ablative procedure (laser, microwave)
—Pharmacologic treatment in the absence of urinary retention and renal insufficiency is an option.

- Interstitial cystitis

—Hydrodistention under anesthesia
—Patient education and empowerment
—Amitriptyline
—Antihistamines
—Intravesical lavage with DMSO

- Bladder calculi

—Removed cystoscopically after manual crushing or lithotripsy
—Open cystolithotomy rarely needed

- Acute bacterial cystitis

—A 3-day course of antibiotic has been shown to be as effective as a 7- to 14-day course, with fewer side effects in women.
—Men with uncomplicated cystitis should be treated with a 7-day course of antibiotic.

- Bladder cancer

—Superficial tumors
  —Intravesical bacillus Calmette-Guérin (BCG)
  —Transurethral resection of bladder tumor (TURBT)
—Invasive tumors
  —Cystectomy

- Urethral syndrome

—Self-limited illness
—Treatment should be supportive and harmless.

- Urethral stricture

—Urethral dilation
—Urethrotomy

 ## Follow-Up

- Prostatitis

—Urine analysis and culture should be performed if signs or symptoms should recur.

- Bladder calculi

—As symptoms dictate

- Bladder cancer

—Urine cytology plus IVP or CT scan

- Acute bacterial cystitis

—Routine urine analysis

- Interstitial cystitis

—Only as necessary

- Urethral syndrome

—As symptoms dictate

- Urethral stricture

—Not considered corrected until stable for at least 1 year after treatment
—Urinary flow rates and urethrograms during follow-up

 ## Miscellaneous

SYNONYMS: N/A

ASSOCIATED CONDITIONS: N/A

NOTES: N/A

ABBREVIATIONS

- TURBT, transurethral resection of bladder tumor

REFERENCES

Hanno P. Interstitial cystitis and related diseases. In: Walsh PC, Retik AB, Vaughan ED, Wein AJ, eds. *Campbell's Urology*, 7th ed. Philadelphia: WB Saunders, 1998.

Meares EM Jr. Acute and chronic prostatitis: Diagnosis and treatment. *Infect Dis Clin North Am* 1987;1:855.

Tanagho EA. Nonspecific infections of the genitourinary tract. In: Tanagho EA, McAnich, eds. *Smith's General Urology*, 14th ed. Norwalk CT: Appleton & Lange, 1995.

Authors: Chris Threatt and Cary N. Robertson

Testis and Genital Pain—Chronic

 Basics

DESCRIPTION

- *Chronic genital pain* is defined as pain without an identified organic cause that includes at least one of the following sites: the perineal area, testicles (orchalgia), scrotum, penis, or urethra.
- Dysuria or suprapubic pain alone is excluded from the definition that may be associated with the other types of pain.
- Recurrent or chronic genital pain is a frequently encountered problem.
- Despite its frequency, little has been written about this entity and generally no physical cause for the problem can be found.

PATHOPHYSIOLOGY

- Data indicate that men with genital pain without organic findings have a high incidence of life stress and psychological disturbance.
- Consistent psychological features in these men are somatization disorder, major depression, anxiety, nongenital chronic pain syndrome, chemical dependency, and a constellation of difficulty establishing relationships, sexual anxiety, and sexual dysfunction.
- One-third of the patients are socially isolated and many experience an important emotional loss at the time of the onset of the pain.
- Somatic fibers from the parietal and visceral layers of the tunica vaginalis and cremaster are carried by the genital branch of the genitofemoral nerve to L1, 2. Other somatic nerve endings are carried from the tunica vaginalis and scrotal skin by the posterior scrotal nerves (S2, 3).
- The testes bring their sympathetic nerve supply with them on their descent from the T10-12 segments. These nerves accompany the internal spermatic vessels. After penetrating the tunica albuginea, they are distributed to the interior of the testis between the seminiferous tubules. The main function of these nerves appears to be supplying arteries and stimulation of the smooth muscles of the tunica albuginea.
- Sympathetic fibers to the vas deferens and epididymis are distinct from those supplying the testis. They arise from the sympathetic outflow of T10-L1 and pass down the sympathetic chains into the pelvic plexus, and from there along the vas deferens to the epididymis. They supply the smooth muscles of the vas deferens and epididymis, but afferent nociceptive fibers also travel in them.
- Patients may complain of perineal or genital pain aggravated by sitting or automobile riding, accompanied by suprapubic pressure or pain and variable urinary symptoms.

—We have coined the term *neuromuscular pelvic floor dysfunction*.
—A syndrome known as pelvic floor tension myalgia, which is characterized by continuous habitual contraction of the muscles of the pelvic floor (levator ani and the short external rotators of the hips), has also been described.

RISK FACTORS

- Infections such as chronic prostatitis or urethritis
- Mass lesions in the scrotum such as testicular tumors, hydrocele, or varicocele may cause a heavy or dragging sensation.
- Significant recent emotional loss
- A previous operation, most commonly vasectomy, has been reported to cause chronic genital pain.

 Differential Diagnosis

- Infection, epididymo-orchitis, also chronic prostatitis and urethritis
- Tumor (testicular tumor)
- Inguinal hernia
- Testicular torsion (acute and intermittent)
- Hydrocele, spermatocele, varicocele
- Trauma (recurrent testicular trauma)
- Previous operation (vasectomy, inguinal herniorrhaphy)
- Referred pain (i.e., nerve root irritation)

 Database

HISTORY

- Patients often have consulted multiple physicians and other urologists.
- Frequently have undergone a variety of treatments: antibiotics and antiinflammatory drugs for various diagnoses, such as prostatitis, with little or no relief. Additionally, a variety of diagnostic tests may have been performed.
- Onset, location, duration, and activities that trigger the pain, such as exercise, sexual intercourse, or ejaculation?
- Obtain a history of the patient's social support and satisfaction with marital or dating relationships; current stresses; stressors coinciding with the onset of pain; assessment of sexual function, including sources of guilt such as paraphiliac fantasies, extramarital sexual activity, or very strong religious views about sexual issues; and assessment of mood and anxiety.

PHYSICAL EXAMINATION

- Penis, scrotum, testis, epididymides, spermatic cords, and inguinal areas for the presence of an inguinal hernia
- Digital rectal examination to evaluate the prostate and rectum
- Examination almost never reveals a discernible abnormality.

Diagnostic Studies

LABORATORY TESTING

- Urinalysis
- Microscopic examination of the expressed prostatic secretion or the urine voided after prostatic massage (VB3). When indicated, culture and sensitivity of the urine or VB3 is obtained.

IMAGING

- To attempt to define the cause of chronic genital pain; include scrotal ultrasound, expiratory urography, and computerized tomography of the abdomen and pelvis.
- The author believes, in the absence of clinical findings, that extensive diagnostic testing is not indicated and may be detrimental by enhancing the patient's concern about the etiology of the pain or increasing his focus on his genitals.
- In some instances, it is reasonable to perform a scrotal ultrasound; it helps eliminate an underlying fear of the physician and patient of missing an occult neoplasm.

SPECIAL STUDIES

- Cystoscopy and urodynamics have been performed to assess men with chronic genital pain. With rare exception, these studies contribute little to the diagnosis of chronic genital pain.

Initial Management

- Medical therapy

—Many medications used; little evidence of utility in most
—Antibiotics: often used, rarely beneficial
—Nonsteroidal antiinflammatory drugs: variable temporary relief
—Alpha-adrenergic blocking agents; some reports of success. The author feels they are seldom beneficial in relieving chronic unexplained genital pain, including in men with so-called prostatodynia and nonbacterial prostatitis.
—The author's opinion is that chronic prostatitis is a vastly overdiagnosed entity, and most of these patients have chronic unexplained genital pain or orchalgia. Most men lack objective criteria consistent with chronic prostatitis.
—Local anesthetic nerve blocks: limited success; rarely long-lasting

- Surgery

—Surgical procedures (epididymectomy or orchiectomy) are rarely successful, and most series indicate persistent pain in a majority of men undergoing surgery. The author believes that, with rare exception, surgical procedures should be avoided.
—Testicular denervation procedures: limited success

- Multidisciplinary approach to the management of chronic genital pain

—Treatment is difficult and time consuming.
—Patients are typically tense, anxious, and concerned about a dangerous condition.
—Initial urologic evaluation to rule out an organic cause and introduce the patient to the multidisciplinary program, arrange referrals, and monitor the patient's progress
—A mental health professional conducts a formalized psychological evaluation.

　　—Includes a brief developmental history, current and lifetime major disorders of mood, anxiety, somatization, chemical dependency, current social support, past and current sexual function, history of sexual trauma or paraphilia, and recent life stress (especially emotional losses)
　　—Written psychological testing is also performed: Brief Symptom Inventory, Male Pain Questionnaire, covering a variety of questions on sexual functioning and the degree of pelvic pain during various sexual and nonsexual activities.
　　—Ongoing psychotherapy as needed is provided, as indicated, often focusing on stress management and treating sexual problems. In some instances, antidepressants may be prescribed.

—An initial physical therapy evaluation

　　—History and examination. Values for pelvic muscle strength are recorded, and pelvic muscle biofeedback is begun.
　　—Exercises are prescribed to increase pelvic muscle strength and voluntary control over pelvic floor muscle contraction.
　　—Maximum contraction is followed by a maximal relaxation.
　　—The patient increases pelvic muscle strength but also learns how to relax the pelvic muscles and control pelvic floor instability.
　　—After 6 months of treatment, ending values for pelvic muscle strength are recorded, and the therapist provides an outcome evaluation.
　　—Physical therapy may assist in pelvic floor muscles or areas of attachment that may be responsible for discomfort observed in this condition.

Follow-Up

- Follow-up visits to the urologist every 2 to 3 months
- A psychologist follows the patient on an as-needed basis and provides required therapy.
- A physical therapist continues to monitor the patient on a regular basis. After 6 months of treatment, ending values for pelvic muscle strength are recorded, and the therapist provides an outcome evaluation.
- It is far too early to know the outcome of this multidisciplinary approach for the management of chronic genital pain. As already emphasized, a large variety of treatments for men with this disorder have almost always been unsuccessful.
- We believe that the described multidisciplinary program for men with so-called neuromuscular pelvic floor dysfunction is a rational means of dealing with and understanding men with this chronic, unrelenting pain disorder.

Miscellaneous

SYNONYMS

- Orchalgia, chronic genital pain, chronic scrotal pain

ASSOCIATED CONDITIONS: N/A

NOTES: N/A

ABBREVIATIONS: N/A

REFERENCES

Costabile RA, et al. Chronic orchalgia in the pain prone patient. *J Urol* 1991;146:1571.

Kursh ED, et al. The dilemma of chronic genital pain. AUA Update Series 16 (Lesson 37):290, 1997.

Schover LR. Psychological factors in men with genital pain. *Cleve Clin J Med* 1990;Nov–Dec: 97.

Segura JW, et al. Prostatosis, prostatitis, or pelvic floor tension myalgia. *J Urol* 1979;122:168.

Author: Elroy D. Kursh

Testicular Mass—Adult and Pediatric

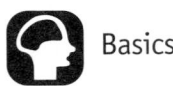 Basics

DESCRIPTION

• Patients sometimes present with a complaint of a testicular mass when in reality they have a mass of the paratesticular structures.

—Epididymal lesions, spermatic cord lesions, varicoceles, inguinal hernias, and lesions of the scrotal skin are commonly labeled "testicular masses."

• Most true testicular lesions require prompt, accurate diagnosis and timely treatment.

PATHOPHYSIOLOGY

• Depends on the underlying etiology of the mass

RISK FACTORS

• History of or current cryptorchidism, trauma, urinary tract infection, sexually transmitted diseases, viral illnesses, urethral instrumentation, and others

 Differential Diagnosis

• Five broad classes of masses are encountered in the testicle: neoplastic, cystic, infectious/inflammatory, congenital/acquired, and traumatic.

NEOPLASTIC LESIONS

• Germ cell tumors

—Germ cell tumors account for 90% to 95% of all testicular malignancies.
—Seminoma
  —Most common tumor of a single-cell type
  —30% to 40% of all adult testicular neoplasms
  —Occurs in 30- to 45-year age group
  —Three different forms (classic, anaplastic, and spermatocytic)
—Embryonal cell carcinoma
  —20% to 30% of all adult testicular neoplasms
  —Occurs in 25- to 35-year age group
—Choriocarcinoma
  —1% to 3% of adult testicular tumors
  —Occurs in 20- to 30-year age group
—Yolk sac carcinoma
  —The adult counterpart is embryonal cell carcinoma.
  —The most common prepubertal germ cell tumor
  —Accounts for 60% of pediatric testicular tumors
  —Occurs in 1- to 4-year-olds, with peak incidence at age 2
—Teratoma
  —1% to 5% of adult testicular tumors
  —Up to 40% of pediatric testicular tumors
  —Occurs primarily in first through third decades of life

—High metastatic potential in adults but low potential in children
—Mixed tumors
  —25% to 40% of all testicular neoplasms
  —The most common combination is teratoma and embryonal cell carcinoma, called teratocarcinoma.

• Gonadal stromal tumors

—Leydig cell tumors
  —The most common non–germ cell tumor of the testis
  —1% to 3% of all testicular neoplasms
  —Bimodal age distribution (5- to 10-year and 25- to 35-year age groups)
  —Has low metastatic potential
—Sertoli cell tumors
  —Less than 1% of all testicular neoplasms
  —Bimodal age distribution (less than 1 year and 25- to 45-year age groups)
  —Has low metastatic potential
—Other possible mesenchymal tumors include angioma, fibroma, leiomyoma, hamartoma, mesothelioma, and neurofibroma.

• Mixed germ cell and stromal tumor

—Gonadoblastoma
  —Occurs in patients with gonadal dysgenesis
  —A majority occur in patients under 30 years of age, but gonadoblastoma has been reported in patients from birth to the eighth decade.
  —Bilateral in 50% of cases secondary to underlying etiology
  —Contains cells similar to seminoma and immature Sertoli cells

• Other neoplasms

—Lymphoma
  —Most common testicular tumor in patients over age 50
  —Approximately 5% of all testicular tumors
  —Asynchronous bilateral involvement can occur.
—Leukemia
  —Common site for relapse in children with acute lymphocytic leukemia
—Adrenal rest tumors
  —Can occur bilaterally in untreated children with congenital adrenal hyperplasia
—Carcinoid
  —Very uncommon
  —One of the few organs in which this can be seen outside of the small bowel
—Metastatic tumors
  —Are theoretically possible from any blood-borne tumor
  —The most commonly reported tumors are from the prostate, lung, and gastrointestinal tract.
  —Other reported sites include the kidney, skin (malignant melanoma), pancreas, bladder (transitional cell carcinoma and sarcoma), and thyroid.

CYSTIC LESIONS

• Simple cysts

—Trauma has been proposed as the predisposing factor.

• Tunica albuginea cysts

—Have been associated with trauma and infection
—Appear as firm masses on the anterolateral testicular surface

• Epidermoid cysts

—The most common testicular cyst
—Account for 1% to 3% of all testicular neoplasms
—Occur in the second through fourth decades of life
—Considered a monodermal development of a teratoma

INFECTIOUS/INFLAMMATORY LESIONS

• Orchitis

—Pyogenic bacteria and viruses are causative agents in most cases.
—Mumps orchitis can be seen in up to 30% of individuals with mumps parotitis, with an onset that is usually 3 to 7 days following the development of the parotitis.
—Tuberculosis and syphilis may also cause orchitis.
—An autoimmune response to spermatozoa can also lead to orchitis in older men.
—Most often seen in concert with epididymitis when the causative agent is bacterial

CONGENITAL/ACQUIRED LESIONS

• Torsion

—Most often seen in prepubertal patients
—May be associated with strenuous activity
—Caused by twisting of the spermatic cord, resulting in occlusion of testicular blood flow

TRAUMATIC LESIONS

• Blunt trauma is the most common form.
• Testicular rupture with hematocele formation can occur if the integrity of the tunica albuginea is violated.
• Testicular hematomas can form if the tunica albuginea remains intact.

Database

HISTORY

• Age of the patient

—Tumor types are age-specific.

—Torsion usually seen in the prepubertal age group

• History of trauma

—Disproportionate hemorrhage to trauma may be a sign of an underlying tumor.

• Description of mass

—Small discrete masses are more commonly neoplastic or cystic.

—Diffuse enlargement is usually seen in infection, torsion, or trauma.

• Associated pain

—Torsion pain is usually described as a sudden, severe, unilateral pain that may be accompanied by nausea and vomiting.

  —Torsion pain may also be described as waxing and waning if the torsion is intermittent.

—Neoplasms rarely are associated with sharp pains and are usually described as a dull ache or painless.

—Orchitis pain may gradually increase as the infectious process causes increased inflammation.

• Previous undescended testicle

—There is a significant increased incidence of malignancy in patients with cryptorchidism.

• Prior scrotal surgery

—Prior orchidopexy for cryptorchidism

• Previous urinary tract infections or current lower urinary tract complaints

—Ascending orchitis ± epididymitis

• Urethral discharge associated with recent sexual activity

—Sexually transmitted disease with concurrent orchitis

• Urethral instrumentation

—Ascending orchitis ± epididymitis

• Other current illnesses

—Mumps, urinary tract infection, sexually transmitted disease, and others

• Other medical problems

—Diabetes mellitus, neurologic disorders, autoimmune disorders, and others

• Other constitutional symptoms

—Weight loss, nausea, vomiting, hemoptysis, shortness of breath, and back pain can all be clues to possible metastatic testicular neoplasm.

—Nausea and vomiting can be present in torsion or orchitis.

PHYSICAL EXAMINATION

• Vital signs

—Elevated temperature can be a marker of infection, tumor necrosis, or testicular necrosis.

—Weight loss in metastatic testicular neoplasms

• Chest/breast

—Gynecomastia can occur with neoplastic disease.

• Abdomen

—Retroperitoneal lymphadenopathy from metastatic tumors can sometimes be palpated.

• Testes

—Confirm that the mass is testicular, and not actually paratesticular.

—Note associated pain on palpation.

  —Neoplastic or cystic processes are usually painless.

  —Active torsion or orchitis is exquisitely tender.

—Discrete lesion vs. diffuse swelling

  —Most early-stage neoplasms or cysts are palpably discrete masses.

  —Orchitis and torsion lead to generalized testicular enlargement.

—Position of mass in testicle

  —May be high riding or in altered position in torsion

  —The bell-clapper deformity sometimes noted in torsion occurs when the testicle is situated in a horizontal lie with the long axis in the anteroposterior direction.

• Scrotum

—Edema and erythema may be seen in torsion or orchitis.

—Evaluate for scars or prior cryptorchidism repair.

• Penis

—Ulcers, induration, or discharge can be seen in orchitis of an infectious (sexually transmitted) etiology

• Epididymis

—Normally located in a posterior position relative to the testicle

  —May be more anterior in torsion

—Pain or swelling helps make the diagnosis of epididymo-orchitis.

—With severe inflammation, it is difficult to demarcate the epididymis and the testicle.

• Extremities

—Retroperitoneal lymphadenopathy from metastatic testicular neoplasms can sometimes lead to lymphatic or venous lower extremity congestion due to obstruction or thrombosis.

• Lymphatics

—Metastatic neoplasms can sometimes be palpated in peripheral lymph nodes.

• Neurologic examination

—The cremasteric reflex is usually absent in torsion.

(continued)

Diagnostic Studies

LABORATORY TESTING

• Urine analysis

—Can aid in the diagnosis of orchitis if evidence of infection is seen
   —Hematuria and proteinuria can be seen with viral infection.
   —Pyuria and bacteriuria are present with bacterial infection.

• Tumor marker screening

—The three primary tumor markers are AFP, hCG, and LDH.
—AFP
   —Oncofetal glycoprotein produced during fetal development and decreases after birth
   —Elevated in most embryonal cell carcinomas and yolk sac carcinomas but never increased in pure seminomas
   —Also elevated in other benign diseases (tyrosinemia, ataxia telangiectasia, hepatitis, or regenerative hepatic disease) and malignancies (liver, pancreatic, lung, and gastric carcinomas)
—hCG (beta-subunit)
   —Glycoprotein normally produced by trophoblastic cells in the placenta to maintain the corpus luteum after conception
   —Elevated in all choriocarcinomas and some embryonal cell carcinomas, yolk sac carcinomas, and seminomas
   —Sometimes elevated in marijuana users and other malignancies (liver, pancreatic, lung, gastric, renal, and bladder carcinomas)
—LDH
   —Glycolytic cellular enzyme with high levels in all muscle types, liver, kidney, and brain
   —Often elevated in bulky metastatic disease
   —Nonspecific marker elevated: multiple malignancies

• Urethral/urine culture

—Diagnosis of infection and identification of offending organism

IMAGING

• Ultrasonography

—The diagnostic procedure of choice for evaluation of testicular lesions
   —Readily available and inexpensive
   —The major downside is that it is operator dependent.
—Gray-scale ultrasound best evaluates testicular neoplasms, cysts, and traumatic injury.
   —Approximate 95% sensitivity for the diagnosis of testicular tumors
   —Specificity for malignancies is lower since ultrasound detects benign lesions as well.
   —Almost all testicular tumors have hypoechoic areas, but overall heterogeneity of the lesion is common.
—Color-flow Doppler is essential for the differentiation of torsion from epididymo-orchitis.
   —Decreased blood flow with torsion
   —Increased blood flow with epididymo-orchitis
   —Can be problematic in neonates and young children with higher false-negative findings.
   —Will also sometimes show increased vascularity in testicular neoplasms

• Radionuclide testicular scan

—Prior to the development of color-flow Doppler, radionuclide scans were the diagnostic procedure of choice.
   —Sometimes difficult to obtain
   —Not sensitive or specific enough to rely on solely
   —Also operator dependent
—Does not provide any more information than color-flow Doppler ultrasound

• Magnetic resonance imaging

—Currently has a minor role in the evaluation of a testicular mass
—Can help evaluate intratesticular masses that are difficult to visualize on ultrasound

SPECIAL STUDIES: N/A

Initial Management

- Of greatest concern is timely diagnosis.
- Testicular neoplasms require surgical removal.

—Radical orchiectomy with high ligation of the spermatic cord through an inguinal incision is the surgical method of removal.
—Testicular biopsy or orchiectomy through a scrotal approach is contraindicated if there is the possibility of neoplasm.

- Cystic lesions are difficult to differentiate from neoplastic lesions and are usually removed as above for testicular neoplasms.
- Testicular torsion requires immediate exploration and repair to salvage an ischemic testicle.

—80% to 100% of testicles can be salvaged if detorsion occurs within 6 hours of onset.
—20% or less are salvaged if detorsion occurs after more than 24 hours from onset.

- Cause-specific as well as supportive care should be applied to cases of orchitis.

—Broad-spectrum antibiotics should be administered if a bacterial source is suspected.
  —Intravenous antibiotics may be required in severe cases.
  —The antibiotic profile should be narrowed when culture and susceptibility data become available.
  —A patient's sexual partners should be treated if sexually transmitted disease is the cause.
—Bed rest, scrotal support, ice bags, and analgesics should also be applied.

- Trauma management is dependent on the severity of the lesion.

—Surgical exploration is warranted if the tunica albuginea is ruptured, significant debridement is required, or uncontrolled bleeding is present.
—Bed rest, scrotal support, ice bags, and analgesics should be applied as well.

 ## Follow-Up

- Neoplasms

—Follow-up should be coordinated with an oncologist.
  —Depending on the clinical and pathologic grade and stage, treatment will involve either surveillance, chemotherapy, or radiotherapy.
—Metastatic work-up includes chest radiograph and abdominal and pelvic computed tomography.
—Regular testicular self-examination is important for evaluation of the remaining testicle.

- Cystic lesions

—Regular testicular self-examination is important for evaluation of the remaining testicle.

- Torsion

—Evaluation in 1 year to check for testicular atrophy and presence of new masses
—Infertility has been noted as a long-term problem.

- Orchitis

—If primary cause resolved, no follow-up needed
—In prepubertal patients, epididymo-orchitis may be due to an underlying urinary tract anomaly, and these patients need structural evaluation of their urinary tracts.
—Infertility has been noted as a long-term problem.

- Trauma: After adequate healing, no follow-up is required.

 ## Miscellaneous

SYNONYMS: N/A

ASSOCIATED CONDITIONS: N/A

NOTES

- See Sections II and III for specific testicular lesions.

ABBREVIATIONS

- AFP, alpha-feto protein; hCG, human chorionic gonadotropin; LDH, lactate dehydrogenase

REFERENCES

Dubinsky TJ, Chen P, Maklad N. Color-flow and power Doppler imaging of the testes. *World J Urol* 1998;16:35.

Junnila J, Lassen P. Testicular masses. *Am Fam Physician* 1998;57:685.

Orland SM, Schlecker BA, Wein AJ. Benign diseases of the testicle and paratesticular tissues. AUA Updates, Series 5, Lesson 24, 1986.

Rowland RG, Foster RS, Donohue JP. Scrotum and testis. In: Gillenwater JY, Grayhack JT, Howards SS, Duckett JW, eds. *Adult and Pediatric Urology*, 3rd ed. St Louis: Mosby, 1996.

Authors: Michael K. Zenni and William A. See

Testosterone—Decreased

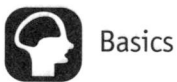 Basics

 Differential Diagnosis

 Database

DESCRIPTION

- Failure of the testes to produce normal levels of testosterone
- Testosterone is the primary androgenic hormone.
- Normal androgenic activity is essential for normal male sexual behavior and function.
- Testosterone in males is responsible for

—Growth and development of male sex organs
—Maintenance of secondary sex characteristics
—Body musculature and fat distribution, etc.

- Testosterone deficiency

—Prepubertal hypogonadism
—Infantile genitalia; lack of virilization
—Abnormal skeletal development (abnormally long legs: delayed epiphyseal closure)
—Decrease/absence of secondary sex characteristics; small, firm testes
—Postpubertal hypogonadism: subtle signs
—Decreased libido, erectile dysfunction, infertility, impaired masculinization
—Decreased facial and body hair (longer intervals between shaving)
—Soft/atrophic testes, osteoporosis

PATHOPHYSIOLOGY

- Normal hypothalamic–pituitary–testes axis

—Hypothalamus secretes GnRH; stimulates the pituitary to secrete FSH and LH
—FSH/LH stimulate testes to produce sperm and androgens.
—Negative feedback of testosterone/metabolites maintains equilibrium.

- Primary hypogonadism

—Testicular dysfunction: inadequate testosterone despite elevated serum FSH/LH

- Secondary hypogonadism

—Hypothalamus or pituitary defect: inadequate FSH/LH to stimulate normal testicular function
—T levels low while FSH/LH levels are low or normal

RISK FACTORS

- Congenital (Klinefelter's, Kallmann's, sickle cell, etc.)
- Stress
- Medications (dopamine antagonist)
- Various diseases, trauma, infections, etc., which involve the hypothalamus, pituitary, or testes
- Obesity

Differential Diagnosis

- Etiology can usually be localized to either the hypothalamus, pituitary gland, or testes.
- Common forms of primary male hypogonadism

—Klinefelter syndrome: congenital disorder with XXY karyotype (1 in 576 male births)
—Impaired T secretion and spermatogenesis
—Small, fibrotic testes (<6 cc) with gynecomastia
—Testicular trauma
—Orchiectomy
—Orchitis
—Drugs
—Decreased production of T: corticosteroids, ethanol, ketoconazole
—Decreased conversion of T to DHT: finasteride
—Androgen receptor blockade: flutamide, spironolactone, cyproterone, cimetidine

- Common forms of secondary male hypogonadism (pituitary vs. hypothalamus)

—Kallmann syndrome (1 in 10,000 males): congenital abnormality in secretion of GnRH, leading to low FSH/LH
—Characterized by anosmia or hyposmia, small testes, and minimal adult male physical traits
—Idiopathic hypogonadotrophic hypogonadism
—Hyperprolactinemia: Prolactin inhibits pituitary secretion of LH or FSH (levels are usually >50 ng/dL).
—Prolactin-secreting pituitary adenomas (prolactinomas)
—Dopamine antagonists (neuroleptics, metoclopramide, etc.): relieve the pituitary cells from the inhibitory effects of endogenous dopamine
—Corticosteroid excess: inhibits GnRH secretion, pituitary response to GnRH, and Leydig cell testosterone production
—Cushing syndrome
—Hemochromatosis: autosomal dominant (0.1% of population): excessive GI iron absorption (iron overload)
—Iron is toxic to pituitary gonadotropes (iron saturation usually >62%).
—Pituitary tumors: pituitary macroadenomas, craniopharyngiomas, and metastatic tumors
—Rare: infections, autoimmune hypophysitis, granulomatous disease, and vascular causes (AV malformations and pituitary hemorrhage)
—Severe systemic illnesses (e.g., end-stage renal disease with associated uremia)
—Drugs
—Decreased secretion of gonadotropins by pituitary: GnRH analogues (Lupron, Zoladex), estrogens, ethanol, corticosteroids, drugs that elevate prolactin (metoclopramide, narcotics, psychotropic drugs)

- Combined primary and secondary hypogonadism: aging males; cirrhosis, sickle cell, obesity

HISTORY

- Developmental abnormalities at birth?
- Rate and extent of virilization at time of puberty?
- Decrease in libido?
- Current status of sexual function (frequency of spontaneous erections and sexual activity, penile tumescence, etc.)?
- Secondary sexual characteristics (beard growth, muscular strength, and overall energy level)
- History of malignancy or granulomatous disease?
- Symptoms suggestive of corticosteroid excess (proximal muscle weakness, skin bruising, etc.)?
- Any complaints of headaches or changes in vision (bitemporal hemianopsia from central sellar mass impinging on optic chiasm)?
- Review all medications.

PHYSICAL EXAMINATION

- Hair on androgen-dependent regions (face, chest, axillae, umbilical area)?
- Hyperpigmented skin changes (iron overload)?
- Skin changes suggestive of corticosteroid excess (striae, etc.)?
- Gynecomastia?
- Measure testes with a Prader orchidometer.

—The normal testicle is ≥15 cc in volume; or ≥3.5 cm in length and ≥2.0 cm in width.
—Less than 6 cc are prepubertal (hypogonadism before puberty).
—Normal size, soft, and atrophic: suggests postpubertal hypogonadism
—Small, fibrotic, firm: suggests Klinefelter syndrome

- Musculoskeletal: signs of muscle atrophy, loss of height, or kyphosis (osteoporosis)

Testosterone—Decreased

 Diagnostic Studies

LABORATORY TESTING

- Initially, morning total serum T should be measured.

—Common T reference ranges for adult men: total 300 to 1200 ng/dL (10.4–41.6 nmol/L); free 9 to 30 ng/dL (0.3–1.0 nmol/L)

- If total T is low and/or there is reduced libido, check serum prolactin.

—Prolactin elevated: Consult with an endocrinologist (pituitary dysfunction).
—Prolactin normal or low: LH level; rule out pituitary or hypothalamic abnormality.
  —High LH/low T: primary hypogonadism
  —LH low or normal, T is low: Evaluate the cause of secondary hypogonadism (consult endocrinologist).
  —Consider iron studies (hemochromatosis), overnight dexamethasone suppression test (Cushing syndrome), and thyroid function tests (especially if < age 50 and no evidence of the aforementioned causes of secondary hypogonadism).

IMAGING

- CT scan or MRI of pituitary to exclude large sellar mass (if suspicious)

—MRI is more expensive but more sensitive in evaluating small pituitary lesions.

SPECIAL STUDIES: N/A

 Initial Management

- T replacement therapy for primary hypogonadism (congenital or acquired) or hypogonadotropic hypogonadism

—Oral preparations (methyltestosterone and fluoxymesterone); not recommended
  —Require large doses (>40 mg/d); dose several times a day (short half-life)
  —Can cause liver toxicity (hepatitis and hepatoma); expensive
—Parenteral preparations (testosterone cypionate and enanthate)
  —Safe, practical, and least expensive; dose adjusted based on clinical response
  —100 mg weekly, 200 mg every other week or every third week, 300 mg every third week, etc.
—Transdermal systems: may cause local skin irritation; more expensive than IM testosterone
  —Scrotal patch: Testoderm (6 mg); associated with elevated DHT; need hairless scrotal area
  —Nonscrotal patch: Androderm (2.5 and 5.0 mg) and Testoderm TTS (5 mg): daily to appendage or torso skin

- Baseline DRE, CBC, lipid profile, and PSA: before T replacement

—T therapy may be associated with lipid abnormalities, polycythemia, azoospermia, sleep apnea, and possible prostate changes.

- Secondary hypogonadism: Treat the underlying cause; consult with an endocrinologist.

—Hyperprolactinemia: Discontinue the drug raising prolactin; follow with a dopamine agonist.
—Pituitary macroadenoma: transsphenoidal resection with or without radiation therapy
—Cushing syndrome: Restore normal corticosteroid levels.
—Hemochromatosis: repeat phlebotomy/chelation therapy with deferoxamine (may still require androgen replacement)

 Follow-Up

- Two to 4 months after initiating replacement therapy

—DRE, PSA, lipid profile, CBC: then and every 6 to 12 months thereafter
—Check T if desired clinical results are not attained.

- Secondary hypogonadism needs endocrinology follow-up.

 Miscellaneous

SYNONYMS: N/A

ASSOCIATED CONDITIONS: N/A

NOTES: N/A

ABBREVIATIONS

- FSH, follicle-stimulating hormone; LH, luteinizing hormone; DHT, dihydrotestosterone; T, testosterone

REFERENCES

Anawalt BD. Endocrinology of male sexual dysfunction. In: Hellstrom WJG, ed. *Handbook of Sexual Dysfunction*. Lawrence, KS: Allen Press, 1998 (*in press*).

Bremner WJ. Endocrinology of the male. In: Becker KL, et al., eds. *Principles and Practice of Endocrinology and Metabolism*, 2nd ed. Philadelphia: JB Lippincott Co, 1995:1032–1146.

Ghusn HF, et al. Evaluation and treatment of androgen deficiency in males. *Endocrinologist* 1991;6:399.

Hellstrom WJ. When and how to treat the androgen-deficient male. *Contemp Urol* 1998 (*in press*).

Vandenberg TL, et al. A guide to androgen replacement therapy. *Contemp Urol* 1997;19:25.

Authors: Sunil K. Purohit and Wayne J.G. Hellstrom

Umbilical Discharge/Mass

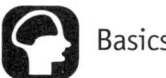 Basics

DESCRIPTION

• The umbilicus is the site of a large number of well-recognized and unusual congenital anomalies.
• Most present during the neonatal period or early infancy.
• Accurate diagnosis is imperative: It varies from trivial to life threatening (peritonitis).
—Most common umbilical lesion: umbilical granuloma

PATHOPHYSIOLOGY

• The umbilical cord develops with the anterior abdominal wall during the second and third weeks of gestation.
• Contents of umbilicus
—Vitelline duct/allantois and their contained vessels
  —The urachus is a tubular structure from the fetal bladder to the umbilicus; it originates from the allantois.
—Primitive mesenchymal tissue (Wharton's jelly)
—Outer covering of amnion
• With failure of vitelline duct/allantois to involute, get persistent remnants (2% incidence)

RISK FACTORS: N/A

 Differential Diagnosis

• Embryonic
—Urachal remnants: most common; comprise spectrum of anomalies
  —Patent urachus (rare, 3 in 1 million), urachal sinus, urachal cyst
  —Infected urachal cysts found in all ages
—Vitelline duct remnant (omphalomesenteric duct)
  —Connects fetal midgut to yolk sac
  —Umbilical sinus, vitelline cyst, or Meckel's (8%–10% of Meckel's have umbilical anomaly)
—Umbilical sinus
—Arterial umbilicalis remnants

• Acquired anomalies
—Umbilical hernia
  —Defect of umbilical ring with sac, which includes inner lining of peritoneum (often adherent to undersurface of umbilical skin)
  —More common in females and Blacks
  —80% close spontaneously (if less than 2 cm). Lesions greater than 2 cm typically do not close and need surgical repair after 3 to 4 years of observation (rarely associated with incarceration).
—Omphalitis: infection of umbilical stump
—Umbilical polyp: excrescence of vitelline duct mucosa retained in umbilicus
  —Resembles granuloma, but does not disappear with silver nitrate
  —Caution: may be associated with persistent vitelline duct or umbilical sinus!!
—Endometriosis: pain and hemorrhagic umbilical discharge during menses
—Sister Mary Josephs' nodule: umbilical metastasis of primary tumors
  —If primary is known, usually from genital or GI tract
—Umbilical granuloma
  —After umbilical cord separation, a small granuloma can develop.
—Others: dermoid cyst, sebum cyst, spontaneous umbilical fistula from Crohn disease/TB/perforated appendix, umbilical hernia, urachal carcinoma

 Database

HISTORY

• When was anomaly detected?
—Most umbilical disorders found antenatal or at birth
—Fistulas can occur later, often associated with inflammatory processes (Crohn) or surgery/percutaneous procedures.
• Has silver nitrate therapy failed?
—Think umbilical polyp/sinus tract.
• Does the discharge appear enteric in nature?
—Suggests persistence of entire vitelline duct
• Association with menses suggests endometriosis.
• Medical history of malignancy or inflammatory bowel disease

PHYSICAL EXAMINATION

• Signs range from silent process to acute abdomen.
• Clinically: local swelling, redness, inflammation, umbilical discharge or bleeding
• Caution: An enlarged or edematous umbilical cord could represent normal cord slough.

Diagnostic Studies

LABORATORY TESTING

• Check any discharging fluid for creatinine to determine if the discharge is urine (patent urachus).

IMAGING

• High-resolution ultrasound

—Suggested by some as best tool for initial assessment
—Accurately determines anatomy of umbilical structures; with compression, can look for small bowel communications/bands
—62% of bladder ultrasounds demonstrate a urachal remnant over the dome of the bladder.

• Fistulography: contrast injected into sinus/tract; unreliable, may miss communicating cysts, may have difficulty cannulating tract

—Note: Urachal sinuses head inferiorly; vitelline duct remnants extend inward towards the peritoneum.

• Voiding cystourethrogram: evaluates for urachal remnant/sinus, and associated bladder outlet obstruction (unlikely that urinary obstruction is directly related to patent urachus)

SPECIAL STUDIES: N/A

 Initial Management

• Umbilical granuloma: topical silver nitrate or diathermy; if not resolved, think of umbilical sinus or polyp.
• Umbilical polyp: If not associated with persistent vitelline duct or umbilical sinus, locally excise.
• Surgical exploration: Inject methylene blue into tract/sinus.

—Infraumbilical incision down to fascia
—If there is no dye or tract below the fascia, close; otherwise, open the fascia along the linea alba and resect.

• Umbilical sinus

—Simple sinus tract: excise
—Patent vitelline duct (enteric contents per umbilicus), needs prompt laparotomy and duct excision: to avoid intussusception/volvulus
—Patent urachus: Resect entire duct via infraumbilical incision (in newborns), or transverse mid-hypogastric incision in older children; remove cuff of bladder with specimen

 Follow-Up

• Based on lesion

 Miscellaneous

SYNONYMS: N/A

ASSOCIATED CONDITIONS: N/A

NOTES

• See also Section II, "Urachal Abnormalities" and "Urachal Carcinoma."

ABBREVIATIONS: N/A

REFERENCES

Bouthroyd A, et al. Ultrasound of the discharging umbilicus. *Pediatr Radiol* 1996;26:362.

Molderey C, et al. Umbilical discharge: A review of 22 cases. *Acta Chir Belg* 1995;3:166.

Walsh PC, Retik AB, Vaughan ED, Wein AJ, eds. *Campbell's Urology*, 7th ed. Philadelphia: WB Saunders, 1998:1543.

Authors: J.C. Trussell and Gabriel P. Haas

Undescended Testicle (Cryptorchidism)

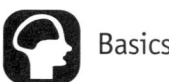 Basics

DESCRIPTION

- Literally means hidden or obscure testis
- Synonymous with incomplete testicular descent
- May be unilateral or bilateral
- Term encompasses palpable, nonpalpable, and ectopic testicles
- Position of testis can be abdominal, inguinal, prescrotal, or gliding
- Incidence is 3% to 5% in full-term boys, and 1.8% at 1 year of age.

PATHOPHYSIOLOGY

- The testis descends to a scrotal position in mammals in order to optimize spermatogenesis.
- The actual mechanisms of descent are unknown at the present time.
- Factors causing proper descent include traction on the testis by the gubernaculum and cremaster muscle, differential growth of the body wall, intraabdominal pressure, maturation of the epididymis being responsible for migration of the testis, and the effect of the genitofemoral nerve.
- Endocrine factors contribute a major role in descent of the testicle.
- Several clinical syndromes with defects in gonadotropin production result in cryptorchidism.
- Accurate mechanisms of androgen influence are not known at present.

RISK FACTORS: N/A

 Differential Diagnosis

- When a child presents with an undescended testicle, the ultimate diagnosis can be classified according to several different categories.
- Testicular retraction

—The most common factor resulting in the inaccurate diagnosis of an undescended testicle
—Common in boys 5 to 6 years old
—Etiology is hyperactive cremaster muscle
—In children from 1 year to 11 years of age, 80% of the fully descended testes can withdraw from the scrotum and leave an empty scrotum behind due to the cremaster reflex.
—If a testicle can be milked down to the bottom of the scrotum, it is considered a retractile testis, and no further treatment is needed.
—This phenomena usually disappears by puberty.

- Canalicular testis

—Testicle located between internal and external inguinal rings
—Tension from external oblique aponeurosis may prevent proper descent here.

- Intraabdominal testes

—Located proximal to the internal inguinal ring

- Gliding testicle

—Testicle is not retractile
—On manipulation, can only bring into upper scrotum
—Immediately retracts after being placed into upper scrotum

- Ectopic testicle

—Five major sites of ectopia are perineum, femoral canal, superficial inguinal pouch, suprapubic area, and contralateral scrotal pouch.
—Etiology is believed to be misdirected gubernacular attachment
—Most common ectopic site is superficial inguinal pouch

- Absent testicle

—Can be bilateral
—Believed to be associated with in utero torsion, vascular insult, or agenesis

- Intersex anomaly

—Children born with bilateral undescended testes and hypospadias or microphallus can actually be virilized females with adrenal hyperplasia.

 Database

HISTORY

- Any prior history of groin or scrotal surgery?
- Has there ever been a testicle present before?

PHYSICAL EXAMINATION

- All general pediatric examinations should include documentation of testicular position.
- The examiner must have warm hands.
- The patient should be supine and relaxed during the examination.

—Document the position of the testicle.
—Determine if there is any hernia, canalicular testicle, or evidence of groin incision.
—Note scrotal skin for degree of rugation.
—Check external genitalia for phallus length and abnormalities.
—Testicular volume should be documented bilaterally with an orchidometer.

Diagnostic Studies

LABORATORY TESTING

- Not usually informative
- Serum FSH levels (see below)

IMAGING

- Generally, radiologic imaging is not reliable.
- Sonography can help identify a testicle located in the inguinal canal, but is of limited use for intraabdominal testes.
- MRI and a CT scan can be useful for intraabdominal testes, but they are often difficult to use on small children and have a high rate of false-negative results.

SPECIAL STUDIES: N/A

 ## Initial Management

- Bilateral undescended testes

—Intersex (females with adrenal hyperplasia) should be ruled out.
—If the boy is less than 9 years old and has bilateral undescended testes, FSH should be measured.
—If FSH is elevated, bilateral anorchia is diagnosed and the work-up can be stopped.
—If FSH is within a normal range, an hCG stimulation test is applied and testosterone is subsequently measured.
—Patients with bilateral anorchia will not make testosterone in response to human chorionic gonadotropin (hCG).

- Retractile testis

—A normal variant; usually disappears by 13 years of age

- Reasons to treat the undescended testicle

—Most pediatric urologists recommend orchiopexy by 1.0 to 1.5 years of age or earlier.
—Goal: to prevent histologic changes that may affect future fertility
—Other: psychosocial reasons and placement of testicle in position more amenable to physical examination to pick up testis cancer

- Pharmacotherapy: avoids anesthesia and is minimally invasive

—hCG is the drug of choice.
—Thought to stimulate Leydig cells of testicle to produce androgens
—The precise mechanism of action is unknown.
—Usually, a maximum 5-week course is undertaken.
—Patients failing hormonal therapy should undergo surgical treatment.

- Surgical therapy

—Surgery immediately performed on ectopic testes, cryptorchids with coexisting hernias, and boys at puberty
  —Standard dartos pouch created with inguinal approach to testicle
—When the standard technique is not applicable, the Fowler-Stephens procedure is used.
—Here the testicle relies on blood flow from the deferential artery and branches from the inferior vesicle artery.
—The spermatic artery and vein are ligated and divided in order to allow maximal testicular mobilization.
—Is often performed in a two-stage fashion

- Laparoscopy

—Laparoscopy can be used to localize nonpalpable, undescended testes.
—Diagnostic laparoscopy is the method of choice to locate the nonpalpable testis.
—If the testis is low in the abdomen, an orchidopexy is performed laparoscopically.
—When a high abdominal testis is located, the first stage of a Fowler-Stephens orchiopexy is performed.
—The second stage of the repair is performed in 6 months.

 ## Follow-Up

- Long-term issues include infertility and tumorigenesis.
- After initial postoperative visits, children should be seen 1 year after surgery to note the location and size of the testes.
- At puberty, boys should be taught how to perform monthly testicular self-examinations.

—The threshold for ultrasound examination and biopsy should be low in these patients.

- Once the boys reach adulthood, issues regarding fertility must be explored with a urologist.

Miscellaneous

SYNONYMS

- Undescended testes, testicular maldescent, ectopic testicle

ASSOCIATED CONDITIONS: N/A

NOTES

- See also Section I, "Ambiguous Genitalia," and Section II, "Intersex Disorders."

ABBREVIATIONS: N/A

REFERENCES

Kogan S, et al. Pediatric andrology. In: Gillenwater JY, Grayhack JT, Howards SS, Duckett JW, eds. *Adult and Pediatric Urology*. St Louis: Mosby, 1996.

Poppas D, Mininberg D. Cryptorchidism. In: Bardin W, ed. *Current Therapy in Endocrinology and Metabolism*. St Louis: Mosby, 1994.

Rajfer J. Congenital anomalies of the testis and scrotum. In: Walsh PC, Retik AB, Vaughan ED, Wein AJ, eds. *Campbell's Urology*. Philadelphia: WB Saunders, 1997.

Rozanski T, Bloom D. The undescended testis: Theory and management. *Urol Clin North Am* 1995;22(1):107–118.

Authors: G. Bino Rucker and Dix P. Poppas

Ureter—Trauma

 Basics

DESCRIPTION

• Ureteral trauma is relatively rare and can be caused by penetrating, blunt, or iatrogenic injury. Disruption of the flow of urine, by stricture, fistula, and/or leakage, may result.

PATHOPHYSIOLOGY

• Ureteral trauma is rare because of the unique anatomy and location of the ureter.

—The retroperitoneal location of the ureter offers a great deal of protection from blunt external trauma.
—The ureter is also very mobile throughout its length, except at the ureteropelvic junction (UPJ) and the ureterovesical junction. Severe flexion/extension injuries in children can cause disruption of the ureter at its point of fixation at the UPJ.
—The small tubular size of the ureter also affords some protection, particularly to penetrating trauma.

• The pelvic portion of the ureter is the most common site of iatrogenic injury.

—The location of the ureter adjacent to the pelvic vessels, uterine vessels, and ligaments, makes it an easy target of pelvic surgeons.

RISK FACTORS

• Penetrating injury to the abdomen, lower chest or back
• Flexion/extension injuries in children
• Pelvic radiation treatment
• Gynecologic surgery (i.e., hysterectomy, tubal ligation, laparoscopy)
• Urologic surgery

—Ureteroscopy (0.5% risk of ureteral stricture in modern series)
—Ureterolithotomy, ureteral reimplantation, cystectomy

• General surgery: colorectal surgery
• Vascular surgery: aortoiliac bypass

 Differential Diagnosis

• Ureteral trauma can be classified based on the mechanism, location, and extent of the injury. The cause of the trauma should be apparent from the patient's history.

—Mechanism: penetrating trauma, blunt trauma, or iatrogenic
—Location: proximal, mid, or distal
—Extent: length and severity of injury

 Database

HISTORY

• History will usually reveal the cause and location of any iatrogenic injury.
• In blunt and penetrating trauma patients, a detailed history of mechanism of injury will help identify patients at risk for ureteral trauma.

—Penetrating trauma to the lower chest, back, abdomen
—Blunt trauma causing significant flexion and/or extension in children

• Prior history of radiation therapy to the abdomen or pelvis can cause ureteral injury and will effect healing of any repair.
• Symptoms can include pain, fever, hematuria, or urinoma causing abdominal distention, inflammation, and possible ileus.
• Urinary fistula may be present.
• Patients can present with "silent" obstruction.

PHYSICAL EXAMINATION

• Penetrating trauma patients should be examined for the proximity of the injury to the ureter.
• Associated injuries to periureteral organs can also be useful in determining the probability of a ureteral injury.
• Physical examination may reveal abdominal distention (due to urinoma), or the presence of a fistula.

Diagnostic Studies

LABORATORY TESTING

• Creatinine may be elevated due to extravasation and reabsorption of urine, or obstruction.
• Urinalysis may reveal hematuria, and UTI should be ruled out.

IMAGING

• Retrograde ureteropyelography is the most useful study in detecting and evaluating ureteral injuries.
• Most trauma patients will have an early CT scan, and ureteral trauma can be demonstrated by extravasation of contrast.
• Ultrasound is generally not useful, except in demonstrating a urinoma, or hydronephrosis.
• Trauma patients should have the presence of a contralateral kidney established prior to repair.

—Either by CT scan, or if the patient is being explored emergently, a "one-shot" IVP

SPECIAL STUDIES

• Whether a fistula originates from the bladder or ureter can be determined by instilling methylene blue or indigo carmine saline through a bladder catheter. If the fistula returns colored fluid, it originates from the bladder.

 Initial Management

• A wide variety of both open and minimally invasive treatment options are available.
• The choice of the most appropriate treatment depends on the extent and location of the injury.
• Open surgical management

—Trauma patients who are being explored for other reasons, long (>2 cm) ureteral strictures, and significant iatrogenic injuries identified intraoperatively are best managed with open surgical repair.
—Principles of open surgical repair of ureteral injuries
  —Debridement of devitalized tissue
  —Water-tight, tension-free anastomosis
  —Isolation of anastomosis from concomitant injuries (omental flap)
  —Drainage of repair; ureteral stenting
—Open repair options
  —Ureteroureterostomy (with renal mobilization to gain length as needed)
  —Ureteroneocystostomy (with psoas hitch and/or Boari bladder flap as needed)
  —Ileal ureter (less desirable in acute trauma setting)
  —Transureteroureterostomy (less desirable in acute trauma setting)
  —Autotransplant (useful for severe, long ureteral strictures)
  —Nephrectomy (for severe damage and presence of normal contralateral kidney)

• Conservative management

—Minor iatrogenic injuries (i.e., clamping, minor suture injury) and minor trauma (minimal extravasation) may be managed with temporary stenting.
—Ureteral strictures <2 cm are best initially managed with ureteroscopic incision and stenting.
  —Endoluminal ultrasound can identify periureteral blood vessels to avoid during endoscopic incision.

 Follow-Up

• Ureteral stents are generally left in place for 2 to 3 weeks after open repair, and 6 to 8 weeks after endoureterotomy.
• IVP several weeks after stent removal will document successful repair.

 Miscellaneous

SYNONYMS: *N/A*

ASSOCIATED CONDITIONS: *N/A*

NOTES: *N/A*

ABBREVIATIONS: *N/A*

REFERENCES

Guerriero WG. Ureteral injury. *Urol Clin North Am* 1989;16:237.

Sagalowsky AI, et al. Genitourinary trauma. In: Walsh PC, Retik AB, Vaughan ED, Wein AJ, eds. *Campbell's Urology*. Philadelphia: WB Saunders, 1997.

Author: Michael J. Conlin

Ureteropelvic Junction Obstruction

 ## Basics

DESCRIPTION

- Ureteropelvic junction obstruction (UPJ) is resistance to urine flow from the renal pelvis into the proximal ureter.
- UPJ obstruction: most common cause of obstruction in children. Incidence: 1:1,000

—Peak incidence is around 5 years of age.
—30% to 50% children with UPJ obstruction now diagnosed prenatally
—Adult UPJ usually diagnosed in third or fourth decade

PATHOPHYSIOLOGY

- Congenital: most common etiology

—A dynamic ureteral segment: present 55% of all pediatric UPJ obstructions
—Intrinsic stenosis: 25% to 50 % of UPJ obstructions associated with functional intrinsic stenosis
—Ureteral valves: rare cause of UPJ
—Lower pole accessory vessels: 10% to 33 % of children with UPJ, up to 50% in adults
—High insertion with kinks, bands/adhesions

- Acquired

—Vesicoureteral reflux (VUR): seen in 15% of children with UPJ
—Inflammation with scarring : trauma, infected urinoma, retroperitoneal fibrosis
—Iatrogenic injury: failed pyeloplasty, ureteroscopic injury
—Malignant neoplasms: TCCa, SCCa, metastatic disease
—Benign neoplasms: fibroepithelial polyps, mesodermal tumors

RISK FACTORS

- Gender

—Male:female ratio (2:1)
—Familial disposition

- Sidedness

—Bilateral obstruction present in 10% to 30% of newborns with UPJ
—Left kidney 2× more affected than right

- Congenital anomalies: 50% of patients with GU anomalies will also have UPJ.

—VUR: 0.5% to 5.0% have concomitant UPJ.
—Horseshoe kidney: 15% associated incidence of UPJ
—Ectopic kidneys: UPJ obstruction seen in 35%

 ## Differential Diagnosis

- Obstructive dilatation

—Impacted urinary calculus
—Fungal balls
—Sloughed papilla
—Intraluminal lesion: neoplasm

- Nonobstructive dilatation

—VUR
—Prune-belly syndrome
—Renal or peripelvic cysts

 ## Database

HISTORY

- Ipsilateral flank pain: chronic, dull vs. acute, severe, sharp, colicky (75% adults, 50% children)

—Intermittent hydronephrosis (Dietl's crisis): intermittent pain associated with nausea and vomiting due to UPJ obstruction associated with high fluid intake and brisk diuresis
—Associated GI symptoms (5% adults, 10%–40% children)
—Vague abdominal pain: often paraumbilical
—Nausea/vomiting

- Gross hematuria (20% adults, 5%–10% children)
- Renal pelvic calculus (20% adults, 5% children)
- UTI (15% adults, 20%–45% children)
- Reduced renal function (5% adults)

PHYSICAL EXAMINATION

- Costovertebral angle tenderness (CVAT)

—More common in adults than in children

- Abdominal or flank mass

—Most common in neonates/small children

- Fever/failure to thrive

—Common in neonates/small children

- Hypertension (HTN)

—Secondary to acute pain/activation of renin–angiotensin pressor system

 ## Diagnostic Studies

LABORATORY TESTING

- Urinalysis (UA)

—Microscopic hematuria (rarely gross)
—Trace proteinuria
—Pyuria and bacteriuria (associated with active infection)

- Serum creatinine

—May be elevated in patients with bilateral UPJ

IMAGING

- Intravenous pyelogram (IVP): most commonly used diagnostic study in both pediatric/adult population

—Delayed opacification of collecting system
—Pyelocaliectasis
—Nonvisualization of ureter/narrowing at the UPJ
—Thinning of renal cortex

- Dynamic renal scintigraphy (DRS): provides differential function/degree of renal obstruction

—Tc-99mm MAG3 preferred agent
—Normal half-life: <15 minutes
—Equivocal half-life: 15 to 20 minutes
—Obstructed half-life: >20 minutes

- Renal ultrasonography: useful in diagnosis of renal masses and detection of dilated ureter to differentiate UPJ from UVJ obstruction; most often used as initial screening study in pediatric age group

SPECIAL STUDIES

- Cystoscopy, retrograde pyelography

—Determines length of ureteral involvement
—A simultaneous temporary indwelling stent can be placed to relieve obstruction.

- Whitaker perfusion study: reserved for equivocal IVP/DRS

—Performed via percutaneous access; contrast instilled at rate of 10 cc/min with measurement of intrarenal pressure during infusion
—Normal, <15 cm/H_2O; equivocal, 15 to 22 cm/H_2O; obstructed, >22 cm/H_2O

- Helical CT evaluation: Three-dimensional reformatting permits visualization of collecting system/associated renal vasculature (crossing vessels).

—Presence of crossing vessels may increase operative complications during endopyelotomy.
—Endopyelotomy success may be lower in UPJ associated with a crossing vessel.

Ureteropelvic Junction Obstruction

 Initial Management

- Restore renal function: especially in patients with bilateral obstruction/patients with absent or poorly functioning contralateral kidney

—Percutaneous nephrostomy drainage/indwelling ureteral stent

- Relieve severe symptoms.

—Temporary percutaneous nephrostomy drainage/indwelling ureteral stent prior to definitive therapy

- Treat pyonephrosis if present.

—Culture-specific antibiotics
—A percutaneous/ureteral stent may be necessary to ensure adequate drainage.

- Expectant treatment

—Asymptomatic adults with normal contralateral kidney/significant comorbidities
—Neonatal hydronephrosis: Obstruction associated with unilateral neonatal hydronephrosis is approximately 15%; a majority of neonates with hydronephrosis can be initially managed nonoperatively.

- Formal operative treatment

—Open procedures: procedures of choice in pediatric age group (flank or dorsal lumbotomy incision)
  —Dismembered (Anderson-Hynes) pyeloplasty: most common open technique with success rate of >90%; appropriate for high insertion, accessory vessels, massively dilated pelvis, or long ureteral involvement. Excision of anatomic and functionally abnormal segment
  —Foley Y-plasty: best applied in high-insertion UPJ
  —Spiral or vertical flap: best applied in UPJ associated with large extrarenal pelves and long proximal ureteral narrowing
  —Ureterocalicostomy: mainly in salvage cases of failed pyeloplasty or UPJ associated with rotational anomalies. A partial lower pole nephrectomy is usually necessary.
  —Nephrectomy: may be necessary in ipsilateral poor renal function and normal contralateral renal function. Indications for nephrectomy: differential renal function <10% to 15%, extensive stone disease and/or chronic infection, multiple failed procedures with significant loss of function
—Endoscopic procedures: procedure of choice in adult age group for both primary/secondary UPJ obstruction
  —Endopyelotomy: antegrade cold-knife incision: Success rates are approximately 80% for both primary/secondary UPJ. Requires percutaneous access. Nephrostomy tube left indwelling 24 to 48 hours, ureteral stent 4 to 8 weeks. Best applied with strictures <2 cm in length. UPJ is associated with renal calculi and children with secondary UPJ obstruction.

—Endopyelotomy: retrograde balloon cautery incision (Acucise) using a cutting balloon catheter. Success rates are approximately 80% for primary/secondary UPJ. The catheter is placed cystoscopically: Endopyelotomy occurs under fluoroscopic guidance. Stent left indwelling 4 to 8 weeks. Best applied in adult patients with primary/secondary UPJ, mild-to-moderate hydronephrosis, stricture <2 cm in length. Used sparingly in pediatric population with reasonable results. Presence of crossing vessels may increase complication rate (bleeding) and decrease success rate.
—Retrograde ureteroscopic incision: requires specialized ureteroscopic equipment, endourologic expertise. Allows direct visualization of the incision/obviates percutaneous access. Success rates in small series approximately 85% to 90%. Stenting required 6 weeks.
—Balloon rupture of UPJ: The balloon is placed over a guidewire across the UPJ from the antegrade or retrograde approach. UPJ is disrupted by inflation of a high-pressure balloon to 24 to 30 F under fluoroscopic guidance. Indwelling stent is left 6 to 8 weeks. Success rates are approximately 70% to 80%. Used mainly in secondary UPJ with <2-cm ureteral strictures. It cannot be used in complete UPJ obliteration.
—Indwelling stent/PCN nephrostomy: reserved for patients who are not candidates for operative Rx. Requires stent/tube change every 8 to 12 weeks. Increased risk of infection, stone formation, ultimate renal damage
—Laparoscopic pyeloplasty: requires proficiency/experienced advanced laparoscopic technique. Approaches: transabdominal/retroperitoneal. Pyeloplasty techniques: dismembered/Y-V plasty. Advantages: decreased postoperative pain, shorter recovery time, improved cosmetic result compared with open surgery. Success rates are >90% (limited series).

 Follow-Up

- Expectant management

—Neonatal UPJ: renal ultrasound or DRS at 1 month, followed at 3 to 6 months. Operative intervention is recommended: symptomatic or if differential renal function >10%, or worsening hydronephrosis.

- Operative treatment

—IVP or DRS postoperatively: 6 weeks to 3 months following repair. 91% of children at 6 to 12 months will have improved DRS. Improved DRS in adults >30 years is rare. IVP usually shows decreased hydronephrosis, prompt excretion.
—Yearly IVP or DRS s/p endopyelotomy: 10% to 13% late failure

 Miscellaneous

SYNONYMS

- Pelvoureteral junction obstruction (PUJ)

ASSOCIATED CONDITIONS: N/A

NOTES: N/A

ABBREVIATIONS

- UPJ, ureteropelvic junction; UVJ, ureterovesical junction; VUR, vesicoureteral reflux; TCCa, transitional cell carcinoma; SCCa, squamous cell carcinoma; CVAT, costovertebral angle tenderness; DRS, diuretic renal scan

REFERENCES

Aslan P, Preminger GM. Retrograde balloon cautery incision of ureteropelvic junction obstruction. *Urol Clin North Am* 1998;25:295–304.

Cartwright PC, Duckett JW, Keating MA, et al. Managing apparent ureteropelvic junction obstruction in the newborn. *J Urol* 1992;148:1224.

Motola JA, Badlani GH, Smith AD. Results of 212 consecutive endopyelotomies: An 8-year followup. *J Urol* 1993;149:453–456.

Novick AC, Streem SB. Surgery of the kidney. In: Walsh PC, Retik AB, Vaughan ED, Wein AJ, eds. *Campbell's Urology*. Philadelphia: WB Saunders, 1998.

Talner LB. Specific causes of obstruction. In: Pollack HM, et al., eds. *Clinical Urography*. Philadelphia: WB Saunders, 1990.

Author: Gary J. Faerber

Urethra—Trauma

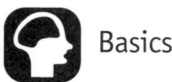 Basics

DESCRIPTION

- Any process that disrupts the water-tight continuity of the urethra
- Uncommon in females; more common in males
- 90% of posterior urethral injuries associated with pelvic fracture

PATHOPHYSIOLOGY

- Anatomy of male urethra

—Penile
—Bulbous
—Membranous
—Prostatic

- Injuries generally divided into regions

—Anterior urethra (bulbous and penile urethra)
—Posterior urethra (membranous and prostatic)

- With blunt trauma, forces are delivered to the urethra that cause tissue injury and destruction.
- With penetrating trauma, the projectile or penetrating object directly injures the urethra, or in the case of a projectile, the blast effect may injure the urethra.
- With pelvic fracture, the membranous urethra is distracted, usually at the departure of the urethra from the bulbospongiosus.
- Iatrogenic
- In children, injury not infrequently involves the prostatic urethra and/or bladder neck.

RISK FACTORS

- Usually associated with either male external genital trauma, perineal straddle, pelvic fracture, and/or perineal laceration. Risk factors for associated bladder neck injuries include children and pubic ramus fracture with displaced pubic fragment.

 Differential Diagnosis

- Studies are to determine if urethral continuity has been injured.
- These studies must be done in association with CT to evaluate the kidneys in the multiple trauma patient and with a trauma CT cystogram or true trauma cystogram to assess for concomitant bladder or bladder neck injuries.

 Database

HISTORY

- Description of the trauma
- Has the patient voided since the trauma?
- Were there symptoms with voiding?

PHYSICAL EXAMINATION

- Pathognomonic: bloody urethral discharge
- In the case of pelvic fracture, often the examination of the prostate is obscured by the pelvic hematoma (high-riding prostate).
- Often associated with findings of external genital trauma, perineal trauma
- If anterior urethral injury is confined by Bucks fascia, classic finding is "sleeve of penis" injury where the ecchymosis and swelling is limited to the penile shaft
- If anterior urethral injury extends beyond Bucks fascia, it may be confined by Colle's fascia and appear as a "butterfly ecchymosis" on the perineum

Diagnostic Studies

LABORATORY TESTING

• With multiple trauma

—CBC, type and cross, electrolytes, BUN, creatinine, urinalysis, urine for culture and sensitivity

IMAGING

• With multiple trauma

—Abdominal and pelvic CT (or "single-shot" excretory urography, as appropriate)
—Retrograde urethrogram (small volumes of contrast using fluoroscopy if possible)
—CT trauma cystogram or true trauma cystogram

• Technique of retrograde urethrogram

—Plain pelvic film to evaluate for pelvic fracture
—Place patient 30 degree oblique; position to aid visualization of the urethra
—A 14 French Foley catheter is passed several cm into the urethra (just beyond fossa navicularis)
—The balloon is gently inflated with 2 to 3 mL water to seal the urethra
—Under fluoroscopy, gently inject approximately 25 mL of diluted contrast into catheter
—A Brodney penile clamp can also be used to inject contrast into the meatus without a catheter

SPECIAL STUDIES

• Cystoscopy in certain cases (often with placement of a stenting or aligning catheter)

 Initial Management

• With suspicion of a urethral injury, a catheter should not be placed until a retrograde urethrogram is performed.
• If a catheter has been placed, the catheter should not be removed; contrast can be placed alongside the catheter using a feeding tube or small IV catheter to evaluate for urethral injury.
• With multiple trauma/pelvic fracture: Stabilize the patient.

—If the patient is unstable with pelvic fracture, should consider external fixation to stabilize the fracture and the patient. If the patient continues to be unstable after external fixation, angiography with angio-occlusion of bleeders or emergent laparotomy with packing of the pelvis
—Place suprapubic catheter (author prefers open suprapubic tube placement)
—If the patient's condition allows, place an aligning urethral catheter (can be done as long as 1 week after trauma).

• With anterior urethral trauma, often a urethral catheter will suffice.

—If in doubt, place a suprapubic tube.
—Penetrating trauma: Immediate reconstruction can be considered.
—Penetrating trauma associated with a projectile, with low-velocity projectiles: Immediate urethral reconstruction is very successful. With high-velocity projectiles: Urethral reconstruction is less reliable because of the unpredictability of the blast injury.

• Broad-spectrum antibiotics in all cases

—Ancef 1 g IV q8h; gentamicin 80 mg IV q8h or 24-hour dosing protocol with kinetic monitoring; piperacillin 3 g IV q6h; ciprofloxacin 400 mg IV q12h or 500 mg po q12h

 Follow-Up

• If immediate urethral reconstruction is accomplished, patients should be appropriately diverted with voiding urethrography at the time of the voiding trial.
• If diverted, diversion for 3 to 4 months

—At 3 to 4 months, retrograde urethrogram with cystogram and voiding urethrogram
—Urethroscopy/cystoscopy at 4 months

• Appropriate reconstruction or endoscopic procedure at 4 to 6 months

 Miscellaneous

SYNONYMS

• Posterior urethral distraction, urethral disruption, urethral tear

ASSOCIATED CONDITIONS: N/A

NOTES

• Classification system used by some authors

—Type I urethral injury: stretching and distortion of the urethra usually due to hematoma
—Type II urethral injury: partial or complete urethral disruption, usually at the prostatic apex
—Type III urethral injury: partial or complete rupture of the prostatomembranous urethra with additional damage to the bulbomembranous urethra and urogenital diaphragm

• See also Section II, "Urethral Stricture."

ABBREVIATIONS: NA

REFERENCES

Carr LK, Webster GD. Posterior urethral reconstruction: Perineal approach. *Urol Clin North Am* 1997;5(2):125–137.

Jordan GH. End to end urethral anastomoses in post traumatic urethral strictures. *Aktuelle Urol* (*in press*).

Mundy AR. Reconstruction of posterior urethral distraction defects. *Urol Clin North Am* 1997; 5(1):139–174.

Author: Gerald H. Jordan

Urethral Discharge

 Basics

DESCRIPTION

- One of the most common complaints in urology
- Must be differentiated from preputial discharge in uncircumcised men
- Young adults, most commonly due to a sexually transmitted disease (gonococcal or nongonococcal)
- Older men, often due to BPH or prostatitis

PATHOPHYSIOLOGY

- Usually represents an episode of acute inflammation of the male urethra

RISK FACTORS

- Multiple sex partners
- Unprotected sexual intercourse (no barrier contraceptive method used)
- Genito-oral intercourse
- No proven relationship with cigarettes, circumcision, caffeinated or alcoholic beverages, striping the urethra, and anal intercourse

 Differential Diagnosis

- Preputial discharge (i.e., from under foreskin)

—Physiologic: retained smegma and/or urine
—Pathologic: balanitis, carcinoma, chemical irritants, syphilis

- Urethral discharge

—Physiologic: phosphaturia, spermatorrhea
—Pathologic: urethritis (gonococcal, nongonococcal), *Chlamydia trachomatis, Ureaplasma urealyticum, Gardnerella vaginalis, Candida albicans,* viral (herpes, cytomegalovirus, human papilloma virus), unknown pathogens, other urinary tract infections, foreign bodies, allergic or sensitivity reactions (use of vaginal douches or lubricants), substance abuse (amphetamines or other stimulants), juvenile urethritis (frequency, dysuria, and blood spotting of the underpants), Reiter disease (see Section III)
—Note: Multiple infections are often seen.

 Database

HISTORY

- Prior history of STD?

—May be recurrence of disease

- Associated symptoms?

—A pricking sensation in the urethra and dysuria are the most common complaints.
—Prostatism suggests post-void dribbling.

- Nature of discharge?

—See "Physical Examination."

- Sexual activity, contraceptive methods, number of sexual partners?

—Identify risk factors for new or recurrent STD.

- History of insertion of foreign bodies in the urethra?

—Not often revealed by the patient

- History of urologic surgery?

—Iatrogenic foreign bodies (i.e., sutures, stones, eroded prosthesis)

PHYSICAL EXAMINATION

- Rectal examination for evidence of BPH or prostatitis
- Penis: glans, foreskin, meatus, urethra

—Inflammation of the urethral mucosa may be seen at the meatus.
—Palpation of the anterior urethra for foreign bodies, masses

- Examination of the discharge with gentle urethral expression if needed

—At least 1 hour after void, preferably 4 hours
  —Gonococcal: Pus is usually profuse, thick, and yellow or gray-brown.
  —Nongonorrheal discharges may be similar in appearance, but often thin, mucoid and scanty.
  —Bloody discharge should suggest a foreign body, stricture, tumor, or prostatitis.

 Diagnostic Studies

LABORATORY TESTING

- Gonococcal urethritis: See Section II: "Gonorrhea."
- Nongonococcal urethritis

—Gram-stained smear of a urethral swab (collected at least 1 hour after last void, preferably 4 hours) containing more than 4 polymorphonuclear leukocytes per oil-immersion field
—Asymptomatic men can have urethral leukocytosis. If urethritis is suspected but urethral inflammation cannot be detected, a urethral swab should be obtained in the early morning before voiding.

- Chlamydial infection: A macron-tipped swab must be used and calcium alginate or cotton swabs avoided. Preliminary results usually take 2 to 3 days. Fluorescing-conjugated monoclonal antibody can be used. It takes 30 minutes to perform and has a sensitivity of 93% and a specificity of 96%.
- Trichomoniasis: Immediately after collecting the urethral discharge, mix with 1 to 2 mL of saline and study microscopically (less accurate in men than in women). Liquid and semisolid medium cultures are more accurate for diagnosis of trichomoniasis.

IMAGING: N/A

SPECIAL STUDIES

- Confirmation that the discharge is arising from the urethra

—Two-glass test: The patient is asked not to void for at least 2 hours, and then passes approximately 20 mL of urine into each of two glasses.
  —If the first glass contains a generalized haze of threads and debris, urethritis is likely.
  —If both glasses are affected, it is more likely that the problem comes from the bladder or upper urinary tract.
  —If there is the presence of phosphate deposits, a uniform haze will be present in both glasses, one that clears when urine is acidified.
—Stamey test (see Section III)
  —Leukocytes or bacteria (or both) only in VB1: anterior urethritis
  —Leukocytes or bacteria (or both) in VB1,2,3: cystitis or upper urinary tract infection
  —Leukocytes or bacteria (or both) in EPS or VB3 only: prostatic source of infection

Initial Management

- Gonococcal urethritis: See Section II: "Gonorrhea."
- Nongonococcal urethritis

—Doxycycline, 100 mg orally, twice daily for 7 days, or
—Azithromycin 1 g, single oral dose, or
—Erythromycin base, 500 mg orally, 4 times daily for 7 days, or
—Erythromycin ethylsuccinate, 800 mg orally, 4 times daily for 7 days
—Important: Always have sexual partners evaluated, and treat with the same regimen.

- Management of persistent or recurrent urethritis

—Question the patient about compliance with treatment and reexposure to infection.
—Reevaluate for less common causes of urethritis, and confirm urethritis.
—Treat any specific cause elucidated.
—If a specific cause is not found or if *Ureaplasma urealyticum* is present, treat with erythromycin base 500 mg qid for 14 days.

- Trichomoniasis

—Metronidazole, 2 g orally as a single dose, to the patient and to the partner, or
—Metronidazole 500 mg, twice daily for 7 days

 ## Follow-Up

- Most cases of nongonococcal urethritis respond promptly to doxycycline.
- Treatment of the sexual partner is imperative.
- Irritative symptoms may remain after eradication of infection, probably due to urethral scarring. These symptoms usually decrease with time.
- Repeat cultures after treatment is established (if previously positive).
- Postgonococcal urethritis: If symptoms continue after adequate treatment of acute gonococcus infection, it probably is due to a secondary organism resistant to the initial medication.
- Complications in men (see also Section II, "Gonorrhea" [complications of])

—Urethral stricture, infertility
—Epididymitis or epididymo-orchitis: less than 35 years of age, probably due to chlamydia; older than 35 years, probably due to coliform infections associated with a history of urologic disease or instrumentation.
—Proctitis: chlamydia in 15% of homosexual men with proctitis

- Complications in women

—Pelvic inflammatory disease, pain, infertility, ectopic pregnancy

 ## Miscellaneous

SYNONYMS: N/A

ASSOCIATED CONDITIONS: N/A

NOTES

- Patients must always be encouraged to undergo testing for other sexually transmitted diseases.
- Of newborns exposed to chlamydia during vaginal delivery, up to 15% contract chlamydial pneumonia and 50% develop chlamydial conjunctivitis.

ABBREVIATIONS: N/A

REFERENCES

Bullock N, et al. Urethral and sexually transmitted disorders. In: *Essential Urology*, 2nd ed. Churchill Livingstone, 1994:291–303.

Berger RE, et al. Sexually transmitted diseases in males. In: Tanagho EA, McAnich, eds. *Smith's General Urology*, 14th ed. Norwalk, CT: Appleton & Lange, 1995:262–275.

Berger RE. Sexually transmitted diseases: The classic diseases. In: Walsh PC, Retik AB, Vaughan ED, Wein AJ, eds. *Campbell's Urology*, 7th ed. Philadelphia: WB Saunders, 1997:663–681.

Authors: David M. Albala and Fernando C. Koleski

Urethral Mass

 Basics

DESCRIPTION

- A urethral mass may be palpable or visualized by endoscopy.
- The significance varies greatly, depending on the clinical scenario.
- Diagnostic work-up is essential due to the potential for serious underlying pathology.
- Biopsy or excision is generally required.

PATHOPHYSIOLOGY

- Anatomic considerations

—The male urethra: approximately 21 cm in length, divided into prostatic, membranous, bulbar, and penile urethra. It terminates at the fossa navicularis and meatus.
—The female urethra: approximately 3 to 5 cm in length; proximal two-thirds considered posterior, distal one-third considered anterior

- The lining of the urethra changes throughout its course in both sexes.

—Male urethra: begins posterior, with transitional cell lining extending through the prostatic urethra, gradual change to a pseudostratified columnar lining in the bulbar and penile urethra, stratified squamous lining near the meatus
—Female urethra: lined proximally (posterior) with transitional cells, distally (anterior) with squamous cells

RISK FACTORS

- Tobacco use, history of sexually transmitted diseases, exposure to tuberculosis, history of other GU tumors (transitional cell carcinoma [TCC]), trauma (e.g., straddle injury, pelvic fracture, or prior catheterization), prior urethral operations, history of stone disease

 Differential Diagnosis

- The etiology of urethral mass varies widely, depending on the patient's age, sex, medical history, and presenting symptoms. In children, a mass may represent congenital disease, including polyps and hemangiomas. In the young adult to middle age, it may represent sequelae of sexually transmitted diseases, while in the adult over 50, it may represent primary or metastatic neoplasm.
- Congenital

—Benign fibroepithelial polyp: originates in the prostatic urethra near the verumontanum, may cause voiding difficulties in children; 50% occur in boys under 5 years old
—Urethral diverticulum: Occasionally congenital in origin, most are secondary to urinary tract infections in females, or secondary to peri-urethral duct obstruction.
—Retention cysts: formed from stricture of the ostia of Cowper's gland ducts, may be congenital or secondary to inflammatory process, lo-

cated in the bulbar urethra, may be palpable through the perineum
—Stricture disease

- Inflammatory

—Condylomata acuminata: sexually transmitted via HPV, generally noted on external genitalia; 4% to 5% of patients will have urethral involvement, increased incidence in second to fifth decade.
—Gonococcal urethritis: The organism is *Neisseria gonorrheae*, gram-negative intracellular diplococcus; culture with Thayer-Martin medium; leads to development of urethral strictures
—Tuberculosis: rare manifestation of disease; all cases associated with proximal involvement of kidneys or bladder; involves the bulbomembranous urethra; stricture and fistula may occur; "watering pot perineum"

- Traumatic

—Stricture disease secondary to urethral rupture, straddle injury, pelvic fracture, previous operation, catheterization
  —Hematoma
  —Foreign body: bullet, shrapnel, self-instrumentation

- Benign neoplasms

—Hemangioma: presents with gross or microscopic hematuria, associated with lesions elsewhere
—Adenomatous polyps: exophytic; occur in prostatic urethra; villoglandular proliferation of prostate tissue
—Squamous papilloma: uncommon lesion of the distal urethra of both sexes
—Transitional cell papilloma: rare neoplasm of the proximal urethra
—Leiomyomas: increased prevalence in females in third to fifth decade; present as palpable mass with retention
—Polypoid urethritis: increased incidence with chronic indwelling catheter
—Nephrogenic adenoma: rare lesion resembling renal collecting tubules; metaplastic response to trauma, infection, or radiation
—Amyloidosis: rare lesion; presents with hematuria with or without obstruction; palpable induration along the urethra; male preponderance
—Caruncle: occurs in postmenopausal women; soft, red tumors occur at the urethral meatus on the posterior lip; post-inflammatory etiology

- Malignant neoplasms

—Primary urethral carcinoma: only GU malignancy more common in females (4:1); represents <1% of all tumors; four subtypes account for 98% of cases
  —Squamous cell (approximately 80% of lesions): more common in proximal and mid-urethra
  —Transitional cell (approximately 15% of lesions): most common in proximal urethra
  —Adenocarcinoma (approximately 4% of lesions): most common in mid-urethra
  —Melanoma (approximately 1% of all lesions): most common in distal urethra

—Rare malignant lesions
  —Clear cell adenocarcinoma: almost exclusively in women over 50 years; increased association with diverticulum
  —B cell lymphoma: appearance similar to caruncle
  —Non-Hodgkin's lymphoma: approximately 7% involve GU source, 10 reported cases of female urethral involvement
  —Cloacogenic carcinoma, adenocystic carcinoma, carcinoid tumor
  —Carcinoma arising in Cowper's gland or Littre's gland
  —Metastatic lesions: TCC bladder, adenocarcinoma of the colon or rectum, and prostate

- Miscellaneous

—Urethral prolapse: presents with irritative voiding symptoms and spotting of blood. Interlabial, well-circumscribed mass most common in young Black girls (ages 5–7)
—Stone impacted in the urethra or within a diverticulum

 Database

HISTORY

- Age and sex of the patient?

—Primary cancer more common in women over age 50

- Sexual history?

—Exposure to HPV, gonorrhea, chlamydia. Patient with history of genital warts more likely to have urethral recurrence
—Gonorrhea is associated with increased risk of stricture disease.

- History of urinary tract infections?

—Associated with urethral diverticulum, urethral caruncle, polypoid urethritis

- Lower urinary tract symptoms?

—Frequency, urgency, hematuria, obstruction, purulent discharge, dysuria

- Presence of pain?

—Advanced primary or metastatic cancer, diverticulum with active infection, stone, gonorrhea

- Constitutional symptoms?

—Fever, weight loss, back pain, groin pain may indicate advanced infection or carcinoma.

- Medical/surgical history?

—A patient with TCC bladder may have urethral recurrence.
—Prior transurethral surgery or pelvic trauma is associated with stricture disease.

- Social history?

—Tobacco use is associated with transitional cell and squamous cell carcinoma.

PHYSICAL EXAMINATION

- General: vital signs, weight, skin color (pallor of anemia)

- Lymph node assessment: cervical, axillary, inguinal

—Metastatic disease from the distal urethra involves the superficial inguinal nodes, proximal urethra spreads to iliac and obturator nodes.
—Abdominal examination: organomegaly, CVA tenderness, palpable bladder

- Extremities: Note presence or absence of edema.
- External genitalia: Inspection may reveal lesions of condyloma acuminata.
- Urethral examination: Careful palpation of the entire length of accessible urethra is essential. Note location, size, consistency, degree of fixation, multiplicity of urethral mass(es).

—The urethral meatus is inspected for discharge, mass, or stricture.
—Diverticulum in females occurs in midurethra. With compression, purulent discharge from meatus may occur.
—Inspect the perineum for fistulous tracts.

 ## Diagnostic Studies

LABORATORY TESTING

- Urinalysis: Examine for nitrites, blood, protein, pH, glucose on dipstick, and pyuria, hematuria, casts, and bacteria on microscopic examination.
- Urine Gram stain and culture: tuberculosis (acid-fast bacteria), cystitis, urethritis
- Urethral swab: culture for gonorrhea, chlamydia, and tuberculosis
- Urine cytology may identify malignancy.

—Urethral washing is helpful in patients postcystectomy for cancer. A 10Fr to 12Fr urethral catheter is placed with saline wash, recovery of effluent.

- Serum creatinine: may detect renal compromise secondary to outlet obstruction

IMAGING

- Retrograde urethrogram: allows for evaluation of the urethra to define intraurethral lesions, strictures, obstruction, diverticula. Location and extent of disease are assessed.
- A voiding cystourethrogram is useful for diverticulum.
- CT scan/MRI: useful for evaluation of the inguinal and pelvic lymph nodes. MRI will detect corporal invasion by carcinoma.

SPECIAL STUDIES

- Cystoscopy: allows direct visualization of the urethral pathology with cold-cup biopsy
- Suprapubic cystotomy and antegrade urethrogram and/or flexible cystoscopy may define length and location of stricture with realignment.

 ## Initial Management

- Management is directed by the pathologic findings. Urethroscopy with direct visualization of an intraurethral lesion along with biopsy will provide the diagnosis.
- Condyloma of the urethra: biopsy and fulguration or Nd:YAG laser or Holmium laser destruction. Intraurethral 5FU cream. Topical treatment for external condylomata podophyllum, podofilox
- Urethral stricture: dilation, direct-vision internal urethrotomy (recurrence approximately 50%, depending on stricture density, length, and multiplicity). Urethroplasty for refractory strictures. Treatment of underlying disease process is essential.
- Urethral prolapse: topical estrogen cream and sitz baths; if persistent or ischemic, may require surgery
- Urethral diverticulum: Surgical excision is necessary for symptomatic relief and control of infection.
- Benign neoplasms: Biopsy is required for diagnosis. May be fulgurated or treated with laser
- Malignant neoplasm

—Male urethra: Treatment depends on the cell type, size, and location.
  —Partial or total urethrectomy and possible penectomy with perineal urethrostomy may be required.
—Female urethra: total urethrectomy. Radiotherapy and chemotherapy are indicated in some cases. Urinary diversion or a suprapubic catheter may be required.
—Treatment should include inguinal node dissection for anterior lesions and pelvic node dissection for proximal lesions. Total cystectomy is indicated for lesions near the bladder neck in both sexes. Survival is related to pathologic stage, tumor location, and size.

 ## Follow-Up

- Condyloma of the urethra: Periodic urethroscopy with retreatment is necessary until all disease is eradicated, without recurrence.
- Urethral stricture: follow-up voiding history with urinalysis and flow rate at 6-month intervals posttreatment, with repeat procedure if there is suspicion of recurrence; retrograde urethrogram or urethroscopy for recurrent symptoms
- Malignant neoplasm

—Transitional cell carcinoma or squamous cell carcinoma with complete urethrectomy: follow-up chest x-ray every 6 months for 5 years, annual CT scan of abdomen and pelvis

- Partial urethrectomy: follow-up urethroscopy with cytology every 3 months for 2 years, every 6 months in follow-up years 3 and 4, and then annually. Chest x-ray every 6 months for 5 years, annual CT scan of the abdomen and pelvis

 ## Miscellaneous

SYNONYMS: N/A

ASSOCIATED CONDITIONS: N/A

NOTES

- See Section II, "Urethra–Abscess (Periurethral Abscess)," "Urethra–Carcinoma, General," and "Urethra–Diverticula, Female."

ABBREVIATIONS: N/A

REFERENCE

Petersen RO. *Urologic Pathology*. Philadelphia: JB Lippincott Co, 1992:395–428.

Authors: Hugh A.G. Fisher and Brian Murray

Urinary Incontinence—Adult Female

 Basics

DESCRIPTION

- Involuntary loss of urine that is objectively demonstrable and is of social and hygienic concern
- Stress incontinence: associated with activities causing abdominal stress (e.g., coughing, sneezing, exercises etc.)
- Urge incontinence: sudden uncontrollable urgency, leading to leakage
- Overflow incontinence: High residual or chronic urinary retention leads to urinary spillage from the distended bladder.
- Total incontinence: constant drainage of urine due to embryologic developmental deficiency of bladder and urethra (e.g., epispadias–exstrophy of bladder or ectopic ureter)

PATHOPHYSIOLOGY

- Sphincteric incontinence: essentially of two types

—Anatomic: due to urethral hypermobility from lack of pelvic support
  —Theory 1: Normally, during increased intraabdominal stress, equal pressure transmission occurs to the proximal urethra, which lies within the abdomen above the plane of fascia and the muscle separating the abdomen from the pelvis. A hypermobile urethra due to loss of pelvic support descends below the plane. The normal pressure transmission mechanism is lost, causing stress incontinence.
  —Theory 2: Hammock theory: Normally, the suburethral support contributed by the endopelvic fascia and anterior vaginal wall provides a stable backboard against which the urethra is compressed during intraabdominal pressure rises. When this suburethral support layer is lax and mobile, any effective compression is not achieved, causing leakage.
—Intrinsic sphincter deficiency (ISD): Impairment of various intrinsic factors are responsible for the normal coaptation and closure of the urethra. Urethral mucosal seal and inherent closure from collagen, fibroelastic tissue, smooth and striated muscles, etc., may be lost secondary to surgical scarring, radiation, or hormonal and senile changes.
—Overflow incontinence: from urinary retention, usually occurs from lower motor paralytic neurogenic bladder disorders
—Total urinary incontinence: in epispadias-exstrophy complex due to absence of bladder neck and urethra. Ectopic ureters in females usually open in the urethra distal to the sphincter urethrae or in the vagina, thereby causing constant leakage.

RISK FACTORS

- Advanced age, menopause, lack of estrogen, multiple parity, difficult vaginal child births, pelvic and vaginal surgeries and radiation therapy, urethral diverticulectomy, genital prolapse, myelodysplasia, alpha-adrenoreceptor-blocking antihypertensives, etc.

 Differential Diagnosis

- Stress incontinence: due to urethral hypermobility or ISD, though in the majority it is mixed or due to both of the factors
- Urge incontinence: can be due to urinary infection, interstitial cystitis, carcinoma in situ, bladder calculi, detrusor overactivity, or neurogenic detrusor hyperreflexia
- Nocturnal enuresis: idiopathic, neurogenic, or obstructive causes
- Continuous leakage: ectopic ureter, urinary fistulas, exstrophy–epispadias complex
- Post-void dribbling: urethral diverticulum, idiopathic, iatrogenic, surgical

 Database

HISTORY

- Age: Stress incontinence is more common in elderly menopausal women. Incontinence dating from childhood indicates congenital causes such as ectopic ureter, epispadias, etc.
- Childbirth: Weakness of the pelvic floor is more likely in multiparous women.
- Amount and nature of leakage: Severity of leakage should be graded by the number of pads used in 24 hours.
- Stress incontinence: occurs in small spurts. Patients remain dry at night in bed.
- Urge incontinence: sudden urge followed by leakage of large amounts
- Continuous slow leakage in between regular voiding indicates ectopic ureter, urinary fistula, etc.
- Pain: Suprapubic pain with dysuria implies urinary infection, interstitial cystitis, etc.
- Medical history

—Cerebrovascular accidents, parkinsonism, multiple sclerosis, myelodysplasia, diabetes, spinal cord injury: can cause neurogenic incontinence
—Radiation to pelvic and vaginal areas: causes ISD, vesical irritative urgency, and low bladder compliance
—A history of smoking and chronic obstructive pulmonary disease can aggravate incontinence.

- Medications

—Sympatholytic alpha-blockers (terazosin, prazocin, doxazocin, clonidine, etc.) can cause or worsen incontinence.
—Sympathomimetic and tricyclic antidepressants such as ephedrine, imipramine, etc., can cause retention with overflow.

- Surgical history: Pelvic and vaginal surgeries can cause weakness of pelvic floor support. Prior antiincontinence surgeries can lead to recurrent incontinence from ISD.

PHYSICAL EXAMINATION

- General neurologic examination

—Mental status, speech, intellectual performance.
—Motor status: gait, generalized or focal weakness, rigidity, tremor
—Sensory status: Impairment of perineal–sacral area sensation helps localize the level of neurologic deficit.
—Reflex: A bulbocavernous reflex implies contraction of the anal sphincter in response to squeezing the clitoris. This reflex tests the integrity of sacral 2,3,4 spinal cord segments.

- Urologic examination

—Abdomen: visible exstrophy–epispadias; incisional scars of previous surgeries
—Suprapubic tenderness: may indicate cystitis
—Palpable distended bladder: chronic urinary retention

- Pelvic examination

—Vaginal examination with empty bladder to check pelvic organs
—Vaginal examination with comfortably full bladder
—The patient is asked to cough or strain to reproduce incontinence.
—Cystocele, if evident, is graded.
—Urethral hypermobility
  —Gauged by palpation of the descent of the proximal urethra on straining
  —Q-tip test: A lubricated Q-tip is inserted to proximal urethra and the patient is asked to strain. A resting or straining angle of greater than 30 degrees is indicative of hypermobility of the urethra.
—Examination of the vaginal vault and posterior vaginal wall for enterocele or rectocele

Diagnostic Studies

LABORATORY TESTING

- Urine analysis

—Specific gravity: Low specific gravity implies renal impairment.
—Dipstick: blood, protein, nitrites, leukocyte esterase
—Crystalluria: suggests urinary calculus disease

- Urine culture: if microscopic and reagent strip tests suggest infection
- Creatinine/BUN: Check renal impairment from associated pathologies.

IMAGING

- Excretory urography: determines status of upper urinary tract, duplicated systems for ectopic ureters, and associated pathologies
- Cystogram and voiding cystourethrogram: preferably done under fluoroscopic monitoring and in combination with videourodynamic studies. Determines presence of trabeculations, diverticula, vesicoureteric reflux, integrity of the sphincteric mechanism, degree and type of incontinence, and associated cystocele

SPECIAL STUDIES

- Urodynamic studies

—Cystometric study of detrusor function: determines bladder compliance, sensations and detrusor responses to filling
  —Useful in patients with history of urgency and urge incontinence, cystometric documentation of detrusor hyperreflexia or detrusor instability has important therapeutic and prognostic implications.
—Urinary flow rate: Good flow rate with minimal post-void residual is characteristic of sphincteric incontinence.
—Valsalva leak point pressure: determines the intraabdominal pressure at which leakage is observed at the meatus or by fluoroscopy. Low leak point pressure implies ISD.

—Videourodynamic studies: sophisticated combination of fluorocystourethrography and urodynamic studies mentioned above.

Initial Management

- Treat correctable causes (UTI, etc.).
- Nonsurgical management: helps about 50% to 65% patients with milder symptoms

—Behavioral therapy: voiding at progressively increasing predetermined intervals
—Biofeedback and pelvic floor exercises (Kegel exercise)
—Electrical stimulation of pelvic floor muscles
—Drug therapy: estrogens, alpha-adrenergic agonists such as ephedrine, pseudoephedrine, phenylpropanolamine, imipramine
—Occlusive and supportive devices, urethral plugs

- Surgical approaches

—Surgical management: provides more successful and sustained outcome
—Periurethral injection of bulking agents: collagen, Teflon, detachable balloon
—Vesicourethral suspension procedures: aim at repositioning and retropubic fixation of bladder neck and proximal urethra
  —Provide high initial success rate, especially as the initial operation. At long-term follow-up, however, the continence rate seems to decline.
  —Abdominal approaches: Marshall-Marchetti-Krantz cystourethropexy, Burch colposuspension, laparoscopic colposuspension
  —Vaginal needle suspension procedures: Raz, Stamey, etc.
  —Urethral compression surgeries
    —Pubovaginal sling suspension: used for coaptation and compression of the incontinent urethra, using autologous fascia or synthetic materials
    —Proven useful especially for ISD patients
    —Lately being recommended for both urethral hypermobility and ISD patients
    —Postoperative de novo urgency, urge incontinence, voiding difficulty, and urinary retention, necessitating intermittent self-catheterization or take-down of the suspension, remain as concerns in up to about 20% of patients.
—Artificial urinary sphincter placement

Follow-Up

- Initial postoperative assessment: Evaluate voiding function with estimation of post-void residual. And need for intermittent catheterization.
- Urgency and urge incontinence: treated with anticholinergics after elimination of urinary tract infection
- Periodic long-term follow-up with outcome-based questionnaire surveys

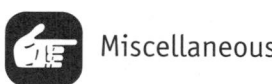

Miscellaneous

SYNONYMS: *N/A*

ASSOCIATED CONDITIONS: *N/A*

NOTES

- See also Section I, "Urinary Incontinence: Pediatric."
- Patient resource: Simon Foundation for Continence, PO Box 815, Wilmette, IL 60091; 847-864-3913.

ABBREVIATIONS

- ISD, intrinsic sphincteric deficiency

REFERENCES

Blaivas JG, Romanzi L. Pubovaginal fascial sling (PVS) for all types of stress incontinence (SUI): Long term follow-up of 251 patients. *J Urol* 1997;157(Pt 2):267(abst 1035).

Delancey JOL. Structural aspects of urethrovesical function in the female. *Neurourol Urodyn* 1988;7:509.

Wein AJ. Neuromuscular dysfunction of the lower urinary tract and its treatment. In: Walsh PC, Retik AB, Vaughn ED, Wein AJ, eds. *Campbell's Urology*, 7th ed. Philadelphia: WB Saunders, 1998.

Author: Sakti Das

Urinary Incontinence—Adult Male

 Basics

DESCRIPTION

- *Urinary incontinence* is defined as involuntary loss of urine through an intact urethra, which is a social or hygienic burden for the patient. Incontinence is caused by bladder or/and sphincter dysfunction.
- Bladder dysfunction due to
—Detrusor overactivity (involuntary detrusor contractions of unknown origin during bladder filling)
  —Hyperreflexia (overactive detrusor due to underlying neurologic condition)
  —Detrusor instability (DI) (overactive detrusor not due to neurologic condition)
—Low bladder compliance
—Acontractile detrusor ("overflow")
- Sphincter dysfunction due to
—Structural deficiency (direct injury by trauma or surgery)
—Functional deficiency (neurogenic)
- Epidemiology
—Prevalence 4% at age 45 ; linear increase to 28% at age 90
—Postprostatectomy incontinence most common in males
  —DI after TURP in 4%, after RRP in 8%
  —Sphincteric incontinence in 1% after TURP, 5% after RRP
  —10% to 32% of men are incontinent after RRP (from patient questionnaires).
  —Half of incontinent patients have coexistent SUI and UI.
- Genetics: N/A
- Staging
—SUI
  —Grade I: incontinence with sudden increase of intraabdominal pressure (cough)
  —Grade II: incontinence with physical stress (walking)
  —Grade III: continuous incontinence
—UI: grade by number of pads used
- Signs and symptoms
—Stress urinary incontinence (SUI)
  —Leakage of urine with cough, sneezing, or physical exertion
  —Cause: sphincter deficiency or stress-induced detrusor overactivity
—Urge incontinence (UI)
  —Involuntary loss of urine associated with strong desire to void
  —Cause: bladder dysfunction

—Unconscious incontinence
  —Incontinence without patient's awareness of stress or urge
  —Cause: sphincteric or bladder dysfunction
—Overflow incontinence
  —Observation of incontinence accompanied by urinary retention
  —Cause: impaired contractility or bladder neck obstruction (BOO) with overactive detrusor or malfunctioning sphincter
—Continuous incontinence
  —Continuous involuntary urine loss
  —Cause: bladder, sphincter malfunction
—Nocturnal enuresis
  —Cause: sphincter or bladder malfunction
—Post-void dribble
  —Cause: retained urine in the urethra due to BPH or in a urethral diverticulum

PATHOPHYSIOLOGY

- Involuntary detrusor contraction (IDC)
—Causes strong desire to void (urge) if aborted by voluntary sphincter contraction
—Causes leakage (UI) if inhibition insufficient
—Mechanism of detrusor overactivity not fully understood

- Low bladder compliance (steep rise of pressure during filling)
—Caused by changes in muscle tone and in extracellular matrix (ECM), mainly in collagen
—Injury to pelvic plexus causes acontractile low-compliance bladder.

- The male urethral sphincter can withstand pressures of 200 cm H_2O before leakage.
—Sphincter consists of
  —Smooth muscle sphincter (proximal)
  —Striated muscle sphincter (distal)
—Leakage of urine occurs when both sphincters are
  —Damaged (prostatectomy and damage to rhabdosphincter): SUI
  —Compromised (prostatectomy and bladder instability): UI
—Also, physical activity can provoke detrusor overactivity (stress hyperreflexia).

- Bladder abnormalities
—Hyperreflexia due to
  —Supraspinal neurologic lesions (CVA, Parkinson disease, brain tumor, MS)
  —Suprasacral spinal lesions (MS, spinal cord injury, spinal dysraphism)
—Instability due to
  —Detrusor dysfunction (cystitis, prostatitis, bladder tumor, stone)
  —Outlet dysfunction (BPH, idiopathic BOO, de novo after prostatectomy)
—Low bladder compliance due to
  —Smooth muscle changes (hypertrophy in BOO)
  —ECM changes (radiation, chronic infection, multiple resections)
  —Neuropathic (pelvic nerve injury due to pelvic fracture, radical pelvic surgery)
—Acontractile detrusor
  —Chronic overstretching, LMN bladder

- Sphincter abnormalities
—Sphincter injury
  —Prostatectomy (simple or radical, TURP)
  —Membranous urethral stricture, and treatment of
  —Radical pelvic surgery or pelvic trauma
—Deficient sphincter innervation
  —Suprasacral neurologic lesion (DSD due to spinal cord trauma)
  —Pudendal nerve injury (pelvic fracture)

Differential Diagnosis

- Differentiation between SUI and UI not always clear (see above)
- Urinary leakage due to genitourinary fistulas

 Database

HISTORY

- Presence of voiding symptoms and symptom severity
- Micturition diary

—Recording of time of each void and voided volume
—Sensation before and during leakage
—Presence and amount of urine leakage

- Pad test

—Regular protective pad change (q6h), with a recording of the weight of each pad
—Alternatively, visual estimation of amount of phenazopyridine-discolored urine

- Medical history pertaining neurologic conditions and conditions associated with diuresis
- History of surgery, radiation, or trauma to prostate, urethra, or pelvic
- Medication contributing to stress incontinence (alpha-blockers, clonidine, phenoxybenzamine)
- Medication contributing to urinary retention and overflow incontinence (tricyclic antidepressants, sympathomimetics, anticholinergics)

PHYSICAL EXAMINATION

- Abdomen and flank (bladder distension, renal masses)
- Genitalia (demonstration of leak)
- Limited neurologic assessment of pelvic dermatomes

—Perianal and perineal sensation (pinprick and touch)
—Anal sphincter tone and control
—Bulbocavernous reflex (visible or palpable contraction of anal sphincter or pelvic muscles in response to squeezing of glans penis or pulling the Foley balloon against the BN)

- Prostatic palpation

—Size, tenderness, nodularity

 Diagnostic Studies

LABORATORY TESTING

- Urinalysis
- Microscopy, urine culture and sensitivity
- BUN, creatinine, electrolytes
- Urine cytology (if bladder cancer suspected)

IMAGING

- Cystourethrogram

—BN configuration
—Integrity of sphincter mechanism
—Site of obstruction
—Bladder trabeculation and diverticulum
—Presence of VUR

SPECIAL STUDIES

- Cystourethroscopy evaluates

—Urethral lesions
—Voluntary sphincter configuration
—BN status
—Bladder size and mucosa

- Urodynamic studies (UDS) are indicated if

—Suspected neurologic disorder
—History of radical pelvic surgery (including RRP)
—Inconclusive diagnosis
—Incontinence not demonstrated on physical examination
—No response to standard treatments
—Surgical therapy failures or recurrences

- UDS tests

—Cystometrogram (measures capacity, compliance, sensation, and UDC)
—Urinary flow and pressure/flow studies (determine BOO)
—Leak point pressure
    —Valsalva leak point pressure is the lowest rectal balloon pressure at which leakage occurs during the Valsalva maneuver with a comfortably full bladder. It measures sphincter tightness during stress and predicts treatment response.
    —Detrusor leak point pressure is determined as the lowest intravesical pressure at which urine leakage occurs during bladder filling. It provides an estimate of bladder compliance.
—Striated sphincter EMG if sphincteric dysfunction or dyssynergia suspected
—Multichannel videourodynamics (connects fluoroscopic events to pressure volume curves)

 Initial Management

GENERAL MEASURES

- Treat underlying condition

—TURP improves detrusor instability in half of patients.
—Allow sufficient time for functional return after surgery (i.e., 6–12 months after RRP).

- Symptomatic relief: diapers, condom catheters, indwelling Foley catheter
- Rehabilitation

—Principles
    —Inhibition of onset IDC
    —Abortion of IDC by sphincter contraction
    —Strengthening of sphincter
    —Conversion of striated muscle fibers from fast to slow twitch
—Determinants of success
    —Motivation and compliance
    —Lifelong treatment

- Pelvic floor exercise (PFE) ± biofeedback

—Voluntary quick, maximal, or sustained contractions of pelvic floor muscle
—Display of auditory or visual correlative of this contraction
—Cure rate: 55% to 85% in SUI and UI

- Behavioral modifications (bladder training to regain detrusor and sphincter control)

—Restriction of fluid
—Prevention of activity causing leakage
—Time voiding
—Voluntary sphincter contractions to abort the IDC
—Cure rate: 50% to 90% in UI

- Electrical stimulation

—Contraction of pelvic floor and sphincter muscle (controls SUI) efferent
    —Higher threshold stimulation of efferent nerves (50–100 Hz)
    —Reflex inhibition of detrusor (controls UUI)
    —Lower threshold stimulation of afferent nerves (5–10 Hz)

- Cutaneous surface electrode

—Transcutaneous electrical nerve stimulation (TENS)
—Interferential electrical stimulation (IFT)

- Anal probe-mounted electrodes

—Chronic (low-threshold) stimulation
    —Best results in DI
—Maximal electrical stimulation
    —Improvement in 40% to 80%; cure in 10%
    —SUI response better than UUI

- Needle electrodes

(continued)

Urinary Incontinence—Adult Male (continued)

MEDICAL

- Drugs used in treatment of overactive bladder
—Agents
  —Musculotropic relaxant (oxybutynin)
  —Anticholinergics (propantheline, hyoscyamine, tolterodine)
  —Tricyclic antidepressants (imipramine): actions
    —Decreased frequency and amplitude of UDC
    —Increased bladder capacity
    —Increased outlet resistance (imipramine only)
    —Warning time between urge and leakage unchanged
  —Contraindications: Narrow-angle glaucoma, myasthenia gravis caution in atony or obstruction of the gastrointestinal tract, bladder outlet obstruction
  —Adverse reactions: decreased secretion, sweating, blurred near vision, urinary hesitancy and retention, constipation, impotence

- Combination treatments
—Pharmacotherapy with time voiding
—Pharmacotherapy with CIC
—Musculotropic or anticholinergic agents with imipramine

- Drug used for treatment of deficient sphincter

—Alpha-adrenergic agonists (ephedrine, pseudoephedrine, phenylpropanolamine)
—Tricyclic antidepressant
  —Mode of action: increased tone of lissosphincter
  —Adverse reactions: CVS (HTN, palpitations, arrhythmia), CNS (insomnia, anxiety, headache, tremor), RS (difficulties with respiration)

SURGICAL

- Injection therapy for SUI

—Bioinjectables for passive occlusion transurethral or antegrade
  —Glutaraldehyde cross-linked (GAX) collagen ($300 for 3 mL)
  —PTFE (Teflon)
  —Silicon particles ($800 for 2.5 mL): only in Europe
—Patients not suitable for injection: excessive scarring, unmanaged detrusor overactivity
—Principles
  —Collagen skin test 4 weeks prior to procedure
  —Submucosal injection into presphincteric area (retrograde) or bladder neck (antegrade)
  —Completion once satisfactory coaptation achieved
—Results
  —Continence achieved in 15% to 25% of patients
  —Improvement achieved in three-fourths of patients
  —Minimal complications (transient urinary retention, diverticulum, or abscess formation)
—Disadvantages
  —Particle migration with Teflon, none with silicone (size-dependent)
  —Multiple injection needed with GAX-collagen; silicone particle more stable
  —Inadequate experience with silicone particles
  —Hypersensitivity to GAX collagen in 3%

- Artificial urethral sphincter (AMS 800) for SUI

—Principle: The inflatable fluid-filled cuff placed around the urethra prevents leakage by urethral compression. Activation of the pump mechanism propels the liquid into an implanted reservoir and opens the passage to urine.
—Absolute and relative contraindications
  —Bladder capacity <150 mL
  —Uncontrollable DI
  —Uncorrected stricture of BN contracture
  —Infection (urinary, genital, or skin)
—Prerequisites
  —Maximum sphincter function return after trauma/surgery
  —Patient's dexterity (for pump handling and CIC)
  —Negative urine culture
—Implanted components
  —Inflatable urethral cuff (4–5 cm for bulbous urethra)
  —Pump with deactivation button
  —Pressure-regulating balloon (60–70 cm H_2O); lower for irradiated pelvis
—Preoperative management: patient counseling and antimicrobial prophylaxis (gentamicin and vancomycin for 24 hours, cephalosporins for 2 weeks)
—Surgery
  —Lithotomy position
  —Cuff positioned around bulbous urethra
  —Insertion of pressure reservoir into the prevesical space
  —Pump implantation into scrotum
  —Establishment of connections
—Postoperative care
  —Ice to scrotum and perineum
  —Foley removal day after surgery, CIC if in retention
  —Activation in 6 weeks (deactivation at night optional)
  —Permanent restrictions (horseback riding, bike riding)
—Results
  —Continence rate: 85% to 100%
  —Revision rate: 20% to 30%
—Early complications
  —Hematoma (drain if large)
  —Retention (due to edema: CIC)
  —Urethral injury (urinoma, infection)
—Late complications
  —Retention (evaluate for stricture or BN contracture)
  —Infection (prophylactic antibiotics for surgery and dentistry)
  —Mechanical failure (10% in 5 years)
  —Cuff erosion, fistula formation
  —Incontinence (mechanical failure, tissue atrophy, insufficient cuff pressure)

- Surgery for overactive bladder and poor compliance

—Enterocystoplasty (bladder augmentation)
  —Satisfactory results in 70% to 95%
  —Raises volume at which IDC occurs
  —Creates low-pressure reservoir
  —Complication (mucus production, UTI, metabolic and electrolyte disturbances)
—Detrusor myomectomy (autoaugmentation)
—Urinary diversion
—Partial sacral rhizotomy: preserves sphincteric function, diminishes reflex contractility

- Neuromodulation via implantation of sacral nerve stimulator

—S3 sacral root stimulation
  —Test stimulation with transcutaneous needle electrode to establish response
  —Implantation of a wire electrode and pulse generator
  —Suitable for treatment of UI
—Results in urge incontinence at 1.5 years: 50% dry; 75% improved by 50%

ALTERNATE THERAPIES: N/A

PATIENT EDUCATION

- Local hygiene to prevent skin breakdown
- Behavioral modifications

—Restriction of fluid
—Prevention of activity causing leakage
—Time voiding
—Voluntary sphincter contractions to abort the IDC

 Follow-Up

- Monitoring

—History: voiding diary, pad test
—Therapist sessions for rehabilitation progress
—Special studies: UDS, cystogram, cystourethroscopy, as needed

- Prevention

—Surgical technique during TURP
  —No resection distal to verumontanum
—Surgical techniques improving post-RRP continence
  —Modified apical dissection (sharp transverse transection of DVC and rectourethralis muscle and their incorporation into anastomosis)
  —Preservation of puboprostatic ligaments
  —Bladder neck sparing (decreases BN contracture, little effect on continence)
  —Anterior bladder tube

 Miscellaneous

SYNONYMS

- Stress urinary incontinence: intrinsic sphincter deficiency; urge urinary incontinence: detrusor instability

ASSOCIATED CONDITIONS: N/A

NOTES

- See also Section I, "Urinary Incontinence—Adult Female."

ABBREVIATIONS

- AUS, artificial urinary sphincter; BN, bladder neck; BOO, bladder neck obstruction; CIC, clean intermittent catheterization; DI, detrusor instability; DSD, detrusor sphincter dyssynergia; DVC, dorsal vein complex; ECM, extracellular matrix; IAP, intraabdominal pressure; IDC, involuntary detrusor contraction; ISD, intrinsic sphincter deficiency; LMN, lower motor neuron; MS, multiple sclerosis; PFE, pelvic floor exercise; PTFE, polytetrafluoroethylene; RRP, radical retropubic prostatectomy; SUI, stress urinary incontinence; UDS, urodynamic studies; UI, urge urinary incontinence

REFERENCES

Blaivas JG. Outcome measures for urinary incontinence. *Urology* 1998;51[2A Suppl]:11.

Blaivas JG, Romanzi LJ, Heritz DM. Urinary incontinence: Pathology, evaluation, treatment overview, and nonsurgical management. In: Walsh PC, Retik AB, Vaughan ED, Wein AJ, eds. *Campbell's Urology,* 7th ed. Philadelphia: WB Saunders, 1998;1059–1093.

Haab F, Yamaguchi R, Leach GE. Postprostatectomy incontinence: Evaluation and management. *Urol Clin North Am* 1996;23(3):447.

Klutke CG, Nadler RB, Tiemann D, Andriole GL. Early results with antegrade collagen injection for post-radical prostatectomy stress urinary incontinence. *J Urol* 1996;156:1703.

Malmsten UG, Milsom I, Molander U, Norlen LJ. Urinary incontinence and lower urinary tract symptoms: An epidemiological study of men aged 45 to 99 years. *J Urol* 1997;158:1733.

Authors: Peter Niemczyk and Carl G. Klutke

Urinary Incontinence—Pediatric

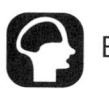 Basics

DESCRIPTION

• A wet child is the most common problem seen by pediatric urologists.
• *Incontinence* is defined as involuntary loss of urine due to an underlying anomaly requiring evaluation and treatment.
• *Enuresis* is defined as involuntary wetting when no underlying anatomic or functional abnormality of the urinary tract is detected.
• Most wetting children will be enuretic. A majority will improve spontaneously. The difficulty is discerning an incontinent from an enuretic child.
• *Nocturnal enuresis* implies nighttime wetting alone; diurnal implies both night and day wetting.
• *Primary enuresis* describes a child who has never been dry; *secondary enuresis* describes one who was dry for at least 6 months before wetting again.

PATHOPHYSIOLOGY

• Daytime control attained before nighttime
• 15% to 20% of 5-year-olds have nocturnal enuresis; 15% of them attain continence each year thereafter.
• 20% of enuretics are diurnal; 10% to 20% also have constipation/encopresis.
• Normal bladder control involves three basic components:

—Intact neurologic system
—Normal anatomy
—Motivated child

• Development of normal control occurs in stages:

—Infantile voiding (0–6 months)
  —Low-pressure filling, reflex detrusor contraction
  —Simultaneous relaxation of external sphincter
  —Complete emptying, uninhibited and frequent voiding
—Transitional voiding
  —Conscious sensation of bladder filling develops (ages 1–2); continence is achieved by gaining control over the external sphincter.
  —Decreased frequency of voiding is in part due to increasing capacity (60 cc from birth plus 30 cc per year up to age 12).
—Adult voiding
  —Supraspinal inhibition of voiding reflex
  —Voluntary inhibition and initiation of voiding

RISK FACTORS

• Urinary tract anomalies
• Developmental delay
• Central nervous system anomalies
• Family history of enuresis

Differential Diagnosis

• Incontinence can be classified as structural, neurogenic, uncomplicated enuresis, or complicated enuresis.
• Structural

—Ureteral duplication with ectopia
—Exstrophy-epispadias complex
—Posterior urethral valves
—Urethral duplication
—Vesical fistula
—Small fibrotic bladder (postsurgery or postradiation)
—Labial adhesions
—Urogenital sinus
—Imperforate anus

• Neurogenic

—Myelodysplasia (meningocele, myelomeningocele, lipomyelomeningocele)
—Occult dysraphisms
  —Lipomeningocele, intradural lipoma, diastematomyelia
  —Tight filum terminale, dermoid cyst/sinus, aberrant nerve roots
  —Anterior sacral meningocele, cauda equina tumor
—Sacral agenesis, spine trauma, cerebral palsy

• Uncomplicated enuresis

—Isolated nocturnal enuresis, normal physical examination, and negative urine culture (very common)
—Incidence of organic pathology no different than population at large
—Radiographic imaging, UDS, and cystoscopy unnecessary

• Complicated enuresis

—No obvious neurologic disorder detected; more serious symptoms present (diurnal enuresis, constipation/encopresis, UTI, slow or intermittent stream, infrequent voiding, urgency and frequency)
—Collectively known as "functional voiding disorders"
—Should be evaluated with KUB, renal and bladder ultrasound (full and empty)
—Use of urodynamics varies according to the physician; most reserve them for cases of associated upper tract and/or bladder deterioration or after empiric therapy has failed.
—Lazy bladder syndrome (infrequent voider)
  —Usually older girls; present with recurrent UTIs; void only 2 to 3 times daily
  —The detrusor becomes hyporeflexic, capacity increases, and sensation of fullness diminishes, all due to misuse of the voluntary sphincter.
  —May have stress or overflow incontinence and often associated encopresis or constipation

—Small-capacity, hypertonic bladder
  —Similar to detrusor hyperreflexia but without a neurologic lesion
  —Etiology similar to infrequent voider; forceful constriction of external sphincter during uninhibited contraction
  —Voluntary sphincter dyssynergia produces bladder outlet obstruction and increased intravesical pressures.
  —Urodynamically, a small-capacity bladder with increased filling pressures noted; results in severe urgency and urge incontinence
  —External sphincter may relax incompletely; results in outflow obstruction and incomplete emptying
  —VUR (vesicoureteric reflux) may also be present; particularly in patients with UTIs.
—Hinman-Allen syndrome (nonneurogenic neurogenic bladder) (occult neuropathic bladder) (see Section III, "Pseudodyssynergia [Hinman Syndrome]")
—Daytime frequency syndrome
  —Typically presents as acute onset of isolated daytime frequency in a previously toilet-trained child without UTI or uropathology
  —Often associated with new stressor in child's life
—Giggle incontinence (enuresis risoria)
  —Complete or partial loss of bladder control occurring with laughing or giggling while awake
  —No known specific cause; suggestions of imbalance between cholinergic and monoaminergic systems proposed
  —Not associated with organic disease; usually begins before puberty and resolves with time
—Unstable bladder
  —Most common cause of daytime incontinence in children
  —Most frequent symptom is urgency with or without urge incontinence
  —Renal and bladder ultrasound and VCUG typically normal; UDS demonstrates uninhibited contractions during filling
  —Characteristic posturing to prevent leakage is common (e.g., Vincent's curtsy).
  —Unlike in a small-capacity bladder, complete relaxation of sphincter occurs, allowing complete emptying during voiding.
  —Also associated with constipation/encopresis, UTIs, and VUR

Database

HISTORY

- Age of child?

—15% of 5-year-olds have nocturnal enuresis.
—1% of adolescents are bedwetters.

- Child male or female?

—Bedwetting is more common in boys than in girls (3:2); daytime frequency and wetting is more common in girls.

- When did symptoms begin; what is the pattern and how severe is it?

—Wetting the bed more than once a night might suggest polyuria.
—Pure nocturnal enuresis does not warrant aggressive investigation.
—Secondary enuresis implies a change from previously normal function and behavior, implying an acquired disorder.
—Primary enuresis implicates an unmasked congenital anomaly that should be sought after.
—Dribbling upon standing in a girl may suggest labial adhesions.

- Associated daytime voiding symptoms (diurnal enuresis, urgency, frequency, weak or intermittent stream, or infrequent voiding)?

—39% of patients with both day and night wetting had symptoms suggestive of bladder instability.
—May suggest a small bladder capacity, bladder instability, acquired voiding dysfunction, or a UTI
—Intermittent stream may indicate detrusor sphincter dyssynergia or urethral obstruction.
—A partially suppressed sudden urge to void suggests bladder instability

- Frequency of bowel movements?

—Enuretic children with more severe diurnal voiding often have chronic constipation and/or encopresis.
—Such findings may signal an underlying, severe voiding dysfunction or an occult neuropathy.

- Relevant psychosocial history?

—Recent stresses (e.g., arrival of new sibling, a move, a new school, or a family death). All may influence child's voiding pattern.
—Environmental factors such as socioeconomic status may impact on enuresis.

- Any tricks to prevent getting wet?

—Many girls will squat down and sit on the heel of one foot (Vincent's curtsy). This is seen in unstable bladder patients.
—Some children cross their legs or jump around, and some boys hold their penises.

- Family history, medical or surgical history?

—There is a strong familial pattern of inheritance with enuresis.
—UTIs may lead to wetting; VUR has been associated with uninhibited bladder contractions.
—Nearly all children with myelodysplasia have diurnal incontinence. Secondary incontinence in a myelodysplastic child may indicate cord tethering.

PHYSICAL EXAMINATION

- General survey

—Mental status, level of development
Abdominal examination
—Abdominal masses can cause extrinsic compression of the bladder, causing incontinence.
—A palpable, low-lying, midabdominal mass could be a distended bladder.

- Back examination

—Dimples, short sacrum, spinal defects, or hairy patches might indicate an underlying dysraphism.
—Flattened buttocks, low gluteal clef, or non-palpable coccyx suggest sacral agenesis.

- Genitourinary examination

—Assess genital and perineal sensation if neuropathy suspected.
—Contusions and bruises could signify abuse.
—Hypospadias and epispadias can be missed in a newborn and present as incontinence.
—Vaginal vault inspection can detect labial adhesions in a child with a history of pooling of urine in the vagina.
—Ectopic ureteral orifice in the perineum is a cause of constant perineal wetness (only in girls).

- Rectal examination

—Can confirm hard stool in vault or absence of anal sphincter tone

- Extremity examination

—Observe the child walking; assess symmetry, coordination, atrophy, and leg muscle strength and size. All are indications of possible neuropathy.

- Neurologic examination

—Reserved for cases of suspected neuropathy based on symptoms and the above examination

- Observation of voiding

—Allows for assessment of stream force, caliber, straining, character, and duration

(continued)

Diagnostic Studies

LABORATORY TESTING

• Urinalysis

—May suggest renal disease: microhematuria or proteinuria
—May suggest endocrinopathy: glucosuria
—A specific gravity of 1.022 or greater signifies normal concentrating ability. Polyurics have much lower values.

• Urine culture

—Although uncommon, infection is a clinically important cause of incontinence.

IMAGING

• KUB with lateral spine film

—May detect spinal anomalies or constipation

• Renal and bladder ultrasonography

—Useful in child with daytime incontinence; finding of major anomaly uncommon
—Recommended in cases with history of UTI, urgency, dysuria, or outlet obstructive symptoms
—Noninvasive study reassures physician, patient, and family of normal urinary tract

• VCUG

—Indicated in cases with UTI, upper tract infection, or hydronephrosis
—Allows evaluation of urethra; rule out stricture, diverticulum, or valves
—Some clinicians recommend the study for all boys with diurnal incontinence.

• Excretory urography

—Performed when ureteral duplication is suspected

• Radioisotope scan

—Assessment of renal function, particularly in duplex kidneys when upper moiety heminephrectomy is being considered

SPECIAL STUDIES

• Urodynamics

—Seldom necessary in patients with nonneurogenic voiding dysfunction
—Advised when bony vertebral anomalies, signs of neurogenic bladder or positive neurologic or neurosurgical history are detected

• Cystoscopy

—Indicated if VCUG demonstrates endoscopically treatable anomaly (e.g., posterior urethral valves)
—No role in evaluation of uncomplicated pediatric enuresis

 Initial Management

• Structural

—The goal of all treatment is to reestablish normal, complete, periodic, spontaneous voluntary voiding with dry periods in between.
—Patients with a duplex upper tract or dysplastic kidney with ectopic ureter can be made dry by an upper pole heminephrectomy or simple nephrectomy.
—Vesical fistulas can be closed, urethral duplications excised, labial adhesions separated, urogenital sinus malformations corrected, and valves ablated.
—Based on UDS findings, patients with most of the remaining conditions will have to live with reasonably long dry periods between IC to empty. Management of these is similar to that for neuropathic conditions.

• Neurogenic

—UDS is the basis for classification and treatment.
—Atonic bladder with adequate urethral resistance; treat with IC
—Compliant bladder with good capacity and poor urethral resistance: Treat with artificial sphincter or fascial sling with or with out IC.
—Poor capacity with adequate urethral resistance: Treat with anticholinergic and smooth-muscle relaxant or augmentation.
—Poor capacity and urethral resistance: Treatment includes combinations of above.

- Uncomplicated (see Section I, "Enuresis—Pediatric")
- Complicated

—Treatment tailored to type of voiding dysfunction and presence or absence of UTI or VUR

—Lazy bladder

—Therapy involves teaching the child proper voiding habits; timed voiding, double voiding, and intermittent catheterization if needed

—Bowel habits must also be corrected.

—Small-capacity bladder

—Anticholinergic therapy and timed voiding are the mainstays of treatment; a majority respond.

—Oxybutynin (Ditropan) 5 mg 2 to 3 times daily is the usual dose for children over 6 years of age.

—Treatment of associated UTI aids in relief of symptoms.

—Hinman-Allen syndrome (see Section III, "Pseudodyssynergia [Hinman Syndrome]")

—Daytime frequency syndrome

—Anticholinergics not useful

—Usually resolves without intervention within 2 to 3 months

—Giggle incontinence

—Methylphenidate (Ritalin) 0.3 to 0.5 mg/kg orally every 4 to 5 hours effective in some children

—Unstable bladder

—Psychological therapy is a mainstay; timed voiding is the basis, with gradually increasing intervals.

—Anticholinergics used in conjunction with timed voiding are quite effective.

—Imipramine may also be beneficial for bladder instability.

—Antibiotic prophylaxis is needed in cases of recurrent UTI; long-term sulfamethoxazole-trimethoprim and nitrofurantoin are well tolerated; the dose should be one-fourth to one-third of the full dose.

 ## Follow-Up

- Structural and neurogenic incontinence requires routine evaluation to rule out upper tract deterioration and to monitor progress.
- Only refractory cases in the functional voiding dysfunction group need routine follow-up; the rest will likely spontaneously resolve.

 ## Miscellaneous

SYNONYMS: N/A

ASSOCIATED CONDITIONS: N/A

NOTES

- See also Section I, "Urinary Incontinence—Adult Male" and "Urinary Incontinence—Adult Female."

ABBREVIATIONS

- VUR, vesicoureteric reflux

REFERENCES

Bauer SB. Pediatric urodynamics: Lower tract. In: O'Donnell B, Koff SA, eds. *Pediatric Urology.* Reed Educational and Professional Publishing Ltd, 1997.

Gonzalez R. Urinary incontinence. In: Kelalis PP, King LR, Belman AB, eds. *Clinical Pediatric Urology,* 3rd ed. Philadelphia: WB Saunders, 1992.

Malone PSJ. The management of urinary incontinence. *Arch Dis Child* 1997;77:175–178.

Rushton HG. Wetting and functional voiding disorders. *Urol Clin North Am* 1995;22:1.

Wojcik LJ, Caldamone AA. Evaluation and management of pediatric daytime incontinence. In: Elder JS, ed. *Topics in Clinical Urology: Pediatric Urology for the General Urologist.* New York: Igaku-Shoin, 1996.

Authors: Allen N. Chiura and Leonard G. Gomella

Urinary Retention—Acute and Chronic

 ## Basics

DESCRIPTION

• Acute urinary retention: distress associated with an uncomfortable distended bladder and the inability to void more than small volumes of urine
• Chronic urinary retention: frequency, weak stream, and incomplete voiding; individuals experience little discomfort from their distended bladder, even though post-void residuals can be large.

PATHOPHYSIOLOGY

• Most commonly occurs in patients with preexisting bladder outlet obstruction
• Infection, bleeding, or overdistension usually is the precipitating event.
• Identify the underlying condition or precipitating event that contributed to retention, especially neurogenic etiologies.
• Catheter drainage results in prompt symptomatic relief.

RISK FACTORS

• General: diabetes, herpes zoster, drugs, psychogenic, recent surgery, especially with epidural or spinal anesthesia (acute retention only)
• Elderly men: benign prostatic hyperplasia (BPH); prostate cancer; history of retention, urologic procedures, or instrumentation; medications, cystoprostatitis; bladder cancer (rare cause)
• Women: neurogenic bladder
• Young patients: neurologic disease (e.g., multiple sclerosis [MS])

 ## Differential Diagnosis

• Generally either bladder outlet obstruction or bladder dysfunction
• Anatomic

—Penis: phimosis, paraphimosis, meatal stenosis, foreign-body constriction
—Urethra: tumor, foreign body, calculus, urethritis, stricture, clot retention, meatal stenosis (female), hematoma
—Prostate: BPH, prostate cancer, bladder neck contracture, prostatitis, prostatic infarction

• Neurologic

—Motor paralytic: spinal shock, spinal cord syndromes (e.g., spina bifida, meningomyelocele)
—Sensory paralytic: tabes dorsalis, diabetes, multiple sclerosis, pernicious anemia
—Syringomyelia
—Herpes zoster, poliovirus
—Herniated disks

• Drugs

—Antihistamines
—Anticholinergics: atropine, belladonna, benztropine mesylate, cyclic antidepressants, phenothiazines, ipratropium bromide
—Antispasmodics
—Tricyclic antidepressants
—Alpha-agonists (induce bladder neck hypertonicity): "cold preparations," ephedrine derivatives, amphetamines
—Narcotics: morphine, meperidine
—Detrusor muscle relaxants: flavoxate, dicyclomine, oxybutynin

 ## Database

HISTORY

• Symptoms of bladder outlet obstruction (weak stream, hesitancy, incomplete voiding, dribbling)?

—BPH is the most common cause in men >50; other causes of obstruction in men include prostate cancer, bladder cancer, urethral structure, and neurogenic bladder.

• Symptoms of irritative voiding (frequency, urgency, dysuria, nocturia)?

—These symptoms may suggest infection or BPH.

• History of urologic procedures or instrumentation?
• History of sexually transmitted diseases or strictures?
• Medications, especially cold medications?
• History of pain?

—Bone pain and weight loss suggest prostate cancer.

• History of spinal cord injury or pelvic trauma?
• History of recent surgery, especially in those with spinal or epidural anesthesia?

PHYSICAL EXAMINATION

• Palpable abdominal mass

—A bladder with >150 mL of urine should be palpable or percussible, depending on the size of the patient.

• Digital rectal examination

—Symmetrically enlarged prostate with BPH; nodularity suggests cancer; boggy, tender, warm prostate suggests prostatitis.

• Neurologic examination

—Complete neurologic examination if suspicion for a neurologic etiology exists
—A directed examination would include testing the anal, bulbocavernosal, knee, and ankle reflexes.
—Anal tone (S2) and levator muscle tone (S3-S4) should be assessed.
—Check sensation over the penis (S2), perianal area (S2-S3), outside of the foot (S2), sole of the foot (S2-S3), and large toe (S3).
—Muscle stretch reflexes and the Babinski reflex are useful in differentiating an upper motor neuron lesion from a lower motor neuron lesion.
—When extremity findings do not parallel perineum findings (i.e., absent sensation and tone in the feet but partial tone or sensation in the perineum), suspect spina bifida or meningomyelocele.

Diagnostic Studies

LABORATORY TESTING

- BUN and creatinine elevated in retention if hydronephrosis present
- With postrenal obstruction, the BUN/creatinine ratio will be increased.
- Urinalysis (dipstick and microscopic analysis)

—Leukocyte esterase or nitrite positivity with pyuria suggests infection.
—Hematuria is suggestive of infection, tumor, or calculi.

- Urine culture if UA suggestive of infection

IMAGING

- An emergency intravenous pyelogram (IVP) is generally not necessary.
- Routine IVP or spinal CT can be done if suspicion for calculi exists.

—Identifies upper tract pathology from chronic retention (rarely needed)

SPECIAL STUDIES

- Cystoscopy: identifies lower urinary tract pathology (urethral stricture, prostatic hypertrophy, bladder malignancy)
- Uroflow: Measuring peak urine flow rate is useful in objectively documenting severity of bladder outlet obstruction. Post-void residual should be determined at the time of initial uroflow.
- Urodynamics: In spinal shock, urodynamics should be done at least 8 weeks after spinal cord injury and then periodically.

 ## Initial Management

- Determine if retention is present by catheterization or ultrasound.

—"Normal" residual immediately after voiding to completion is generally <30 mL in adults, but can vary slightly.

- Initial management is to provide urinary drainage by the least invasive technique available.
- Urethral catheter

—The usual approach is with a standard urethral catheter (for men, a 16Fr to 18Fr Foley may be used).
—Men with BPH may need a larger caliber catheter to help separate hypertrophied lateral lobes; a curved-tip Coudé catheter may facilitate negotiating the median lobe of the prostate.
—If a catheter is successfully passed, the bladder should be decompressed slowly (approximately 300 mL/h) to minimize urothelial bleeding.

- Percutaneous suprapubic tube

—Generally placed when a urethral catheter cannot be passed or in cases of acute bacterial cystoprostatitis in men.
—Relative contraindications: previous lower abdominal surgery; small, contracted neurogenic bladder, coagulopathy; known bladder tumor
—Insertion requires at least 200 to 300 cc urine in an easily percussible bladder; if percussion is difficult, use bladder ultrasound.

- Filiforms and followers if catheter will not pass easily

—Filiforms are long, thin fiberglass probes with straight or spiral tips, inserted per the urethra, that can often negotiate narrow strictures.
—Followers are tapered, stiff catheters that screw into the end of the filiform and can follow the filiform through the stricture into the bladder.
—Progressively larger caliber followers are used to dilate a strictured area to allow passage of a standard Foley catheter.
—An open-tipped catheter can be placed over a Councill stylet and follow the filiform into the bladder; the stylet and filiform can then be removed, leaving the catheter in the bladder.

- Cystourethroscopy

—The filiform can be passed through a stricture under direct vision using a cystoscope.

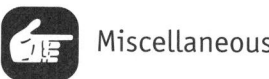 ## Follow-Up

- Monitoring

—Patients may require monitoring and fluid replacement for postobstructive diuresis (>200 mL/h), especially after chronic or prolonged retention and when BUN and creatinine are significantly elevated.
—Relief of chronic or prolonged obstruction may result in major hemorrhage secondary to bladder mucosal disruption.
—Significant hypotension may occur secondary to a vasovagal response.
—Patients with signs of serious infection or decreased renal function should be admitted.

- Prevention

—Chronic retention may be managed with clean intermittent catheterization.
—Work-up of the underlying cause or precipitating event should be done.

Miscellaneous

SYNONYMS: N/A

ASSOCIATED CONDITIONS: N/A

NOTES

- See also Section II, "Postobstructive Diuresis" and "Bladder Outlet Obstruction."

ABBREVIATIONS

- MS, multiple sclerosis

REFERENCES

Bushman W, et al. Standard diagnostic considerations. In: Gillenwater JY, Grayhack JT, Howards SS, Duckett JW, eds. *Adult and Pediatric Urology*, 3rd ed. St Louis: Mosby, 1996.

Harwood-Nuss AL, et al. Urologic emergencies. In: Rosen, et al., eds. *Emergency Medicine: Concepts and Clinical Practice*. St Louis: Mosby, 1998.

Macfarlane MT. Urinary retention. In: Satterfield TS, et al., eds. *Urology*. Baltimore: Williams & Wilkins, 1995.

Tanagho EA, et al. Neuropathic bladder disorders. In: Tanagho EA, et al., eds. *Smith's General Urology*. Norwalk, CT: Appleton & Lange, 1995.

Authors: Leah Perez McMann and J. Brantley Thrasher

Urinary Tract Infection—Adult Female

 Basics

DESCRIPTION

- Urinary tract infection (UTI): symptomatic urothelial inflammation due to microbial invasion; characterized by bacteriuria and pyuria
- Uncomplicated UTI: infection in a normal patient without any structural or functional urinary tract abnormalities (i.e., isolated or recurrent bacterial cystitis, acute pyelonephritis); comprises the vast majority of female patients with UTI
- Complicated UTI: infection in a pregnant, diabetic, renal transplant, frail elderly, or immuno-compromised patient, with or without anatomic or functional urinary tract abnormalities
- Patterns of UTI

—Isolated infection: first UTI or UTI occurring at least 6 months after a previous infection
—Unresolved infection: failure of the initial treatment course to eradicate bacteria from the urine, usually due to preexisting or acquired antimicrobial resistance, noncompliance, or insufficient antibiotic dosing, or from disorders that decrease drug bioavailability (i.e., azotemia, urinary calculus)
—Reinfection: most common cause of recurrent UTIs. Following resolution of a UTI, a new infection with a different organism or different coliforms ascending from rectum to vagina
—Bacterial persistence: recurrent UTI following sterilization of the urine and resolution of a prior UTI, caused by the same bacteria as the preceding infection, usually arising from an underlying abnormality (i.e., renal stone)
—Relapse (or bacterial persistence): recurrent UTI caused by an identical bacteria within 2 weeks of completing antibiotic treatment

PATHOPHYSIOLOGY

- Urinary pathogens

—Community-acquired UTI: *E. coli* most common (85%); also *Proteus, Klebsiella, Enterococcus faecalis,* and *Staphylococcus saprophyticus* (young females)
—Nosocomial UTI: *E. coli* most common (50%), also *Enterococcus, Klebsiella, Citrobacter, Serratia, Pseudomonas,* and *Providencia.*

- Routes of infection

—Ascending route: most common in normal females; fecal flora spread from perianal area into bladder; may ascend into the upper urinary tracts (causing pyelonephritis) if reflux is present
—Hematogenous route: uncommon, occurs in *Staphylococcus aureus* bacteremia or candidal fungemia.

- Bacterial virulence vs. host resistance

—Increased bacterial virulence in *E. coli* strains with hemolysin to serologic O groups (01,04,06,018, and 075), K antigens, and certain types of surface adhesin molecules
—>90% of *E. coli* responsible for pyelonephritis express P fimbriae.

—Type 1 (mannose sensitive) fimbriated *E. coli* are responsible for most cases of bacterial cystitis.
—Increased epithelial cell receptivity for *E. coli* in patients with HLA-A3 antigen expressions, Lewis blood group Le (a+b-) (nonsecretor) phenotypes
—Increased binding of *E. coli* to vaginal fluid at alkaline pH (postmenopausal conditions)
—In premenopausal woman, estrogen promotes vaginal *Lactobacillus* colonization.
　—Lactobacilli lower vaginal pH and inhibit adherence of pathogenic bacteria by competing for epithelial receptor sites, and by secreting biosurfactant substances.
—In postmenopausal women, loss of estrogen is associated with increased bacterial adherence.

RISK FACTORS

- Facilitated bacterial ascent into bladder

—Sexual intercourse, diaphragm and/or spermicidal contraceptive containing nonoxynol-9, intermittent or indwelling catheter use, fecal soilage of perineum

- Anatomic/functional urinary tract abnormalities

—Urinary obstruction, neurogenic/diabetic bladder, vesicoureteral reflux, urinary tract calculi, urethral/bladder diverticula, cystocele

 Differential Diagnosis

- Acute bacterial cystitis

—Bladder tumor: older aged patients with hematuria, urgency/frequency; standard evaluation includes urine cytology, cystoscopy, upper tract imaging
—Bladder calculus: usually associated with urinary stasis
—Vaginitis: characterized by pruritus, vaginal discharge/odor, dyspareunia
—Urethritis: urethral discharge, dysuria, pruritus, initial hematuria, history of STD risk factors or urethral instrumentation; microscopy and culture of initial 10 mL of voided urine and urethral swab may show pyuria and causative organism.
—Interstitial cystitis: chronic urgency, frequency, and pain with bladder filling, which decreased in severity after voiding; diagnosis of exclusion; typically have decreased bladder capacity with glomerulations or Hunter's ulcer on cystoscopy following hydrodistention under anesthesia

 Database

HISTORY

- Does the patient have typical or atypical symptoms?

—Typical symptoms of bacterial cystitis include urinary frequency, urgency, dysuria, small-volume voiding, nocturia, or suprapubic/lower abdominal pain or "pressure."

—Atypical symptoms (fever, flank pain, and chills) may indicate acute pyelonephritis.
—Vaginal discharge, foul vaginal odor, and pruritis suggest vaginitis or urethritis.
—Gross or microhematuria that does not resolve may be due to urinary tract tumor or stones.

- Any risk factors for UTI (as above)?

—Identify correctable factors that facilitate bacterial ascent into the bladder.
—Identify any anatomic or functional urinary tract abnormalities that may be complicating factors.

- Is the patient community-dwelling or institutionalized?

—Expect different urinary pathogens in nosocomial than in community-acquired UTI.

- How often does the patient get UTIs?

—More than two UTIs in a 12-month period should raise suspicion of underlying structural or functional urinary tract abnormality, relapsing infection, or reinfection.
—How were the UTIs treated, and what were the treatment results?
—Determine if the infection was treated appropriately; if the infection responded appropriately; if the infection is likely to respond to or be resistant to a particular empiric antibiotic.
　—Determine if the patient was compliant with the prescribed antibiotic course.
—What were the previous urine culture results?
　—Establish a pattern of infection; the patient may have a relapse with the same organism (bacterial persistence) or reinfection with a different organism.
—Medical/surgical history, including childhood UTIs and current medications
　—Identify any complicating structural or functional urinary tract abnormalities or immuno-compromising factors.
　—Determine if the patient has had a recent hospitalization which might have lead to infection with nosocomial rather than community organisms.
　—The patient may have had recent urinary tract catheterization or instrumentation, which may have lead to a UTI.
　—Medications, (such as an antacid), may decrease the efficacy of a previously prescribed antibiotic, or the patient may be on a medication, which will affect future antibiotic selection.
—Gynecologic history, including STDs
　—Loss of estrogen in postmenopausal women is associated with increased bacterial adherence in the vagina.
　—A history of STDs should raise suspicion of urethritis or vaginitis in patients with appropriate symptoms.

PHYSICAL EXAMINATION

- Bladder distention/suprapubic tenderness indicate urinary retention, which may promote UTIs due to urinary stasis.
- Flank tenderness suggests pyelonephritis or possible upper tract obstruction.

—Abdominal tenderness and peritoneal signs may indicate other intraabdominal pathology.

—Vaginal/urethral discharge may be present in patients with vaginitis or urethritis.

—Vaginal mucosal atrophy may reflect estrogen status in perimenopausal women.

—An anterior vaginal wall mass with purulent urethral discharge expressed during palpation can be seen with urethral diverticulum.

—A large cystocele should raise a suspicion of incomplete voiding stasis.

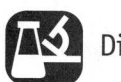 ## Diagnostic Studies

LABORATORY TESTING

• Urinalysis

—Test for patients with urinary symptoms

—Dipstick: leukocyte esterase (50% positive predictive value, 92% negative predictive value), nitrate (sensitivity 35%–85%), false negatives common in setting of low dietary nitrate, diuretics, *Staphylococcus, Enterococcus, Pseudomonas*

—Microscopy (if positive dipstick): pyuria $\geq$ 10 WBCs/(μL urine, bacteriuria $\geq$ 1 organism per oil immersion field of uncentrifuged urine correlates with $\geq 10^5$ CFU/mL ($\cong$90% sensitivity/specificity). Bacterial counts of at least 30,000/mL are necessary for detection.

• Urine culture

—"Gold standard" $\geq 10^5$ CFU/mL urine; however, this limit excludes 30% to 50% of women with classic symptoms of acute bacterial cystitis. Treatment is indicated if $\geq 10^2$ CFU/mL in a symptomatic patient.

—Obtain prior to treatment if atypical symptoms (suspected pyelonephritis), negative pyuria/hematuria/bacteriuria on urinalysis, recent antibiotic use, symptom duration >7 days, age >65, diabetes, pregnant, immunosuppressed, recent urinary tract instrumentation, indwelling catheter

IMAGING

• Reserve for cases of suspected complicated UTI
• Indications: persistent fevers after 72 hours of treatment, *Proteus* in urine culture with urine pH $\geq$8.0 (associated with struvite calculi), bacterial persistence, unexplained hematuria, suspected upper tract obstruction, history of calculi, neurogenic bladder dysfunction, analgesic abuse, diabetes
• KUB: quick and easy screening study for suspected urolithiasis (radiopaque); use in addition to ultrasound to detect ureteral stones, note any gas in the renal shadow (emphysematous pyelonephritis).
• Renal ultrasound: most appropriate initial study to rule out suspected hydronephrosis, abscess, bladder or renal stones
• IVP: appropriate initial study if hematuria, flank pain, or analgesic abuse present, or to further evaluate hydronephrosis detected by ultrasound
• Noncontrast spiral CT: alternative screening study when IV contrast contraindicated
• CT scan $\pm$ IV contrast: further evaluation of sus-

pected acute focal bacterial nephritis or renal abscess, renal mass, or radiolucent renal calculus
• Voiding cystourethrogram: used to detect vesicoureteral reflux in patients with a history of reflux or neurogenic bladder, or to evaluate the uncommon patient with a urethral diverticulum

SPECIAL STUDIES

• Cystoscopy: if urine cultures grow unusual organisms, persistent bacteriuria, or hematuria in the absence of infection
• Urodynamic testing: indicated for urinary retention, or voiding difficulty with history of diabetes, or neurologic disease

 ## Initial Management

• Acute uncomplicated bacterial cystitis

—Urinalysis, 3-day course of trimethoprim-sulfamethoxazole 160 mg/800 mg bid, nitrofurantoin 100 mg tid, or fluoroquinolone (more costly) if allergic

• A 3-day course of antibiotics has better efficacy with fewer recurrences than does single-dose therapy, and has similar efficacy as a 7-day course, with fewer side effects.

 ## Follow-Up

• Isolated uncomplicated UTI

—If symptoms resolve after a 3-day course of antibiotics, no further evaluation/treatment is needed unless UTIs occur more frequently than twice per year.

—If symptoms do not resolve by the end of treatment, or if symptoms initially resolve but recur within 2 weeks

—Obtain posttreatment culture

—Assume infecting organism is not susceptible to the initial antibiotic and begin a 7-day course of another antibiotic

—Identify and address risk factors: Determine whether recurrence is related to sexual activity and/or contraceptives.

—Rule out possible complicated infection: Use urinary tract imaging as indicated to uncover structural or functional abnormalities that may require urologic intervention, and treat with appropriate antibiotic regimen.

—If posttreatment urine culture shows the same organism as the pretreatment culture (i.e., unresolved bacteriuria), check sensitivities for antibiotic resistance, rule out azotemia, and rule out underlying structural/functional urinary tract abnormality.

• Recurrent uncomplicated UTI

—Give a 3-day course of antibiotics (as in acute uncomplicated bacterial cystitis).

—Consider a 7- to 10-day treatment course if an unusual organism is present, or if the patient has a neurogenic bladder or other structural/functional urinary tract abnormality, or is immunocompromised.

—Determine whether UTIs are temporally related to a specific point in the menstrual cycle; consider selective prophylactic antibiotic use (one pill per day) during the susceptible time period.

—Determine whether UTIs are temporally related to intercourse; treat as follows.

—Sex-related (UTI occurs within 24–48 hours after intercourse)

—Give pre- or postcoital antibiotic prophylaxis with one pill (nitrofurantoin, TMP/SMX, first-generation cephalosporin, penicillin, fluoroquinolone).

—Instruct the patient to void following sex.

—Consider an alternative method of contraception (if patient using diaphragm and/or spermicidal jelly containing nonoxynol-9).

—Reevaluate the patient periodically.

—Non–sex-related, infrequent UTIs

—"Self therapy" with a 3-day course of antibiotics with the first symptoms of cystitis

—The patient collects a midstream urine culture at home prior to taking the antibiotic, and may store the specimen in a refrigerator up to 24 hours prior to delivering it to a lab.

—The advantage of self-therapy: rapid treatment of infection with decrease in the severity and time course for symptoms.

—Non–sex-related, more than three recurrences per year

—Chronic prophylaxis with single suppressive antibiotic dose each night or every other night

—Rule out structural/functional abnormalities with appropriate radiologic imaging studies if breakthrough UTIs occur.

—Reevaluate patient every 6 months; usually will be able to change to self-therapy after 6 months

 ## Miscellaneous

SYNONYMS: *N/A*

ASSOCIATED CONDITIONS: *N/A*

NOTES: *N/A*

ABBREVIATIONS: *N/A*

REFERENCES

Hooten TM, et al. Management of acute uncomplicated urinary tract infection in adults. *Med Clin North Am* 1991;75(2):339–357.

Moldwin RM, et al. Three treatment choices for recurrent cystitis. *Emerg Med* 1992;30–46.

Pappas PG. Laboratory in the diagnosis and management of urinary tract infections. *Med Clin North Am* 1991;75(2):313–325.

Safir MH, et al. Urinary tract infection: Simple and complicated. AUA Update Series, Lesson 10, Volume XVI, 1997.

Authors: Michael G. Desautel and Robert M. Moldwin

Urinary Tract Infection—Adult Male

 Basics

DESCRIPTION

- Inflammatory changes in the UT secondary to the presence of an invasive infectious agent
- Uncomplicated UTI: normal UT, and usually clears with antibiotics (rare in males)
- Complicated UTI: functional or anatomically abnormal UT, or catheterized male (usually febrile)
- Occurs in 0.1% in younger men and 5% to 20% in men over 80 years

PATHOPHYSIOLOGY

- Interaction of host defense mechanism, inoculum size, and virulence
- Three routes of infection:
—Ascending: urethra to bladder (catheters, VUR, vaginal or fecal spread)
—Hematogenous: oral, IV, bacteremia, or fungemia (enhanced by renal obstruction)
—Lymphatic: unusual, can be caused by RP abscess or direct extension
- Pathogens
—*E. coli* (70%–90%), *Klebsiella, Pseudomonas, Enterobacter, Proteus, Enterococcus, Candida,* and *Mycobacteria* (usually complicated)
—Virulence
　—*E. coli* has been studied most extensively.
　—Uropathogenic clones adhere to the uroepithelium.
　—O antigens (80% uropathogenic strains): inflammatory and toxic effects
　—K antigens (antiphagocytic), hemolysins, and resists bactericidal effects
　—Adhesin system: P. pili (type 2), P. fimbriae (harder to phagocytize), Gal-gal adhesins, Pap (pyelonephritis-associated pili). P. fimbriae attach to the urothelium via glycolipids (globoseries). PMNs only possess mannose radicals that bind type 1 pili (not type 2).
—Host defenses
　—Urine inhibitors: urea, salts, low pH, high osmolality, and organic acids; with high osmolality and low pH, phagocytosis is decreased.
　—Bladder mucosa: Tamm-Horsfall protein, bladder MPS layer, and low-molecular-weight oligosaccharides add to the antibacterial activity.
　—Flow and micturition aid in the elimination of bacteria.
　—Immune effects
　　—Uroepithelial cells secrete IL-8 (attracts PMNs). The cytokines IL-1, TNF, and IL-6 are produced, which also attract PMNs.
　　—IgM and IgG produce antibodies to P. fimbriae, O, and A antigens.
　　—High IgA levels appear to protect from pyelonephritis.
　　—CD4+ and CD8+ in submucosa may increase IL-6.

RISK FACTORS

- Uncomplicated UTI
—Homosexuality, anal intercourse, intercourse with infected female partner, lack of circumcision, and highly virulent strains of bacteria

- Complicated UTI
—Urinary tract obstruction, stasis of urine, VUR, urologic manipulation, diabetes, elderly age, catheters, stents, fistulas, NGBD, SCI, chronic diseases, impaired host responses, calculi, unusual pathogens, abnormal UT, and childhood UTIs

 Differential Diagnosis

- Uncomplicated UTIs
—Bacteriuria
　—Bacteria present in urine without symptoms and >10,000 CFU/mL on two consecutive samples
　—Increases with age (>5% if over 65 years), institutionalized elderly (15% to 35%)
　—>75% of ambulatory men clear spontaneously; *E. coli* is harder to clear.
　—Causes include increased residual, decreased concentration ability of the kidney, and bactericidal activity of prostatic secretions, chronic diseases, indwelling catheters, and condom catheters.
　—The nidus is commonly the prostate.
　—More commonly, bacteriuria converts to symptomatic disease in men.
　—Infectious urethritis: usually associated with multiple sex partners, due to gonorrhea, chlamydia, herpes simplex, and *Trichomonas;* purulent meatal discharge and erythema of meatus
　—Noninfectious urethritis: usually traumatic following sex or chemical irritants (soaps, etc.)
- Complicated UTIs
—Prostatitis: 50% lifetime risk
　—Acute bacterial: urinary symptoms associated with high fever and tender, swollen, hot prostate. Do not massage; can progress to abscess. Abscess requires drainage (transurethral, transperineal, or transrectal).
　—Chronic bacterial: urinary symptoms with recurrent bacteriuria with same pathogen. It can be due to prostatic calculi and pyuria noted on massage. It requires 6 weeks to 3 months of antibiotics.
　—Nonbacterial: urinary symptoms with no bacteria but pyuria on EPS. Eight times more common than bacterial prostatitis
—Gastrointestinal fistulas: multiple bacteria, persistent; may have pneumaturia
—Acute pyelonephritis: urinary symptoms associated with chills, fever, and flank pain (50% of patients have same symptoms and have lower UTI only). Can be confused with appendicitis and diverticulitis.
—Acute focal pyelonephritis: similar to above but with more severe symptoms. Usually diabetic and septic or bacteremic
—Renal abscess: usually ascending infection complicated by calculi, obstruction, or abnormal UT. High fever and chills occur, and it can be hematogenously spread as well. Diabetes increases the risk.

—Emphysematous pyelonephritis: 90% are diabetic with gas-forming organisms (*E. coli, Klebsiella, Proteus, Candida,* and *Aerobacter aerogenes*). Sepsis with high fever and gas in parenchyma; usually requires nephrectomy
—Pyohydronephrosis: obstructed upper UT with infection (50% associated with calculi); requires drainage
—Renal tuberculosis: usually in men under 50 years. Hematuria, flank pain, and colic occur (usually asymptomatic if lower UT uninvolved). Sterile acid pyuria, acid-fast smear may be negative. Can be associated with draining cutaneous sinuses, renal failure, epididymitis, nodular seminal vesicles, and hypertension
—Xanthogranulomatous pyelonephritis: Lipid-laden macrophages cause color. Usually due to obstruction from calculi. Flank pain, fever, chills, weight loss, and UT symptoms. Anemia, leukocytosis, and pyuria can occur.
—Malakoplakia: histiocytes with Michaelis-Guttman bodies. Marked enlargement of kidney with UTI. Fever, flank pain, and palpable mass with solid or cystic lesions on EU, CT, or US

 Database

HISTORY

- Dysuria, frequency, suprapubic pain, urgency: suggests prostatitis
- Flank pain, cloudy urine, gross hematuria
- Any recent urologic manipulation?
- Childhood febrile illnesses: can be associated with possible VUR
- Impaired host response (transplant, HIV, immunosuppression, IV drug, etc.)
- History of calculi: Suspect hydronephrosis, XGP.
- History of diabetes: Suspect renal abscess, emphysematous pyelonephritis, acute/focal pyelonephritis.
- Persistent or relapsing infection ± unusual pathogens): suggests obstruction, calculi, NGBD, fistula, high residual urine, prostatitis
- High fever with flank pain and chills: acute or focal pyelonephritis, renal abscess, XGP
- Medications: anticholinergics, antispasmodics, antihistamines, antidepressants, others

PHYSICAL EXAMINATION

- Suprapubic tenderness/fullness: increased residual urine
- Flank tenderness or mass: CVA tenderness associated with pyelonephritis
- Draining fistulous tracts: renal TB
- Swollen, tender, indurated or hot prostate, with pyuria or +EPS: acute prostatitis
- Penile discharge meatal erythema: urethritis.
- Is patient circumcised? May increase chance of UTI
- Hepatomegaly, weight loss, hypertension, and hematuria: suggests XGP, renal TB

Diagnostic Studies

LABORATORY TESTING

• Urine collection: Retract foreskin (if present) and clean the area. Midstream specimen (bladder), initial (urethra), following massage (prostate). Straight catheterization or suprapubic aspiration if unable to void
—Urine analysis/dipstick
 —Color: yellow, amber, or red (RBCs)
 —Clarity: usually clear but can be cloudy (WBCs).
 —pH: usually 5.0 to 8.0. If high pH (>8.0), a urea-splitting organism (i.e., *Proteus*) may be present.
 —Glucose: ?diabetic
 —Nitrite test: if positive, helpful; but many false negatives
 —Leukocyte esterase test: many false negatives and false positives. 71% sensitivity, 83% specificity for UTI
 —RBCs: may be dipstick positive if urine specific gravity <1.007, with negative microscopy, due to cell lysis
—Urinalysis/microscopy
 —Bacteriuria is usually noted if >100,000 CFU/mL.
 —>10 WBCs/μL (unspun), or >2 WBCs/μL (spun)
 —>5 WBCs/hpf (0.5 sensitivity) or >10 WBCs/hpf is more reliable. Hematuria may be present.
—Urine culture
 —≥10,000 CFU/mL (midstream clean catch), or ≥100 to 1000 CFU/mL (catheterized)
 —CLED agar/EZSTREAK methods are 98% sensitivity and 99% specificity.
—Other laboratory tests
 —A slide centrifuge Gram stain is very sensitive for ≥10,000 CFU/mL.
 —Uriscreen (catalase tube test) works well and may be better for *Candida* detection.
 —Amplification assay (LCx, COBAS Amplicor, AMPCT): All work well for chlamydia.
 —PCR is also reliable for chlamydia.

IMAGING

• Uncomplicated UTI: imaging generally not helpful or needed
• Complicated UTI
—Excretory urography: most helpful to denote hydronephrosis, calculi, strictures, gas
—Ultrasound with KUB: can denote calculi, debris (hydronephrosis from pyohydronephrosis), cavitation (TB), gas, abscess, or infected cysts
—CT scan/MRI: most helpful for diagnosing pyelonephritis (patchy uptake, wedge defect), renal abscess, cavitation (TB), debris (hydronephrosis vs. pyohydronephrosis), malakoplakia, solid masses from infected cysts
—Gallium-67: may be helpful for diagnosing pyelonephritis or abscess in rare cases

SPECIAL STUDIES

• Cystoscopy: helpful for diagnosing obstructing prostates, bladder stones, increased residuals (when indicated), fistula

Initial Management

• Empiric therapy is listed below; modify therapy based on clinical response and/or cultures.
• Uncomplicated UTIs: In men they are extremely uncommon (5 in 10,000 men/yr). If under 40 years, may consider single-dose therapy; generally, 7 to 14 days is recommended. If infection persists or recurs, treatment for 4 to 6 weeks is recommended (to clear prostatitis), along with further work-up.
—Empiric treatment
 —TMP/SMX: low cost, low resistance, but moderate side effects (rash, GI upset). Poor sensitivity for *Pseudomonas* and *Enterococcus*
 —Nitrofurantoin: low cost, low resistance, and low side effects. Poor tissue levels, poor choice in men, as they frequently have complicated UTIs. Poor sensitivity for *Pseudomonas* and *Proteus*
 —Amoxicillin/ampicillin: increased resistance to urinary pathogens. When combined with clavulanate, high cost, less resistance. Frequent side effects
 —Fluoroquinolones: low resistance but high cost. High number of GI side effects and drug interactions (methylxanthines). Probably no more effective than other antibiotics for uncomplicated UTIs

• Complicated UTIs: usually require antibiotics and x-ray studies (CT, US, EU, MRI, or VCUG).
—UTI in men with a catheter/SCI/high residuals: high fever, change to intermittent catheterization or solve voiding problem
 —Usually IV ampicillin with aminoglycoside. Can use IV fluoroquinolone or third-generation cephalosporin. IV therapy until afebrile for 24 hours, then orally for 7 to 14 days
—UTI following urologic procedures/intermittent catheterization/SCI/NGBD: no fever
 —Oral TMP/SMX or fluoroquinolones for 7 to 14 days
—UTI with prostatitis
 —Oral fluoroquinolone for 4 to 12 weeks; alternatively, TMP/SMX or carbenicillin
—UTI in immunosuppressed patient: no fever
 —Fluoroquinolone for 6 weeks, or alternatively, 6 weeks of TMP/SMX
—Acute pyelonephritis/focal pyelonephritis/pyohydronephrosis/abscess/emphysematous pyelitis
 —IV ampicillin or TMP/SMX and aminoglycoside, or alternatively, cephalosporin (if renal insufficiency)
 —Treat a minimum of 14 days, longer if culture remains positive.
 —For abscess, antibiotics, open or percutaneous drainage if necessary.
 —For pyohydronephrosis, drainage and consequent removal of source, if required
 —Emphysematous pyelonephritis: IV ampicillin and an aminoglycoside with fluid resuscitation and usually nephrectomy

—Renal tuberculosis
 —IV therapy with combination of INH, rifampin, ethambutol, cycloserine, or streptomycin
 —Surgery when indicated
—Xanthogranulomatous pyelonephritis: Stabilize with IV ampicillin and an aminoglycoside, followed by nephrectomy.
—Malakoplakia: long-term treatment with TMP/SMX or fluoroquinolones and surgical repair; poor prognosis

Follow-Up

• Uncomplicated UTIs
—If symptoms disappear, repeat U/A and cultures at 1 to 2 weeks and 4 to 6 weeks post-therapy.
—If symptoms persist, follow complicated UTI guidelines; >85% are cured by 5 to 9 days.

• Complicated UTIs
—1 to 2 weeks and 4 to 6 weeks after initial therapy, U/A, reculture, and examine.
—Some patients may require additional studies (cystoscopy, localizing studies) or x-rays.
—Cure rates are >90% at 1-week follow-up but fall to 70% at 3 to 6 weeks.

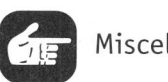

Miscellaneous

SYNONYMS: N/A

ASSOCIATED CONDITIONS: N/A

NOTES

• Simple cystitis in males is not usually seen except in conjunction with prostatitis.

ABBREVIATIONS

• EPS, expressed prostatic secretion; EU, excretory urography; NGBD, neurogenic bladder disease; MPS, mucopolysaccharide; TMP/SMX, trimethoprim-sulfamethoxazole; UT, urinary tract; VCUG, voiding cystourethrogram; VUR, vesicoureteral reflux; XGP, xanthogranulomatous pyelonephritis

REFERENCES

Hooton TM. Diagnosis and treatment of uncomplicated urinary tract infection. *Infect Dis Clin North Am* 1997;11:551.

Kaplan DM. Advances in the imaging of renal infection. *Infect Dis Clin North Am* 1997;11:681.

Nicolle LE. Asymptomatic bacteriuria in the elderly. *Infect Dis Clin North Am* 1997;11:647.

Rubin RH, et al. Evaluation of new anti-infective drugs for the treatment of urinary tract infection. *Clin Infect Dis* 1992;15[Suppl 1]:S216.

Sobel JD. Pathogenesis of urinary tract infection. *Infect Dis Clin North Am* 1997;11:531.

Author: Evan B. Krisch

Urinary Tract Infection—Pediatric

 Basics

DESCRIPTION

• Inflammatory changes in the urinary tract caused by the presence of an invasive infectious agent
• In children less than 1 year old, is four times more common in boys than in girls
• In children greater than 1 year old, is two to three times more common in girls than in boys

PATHOPHYSIOLOGY

• Most common pathogen is *E. coli*
—P. fimbriae are associated with higher virulence and increased incidence of cystitis and pyelonephritis
• Humoral and cellular responses to the infectious agent result in inflammation of the urinary tract.
—Inflammation peaks 3 to 5 days from initiation of infection.
—Renal scarring from inflammatory response results in hypertension, and potentially proteinuria and progressive renal failure.
• In children, infections are often due to congenital anomalies.
• May see increased incidence during toilet training in young girls

RISK FACTORS

• Infants: more common during first year of life, especially first 3 months, than at other times of childhood
• Sex: more common in females after first year of life
• Circumcision: Noncircumcised males have increased periurethral colonization, leading to increased infection and recurrence risk.
• Bottle feeding: Studies suggest that breast feeding confers immunogenic protection.
• Familial: higher risk of recurrent UTIs in families
• Neurogenic bladder: much higher incidence of bacteriuria and pyuria and subsequent renal scarring
• Anatomic abnormalities of the urinary tract (i.e., reflux, ureterocele, etc.)

 Differential Diagnosis

• Presentation vague, thus may present similarly to many other types of infections
—Urine culture and DMSA scan will be useful tools to differentiate urinary tract infections from other sources of infection.
• Hemorrhagic cystitis is often associated with adenovirus infection.
• Given the serious consequences of renal damage, a high index of suspicion and a low threshold for early treatment must be maintained.

 Database

HISTORY

• Vague in infants
—Fever (67%), irritable (55%), poor feeding (38%), vomiting (36%), diarrhea (31%), abdominal distention (8%), jaundice (7%)
• Older children may indicate dysuria, incontinence, lower abdominal pain, voiding dysfunction, nocturnal and/or diurnal diuresis, urgency.
• Inquire about previous urinary tract infections, surgery.
• Familial history of infections or GU anomalies

PHYSICAL EXAMINATION

• Occasionally, a palpable renal mass may be found, with severe hydronephrosis.
• Older children may have suprapubic, flank, abdominal and/or upper quadrant tenderness.
• Rule out epididymitis via a testicular examination.
• Rarely any specific findings in infants

Diagnostic Studies

LABORATORY TESTING

• Urinalysis

—First void in the morning is most accurate for evaluation of nitrite, leukocyte esterase
—Nitrite positive and leukocyte esterase positive with bacteria seen on microscopy positively identifies UTI
—Nitrite negative and leukocyte esterase negative correctly identifies lack of UTI
—More than 10 WBCs/μL and bacteria on microscopy suggest clinical infection.

• Urine culture best establishes UTI.

—The method of obtaining urine sample is critical for accuracy.
  —Suprapubic aspirate is most accurate.
  —Midstream sample via catheterization is a reasonable alternative.
  —Midstream-voided samples can only be used with circumcised boys and older girls.
—More than 100,000 CFU/mL indicates clinical UTI.
—In febrile children <2 years old, >50,000 CFU/mL is consistent with a clinical UTI.

• C-reactive protein, erythrocyte sedimentation rate, and CBC are not reliable indicators of infection.

IMAGING

• Abdominal ultrasound is the initial screening test in febrile UTI.
• A DMSA renal scan may reveal renal inflammation otherwise not readily apparent.

—If a UTI is already suspected and will be treated, this scan is unnecessary.

SPECIAL STUDIES: N/A

 ## Initial Management

• Early detection is key to preventing renal damage: Keep a high index of suspicion.
• In systemically ill, young infants (<3 months old), 2 to 3 days of broad-spectrum antibiotics are indicated.

—Ampicillin/gentamicin or third-generation cephalosporin
—Upper UTI with *Pseudomonas aeruginosa* may require a quinolone.
  —Quinolones have shown cartilage toxicity in animal studies, and should not be used.
—The patient will likely need to be admitted to hospital to ensure hydration.
—Continue antibiotics until the patient is afebrile and the urine is sterile.

• School-age children without systemic signs can be treated with 3 to 5 days of oral broad-spectrum antibiotics, such as trimethoprim-sulfamethoxazole, nitrofurantoin, amoxicillin/clavulanate, cephalexin, and cefixime.

 ## Follow-Up

• Prophylactic antibiotics

—Nitrofurantoin (in children without G6P deficiency), trimethoprim-sulfamethoxazole (except in those <3 months old), and cephalexin should follow the initial antibiotic treatment, continued through the radiologic evaluation.

• Imaging

—Given the susceptibility of pediatric kidneys to scarring with infection, a full radiologic evaluation should be performed after the first episode of infection in children.
—VCUG
  —Nuclear study is more sensitive for reflux.
  —Contrast study is superior in detecting structural anomalies such as obstruction, ureterocele, urethral abnormalities, and dysplasia.
—A DMSA scan is the best scan to determine renal scarring.
  —If scarring is present, consider a nephrology consult to monitor for evaluation of hypertension, proteinuria, and renal insufficiency.

• Contact the primary care provider to ensure that adequate follow-up can be maintained.

 ## Miscellaneous

SYNONYMS: N/A

ASSOCIATED CONDITIONS: N/A

NOTES

• See also Section I, "Urinary Tract Infection—Adult Female" and "Urinary Tract Infection—Adult Male."

ABBREVIATIONS

• DMSA, technetium-99m dimercaptosuccinic acid

REFERENCES

Jakobsson B, Esbjorner E, Hansson S. Minimum incidence and diagnostic rate of first urinary tract infection. *Pediatrics* 1999;104(2 Pt 1):222–226.

Ross JH, Kay R. Pediatric urinary tract infection and reflux. *Am Fam Physician* 1999;59(6):1472–1478, 1485–1486.

Authors: Jerome R. Zink and Leonard G. Gomella

Weak Urinary Stream

 Basics

DESCRIPTION

- Decreased force of urinary stream

—Can be measured objectively with uroflowmetry
—Can be a subjective finding on history

PATHOPHYSIOLOGY

- Most commonly caused by bladder outlet obstruction (BOO) or increased outlet resistance
- Rare in female patients
- Most common cause of outlet obstruction is benign prostatic hyperplasia (BPH) in elderly males

—Low bladder pressure–low urinary flow

- Found in urodynamic study of young men with obsessional behavior who are otherwise normal

—Poor detrusor contraction

- Neurologic conditions such as Parkinson's, multiple sclerosis

RISK FACTORS

- Elderly men (prostatism)
- Prior urethral instrumentation or prostatic surgery
- History of gonorrhea, sexually transmitted diseases(strictures)
- Obsessional behavior (low pressure–low flow)
- Parkinson's, multiple sclerosis

 Differential Diagnosis

- Benign prostatic hyperplasia
- Prostate carcinoma
- Urethral stricture
- Bladder neck contracture
- Obstructing bladder calculus
- Low pressure–low flow
- Underactive detrusor contraction
- Urinary tract infection or prostatitis may mimic symptoms of outlet obstruction.

 Database

HISTORY

- Age: BPH and prostate cancer more likely in older men
- Sex: rare in women
- Symptom score (Note: not useful in evaluation of voiding patterns in women)

—American Urological Association Symptom Score/International Prostate Symptom Score
　—Indicators of obstructive symptoms: slow to start stream, hesitancy, weak urinary stream, incomplete emptying
　—Indicators of irritative symptoms: frequency, urgency, nocturia

- Medications

—Alpha-blockers, 5-alpha reductase inhibitors: alleviate bladder outlet obstruction
—Sympathomimetics (ephedrine, phenylephrine): contribute to outlet obstruction, weak stream

- Medical problems: neurologic disorders (multiple sclerosis, Parkinson's, spine trauma)
- Urethritis, gonorrhea, or straddle injury: urethral strictures
- Surgical history

—Prior prostate surgery: bladder neck contracture, adenoma regrowth
—Urethral instrumentation: iatrogenic urethral strictures
—Spine surgery: for neurologic injury

PHYSICAL EXAMINATION

- Digital rectal examination: Palpate the prostate for enlargement, induration, or nodules.

—Genital examination: Check for meatal stenosis, prior hypospadias surgery.

- Abdominal examination
- Palpate for suprapubic mass (distended bladder)
- Inguinal examination for hernias

 Diagnostic Studies

LABORATORY TESTING

- Urinalysis
- PSA

IMAGING

- Bladder ultrasound to evaluate for residual urine

SPECIAL STUDIES

- Voiding diary: The patient keeps a record of the time and volume voided in a period of 24 hours or more.

—Helps to obtain objective verification of patient's voiding complaints

- Urodynamic studies

—Uroflowmetry with bladder ultrasound (bladder volume index) or post-void residual (PVR)
—Voided volumes should be above 150 mL for a valid study.
—Maximum flow (Q max) is the most valuable measurement.
　—>15 cc/s normal; 10 to 15 cc/s equivocal
　—<10 cc/s slow; likely BOO
—Cystometry
　—Indicated in patients with associated bladder dysfunction such as urgency and frequency
　—Helps to distinguish detrusor instability (may be present in advanced outlet obstruction)
—Pressure–flow studies
　—High pressure–low flow suggests bladder outlet obstruction.
　—Low pressure–low flow suggests poor detrusor contraction secondary to neurologic causes or detrusor muscle decompensation.
　—Abrams-Griffith nomogram: may distinguish true BOO patients
—Cystoscopy: identifies meatal stenosis, urethral strictures, prostatic lobe coaptation, bladder trabeculation, cellules and diverticula, bladder stones (ball-valve effect or presence suggests BOO)

Initial Management

- Indications for treatment

—Absolute indications include associated azotemia, hydronephrosis, bladder decompensation, and overflow incontinence.

—Relative indications: episodes of acute urinary retention, recurrent urinary tract infections with increased residual, bladder instability, severe recurrent hematuria, and significant symptoms

- Benign prostatic hypertrophy

—Alpha-blocker therapy
  —Relaxes smooth muscles of the bladder outlet
  —"First-dose phenomenon": Side effects include faintness, dizziness, palpitation, and syncope due to acute postural hypotension; therefore, doses are gradually increased.
  —Commonly prescribed alpha-blockers
    —Terazosin (Hytrin): 1 to 8 mg qid
    —Doxazosin (Cardura): 1 to 8 mg qid
    —Tamsulosin (Flomax): 0.4 mg to 0.8 mg qid; no reported first-dose phenomenon

—5-alpha reductase inhibitor (finasteride)
  —May take up to 6 months to see effect; helpful in larger glands; 5 mg po qid

- Surgical management

—Prostatic enlargement
  —Open prostatectomy: suprapubic, retropubic, perineal approach; consider for large glands (> 80–100 g)
  —Transurethral prostatectomy (TURP): "gold standard"
  —Transurethral incision of prostate (TUIP) or bladder neck: effective in smaller glands (< 30 g)
  —Transurethral electrovaporization
  —Laser techniques: noncontact coagulative necrosis; contact laser vaporization; holmium laser resection; interstitial laser coagulation
  —Microwave therapy (TUMT): minimally invasive, local anesthesia procedure
  —Prostatic stent prosthesis: encrusts, causes irritating symptoms; for poor surgical candidates

—Urethral strictures
  —Urethral dilation; visual internal urethrotomy
  —Urethroplasty with primary anastomosis, free or island grafts: gold standard with highest success rate

—Bladder neck contracture
  —Bladder neck incision, dilation, vaporization
  —Y-V plasty of bladder neck

—Bladder stones
  —Transurethral stone extraction with endoscopic lithotripsy
  —Cystolitholapaxy; cystotomy

—Prostate cancer
  —Limited channel TURP in advanced disease to alleviate obstruction
  —Radical prostatectomy (perineal, retropubic)
  —Radiation (external or brachytherapy): Note, brachytherapy may worsen obstructive symptoms for up to 1 to 2 years.
  —Hormonal ablation (orchiectomy, LH-RH agonists, antiandrogens

—Low detrusor pressure: no definitive therapy; treat primary etiology

—Neurologic disease: treat primary neurologic etiology

Follow-Up

- Annual PSA and digital rectal examination
- Periodic symptom score uroflowmetry with bladder ultrasound to detect elevated residuals

Miscellaneous

SYNONYMS

- Bladder outlet obstruction

ASSOCIATED CONDITIONS: N/A

NOTES: N/A

ABBREVIATIONS

- BOO, bladder outlet obstruction

REFERENCES

Abrams PH, Griffith DJ. The assessment of prostatic obstruction from urodynamic measurements and from residual urine. *Br J Urol* 1979;51:129.

Wein AJ. Neuromuscular dysfunction of the lower urinary tract. In: Walsh PC, Retik AB, Vaughan ED, Wein AJ, eds. *Campbell's Urology*. Philadelphia: WB Saunders, 1998:969–1000.

Authors: Gregory L. Chen and Demetrius H. Bagley

SECTION II
Urologic Diseases and Conditions

Acute Tubular Necrosis

 Basics

DESCRIPTION

- Most common type of intrarenal acute renal failure (ARF), usually due to prolonged ischemia or administration of nephrotoxins

EPIDEMIOLOGY

- Incidence of ARF is 209 per million population.
- Breakdown of ARF: acute tubular necrosis (ATN) 45%, prerenal causes 21%, acute or chronic renal failure 13%, urinary tract obstruction 10%, glomerulonephritis or vasculitis 4%, acute interstitial nephritis 2%, atheroemboli 1%

GENETICS

- No known genetic link

STAGING: N/A

SIGNS AND SYMPTOMS

- Decreased urine output

—Can be nonoliguric, oliguric >500 mL/d, or anuric. Mortality increases from 20% to 60% to 80% if the patient is oliguric or anuric.

- Signs of underlying disorder

—Signs of sepsis or of hypotensive events secondary to trauma, cardiac disease, surgery with excessive blood loss, or interruption of blood supply to kidneys

PATHOPHYSIOLOGY

- Acute tubular injury

—Secondary to ischemia, toxins, radiocontrast agents, hemoglobinuria, myoglobinuria

- The ischemic form is the most common, and the reductions in glomerular filtration rate (GFR) are secondary to vascular and tubular factors.

—Ischemia from reductions in GFR from decreased renal plasma flow or dilatation of the efferent arteriole. After return of normal blood flow, ATN persists secondary to tubular changes.
—Tubular factors: backleak and tubular obstruction. Tubular obstruction secondary to a sloughed brush border, cellular debris, Tamm-Horsfall protein, and decreased filtration pressure contribute to obstruction and maintenance of ATN.

CAUSES/RISK FACTORS

- Decreased renal perfusion from

—Prolonged hypotension, surgical interruption of blood flow, nonsteroidal antiinflammatory agents, angiotensin-converting enzyme inhibitors, cyclosporin

- Nephrotoxic agents

—Radiocontrast media (low osmolality is safer), aminoglycosides, cisplatinum, amphotericin, drug intoxications with acetaminophen or ethylene glycol

COMPLICATIONS

- Fluid overload, electrolyte disturbances, metabolic acidosis

—Hypertension, edema, acute pulmonary edema, hyponatremia, hyperkalemia, hypermagnesemia, hypercalcemia, hyperphosphatemia, hyperuricemia

- Uremic signs and symptoms

—GI: nausea, vomiting, GI bleed; neurologic: encephalopathy, coma, seizures, peripheral neuropathy; cardiac: pericarditis uremic pneumonitis; hematologic: bleeding, anemia; immunologic: impaired granulocyte/lymphocyte function

DIFFERENTIAL DIAGNOSIS

- Prerenal azotemia
- Postrenal azotemia
- Other forms of renal azotemia
- Glomerulonephritis, disseminated intravascular coagulopathy, arterial or venous obstruction, intrarenal precipitation

 Database

HISTORY

- Specific attention to

—Hypotensive episodes, blood transfusions, intravenous contrast exposure

- Meticulous listing of medications to include dosage to assure appropriate dosing for level of renal function

—Make sure other medications which depend on renal metabolism are also given at appropriate doses to avoid side effects.

PHYSICAL EXAMINATION

- Evaluate the volume status of the patient.

—Evaluate neck veins and auscultation of heart and lungs; assess extremities and the presacral area for edema.

- General examination

—Evaluate for bladder distention and assess for signs of vasculitis or cutaneous rashes.

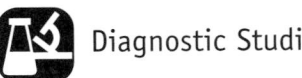 Diagnostic Studies

LABORATORY TESTING

- Serum tests

—BUN/plasma creatinine ratio: The ratio is normal at 10 to 15:1 in ATN, but >20:1 in prerenal disease due to the increase in passive reabsorption of urea, the ratio may also be increased with GI bleed, muscle breakdown, and administration of corticosteroids or tetracycline.
—Rate of rise of plasma creatinine: rise of greater than 0.3 to 0.5 mg/dL in ATN vs. slower rise with fluctuations with prerenal disease

- Urine tests

—Urinalysis: muddy brown granular and epithelial cell casts and free epithelial cells secondary to sloughing of the tubular epithelium vs. near-normal in prerenal disease
—Urine sodium concentration: high >40 mEq/L due to tubular injury vs. <20 mEq/L in prerenal disease in an attempt to conserve sodium
—Fractional excretion of sodium: above 2% in ATN while less than 1% in prerenal disease, measured as urine NA divided by plasma NA times plasma CR divided by urine CR
—Urine osmolality: urine osmolality <450 mOsmol/kg in ATN secondary to loss of concentrating ability; >500 mOsmol/kg in prerenal disease
—Urine creatinine concentration divided by plasma creatinine concentration: ratio is <20 in ATN while >40 in prerenal disease, reflecting loss of tubular water reabsorption

IMAGING

- Renal ultrasonography

—Sensitive test to determine obstruction. Doppler can detect blood flow in different vessels.

- Functional studies

—Nuclear scans can determine perfusion or tubular secretion; MRI can give some functional information while providing anatomic information.

SPECIAL STUDIES: N/A

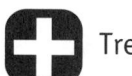 ## Treatment

GENERAL MEASURES

- Define and treat the underlying cause.
- Prophylaxis and treatment of complications of ARF
- Early nephrology consultation

MEDICAL

- Management of fluid disturbances

—Maintain a euvolemic state by restricting total fluids to no more than urine output plus insensible losses.
—High-dose loop diuretics (1–3 g/d) may convert oliguric to nonoliguric ATN in some patients; it has not been determined that this conversion decreases the duration of ATN or mortality. Dopamine may increase urine output, but its benefit is in question.

- Management of electrolyte disturbances

—Electrolyte disturbances can be minimized by prophylactic institution of a low-potassium, low-protein diet accompanied by fluid restriction and oral phosphate binders.
—Hyperkalemia is the most common and most dangerous abnormality and should be treated aggressively with calcium supplementation until potassium levels can be reduced with combinations of insulin and glucose or potassium-binding resins.

SURGICAL

- Consideration for dialysis access if renal failure severe

ALTERNATIVE THERAPIES

- Hemodialysis (HD), peritoneal dialysis (PD), and continuous arteriovenous hemofiltration (CAVH)

—CAVH: need ICU, limited mobility, need anticoagulation, removes fluid well but slow correction of electrolyte abnormalities
—PD: no anticoagulation needed but slower correction of electrolyte abnormalities
—HD: expensive, anticoagulation necessary, vascular access necessary but allow rapid correction of fluid and electrolyte abnormalities

PATIENT EDUCATION: N/A

 ## Follow-Up

MONITORING

- Duration

—Renal failure phase usually lasts 7 to 21 days if the primary insult (ischemia, nephrotoxin) can be corrected. Recovery is usually heralded by a progressive increase in urine output and a return of BUN and CR to the previous baseline.

- Recovery of renal function

—Irreversible loss of renal function can occur if the combination of preexisting renal disease and prolonged ARF secondary to repeat ischemic insults and/or nephrotoxin administration
—If the patient survives, baseline CR is usually only 1 to 2 mg/dL above baseline.
—Those patients that need dialysis and have bioincompatibility with the dialysis membrane or have repeat episodes of hypotension have a worse prognosis.

PATIENT SURVIVAL

- Slight improvements in survival in those patients with ATN requiring dialysis in an ICU setting

—The Mayo Clinic report comparing 1977–79 with 1991–92 showed high survival both in hospital (52% vs. 32%) and at 1 year (30% vs. 21%).

- Major causes of death are infection and underlying disease, not renal failure.

—Patients at risk are generally very ill, with evidence of multiple organ dysfunction.

PREVENTION: N/A

 ## Miscellaneous

SYNONYMS: N/A

ASSOCIATED CONDITIONS: N/A

NOTES

- See Section I, "Renal Failure—Acute."

ABBREVIATIONS: N/A

REFERENCES

Edelstein CL, Alkhunazi A, Yagoob MM, et al. Etiology, pathogenesis, and management of renal failure. In: Walsh PC, Retik AB, Vaughan ED Jr, eds. *Campbell's Urology,* 7th ed. Philadelphia: WB Saunders, 1998.

Rose BD. Diagnosis of acute tubular necrosis and prerenal disease. *UpToDate Med* 1996; 6(2) online.

Rose BD. Prognosis of acute tubular necrosis. *UpToDate Med* 1996;6(2) online.

Rose BD. Duration and possible therapy of acute tubular necrosis. *UpToDate Med* 1996;6(2) online.

Author: Burkhardt H. Zorn

Addison Disease

 Basics

DESCRIPTION

• Condition caused by primary adrenal insufficiency

EPIDEMIOLOGY

• Rare, with a death rate of approximately 0.3/100,000
• In the Third World, most cases result from infections (TB most common).
• In developed countries, the most common cause is autoimmune with antiadrenal antibodies in 70% of cases.

GENETICS

• Type II autoimmune polyglandular syndrome (Schmidt syndrome)

—Onset between 20 and 50 years; women > men; associated with HLA alleles B8, DR3, and DR4
—Consists of Addison disease, autoimmune thyroid disease (Grave disease or Hashimoto's thyroiditis), insulin-dependent diabetes mellitus, ovarian and testicular failure, vitiligo, and pernicious anemia

• Can occur as part of hereditary disorder marked by progressive myelin degeneration in the brain (adrenoleukodystrophy) or spinal cord (adrenomyelodystrophy)

STAGING: N/A

SIGNS AND SYMPTOMS

• Symptoms

—Weakness, fatigue, weight loss, anorexia, nausea and vomiting, and vague gastrointestinal complaints occur in the majority of patients.
—Chronicity results in nonspecific signs and symptoms that result primarily from chronic volume depletion; therefore, a diagnosis is often not made until stress induces an increased requirement for glucocorticoids that leads to adrenal crisis.

• Signs

—Hyperpigmentation concentrated in the palmar creases, pressure points, mucous membranes, and areolas
—Orthostatic hypotension

PATHOPHYSIOLOGY

• Commonly results from atrophy or replacement of the adrenal glands

—Decreased production of cortisol, aldosterone, and adrenal androgens
—The pituitary compensates by increased production of ACTH and hyperpigmentation of skin and mucous membranes.

• Severe volume deficiency and prerenal azotemia lead to orthostatic hypotension, dizziness, or syncope, and eventually to lethargy and disorientation.
• The acute form produces vascular collapse and, if not recognized and treated promptly, death.

CAUSES/RISK FACTORS

• Autoimmune
• Idiopathic

—Autoimmune polyglandular syndromes type I (triad of hypoparathyroidism, adrenal insufficiency, and mucocutaneous candidiasis that presents in childhood) and type II (see above)
—Infection: tuberculosis, HIV infection, histoplasmosis, blastomycosis, and coccidiomycosis

• Infiltrative: amyloidosis, sarcoidosis, adrenoleukodystrophy (see above), adrenomyodystrophy (see above)
• Spontaneous adrenal hemorrhage secondary to meningococcemia, disseminated intravascular coagulation, or anticoagulant therapy
• Lymphoma, bilateral adrenal metastases, or, in AIDS patients, Kaposi's sarcoma
• Iatrogenic

—Cessation of chronic glucocorticoid therapy, failure to increase glucocorticoid replacement therapy during times of stress
—Pituitary irradiation or surgical adrenalectomy
—Medications: ketoconazole, aminoglutethimide, and etomidate

COMPLICATIONS

• Acute adrenal insufficiency results from failure to recognize Addison disease during times of stress, cessation of glucocorticoid replacement therapy during operative stress or trauma, or failure to increase glucocorticoid replacement therapy during stress.
• Patients are commonly replaced with excessive doses of glucocorticoids and inadequate doses of mineralocorticoids. Overtreatment with glucocorticoids results in insidious weight gain, cushingoid appearance, and osteoporosis; and inadequate mineralocorticoid replacement causes orthostatic hypotension, dizziness, and syncope.

DIFFERENTIAL DIAGNOSIS

• Primary adrenal insufficiency (Addison's)
• Secondary adrenal insufficiency

—Pituitary failure: low or absent serum levels of ACTH, and may be due to panhypopituitarism, Sheehan syndrome (pituitary injury due to severe postpartum hemorrhagic or infectious shock), pituitary apoplexy, or isolated corticotropin deficiency
—Familial glucocorticoid deficiency: unresponsiveness to corticotropin due to mutations in the glucocorticoid receptor
—Patients have excess mineralocorticoids, but fail to develop cushingoid features.
—Isolated corticotropin-releasing deficiency

• Tertiary adrenal insufficiency: adrenal suppression due to use of glucocorticoids

 Database

HISTORY

• Symptoms are generally nonspecific; a high index of suspicion must be maintained to diagnose Addison disease prior to the development of adrenal crisis.
• Preoperative history: careful questioning for current or past steroid use
• Abdominal pain may result from unilateral or bilateral adrenal hemorrhage.

PHYSICAL EXAMINATION

• Hypotension, tachycardia, orthostatic hypotension
• Hyperpigmentation of the palmar creases, mucous membranes, pressure points, and areolas

Diagnostic Studies

LABORATORY TESTING

• Electrolyte disturbances: hyperkalemia, hyponatremia, hypercalcemia, eosinophilia, lymphocytosis, hypoglycemia, metabolic acidosis, azotemia (all occur in < half of patients)
• Serum ACTH and cortisol levels (see below)

IMAGING

• If adrenal infarction or hemorrhage is suspected, CT or MRI is appropriate.

SPECIAL STUDIES

• Cosyntropin stimulation test

—Plasma cortisol and ACTH obtained before 0.25 mg cosyntropin IV
—If the patient is in adrenal crisis, stress doses of dexamethasone (4 mg q8h) are administered along with aggressive volume restoration.
—60 minutes after cosyntropin administration, plasma cortisol is obtained.
—Diagnosis of Addison disease: Cortisol levels fail to reach 18 μg/dL after 60 minutes or, if the serum cortisol level is <18 μg/dL at 60 minutes, serum cortisol fails to increase at least 8 μg/dL.

• ACTH >52 pg/mL is consistent with adrenal failure; if ACTH is low (<9 pg/mL), adrenal function is either normal or secondary adrenal insufficiency exists.

 Treatment

GENERAL MEASURES: N/A

MEDICAL

• Glucocorticoid replacement: 15 to 20 mg of hydrocortisone qAM and 5 mg at about 4 PM (mimics the physiologic secretion of cortisol)
• Mineralocorticoid replacement: varies greatly, initiated with 100 μg/d fludrocortisone (Florinef) and adjusted to keep standing plasma renin secretion between 1 and 3 ng/mL/h
• Minor stress (minor illness) double hydrocortisone dose for as short a period as possible.
• Major stress (surgery requiring general anesthesia or major trauma): Hydrocortisone should be administered 150 to 300 mg daily in three divided doses and tapered rapidly during recovery to normal replacement (see drugs in Section V).

SURGICAL: N/A

ALTERNATIVE THERAPIES: N/A

PATIENT EDUCATION

• A Medic-Alert bracelet should be worn at all times, and patients should be instructed in the use of intramuscular emergency hydrocortisone injections.

 Follow-Up

MONITORING

• Acid-base status should be monitored to assure maintenance of normal bone density. Mineralocorticoid replacement should be monitored to assure normal acid-base and volume status.

PREVENTION: N/A

 Miscellaneous

SYNONYMS

• Adrenal insufficiency, hypoadrenalism

ASSOCIATED CONDITIONS

• See "Synonyms."

NOTES: N/A

ABBREVIATIONS: N/A

REFERENCES

Mohler JL, Michael KA, Freedman AM, McRoberts JW, Griffen WO Jr. The evaluation of postoperative adrenal corticoid function. *Surg Gynecol Obstet* 1985;161:445–449.

Vaughan ED Jr, Blumenfeld JD. The adrenals. In: Walsh PC, Retik AB, Stamey TA, Vaughan ED Jr. *Campbell's Urology*, 6th ed. Philadelphia: WB Saunders, 1992:2381–2384.

Author: James L. Mohler

Adenomatoid Tumors (Testis/Epididymis)

 Basics

DESCRIPTION

• Adenomatoid tumors are the most common neoplastic processes involving the testicular adnexal and spermatic cord structures.

EPIDEMIOLOGY

• May occur in females; >70% found in males
• Age: 20 to 30 years (range: 20–80 yr)

GENETICS: N/A

STAGING: N/A

SIGNS AND SYMPTOMS

• Scrotal mass, typically painless

PATHOPHYSIOLOGY

• Grossly may arise anywhere within the epididymis, but most commonly involves the distal epididymis, adjacent to the lower pole of the testes

—Sometimes found in tunica albuginea of the testes, and spermatic cord
—Small and well circumscribed

• Microscopic

—Uniformly benign: None has ever been reported to metastasize; local invasion of adjacent structures has occasionally been observed.
—Mixed epithelial and stromal elements
  —The epithelial element is eosinophilic and has a vacuolated cytoplasm.
  —Irregular, somewhat branched-appearing tubular structures appear within the tumor, a coalescence of the cellular vacuoles, which form a false lumen.
  —Based on the presence of microvilli on the free surface of the cells and the presence of mucopolysaccharides, these cells are of mesothelial origin.

CAUSES/RISK FACTORS: N/A

COMPLICATIONS: N/A

DIFFERENTIAL DIAGNOSIS

• Benign tumors of the epididymis

—Leiomyoma
—Papillary cystadenoma (associated with von Hippel-Lindau syndrome)
—Embryomas
—Cholesteatomas
—Teratomas
—Lipomas
—Hamartomas
—Dermoid cyst
—Adrenal cortical adenomas

• Malignant tumors of the epididymis

—Sarcoma (rhabdomyosarcoma, leiomyosarcoma, fibrosarcoma, liposarcoma)
—Melanotic neuroectodermal tumor of the epididymis

• Extension of primary testicular tumor
• Metastatic tumors of the epididymis

—Urologic (prostate, kidney)
—Gastrointestinal (stomach, colon, carcinoid, pancreas)

• Other lesions of the epididymis

—Granuloma (sperm, TB)
—Spermatocele
—Epididymitis
—Sarcoid
—Epidermoid inclusion cyst
—Epididymal abscess

 Database

HISTORY

• Duration of scrotal mass, change in size over time
• Prior malignancy or scrotal surgery
• Symptoms

—Pain or aching sensation
  —Radiation of pain
  —Conditions that ameliorate or exacerbate discomfort

PHYSICAL EXAMINATION

• Scrotum and scrotal contents

—Inspection: symmetry, varicocele
—Palpation: localization of the mass outside of the testes and within the epididymis; fluctuans (hydrocele, spermatocele); examination of the cord structures with and without Valsalva to rule out hernia, or extension to the cord
—Transillumination: to identify the presence of a clear, fluid-filled mass

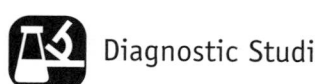 Diagnostic Studies

LABORATORY TESTING

- No specific laboratory tests
- If suspicious for testicular tumor, beta hCG, AFP, and LDH should be obtained prior to inguinal exploration.

IMAGING

- Ultrasound

—Delineates the extent of the adenomatoid tumor and distinguishes it from other tumors of the testes and paratesticular tissues, including testicular cancer, epididymitis, spermatocele

SPECIAL STUDIES: N/A

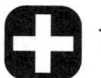 Treatment

GENERAL MEASURES

- The patient should be informed regarding the diagnosis and the intended treatment.
- The patient must realize that an orchiectomy may be indicated based on clinical judgment at the time of surgery, even in the absence of malignancy.
- Frozen-section diagnosis of adenomatoid tumor is not always certain, and when doubt exists regarding the malignant potential of a testicular or paratesticular mass, orchiectomy is the safest course of action.

MEDICAL: N/A

SURGICAL

- Because testicular cancer or papillary cancer of the epididymis cannot be ruled out prior to exploration, an inguinal approach with proximal vascular control is the standard of care.
- Once the testes is delivered, the surgeon may elect to perform biopsy with frozen section to confirm the diagnosis of adenomatoid tumor.
- If there is any doubt regarding the benign nature of the mass, then radical orchiectomy is the prudent treatment.

ALTERNATIVE THERAPIES: N/A

PATIENT EDUCATION: N/A

 Follow-Up

MONITORING

- After excision, no special monitoring is indicated.
- Teach testicular self-examination, to provide early detection of testicular cancer.
- No increased risk of testicular cancer

PREVENTION

- No known method of prevention

 Miscellaneous

SYNONYMS: N/A

ASSOCIATED CONDITIONS

- None known

NOTES

- See also Section I, "Testicular Mass—Adult."

ABBREVIATIONS: N/A

REFERENCES

Frates MC, Benson CB, DiSalvo DN, Brown DL, Laing FC, Doubilet PM. Solid extratesticular masses evaluated with sonography: Pathologic correlation. *Radiology* 1997;204(1):43–46.

Manson AL. Adenomatoid tumor of testicular tunica albuginea mimicking testicular carcinoma. *J Urol* 1988;139(4):819–820.

Tammela TL, Karttunen TJ, Maarainen HP, Hellstrom PA, Mattila SI, Kontturi MJ. Intrascrotal adenomatoid tumors. *J Urol* 1991;146(1):6105.

Author: James F. Donovan, Jr.

Adrenal Adenoma

 Basics

DESCRIPTION

• A benign adrenal cortical neoplasm that may or may not have endocrine activity, generally less than 4 cm in size

EPIDEMIOLOGY

• Rare, usually observed in adults 20 to 60 years of age
• Autopsy incidence of benign adrenal tumors ranges from 1.4% to 8.7%.

GENETICS: N/A

STAGING: N/A

SIGNS AND SYMPTOMS

• Most adenomas are nonfunctional.
• Often discovered incidentally on radiologic studies
• Clinical manifestations result from hormone production.
• Cortisol production causes Cushing syndrome from excess glucocorticoid.

—25% of cases not due to an exogenous source are caused by adrenal neoplasm (adenoma or carcinoma).
  —"Moon" facies and central/truncal obesity or "buffalo" hump
  —Severe muscle wasting common
  —Hirsutism in women and prepubertal boys
  —New-onset diabetes mellitus/hyperglycemia
  —Menstrual abnormalities/sexual dysfunction
  —Osteoporosis
  —Edema

• Aldosterone production

—Primary hyperaldosteronism or Conn syndrome may be caused by adenoma.
—Accounts for 1% of hypertensive patients
—Headaches, polyuria, paresthesia
—The hallmark is hypertension with hypokalemia and without edema.

PATHOPHYSIOLOGY

• Adenoma may consist of cells of either zona glomerulosa (aldosterone) or zona fasciculata (cortisol).
• Generally less than 2 cm in diameter
• Most are unilateral.

CAUSES/RISK FACTORS: N/A

COMPLICATIONS

• Associated with the production of cortisol and/or aldosterone

—Hypertension
—Protein wasting
—Growth arrest in children
—Poor wound healing
—15% with Cushing syndrome develop urinary calculi secondary to hypercalciuria.

DIFFERENTIAL DIAGNOSIS

• Functional

—Adrenal adenoma
—Adrenocortical carcinoma
  —80% functional
—Pheochromocytoma

• Nonfunctional

—Adrenal adenoma
—Metastatic tumors to the adrenal: breast, melanoma, renal cell
—Adrenocortical carcinoma
—Neuroblastoma
—Pheochromocytoma
—Myelolipomas
—Adrenal cysts

 Database

HISTORY

• Recent hair growth
• Oligomenorrhea
• Easy bruising
• Personality changes
• Excessive acne
• Polyuria/polydipsia
• Weakness
• Hypertension

PHYSICAL EXAMINATION

• Findings may suggest a functioning adenoma.
• Central obesity
• Hypertension with or without edema
• Purple striae

Diagnostic Studies

LABORATORY TESTING

• Provides proof of biochemical function

—Electrolytes: hypokalemia, hypernatremia, alkalosis with aldosteronism
—Plasma catecholamines (norepinephrine, epinephrine, and dopamine): elevated with pheochromocytoma
—Cushing syndrome: excess glucocorticoids

• Dexamethasone suppression test
—Based on premise that pituitary ACTH secretion is regulated with negative feedback inhibition by adrenal cortisol
—Normal individuals, dexamethasone 0.5 mg orally every 6 hours for 2 days: significant fall in 17-hydroxycorticosteroid, urinary free cortisol, or plasma cortisol (<5 mg/dL); "low-dose" test
—"High-dose" dexamethasone with 1 mg orally between 11 PM and midnight; check plasma cortisol between 8 and 9 AM.
—An individual with Cushing syndrome shows the inability/resistance to suppression of cortisol.
—"Low-dose" dexamethasone is primarily reserved for patients with equivocal 24-hour urinary cortisol.
—Elevated 17-ketosteroid and DHEA with virilization: more common with adrenal carcinoma causing Cushing syndrome

• Urine tests

—24-hour urinary cortisol: the most reliable index of cortisol secretion
—Elevated urinary metanephrines and catecholamines: pheochromocytoma

IMAGING

• Adenoma: usually solitary, and associated with atrophy of opposite gland

—MRI useful in identifying and characterizing neuroendocrine adrenal tumors
—Adrenal adenoma: slightly hypodense or iso-intense relative to liver/spleen on T1 images, and slightly hyper-intense or iso-intense on T2 images
—Most are larger than 2 cm and are solitary.
—Atrophy of contralateral adrenal gland common
—Adrenal cortical carcinoma
—Generally hypointense on T1 and hyperintense on T2-weighted images
—Often indistinguishable from adenoma except for size (>5 cm)

• CT: 1.5- to 3.0-mm cuts also reportedly accurate
• Size criteria imperative: Nonfunctional solid lesions >5 cm should be removed (increased chance of malignancy).

SPECIAL STUDIES

• Iodinated cholesterol agents for adrenal cortical scanning no longer routinely employed

—Differentiate functional adrenal tissue from retroperitoneal masses
—Identify residual cortical tissue.
—Not useful for diagnosis of adrenal carcinoma

• Fine-needle adrenal biopsy guided by CT or US

Treatment

GENERAL MEASURES

• Determine if functional
• CT scan or MRI to determine size
• Small (<4 cm), nonfunctional lesions do not need treatment.
• Exploration for all lesions >5 cm on imaging study
• Adrenalectomy: treatment of choice if removal is necessary
• Preoperative preparation based on biochemical status of tumors

MEDICAL

• Aminoglutethimide: blocks conversion of cholesterol to pregnenolone
• Metapyrone: blocks conversion of 11-deoxycortisol to cortisol
• Ketoconazole: blocks cytochrome P-450

SURGICAL

• Adrenal adenoma causing Cushing syndrome: surgical removal
• Solid, nonfunctioning adrenal masses between 3 and 5 cm are controversial since a majority are benign.
• The proper surgical approach appears to depend on

—Size of mass; body habitus of patient; underlying cause of adrenal pathology; surgeon preference

• Options for approach

—Eleventh rib (left or right); thoracoabdominal (large masses); posterior (small lesions); laparoscopic

ALTERNATIVE THERAPIES: N/A

PATIENT EDUCATION: N/A

Follow-Up

MONITORING

• Nonfunctional small adrenal lesions: Observe with follow-up by CT or MRI.
• Functional lesions: monitored for activity if surgical removal is deferred

PREVENTION: N/A

Miscellaneous

SYNONYMS: N/A

ASSOCIATED CONDITIONS: N/A

NOTES

• See Section I, "Adrenal Mass."

ABBREVIATIONS

• ACTH, adrenocorticotropic hormone; DHEA, dehydroepiandrosterone

REFERENCES

Blumenfeld JD, Schlussel J, Sealey JE, et al. Diagnosis and treatment of primary hyperaldosteronism. *Ann Intern Med* 1994;121:877–882.

Daitch JA, Goldfarb DA, Novick AC. Cleveland Clinic experience with adrenal Cushing's syndrome. *J Urol* 1997;158(6):2051–2055.

Vaughan ED Jr, Blumenfeld JD. The adrenals. In: Walsh PC, Retik AB, Vaughan ED, Wein AJ, eds. *Campbell's Urology*, 7th ed. Philadelphia: WB Saunders, 1997:2915–2972.

Winfield HN, Hamilton BD, Bravo EL, Novick AC. Laparoscopic adrenalectomy: The preferred choice? A comparison to open adrenalectomy. *J Urol* 1998;160(2):325–329.

Authors: K. Shane Geib and Michael J. Manyak

Adrenal Cortical Carcinoma

 Basics

DESCRIPTION

• Primary malignancy arising in the adrenal cortex

EPIDEMIOLOGY

• Adrenal cortical carcinoma (ACC) is rare; incidence of 0.5 to 2.0 per million population per year
• About 80 to 130 cases in the United States annually
• More common in women and on left side, but of little diagnostic significance
• Bimodal occurrence: initial peak in children <5; second peak in adults 30 to 40

GENETICS

• Linked to Beckwith-Wiedemann syndrome in about 15% with ACC
• Loss of heterozygosity at locus 11p15.5
• Overexpression of insulin-like growth factor-II (IGF); IGF-II gene maps to same locus

STAGING

• See Appendix: TNM Classifications.

SIGNS AND SYMPTOMS

• Either due to functioning tumor or advanced malignancy
• Most common is excess cortisol production (Cushing syndrome) in 50% to 60%, then virilization (20%), or mixed syndromes (20% to 30%)
• Hyperaldosteronism rare
• Signs of Cushing syndrome: moon facies, truncal obesity, buffalo hump, glucose intolerance, and hypokalemia
• Nonfunctioning tumors: pain, nonspecific gastrointestinal complaints, weight loss, fatigue, and abdominal mass
• Average time between onset of symptoms and diagnosis of ACC: 9 months
• Cushing syndrome in children suggested by generalized weight gain and delayed growth
• Aldosterone-producing ACC: hypertension and hypokalemic alkalosis
• Other signs and symptoms of hypokalemia: muscle cramps, polyuria, nocturia, headache, weakness

PATHOPHYSIOLOGY

• Extremely difficult to distinguish benign from malignant adrenal tumors in absence of metastatic disease
• Role of percutaneous needle biopsy limited for this reason
• Pathologic features such as mitotic activity, grade, vascular invasion, various architectural features, and tumor size have not correlated well with prognosis.
• Most (60% to 70%) ACCs are functioning, although this is related to the extent of work-up (cortisol most common, aldosterone).

CAUSES/RISK FACTORS: N/A

COMPLICATIONS

• Fever due to tumor necrosis
• Anemia from hemorrhage into the tumor
• Adrenal crisis in patients who undergo surgery for functioning tumors without adequate steroid prep

DIFFERENTIAL DIAGNOSIS

• Functioning adrenal masses

—Adenoma, aldosteronoma, pheochromocytoma

• Nonfunctioning adrenal masses

—Hemorrhage, cyst, metastatic tumor, neuroblastoma

• Other: renal cell carcinoma

 Database

HISTORY

• Abdominal complaints?

—Symptoms due to a palpable mass are often seen at presentation.
—The patient is often aware of a mass or lump in the upper quadrant.

• Constitutional symptoms?

—Weight loss, malaise, weakness, nausea or vomiting usually associated with poor prognosis

• Change in appearance, unexpected weight gain?

—Suggests functioning ACCs

• Polyuria and polydipsia?

—Possible glucose intolerance or frank diabetes (Cushing syndrome)

PHYSICAL EXAMINATION

• Palpable abdominal mass
• Signs of Cushing syndrome (functional ACCs): violaceous striae, moon facies, truncal obesity, buffalo hump, glucose intolerance, hyperpigmentation

Diagnostic Studies

LABORATORY TESTING

- The initial screen for function in an adrenal mass should include serum electrolytes, serum catecholamines, and a 24-hour urinary free cortisol.
- 24-hour urinary free cortisol: most sensitive measure of excess cortisol production
- Urine levels of cortisol metabolites including 17-hydroxycorticosteroids and 17-ketosteroids may be elevated.
- Other biochemical abnormalities

—Loss of circadian rhythm of cortisol secretion
—Loss of suppressibility of pituitary–adrenal axis
—Low levels of ACTH (due to high cortisol level)

- When an adrenal mass is present and function is demonstrated, additional tests, such as the dexamethasone suppression test, are rarely indicated.

IMAGING

- CT scan of the abdomen: initial study in patients with suspected ACC

—Benign tumors by CT: homogenous appearance, generally <4 to 6 cm, smooth and round or oval contour, and well-delineated margins
—Primary ACCs: irregular contour, invasion of surrounding structures, and nonhomogeneous internal architecture

- MRI of limited value in diagnosis of ACC

—ACCs generally isodense to the liver on T1-weighted images, and hyperintense (brighter white) on T2-weighted images.
—MRI coronal cuts to determine liver invasion or vena caval tumor thrombus

SPECIAL STUDIES: N/A

 Treatment

GENERAL MEASURES

- The prognosis for patients with ACC is poor.
- 70% or more of patients have advanced disease at presentation.
- The prognosis equally poor for functioning and nonfunctioning ACCs.
- Stage at diagnosis is the most important prognostic variable.
- Median survival is <3 years.
- Mean survival of 3 months with unresectable disease

MEDICAL

- Often the first and only treatment of ACC, due to high rate of advanced disease at presentation
- Mitotane (op-DDD), an analog of the insecticide DDT, is the treatment of choice for metastatic ACC.

—Objective regression in tumor size in 35%
—Dosage escalated to tolerance, which is limited
—Late CNS toxicity, particularly depression, often significant
—Both glucocorticoid and mineralocorticoid replacement necessary

- Cytotoxic chemotherapy trials limited by small number of cases

—Cisplatin and etoposide (VP 16) have shown synergistic antitumor activity against ACC.

- Inhibitors of steroid synthesis (metyrapone, aminoglutethimide, and ketoconazole) may be useful in controlling symptoms of glucocorticoid excess.

SURGICAL

- High rate of unresectability; complete surgical resection the only curative therapy
- Adrenal masses with endocrine activity should be resected.
- Adrenal masses >6 cm: high rate of malignancy and should also be resected
- Anterior approach (chevron or subcostal incision) for the rare low-stage ACC
- For more usual advanced ACCs, a thoracoabdominal incision provides optimal exposure.
- En bloc nephrectomy often necessary
- Invasion of vena cava or caval tumor thrombus managed as for renal cell carcinoma
- Extent of caval involvement often determines resectability.
- "Debulking" of ACC of dubious value, at best
- Important to give preoperative steroid preparation for functioning ACCs to avoid adrenal crisis
- While aggressive surgical resection of locally recurrent or metastatic ACC, 5-year survival only 10% to 20% in these patients

ALTERNATIVE THERAPIES: N/A

PATIENT EDUCATION: N/A

 Follow-Up

MONITORING

- Follow-up after resection of ACC: periodic visits for symptom screening and physical examination
- Chest x-ray and CT scans should be done periodically to monitor for local and pulmonary recurrences.
- Serum and urinary steroid levels appropriate for clinical presentation should also be monitored.
- Follow-up should be long-term, since late recurrence of ACC (after 10 or more years) is not uncommon.

PREVENTION: N/A

 Miscellaneous

SYNONYMS

- Adrenocortical carcinoma

ASSOCIATED CONDITIONS

- Cushing syndrome (functioning tumors)
- Beckwith-Wiedemann syndrome

NOTES

- See also Section I, "Adrenal Mass."

ABBREVIATIONS

- ACC, adrenal cortical carcinoma

REFERENCES

Bukowski RM, Klein EA. Management of adrenal neoplasms. In: Vogelzang NJ, et al., eds. *Comprehensive Textbook of Genitourinary Oncology*. Baltimore: Williams & Wilkins, 1996.

Haas GP, et al. Nonsurgical treatment of adrenocortical cancer. In: Raghavan D, et al., eds. *Principles and Practice of Genitourinary Oncology*. Philadelphia: Lippincott-Raven, 1997.

Katz MD, et al. Adrenal cancer: Endocrinology, diagnosis and clinical staging. In: Raghavan D, et al., eds. *Principles and Practice of Genitourinary Oncology*. Philadelphia: Lippincott-Raven, 1997.

Author: Robert P. Huben

Adrenal Hemorrhage

 Basics

DESCRIPTION

• Adrenal hemorrhage (AH) is a collection of blood producing a mass effect in one or both adrenal glands with or without adrenal necrosis and insufficiency.

EPIDEMIOLOGY

• Detected with increasing frequency
• Up to 30% of selected neonatal intensive care patients
• 14% to 22% of newborns at autopsy
• Up to 15% at autopsy of adult patients dying in shock
• Male to female ratio 3:2 in bilateral adrenal hemorrhage (BAH)
• 75% right-sided in unilateral AH

GENETICS: N/A

STAGING: N/A

SIGNS AND SYMPTOMS

• Neonatal: Unilateral AH may be an incidental finding of imaging an abdominal mass, unexplained jaundice, or anemia.
• General: fever, flank or abdominal pain, tachycardia, nausea, vomiting, respiratory distress, weakness

PATHOPHYSIOLOGY

• Anatomic and physiologic considerations: enlarged; very vascular glands in newborn
• Adrenal: high blood flow via many arteries, with limited, high-resistance venous outflow; "vascular dam."
• Pathology: hemorrhage and hemorrhagic necrosis
• Mechanisms: multiple mechanisms; stress, sepsis, anticoagulation-related hypotension, vascular spasm, adrenal venous thrombosis, heparin-associated thrombocytopenia

—Chronic adrenal stimulation (burns, sepsis, etc.); produces necrosis and hemorrhage
—Catecholamine concentration may induce venous obstruction and thrombosis.
—Heparin-induced thrombocytopenia

CAUSES/RISK FACTORS

• High-stress conditions
• Birth trauma, large birth weight
• Severe sepsis, Waterhouse-Friderichsen syndrome, meningococcal sepsis
• Surgical causes: open heart surgery, joint replacement, burns
• Obstetric causes: preeclampsia, hyperemesis gravidarum
• Other: coagulopathy, thromboembolic disease (35%); primary antiphospholipid antibody, ACTH therapy, heparinization, trauma, orthotopic liver transplantation, renal vein thrombosis, hypothrombinemia, hypotension-shock, CMV, corticosteroid therapy

COMPLICATIONS

• Cardiovascular collapse and death secondary to adrenal insufficiency (mortality 15%, current series)
• Chronic adrenal insufficiency (rare in neonates; common in adults with BAH)
• Abscess
• Hyperbilirubinemia

DIFFERENTIAL DIAGNOSIS

• Neonate: neuroblastoma, adrenal cyst, Wilms' tumor, cortical renal cyst, obstructed upper renal moiety
• Adult/general: sepsis, postoperative bleeding, cardiovascular collapse (not of adrenal insufficiency), adrenal malignancy, or hyperplasia or metastases

 Database

HISTORY

• Stress or highly stressful illness: birth trauma, trauma, burns, heparin therapy, surgery (cardiac or orthopedic), complicated pregnancy with clinical deterioration of unclear etiology (variable timing: 2 to 10 days postevent).

PHYSICAL EXAMINATION

• Provides few clues; findings are nonspecific.
• Fever is frequently present (50%).
• Pain is common in adult patients (back, abdomen, or flank; 66%).
• Abdominal examination is strikingly unremarkable in adults (guarding in 15%).
• In neonates, a flank or abdominal mass may be palpable.
• Hypotension is usually absent prior to cardiovascular collapse if adrenal insufficiency ensues.
• Tachycardia
• Obtundation, weakness, lethargy (12%)

Diagnostic Studies

LABORATORY TESTING

- CBC: dropping hematocrit, hemoglobin; common
—Eosinophilia; rare
- Electrolyte abnormalities; hyponatremia, hyperkalemia 56% of BAH
- Serum cortisol (may be normal)
- Serum catecholamines, serum bilirubin

IMAGING

- Excretory urography: old study showing renal displacement by a suprarenal lucency
- Renal ultrasound: good initial study; echogenic mass evolves into cystic mass with subsequent lysis and degeneration; shrinkage and calcification (shell-like) over 6 to 8 weeks
- CAT scan: adrenal enlargement with increased tissue attenuation
- MRI: useful in differentiating hemorrhage from tumor. An initially enlarged adrenal has an intermediate-intensity center and a high-intensity outer ring; 5 to 6 weeks later, the hematoma shrinks and inner intensity increases while outer intensity decreases.

SPECIAL STUDIES

- Cortrosyn stimulation test: 250 μg of synthetic ACTH (cosyntropin) IV; serum cortisol is drawn prior to and 1 hour postinjection.
- A nonstressed response would be an increase of 7 μg/dL cortisol or a peak greater than 20 μg/dL.

 ## Treatment

GENERAL MEASURES

- Replacement of fluids, electrolytes, and blood if hemorrhage is significant

MEDICAL

- Steroid replacement as soon as adrenal insufficiency is suspected
- IV dexamethasone (will not interfere with Cortrosyn test)
- Long-term steroid replacement rarely required in neonates; often required in adults that survive BAH

SURGICAL

- Exploration for uncontrollable hemorrhage, uncertain diagnosis, or abscess formation

ALTERNATIVE THERAPIES: N/A

PATIENT EDUCATION

- Potential need for long-term steroid supplementation

 ## Follow-Up

MONITORING

- Intensive care setting initially; serial H/H, electrolytes
- Serial imaging: CT, ultrasound, or MRI to demonstrate shrinkage of mass

PREVENTION: N/A

 ## Miscellaneous

SYNONYMS: N/A

ASSOCIATED CONDITIONS

- Birth trauma, primary antiphospholipid syndrome, meningococcal septicemia

NOTES: N/A

ABBREVIATIONS

- AH, adrenal hemorrhage; BAH, bilateral adrenal hemorrhage

REFERENCES

Felc Z, Zlata X. Ultrasound in screening for neonatal adrenal hemorrhage. *Am J Perinatol* 1995; 12(5):363.

McCroskey RD, et al. Antiphospholipid antibodies and adrenal hemorrhage. *Am J Hematol* 1991; 36:60–62.

Rao R, et al. Bilateral massive adrenal hemorrhage. *Med Clin North Am* 1995;79(1):107.

Siu SC, et al. Adrenal insufficiency from bilateral adrenal hemorrhage. *Mayo Clin Proc* 1990;65: 664–670.

Author: Mark V. Jarowenko

Adrenal Medullary Neuroblastoma

 Basics

DESCRIPTION

• Tumor arising from the adrenal medulla or other paraganglionic tissues of neural crest origin

EPIDEMIOLOGY

• Neuroblastoma in general

—Tumor of childhood with a few adult cases reported

—7% to 8% of all childhood malignancies

—Most common malignant tumor in infancy and most common extracranial solid tumor of childhood

—US annual incidence: 10 per one million live births

—No sex-related difference in incidence

—75% of cases occur by fourth year of life.

—37% of neuroblastomas arise from the adrenal medulla.

GENETICS

• Numerous karyotypic abnormalities: chromosomal deletions, translocations, gene amplification

—Deletion of short arm of chromosome 1: 70% to 80% of patients

• 20% of cases are familial: inheritance pattern is postulated to be autosomal dominant.

STAGING

Evans Staging System

Stage I	Tumor confined to organ of origin
Stage II	Tumor extending in continuity beyond the organ or structure or origin, but not crossing the midline. Regional nodes on the ipsilateral side may be involved
Stage III	Tumor extending in continuity beyond the midline. Regional nodes may be involved bilaterally
Stage IV	Remote disease involving skeleton, organs, soft tissues, or distant nodes
Stage IVS	Patients who would otherwise be stage I or II but have remote disease confined to liver, skin, and/or bone marrow

International Neuroblastoma Staging System

Stage I	Localized tumor with complete gross excision, with ipsilateral nodes negative for tumor microscopically
Stage IIA	Localized tumor with incomplete gross excision, with ipsilateral nonadherent nodes negative for tumor
Stage IIB	Localized tumor with or without complete gross excision, with ipsilateral nonadherent nodes positive for tumor
Stage III	Unresectable unilateral tumor infiltrating across the midline, with or without regional node involvement
Stage IV	Any primary tumor with dissemination to distant nodes and other organs/structures except those defined in stage IVS
Stage IVS	Localized primary tumor (as I, IIA, IIB) with dissemination limited to skin, liver, and/or bone marrow

SIGNS AND SYMPTOMS

• Ill-appearing, fever, malaise, weight loss
• Abdominal pain, abdominal mass, typically firm and irregular, often extending across midline
• Paroxysmal hypertension, palpitation, flushing, headache
• Watery diarrhea (VIP-secreting tumors)
• Acute myoclonic encephalopathy (myoclonus, multidirectional eye movements, and truncal ataxia)
• Bone pain (bone metastasis)
• Proptosis and periorbital ecchymosis (periorbital metastasis)
• Subcutaneous nodules (skin metastasis)
• Pallor (bone marrow metastasis)

PATHOPHYSIOLOGY

• Gross pathology: variable appearance, depending on the degree of stromal elements; usually pale gray to light red tumors; areas of necrosis, hemorrhage, cyst formation, and calcification are common
• Histology: one of the small blue cell tumors; arrangement of cells in pseudorosette pattern is characteristic but present in only 50% cases; lobular growth pattern
• Electron microscopy: neurosecretory granules representing accumulations of catecholamines present in cytoplasm

CAUSES/RISK FACTORS

• Causes: unknown; but a genetic influence is apparent (see "Genetics" above)
• Risk factors: Prenatal exposure to alcohol may increase the risk.

COMPLICATIONS

• Usually specific to sites of metastasis: bone fracture in bone metastasis; anemia in bone marrow metastasis; coagulopathy in liver metastasis

DIFFERENTIAL DIAGNOSIS

• Wilm's tumor
• Adrenal medullary tumors: pheochromocytoma, ganglioneuroma, ganglioneuroblastoma
• Adrenal cortical tumors: adrenal cortical carcinoma, adenoma, sarcoma
• Retroperitoneal sarcomas
• Metastasis to adrenal gland

 Database

HISTORY

• Unexplained fever, anorexia, weight loss, malaise, diarrhea, bone pain, flushing, headache, palpitation
• Family history of neuroblastoma

PHYSICAL EXAMINATION

• Pallor, hypertension
• Abdominal mass: typically firm, irregular, fixed
• Bluish subcutaneous nodules (skin metastasis)
• Proptosis and periorbital ecchymosis (periorbital metastasis)
• Myoclonus, rapid multidirectional eye movements, and truncal ataxia

Diagnostic Studies

LABORATORY TESTING

• Serum

—Neuron-specific enolase: elevation in >90% cases with metastasis

—Ferritin level: elevation in 40% to 50% cases with advanced stage (elevation is a poor prognostic sign)

—Hemoglobin/hematocrit: low in cases with bone marrow metastasis

—Coagulation profile: abnormal in liver metastasis

—Norepinephrine level: not usually elevated

• Urine

—24-hour urine VMA and HVA: elevation (>3 standard deviations above the mean per milligram for age) of one or both in 90% of patients

IMAGING

• Abdominal plain film: speckled pattern of calcification in 50% cases

• Ultrasound: suprarenal mass; good for assessing IVC involvement

• IVP: inferior displacement of kidney by a suprarenal mass; usually not obtained for diagnostic evaluation

• CT: suprarenal mass often with calcification; inferior displacement of kidney

• MRI: suprarenal mass; good for assessing IVC involvement and relationship of tumor to great vessels; spine bone scan/bone plain film skeletal survey: good for assessing cortical bone metastasis

• MIBG scan: good for assessing extent of disease in bones and soft tissues

• Chest x-ray to rule out lung metastasis (although rare)

SPECIAL STUDIES

• Bone marrow aspiration and marrow biopsy in all patients to rule out bone marrow involvement

• Pathologic tissue diagnosis based on standard methods, including ultrastructural studies

 ## Treatment

GENERAL MEASURES

• Therapy based on stage of disease

—Surgical excision if disease is localized

—If excision is not feasible, chemotherapy to reduce tumor size, followed by surgical excision

MEDICAL

• Chemotherapeutic agents for advanced stages (III, IV) include cyclophosphamide, doxorubicin, cisplatin, epipodophyllotoxins, vincristine, and dicarbazine (as single agent or in combination)

SURGICAL

• Resection in stages I and II: can be considered as part of multimodal therapy in stage IVS

• Controversial role in stages III and IV; may be performed after initial chemotherapy

ALTERNATIVE THERAPIES

• Radiotherapy

—Intraoperative radiation to achieve local tumor control in unresectable disease

—May be cytoreductive in stages III and IV before secondary resection or for palliation of metastasis

—Autologous bone marrow transplant: performed after chemotherapy and total body irradiation in stage IV

PATIENT EDUCATION

• http://cancer.med.upenn.edu/disease/neuroblast

• http://noah.ouny.edu/cancer/nci/cancernet/200530.html

• http://nuomedweb.tch.harvard.edu/Patient/Tumor/neuroblastoma.html

• http://www.stayhealthy.com

 ## Follow-Up

MONITORING

• Urinary VMA and HVA levels (every 3 months for 2 years), CT scan and/or MRI of abdomen (every 6 months for 2–5 years), and MIBG scan (every year) are usually used to detect recurrence after treatment.

• 1% to 2% cases: spontaneous regression or maturation into benign ganglioneuroblastoma and ganglioneuroma; usually in first year of life; usually with stage IVS disease

• Adrenal origin: The survival rate tends to be worse than in those with nonadrenal origin.

• Favorable prognostic factors: young age at diagnosis (<1 yr), low stage (I or II), favorable histology (high degree of differentiation), DNA aneuploidy, normal serum ferritin level (<150 ng/mL), normal serum neuron-specific enolase level (<100 ng/mL), low number of copies of

N-myc oncogene copies (<10) in cytogenetic study

• Stage IVS patients tend to have >80% survival rate.

• Survival for 2 years without evidence of disease is usually equivalent to cure.

PREVENTION

• Current genetic studies may lead to future gene therapy, allowing correction of the genetic defect.

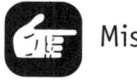 ## Miscellaneous

SYNONYMS

• Neuroblastoma

ASSOCIATED CONDITIONS

• Neurofibromatosis, Hirschsprung disease; an increased incidence of brain and skull defects has been reported.

NOTES

• See also Section I, "Adrenal Mass."

ABBREVIATIONS

• VIP, vasoactive intestinal peptide; VMA, vanillylmandelic acid; HVA, homovanillic acid; IVC, inferior vena cava; MIBG, ^{123}I-metaiodobenzylguanidine

REFERENCES

Brodeur GM, et al. Revision of the international criteria for neuroblastoma diagnosis, staging, and response to treatment. *J Clin Oncol* 1993; 11:1466.

Evans AE, et al. A proposed staging system for children with neuroblastoma. *Cancer* 1971; 27:1799.

Ritchey MC, et al. Pediatric urologic oncology. In: Gillenwater JY, Grayhack JT, Howards SS, Duckett JW, eds. *Adult and Pediatric Urology*, 3rd ed. St Louis: Mosby, 1996.

Seeler RA, et al. Ganglioneuroblastoma and fetal hydantoin-alcohol syndromes. *Pediatrics* 1979;63:S24.

Authors: Thomas H.S. Hsu, Jonathan Ross, and Eric A. Klein

Adrenogenital Syndrome

 Basics

DESCRIPTION

- Most common cause of ambiguous genitalia caused by an inborn error of metabolism involving cortisol synthesis. Caused by a defect in any one of five enzymes involved in the cortisol biosynthetic pathway (21-hydroxylase, 11-hydroxylase, 3-hydroxysteroid dehydrogenase, 20,22-desmolase, or 17-hydroxylase), which may result in congenital adrenal hyperplasia (CAH)

EPIDEMIOLOGY (21-hydroxylase deficiency)

- Incidence

—Classic form: 1:15,000 to 1:10,000
—Milder, nonclassic form: 1:500

- Prevalence: accounts for 95% of patients with CAH
- Sex

—Females: variable degrees of masculinization; 50% salt-losing crisis
—Males: normal genitalia; 50% salt-losing crisis

- Age: female pseudohermaphroditism recognized as newborn; salt-losing crisis between 6 and 14 days of age
- Race: Including the nonclassic form, CAH is the most common autosomal recessive inherited disease in Caucasians.

GENETICS

- Autosomal recessive

—21-hydroxylase: gene locus on chromosome 6 within the HLA complex
—11B-hydroxylase: gene locus on chromosome 8
—3-hydroxysteroid dehydrogenase: gene locus on chromosome 1
—20,22-desmolase: mutation of steroidogenic acute regulatory protein (StAR)
—17-hydroxylase: gene locus on chromosome 10

STAGING: N/A

SIGNS AND SYMPTOMS

- 21-hydroxylase: females with variable degree of masculinization; males have normal genitalia; both have 50% salt-losing crisis with dehydration and shock
- 11-hydroxylase: ambiguous genitalia in female; mild salt wasting in infancy or hypertension in childhood
- 3-hydroxysteroid dehydrogenase: mild virilization in female; pseudohermaphroditism in male; severe salt wasting
- 20,22-desmolase: All patients are phenotypic female (regardless of karyotype).
- 17-hydroxylase: female infantilism; male pseudohermaphroditism; hypertension

PATHOPHYSIOLOGY

- Enzyme disorder in which the conversion of cholesterol to cortisol is impaired. The loss of cortisol feedback on the pituitary leads to high levels of ACTH and results in adrenal hyperplasia. Depending on the site of enzymatic block, precursors may be shunted to mineralocorticoid or sex steroid production

—21-hydroxylase
—Type I: defect limited to zona fasciculata; normal aldosterone levels
—Type II: defect involves granulosa, causing deficiency of mineralocorticoid; leads to salt/water loss
—11-hydroxylase: accumulation of deoxycorticosterone (DOC), a potent mineralocorticoid; leads to hypertension and masculinization
—3-hydroxysteroid dehydrogenase: high levels of dehydroepiandrosterone (DHEA) converted to testosterone
—20,22-desmolase: All steroid hormone production is prevented.
—17-hydroxylase: prevents production of cortisol and sex steroids; mineralocorticoid production is high

CAUSES/RISK FACTORS

- Autosomal recessive inheritance (see "Genetics")

COMPLICATIONS

- For untreated females

—Premature pubic and axillary hair development
—Rapid somatic maturation, premature epiphyseal closure, short adult stature
—No breast development or menstruation until excessive androgen production is suppressed

- For untreated males

—Sexual and somatic precocity within first 2 years of life
—Premature epiphyseal closure, short adult stature

- Untreated males and females with salt-losing variant

—Progressive weight loss, dehydration within first few weeks of life

DIFFERENTIAL DIAGNOSIS

- Female pseudohermaphroditism

—From 21-hydroxylase or 11-hydroxylase deficiencies
—Rule out males with hypospadias and bilateral undescended testes.

- Male pseudohermaphroditism

—Adrenogenital causes (3-hydroxysteroid dehydrogenase, 17-hydroxylase); extremely rare
—Rule out other forms of male pseudohermaphroditism (true hermaphrodite, partial androgen insensitivity, 5-reductase deficiency).

- Apparently normal male with salt-losing variant

—From 21-hydroxylase deficiency
—Severe vomiting may mimic pyloric stenosis.

 Database

HISTORY

- Family history

—Abnormal sexual development
—Unexplained infant deaths (possible metabolic cause)

PHYSICAL EXAMINATION

- Female pseudohermaphrodite from 21-hydroxylase or 11-hydroxylase deficiencies

—Enlarged clitoris
—Sometimes may be indistinguishable from a normal newborn male penis
—If both gonads are not palpable, suspect a diagnosis of CAH, no matter how much the phallus resembles a penis.
—Fusion and rugosity of labioscrotal folds resembling a scrotum without gonads
—Areolar hyperpigmentation
—Uterus and vagina are present; the vagina usually enters a common urogenital sinus.
—No testis

Diagnostic Studies

LABORATORY TESTING

- Serum electrolytes
—Detect electrolyte disturbance (hyperkalemia)
- Karyotype
—Especially to rule out 46,XX female pseudohermaphrodite
- Plasma 17-hydroxyprogesterone
—Elevated greater than 100-fold in 21-hydroxylase deficiency (also elevated in 3-hydroxysteroid dehydrogenase deficiency)
- Additional specific tests to determine other forms of CAH
—11-hydroxylase deficiency: elevated serum 11-deoxycortisol and DOC
—3-hydroxysteroid dehydrogenase deficiency: high serum ratio of 17-hydroxypregnenolone/17-hydroxyprogesterone
—17-hydroxylase deficiency: high levels of serum mineralocorticoid

IMAGING

- Female pseudohermaphrodite
—Genitogram: demonstrates urogenital sinus, urethra, bladder, vagina, cervix, uterus
—Ultrasound: demonstrates uterus
—Cystovaginoscopy
  —Usually not part of initial diagnostic study
  —Augments the findings from genitogram
  —Important in providing distance from the bladder neck to the vaginal entry into urogenital sinus; enables planning for type of vaginoplasty

SPECIAL STUDIES: N/A

 Treatment

GENERAL MEASURES

- It is important to diagnose the condition in the newborn to provide correct gender assignment and prevent possible metabolic consequences.
- Introduction of the family to a team of care providers, including pediatric urologist, primary physician, geneticist, endocrinologist, and possibly psychiatrist, will help establish a long-term relationship.
- Newborn genotypic females with ambiguous genitalia have normal female internal structures and should be raised as girls.

MEDICAL

- Cortisone replacement
—Supplies deficient hormone; suppresses pituitary ACTH secretion, adrenal androgen production, virilization
—Prevents rapid somatic growth and premature epiphyseal closure
—Permits normal gonadal development
—Corrects salt/water loss or hypertension
—Hydrocortisone: 10 to 15 mg daily
- Fluorohydrocortisone
—Mineralocorticoid replacement in children who are salt losers
—May even be beneficial in non–salt-losing patients by reducing cortisone requirements
—Fluorohydrocortisone: 0.05 to 0.10 mg daily

SURGICAL

- Feminization genitoplasty
—Clitoral reduction
—Usually performed at 6 months of age to correct the phallic structure which is disturbing to parents
—Anesthesia risk minimized by 6 months
—At surgery, the enlarged erectile clitoral bodies are reduced while preserving the neurovascular innervation.
- Vaginoplasty
—Usually performed at the time of clitoral reduction
—The vagina is detached from its entrance into the urogenital sinus, and a new separate vaginal opening is created.
—For severe forms, where the vagina enters the urogenital sinus high near the bladder neck, the vaginoplasty is postponed until the child is older.

PATIENT EDUCATION

- Address the need for medical management and issues concerning sexual development.

 Follow-Up

MONITORING

- Long-term cortisone replacement should be administered under the supervision of a pediatric endocrinologist.
- In children with salt loss, most tend to outgrow their need for fluorohydrocortisone by the time they are 6 years old.

PREVENTION

- Prenatal diagnosis of CAH in the at-risk fetus is possible in the first trimester
—HLA typing or DNA analysis
—Chorionic villus cells provide diagnosis by 8 to 10 weeks' gestation.
—Cells from amniotic fluid provide diagnosis at 16 to 17 weeks' gestation.
—Treatment of mothers with dexamethasone (20 g/kg/d), which crosses placenta, may suppress fetal secretion of ACTH, thereby preventing virilization of female genitalia.
—Potential problems with dexamethasone therapy
  —Heterogenous response: There is no response in about one-third.
  —The ideal time for instituting treatment is 5 to 6 weeks of gestation (prior to availability of fetal diagnosis).

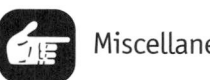 Miscellaneous

SYNONYMS

- Congenital adrenal hyperplasia, female pseudohermaphrodite, male pseudohermaphrodite

ASSOCIATED CONDITIONS: N/A

NOTES

- See also Section I, "Ambiguous Genitalia."

ABBREVIATIONS

- ACTH, adrenocorticotropic hormone; CAH, congenital adrenal hyperplasia; DHEA, dehydroepiandrosterone; DOC, deoxycorticosterone; StAR, steroidogenic acute regulatory protein

REFERENCES

Newman K., Randolph J, Anderson K. The surgical management of infants and children with ambiguous genitalia. Lessons learned from 25 years. *Ann Surg* 1992;215:644–653.

Pang S. Congenital adrenal hyperplasia. *Endocrinol Metab Clin North Am* 1997;26:853–891.

Authors: Harry P. Koo and David A. Bloom

Amyloidosis—Genitourinary

 Basics

DESCRIPTION

- Amyloidosis results from the deposited insoluble, fibrous amyloid proteins in the extracellular spaces of organs and tissues.
- Amyloidosis is classified according to the biochemical nature of the fibril-forming protein.
- Multiple clinical and biochemical distinct forms of amyloid exist.
- Over 14 different classifications of amyloid are classified generally under systemic amyloidosis (which include biochemically distinct forms that are neoplastic, inflammatory, genetic, or iatrogenic in origin) and under localized or organ-limited amyloidosis, which occurs in isolated organs without evidence of systemic involvement.

EPIDEMIOLOGY

- Mean age is 65 years at diagnosis.
- Incidence is 9 per million per year.

GENETICS

- Familial clustering suggested (familial Mediterranean fever)

STAGING: N/A

SIGNS AND SYMPTOMS

- General, highly variable depending on the organ systems involved

—Fatigue, weight loss, gastroparesis, malabsorption, pseudointestinal obstruction
—Dyspnea, CHF
—Polyarteritis, soft-tissue swelling

- Kidney: associated with multisystem amyloidosis, proteinuria, nephrotic syndrome, renal insufficiency

—May be organ specific or as part of systemic amyloidosis

- Bladder: hematuria, irritative voiding symptoms. Polypoid or ulcerative are masses often confused with cancer.
- Ureteral: obstructive symptoms, anuria when bilateral involvement, hematuria
- Urethral obstructive symptoms: hematuria
- Adrenal: signs and symptoms of adrenal insufficiency

PATHOPHYSIOLOGY

- All forms of amyloidosis involve the extracellular deposit of protein, characteristic fibrillar aggregates, which interfere with the tissue structure and function.
- Amyloid fibrils are derived from different unrelated proteins in different forms of the disease.
- Amyloid fibrils share many common properties, including the capacity to bind the normal plasma protein, serum amyloid P component (SAP).
- Tissue staining with Congo red to identify amyloid; electron microscopy is definitive tool
- Primary amyloidosis: plasma cell disorders (multiple myeloma)
- Secondary amyloidosis: associated with chronic inflammatory diseases (i.e., rheumatoid arthritis, osteomyelitis, TB, etc.)
- Patients on hemodialysis can have amyloid accumulation in the kidney.

CAUSES/RISK FACTORS

- Chronic inflammatory disorders
- Chronic infectious disease (TB)
- Neoplastic disorders
- Familial disorders
- Hemodialysis

COMPLICATIONS

- Renal: nephrotic syndrome
- Bladder: hematuria
- Ureter: obstruction, anuria
- Urethra: obstruction, hematuria

DIFFERENTIAL DIAGNOSIS

- Bladder: carcinoma of the bladder
- Ureter: stone disease, carcinoma
- Urethral stricture, carcinoma
- See also causes of nephrotic syndrome and renal failure

 Database

HISTORY

- History of hemodialysis?
- Chronic illnesses?
- Family members affected?

PHYSICAL EXAMINATION

- No specific physical findings
- If nephrotic syndrome, may see edema

Diagnostic Studies

LABORATORY TESTING

- Anemia common
- Renal failure in 50% at initial presentation
- Proteinuria in up to 80%
- Serum/urine electrophoresis will demonstrate monoclonal protein levels.

IMAGING

- Ultrasound/IVP/CT may demonstrate ureteral obstruction.

SPECIAL STUDIES

- Cystoscopy, biopsy bladder
- Biopsy of other organ systems
- Diagnosis by biopsy and special studies

—Electron microscopy
—Special stains, Congo red

 ## Treatment

GENERAL MEASURES

- Therapy should be directed at the underlying disorder.
- Hemodialysis for amyloidosis has no definite therapy, except for transplantation.

MEDICAL

- Plasma cell disorder therapy

—Medphalan, prednisone
—Colchicine may slow amyloid deposition.

SURGICAL

- Bladder lesions: transurethral resection
- Urethra: excision
- Ureters: excision, stenting/diversion
- Renal transplantation
- Splenectomy may help slow amyloid deposition.

ALTERNATIVE THERAPIES: N/A

PATIENT EDUCATION: N/A

 ## Follow-Up

MONITORING

- Based on site of involvement: cystoscopy, urethroscopy, ureteroscopy
- Imaging: ultrasound, IVP
- Primary amyloidosis: Once renal failure develops, prognosis is usually <1 year.

—Overall prognosis is 12 to 14 months.

- Secondary amyloidosis: prognosis better, related to primary disease

PREVENTION

- Reduce risk factors of the underlying disease.

 ## Miscellaneous

SYNONYMS: N/A

ASSOCIATED CONDITIONS: N/A

NOTES: N/A

ABBREVIATIONS: N/A

REFERENCES

Adler S, et al. Sensory glomerular disease. In: Brenner B, ed. *The Kidney*. Philadelphia: WB Saunders, 1996, pp. 1536–1541.

Kyle RA. Clinical aspects of multiple myeloma and related diseases including amyloidosis. *Pathol Biol* 1999;47(2):148–157.

Author: Joseph Mowad

Anorectal Malformations

 Basics

DESCRIPTION

• Anorectal malformations (ARMs): congenital anomalies characterized by absence of anus or of anus and distal rectum and, often, by an anomalous connection (fistula) between the bowel and either the perineal skin or the urinary tract in males or the genital tract in females
• Urogenital sinus: common channel into which both urethra and vagina open
• Cloaca: complex malformation resulting from the combination of an anorectal agenesis and an urogenital sinus

EPIDEMIOLOGY

• Incidence: 1 in 5000 live births (varies from 1:1800 to 1:10,000)
• Male:female ratio: 3:2
• High lesions more frequent in males; low lesions in females

GENETICS

• ARMs often occur as isolated malformations.
• More than 25 families with multiple affected members reported in literature
• Pattern of inheritance is unclear.
• ARMs may be part of a syndrome.

—VACTERL syndrome (vertebral, anorectal, cardiac, tracheoesophageal, renal)
—Currarino triad (anorectal stenosis, presacral mass, sacral bony anomaly): autosomal dominant
—Townes-Brocks syndrome (imperforate anus, sensorineural deafness, bony anomalies of the hand)
—Cat-eye syndrome (hypertelorism, coloboma, microphthalmia, imperforate anus): acrocentric chromosome of group G

STAGING

• The most recent accepted classification of ARMs is the "Wingspread" classification (1984).

—ARMs are classified into high, intermediate, and low, depending on the relationship of the terminal bowel or fistula to the pelvic diaphragm.
  —High anomalies in the male
    —Rectal atresia
    —Anorectal agenesis with rectovesical or rectoprostatic fistula
    —Anorectal agenesis without fistula
  —High anomalies in the female
    —Rectal atresia
    —Anorectal agenesis with rectovaginal fistula
    —Anorectal agenesis without fistula
  —Intermediate anomalies in the male
    —Anal agenesis without fistula
    —Anal agenesis with rectobulbar fistula
—Intermediate anomalies in the female
  —Anal agenesis without fistula
  —Anal agenesis with rectovaginal or rectovestibular fistula
—Low anomalies in the male
  —Anocutaneous fistula
  —Anal stenosis
—Low anomalies in the female
  —Anovestibular fistula
  —Anocutaneous fistula
  —Anal stenosis
  —Urogenital sinus may occur.
—Isolated
  —As a component of ambiguous genitalia in intersexual conditions
  —Together with imperforate anus as a cloacal malformation

SIGNS AND SYMPTOMS

• Most anorectal anomalies are detected after birth at the physical examination of newborn.
• Rectal atresia with an apparently normal anus and anorectal stenosis may be discovered later.
• If untreated, an imperforate anus causes symptoms of intestinal obstruction; the presence of a sizable perineal or vaginal fistula delays the onset and reduces the severity of symptoms.
• Meconium may be observed at the perineal or vaginal fistula site or at the urethral meatus in males with high/intermediate anomalies.
• A short sacrum, a flat perineum, and poor muscular contraction suggest a high anomaly.
• A normal sacrum, a well-conformed perineum, and a perineal midline raphe suggest a low anomaly.
• A single perineal opening with small external genitalia in a female point to the presence of a cloaca.
• A midline low abdominal mass in a female affected by a cloaca is due to a hydrometrocolpos.
• A single perineal orifice anterior to a normal anus implies the presence of an isolated urogenital sinus. External genitalia are often anomalous.
• An isolated urogenital sinus may be discovered late in life; it may be asymptomatic or cause

—Urinary incontinence due to short urethra
—Urinary retention
—Hydrometrocolpos or hematocolpos at puberty

PATHOPHYSIOLOGY

- The external sphincter complex is normal in low and intermediate anomalies and hypoplastic in high malformations.
- The internal sphincter is rudimentary.
- Associated malformations

—Vertebral anomalies
- Affect 30% to 50% of patients
- Spinal dysraphism (tethered cord, lipoma, or syringohydromyelia) in 17% of low, in 34% of high, and in 47% of cloacal anomalies
- The lumbosacral spine is frequently abnormal; complete or partial sacral agenesis is the most common vertebral anomaly.
—Skeletal anomalies
- Radial aplasia (2% to 4%)
—Gastrointestinal anomalies
- Esophageal atresia (6% to 10%)
- Duodenal atresia (1% to 2%)
- Hirschsprung disease and related conditions (incidence is debated)
—Cardiovascular anomalies
- Incidence: 12% to 22%. Tetralogy of Fallot and ventricular septal defects most common
—Genitourinary anomalies: most common associated anomalies (20% and 60% in low and high anomalies, respectively)
- Vesicoureteric reflux (VUR) (33% to 59%)
- Renal agenesis and dysplasia (39%)
- Cryptorchidism (10%)
- Hypospadias (6%)
- Neurogenic bladder secondary to sacral malformations
- Female genital abnormalities
- Overall incidence (high anomalies): 30% to 40%
- Bicornuate uterus or uterus Didelphis
- Vaginal septum
- Urogenital sinus
- Frequently found in intersexual states or associated with an anorectal malformation as a cloacal anomaly, rarely as an isolated malformation
- When the urethra and vagina join close to the bladder neck, the urogenital sinus is long (>3 cm) and urinary continence is often compromised.
- When the urethra and vagina join distally, the urogenital sinus is short (<3 cm).
- The urethra and vagina share a tract of common wall. Genital anomalies are frequently associated.

CAUSES/RISK FACTORS

- Two embryologic theories:

—Classical theory: ARMs are due to a failure of the urorectal septum in its downgrowth to fuse with the lateral Rathke's folds and divide the cloacal membrane into an anterior urogenital and a posterior anal membrane.
—Modern theory: ARMs are due to an anomaly of the dorsal cloacal membrane that doesn't reach the tail gut, but is displaced anteriorly by a mesenchymal mass. The size of the mass will determine whether the ARMs will be low or high.

COMPLICATIONS

- Mortality is related to associated malformations; it ranges from 5% for low to 15% for high malformations.
- Voiding dysfunctions (7%–18%) are either secondary to sacral agenesis or present after rectal surgery due to iatrogenic nerve damage.
- Giant hydrocolpos may cause respiratory distress in the newborn.
- UTI may be caused by the vesicoureteric reflux and/or the presence of a communication between intestine and the urinary tract.
- Hyperchloremic acidosis is due to the presence of urine in the bowel, causing absorption of chloride ions and excretion of bicarbonate by the intestinal wall.
- Constipation: most frequently after repair of low anomalies (30%–60%); improves with age

—Much less frequent in high anomalies (20%–30%)

- Fecal incontinence

—Continence is related to the type of anomaly, the coexistence of sacral defects, and the surgical technique used for repair.
—Continence after repair of low anomalies is achieved in 90% of patients.
—Intermediate and high anomalies: Continence ranges from 25% to 65% after posterior sagittal anorectoplasty (PSARP).
—Obstetric complications are reported in females with cloacal and high anorectal anomalies associated with vaginal or uterine malformations.

DIFFERENTIAL DIAGNOSIS

- Differential diagnosis between a low and a high anomaly is mandatory in the newborn to decide proper management.
- A perineal fistula in the male is always associated with a low anomaly.
- It may take 24 hours before gas or meconium appears in the perineum through an often tiny orifice.
- Meconium in the urine deposes for a high malformation.
- In the female

—Single perineal opening with small external genitalia: cloaca
—Two perineal orifices: high malformation
—Three perineal orifices: low or intermediate malformation (imaging required)

Database

HISTORY

- Birth rate and maternal age are noninfluent.
- Maternal ingestion of thalidomide or of oral contraceptives has been implicated in multiple anomalies syndromes, including ARM.

PHYSICAL EXAMINATION

- Careful inspection of perineum and external genitalia, recording number and position of orifices
- Inspection and palpation of sacrum
- Look for a midline abdominal mass (distended bladder or hydrometrocolpos in the female?).
- Observe the newborn while it is voiding (good stream or dribbling?).
- Search for associated malformations.

—Insert a nasogastric tube to rule out esophageal atresia.
—Palpation of femoral pulses and auscultation of cardiac murmurs
—Palpation of both kidneys
—Obvious skeletal malformations

(continued)

Anorectal Malformations (continued)

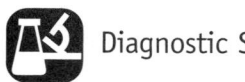 Diagnostic Studies

LABORATORY TESTING

- Urinalysis

—Meconium or squamous cells in the urine indicate a urinary–intestinal communication in males.

IMAGING

- Radiologic studies to assess the level of malformation

—Invertogram (24 hours after birth)
  —Child in inverted position for 3 minutes
  —A lateral radiograph centered on the trochanters with extended hips is taken.
  —Two landmarks: the P-C line from the center of the pubis to the inferior margin of the coccyx and the inferior point of ischial shadow (I point).
  —If the gas shadow of the terminal colon ends above the P-C line, the malformation is high; if it ends between the P-C line and the I point, it is intermediate; and if distally to the I point, it is low.
  —If the child is crying or straining, the gas shadow may appear more proximal.
  —A lateral pelvic cross-table radiograph with the baby prone and the hips raised may give the same information: If the gas shadow and the skin are more than 1 cm apart, the malformation is high.
  —Kidney and bladder ultrasound and micturating cystourethrogram to detect associated urinary malformations

- Ultrasound and x-ray of spine to show vertebral anomalies
- High malformations, before definitive surgery

—Pelvic CT scan and NMR to clarify muscular anatomy
—Distal colostogram

- Cloaca and urogenital sinus

—Genitography
  —Internal genitalia may be studied with an ultrasound CT scan and NMR imaging.

SPECIAL STUDIES: N/A

 Treatment

GENERAL MEASURES

- Before initial surgery, the baby has an intestinal obstruction, therefore

—No oral feeding
—Intravenous fluids
—Nasogastric suction

- Treatment of constipation after definitive surgery

—Bowel wash-outs

- Treatment of incontinence: enemas and colonic wash-outs; biofeedback

MEDICAL

- IV antibiotics at surgery and 2 to 3 days after
- Maintain on oral suppressive chemoprophylaxis until VUR is ruled out.
- Oral Lactulose for constipation (doses vary according to individual response)

SURGICAL

- Low anomalies are treated in the newborn.
- Cut-back of the fistula with skin mucosal suture
- Limited posterior sagittal anorectoplasty
- Anterior transposition of an anteriorly placed anus
- Intermediate and high anomalies require a colostomy in the newborn.
- The colostomy should be placed in the descending colon and the stoma divided.
- Definitive treatment (from 2–12 months of age)
- Most high ARMs may be treated with a posterior sagittal anorectoplasty (Pena and De Vries procedure)
- 10% and 50% of cloacae require laparotomy to mobilize the rectum.
- Posterior sagittal anorectoplasty (PSARP) involves the following steps:

—Electrical stimulation to identify external sphincter
—Incision from midsacrum to the anal site, dividing all posterior muscles strictly in the midline
—Identification and incision of posterior wall of the rectal pouch
—Identification and dissection of the fistula from the rectum
—Closure of the fistula and mobilization of rectal pouch
—Closure of striated muscular complex anteriorly and over the rectal pouch
—Anoplasty

- The goal of the treatment of a persistent cloaca is to separate the rectum from the vagina and then the vagina from the urinary tract and mobilize the two structures in order to reach the perineum.

—The operation is done through a posterior sagittal approach.
—The rectum is separated from the vagina.
—The vagina is detached from the urogenital sinus (they share a tract of common wall).
—If the common channel is short (<3 cm), the urogenital sinus may be mobilized as a whole and brought to the perineum (total urogenital sinus mobilization).
—Otherwise, the urogenital sinus is used as the urethra.
—If the vagina is high and cannot reach the perineum, a segment of bowel may be used to reconstruct the vagina.
—The main genital anomalies must be repaired at this time.

- Both genital and anorectal reconstructions are accomplished as a single procedure.

ALTERNATIVE THERAPIES: N/A

PATIENT EDUCATION

- To avoid anal stenosis, parents must regularly dilate the new anus.
- Start dilatations 2 weeks after surgery.
- Dilatations are performed twice a day.
- Every week, the diameter is increased by 1 mm until the desired size is reached.
- Optimal size depends on the patient's age.
- The frequency of dilatations may subsequently be reduced.
- Once the desired caliber is reached, the colostomy is closed.
- Also, the new vaginal orifice of cloacae or urogenital sinus requires regular dilatations.

 Follow-Up

MONITORING

- Length and frequency of follow-up is related to complexity of malformations and to the problems arising after reconstruction (constipation and incontinence).
- Hematocolpos may affect cloacae at puberty.

PREVENTION: N/A

 Miscellaneous

SYNONYMS: N/A

ASSOCIATED CONDITIONS

- See "Pathophysiology."

NOTES

- See also Section II, "Exstrophy—Cloacal."

ABBREVIATIONS

- ARM, anorectal malformations; VACTERL, vertebral, anorectal, cardiac, tracheoesophageal, renal (or radial) anomalies; VUR, vesicoureteric reflux; PSARP, posterior sagittal anorectoplasty

REFERENCES

Brock WA, Pena A. Cloacal abnormalities and imperforate anus. In: Kelalis P, King L, Belman B, eds. *Clinical Pediatric Urology*, 3rd ed. Philadelphia: WB Saunders, 1992:920–942.

Freeman NV. Anorectal malformations. In: Freeman, L, et al., eds. *Surgery of the Newborn*. Edinburgh: Churchill Livingstone, 1994:71–198.

Authors: Douglas A. Canning and Emilio Merlini

Autonomic Dysreflexia

 Basics

DESCRIPTION

• Autonomic dysreflexia (AD) can cause rapid, extreme blood pressure elevation, bradycardia, headache, sweating, and piloerection in patients with spinal cord lesions at and above the sixth thoracic nerve level (T6).

EPIDEMIOLOGY

• AD occurs intermittently in as many as 90% of complete cervical spinal cord–injured patients.
• Any patient with spinal cord injury (SCI) or severe neurologic disease (e.g., transverse myelitis, etc.) at or above T6 is at risk.
• More common (>4:1) in men than in women due to increased bladder outlet resistance. Age and race are not important.

GENETICS: N/A

STAGING: N/A

SIGNS AND SYMPTOMS

• Rapid, often extreme blood pressure elevation, headache, sweating, and piloerection. Systolic BP values of 250 to 300 can be encountered.

PATHOPHYSIOLOGY

• Triggered by internal stimulation such as bladder or bowel distension and leads to reflexive sympathetic discharge. SCI above the level where sympathetic fibers leave the spinal cord prevents central inhibition and modulation of vascular constriction.

CAUSES/RISK FACTORS

• Lack of an effective bladder or bowel program increases the risk of AD. Complete bladder emptying at least 4 times daily should be assured through intermittent catheterization or other means.

COMPLICATIONS

• Stroke from extreme BP elevation
• In less severe cases, patients report lethargy and nonspecific ill feelings.

DIFFERENTIAL DIAGNOSIS

• Significant BP elevation is diagnostic.
• Patients with cervical or high thoracic SCI normally have low BP (systolic 80–90). The less emergent symptoms are likewise diagnostic.

 Database

HISTORY

• History of complete or nearly complete SCI or other severe neurologic disease above the T6 level
• The intermittent nature of AD causes the symptoms of headache, sweating, and piloerection to be very important.

PHYSICAL EXAMINATION

• Physical examination findings may not be present at the time of the examination.
• Blood pressure during a symptomatic episode compared with baseline BP.
• Bladder catheterization and a rectal examination to check for fecal impaction should be performed immediately.

 Diagnostic Studies

LABORATORY TESTING

• AD should be diagnosed and treated simultaneously.
• Urinalysis and urine culture are indicated to determine the presence of infection, which can trigger AD in some patients.

IMAGING

• Ultrasound may demonstrate a distended bladder.

SPECIAL STUDIES

• Urodynamic testing

—With continued AD on an appropriate bladder- and bowel-emptying regimen, should undergo urodynamic testing to detect possible loss of bladder wall elasticity and high bladder storage pressure

Treatment

GENERAL MEASURES

• Initial treatment is directed to removal of the triggering stimulus by bladder drainage or bowel decompression.
• BP normalizes almost immediately following removal of the triggering stimulus.

MEDICAL

• Treat symptomatic UTI with appropriate antibiotics.
• The unusual patient requires antihypertensive medication. Nifedipine 5 to 10 mg SL has been described but is controversial.
• Chronic dysreflexia can be treated with alpha-blockade. Begin with 1 mg prazosin bid to tid. Long-acting alpha-blockers can be considered once a stable dosage is obtained.

SURGICAL

• SCI patients who develop high bladder storage pressure due to loss of bladder wall elasticity require surgical treatment.
• Sphincterotomy or intraurethral stent procedures allow low-pressure bladder emptying into a condom catheter.
• Bladder augmentation using bowel or other material lowers bladder pressure if the patient wants to remain continent.

ALTERNATIVE THERAPIES: N/A

PATIENT EDUCATION

• Patients should be taught the mechanism and significance of dysreflexia. Symptoms should prompt patients to empty their bladder and bowel. Patients should alert their physician about recurrent symptoms.

 ## Follow-Up

MONITORING

• History asking about AD symptoms and BP at every appointment.

PREVENTION

• Frequent (at least 4 times daily) clean, intermittent catheterization and a regular bowel program for every SCI patient

 ## Miscellaneous

SYNONYMS: N/A

ASSOCIATED CONDITIONS

• Spinal cord injury

NOTES

• See also Section II, "Spinal Cord Injury—Urologic Considerations."

ABBREVIATIONS

• AD, autonomic dysreflexia; SCI, spinal cord injury; T6, sixth thoracic spinal cord level

REFERENCES

Eltorai IM, Wang DH, Lacerna M, Comarr AE, Montroy R. Surgical aspects of autonomic dysreflexia. *J Spinal Cord Med* 1997;20(3):361–364.

LaFavor KM, Ang R. Managing autonomic dysreflexia through the use of clinical practice guidelines. *SCI Nurs* 1997;14(3):83–86.

McGuire EJ, Rossier AB. Treatment of acute autonomic dysreflexia. *J Urol* 1983;129(6):1185–1186.

Author: Douglas F. Milam

Balanitis and Balanoposthitis

 Basics

DESCRIPTION

- *Balanitis* is inflammation of the glans penis and is generally only seen in uncircumcised individuals.
- *Balanoposthitis* is inflammation of the foreskin and glans penis, occurring in uncircumcised individuals.

EPIDEMIOLOGY

- Most common in boys less than 5 years of age but can occur at any age

GENETICS: N/A

STAGING: N/A

SIGNS AND SYMPTOMS

- Balanitis

—Edematous, red, painful glans penis; urethral discharge; discharge from between the prepuce and the glans; dysuria; and often difficulty in voiding (secondary to discomfort)

- Balanoposthitis

—Swollen, red, and painful foreskin and glans penis + symptoms of balanitis as above

PATHOPHYSIOLOGY

- Both occur by means of the intertrigo syndrome (a condition in which damp, moist areas are particularly predisposed to inflammatory changes).
- Poor hygiene technique compounded with this degree of dampness predispose to secondary "opportunistic" bacterial or fungal infiltration.
- The pathophysiology is usually different in young boys compared with men.

—Boys tend to have bacterial invasion, whereas men suffer from a combination of intertrigo, irritant dermatitis, maceration injury, and bacteria or candidal overgrowth.

- Balanitis xerotica obliterans (BXO) is a specific form of balanitis.

—There is a loss of elastin and a replacement by collagen.
—The penile skin around the urethral meatus becomes white, featureless, and contracted, causing meatal stricturing.
—The lesion may spread to the prepuce, and the coronal sulcus may be lost, and in extreme cases the entire end of the penis becomes whitened and fibrotic, with complete obliteration of distinction between glans, prepuce, and shaft.

CAUSES/RISK FACTORS

- Noncircumcised boys and men: poor hygiene, STD exposure, diabetics, immunocompromised patients

COMPLICATIONS

- Scarring and subsequent phimosis, penile shaft cellulitis, or abscess formation

DIFFERENTIAL DIAGNOSIS

- Balanitis/balanoposthitis
- Fixed drug eruption (allergy)
- Contact dermatitis
- Squamous cell carcinoma of the penis
- Carcinoma in situ (CIS) of the penis (erythroplasia of Queyrat)
- Zoon's balanitis
- Psoriasis
- HPV

 Database

HISTORY

- Use of topical allergens/irritants, prior episodes and treatment, sexual contacts or STDs, voiding symptoms (dysuria, hesitancy, and frequency), hygiene techniques, systemic diseases (diabetes, malignancy, etc.), foreskin retractability

PHYSICAL EXAMINATION

- Genital examination

—Inspection (ulcers, lesions, visible pus),
—Palpation (tenderness, induration, mass effect)

- Lymph nodes: Inspect and palpate the bilateral inguinal nodes (should not be enlarged).

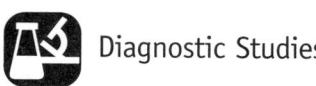 Diagnostic Studies

LABORATORY TESTING

- Swab of glans/foreskin for viral, bacterial, and fungal culture
- KOH and Tzanck preparation for men
- Biopsy lesion in select cases

IMAGING: N/A

SPECIAL STUDIES: N/A

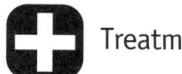 Treatment

GENERAL MEASURES

- Meticulous personal hygiene, keeping the glans and foreskin clean and dry
- Exposing glans to air as often as possible
- Cleaning with soap and water routinely

MEDICAL

- Treat the underlying cause.
- Care of penile hygiene, including retraction of prepuce where possible
- Systemic antibiotics may work quickly but are seldom needed.
- Topical antifungals (Nystatin)
- Topical antibiotics
- Topical steroids (Betnovate 0.5%, hydrocortisone 0.1%)
- Castellani's paint (drying agent)
- Barrier ointment (petrolatum jelly)

SURGICAL

- Circumcision is reserved for recurrent cases or phimosis that has failed conservative treatment.
- Care of meatal narrowing or stricture in BXO

—Self-dilation
—Dilation by urologist

ALTERNATIVE THERAPIES: N/A

PATIENT EDUCATION

- Need for excellent personal hygiene is mandatory: Retract the foreskin for each void and clean the prepuce and glans twice per day.

 Follow-Up

MONITORING

- After an acute episode and treatment is implemented, the patient should be seen within 4 to 6 weeks, unless problems occur, in which case he should be seen sooner to alter treatment.

PREVENTION

- Good personal hygiene
- Good diabetic/systemic disease control

 Miscellaneous

SYNONYMS: N/A

ASSOCIATED CONDITIONS

- Diabetes

NOTES

- See Section II, "Balanitis Xerotica Obliterans."

ABBREVIATIONS: N/A

REFERENCES

Birley HD, et al. Clinical features and management of recurrent balanitis; association with atopy and genital washing. *Genitourin Med* 1993;69:400–403.

Walsh PC, Retik AB, Vaughan ED Jr, Wein AJ, eds. *Campbell's Urology*, 7th ed. Philadelphia: WB Saunders, 1997:726,3324–3325.

Authors: Gregory R.J. Leal and Jeremy P.W. Heaton

Balanitis Xerotica Obliterans

Basics

DESCRIPTION

• Balanitis xerotica obliterans (BXO) is an inflammatory lesion of the glans and foreskin. It is now considered to be synonymous with lichen sclerosus et atrophicus (LSA). The term *BXO* is used when the skin of the genitalia is effected.

EPIDEMIOLOGY

• Caucasian patients: 1% to 3%. LSA is reported in native Africans, Asians, and other dark-skinned races.

GENETICS

• None identified

STAGING: N/A

SIGNS AND SYMPTOMS

• Itching and loss of sensation of the glans penis
• Erections are painful.
• Inevitably associated with meatal stenosis or distal urethral stricture; complaints of urethral discharge
• Decreased force of stream, and/or dysuria
• Uncommonly, patients initially present in retention.
• Lesions are atrophic white areas on the glans and preputial skin.
• In early cases, changes are confined to the meatal area.
• Advanced cases: There is retrusion along with stenosis of the meatus and obliteration of the glandular coronal margin.
• In uncircumcised patients, severe phimosis and balanoposthitis are common.

PATHOPHYSIOLOGY

• Early: thinned epithelium with flattening of the rete pegs and hyperkeratosis. The adventitial dermis has a dense neutrophil infiltrate.
• Later: As with early cases, however, the inflammatory dermal infiltrate becomes composed of lymphocytes and plasma cells. The epidermis becomes severely atrophic, with complete loss of the rete pegs.
• Clinical association with autoimmune phenomenon and with Class II antigens suggests an immunologic factor in the development of BXO.

CAUSES/RISK FACTORS

• Uncertain. It is an inflammatory process.
• Often seen in uncircumcised males with severe phimosis and balanitis
• Suggestion of association with autoimmune disease
• Trauma, chronic antigenic stimuli, and infection as causative
• More frequently in Caucasians

COMPLICATIONS

• Severe distal urethral obstruction that becomes long segment urethral stricture over time
• May predispose to squamous cell carcinoma of the penis
• Possibly, the relief of the distal obstruction early may prevent subsequent, more severe urethral stricture disease.

DIFFERENTIAL DIAGNOSIS

• Leukoplakia
• Bowen disease
• Erythroplasia of Queyrat
• Squamous cell carcinoma of the glans or preputial skin

Database

HISTORY

• If circumcised, at what age, and were there "complications" with the circumcision?
• If the patient is not circumcised, can he retract his foreskin?
• Has he had irritation of the glans penis and painful erections?
• Does the patient have voiding obstructive or irritative symptoms?

PHYSICAL EXAMINATION

• Early: the presence of atrophic pearly white scars near/surrounding the meatus. Is there meatal stenosis?
• Later: atrophic, painful, pearly white scarring of the glans, usually to include the meatus. Complete replacement of glandular and preputial skin with atrophic, pearly white skin, retrusion and stenosis of the meatus, and obliteration of the coronal margin. Note: In later cases, the skin is at times denuded and severely inflamed.

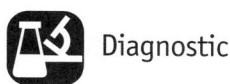 Diagnostic Studies

LABORATORY TESTING

• Urinalysis, urine culture and sensitivity

IMAGING

• Retrograde urethrogram and voiding urethrogram

—Classic finding: irregular stenosis of the distal urethra, with typical intravasation of contrast into the dilated glands of Littre. Often, the proximal anterior urethra is spared.

SPECIAL STUDIES

• In late or severely inflamed cases, biopsy of the glans. Try to place the biopsy across the margin of involved and "uninvolved tissue."
• Urethroscopy: Oftentimes a pediatric cystoscope is necessary.

 Treatment

GENERAL MEASURES

• BXO is a benign condition, but it is considered by many to be premalignant. The question arises as to whether BXO is truly premalignant. However, squamous cell carcinoma of the glans, in some cases, appears grossly very similar to BXO and may be thus misdiagnosed.
• Biopsy is usually necessary to confirm a diagnosis of BXO.

MEDICAL

• Local application of triamcinolone cream, estrogen cream, or testosterone cream

SURGICAL

• In early cases, reconstruction of the fossa navicularis, using flap techniques or extragenital graft techniques
• In later cases, graft resurfacing of the glans, with long segment urethral reconstruction
• Meatal dilation, meatotomy, urethral dilation, and internal urethrotomy are seldom effective.
• Children: circumcision, if appropriate
• Adults with phimosis, circumcision

ALTERNATIVE THERAPIES: N/A

PATIENT EDUCATION

• Note potential consideration as a premalignant lesion and for urethral stricture disease

 Follow-Up

MONITORING

• Interval examination of the glans with biopsy if suspicious
• If urethral reconstruction, follow up with endoscopy and/or urethroscopy to assess results and durability of reconstruction.
• In the patient in whom inflammation does not respond to local application of steroids, biopsy must be performed.
• In patients followed "conservatively," interval contrast evaluation of the urethra must be performed.

PREVENTION: N/A

 Miscellaneous

SYNONYMS

• Lichen sclerosus et atrophicus

ASSOCIATED CONDITIONS

• Urethral stricture, phimosis

NOTES: N/A

ABBREVIATIONS

• BXO, balanitis xerotica obliterans; LSA, lichen sclerosus et atrophicus

REFERENCES

Akporiaye LE, Jordan GH, Devine CJ. Balanitis xerotica obliterans (BXO). AUA Update Series, Lesson 21, Volume XVI, 1997.

Datta C, Dutta SK, Chaudauri A. Histopathological and immunological studies in a cohort of balanitis xerotica obliterans. *J Indian Med Assoc* 1993; 916:146–148.

Garat JM, Chechile G, Algaba F, et al. Balanitis xerotica obliterans in children. *J Urol* 1986;136: 436–437.

Jordan GH. Reconstruction of the fossa navicularis. *J Urol* 1987;138:102–104.

Meffert JJ, Davis BM, Grimwood RE. Lichen sclerosus. *J Am Acad Dermatol* 1995;32:393–416.

Staff WA. Urethral involvement in balanitis xerotica obliterans. *Br J Urol* 1970;47:234–239.

Author: Gerald H. Jordan

BCG Sepsis

Basics

DESCRIPTION

• BCG sepsis, the most serious complication of intravesical BCG therapy for bladder cancer, is usually caused by intravascular absorption of BCG organisms and is associated with circulatory collapse, acute respiratory distress, and disseminated intravascular coagulopathy.

EPIDEMIOLOGY

• Incidence of BCG sepsis is 0.4% (decreasing with increased awareness of preventive measures).
• At least 10 reported deaths have been directly related to intravesical BCG.
• Other adverse side effects include fever (2.9%), hematuria (1.0%), arthralgia (0.5%), prostatitis (0.9%), epididymitis (0.4%), pneumonitis/hepatitis (0.8%), ureteral obstruction (0.3%), and rash (0.3%).

GENETICS: N/A

STAGING: N/A

SIGNS AND SYMPTOMS

• High fever
• Shaking chills
• Mental confusion
• Shortness of breath
• Hypotension
• Disseminated intravascular coagulopathy
• Respiratory and liver failure

PATHOPHYSIOLOGY

• BCG is an attenuated strain of *Mycobacterium bovis,* and is instilled intravesically to prevent recurrences and delay progression in patients with carcinoma in situ and superficial TCC of the bladder.
• BCG contains dead microorganisms, subcellular debris, and living microorganisms that maintain immunologic properties and antibiotic sensitivities similar to those of their parent strain.
• BCG related side effects normally include local (bladder-related) and systemic (flu-like) symptoms. Ninety-five percent of patients tolerate BCG therapy without any major adverse reactions.
• BCG sepsis requires systemic absorption of live attenuated *Mycobacterium bovis* organisms, which may gain access through disrupted bladder urothelium following a recent TUR or severe cystitis or following a traumatic catheterization immediately prior to BCG instillation.

CAUSES/RISK FACTORS

• Systemic absorption of live attenuated BCG organisms
• BCG administration within 7 to 10 days of TUR, in the presence of gross hematuria, or following a traumatic catheterization

COMPLICATIONS

• Profound sepsis and death

DIFFERENTIAL DIAGNOSIS

• Initially indistinguishable from urosepsis (gram-negative sepsis)

Database

HISTORY

• Recent administration of intravesical BCG immunotherapy
• Traumatic catheterization, severe cystitis, recent TUR, or gross hematuria prior to BCG
• A history of high fever, chills, and flu-like symptoms following BCG administration is common, and patients with a prior sensitization to BCG may be particularly susceptible.
• Lower urinary tract symptoms may be present (frequency, urgency, hesitancy, and dysuria).
• A medical history of superficial bladder cancer is the usual indication for BCG administration.
• Prior TB, HIV/AIDS, or immunocompromised conditions are relative contraindications to BCG. Patients with a history of TB are able to receive BCG therapy; however, active TB infection is an absolute contraindication to therapy.
• Current medications, including the use of any antibiotics and corticosteroids. Steroid use is a relative contraindication to BCG therapy.

PHYSICAL EXAMINATION

• High fever
• Hypotension
• Tachycardia
• Shock

Diagnostic Studies

LABORATORY TESTING

- Complete blood count with differential

—White blood cell count may be elevated and platelet count lowered.

- Serum electrolytes and creatinine

—Renal insufficiency may be present due to underlying disease of renal hypoperfusion.

- Liver function studies

—May be elevated secondary to TB hepatitis, shock

- Coagulopathy and DIC Screen

—PT and PTT, fibrinogen, and fibrin degradation products, as well as D-dimer.

- Urinalysis (hematuria, pyuria)
- Urine and blood cultures, including routine urine (gram-negative) and mycobacterial cultures

IMAGING

- Chest x-ray

SPECIAL STUDIES

- Urine and blood should be sent for acid-fast bacilli (AFB) staining and *Mycobacterium bovis* cultures.

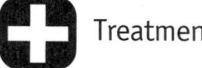 ## Treatment

GENERAL MEASURES

- Initial management includes inpatient admission for intravenous fluid resuscitation with normal saline and/or colloid to restore intravascular fluid volume.
- Invasive monitoring, usually in an intensive care unit

—Central venous pressure measurements
—Foley catheter insertion may be necessary.

- Treatment includes prompt administration of broad-spectrum antibiotics for standard urinary organisms (both gram-positive and -negative organisms)
- Antituberculosis therapy
- Intravenous steroids
- Correction of any coagulopathy with fresh-frozen plasma (FFP) and vitamin K may be necessary.

MEDICAL

- Patients with fever persisting more than 48 hours following intravesical BCG therapy and not responding to antipyretics should be started on oral isoniazid 300 mg daily plus pyridoxine 50 mg daily.
- Patients with fever >38.5°C and severe systemic symptoms should be treated with isoniazid 300 mg, rifampin 600 mg, and pyridoxine 50 mg daily.
- Corticosteroids (initially IV hydrocortisone 100 mg every 8 hours, and ultimately po prednisone 40 mg daily) should be included as part of the initial management of patients with BCG sepsis.
- Ethambutol 1200 mg and cycloserine 200 to 500 mg twice daily should be added in patients who do not respond to initial drug therapy.

SURGICAL: N/A

ALTERNATIVE THERAPIES: N/A

PATIENT EDUCATION

- Patients with a history of BCG sepsis should not receive any further BCG.
- Prior to BCG therapy, those patients with high fever, gross hematuria, or a TUR within 7 days, or those who experience a traumatic catheterization should alert their physician and nursing personnel.
- Following BCG administration, patients should alert their physician if they experience a fever >38.5°C, and particularly if fever persists for greater than 48 hours.

 ## Follow-Up

MONITORING

- While the optimal duration of antituberculosis therapy following BCG sepsis is unknown, a 6-month course is currently recommended.
- Steroids are tapered slowly over a period of approximately 6 weeks.

PREVENTION

- BCG should not be administered within 14 days following tumor resection, and it should be withheld in the presence of gross hematuria or a traumatic catheterization.
- BCG should be administered only under gravity flow and never under pressure.
- BCG should never be administered to patients with a history of BCG sepsis.
- Contraindications to BCG administration include active TB, pregnancy, active urinary tract infection, leukemia, and Hodgkin disease; nor should it be administered to AIDS/HIV-positive patients or transplant recipients, because of their immunocompromised conditions.
- There is no evidence that BCG is contraindicated in patients with valvular heart disease or joint prosthesis, although antibiotic prophylaxis as recommended by the American Heart Association should be given, as is standard, in such patients undergoing urethral instrumentation.

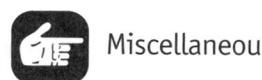 ## Miscellaneous

SYNONYMS

- BCGosis

ASSOCIATED CONDITIONS: N/A

NOTES

- Consultation with an infectious disease specialist is encouraged, particularly in monitoring side effects of antituberculosis medications, such as hepatotoxicity in isoniazid therapy.

ABBREVIATIONS

- BCG, bacille Calmette-Guérin; TCC, transitional cell carcinoma

REFERENCES

Berry DL, et al. Local toxicity patterns associated with intravesical bacillus Calmette-Guerin: A Southwest Oncology Group study. *Int J Urol* 1996;3: 98–100.

Koukol SC, et al. Drug therapy of bacillus Calmette-Guerin sepsis. *Urol Res* 1995;22:373–376.

Lamm DL. Complications of bacillus Calmette-Guerin immunotherapy. *Urol Clin North Am* 1992;19:565.

Author: Michael S. Cookson

Bladder Calculi

 Basics

DESCRIPTION

• Presence of calculus material in the bladder that does not pass with normal micturition

EPIDEMIOLOGY

• Incidence: Bladder stones are uncommon in developing countries and are often related to bladder outlet obstruction or foreign bodies within the bladder
• In undeveloped countries, they occur in children, more commonly in boys under the age of 10. These stones are generally related to poor nutrition, specifically a low-protein diet.

GENETICS: N/A

STAGING: N/A

SIGNS AND SYMPTOMS

• Presentation: Bladder stones may be completely asymptomatic.
• Symptoms: suprapubic pain, dysuria, stranguria, gross hematuria, intermittent stream, hesitancy, frequency, urgency, nocturia, pain radiating to the tip of the penis
• Signs: microscopic hematuria, pyuria, bacteriuria, crystalluria, palpable mass

PATHOPHYSIOLOGY

• Bladder stones may form primarily within the bladder or in the kidney and pass into the bladder, where they grow.
• Stone composition: Ammonium acid urate is a common type of bladder stone and may be pure or admixed with other mineral components. Bladder stones can be uric acid, calcium oxalate, and calcium phosphate as well.
• Size: In most people, if the stone is small enough to pass through the ureter, it will continue on through the urethra. However, once remaining in the bladder, for whatever reason, the stone may continue to grow to completely fill the bladder.
• There may be single or multiple stones. Some may be very hard and laminated. Shapes vary from elliptical to jack stones. Some will have a faceted surface.
• Stones may be free floating or fixed to the bladder wall

CAUSES/RISK FACTORS

• Bladder outlet obstruction is the most common cause of bladder stones.

—A combination of an increased post-void residual and an elevated bladder neck results in the formation of stones in static urine, which cannot overcome gravity to get over the intravesical prostate and out through the urethra.
—Foreign bodies within the bladder act as a nidus for stone formation.

—Iatrogenic: stents, staples, metal from endourologic instruments, suture material, retained sponges, shattered latex balloons, etc.
—Noniatrogenic: objects placed into the bladder by the patient

COMPLICATIONS

• Often related to intermittent obstruction of the bladder neck
• Gross hematuria, recurrent bacterial cystitis, suprapubic pain, chronic cystitis, potential risk for development of squamous cell carcinoma

DIFFERENTIAL DIAGNOSIS

• Bacterial cystitis
• Prostatism
• Urethral stricture, bladder neck contracture
• Carcinoma in situ
• Ureterocele
• Fungal bezoar
• Neurogenic bladder
• Interstitial cystitis

 Database

HISTORY

• History of suprapubic pain, hematuria, bladder outlet obstructive symptoms or infection
• Previous surgery (bladder, prostate, urethral)

PHYSICAL EXAMINATION

• Abdominal examination: Percuss the top of the bladder to look for distension. Palpate for abdominal or suprapubic or costovertebral angle tenderness. Examine for previous surgical scars.
• Pelvic examination: bimanual examination for bladder mass, check for IUD; assess cervical motion tenderness, and look for urethral or vaginal inflammation or fistulas.

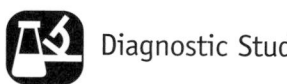 Diagnostic Studies

LABORATORY TESTING

- Urinalysis

—Dipstick: A bladder stone could result in the presence of leukocyte esterase, nitrites, and blood.
—Microscopic: Look for the presence of red cells (micro- or gross hematuria), white cells (pyuria), and bacteria; crystalluria may be present.

- Urine culture and sensitivity: to document and treat associated infections

IMAGING

- A plain radiograph (KUB) will often demonstrate radiopaque bladder stones; however, uric acid and ammonium acid uratestones are radiolucent.
- A voiding cystourethrogram or intravenous urography would reveal a filling defect in the bladder, even for a radiolucent stone; if the filling defect moves when the patient is repositioned, it is a stone. Also, other bladder abnormalities, such as a diverticulum or ureterocele, can be seen with these studies.
- Pelvic ultrasound: readily diagnoses the presence of a bladder stone
- Computed tomography is highly sensitive and specific for calculi anywhere within the urinary tract.

SPECIAL STUDIES

- Cystoscopy is ideal for visualizing stones, to assess their number, size, and position.

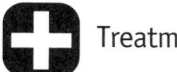 Treatment

GENERAL MEASURES

- Bladder stones should be removed, and if bladder outlet obstruction is a causative factor, the patient should be counseled to have definitive treatment for the obstruction.

MEDICAL

- Dissolution of bladder stones is possible if the stones are composed of pure uric acid.

—Alkalization therapy to raise the urine pH to approximately 6.5 may dissolve the stone; however, overalkalization can lead to a deposit of calcium phosphate on the surface of the stone. Use potassium citrate (Polycitra K, Urocit K) 60 mEq/d po.

SURGICAL

- Three approaches to the bladder can be used to treat bladder stones:

—Retrograde urethroscopic: (Cystolitholapaxy) Cystoscopy is used to visualize the stone, an energy source is used to fragment the stone, and the fragments are irrigated through the cystoscope. Energy sources include the following:
  —Mechanical: The lithotrite, a hand-activated device like pliers, crushes the stone in its jaws. The lithoclast, a device that uses a pneumatic piston, breaks the stone through direct contact.
  —Electrohydraulic lithotripsy: An electrical shock wave near the stone creates a plasma energy that fragments the stone.
  —Laser: Pulsed-dye and holmium-YAG lasers are used to break bladder stones.
—Open: An open cystotomy is done to remove the stone (or stones) intact. If the stone is due to a grossly enlarged prostate (>100 g), a suprapubic prostatectomy can be done simultaneously.
—Percutaneous: Percutaneous suprapubic access is obtained in a fashion similar to that for percutaneous renal access. A rigid nephroscope, graspers, and ultrasonic lithotripsy with suction are used to rapidly evacuate the stone.

ALTERNATIVE THERAPIES: N/A

PATIENT EDUCATION: N/A

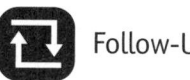 Follow-Up

MONITORING

- Periodic evaluation to rule out residual/recurrent stones

PREVENTION

- Treatment of the underlying cause of the stone is essential.

—Stone analysis is performed. Directed medical therapy is initiated as necessary.
—Encourage hydration; utilize intermittent catheterization to avoid an indwelling catheter.
—Treat bladder outlet obstruction.

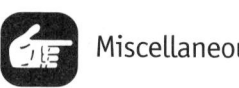 Miscellaneous

SYNONYMS

- Bladder stones, bladder calculi, vesical stones

ASSOCIATED CONDITIONS

- Bladder outlet obstruction

NOTES: N/A

ABBREVIATIONS: N/A

REFERENCES

Dhanamitta S, et al. Research report on bladder stone disease, Thailand. In: van Reem R, ed. *Idiopathic Urinary Bladder Stone Disease*. Washington, DC: Department of Health, Education, and Welfare, DHEW Publication No 77-1063, 1977: 151–171.

Short KL, Amin M, Harty JI, et al. Comparison of recurrence rates of calculi of the bladder in patients with indwelling catheters following vesicolithotomy, litholapaxy, and electrohydraulic lithotripsy. *Surg Gynecol Obstet* 1984;159:247.

Valyasevi A, Dhanamitta S. A general hypothesis concerning the etiological factors in bladder stone disease. In: van Reem R, ed. *Idiopathic Urinary Bladder Stone Disease*. Washington, DC: Department of Health, Education, and Welfare, DHEW Publication No 77-1063, 1977:135–180.

Author: Kevin R. Anderson

Bladder Cancer—Adenocarcinoma

Basics

DESCRIPTION

- Adenocarcinoma of the urinary bladder is an uncommon and often aggressive urologic malignancy.
- It is frequently muscle invasive or metastatic at the time of diagnosis and therefore carries a poor prognosis.

EPIDEMIOLOGY

- 0.5% to 2.0% of all primary bladder malignancies
- Can arise from the urachus or the nonurachal epithelium, or in association with exstrophy of the bladder
- A majority of nonurachal-, nonexstrophy-associated adenocarcinomas occur in men and frequently have an associated history of long-term inflammation or infection.
- Urachal cancers: <1% of primary bladder cancers; 20% to 39% of vesical adenocarcinomas

GENETICS

- In tissue recombinant studies, adenocarcinoma can be produced from bladder transitional epithelium under the appropriate hormonal and mesenchymal stimulus.

STAGING

- See Appendix for the TNM staging system for bladder cancer.

SIGNS AND SYMPTOMS

- Painless hematuria

—Cancer is found in up to 10% of patients with microscopic hematuria.
—Amount of blood does not predict the probability of cancer.

- Irritative voiding symptoms: frequency, urgency, dysuria

—Seen in approximately one-third of patients with bladder cancer
—More often in patients with carcinoma in situ and invasive cancer

- Mucosuria: passage of mucus

PATHOPHYSIOLOGY

- Classification: Three groups are related to the site of tumor origin:

—Primary adenocarcinoma of bladder
—Urachal adenocarcinoma
—Extravesical adenocarcinoma (metastasis)

- Primary vesical adenocarcinoma
- It can occur anywhere in the bladder, but the dome and the trigone of the bladder are common.

—Most common type of cancer in bladder exstrophy
—All histologic variants of enteric carcinoma may occur in the bladder.
—Papillary or solid; most are mucin producing

—Most are poorly differentiated and invasive at the time of diagnosis.
—Poor response to radiotherapy and cytotoxic chemotherapy

- Urachal carcinoma: rare

—For classification as a urachal carcinoma, there must be

—Clear demarcation between the tumor and adjacent bladder mucosa
—Tumor location within the wall of the bladder (beneath normal urothelium)
—Possible production of mucoid drainage from the umbilicus
—May produce stippled calcifications on plain films
—The prognosis is worse for urachal carcinoma than for primary adenocarcinoma of the bladder.
—Urachal carcinoma demonstrates more extensive infiltration of the bladder wall than expected, and for this reason, radical cystectomy is preferred over partial cystectomy, although the latter is still an option.
—Tumors are relatively chemo- and radioresistant.
—Urachal carcinomas are not always adenocarcinomas (most common type); others include transitional cell carcinoma, squamous cell carcinoma, and rarely sarcoma.

- Metastatic lesions: rare (only 0.26% of cases)

—Adenocarcinomas from the colon, stomach, breast, ovary, endometrium, and prostate can metastasize to the bladder.
—Local invasion of a colonic primary tumor is more common than metastasis.
—Bladder adenocarcinoma is histologically indistinguishable from adenocarcinoma of the colon.

CAUSES/RISK FACTORS

- Chronic irritation, inflammation, or infection
- Bladder exstrophy
- Schistosomiasis

COMPLICATIONS

- Ureteral obstruction from local spread of tumor
- Metastasis to pelvic lymph nodes, liver, lung, mediastinum, and bone

DIFFERENTIAL DIAGNOSIS

- See Section II, "Bladder Tumors—Benign and Malignant, General."
- Metastasis from colon, prostate, or other adenocarcinoma

Database

HISTORY

- See "Signs and Symptoms": hematuria, mucosuria.
- Foreign travel: schistosomiasis
- Weight loss, flank pain, umbilical discharge (rare)
- Chronic infection
- History of exstrophy or other bladder pathology
- History of colon cancer or other malignancy: risk of metastatic lesion

PHYSICAL EXAMINATION

- Pelvic mass by bimanual/rectal examination
- Lower extremity edema: suggests retroperitoneal adenopathy
- Digital rectal examination: presence of blood in stools

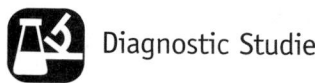 Diagnostic Studies

LABORATORY TESTING

- Urine studies: urinalysis, culture and sensitivity, urine cytology
- Serum electrolytes: BUN/creatinine, liver function tests

IMAGING

- IVP: It can provide anatomic detail of the upper urinary tract, with delineation of filling defects in the bladder; however, it is not helpful in staging: Only 60% of bladder tumors are detected with IVP.
- CT scan: imaging method of choice for staging of bladder tumors; useful for detecting presence of pelvic lymphadenopathy and extravesical tumor extension

—Sensitivity of 64% to 94%, specificity of 62% to 100%, and accuracy of 80% to 7%

SPECIAL STUDIES

- Diagnostic cystoscopy and biopsy

—Essential for definitive diagnosis
—Bloody efflux from ureteral orifices suspicious for upper tract pathology

 Treatment

GENERAL MEASURES

- Site of origin and tumor behavior are factors important in determining treatment.
- Histologic cell type is less likely to affect prognosis, with the exception of signet ring tumors. Signet ring tumors are aggressive, and radical surgical excision should be considered. As many as half of patients with the signet cell variant will succumb to their disease within 1 year.
- Adenocarcinoma of the bladder is generally unresponsive to radiation and chemotherapy. Radical cystectomy with excision of the urachus and umbilicus is usually required if a urachal primary is suspected.
- Adjuvant chemotherapy or radiotherapy may be used, but surgery remains the most consistently effective treatment.

MEDICAL

- Some response to standard regimens such as combination methotrexate, vinblastine, Adriamycin, cisplatinum (MVAC)
- Recently, combination vinblastine, ifosfamide, gallium (VIG) has shown activity.

SURGICAL

- Radical cystectomy remains the gold standard.

ALTERNATIVE THERAPIES: N/A

PATIENT EDUCATION

- American Cancer Society: 1-800-ACS-2345; www.cancer.org
- National Cancer Institute: 1-800-4-CANCER; www.nci.nih.gov
- United Ostomy Association: 1-800-826-0826; www.uoa.org

 Follow-Up

MONITORING

- Five-year mortality of up to 50%

PREVENTION: N/A

 Miscellaneous

SYNONYMS: N/A

ASSOCIATED CONDITIONS

- Exstrophy of the bladder, schistosomiasis

NOTES

- See also Section II, "Bladder Tumors—Benign and Malignant, General" and "Urachal Carcinoma."

ABBREVIATIONS: N/A

REFERENCES

Burnett AL, Epstein JI, Marshall FF. Adenocarcinoma of the urinary bladder. *Urology* 1991;37: 315.

Walsh PC, Retik AB, Stamey TA, Vaughan ED, eds. *Campbell's Urology,* 6th ed. Philadelphia: WB Saunders, 1992.

Authors: V. Keith Jimenez and Thomas E. Keane

Bladder Cancer—Squamous Cell Carcinoma

 Basics

DESCRIPTION

• Squamous cell cancer (SCC) of the bladder is a malignant tumor of epithelial origin with cells capable of producing keratin or demonstrating intercellular bridges.

EPIDEMIOLOGY

• 5% of all neoplastic bladder tumors
• Increased incidence in spinal cord injury (SCI) patients (2.5% to 10.0% develop SCC)
• Endemic regions of *Schistosoma hematobium* infection (Egypt, Sudan, Saudi Arabia, Africa)

—Most common cancer in men in these regions
—Presents at 40 to 50 years
—Up to 80% *Schistosoma*-related bladder cancers are SCC.

GENETICS

• Frequent chromosome alterations at the 9p allele
• Mutations of the tumor suppressor gene CDKN2 common; three times higher than TCC
• Psoriasin (calcium-binding protein) expressed and externalized into urine by keratinocytes of SCC

—Detected by immunoassay
—Experimental at this point; concern of false positives in states of squamous metaplasia and TCC with squamous differentiation

STAGING

• TMN staging similar to TCC (See Section VII)
• Histologic grading from 1 to 3 based on degree of differentiation according to WHO classification scheme

SIGNS AND SYMPTOMS

• Hematuria: 60% to 70%
• Irritative voiding complaints: 35% to 50%
• Chronic UTI
• Upper tract obstruction: 10% to 20%
• Back/pelvic pain
• Acute retention
• Weight loss

PATHOPHYSIOLOGY

• Grossly appears as solitary, sessile, necrotic/ulcerated lesion
• Detection by biopsy in areas of chronic inflammation not uncommon in high-risk patients
• Most tumors are well to moderately differentiated in the schistosomal population, while in other populations moderate to poorly differentiated tumors predominate.
• A majority are invasive at the time of diagnosis.
• Pelvic lymph node involvement is seen in 10% to 20% of cases.
• Focal areas of squamous differentiation in high-grade TCC are common.
• Histologic characteristics of pure SCC: squamous "pearls," intercellular bridges, keratotic cellular debris
• A rare variant of pure SCC is verrucous carcinoma.

—Grossly appears as white, exophytic mucosal lesion
—Cells demonstrate minimal atypia; there is little tendency towards metastatic disease but foci of SCC may occasionally be found.

CAUSES/RISK FACTORS

• Risk factors

—Urothelial irritants: chronic cystitis, bladder stones, long-term indwelling catheter
—Smoking: increases risk several-fold over general population
—Squamous metaplasia: urothelium transformed into stratified squamous epithelium; not considered premalignant; associated with inflammation of the bladder and seen in 17% to 25% of SCC cases
—Leukoplakia: considered premalignant condition; increased risk for SCC, more so than TCC; histologically distinguished from squamous metaplasia by presence of keratin
—Bilharziasis: Schistosomal eggs cause a foreign-body reaction in the bladder wall, initiating "bilharzial granulomas," which coalesce, forming nodules. A foreign-body reaction results in squamous metaplasia and eventual fibrosis/necrosis and calcification associated with bladder contraction, as well as ureteral and urethral strictures, resulting in obstruction. Susceptibility to bacterial infection and subsequent reduction of nitrates are thought to promote carcinogenesis.
—Pelvic XRT: Most cases involve gynecologic primary; usual latency period of 10 years or longer
—Cyclophosphamide: metabolites acrolein and phosphoramide mustard mutagenic; associated with long-term ingestion
—Condyloma (HPV) infection: Association with SCC is not established, but sporadic case reports exist.

COMPLICATIONS

• Local/regional spread: frequently present; typically occurs within 12 months of primary surgical therapy; most common mode of recurrence and principal cause of death
• Metastatic disease primarily involves the lung, liver, and bone.
• Ureteral obstruction
• Tumor implantation of suprapubic cystostomy tract; uncommon, associated with advanced disease

DIFFERENTIAL DIAGNOSIS

• TCC with squamous differentiation
• Inflammatory conditions: chronic cystitis, squamous metaplasia, leukoplakia, hemorrhagic cystitis
• Lymphoepithelioma-like carcinoma: poorly differentiated malignant cells arranged in a syncytial pattern and characteristic lymphocytic infiltrate; syncytial pattern may resemble SCC

—Often invasive and may be seen as a component of TCC
—Treatment of pure lymphoepithelioma-like carcinoma: transurethral resection and MVAC chemotherapy; generally has good prognosis

• In females, direct extension of cervical SCC to the bladder occurs infrequently.

Database

HISTORY

- History of SCI: period of indwelling catheter, external collecting device, or clean intermittent catheterization
- New-onset hematuria/irritative symptoms
- Chronic cystitis
- Smoking history
- Country of origin of patient if suspect schistosomal infection

PHYSICAL EXAMINATION

- Abdominal and bimanual examination to aid in clinical staging
- Assess for inguinal adenopathy.

 Diagnostic Studies

LABORATORY TESTING

- Urinalysis (hematuria, pyuria, bacteriuria) and culture if indicated
- BUN, creatinine

IMAGING

- CT scan to detect lymph node enlargement, urinary obstruction, and assess extravesical spread of tumor
- CXR to rule out metastasis to lungs
- Bone scan only in setting of bone pain or elevated alkaline phosphatase

SPECIAL STUDIES

- Cystoscopy and biopsies of suspicious lesions
- Flow cytometry: nondiploid DNA pattern associated with worse prognosis within each grade/stage of SCC compared with diploid pattern

 Treatment

GENERAL MEASURES

- Clinical understaging is common (35%).
- Tumor grade/stage and lymph node status most important prognostic variables

MEDICAL

- Radiotherapy: disappointing 5-year survival rates for T2 (15%) and T3 (5%) disease when XRT used as sole therapy
- Chemotherapy: not enough information to advocate use as primary or adjuvant therapy in SCC of the bladder

SURGICAL

- Radical cystectomy and pelvic lymph node dissection: larger series report similar prognosis stage for stage for SCC compared with TCC; 35% to 48% 5-year survival for all stages combined; 65% to 75% P1 and P2 disease; 15% to 35% P3 and P4 disease
- Preoperative XRT/radical cystectomy: One randomized study showed improved survival in patients with high-stage disease treated preoperatively with 2000 rads.
- Partial cystectomy: not standard therapy but may be considered only in select patients with small tumors and no evidence of local spread

ALTERNATIVE THERAPIES: N/A

PATIENT EDUCATION

- Compliance with long-term surveillance in patients with indwelling catheter necessary to optimize detection

 Follow-Up

MONITORING

- Controlled studies needed to determine most effective patient monitoring in SCI patients; unclear whether annual cystoscopy improves detection rate or survival from SCC

—Single voided cytologies are generally not helpful in the diagnosis, especially in the setting of concurrent inflammatory conditions.
—Multiple cytologies with an experienced cytopathologist may improve detection, but as many as 25% may go unrecognized with cytologies alone under these circumstances.
—Cystoscopy on an annual basis or for investigation of recurrent UTIs, irritative symptoms, or hematuria, and biopsy of suspicious lesions is the preferred management in patients with a long history of indwelling catheters or routine catheterization regimens.

PREVENTION

- Theoretically, changing from an indwelling catheter to clean, intermittent catheterization may decrease the incidence of SCC, but the presence of chronic infection probably plays a more significant role.

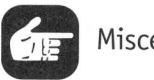 Miscellaneous

SYNONYMS: N/A

ASSOCIATED CONDITIONS

- SCI or neurogenic bladder, schistosomal bladder infection, leukoplakia, squamous metaplasia

NOTES

- See also Section II, "Bladder Tumors—Benign and Malignant, General."

ABBREVIATIONS

- SCC, squamous cell cancer; SCI, spinal cord injury; MVAC, methotrexate, vinblastine, Adriamycin, cisplatin–based chemotherapy; TCC, transitional cell carcinoma

REFERENCES

Ghoneim MA, El-Mekresh MM, El-Baz MA, et al. Radical cystectomy for carcinoma of the bladder: Critical evaluation of the results in 1,026 cases. *J Urol* 1997;158:393–399.

Richie JP, Waisman J, Skinner DG, et al. Squamous carcinoma of the bladder: Treatment by radical cystectomy. *J Urol* 1976;115:670–672.

Rundle JSH, Hart AJL, McGeorge A, et al. Squamous cell cancer of bladder. A review of 114 patients. *Br J Urol* 1982;54:522–526.

Authors: Michael P. Gardner and Robert A. Stephenson

Bladder Cancer—TCC, Invasive (T2/3/4)

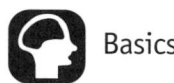 Basics

DESCRIPTION

• TCC accounts for >90% of BC; other etiologies include squamous cell cancer and adenocarcinoma.

EPIDEMIOLOGY

• Incidence: 100,000 persons/yr; increases with age and is higher in men:women (3:1); White males:Black males (2:1); White females:Black females (1.5:1)
• Median age at diagnosis: 69 (men) and 71 (women)

GENETICS

• Hereditary patterns: autosomal dominant and multifactorial polygenic
• Cytogenetic abnormalities: loss of chromosome 9q (superficial); loss of chromosomes 17p, 5q, and 3p; tumor suppressor gene *p53* mutation; and overexpression of p53 protein-invasive

STAGING

• See TNM classification in the Appendix.

SIGNS AND SYMPTOMS

• Painless hematuria
• Voiding irritative symptoms

—Frequency, urgency, and dysuria

• Advanced invasive/metastatic disease

—Loin and bone pain; weight loss, pelvic fullness/mass, and inguinal adenopathy

PATHOPHYSIOLOGY

• TCC growth patterns: papillary (70%), nodular (10%), and sessile or mixed (20%)
• Invasive tumors (T2–T4) arise from both papillary and sessile precursors.
• Grading (WHO)

—1: superficial, normal fibrovascular cores and intact umbrella cells
—2: shorter and broader fibrovascular cores, more cellular crowding, and thicker urothelium
—3: disoriented nuclei; enlarged, hyperchromatic, and pleomorphic cells

• Prognostic factors

—Disease-free survival correlates best with pathologic rather than clinical stage.
—Survival rates (5-year): Survival with T1–T2b lesions ranges from 52% to 70% (negative lymph node metastases), and from 4% to 33% in patients with positive lymph nodes. Survival with ureteral involvement is 40% compared with 60% without involvement. Prostate involvement is ≤20%.
—Patients with CIS of the prostatic urothelium without stromal invasion have survival rates dependent on the stage of the primary bladder tumor.
—Recurrent superficial BC will become invasive in 10% to 15%.

• Spread

—Metastasis occurs via hematogenous and/or lymphatic routes (obturator and external iliac lymph node involvement in 20% to 66% in invasive disease).
—50% of all muscle-invasive BC may have distant micrometastases at the time of presentation.

CAUSES/RISK FACTORS

• Cigarette smoking, occupational chemical exposure (dye, textile, rubber, and leather), dietary factors (coffee drinking, artificial sweetener, high-fat diet), analgesic abuse (phenacetin), cyclophosphamide, chronic bladder infection, pelvic radiation, and cytotoxic agents
• Possible carcinogens

—Aromatic amines, aflatoxins, benzidine, *N*-nitroso compounds, 2-naphthylamine, and 4-aminobiphenyl.

COMPLICATIONS

• Generally due to invasion and advancement of disease into other organs or due to treatment of disease

—Malnutrition, infection, etc.

• Surgical: See "Treatment," complication of RC (bleeding, infection, impotence).

—Nerve-sparing RC does not affect local recurrence or survival rates.
—Tumor cells' spillage and implantation within the pelvis and/or wound with partial cystectomy (20% cases)

DIFFERENTIAL DIAGNOSIS

• Differential for hematuria: upper tract urothelial tumors, lithiasis, prostate diseases (men) (see Section I, "Hematuria–Adult [Gross and Microscopic]")
• Gynecologic and other pelvic tumors: ovary, colon, pelvic, etc.

 Database

HISTORY

• History of

—Exposure to risk factors, especially smoking
—Previous bladder tumor

• Family history of

—Bladder tumor and other malignancies

PHYSICAL EXAMINATION

• General

—Loss of weight, abdominal/pelvic masses, and/or lymphadenopathy

• DRE/bimanual pelvic examination (women)

—Abnormal examination due to contiguous invasion
—Urethral pain, bloody urethral discharge indicate prostate or urethral involvement.

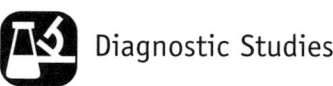 Diagnostic Studies

LABORATORY TESTING

• Blood

—CBC, electrolytes, LFT
—Elevated alkaline phosphatase suggests liver or bone involvement.

• Urine

—Urinalysis: Most have microscopic or gross hematuria.
—Cytology: accurate (95%) for high-grade carcinoma or CIS; poor for low-grade cancers. Markers (telomerase, NP22) are still experimental.

IMAGING

• IVU prior to cystoscopy and biopsy to evaluate for obstruction, tumor (15%–20% also have upper tract tumors)
• Retrograde pyelogram evaluates the upper tracts if IVU is questionable.
• CT scan or MRI prior TURBT (avoid artifact)
• Chest x-ray (rule out metastases)

SPECIAL STUDIES

• TURBT establishes the diagnosis.
• Flow cytometry

—Accurate in diagnosis of CIS
—DNA ploidy correlates with prognosis (progression, recurrence, and survival rate).

• Quantitative fluorescent image analysis: increased sensitivity for superficial lesions (76%); computerized cytologic technique to evaluate DNA content

Treatment

GENERAL MEASURES

- Careful preoperative evaluation and treatment of comorbid conditions
- High-grade T1 lesions may behave like invasive cancer, requiring aggressive treatment.
- Patient and his/her family education
- Radical cystectomy generally considered gold-standard therapy for invasive disease

MEDICAL

- Chemotherapy

—Neoadjuvant/adjuvant: A combination of different agents has similar response rates: MVAC (methotrexate, vinblastine, Adriamycin, and cisplatinum), CMV (MVAC without Adriamycin), and CISCA (cisplatinum, Adriamycin, and cyclophosphamide). New agents include Taxol and carboplatin.
—Intravesical chemotherapy (superficial disease): bacille Calmette-Guérin (potentiates antineoplastic cytokines), thiotepa (alkylating antineoplastic), mitomycin C (antitumor antibiotic), Adriamycin (also used systemically)

SURGICAL

- Radical cystectomy

—Indications: High-risk T1 and >T2 stage diseases, clinically localized to the pelvis are the best candidates.
—PLND will stage and identify candidates for adjuvant chemotherapy; it is questionable whether it has any curative role.
—Wide tumor excision and PLND provide the best chances for local control.
—Prognostic factors: clinical tumor stage, grade, and size. Poor prognosis: ≥T3a/P3a, high grade, age >65 years, irritative voiding symptoms, Hb <12 g/dL, obstructive hydronephrosis, creatinine >1.5 mg/dL, prior DXRT or nephroureterectomy

- Partial cystectomy

—Criteria: resectable solitary lesion with 2-cm margin; negative random biopsies. 5-year survival rates: stage B, 40% to 53%; stage C, 12% to 33%
—Usually, recurrence within first 2 years after surgery

- TURBT

—Palliative measure (control local disease) in elderly patients with significant comorbidity

- Urethrectomy

—Indication: at the time of the initial surgery, involvement of the prostatic urethra or stroma by either direct tumor extension or with CIS; delayed urethrectomy: final pathology reveals positive urethral margin
—Risk of urethral recurrence ranges from 17% to 40%.

- Urinary diversion

—Continent: Indiana and Kock pouches and their variations. Orthotopic diversion to urethra in patients with no urethral disease
—Incontinent: The ileal conduit is most common.

ALTERNATIVE THERAPIES

- Radiation

—DXRT is inferior to radical cystectomy alone for invasive bladder cancer.
—PO-XRT objectives: (1) prevent intraoperative seeding of cancer cells, (2) treat local extravesical disease, and (3) tumor downstaging. Dosage: radical cystectomy immediately after 2000 cGy/1 wk, or 5000 cGy/5 wk with cystectomy 4 weeks later. Higher doses are associated with increased toxicity. There is no survival advantage over cystectomy alone (VA study, SWOG, and NSABG).
—Bladder preservation protocols: The RTOG study was designed to determine whether XRT + chemotherapy is comparable to RC alone or with neoadjuvant chemotherapy.

PATIENT EDUCATION

- Discuss treatment options and types of urinary diversion.

—Contact a stoma therapy nurse.

 ## Follow-Up

MONITORING

- Upper tract

—Ultrasound, IVU, or retrograde pyelogram at least once a year for the first 5 years (more necessary with higher grade and/or stage cancers)

- Lower tract evaluation

—Cystoscopy and cytology every 3 months for the first 2 years; then every 6 months for 3 years, and yearly thereafter.

- When urethra is preserved

—Urethroscopy/urethral cytologic washings (barbotage) every 3 to 6 months (orthotopic neobladder)
—If sign of recurrence: perform urethrectomy

PREVENTION

- Avoid exposure to risk factors, especially chemicals and cigarette smoking.

 ## Miscellaneous

SYNONYMS

- Radical cystectomy is radical cystoprostatectomy in men, and anterior exenteration in women.

ASSOCIATED CONDITIONS

- Other pelvic malignancies: prostate and gynecologic cancer

NOTES

- See Section II for other bladder cancer topics.

ABBREVIATIONS

- BC, bladder cancer; NSABG, National Surgical Adjuvant Bladder Group; PLND, pelvic lymph node dissection; RC, radical cystectomy; DXRT, radiotherapy, definitive; PORT, postoperative radiotherapy; RTOG, Radiation Oncology Group; SWOG, Southwest Oncology Group; TCC, transitional cell carcinoma; TURBT, transurethral resection bladder tumor; VA, Veterans Administration; WHO, World Health Organization

REFERENCES

Hudson M, Catalona W. In: Gillenwater JY, Grayhack JT, Howards SS, Duckett JW, eds. *Adult and Pediatric Urology*, 3rd ed. St Louis: Mosby, 1996:1379–1464.

Messing E, Catalona WJ. In: Walsh PC, Retik AB, Vaughan ED, Wein AJ, eds. *Campbell's Urology*, 7th ed. Philadelphia: WB Saunders, 1998:2329–2382.

Authors: Fernando J. Kim and Robert C. Flanigan

Bladder Cancer—TCC, Metastatic (N+, M+)

 ## Basics

DESCRIPTION

- Lymphatic and hematogenous spread of TCC from the bladder

EPIDEMIOLOGY

- 12,100 deaths in the United States (8,100 male and 3,900 female) in 1999 from bladder cancer.
- Majority of deaths from metastasis
- Most die within 2 years.

GENETICS

- Epidemiologic evidence for hereditary causes does not presently exist.

STAGING

- AJCC-UICC TNM classification: see Section VII.
- Jewett classification

—D1: regional or pelvic lymph node metastases
—D2: metastases to distant sites

- Staging is important for assigning prognosis and treatment.

SIGNS AND SYMPTOMS

- Local disease

—Hematuria, irritative voiding symptoms

- Advanced disease

—Weight loss, fever, leg edema, flank pain, pelvic mass, abdominal or bone pain

- Paraneoplastic symptoms with metastases (hypercalcemia, leukemoid reaction, eosinophilia)

PATHOPHYSIOLOGY

- The pattern of spread is usually ordered.
- Regional lymph nodes

—Anterior and lateral perivesical lymph nodes, hypogastric lymph nodes, obturator lymph nodes, external iliac lymph nodes, lateral sacral lymph nodes

- Distant lymph nodes

—Common iliac lymph nodes, paraaortic lymph nodes, inguinal lymph nodes

- Common distant metastases

—Bone, lung, liver, skin

- Uncommon distant metastases

—Brain, meninges, intraperitoneal organs

CAUSES/RISK FACTORS

- Cancer extending beyond lamina propria and muscularis mucosa into lymphatics and blood vessels
- High-grade tumor

COMPLICATIONS: N/A

DIFFERENTIAL DIAGNOSIS: N/A

 ## Database

HISTORY

- Symptoms of metastatic cancer

—Weight loss, fever, flank pain, abdominal pain, bone pain, pelvic pain

PHYSICAL EXAMINATION

- Fever, pallor, palpable abdominal mass, pelvic mass on bimanual examination, flank tenderness, lower extremity edema

 ## Diagnostic Studies

LABORATORY TESTING

- Renal function tests: creatinine, blood urea nitrogen
- Renal impairment secondary to ureteral obstruction
- Complete blood count revealing anemia
- Coagulation profile revealing coagulopathy secondary to liver metastases

IMAGING

- Assessment of lymph node metastases by bipedal lymphography replaced by CT scan and MRI

—CT and MRI equally effective as lymphography, with accuracy rates 70% to 96%
—Contrast-enhanced CT scans improve accuracy of staging.
—Does not detect micrometastasis; only detects lymph node enlargement
—May perform CT-guided FNA if uncertain

- Bone scan for detection of osseous metastases

—CT scan and/or MRI for further evaluation of indeterminate osseous lesions

- CXR to determine the presence of lung metastases

SPECIAL STUDIES

- Mutations of tumor suppressor genes *P53* and *RB* have been linked to aggressive bladder cancer and risk of metastasis.

 ## Treatment

GENERAL MEASURES

- The goal should be cure, not just palliation.
- Chemotherapy is the mainstay of treatment.
- Many studies describe various response rates.

—Low-volume disease fairs better than high-volume disease.
—Patients with nodal and soft-tissue metastases do better than patients with visceral metastases.

- Patients with a poor performance status also do poorly
- Attempts at improving response rates with higher dose chemotherapy by using hematopoietic growth factors have not been promising (response rate improved but median survival unchanged).

MEDICAL

- Cisplatin and methotrexate: most active single agents

—Subjective tumor regression in 20% to 30% of patients
—Most are only partial regression.

- Platinum-based combination regimes are most common.

—MVAC (methotrexate, vinblastine, Adriamycin [doxorubicin], cisplatin) and CMV (cisplatin, methotrexate, vinblastine) have been the most commonly used regimes.

- MVAC

—Considered standard therapy over the past 10 years
—Four cycles of therapy are the minimum required.
—Most common side effects: mucositis, renal insufficiency, myelosuppression, sepsis
—Objective complete response range: 30% to 50% in early studies
—Recent larger studies have shown complete response rates of 13%.
—Long-term survival is uncommon (10%).
—Bone and liver metastases are less responsive than lymph node or lung metastases, with liver metastases responding the poorest.

- CMV (cisplatin, methotrexate, vinblastine)

—A median of 6 cycles (range: 4 to 10) obtained a complete response.
—28% complete response, 28% partial response
—Toxicity similar to that of MVAC
—Carboplatin-based regimes are used for patients who cannot receive MVAC or CMV, such as patients with renal insufficiency or elderly patients with other comorbidities.

- Paclitaxel (Taxol)

—Antimicrotubular agent
—Most common side effects: mucositis, neuropathy, granulocytopenic fevers
—Objective response rate of 42% in early studies, with responses in liver metastases as well

- Ifosfamide

—Analog of cyclophosphamide
—20% response rate in patients refractory to previous systemic chemotherapy

- Gallium nitrate

—Heavy metal–based compound
—Most common side effects: hypocalcemia, hypomagnesemia, nephrotoxicity, visual disturbances
—17% response rate in patients refractory to previous systemic chemotherapy
—A phase II trial of combining vinblastine, ifosfamide, and gallium nitrate (VIG) had a 41% complete response rate and a 26% partial response rate.

- Gemcitabine (2′,2′-difluouro-2′-deoxycytidine)

—A novel deoxycytidine analog with a broad spectrum of antitumor activity
—Overall response rate of 27%, with responses in liver metastases as well
—Most common side effects: leukopenia, thrombocytopenia, nausea/vomiting
—Recent phase II trials are assessing combinations of cisplatin or carboplatin with gemcitabine or paclitaxel. These appear to be very active.

- Randomized trials of newer combinations with MVAC are ongoing.

SURGICAL

- Palliation for hemorrhagic cystitis or bladder tumor

—Intravesical therapy, laser treatment, percutaneous hypogastric artery embolization, palliative cystectomy

ALTERNATIVE THERAPIES

- Systemic immunotherapy is under investigation.

—Radiation therapy to relieve pain from bone metastases

PATIENT EDUCATION

- American Cancer Society: 1-800-ACS-2345; www.cancer.org
- National Cancer Institute 1-800-4-CANCER; www.nci.nih.gov
- United Ostomy Association 1-800-826-0826; www.uoa.org
- Bladder Health Council, c/o American Foundation for Urologic Disease: 800-242-2383

 Follow-Up

MONITORING

- Overall, prognosis of metastatic disease is poor (most die within 2 years).

—CT scan, MRI

PREVENTION

- The focus is prevention of initial occurrence.

—Elimination of agents linked to bladder cancer (i.e., smoking, drugs, industry-related carcinogens)

 Miscellaneous

SYNONYMS: N/A

ASSOCIATED CONDITIONS: N/A

NOTES: N/A

ABBREVIATIONS

- AJCC-UICC, American Joint Committee on Cancer–Union Internationale Contre le Cancer; FNA, fine-needle aspiration; MVAC, methotrexate, vinblastine, Adriamycin (doxorubicin), cisplatin; CMV, cisplatin, methotrexate, vinblastine; CISCA (CAP), cisplatin, cyclophosphamide, doxorubicin; VIG, vinblastine, ifosfamide, gallium nitrate

REFERENCES

Fagbeni SO, Stadler WM. New chemotherapy regimes for advanced bladder cancer. *Semin Urol Oncol* 1998;16:1, 23.

Hudson MA, Catalona WJ. Urothelial tumors of the bladder, upper tracts, and prostate. In: Gillenwater JY, Grayhack JT, Howards SS, Duckett JW, eds. *Adult and Pediatric Urology,* 3rd ed. St Louis: Mosby, 1996:1379–1435.

Husband JE. Bladder cancer radiologic investigation. In: Raghavan D, Scher HI, Leibel SA, Lange P, eds. *Principles and Practice of Genitourinary Oncology.* Philadelphia: Lippincott-Raven, 1997:261–268.

Loehrer PJ, De Mulder PHM. Management of metastatic bladder cancer. In: Raghavan D, Scher HI, Leibel SA, Lange P, eds. *Principles and Practice of Genitourinary Oncology.* Philadelphia: Lippincott-Raven, 1997:299–305.

Messing EM, Catalona W. Urothelial tumors of the urinary tract. In: *Campbell's Urology,* 7th ed. Walsh PC, Retik AB, Vaughn ED Jr, Wein AJ, eds. Philadelphia: WB Saunders, 1997:2329–2382.

Parker SL, Tong T, Bolden S, Wingo PA. Cancer statistics, 1997. *CA* 1997;47:1.

Authors: Peter A. Pinto, Gary H. Weiss, and Mark Hoffman

Bladder Cancer—TCC, Superficial (CIS, Ta, T1)

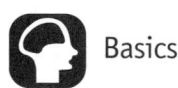 Basics

DESCRIPTION

• A malignant neoplasm originating from the surface lining (uroepithelium) of the bladder, the most common form of which is transitional cell carcinoma (TCC). When the cancer is confined to the mucosa and/or submucosa of the bladder, it is referred to as "superficial."

EPIDEMIOLOGY

• Fourth most common cancer in men; eighth most common in women (male:female ratio: approximately 3:1)
• Highest incidence: men >60 and women >70
• Ethnic predominance: White>Black>Latino

GENETICS

• No clear familial clustering
• Rare hereditary form in association with Muir-Torre syndrome (a familial multicancer syndrome characterized by sebaceous tumors and visceral malignancy)

STAGING

• See the Appendix for TNM classification.
• Classifications

—Carcinoma in situ (CIS): a flat surface–spreading variant of TCC comprised of highly anaplastic cells; equivalent to severe dysplasia
—Stage Ta: confined to the surface mucosa. May be of either low, intermediate or high grade (grades 1–3, respectively)
—Clinical staging may underestimate true pathologic staging by 20% to 30%, especially for larger, deeper, higher grade tumors such as T1, Gr 3.

SIGNS AND SYMPTOMS

• 85% present with either gross or microscopic hematuria, usually painless and often intermittent.
• Less commonly (approximately 20%) associated with irritative symptoms of dysuria, frequency, and urgency (suspect CIS)
• Occasionally discovered during unrelated radiographic evaluation, especially pelvic ultrasound

PATHOPHYSIOLOGY

• Natural history

—5-year recurrence rate: approximately 60%; similar for all grades
  —Most recurrences in first 6 months after resection
  —Recurrence within the first 24 months is associated with reduced long-term recurrence (approximately 10%), however, tumors may recur even years later.
  —Recurrences >4 years continue to have recurrences until death or cystectomy.
  —No relationship between recurrence and progression

—Progression influenced by stage and grade
  —Stage Ta, Gr 1: 2% to 5%; Gr 2: 10% to 15%
  —Stage T1, Gr 2: 20% to 30%; Gr 3: 30% to 50%
  —CIS: 50% to 80% (worse when associated with visible tumor ["secondary CIS"])
—Fatality rate from superficial TCC: approximately 20% at 20 years from onset

• Other clinical/histologic features associated with greater risk of progression and (to a lesser extent) recurrence

—Architecture: nodular/sessile/broad based > papillary
—Multifocal > solitary; size >5 cm
—Lymphatic and/or vascular invasion; high blood vessel density (angiogenesis)

• Molecular tumor markers associated with higher risk of progression

—p53-positive staining/retinoblastoma (RB)-negative staining/epidermal growth factor receptor positivity
—E-cadherin loss

CAUSES/RISK FACTORS

• Tobacco smoking, especially cigarettes

—Dose relationship between number of pack-years and bladder cancer risk
—Quitting smoking decreases risk but never returns to level of nonsmoker
—Latency often >20 years from time of exposure

• Occupational exposure

—Organic chemicals, especially aromatic (aryl)-amines such as naphthalenes, benzidine, aniline dyes, and 4-aminobiphenyl
—High-risk occupations: petroleum chemical/rubber workers, hairdressers, textile workers, truck drivers, aluminum electroplaters

• Medications

—Phenacetin-containing analgesics
—Cyclophosphamide (Cytoxan); when given in chronic low-dose form

• Radiotherapy to the pelvis

COMPLICATIONS

• Ureteral obstruction: Tumor blocks ureteral orifice, but more likely suspect muscle invasion.
• Urinary retention from gross hematuria or prolapsing bladder neck tumor

DIFFERENTIAL DIAGNOSIS

• Urinary tract infection (especially in women): common cause of delayed diagnosis
• Interstitial cystitis/urethral syndrome/chronic prostatitis (mistaken cause of chronic irritative complaints)
• Radiation cystitis
• Bladder stones
• Rarely: other benign or malignant diseases of the bladder or prostate, including metastatic cancer

 Database

HISTORY

• Age and sex of patient?

—Most common in men >50; males > females

• When did you first have blood in the urine? Was is visible (gross) or invisible (microscopic)? Was there any associated pain?

—Painless gross hematuria is the most common presenting sign of bladder cancer, even if intermittent.

• Irritative bladder symptoms present? (e.g., dysuria, urgency, frequency)

—Occasionally associated with bladder cancer, especially CIS

• Smoking history? (Record age of onset, total years, packs per day, years since quitting.)

—Cigarette smoking is the leading cause of bladder cancer, with risks proportional to duration and amount. A long latency (>20 years) is common.

• Occupational risk factors?

—Naphthylamine, benzidine, aniline dyes, and 4-aminobiphenyl (often in rubber, dye, petroleum industries)

PHYSICAL EXAMINATION

• Rarely abnormal for superficial TCC

 Diagnostic Studies

LABORATORY TESTING

• Urinalysis, including standard dipstick and microscopic evaluation for RBCs
• Urine cytology: Three separate determinations increase sensitivity.

—Very high specificity but low overall sensitivity. Positive readings are nearly always genuine, but negative or atypical results do not exclude TCC. Best at detecting high-grade TCC and CIS

• Other urinary tests (e.g., DNA ploidy, BTA-Stat, NMP-22, FDP, DD23) may be useful for monitoring tumor recurrences.

IMAGING

• Excretory urography/intravenous pyelogram (IVP)

—Exclude coincident upper tract TCC in patients with bladder cancer (approximate 2% incidence).

• Abdominal/pelvic ultrasound

—Excluding hydronephrosis. Occasionally images bladder tumors. Especially useful in low-risk patients (e.g., younger women) with unexplained hematuria when combined with cystoscopy

• Abdominal CT with contrast

—Study of choice when initially evaluating gross painless hematuria in high-risk patients with sus-

pected TCC or prior to tumor resection in high-volume, aggressive-appearing bladder tumors suspected of being invasive

SPECIAL STUDIES

• Cystoscopy: "gold standard" for evaluating lower tract bladder lesions

—In office, under local anesthesia at time of initial presentation. If TCC strongly suspected, however, may be combined with biopsy/TURBT as single definitive procedure under anesthesia

• Retrograde pyelography is used for equivocal IVP or CT or in cases of contrast allergy to rule out coincident upper tract lesions.

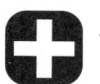 Treatment

GENERAL MEASURES

• Goals: Remove all visible tumor, if possible; reduce recurrences; and prevent disease progression.

MEDICAL

• Intravesical therapy

—General
  —Adjuvant to surgery to reduce tumor recurrence, or as a definitive treatment to eliminate small-volume residual disease and/or inaccessible disease such as CIS
  —Usually administered as an induction course of 6 to 8 weekly sequential treatments via Foley catheter and retained for 2 hours
—Intravesical chemotherapy
  —Drugs: (United States and elsewhere) thiotepa, doxorubicin (Adriamycin), mitomycin, valrubicin; (outside of United States) epirubicin, ethoglucid
  —In addition to induction regimen, effective as single dose given within 24 hours of tumor resection; role of maintenance chemotherapy uncertain
  —Marginal (7%–14%) reduction in long-term recurrence rate; no evidence for effectiveness in preventing tumor progression
—Intravesical immunotherapy
  —Drugs: BCG (a live suspension of the attenuated *Mycobacterium bovis* vaccine strain: bacillus Calmette-Guérin), interferon-alpha (IFN-α)
  —BCG administered no sooner than 10 days after tumor resection as 6-week induction course. Repeat induction courses and maintenance courses are likely beneficial.
  —BCG is the single most effective intravesical agent, with complete response rates of approximately 55% to 75% for residual disease and CIS, respectively. It is 3× more effective than chemotherapy for prophylaxis. Two-thirds of responses persist for 5 years.
  —BCG is generally used more cautiously than chemotherapy due to a low (<5%) but serious risk of systemic BCG infection (BCGosis), especially if administered in a setting of recent surgery or traumatic catheterization (see Section II, "BCG Sepsis").

—IFN-α may be useful as a low-toxicity, second-line agent for BCG failures or in combination with other agents.
  —BGG-IFNα under study for combination therapy

SURGICAL

• Transurethral resection of bladder tumor (TURBT or TURB)

—First-line treatment for all visible tumors; diagnostic and therapeutic

• Bladder biopsies (peritumoral and "random")

—Helpful in cases of large, multiple, or high-grade tumors to assess for presence of dysplasia and CIS (field disease)

• Laser or electrofulguration

—Useful for elimination of recurrent, small-volume, low-grade, papillary tumors (especially papillomas); can be performed under local anesthesia

• Radical cystectomy

—Sometimes appropriate for recurrent T1, Gr 3 disease or multifocal CIS that has failed to respond to one or two courses of BCG therapy, respectively.
—Rarely, may be necessary for extensive unresectable superficial disease

ALTERNATIVE THERAPIES

• Photodynamic therapy (PDT)

—Appropriate for select cases of multifocal CIS refractory to other modalities

PATIENT EDUCATION

• Patients should be counseled that bladder cancer is best regarded as a lifelong disease requiring frequent and scheduled monitoring.

 Follow-Up

MONITORING

• Cystoscopic and cytologic monitoring every 3 months for 2 years, then every 6 months for 2 years, and then annually thereafter. Schedule resets with each recurrence. Intervals may be extended sooner for low-risk tumors.
• Bladder biopsies recommended at first post-therapy cystoscopy for high-grade tumors, then as necessary, depending on cytology results and cystoscopic appearance.
• Upper tract surveillance studies (IVP or retrograde pyelogram) are suggested every 2 to 3 years for high-grade bladder tumors and CIS.

PREVENTION

• Immediate smoking cessation reduces recurrence/progression rate.
• Daily megadoses of antioxidant vitamins (A, 32,000 IU; C, 2000 mg; E, 400 IU) may reduce recurrence rate, especially after a successful BCG response.

 Miscellaneous

SYNONYMS

• Bladder tumor, papilloma (Ta, Gr 1), severe dysplasia (CIS)

ASSOCIATED CONDITIONS

• Other smoking-related illnesses

NOTES

• See also bladder cancer—related topics in Section II; "BCG Sepsis" (in Section II); Section III, "WHO Classification of Bladder Tumors."

ABBREVIATIONS

• BT, bladder tumor; CIS, carcinoma in situ; PDT, photodynamic therapy; TCC, transitional cell carcinoma; TURB(T), transurethral resection of bladder tumor

REFERENCES

Crawford ED. Diagnosis and treatment of superficial bladder cancer: An update. *Semin Urol Oncol* 1996;14:1–9.

Heney NM. Natural history of superficial bladder cancer: Prognostic features and long-term disease course. *Urol Clin North Am* 1992;19:429–433.

Lamm DL, van der Meijden APM, Akaza H, et al. Intravesical chemotherapy and immunotherapy: How do we assess their effectiveness and what are their limitations and uses? *Int J Urol* 1995;2[Suppl 2]:23–35.

Scher HI, Shipley WU, Herr HW. Cancer of the bladder. In: DeVita VT, Hellman S, Rosenberg SA, eds. *Cancer: Principles and Practice of Oncology.* Philadelphia: Lippincott-Raven, 1997:1300–1321.

Author: Michael A. O'Donnell

Bladder Diverticulum

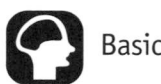 Basics

DESCRIPTION

• An outpouching of urothelium through the muscular wall of the bladder; may be congenital (primary) or acquired (secondary)

EPIDEMIOLOGY

• Congenital: peak incidence less than 10 years old

—More common in males than in females
—May be incidental finding in adulthood

• Acquired: peak incidence greater than 60 years old

—Almost exclusively males
—May occur in children with high voiding pressures

GENETICS

• Unknown

STAGING: N/A

SIGNS AND SYMPTOMS

• Direct symptoms are uncommon.

—Lower abdominal distention
—Iliac fossa pain during voiding
—Double voiding

• Secondary to complicating factors

—Urinary tract infections
—Stones
—Obstruction

• Commonly asymptomatic and/or incidental finding

PATHOPHYSIOLOGY

• Congenital

—Weakness or malformation of bladder wall in area of ureterovesical hiatus
—May have normal voiding dynamics and pressures

• Acquired

—Secondary to high bladder pressures, bladder outlet obstruction
   —Also common in area of ureterovesical junction
   —May be at junction of bladder base and distensible portion of bladder
—Iatrogenic
   —After ureteral reimplant
   —In any area of bladder after surgical cystotomy if inadequate closure of bladder muscle

CAUSES/RISK FACTORS

• Congenital

—May have no risk factors

• Acquired: high bladder pressure and/or outlet obstruction

—Prostatic hypertrophy or malignancy
—Urethral stricture disease
—Neurogenic voiding dysfunction
—Cystostomy

COMPLICATIONS

• Urinary tract infection

—Standard irritative symptoms
—Difficult to eradicate secondary to residual urine
—Spontaneous perforation may be fatal.

• Calculus formation

—Stasis and/or infection

• Ureteral or urethral obstruction

—Extrinsic compression by diverticulum

• Vesicoureteral reflux
• Extraurinary compression or obstruction

—Rectum
—Pelvic veins

• Carcinoma in the diverticulum

—75% to 80% TCC; 20% to 25% squamous cell cancer
—2% to 7% incidence
—Peak incidence: 65 to 75 years old
—Prolonged contact of carcinogens secondary to stasis

DIFFERENTIAL DIAGNOSIS

• Bladder outlet obstruction
• Urinary tract infection
• Pelvic mass of any etiology

 Database

HISTORY

• Usually nonspecific

—Irritative symptoms: frequency, urgency, dysuria
—Obstructive symptoms: decreased stream, double voiding, sense of incomplete bladder emptying

• Pelvic pain

PHYSICAL EXAMINATION

• Abdominal/pelvic distention
• Palpable or percussible mass

Diagnostic Studies

LABORATORY TESTING

- Urinalysis and culture
—Hematuria
—Infection
—Electrolytes and creatinine

IMAGING

- Voiding cystourethrogram
—Study of choice
—Voids contrast into diverticulum
—Multiple views needed to see all surfaces
- Intravenous urography
—May demonstrate diverticulum
—May suggest presence of diverticulum by bladder wall distortion
- CT scanning
—Defines relationship to other pelvic structures

SPECIAL STUDIES

- Cystourethroscopy
—The entire surface of the diverticulum must be visualized.
—Location of ureteral orifices should be identified.
- Urine cytology
—Voided
—Bladder washings at time of cystoscopy

 Treatment

GENERAL MEASURES

- Surgical indications
—Chronic infection
—Stones
—Premalignant changes or carcinoma
- Controversy regarding management of asymptomatic, uncomplicated diverticula
—Excision vs. surveillance
—Age
—General health
—Other procedures
　—Relief of bladder outlet obstruction

MEDICAL

- Antibiotics

SURGICAL

- Reduction of bladder outlet obstruction
—To treat etiology of acquired diverticula
—TURP/TUIP/alternative transurethral measures
　—For simple diverticulum with subsequent surveillance
—Suprapubic prostatectomy with bladder diverticulectomy
- Surgical management of diverticulum
—Transurethral resection of diverticular neck
　—Adjunct to TURP, etc., if poorly draining diverticulum
　—To open neck to visualize interior of diverticulum
—Transvesical approach
　—Inversion of mucosa, excision of neck, and closure of bladder defect; especially small diverticula
　—Submucosal excision of inner mucosal lining from outer fibrous shell
—Extravesical approach
　—Usually in combination with transvesical identification of diverticulum
　—Allows packing of diverticulum and/or bimanual dissection
　—Especially for large lesions
- Laparoscopy
—Recently described

ALTERNATIVE THERAPIES

- Surveillance
—Urinary cytology every 6 to 12 months
—For asymptomatic, uncomplicated diverticula

PATIENT EDUCATION: N/A

 Follow-Up

MONITORING

- Surveillance: see above

PREVENTION: N/A

 Miscellaneous

SYNONYMS: N/A

ASSOCIATED CONDITIONS

- Bladder outlet obstruction, urethral stricture disease, neurogenic voiding dysfunction

NOTES: N/A

ABBREVIATIONS

- TURP, transurethral resection of prostate; TUIP, transurethral incision of prostate

REFERENCES

Das S. Laparoscopic removal of bladder diverticulum. *J Urol* 1992;148:1837–1839.

McLean P, Kelalis PP. Bladder diverticulum in the male. *Br J Urol* 1968;40:321.

VanArsdalen KN, Wein AJ. Bladder diverticulectomy. In: Droller MJ, ed. *Surgical Management of Urologic Disease—An Anatomic Approach.* St Louis: Mosby–Year Book, 1992;629–639.

Author: Keith VanArsdalen

Bladder Neck Contracture

 Basics

DESCRIPTION

• Physical and functional obstruction at the bladder neck outlet, consisting of two types:

—Organic fibrosis secondary to surgery or trauma, chronic inflammation or infection
—Physiologic: smooth sphincter dyssynergia (SSD): increased smooth muscle tone at BN and internal sphincter

EPIDEMIOLOGY

• Organic fibrosis type: often seen after prostate surgery (i.e., TURP, open prostatectomy, RRP), >60 years of age, males > females; can see in females with history of bladder neck surgery or trauma. Race, socioeconomic status not a factor
• Smooth sphincter dyssynergia (SSD): men often <60 years of age, long-standing symptoms of bladder outlet obstruction (BOO) type. Rarely see in females

GENETICS: N/A

STAGING: N/A

SIGNS AND SYMPTOMS

• Obstructive voiding symptoms: often gradual in onset

—Hesitancy, stranguria
—Decreased flow
—Nocturia
—Incomplete voiding

• Irritative

—Frequency
—Urgency

• Asymptomatic

—Organic fibrosis type: often without symptoms until BOO is severe
—SSD often symptomatic: symptoms similar to prostatitis

PATHOPHYSIOLOGY

• Organic fibrosis: abnormal collection of fibrotic collagenous tissue at BN. Lack of epithelial cells. Typically develops postoperatively
• SSD: pathophysiology uncertain; possible increased sympathetic nervous system function, increased sensitivity of alpha-1 receptors, resulting in increased smooth muscle contraction tone

CAUSES/RISK FACTORS

• Organic fibrosis: trauma to the BN area, causing abnormal deposit of scar tissue

—TURP: 3% to 10% overall incidence. Increased with TURP of small glands up to 20%; small prostate glands do not protect BN from TUR injury. Large glands push BN out of harms' way.
  —Excessive resection into the trigone inhibits epithelial migration to BN before scar tissue formation.

—RRP: 2% to 15% incidence. Excessive leakage at anastomotic site, poor urethra mucosa–bladder neck mucosal interface. Suture reaction or tight anastomosis formation
—Prolonged irritation and inflammation: excessive catheter time, foreign body (i.e., suture, Gore-Tex, mesh from BN suspensions), chronic infection
—Radiation: especially if TURP in time (3 months) close to initiation of radiation treatment

COMPLICATIONS

• Chronic BOO with secondary urinary retention
• Vesicolithiasis
• Pelvic pain

—Detrusor muscle dysfunction. Hyperactivity, increased bladder pressure, seen in early stage of obstruction. Decompensation of detrusor with atony and retention, in end-stage obstruction, rare

• Renal failure: rarely seen
• Increased risk for infection thought secondary to increased PVR
• Incontinence

—Overflow: detrusor decompensation
—Urgency: detrusor hyperactivity

• Hematuria

—Usually microscopic but gross can be seen. Rarely presents with severe hemorrhage

DIFFERENTIAL DIAGNOSIS

• BPH with BOO
• Urethral stricture: history of urethritis, GC infection, catheter use, instrumentation
• Neurogenic bladder: history of laminectomy, spinal trauma, MS, CVA, Parkinson disease, herpes infection
• Prostatitis: swollen, tender prostate; fever; abnormal urine/bacteria in urine
• Bladder cancer: A large tumor at BN can cause BOO.
• Bladder stone, foreign body (FB): often history of intermittent BOO. History of stone disease. History of bladder suspension surgery
• Psychogenic: psychiatric history
• Drugs: sympathomimetic drugs, anticholinergic drugs, narcotics, antihistamines, neuroleptic drugs
• Locally advanced prostate cancer: abnormal DRE, elevated PSA

 Database

HISTORY

• Age and sex of the patient?

—Rare in females
—Older males (>60 years): organic fibrosis most common type BNC, post TURP or open prostatectomy. Ask if the patient has had urologic surgery.
—Younger males (<60 years): SSD type of BOO most likely type of BNC (functional)

• History of previous surgery or trauma?

—History of TURP, RRP, open prostatectomy: often voided well initially after procedure, but symptoms occurred later

• History of gross hematuria?

—Rule out stones, GU malignancies (see "Differential Diagnosis")

• History of pelvic radiation?

—See "Differential Diagnosis."

• Current medication?

—See "Differential Diagnosis."

• History of infections or venereal disease?

—See "Differential Diagnosis."

PHYSICAL EXAMINATION

• Palpation of lower abdomen; rule out bladder distention
• DRE: post TURP, prostate often small with increased firmness; may also note asymmetry. Large, irregular, firm prostate: rule out cancer. Boggy, tender prostate: suggests prostatitis
• Neurogenic bladder

—Poor rectal tone may suggest bladder atony and neurologic disease. Bulbocavernosal reflex checks S_2-S_3-S_4 reflex arc; if abnormal, may indicate neural pathology

• Palpation of penile urethra

—Discharge, tenderness, or firmness of the urethra may indicate urethritis, urethral stricture, or FB.
—Examine the meatus to rule out meatal stenosis.
—Blisters on genitalia suggests herpes infection.

Diagnostic Studies

LABORATORY TESTING

- Urine

—Urine analysis: with organic fibrosis type BNC, can see microhematuria, pyuria. Often normal. Rule out infection: positive nitrate dipstick, positive Gram stain or culture. Excessive pyuria suggests urethritis, prostatitis, FB, stone, or tumor.
—Cytology: negative with BNC; positive suggests tumor

- Serum chemistry

—Serum creatinine: usually normal with BNC. Elevation suggests upper tract obstruction or intrinsic renal disease.
—PSA: usually normal in BNC. If patient S/P, RRP should be undetectable. Elevation seen in prostatitis/urethritis, some BPH, and cancer of prostate. Catheterization may also cause a temporary rise.

IMAGING

- KUB may help rule out bladder stone, FB.
- EXU: BNC often causes thickened bladder, ↑ PVR. Rarely see upper tract obstruction. Look for enlarged prostate shadow: BPH, prostatitis. End-stage BOO: may see large flacci-type bladder, possible hydroureter. Neurogenic bladder: may see Christmas tree bladder with upper tract dilation
- CAT/MRI usually not helpful unless suspect malignancy
- Retrograde urethrogram: BNC ("toothpaste sign") caused by small bladder opening, causing layering of contrast material as it enters bladder. Look for urethral strictures.

SPECIAL STUDIES

- Cystoscopy: Gold study to make organic fibrosis–type BNC diagnosis. Will rule out urethral stricture. BNC may appear as an elevated posterior elevation of bladder neck or a diaphragm-type contrast. Use with the opening superior and midline.
- Urodynamics: measures capacity, compliance, detrusor function and pressures, flow of stream, and sensation

—Simple flow study: BNC: often see poor flow (<15 cc/s). May see poor upstroke of flow pattern and abdominal straining pattern. Post-void residual is normal to elevated.
—Pressure flowmetry: measures flow and detrusor pressure generated during voiding. Low flow and elevated pressure (>40 cm H_2O pressure) indicate obstruction.
   —The video component will show narrowing at the contracture site.
—Cystometrogram (CMG): may show decreased compliance; instability often present (uninhibited detrusor contractions); end-stage obstruction may show a decompensated detrusor pattern (large capacity, poor detrusor contractions, elevated PVR).

 ## Treatment

GENERAL MEASURES

- If patient presenting with acute urinary retention, may need Foley or suprapubic catheter

MEDICAL

- Not helpful with organic fibrosis type; helpful with SSD type

—SSD: Alpha-blocker medication is beneficial. Tamsulosin (Flomax) 0.4 mg qhs; terazosin (Hytrin) 1 mg, increasing to 5 mg qhs; doxazosin (Cardura) 1 mg, increasing to 4 mg qhs
   —Possible adverse effects: orthostatic hypotension, lethargy, nasal congestion, dry mouth, constipation; 10% of patients have side effects.

SURGICAL

- Endoscopic incision of BNC: cold knife, laser, or electrocautery (Collins knife) acceptable

—Incision made at 4 and 8 o'clock positions of BNC; cut down until fat noted at incision area. Catheter drainage of the bladder for 24 hours postprocedure. Usually done as an outpatient. >90% success rate in relieving BNC. Applies to BNC secondary seen after TURP, open prostatectomy

- Dilation: may be successful, especially with BNC after RRP; less successful with BNC from TURP or trauma
- If dilation unsuccessful, cold knife incision at 6 o'clock position often successful in post-RRP BNC. Steroid injections controversial. Laser use (KTP/532, Nd:YAG) theoretically may give rise to less recurrent scar formation.

ALTERNATIVE THERAPIES

- Balloon dilation: rarely done. Holmium laser ablation of BNC

PATIENT EDUCATION

- *Benign Prostatic Hyperplasia: Diagnosis and Treatment*. Clinical Practice Guideline No. 8. U.S. Department of Health and Human Services, 1994.

 ## Follow-Up

MONITORING

- Every 3 to 4 months for 1 year, then every year to rule out recurrent stricture. Simple flow study with PVR usually adequate. Flexible cystoscopy if suspicious of recurrent BNC

PREVENTION

- Consider TUIP instead of TURP for small glands (<30 g).
- Consider BN incisions at 5 and 7 o'clock after TURP in small-gland TURP.
- Steroid injection of BN is controversial.
- Watertight, urethral mucosa to bladder neck mucosa anastomosis with RRP
- Minimize catheter drainage time.
- If excessive pelvic hematoma occurs after RRP: early drainage beneficial
- Wedge resection of posterior BN during open simple prostatectomy

 ## Miscellaneous

SYNONYMS

- Bladder neck stricture, bladder neck narrowing

ASSOCIATED CONDITIONS: N/A

NOTES

- See also Section II, "Bladder Outlet Obstruction."

ABBREVIATIONS

- BN, bladder neck; BNC, bladder neck contracture; BOO, bladder outlet obstruction; CVA, cerebral vascular accident; FB, foreign body; MS, multiple sclerosis; PVR, post-void residual; RRP, radical retropubic prostatectomy; SSD, smooth sphincter dyssynergia; TUIP, transurethral incision of prostate; TURP, transurethral resection of prostate

REFERENCES

Grayhack JT, Kozlowski JM. Benign prostatic hyperplasia. In: Gillenwater JY, Grayhack JT, Howard SS, Duckett JW, eds. *Adult and Pediatric Urology*, 3rd ed. St Louis: Mosby–Year Book, 1996.

Green LF. Postoperative contracture of the vesical neck. AUA Update, Vol II, Lesson 32, 1983.

Mebust WK. A review of TURP complications and the AUA National Cooperative Study. AUA Update, Vol 8, Lesson 24, 1989.

Author: Michael J. Wehle

Bladder Neck Hypertrophy

 Basics

DESCRIPTION

• Bladder neck hypertrophy (BNH) is a frequently misdiagnosed cause of urinary tract symptoms and voiding difficulty in young men.

EPIDEMIOLOGY

• Men, usually 20 to 60 years old
• Very rare in women
• Symptom history often lasting years prior to diagnosis
• History of misdiagnosis as chronic prostatitis, neurogenic bladder dysfunction, psychogenic voiding dysfunction

GENETICS

• Unknown

STAGING: N/A

SIGNS AND SYMPTOMS

• Obstructive and irritative

—Urgency, frequency, nocturia, dysuria, delay, decreased force of stream, dribbling
—Difficulty voiding in young men after an operation
—History of difficulty voiding in company of others

• Nonspecific pelvic pain
• Patients commonly deny a decreased flow of stream.
• Mimics chronic nonbacterial prostatitis/prostatodynia

PATHOPHYSIOLOGY

• Historical

—Fibrosis (Marion); developmental disorder of bladder neck musculature (Turner-Warwick)

• Current hypothesis (backed by neuropathologic study)

—Sympathetic nervous dysfunction
—Functional obstruction with bladder neck contraction during micturition

• Trapped prostate

—When BPH occurs in conjunction with bladder neck hypertrophy, the bladder neck prevents inward prostate growth.
—Results in obstructive small prostate

CAUSES/RISK FACTORS

• Obstruction due to bladder neck hypertrophy is caused by

—Bladder neck smooth muscle contraction during micturition

COMPLICATIONS

• Bladder decompensation

—Poor detrusor function, high residual urine, UTI

DIFFERENTIAL DIAGNOSIS

• Benign prostatic hyperplasia
• Bladder neck contracture

—History of prior prostatectomy or bladder neck surgery
—History of chronic inflammation and fibrosis

• Relative bladder neck obstruction

—Result of inadequate detrusor contraction/inability to open a normal bladder neck
—Common finding in women with voiding dysfunction
—Diagnosis confirmed by urodynamics

• Postoperative urethral stricture

—Can cause bladder neck hypertrophy that is not obstructive (global detrusor response to distal obstruction)
—Stricture management resolves BNH.
—If performed, bladder neck surgery may lead to incontinence after subsequent urethroplasty.

• Neurogenic bladder

—Generally associated with history of neurologic event/disorder
—Striated sphincter dyssynergia differentiated by videourodynamics (obstruction at membranous urethra, bladder neck funneling preserved)

• Psychogenic voiding dysfunction/"anxious bladder"

—Young men with a similar symptom complex but without measurable flow or bladder neck funneling abnormalities
—Poor response to surgical therapy/avoid empiric surgical therapy

 Database

HISTORY

• Age and sex?

—Disorder with onset in relatively young men

• Voiding symptoms?

—Obstructive/irritative symptoms; many patients virtually asymptomatic
—Difficulty voiding in company of others (should lead to further evaluation to rule out bladder neck obstruction)

• Quality of urinary stream?

—Decreased urinary flow rates in all patients; frequently denied (due to lifelong symptom pattern)

• History of UTI/prostatitis/gonococcal (GC) urethritis?

—Commonly misdiagnosed as chronic nonbacterial prostatitis (due to overlap of obstructive and irritative symptoms)
—Residual urine in later stages may set up for infection.
—GC a common cause of urethral stricture disease.

• Significant medical or surgical history?

—Medical conditions associated with neurogenic bladder
—Prior abdominal, pelvic, or back surgery (differential diagnosis)

• Prior endoscopic urologic evaluation/catheterization/surgery?

—Results, and possibility of postoperative stricture

• Current medications?

—Anticholinergic side effects, adrenergic agonists (decongestants)

PHYSICAL EXAMINATION

• Blood pressure

—Side effects of potential medical therapy with alpha-blockers

• Abdominal examination

—Bladder distention, scars from previous surgery

• Urogenital examination

—Palpable urethral stricture, meatal stenosis

• Digital rectal examination

—Prostate size, character, nodularity, tenderness
—Prostate may be large or small

• Neurologic examination

—Sensory, motor reflexes; pelvic reflexes; gait (neurogenic bladder)

Diagnostic Studies

LABORATORY TESTING

• Serum creatinine

—Evaluate for renal parenchymal sequela of obstruction.

• Serum electrolytes

IMAGING

• Ultrasound

—Evaluate for upper tract involvement in obstruction.
—Can evaluate post-void residual

• Intravenous pyelogram

—Evaluate for upper tract involvement in obstruction; more invasive than ultrasound

SPECIAL STUDIES

• Cystoscopy

—Evaluate other causes of obstruction (prostate, stricture) and bladder/bladder neck contour
—Cannot make diagnosis based on cystoscopic view of bladder neck
  —Apparently hypertrophied bladder necks may be deemed non-obstructive using urodynamic evaluation.
  —Functional obstruction can occur in the absence of any endoscopic change.

• Voiding flow-rate study

—Decrease in peak flow rate
—Not sufficient for evaluation without videourodynamics (usually concurrent)

• Urodynamic evaluation (synchronous video pressure-flow–cystourethrography)

—Essential for diagnosis
—Findings
  —Elevated detrusor pressure during voiding
  —Decreased urinary flow rate
  —Poor funneling of the bladder neck during voiding (failure to open)
—Electromyography not necessarily indicated in neurologically intact patients

 Treatment

GENERAL MEASURES

• Relief of bladder neck obstruction without compromising continence
• Urodynamically significant obstructing bladder neck should be identified prior to surgical therapy.

MEDICAL

• Alpha-adrenergic blockade

—Reasonable initial therapy based on pathophysiology
—Poor long-term outcomes
—Confounded by poor long-term compliance due to poor early symptom relief
—67% improvement in subset of patients who continued long-term α-blocker therapy in one study
—Avoids potential risk of retrograde ejaculation
—Agents (nonselective vs. selective): need to use high doses for effect
  —Terazosin (Hytrin) 1 to 20 mg po qd
  —Doxazosin (Cardura) 1 to 8 mg po qd
  —Tamsulosin (Flomax) 0.4 to 0.48 mg po qd; GU selective
—These agents may cause orthostatic hypotension (especially initial dose) and rare retrograde ejaculation.

• Anxiolytics

—Reduce anxiety/focus on voiding and may relax external striated sphincter
  —Diazepam (Valium) 2 to 5 mg po bid/qid

SURGICAL

• Bladder neck incision

—Gold standard treatment
  —87% complete symptom resolution in one study
—Performed endoscopically from the proximal bladder neck to the proximal verumontanum
  —Using electrocautery/laser/Collins knife
  —Unilateral at the 5 or 7 o'clock position vs. bilateral
  —Unilateral associated with much lower incidence of retrograde ejaculation
—May relieve trapped prostate, or may be combined with limited transurethral resection of the prostate
—Complications
  —Retrograde ejaculation (27% if bilateral incision in one study, 0% with unilateral incision in two studies); counsel in young patients with fertility concerns
  —Bleeding, risks of anesthesia
  —Incontinence, especially in women (poor distal urethral mechanism)
  —Theoretical risk of postoperative stricture

• Y-V vesicoplasty (historical interest only)

ALTERNATIVE THERAPIES: N/A

PATIENT EDUCATION

• Natural history and chronic nature of disease

—Eventual bladder decompensation may result.

• Importance of long-term medical compliance if medical therapy undertaken

 Follow-Up

MONITORING

• Periodic reevaluation of obstruction

—History, uroflow, post-void residual
—Repeat urodynamics not necessarily indicated unless response equivocal

• Regular follow-up reasonable for patients on α-blocker therapy

—Ensure compliance and relief of obstruction vs. possible need for surgery.

PREVENTION

• Early diagnosis diminishes complications.

Miscellaneous

SYNONYMS

• Primary bladder neck obstruction, functional bladder neck obstruction, bladder neck dysfunction, bladder neck dyssynergia, Marion disease

ASSOCIATED CONDITIONS: N/A

NOTES

• See also Section II, "Bladder Outlet Obstruction."

ABBREVIATIONS

• BNH, bladder neck hypertrophy

REFERENCES

Bates CP, et al. The nature of the abnormality in bladder neck obstruction. *Br J Urol* 1975;47:651–656.

Marion G. Surgery of the neck of the bladder. *Br J Urol* 1933;5:351–380.

Trockman BA, et al. Primary bladder neck obstruction: Urodynamic findings and treatment results in 36 men. *J Urol* 1996;156:1418–1420.

Turner-Warwick R, et al. A urodynamic view of the clinical problems associated with bladder neck dysfunction and its treatment by endoscopic incision and trans-trigonal posterior prostatectomy. *Br J Urol* 1973;45:44–59.

Webster GD, et al. The evaluation of bladder neck dysfunction. *J Urol* 1980;123:196–198.

Authors: Robert R. Byrne and Craig F. Donatucci

Bladder Outlet Obstruction

 Basics

DESCRIPTION

• *Bladder outlet obstruction* (BOO) is strictly defined as a sustained detrusor contraction of over 40 to 50 cm H_2O, associated with a uroflow of less than 12 to 15 mL per second.

EPIDEMIOLOGY

• Most common cause in men: BPH
• Most common cause in women is iatrogenic from urethropexy or sling procedures

GENETICS: N/A

STAGING: N/A

SIGNS AND SYMPTOMS

• Male: hesitancy, straining, decreased stream, post-void dribbling

—Signs and symptoms of prostatism predominate for BOO in men.

• Female

—Vague symptoms that cannot distinguish BOO from poor detrusor contractility to any consistent degree

PATHOPHYSIOLOGY

• Outflow obstruction leads to detrusor hypertrophy and classic symptoms of BOO.

CAUSES/RISK FACTORS

• Depends on the etiology (see above)

—Not all men with BPH have prostatic obstruction. The incidence of urinary retention in BPH is less than 5%.
—Advancing age, lower urinary tract surgery
—Anticholinergic and adrenergic medications

COMPLICATIONS

• Bladder instability; flaccid bladder
• Urinary retention with the possibility of a post-obstructive diuresis
• UTIs and stones secondary to urine stagnation
• Bladder diverticula
• Compromised renal function

DIFFERENTIAL DIAGNOSIS

• Urinary retention or large post-void residual volumes in women more commonly are the result of a poor detrusor contractility rather than BOO.
• Poor detrusor contractility must also be ruled out in men.
• Male

—Benign prostatic hyperplasia with prostatic obstruction
—Urethral strictures, usually from previous instrumentation, trauma, or surgery (e.g., bladder neck contracture after radical prostatectomy)
—Infection (caruncle, prostatitis, intraurethral wart)
—Neoplasm at bladder neck or urethra
—Urethral valve: more common in children
—Foreign body
—Neurologic (detrusor sphincter dyssynergia, pseudodyssynergia, diabetes mellitus)
—Meatal stenosis
—Primary vesicle neck obstruction (bladder neck hypertrophy)

• Female

—Same as in men, with the exception of prostatic etiologies
—Extrinsic compression from benign or malignant growths of the uterus, ovaries, or vagina
—Cystocele
—Periurethral diverticulum
—Other infections, such as Skene's duct abscess and labial caruncle

 Database

HISTORY

• Gastrointestinal, gynecologic, urologic (including frequency, strength of stream, straining, urgency, hesitancy, urge incontinence, post-void dribbling, trauma) and neurologic history

—Medications (e.g., psychotropics)

• Past surgery or catheterizations
• Voiding diary
• AUA symptom scores: mild (score: ≤7); moderate (score: 8–19); severe (score: 20–35)

PHYSICAL EXAMINATION

• Abdominal for distended bladder
• Genitourinary

—Rectal: prostate size, tenderness, consistency

• Neurologic examination to screen for gross deficits

Diagnostic Studies

LABORATORY TESTING

- Urinalysis: usually normal
- Determine baseline renal function.

IMAGING

- Uroflow and post-void residual ultrasound

—These are good screening procedures, but not specific to distinguish between prostatic obstruction, detrusor instability, and impaired detrusor contraction.

SPECIAL STUDIES

- Full urodynamic study

—This is how the definition was established for BOO.

—This definition is mainly for men (see above).

—In women it is more vague, but the consensus is voiding pressures of 50 cm H_2O with flow rates less than 15 mL per second.

- EMG: useful in women and men with neurogenic etiologies

 ## Treatment

GENERAL MEASURES

- Treatment is based on specific etiology.
- "Watchful waiting" for patients with mild symptoms and no significant side effects (retention, UTI, etc.)
- BPH is often initially managed with medical therapy.

—Surgical intervention for complicated clinical conditions (renal insufficiency secondary to BOO, calculi, etc.)

MEDICAL

- Postobstructive diuresis

—Usually self-limited and is corrected by the patient drinking water freely, allowing the osmoreceptors to be reset and control ADH secretion

- Foley catheter to monitor fluid management

—Replacement with IV fluids of one-half normal saline with potassium. The fluid replacement should be 0.5 cc for every 1 cc of urine output. Strict monitoring of serum electrolytes every 4 to 6 hours during diuresis

- Oral agents for BPH: See Section II, "Prostate—Benign Hyperplasia."

SURGICAL

- See Section II, "Prostate—Benign Hyperplasia," for options.
- Urethral stricture: managed with dilation or visual internal urethrotomy
- Sphincterotomy for medically failed detrusor sphincter dyssynergia

ALTERNATIVE THERAPIES

- Prostatic stents

PATIENT EDUCATION

- Awareness of signs and symptoms of BOO

—Voiding diary to help track condition and/or therapy

 ## Follow-Up

MONITORING

- Normalization of serum creatinine if elevated secondary to renal compromise due to obstruction

—Follow the course of etiology to be aware or prevent recurrence.

PREVENTION

- Correction of high-pressure voiding can protect upper tracts and bladder from further damage.

 ## Miscellaneous

SYNONYMS

- Obstructive uropathy, lower urinary tract symptoms

ASSOCIATED CONDITIONS

- Inguinal hernia due to high-pressure voiding

NOTES

- See also Section II, "Prostate—Benign Hyperplasia," "Detrusor—Sphincter Dyssynergia," and "Urethral Stricture."

ABBREVIATIONS

- BOO, bladder outlet obstruction

REFERENCES

Blaivas JC. Obstructive uropathy in the male. *Urol Clin North Am* 1996;23(3):373–384.

Carr LK, Webster GD. Bladder outlet obstruction in women. *Urol Clin North Am* 1996;23(3):385–390.

Faerber GJ. Urinary retention and urethral obstruction. In: Kursh ED, McGuire E, eds. *Female Urology.* Philadelphia: JB Lippincott Co, 1994.

Authors: Pasquale Casale and Leonard G. Gomella

Bladder Tumors—Benign and Malignant, General

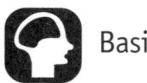 Basics

DESCRIPTION

- Bladder tumors range from benign-behaving, superficial low-grade papillary lesions to aggressive, invasive high-grade malignancies.

EPIDEMIOLOGY

- For malignant tumors, approximately 50,000 new cases per year; 11,000 deaths per year; no data on benign tumors.
- Fourth most common cancer in men; eighth most common cancer in women
- 3× more common in men than in women
- 2× more common in White men compared with Black men
- 1.5× more common in White women compared with Black women
- Median age: 69 in men, 71 in women
- Lifetime risk: 2.8% for White men, 0.9% for Black men, 1.0% for White women, and 0.6% for Black women
- Tumors in adults <30 tend to be well differentiated and more indolent.

GENETICS

- Generally not hereditary
- Familial clusters have been reported.

STAGING

- See the Appendix for TNM classification.

SIGNS AND SYMPTOMS

- Intermittent painless hematuria (85% of patients)
- Bladder irritability, frequency, urgency, and dysuria (one-third of patients)
- Flank pain from ureteral obstruction
- Lower extremity edema secondary to pelvic lymph nodal metastasis
- Pelvic mass
- Systemic symptoms of weight loss and abdominal or bone pain occur with metastatic disease.

PATHOPHYSIOLOGY

- Benign lesions

—Epithelial hyperplasia
—Squamous metaplasia: found in 50% women and 10% men; benign
—Von Brunn's nests
—Cystitis cystica
—Cystitis follicularis
—Cystitis glandularis: ? precursor for adenocarcinoma
—Mild-to-moderate dysplasia: requires follow-up but no particular treatment
—Inverted papilloma: associated with transitional cell carcinoma (TCC) elsewhere
—Nephrogenic adenoma
—Vesical leukoplakia: may progress to squamous cell carcinoma (SCC) in 20%
—Pseudosarcoma (postoperative spindle cell nodule)

—Condyloma acuminata of the urethra and rarely bladder or ureters

- Urothelial carcinoma

—Carcinoma in situ (CIS): may appear as a velvety patch on endoscopy but often is undetectable to the naked eye
    —Usually poorly differentiated (high-grade) TCC confined to the urothelium
    —Urine cytology results are positive 80% to 90% of the time.
    —May be asymptomatic
    —Symptoms: frequency, urgency, and dysuria; may be confused with other genitourinary conditions
    —Rare in association with well-differentiated (low-grade), superficial bladder tumors
    —Present in 25% or more of patients with high-grade tumors
    —40% to 83% progress to muscle invasion if treated with endoscopic resection alone.
    —CIS is found with 20% to 75% of high-grade, muscle-invasive cancers.
    —A high proportion have deletions or mutations of the *p53* gene
—Transitional cell carcinoma
    —90% of bladder cancers
    —70% are papillary, 10% are nodular, and 20% are mixed.
    —Most common arise in the trigone/bladder base or lateral walls
    —May contain spindle cell, squamous cell, or adenocarcinomatous elements
    —Grade based on degree of anaplasia of tumor cells
    —Divided into well differentiated, moderately differentiated, and poorly differentiated
    —Strong correlation between grade and stage
    —The most well-differentiated and moderately differentiated tumors are superficial tumors, and the most poorly differentiated tumors are muscle invasive.
    —Low-grade, superficial tumors appear to have the loss of suppresser genes on chromosome 9
    —High-grade, invasive tumors appear to have *p53* abnormalities.
—Squamous cell carcinoma
    —3% to 7% of bladder cancers in United States; 75% of bladder cancers in Egypt
    —80% of SCCs in Egypt associated with chronic infection with *Schistosoma haematobium;* called bilharzial bladder cancers
    —Bilharzial cancers tend to be exophytic, nodular, fungating lesions that are well differentiated and have a low incidence of lymph node or distant metastases.
    —Nonbilharzial SCCs are usually caused by chronic irritation from urinary calculi, long-term indwelling catheters, chronic urinary infections, or bladder diverticuli.
    —5% of paraplegics develop SCC of the bladder.
    —Prognosis is poor, as most present with advanced disease.
—Adenocarcinoma
    —<2% of bladder cancers
    —Associated with bladder exstrophy cystitis glandularis
    —Can arise as a urachal adenocarcinoma

—Most poorly differentiated and invasive
—Most common type associated with ureterosigmoidostomy

CAUSES/RISK FACTORS

- Occupational exposure to chemicals (aniline dyes, aromatic amines, 2-naphthylamine, and benzidine), combustion gases and soot from coal, aldehydes such as acrolein

—Long latent period (30–50 years)
—Occupations at risk: autoworkers, painters, truck drivers, drill press operators, leather workers, rubber workers, metal workers, machinists, dry cleaners, paper manufacturers, rope makers, dental technicians, barbers and beauticians, physicians, apparel manufacturers, and plumbers

- Smoking increases risk by factor of 4; takes 20 years after cessation to reduce risks to baseline
- Abuse of the analgesic phenacetin (5–15 kg over a 10-year period)
- Chronic cystitis resulting from indwelling catheters or calculi increase the risk of squamous cell carcinoma.
- *Schistosoma haematobium* cystitis predisposes to bladder cancer.
- Pelvic irradiation
- Cyclophosphamide (Cytoxan) increase risk by factor of 9; short latency of 6 to 13 years
- Prognostic factors

—Recurrence: tumor multiplicity (number and/or frequency)
—Progression: grade, stage, and ABH blood group

COMPLICATIONS

- Hematuria with clot formation, leading to urinary retention
- Bladder perforation after TURBT
- Absorption of excess irrigating fluid
- Progression to higher grade or invasive cancer
- Metastases
- Infections

DIFFERENTIAL DIAGNOSIS

- Interstitial cystitis
- Chronic bacterial/abacterial cystitis
- Endometriosis of bladder
- Metastatic lesions from occult or known primary

Database

HISTORY

- Occupational exposure, smoking history
- History of chronic indwelling catheter, pelvic irradiation, Cytoxan chemotherapy
- Hematuria, dysuria, frequency, urgency
- Flank pain, abdominal pain, bone pain (in advanced disease)
- Weight loss (rare, except in advanced disease)
- Family history

PHYSICAL EXAMINATION

- Pelvic mass (large invasive tumors) (bimanual examination under anesthesia)
- Costovertebral angle tenderness (ureteral obstruction)

 Diagnostic Studies

LABORATORY TESTING

- Urinalysis for hematuria
- Microscopic cytology from bladder washings or voided urine (former more useful)

—Better at identifying high-grade tumors (i.e., CIS)
—Not cost effective in screening for bladder cancer, except in high-risk populations

- Flow cytometry

—Measures DNA content
—Diploid tumors tend to be of low grade and low stage, and have a better prognosis.
—Aneuploidy is a common feature of high-grade tumors.
—Generally, cytology alone is clinically just as good.

IMAGING

- Intravenous pyelogram (IVP) and retrograde pyelograms to identify upper tract tumors and large bladder tumors

—Ureteral obstruction on IVP associated with a bladder cancer is usually a sign of muscle-invasive disease.

- CT scan and chest x-ray are used in staging muscle-invasive disease.

SPECIAL STUDIES

- Cystoscopy with bimanual examination: gold standard for identifying tumors of the bladder

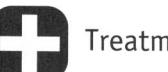 Treatment

GENERAL MEASURES

- Treatment based on stage

—Superficial: primarily transurethral resection
—Muscle invasive, but not metastatic: primarily radical cystectomy

MEDICAL

- Intravesical therapies are used to decrease tumor recurrence in those at high risk (i.e., those with multiple tumors, high-grade tumors, or CIS).

—Bacille Calmette-Guérin (BCG): an attenuated strain of *Mycobacterium bovis* that works by stimulating an immune reaction in the bladder
  —Most effective intravesical therapy
  —Used as prophylaxis in tumor-free patients
  —Used to treat residual tumor in patients with papillary tumors
  —Used to treat CIS
—Triethylenethiophosphoramide (thiotepa): an alkylating agent that acts by cross-linking nucleic acids and proteins
  —Used as prophylaxis against tumor recurrence
  —Causes myelosuppression in 15% to 20% of patients
  —Works best in low-grade tumors
—Mitomycin C: an antibiotic chemotherapeutic agent that acts by inhibiting DNA synthesis
  —More effective in treating high-grade tumors
—Doxorubicin (Adriamycin): an antibiotic chemotherapeutic agent
  —No significant difference in response with low-grade vs. high-grade tumors
  —Valrubricin recently approved for CIS (Adriamycin analogue)
—α-Interferon: for BCG failures

- Neoadjuvant systemic chemotherapy may be useful in locally advanced tumors.

—Specific regimen used: MVAC (methotrexate, vinblastine, Adriamycin, and cisplatin)

- Radiation therapy may be used as a bladder-preserving treatment for invasive bladder cancer, but generally is not as effective.

SURGICAL

- TURBT: primary therapy for superficial bladder cancers and first step in diagnosing invasive tumors
- Radical cystectomy: primary treatment in localized muscle-invasive bladder tumors
- Partial cystectomy: may be used in select patients without evidence of CIS or multiple tumors in whom an adequate margin can be obtained

ALTERNATIVE THERAPIES

- Photodynamic therapy (PDT): photosensitizing dye and laser light (630 nm) combination to destroy cancerous tissue

—Indicated in immunotherapy (BCG) and/or chemotherapy failures

- High-dose vitamins (40,000 U vitamin A, 100 mg vitamin B6, 200 mg vitamin C, 400 U vitamin E, and 90 mg zinc) to reduce recurrence rate
- Keyhole-limpet hemocyanin (KLH): oral immune modulator

PATIENT EDUCATION

- The need for surveillance
- Smoking cessation

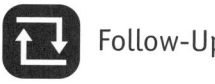 Follow-Up

MONITORING

- Cystoscopy every 3 months for 2 years, then every 6 months for 2 years, and then once a year indefinitely

PREVENTION

- Minimize chemical exposures.
- Stop smoking.
- Avoid use of chronic indwelling catheters.

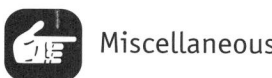 Miscellaneous

SYNONYMS: N/A

ASSOCIATED CONDITIONS: N/A

NOTES

- See also Section II, "Bladder Cancer—TCC, Superficial" and Bladder Cancer—TCC, Invasive."

ABBREVIATIONS

- CIS, carcinoma in situ; SCC, squamous cell carcinoma; TCC, transitional cell carcinoma; TURBT, transurethral resection of bladder tumor

REFERENCES

Huson MA, Catalona WJ. Urothelial tumors of the bladder, upper tracts, and prostate. In: Gillenwater JY, Grayhack JT, Howards SS, Duckett JW, eds. *Adult and Pediatric Urology,* 3rd ed. St Louis: Mosby, 1996:1379–1435.

Messing EM, Catalona WJ. Urothelial tumors of the urinary tract. In: Walsh PC, Retik AB, Vaughan ED, Wein AJ, eds. *Campbell's Urology,* 7th ed. Philadelphia: WB Saunders, 1998:2327–2383.

Nseyo UO, Lamm DL. Immunotherapy for bladder cancer. *Semin Oncol* 1997;23:598.

Authors: David M. Hall and Unyime O. Nseyo

Bowen Disease and Erythroplasia of Queyrat

 Basics

DESCRIPTION

• Erythroplasia of Queyrat (EQ) is a squamous cell carcinoma in situ (CIS) of the glans penis. Bowen disease is squamous cell CIS of the penile shaft and scrotum instead of the glans penis.

EPIDEMIOLOGY

• Carcinoma of the penis occurs in less than 1% of all malignancies in the American male, with EQ comprising only a fraction of these cases.
• Most common in Caucasian males
• Median age 50
• Greater than 90% of cases in uncircumcised males

GENETICS

• A positive family history is rare with EQ or Bowen disease.

STAGING

• By definition, the lesion is confined to the epithelium without local invasion or distant metastasis.

SIGNS AND SYMPTOMS

• Painful, itching, and red penile glans lesion
• Crusting, scaling, and bleeding plaque

PATHOPHYSIOLOGY

• Lesion confined to the epithelium, exhibiting cytologic changes of malignancy

—Cellular atypia and pleomorphism, mostly in keratinocytes
—Nuclear hyperchromicity and mitotic figures

• Thin granular layer, elongation of rete ridges
• Parakeratosis, hyperkeratosis, papillomatosis, acanthosis
• Chronic inflammatory infiltrate in the dermis

CAUSES/RISK FACTORS

• Almost exclusively in uncircumcised men

—Phimosis present in 75% of cases
—Smegma thought to be carcinogenic

• Infection with human papillomavirus (HPV) is a common association. HPV type 16 DNA has been isolated from biopsies of Bowen disease. Its presence in EQ has not yet been established, but it may play a role in disease progression.
• Men whose sexual partners have cervical neoplasia are more likely to develop penile neoplasia.

—This is possibly due to HPV as a common pathogen.

• Sexual promiscuity and poor genital hygiene

COMPLICATIONS

• Malignant transformation in 10% to 33% of patients with CIS of penis

DIFFERENTIAL DIAGNOSIS

• Invasive carcinoma

—Ruled out by deep biopsy

• Bowen disease of the penis

—Squamous cell CIS of penile shaft and scrotum instead of glans penis
—Grey-white, solitary plaque
—Age greater than 35
—Historically thought to be associated with visceral malignancies (not seen with EQ)
　—Recent studies have found no association between Bowen disease of the penis and internal malignancies.
—Associated with HPV-16 infection of penis
—Weak association with uncircumcised status
—Greater chance of progression to invasive carcinoma than EQ
—Histologically almost identical to EQ

• Bowenoid papulosis

—Histologically similar to squamous cell CIS of penis, but with benign course
—Appear as multiple rather than solitary, reddish to brown pigmented lesions
—Younger patients affected, typically 20 to 35 years old
—Strong association with HPV

• Balanitis circinata

—Dry and scaling lesions on glans and corona of circumcised or uncircumcised males
—Associated with Reiter syndrome
—Can be moist and erythematous in uncircumcised males

• Candidal balanitis

—Reddened and edematous lesion found in uncircumcised diabetics
—Patients unresponsive to antifungal therapy should undergo biopsy to rule out CIS.

• Zoon's balanitis (balanitis plasmacellularis circumscripta)

—A red, raised lesion occurring in elderly, uncircumcised men
—Biopsy generally required to distinguish from CIS
—Epidermal thinning, hemosiderin deposition, and leukocyte infiltration of the dermis

• Penile psoriasis

—A well-demarcated, raised, red to whitish lesion that tends to scale
—Usually accompanied by lesions at other sites

• Fixed drug eruptions (dermatitis medicamentosa)

—Can appear as recurring erythema or bulla on the penis

• Others include lichen planus, herpes simplex, and secondary syphilis.

 Database

HISTORY

• Age

—The median age for EQ is 50 (younger for Bowen disease and bowenoid papulosis).

• Sexual history

—Having multiple sexual partners increases the likelihood of HPV-16 infection associated with Bowen disease and bowenoid papulosis, not EQ.

• History of phimosis

—Increases likelihood of EQ

• History of chronic sun exposure of genitals or of arsenic poisoning

—Associated with Bowen disease not EQ

• History of nonhealing lesion on glans after treatment with topical antifungals

PHYSICAL EXAMINATION

• Appearance and location of lesion(s)

—EQ: solitary red plaque on glans
—Bowen disease: solitary thick, gray-white, crusting plaque on shaft or scrotum
—Bowenoid papulosis: multiple reddish-brown, papular lesions on penis

• Presence of ulceration

—Increased likelihood of invasive carcinoma rather than CIS

• Examine the inguinal nodes.

Diagnostic Studies

LABORATORY TESTING

• DNA testing for HPV-16 of biopsy specimen

—HPV-16 associated with Bowen disease and bowenoid papulosis, not EQ

IMAGING

• Chest x-ray

—Not necessary for EQ (Bowen disease, as is possibly associated with internal malignancy)

• MRI or CT of pelvis if invasive carcinoma present

SPECIAL STUDIES

• Definitive diagnosis only made by biopsy and histopathologic examination

Treatment

GENERAL MEASURES

• In general, surgical excision is the preferred method of treatment.
• Circumcision is recommended to decrease the likelihood of recurrence.
• Management of CIS of the penis is related to the surface area and the size of the lesion.

—The efficacy of invasive treatment should be weighed against the degree of disfigurement caused by that modality.

• Regardless of treatment modality, a biopsy of the lesion and deeper tissue is absolutely required for an accurate diagnosis.

MEDICAL

• Daily application of 5% 5-fluorouracil cream

—Effective on large lesions not amenable to surgery or laser
—Rubber condom to occlude cream, prolong contact time
—A concurrent topical anesthetic reduces irritation symptoms.

• Used in recurrent lesions

SURGICAL

• Small lesions: complete surgical excision

—Complete surgical excision most effective modality of treatment
—Obtain 5-mm margins.
—Obtain deep subcutaneous tissue to rule out invasive disease.

• Larger lesions not amenable to complete surgical excision without disfigurement: laser

—Neodymium:YAG preferred over CO_2 laser due to depth of penetration

• Larger lesions not amenable to laser due to risk of disfigurement

—Mohs micrographic surgical excision

ALTERNATIVE THERAPIES

• Radiation

—Treatment of large lesions not amenable to complete surgical excision or laser due to risk of disfigurement
—Treatment of recurrent lesions

PATIENT EDUCATION

• Proper hygienic practices for uncircumcised males

—Retract foreskin daily to cleanse glans penis and remove smegma.

• Helpful web sites:

—www.graylab.ac.uk/cancernet/101082.html
—www.healthanswers.com/database/ami/converted/001300.html

Follow-Up

MONITORING

• No clear guidelines for follow-up have been established.
• In general, patients must be reexamined on a regular basis for recurrence.

—Consider rebiospy of recurrent lesions to rule out transformation to invasive carcinoma.

PREVENTION

• Daily cleansing of the glans penis
• Circumcision protects against EQ.

—Prophylactic circumcision controversial due to high cost-to-benefit ratio.

Miscellaneous

SYNONYMS

• EQ: carcinoma in situ of the glans penis

ASSOCIATED CONDITIONS

• Lichen planus, balanitis xerotica sclerosis

NOTES

• See also Section I, "Penis—Lesion," and Section II, "Penis Cancer—General."
• CIS of the clitoris may also be referred to as EQ.

ABBREVIATIONS

• EQ, erythroplasia of Queyrat; HPV, human papillomavirus

REFERENCES

Gerber GS. Carcinoma in situ of the penis. *J Urol* 1994;151:829.

Grossman HB. Premalignant and early carcinomas of the penis and scrotum. *Urol Clin North Am* 1992;19:221.

Schellhammer PF. Premalignant lesions and non-squamous malignancy of the penis and carcinoma of the scrotum. *Urol Clin North Am* 1992;19:131.

Authors: S. Adam Ramin, Darren D. Bray, and Herbert C. Ruckle

Calyceal Diverticulum

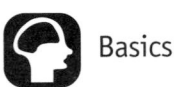 Basics

DESCRIPTION

- Calyceal diverticula are smooth-walled, nonsecretory cavities within renal parenchyma.

EPIDEMIOLOGY

- No sex predominance
- No kidney predominance; bilateral in 3% of cases; rare in children

GENETICS: N/A

STAGING: N/A

SIGNS AND SYMPTOMS

- Flank pain, hematuria, urinary tract infection

PATHOPHYSIOLOGY

- Calyceal diverticula are believed to be congenital in origin.
- The lining is transitional cell epithelium.
- Passive retrograde filling from adjacent collecting system through a narrow infundibulum
- Stasis of urine will predispose to infection and calculus formation.
- Calculi are concomitant in 9.5% to 39.0% of cases.
- Calculi rarely pass spontaneously because of the narrow infundibulum of the diverticulum.

CAUSES/RISK FACTORS

- None known

COMPLICATIONS

- Urinary tract infection and obstruction of the diverticular neck may lead to sepsis, abscess formation, or hypertension.
- Spontaneous hemorrhage and rupture of calyceal diverticulum has been reported.

DIFFERENTIAL DIAGNOSIS

- On plain x-ray, calculi may represent routine calcification within the kidney. Contrast studies, such as intravenous pyelogram, are required to diagnose accurately.
- In areas where tuberculosis is prevalent, renal cortical cavitation secondary to renal tuberculosis should be considered. The radiologic appearances may be similar.
- Cystic renal disease: Ultrasound evaluation of the kidney may reveal a cystic structure. Contrast studies should differentiate between a simple renal cyst and calyceal diverticulum.
- Renal abscess: If infected, the calyceal diverticulum may represent localized abscess or a lobar nephronia. Investigations such as CT scanning can differentiate adequately.

 Database

HISTORY

- Age and sex of patient
—Uncommon in the pediatric age group, but possible
—Usually present in the age spectrum paralleling the prevalence of urolithiasis

- Diagnostic criteria: Presentation could be similar to a renal colic. Classic flank pain with radiation to the loin
- Microscopic hematuria secondary to presence of calculi within the diverticulum
- Pyuria secondary to the diverticulum and/or inflammatory process
- The initial diagnosis may be unrelated to the final diagnosis, since plain x-ray may only reveal kidney calculus/calculi.
- Fever and chills may be associated with infection and/or abscess formation.
- If infection is left undrained or untreated, the patient could present with impending sepsis or frank sepsis.

PHYSICAL EXAMINATION

- Presentation could mimic renal colic or, rarely, a renal abscess.
- Classic loin-to-groin pain

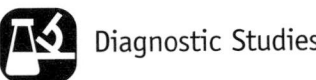 Diagnostic Studies

LABORATORY TESTING

- Urine analysis may be suggestive of hematuria and/or infection.
- Renal function tests, such as creatinine and blood nitrogen, are obtained as a baseline.

IMAGING

- Plain x-ray of the abdomen
- Contrast studies such as intravenous pyelogram
- CT scan of the kidneys
- Renal scan, if indicated

SPECIAL STUDIES

- Cystoscopy and retrograde pyelogram

Treatment

GENERAL MEASURES

• Asymptomatic/incidental calyceal diverticula can be observed.
• Invasive treatment, such as the percutaneous approach, is recommended only in patients who are symptomatic.
• If imaging studies show a wide neck to the diverticulum with small calculi (small stone burden), then initial ESWL is recommended.
• ESWL is not recommended if acute infection is present.
• If ESWL is unsuccessful, then use percutaneous management.

MEDICAL

• Only to treat infection

SURGICAL

• Percutaneous calyceal diverticulectomy

—Cystoscopy and retrograde pyelogram are performed.
—Risks include standard operative risks and inability to obtain adequate access if the calyceal diverticulum is relatively small.
—A 5Fr open-ended catheter is placed into the renal pelvis so as to inject contrast and/or air to adequately localize the diverticulum for direct percutaneous puncture.
—The patient is placed prone on an operating room table with imaging capabilities.
—A Hinck needle is inserted percutaneously into the calyceal diverticulum.
—A guidewire is introduced through the Hinck needle and curled within the calyceal diverticulum.

—The tract is dilated to 28 or 30Fr, and an Amplatz sheath is placed.
—Remove stones (if small, extract; if large, fragment [ultrasonic, electrohydraulic, or holmium laser lithotriptors]).
—After stone removal, the diverticulum is fulgurated (holmium laser or a roller-ball electrode).
—The kidney is stented with a double pigtail stent.
—The diverticulum and the kidney are drained with a "nephrostomy tube." (We use a Foley catheter with the tip of the balloon cut off so that the balloon is inflated to the size of the diverticulum. The nephrostomy tube balloon snugly fills the ablated diverticulum; when removed 24 to 48 hours later, the diverticulum collapses.)

• Open surgical intervention in lieu of percutaneous nephroscopic treatment is rarely needed these days, though complications such as bleeding, frank abscess formation, etc., may warrant such invasive methods.

ALTERNATIVE THERAPIES: N/A

PATIENT EDUCATION: N/A

 Follow-Up

MONITORING

• The stent is removed 2 to 3 weeks after contrast study confirms ablation of the cavity and healing of the percutaneous tract.
• Follow up with plain x-rays and other imaging studies (ultrasound, intravenous pyelogram, etc.) to determine recurrence.

PREVENTION: N/A

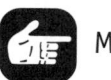 Miscellaneous

SYNONYMS: N/A

ASSOCIATED CONDITIONS: N/A

NOTES: N/A

ABBREVIATIONS

• ESWL, extracorporeal shock wave lithotripsy

REFERENCES

Bellman GC, Silverstein JI, Blickensderfer S, Smith AD. Technique and follow-up of percutaneous management of calyceal diverticula. *Urology* 1993;42:21–25.

Choudhury SR, Maji BP. Calyceal diverticula. *J Indian Med Assoc* 1992;90:159–161.

Ellis JH, Patterson SK, Sonda LP, Platt JF, Sheffner SE, Woolsey EJ. Stones and infection in renal calyceal diverticula: Treatment with percutaneous procedures. *AJR* 1991;156:995–1000.

Hulbert JC, Reddy PK, Hunter DW, Castaneda-Zuniga W, Amplatz K, Lange PH. Percutaneous techniques for the management of calyceal diverticula containing calculi. *J Urol* 1986;135:225–227.

Psihramis KE, Dretler SP. Extracorporeal shock wave lithotripsy of calyceal diverticula. *J Urol* 1987;138:707–711.

Authors: R. Thomas and M. Monga

Candidiasis—Cutaneous, External Genitalia

 Basics

DESCRIPTION

• A superficial skin infection with a *Candida* fungus

EPIDEMIOLOGY

• *Candida albicans* is the most common *Candida*.
• Other important *Candida* species include *C. guilliermondi, krusei, parapsilosis, stellatoidea, tropicalis, pseudotropicalis,* and *C. (Torulopsis) glabrata*.
• *C. albicans* is a normal commensal organism found in the gastrointestinal tract, female genital tract, and oropharynx.
• *Candida* rarely colonize normal skin, but colonize damaged skin and skin of the elderly.
• Isolated from soil, food, hospital environment, and animals

GENETICS: N/A

STAGING: N/A

SIGNS AND SYMPTOMS

• Involvement of the distal urethra, scrotum, inguinal region, glans penis of uncircumcised male
• Itching, burning, discharge, dryness, and dysuria in females (vulvovaginitis)
• Found in warm, moist areas such as the perineum

—Begins as vesicopustules that enlarge and rupture
—Progresses to maceration and erythema
—Distinct border, often with satellite lesions
—Vaginal discharge usually white, thick, and cottage cheese-like or thin and yellow
—Can cause rash around postoperative wounds, ileostomies, or cutaneous pyelostomies

PATHOPHYSIOLOGY

• Small (4–6 μm), oval, thin-walled cells
• Exist in three morphologic forms: yeast, pseudohyphae, hyphae

CAUSES/RISK FACTORS

• Diabetes mellitus
• Broad-spectrum antibiotic administration
• Steroid therapy
• Oral contraceptive use
• Pregnancy
• Immunosuppression/HIV with neutropenia

COMPLICATIONS

• Disseminated candidiasis

—Usually in neutropenic patients, transplant recipients, postsurgical patients, and burn victims
—Mortality approaches 50%.
—Bacterial superinfection

DIFFERENTIAL DIAGNOSIS

• Superficial bacterial infection or cellulitis
• Drug reaction

—Contact dermatitis
—Psoriasis
—Herpes simplex

 Database

HISTORY

• Poor hygiene
• Use of broad-spectrum antibiotics or steroids
• History of HIV, malignancy requiring chemotherapy, diabetes mellitus

PHYSICAL EXAMINATION

• Involvement of distal urethra, scrotum, inguinal region, glans penis of uncircumcised male
• Itching, burning, discharge, dryness, and dysuria in females (vulvovaginitis)
• Found in warm, most areas such as perineum

—Begins as vesicopustules that enlarge and rupture
—Progresses to maceration and erythema
—Distinct border, often with satellite lesions
—Vaginal discharge usually white, thick, and cottage cheese-like or thin and yellow
—Around postoperative incisions, ileostomies, or cutaneous pyelostomies

Diagnostic Studies

LABORATORY TESTING

- Scrapings of affected area or wet-mount preparation of discharge

—Microscopic examination with potassium hydroxide or Gram stain
—Identify hyphae and pseudohyphae.
—Latex agglutination test in equivocal cases

IMAGING: N/A

SPECIAL STUDIES: N/A

 Treatment

GENERAL MEASURES

- Keep affected areas dry and exposed to air.

MEDICAL

- Apply topical antifungal powders or creams.

—Nystatin 100,000 U/d
—Miconazole cream four times a day
—For vulvovaginitis, apply antifungal vaginal troches or creams; apply one of the following:
　—Nystatin 100,000 to 200,000U/d for 1 to 2 weeks
　—Clotrimazole troches or cream 100 mg/d for 3 to 7 days
　—Miconazole cream 50 mg daily for 3 to 7 days
　—Other imidazoles: butoconazole, terconazole, tioconazole also effective
　—Oral fluconazole (single 150-mg dose) is as effective as intravaginal clotrimazole.
　—Treatment of the partner is recommended, although not proven to prevent recurrences.

SURGICAL: N/A

ALTERNATIVE THERAPIES

- Women with chronic *Candida* vaginitis that respond only partially to topical antifungals may require long-term ketoconazole.

—Ketoconazole 400 mg daily for 2 weeks, followed by 100 to 200 mg daily by mouth for 6 months, has maintained 95% of patients disease-free for 6 months.
　—Use as last resort; risk of toxicity, including hormonal and liver dysfunction
　—Recurrence will develop with cessation of therapy.
—Boric acid powder (600-mg capsules) inserted vaginally for 2 weeks as cost-effective therapy

PATIENT EDUCATION

- Keep the area clean and dry.
- Proper control of diabetes, if indicated

 Follow-Up

MONITORING

- Treat with a return of signs and symptoms.

PREVENTION

- Keep perineal and peristomal areas clean and dry.
- Avoid moisture-retaining fabrics such as nylon undergarments.
- Minimize duration and excessive use of broad-spectrum antibiotics.

 Miscellaneous

SYNONYMS

- Thrush, *Monilia,* yeast

ASSOCIATED CONDITIONS

- Diabetes mellitus, use of broad-spectrum antibiotics, steroids, chemotherapy, neutropenia

NOTES: N/A

ABBREVIATIONS: N/A

REFERENCES

Crislip MA, Edwards JE Jr. Candida albicans and related species. In: Gorbach SL, Bartlett JG, Blacklow NR, eds. *Infectious Disease.* Philadelphia: WB Saunders, 1992:1887–1895.

Wise G. Infections of the urinary tract. In: Walsh PC, Retik AB, Wein A, Vaughn ED Jr, eds. *Campbell's Urology,* 7th ed., vol 2. Philadelphia: WB Saunders, 1997.

Authors: Gregory L. Chen and Demetrius H. Bagley

Candidiasis—Genitourinary (Noncutaneous)

 Basics

DESCRIPTION

- Most common fungal pathogen of genitourinary tract; colonization vs. infection is unclear and controversial; infection is opportunistic and nosocomial, usually immunocompromised patient

EPIDEMIOLOGY

- Organism is normal human commensal of oral cavity, gastrointestinal tract, vagina, external genitalia, perineum, and skin
- <1% of properly collected urine cultures yield *Candida* (asymptomatic colonization).
- Asymptomatic candiduria in 14% of boys and 39% of girls receiving antibiotics for URI
- Candiduria in 11% of men and 30% of women inpatients receiving antibiotics
- Females are predisposed (57% of cases), probably due to anatomy.
- 14% of patients are diabetics.
- *Torulopsis glabrata* (formerly *Candida glabrata*) found in 5% to 30% of isolates; second most common yeast
- Isolation of *Candida/Torulopsis* from urine is *abnormal* and warrants investigation.

GENETICS

- No known association

STAGING: N/A

SIGNS AND SYMPTOMS

- Lower tract infection or colonization (asymptomatic candiduria, urethritis, cystitis)

—Commonly asymptomatic
—Urgency, frequency
—Passage of debris per urethra
—Perineal or vulvar candidiasis (may be present); erythema with satellite lesions

- Disseminated, systemic (renal candidiasis)

—Fever
—Chills
—Flank pain
—Critically ill picture
—Retinal exudates

PATHOPHYSIOLOGY

- Breakdown of normal host mechanical barriers (intact integument and mucosal membranes)
- Prime host defense: cellular immunity (T-lymphocytes)
- Humoral response plays minor role: phagocytosis inhibited by hyphal length
- Lower tract infection

—Retrograde infection of yeast from perineum
—May invade genital ducts retrograde via ejaculatory ducts to seminal vesicles, vas deferens, epididymis, and testis (rare)

- Upper tract infection

—Stone, suture, or stent may serve as nidus
—Ascending or hematogenous dissemination with bezoar (fungal ball) formation
—Kidney most common organ in disseminated candidiasis (82%)
—GI tract: usual source of disseminated disease (translocation)
—Multiple intrarenal abscesses and papillary necrosis
—Tenacious bezoar of fungal elements, matrix, and cellular debris forms a cast of the collecting system.
—Obstructive uropathy results; renal failure, sepsis, death

- Genital candidiasis

—Cutaneous irritation, cellulitis, or balanoposthitis
—Ascending epididymo-orchitis with abscess formation

CAUSES/RISK FACTORS

- Glycosuria >150 mg/mL

—*Candida* is found in 35% of diabetics with glycosuria vs. 9% of nonglycosuric diabetics.

- Antibiotic therapy

—Eradicates bacteria competing with fungi
—Longer duration of therapy (mean: 16 days)
—Especially quinolones

- Urinary catheterization

—Greater risk with longer duration of catheter (mean: 12 days)
—8% of ureteral stent biofilms yield *Candida*.

- Immunocompromised conditions, AIDS, transplant recipients, long-term antibiotics, chronic steroids, diabetes, malignancies, chemotherapy, IV drug abuse, premature infants, parenteral nutrition, obstructive uropathy, indwelling catheters in the urinary tract, prosthetics, vascular catheter or other foreign bodies

COMPLICATIONS

- Acute and chronic cystitis
- Prostatitis/abscess
- Epididymo-orchitis/abscess requiring orchiectomy
- Renal failure/abscess requiring nephrectomy
- Sepsis, death

DIFFERENTIAL DIAGNOSIS

- Bacterial cystitis
- Transitional cell carcinoma of bladder or renal pelvis
- Other fungal diseases (*Aspergillus*, etc.)
- Cystitis follicularis
- Nephrolithiasis
- Blood clots
- Sloughed papilla/papillary necrosis
- Squamous cell carcinoma
- Interstitial cystitis

 Database

HISTORY

- Assess for current or past risk factors (immunosuppression, diabetes, etc.).
- Assess for oliguria (obstruction from lower tract bezoar).
- Passage of flocculent debris per urethra
- Evaluate for symptoms of systemic candidiasis: fevers, chronic debilitation.

PHYSICAL EXAMINATION

- Assess for renal candidal involvement.

—Costovertebral angle tenderness, tender or palpable upper abdominal mass

- Genital/perineal skin for excoriation, erythema, satellite lesions
- Testes, epididymis, and prostate for tenderness, fluctuant masses
- Palpate and percuss the bladder to rule out retention.
- Suspicious debris in catheter tubing
- Funduscopic

—Retinal patches/exudates as sign of disseminated candidiasis

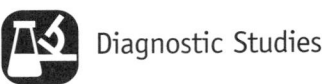 Diagnostic Studies

LABORATORY TESTING

- UA and culture

—*Candida*: budding yeast and pseudohyphal forms seen on microscopic; colony count >15,000/mL may distinguish significant infection (controversial); lab must perform speciation and sensitivity—resistance is well known.
—*Torulopsis*: yeast without hyphae
—Pyuria

- Serum precipitating antibodies (does not localize infection)
- PCR amplification of *Candida* DNA (more sensitive for candidemia than are blood cultures)
- Renal function tests (creatinine and blood urea nitrogen)

IMAGING

- Renal US

—Fungal balls/bezoars are hyperechoic; hydronephrosis may be present; cortex may be thinned and hyperechoic in renal candidiasis.

- IVP, nephrostogram, or retrograde pyelogram

—Filling defect in upper tract; hydronephrosis; possibly poor drainage and poor function with delayed excretion of contrast

SPECIAL STUDIES

- Nuclear renal scintigraphy

—Evaluate differential renal function if upper tract bezoars and compromised function

- Cystoscopy
—Fungal ball: "snowstorm effect"
—Intense inflammatory reaction, with white exudate on urothelium
—Biopsy shows invasive fungal elements.

Treatment

GENERAL MEASURES

- Remove or change urinary catheters.
- Discontinue unnecessary broad-spectrum antibiotics and steroids.
- Improve nutritional status.
- Repeat urine culture—funguria may be transient.
- Obtain infectious disease consultation.

MEDICAL

- First line of therapy for systemic or renal candidiasis
- Fluconazole (Diflucan)

—Dose: 50 to 100 mg po for at least 7 to 14 days
—80% excreted in urine, serum half-life of 30 hours
—90% success rates in candidal UTIs; case reports of success in renal candidiasis
—Potentiates oral hypoglycemics, warfarin
—Minor adverse effects: nausea, diarrhea, abdominal pain, vomiting, rash—up to 16%
—Resistance to non-*C. albicans* species and *T. glabrata*—use caution
—Much less toxic than others below
—Continue for several days after any antibacterial antibiotics have been discontinued.
—Mortality decreased in elderly patients (22%) vs. local amphotericin B irrigation alone (41%); benefit of systemic treatment?

- Amphotericin B (intravenous)

—Formerly was principal medication for systemic candidiasis; now seldom used IV due to toxicity
—Renal and bone marrow toxicity
—100 to 200 mg divided over 7 to 10 days
—Adverse reactions: anaphylaxis, fever, arrhythmias, electrolyte (K, Mg) imbalance

- Irrigation

—Fluconazole: 1 mg/mL in normal saline instilled bid (50 mL per urethral catheter) for 20 minutes and then drain; 85% success in eradicating *Candida* UTIs after 6 days; for upper tract, instill 10 mL per nephrostomy; no reports of continuous fluconazole irrigation
—Amphotericin B: 50 mg/1000 mL sterile water at 40 mL/h for 48 hours continuous bladder irrigation; continuous irrigation more effective than intermittent (80% vs. 30%) and easier to administrate; protect from UV light
—Continuous renal irrigation under low-pressure manometer control at 25 cm H_2O and 40 mL/h

- Urinary alkalinization (anecdotal experience)
- Others

—Flucytosine: oral dose 100 to 150 mg/kg/d divided qid; produces resistant organisms, liver and bone marrow toxicity; no longer popular
—Ketoconazole: poor urinary excretion; affects steroidogenesis in humans (cytochrome P-450); liver toxicity; minor role
—Miconazole, nystatin, or clotrimazole cream bid for genital, perineal, or crural infections

SURGICAL

- Endourology

—Percutaneous debulking if medical and irrigation therapy fails or disease progresses
—Follow up percutaneous irrigation with antifungal medication until culture negative
—Second-look percutaneous nephroscopy/debulking

- Nephrectomy if above treatment fails and/or poor renal unit function
- Instrumentation without prior antifungal treatment may induce fungemia—prophylactic treatment critical

ALTERNATIVE THERAPIES: N/A

PATIENT EDUCATION

- Control diabetes.
- Appropriate-interval change of indwelling catheters (monthly or less)

Follow-Up

MONITORING

- UA and urine fungal culture weekly after eradication of *Candida* until risk factors for recurrence minimized; must have ceased all antibacterial antibiotics for several days

—Repeat monthly for 6 months, then quarterly

- Renal US

—One month after eradication; then every 6 months for 1 year

PREVENTION

- Avoid risk factors.

Miscellaneous

SYNONYMS

- *Monilia*, thrush, yeast

ASSOCIATED CONDITIONS: N/A

NOTES

- See also Section II, "Candidiasis—Cutaneous, External Genitalia."

ABBREVIATIONS

- AIDS, acquired immunodeficiency syndrome; *C. albicans, Candida albicans; T. glabrata, Torulopsis glabrata;* UA, urinalysis; UTI, urinary tract infection; PCR, polymerase chain reaction; DNA, deoxyribonucleic acid

REFERENCES

Gubbins PO, et al. Candidal urinary tract infections: A comprehensive review of their diagnosis and management. *Pharmacotherapy* 1993; 13(2):110.

Irby PB, et al. Fungal bezoars of the upper urinary tract. *J Urol* 1990;143:447.

Trinh T, et al. Continuous versus intermittent bladder irrigation of amphotericin B for the treatment of candiduria. *J Urol* 1995;154:2032.

Wise GJ, et al. Fungal infections of the genitourinary tract. *J Urol* 1993;149:1377.

Author: Pierce B. Irby

Chancroid

 Basics

DESCRIPTION

• A sexually transmitted condition characterized by painful genital ulcers

EPIDEMIOLOGY

• Worldwide in distribution
• In industrialized countries, sporadic outbreaks occur in disadvantaged urban populations.

GENETICS

• Unknown

STAGING: N/A

SIGNS AND SYMPTOMS

• Painful, usually multiple ulcers on the genitalia of men or women

—Adjacent areas can become involved: autoinoculation.

• Regional lymph nodes may be involved.

—Suppuration (bubo formation) may occur.

PATHOPHYSIOLOGY

• The causative microorganism is the gram-negative bacillus *Haemophilus ducreyi*.

—Bacterium inoculated into abraded skin or mucous membranes during sexual contact

• Three histologic zones noted in pathologic specimens

—Biopsies rarely indicated in current management

CAUSES/RISK FACTORS

• *H. ducreyi* virtually always spread by sexual contact

—Commercial sex workers (prostitutes) an important reservoir of infection

• Recent outbreaks in the United States have occurred in urban areas.

—"Crack" cocaine use with exchange of sex for drugs is at the center of many recent outbreaks.

COMPLICATIONS

• Local destruction and secondary infection

—Phimosis may occur.

DIFFERENTIAL DIAGNOSIS

• Primary syphilis (chancre)
• Genital herpes simplex viral infection
• Granuloma inguinale (donovanosis)
• Lymphogranuloma venereum
• Genital trauma

 Database

HISTORY

• Recent sexual contact

—Prostitutes or other high-risk partners

• Painful genital ulceration

—Tender regional lymph nodes

• History of other STD

PHYSICAL EXAMINATION

• Ulcers are not indurated.

—Undermined edges are characteristic.

• Lymph nodes are enlarged and tender.

—Suppuration (bubo formation) may occur.

 Diagnostic Studies

LABORATORY TESTING

• Gram-stained smears from the base of the ulcer may show short gram-negative rods in the classical "school of fish" or "railroad tracks" arrangement.

—Use of Gram-stained smears neither sensitive nor specific

• Cultures for *H. ducreyi* require special media that are not readily available and not more than 80% sensitive.

—Polymerase chain reaction (PCR) tests have been developed and may soon become commercially available. PCR testing should greatly improve our ability to accurately diagnose chancroid

IMAGING: N/A

SPECIAL STUDIES

• Rule out other common causes of genital ulcers.

—Syphilis (dark-field microscopy, rapid plasma reagin [RPR] test)
—Genital herpes (Tzanck smear, culture or antigen detection test)

Treatment

GENERAL MEASURES

• HIV test

—Patients with chancroid are at increased risk for HIV.

• Sexual partners

—All recent sex partners should be examined and treated.

MEDICAL

• Effective regimens

—Azithromycin: 1.0 g orally as a single dose
—Erythromycin base: 500 mg orally four times a day for 7 days
—Ceftriaxone: 250 mg intramuscularly as a single dose
—Ciprofloxacin: 500 mg orally twice a day for 3 days

• Ampicillin, sulfonamides, and tetracyclines are *not* effective.

SURGICAL

• Percutaneous aspiration of suppurative lymph nodes

ALTERNATIVE THERAPIES: N/A

PATIENT EDUCATION

• Encourage "safe sex."

—Condoms, avoidance of high-risk partners

 ## Follow-Up

MONITORING

• Reexamine 3 to 7 days after initiation of treatment.

—If healing has not begun, consider another diagnosis, a resistant strain of *H. ducreyi,* noncompliance with treatment, or coinfection with HIV.

• Check HIV test results.

—Single-dose treatments are less effective in HIV-infected patients.

PREVENTION

• Barrier methods of contraception

—Latex condoms

• Selection of sexual partners

—Avoid commercial sex workers and other high-risk individuals.

 ## Miscellaneous

SYNONYMS

• Soft chancre, uncus molle

ASSOCIATED CONDITIONS

• HIV infection

NOTES

• See also Section I, "Penis—Lesion" and "Groin Mass."

ABBREVIATIONS: N/A

REFERENCES

Centers for Disease Control and Prevention. 1998 Guidelines for treatment of sexually transmitted diseases. *Morb Mortal Wkly Rep* 1998; 47[No. RR-1]:18–20.

Dillon SM, Cummings M, Rajagopalan S, McCormack WM. Prospective analysis of genital ulcer disease in Brooklyn, New York. *Clin Infect Dis* 1997;24:945–950.

Author: William M. McCormack

Chlamydial Sexually Transmitted Diseases

 Basics

DESCRIPTION

• *Chlamydia trachomatis* is transmitted by vaginal, oral, or anal sexual activity and is most common in young, sexually active people.

EPIDEMIOLOGY

• Multiple serotypes: L1, L2, and L3 associated with LGV; infect lymphoid cells and replicate most efficiently in macrophages

—LGV: common in areas of Africa, Asia, and South America; rare in United States

• Serotypes D through K: infect mucosal surfaces; associated with urogenital infections such as NGU, epididymitis, cervicitis, salpingitis, and others (proctitis, pharyngitis, conjunctivitis, and infantile pneumonia)

—*C. trachomatis* is responsible for 30% to 50% of cases of NGU.
—STDs tend to affect poor, inner-city, and minority groups; *Chlamydia* often affects patients of higher socioeconomic status than does GC.
—Urethritis in homosexual men: more likely GC than *Chlamydia*
—GC and syphilis, primarily in southern states; chlamydial more geographically widespread
—6:1 female-to-male detection rate (because most males asymptomatic)
—Incidence increased 55% between 1984 and 1995 due to reporting and screening efforts.

GENETICS: N/A

STAGING: N/A

SIGNS AND SYMPTOMS

• Urethritis

—Men: usually asymptomatic; occasionally dysuria and frequency. Any discharge will be scant and mucoid.
—Women: Dysuria and frequency are usually more pronounced due to concomitant cystitis, but vaginal symptoms generally precede these complaints.

• Vaginitis: pain, itching, and discharge; progression to pelvic and abdominal pain due to PID in more severe cases
• Scrotal discomfort: pain and swelling from epididymitis and orchitis (retrograde infection from urethra)
• Ulceration from LGV

—Initial stage: transient inconspicuous genital ulcer
—Tertiary phase: rare, painful, inflamed ulcers; rarely fistula formation, genital elephantiasis

• Secondary LGV characterized by inguinal adenopathy or "bubo" formation
• Arthritis symptoms may present due to Reiter syndrome.

PATHOPHYSIOLOGY

• Infection often occurs in combination with *Neisseria gonorrhoeae;* therefore, many cases of postgonococcal urethritis syndrome are due to *C. trachomatis.*
• *C. trachomatis* is an obligate intracellular parasite of columnar epithelium.
• The pathogenesis of LGV is divided into three distinct phases:

—Primary: inconspicuous genital ulcer
—Secondary: bubo formation
—Tertiary: strictures, fistula, and genital elephantiasis

• Non-LGV serotypes: less complex pathogenesis

—Males: initial urethral mucosal infection; occasional spread to the epididymis and testes
—Females: initial vulvovaginitis; may spread to urethra, bladder, or fallopian tubes
    —Newborn transmission during childbirth can cause severe problems for the infant.

• Postinflammatory strictures: 1 to 30 years after the infection

—Non-LGV serotypes: strictures in male urethra and female fallopian tubes
—LGV: lymphatic vessel strictures more common

CAUSES/RISK FACTORS

• Unprotected vaginal, oral, or anal intercourse with infected partner
• Young adolescents are more susceptible (more extensive GU columnar epithelium and less responsible sexual activity).
• Cigarette smoking, substance abuse, and circumcision may increase risk of infection.

COMPLICATIONS

• Urethral strictures: Early antibiotic therapy may lessen strictures.
• Infertility: female tubal damage: 1 in 25 with mild salpingitis, and 1 in 3 with severe salpingitis
• Chronic pain: due to chlamydial PID

—Maternal/fetal complications: Chlamydial PID increases ectopic pregnancy 7×. Infant problems: otitis media, conjunctivitis, nasopharyngitis, and pneumonia; chorioamnionitis, premature rupture of membranes, stillbirth, spontaneous abortions, low birth weight, and premature delivery

• HIV risk: Chlamydial infections may increase the efficiency of HIV transmission.
• Reiter syndrome

—1% to 2% of patients with NGU, onset usually 1 to 4 weeks after urethritis; syndrome classic triad: urethritis, arthritis, and uveitis; ? idiosyncratic immune response

DIFFERENTIAL DIAGNOSIS

• Urethritis

—Gonorrhea
—*Mycoplasma*
    —*M. hominis* and *M. genitalium* are often isolated in men with NGU and can be a source of maternal/fetal complications, but they are not thought to cause urethritis.

—Ureaplasma urealyticum: usually a diagnosis of exclusion
—*Trichomonas vaginalis*
—Fungus
—Intraurethral warts
—Bacterial urethritis: coliform bacteria urethritis after anal intercourse
—Urethral foreign body or trauma
—Urethritis: may be associated with diseases (Wegener's granulomatosis and Stevens-Johnson syndrome)

• Orchitis
• Ulcers

—Syphilis ulcer characteristics (painless, firm, nonpurulent, sharply demarcated, usually solitary), dark-field examination and serologic tests (RPR, VDRL, FTA-ABS, MHA-ABS)
—Herpes ulcer characteristics (multiple painful vesicles), recurring pattern, viral culture, antigen activation, Tzanck smear, and fluorescent antibody smear
—Chancroid: diagnosed by selective media culture and ulcer characteristics (multiple, ragged, irregular, tender, pustule; may coalesce)
—Granuloma inguinale (donovanosis): diagnosed by crush preparation and ulcer characteristics (red, firm, elevated papule)
—Traumatic ulcers or fixed drug reactions depend primarily on history for diagnosis.

 Database

HISTORY

• Urinary symptoms to suggest *Chlamydia?* Dysuria, frequency, discharge
• Vaginal symptoms? Dyspareunia, itching, discharge, ulcers
• Scrotal symptoms? Scrotal pain, swelling, or ulcers
• Risky sexual behavior? Multiple partners, no condom use
• Prior STDs or infertility?
• Substance abuse?
• Medications, recent antibiotics, or allergies?

PHYSICAL EXAMINATION

• General: Culture swabs should be available in order to obtain samples during the examination.
• Temperature may be elevated with secondary LGV.
• Abdominal examination

—Lower abdominal tenderness with PID
—Inguinal adenopathy: Bubo formation with secondary LGV is usually unilateral, loculated, and often suppurative.

• Genital examination

—Discharge (urethral or vaginal) amount, color, viscosity
—Ulcers
—The typical ulcer of primary LGV is 2 to 10 mm in diameter and is firm and painless, with low, elevated borders.
—Palpation of the urethra for masses

Chlamydial Sexually Transmitted Diseases

 Diagnostic Studies

LABORATORY TESTING

- Diagnostic testing is difficult due to the obligate intracellular growth of the organism, making routine culture impossible.
- Urethral swabs

—Urethral swabs (not a sample of discharge): Obtain at least 4 hours after urination; an early-morning sample before urination is optimal and useful in some patients in whom diagnosis has been elusive.
—Use a calcium alginate swab (cotton swabs bacteriocidal).
—Samples for both Gram stain and culture taken from 2 to 4 mm inside the urethra
—Initial Gram stain reveals many polymorphonuclear leukocytes but no organisms.
—Samples for culture are placed directly into culture media and transported promptly to the laboratory.
—Swabs can be inoculated onto cultured cell monolayers, and the chlamydial inclusions are subsequently detected in the infected cells with stains. This method of diagnosis requires specially trained and equipped laboratory personnel and is slow and expensive.

- Nonculture techniques: yield more false positives but are rapid and less complex than cultures.

—Papanicolaou's stain can reveal chlamydial inclusions in clinical specimens.
—Direct fluorescent antibody rapidly identifies *C. trachomatis* elementary bodies using chlamydia-specific monoclonal antibodies conjugated to a fluorescent stain.
—Enzyme immunoassay is a rapid colorimetric test for *Chlamydia*.
—PCR: newest test, positive in approximately 6% of cases negative by culture

- Frei test: historical importance; no longer utilized
- Serologic tests: high false-positive rate; sometimes useful for LGV or infantile infections
- CBC: leukocytosis in secondary LGV

IMAGING

- No studies diagnostic of *C. trachomatis* infection; tests used in evaluation of sequelae of the disease
- Urethrogram: strictures
- Ultrasound/nuclear scans: differentiate epididymoorchitis from torsion

SPECIAL STUDIES

- Use cysto for strictures, but routine instrumentation should be avoided in uncomplicated cases to limit epididymal spread.

 Treatment

GENERAL MEASURES

- Identification and treatment of sexual partners
- Any patient being treated for gonorrhea should have simultaneous treatment for *Chlamydia* due to the high incidence of concomitant infection.

MEDICAL

- For urethral or vaginal *C. trachomatis* (non-LGV serotypes), administer one of the following:

—Tetracycline hydrochloride 500 mg po qid for at least 7 days
—Doxycycline 100 mg po bid for at least 7 days
—Azithromycin 1 g po as a single dose
—Ofloxacin 300 mg po bid for at least 7 days
—Erythromycin 500 mg po qid for at least 7 days if tetracyclines contraindicated or poorly tolerated or in pregnant women

- LGV

—Tetracycline hydrochloride 500 mg po qid for at least 14 days
—If tetracyclines are contraindicated or poorly tolerated: erythromycin 500 mg po qid for at least 7 days, or doxycycline 100 mg po bid for at least 14 days, or sulfamethoxazole 1 g po bid for at least 14 days

SURGICAL

- Lymph node aspiration

—Suppurative adenopathy during the secondary stages of LGV may require intervention. Aspiration with a large-bore needle through adjacent healthy skin is the optimal treatment. Formal incision and drainage is not recommended due to the potential for prolonged drainage and poor healing.

- Strictures

—Urethral strictures due to *Chlamydia* urethritis or the tertiary phase of LGV
　　—Dilation, endoscopic management (see Section II, "Urethral Stricture")
　　—Open urethroplasty: for long, recurrent strictures or with fistula formation

ALTERNATIVE THERAPIES

- Topical antibiotics and antiseptics may have a role in prevention but are not recommended for treatment of established infections.

PATIENT EDUCATION

- Patients should be educated on the long-term sequelae of the disease, such as strictures, infertility, and maternal/fetal complications.
- Web sites

—http://www.valleymotors.com/~epi1/chlamy.htm
—http://www.columbia.edu/cu/healthwise/0959.html
—http://www.uhs.uga.edu/chlamydia.html

 Follow-Up

MONITORING

- None is recommended for patients whose symptoms resolve with antibiotic treatment. Patients should be seen for follow-up initially to confirm adequacy of treatment.

PREVENTION

- Sexual abstinence, monogamous sexual relationships, and use of condoms are successful measures in avoiding infection.
- Postcontact oral antibiotics or topical antiseptics and antibiotics may prevent infection.
- Compulsive identification and treatment of sexual partners is important to avoid reinfection.

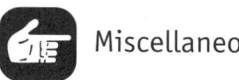 Miscellaneous

SYNONYMS

- Lymphogranuloma venereum is also known as climatic bubo, strumous bubo poradenitis inguinalis, Durand-Nicolas-Favre disease, and lymphogranuloma inguinale.

ASSOCIATED CONDITIONS

- Proctitis, pharyngitis, conjunctivitis (infant and adult), and infantile pneumonia

NOTES: N/A

ABBREVIATIONS

- STD, sexually transmitted disease; GC, gonorrhea; LGV, lymphogranuloma venereum; NGU, nongonococcal urethritis; PID, pelvic inflammatory disease

REFERENCES

Berger RE. Sexually transmitted diseases: The classic diseases. In: Walsh PC, Retik AB, Vaughan ED, Wein AJ, eds. *Campbell's Urology*, 7th ed. Philadelphia: WB Saunders, 1998.

Krieger JN. Urethritis in men: Etiology diagnosis, treatment, and complications. In: Gillenwater JY, Grayhack JT, Howards SS, Duckett JW, eds. *Adult and Pediatric Urology*, 2nd ed. St Louis: Mosby–Year Book, 1991.

Kuhn GJ, et al. Diagnosis and follow-up of Chlamydia trachomatis infections in the ED. *Am J Emerg Med* 1998;16:157–159.

Quinn TC, et al. Epidemiologic and microbiologic correlates of Chlamydia trachomatis infection in sexual partnerships. *JAMA* 1996;276:1737–1742.

Authors: Martha K. Terris and Howard N. Winfield

Chordee

 Basics

DESCRIPTION

- Any noted curvature of the penis during erection

EPIDEMIOLOGY

- Associated predominantly with hypospadias (35%), but may be isolated finding
- Congenital in nature, it is found in 44% of fetuses through the second trimester, suggesting that chordee is a normal part of penile development.
- Associated with epispadias, with curvature being dorsal in nature

GENETICS

- May be found in syndromes associated with hypospadias
- Also seen in small percentage of siblings where father or brother has hypospadias with chordee

STAGING: N/A

SIGNS AND SYMPTOMS

- Variable degrees of penile bend upon erection
- The predominant bend is ventral but can also be dorsal or lateral.

PATHOPHYSIOLOGY

- Chordee with hypospadias secondary to skin tethering

—Decreased elasticity of one or more of the penile fascial layers, causing corporal body disproportion
—Fibrous spongiosum tissue

- Chordee without hypospadias

—Absent or fibrous spongiosum tissue
—Skin tethering and/or abnormality of the superficial fascia in and beneath the skin
—Hypoplastic and/or foreshortened urethra
—Corporal disproportion

CAUSES/RISK FACTORS

- Congenital
- Induced by prior surgery (i.e., foreshortened ventral skin)

COMPLICATIONS

- Unless corrected, potential difficulty with achieving sexual intercourse
- After surgery, may develop recurrent or persistent chordee

DIFFERENTIAL DIAGNOSIS

- Penile curvature: pediatric

—Hypospadias (ventral curvature)
—Epispadias (dorsal curvature)
—Chordee without hypospadias
—Skin disproportion
—Tethering caused by urethral plate and dysplastic underlying spongiosum
—Corporal body disproportion

 Database

HISTORY

- Presence of hypospadias in infant and/or family
- Visualization of penile bend during erection
- History of circumcision or other surgery

PHYSICAL EXAMINATION

- Observe the patient's erection, if possible, to determine extent and direction of penile curvature.
- General penile appearance variable and may suggest chordee
- Presence of hypospadias
- Presence of incomplete foreskin
- Penoscrotal web
- Hypoplastic ventral penile skin/urethra

Diagnostic Studies

LABORATORY TESTING: N/A

IMAGING: N/A

SPECIAL STUDIES

- Artificial erection test: to be done only under general anesthesia in infant or child at time of definitive surgery. Infusion of isotonic saline into corporal body with tourniquet at base of penis

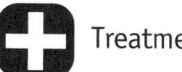 Treatment

GENERAL MEASURES

- Specific treatment depends on the causes of the chordee.
- Surgery is the standard approach.

MEDICAL: N/A

SURGICAL

- Correction of chordee after infant reaches 6 months of age, providing there are no contraindications to anesthesia. After penile skin release, induce the artificial erection test.
- Chordee secondary to skin tethering/dartos abnormality requires skin release and dissection of abnormal tissue anterior to the urethra.
- Chordee secondary to fibrous or absent spongiosum tissue requires deeper dissection with urethral mobilization and/or transection (if foreshortened urethra).
- Chordee secondary to corporal body disproportion involves incising the tunica albuginea on the ventral surface of the penis, in a transverse direction over the point of maximal curvature; cover the defect with either a free dermal or tunica vaginalis graft.
- An alternative to the latter two surgical techniques is to plicate the tunica albuginea dorsally or laterally as needed to reverse the chordee. It is important to avoid the nerve complex dorsally.

ALTERNATIVE THERAPIES: N/A

PATIENT EDUCATION

- Provide appropriate drawings to the family to explain chordee and its ramifications.

 Follow-Up

MONITORING

- Two weeks' postoperative visit, 3-month follow-up, 1-year follow-up; follow up at puberty.

PREVENTION: N/A

 Miscellaneous

SYNONYMS: N/A

ASSOCIATED CONDITIONS

- Hypospadias, epispadias

NOTES

- See also Section I, "Penis—Curvature and/or Pain," and Section II, "Hypospadias."

ABBREVIATIONS: N/A

REFERENCES

Devine CJ Jr, Horton CE. Chordee without hypospadias. *J Urol* 1973;110:264.

Gittes RF, McLaughlin AP III. Injection technique to induce penile erection. *Urology* 1974;4:473.

Hendren WH, Keating MA. Use of dermal graft and free urethral graft in penile reconstruction. *J Urol* 1988;140:1265.

King LR. Hypospadias—A one stage repair without skin graft based on a new principle: Chordee is sometimes produced by the skin alone. *J Urol* 1970;103:660.

Nesbit RM. Congenital curvature of the phallus: Report of three cases with description of corrective operation. *J Urol* 1965;93:230.

Authors: Mark R. Zaontz and Michael G. Packer

Chyluria

 Basics

DESCRIPTION

- The presence in urine of chyle, a combination of lymphatic fluid and triglycerides

EPIDEMIOLOGY

- Most common in areas of endemic parasitic filariasis
- Rare in developed countries

GENETICS: N/A

STAGING: N/A

SIGNS AND SYMPTOMS

- Passage of milky white or gelatinous urine
- May cause renal colic: rarely urinary retention

PATHOPHYSIOLOGY

- Obstruction of suprarenal lymphatics
- Results in rupture of lymphatic vessel into calyceal fornix, forming intrarenal lymphatic-urinary fistula

CAUSES/RISK FACTORS

- Parasitic chyluria: most common

—Filariasis resulting from *Wuchereria bancrofti* infection; rarely from *Brugia malayi* or *B. timori.*

- Mosquitoes serve as vectors.
- Filarial infections are endemic in nearly all tropical regions.

—Prevalence varies: sporadic in Puerto Rico; nearly 50% in parts of India.

- Nonparasitic chyluria

—Retroperitoneal tumors, tuberculosis, trauma, or spontaneous rupture of congenital lymphatic malformation

COMPLICATIONS

- Hypoalbuminemia and anasarca from massive protein loss
- Underlying filariasis may cause epididymitis, hydrocele, and elephantiasis of the penis/scrotum.

DIFFERENTIAL DIAGNOSIS

- Appearance of urine is usually diagnostic; urinary chemistries are confirmatory.
- Phosphaturia, most common cause of cloudy urine
- Pyuria

 Database

HISTORY

- Country of origin of patient?
- Travel to any tropical regions?
- History of tuberculosis exposure/infection?
- History of trauma?

PHYSICAL EXAMINATION

- Lymphadenitis/lymphangitis, genital edema, hydrocele

—Lymphatic filariasis

- Palpable abdominal or flank mass

—Retroperitoneal tumor

 Diagnostic Studies

LABORATORY TESTING

- Urinalysis
- Postprandial urinary triglycerides
- Peripheral blood eosinophilia; may be indication of parasitic infection
- Evaluate for tuberculosis if clinically indicated (tuberculin test, urine stain and culture for acid-fast bacillus).

IMAGING

- Abdominal/pelvic CT

—Exclude a retroperitoneal mass.

- Pedal lymphangiography

—Demonstrates abnormal lymphatics and entrance of contrast material into renal collecting system

- Retrograde pyelography

—Rarely warranted as diagnostic study; may show diffuse pyelolymphatic backflow

SPECIAL STUDIES

- Serodiagnostic tests for *W. bancrofti* are available from the Centers for Disease Control and Prevention.
- Examination of peripheral blood for microfilariae, using Giemsa stain

Treatment

GENERAL MEASURES

- Bed rest and/or use of an abdominal binder to increase intraabdominal pressure may allow spontaneous closure.
- Medium-chain fatty-acid diet

—Transported from gut by portal system, not by chylomicrons

MEDICAL

- Treat the underlying infection.

—Rarely sufficient; chyluria is late manifestation of disease

SURGICAL

- Nephrolysis

—Stripping and ligation of all lymphatic vessels to the kidney and upper ureter; open or laparoscopic technique
—Success rates of 88% to 98% reported

- Endoscopic coagulation of fistula
- Lymphangiovenous anastomosis with ligation of renal lymphatics
- Renal autotransplantation
- Nephrectomy

ALTERNATIVE THERAPIES

- Silver nitrate (1%) instillation into the affected collecting system causes sclerosis of lymphatic fistulas.

—Success rate of 48% reported

PATIENT EDUCATION: N/A

 ## Follow-Up

MONITORING

- Treatment failures readily apparent
- Reevaluate if chyluria recurs following treatment; consider the contralateral kidney as the source.

PREVENTION: N/A

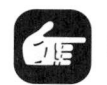 ## Miscellaneous

SYNONYMS: N/A

ASSOCIATED CONDITIONS

- Filariasis

NOTES: N/A

ABBREVIATIONS: N/A

REFERENCES

Diamond E, Shapira HE. Chyluria—Review of the literature. *Urology* 1985;26:427.

Gomella LG, Shenot PJ, Abdel-Meguid TA. Extraperitoneal laparoscopic nephrolysis for the treatment of chyluria. *Br J Urol* 1998;81:320.

Yagi S, Goto T, Kawamoto K, et al. Endoscopic treatment of refractory filarial chyluria: A preliminary report. *J Urol* 1998;159:1615.

Author: Patrick J. Shenot

Condylomata Acuminata (Venereal Warts)

 Basics

DESCRIPTION

- Anogenital lesions caused by the transmission of human papilloma virus (HPV)

EPIDEMIOLOGY

- Approximately 1% of sexually active adults in the United States (1.4 million)
- Highest prevalence: 18- to 28-year-olds
- HPV DNA can be detected in 10% to 15% of the U.S. population (26–39 million).
- 70% of men with same viral subtype as infected female partner

GENETICS: N/A

STAGING: N/A

SIGNS AND SYMPTOMS

- Signs

—Soft, fleshy, and vascular lesions, which usually appear on moist surfaces
—Lesions marked by a raised, granular surface, often with multiple finger-like projections
—Central venule seen within each projection with magnification

- Symptoms

—Nonhealing, painless penile lesion
—Associated symptoms may include penile pruritis, urethral discharge, and a bloody ejaculate.
—Hematuria and/or obstruction may be present with urethral lesions.

PATHOPHYSIOLOGY

- HPV is a double-stranded, circular DNA genome consisting of approximately 8000 base pairs. Subtypes 6 and 11 are associated with the majority of genital warts.
- Transmission

—Sexual contact is the primary cause.
—Autoinoculation of HPV from nongenital skin warts
—Maternal to neonatal, producing laryngeal papillomatosis

- The incubation period is difficult to define because most infections are latent or subclinical.

—New onset of visible lesions, following sexual contact with an infected partner, usually arise 2 to 3 months following exposure.

- Natural history is variable, with occasional spontaneous regression.
- Subclinical infection often persists, and recurrences are frequent.

CAUSES/RISK FACTORS

- Increased risk with number of sex partners, frequency of sexual activity, and presence of condyloma on partners
- Immunocompromised status
- Cigarette smoking may be associated with an increased risk.

COMPLICATIONS

- Urethral transitional cell carcinoma is rare.
- Suggested association with cervical cancer

DIFFERENTIAL DIAGNOSIS

- Herpes simplex virus
- Molluscum contagiosum
- Seborrheic keratosis
- Nevi
- Pearly penile papules
- Buschke-Lowenstein tumor
- Squamous cell carcinoma/basal cell carcinoma
- Bowenoid papulosis
- Malignant melanoma
- Condyloma latum (syphilis)

 Database

HISTORY

- Age and sex of patient

—Highest age prevalence in 18- to 28-year-olds

- History of recent sexual exposure

—Visible warts usually seen within 2 to 3 months of exposure

- Number of partners and frequency of sexual intercourse

—Increased risk of becoming infected with increased frequency or number of partners

- Must check for associated STDs
- Practice of anal intercourse

—Careful inspection of anal region for warts

- Immunocompromised

—Multiple verrucae vulgares, verrucae planae, and extensive condylomata occur more frequently in patients with HIV.

- Associated urethral symptoms of hematuria or obstruction

—Cystoscopy to rule out a urethral lesion

PHYSICAL EXAMINATION

- Classic condyloma acuminata appears as multiple coalescing lesions.
- Lesions are pinkish red–grayish white cauliflower-like lesions found on moist surfaces.
- With magnification, a central venule can be seen within each projection.
- Male: penis, perineum, perianal region, suprapubic area, and scrotum
- Female: vaginal introitus, vulva, perineum, perianal region, and cervix
- Magnification to identify less visible lesions

 Diagnostic Studies

LABORATORY TESTING

- HPV cannot be readily grown in culture.
- Cytologic testing with Pap smear: Exfoliated genital cells are stained and examined for koilocytosis and neoplasia.

—Specificity, 90%; sensitivity, 15% to 50%

- Histologic analysis from biopsy specimens
- Serologic assays not useful in screening for HPV infection, but may provide prognostic information for patients with abnormal Pap smears
- HPV DNA detection techniques can determine viral subtype.

IMAGING: N/A

SPECIAL STUDIES

- Magnification of the genital region after application of 3% to 5% acetic acid for 5 minutes allows visualization of nonvisible lesions, but has low specificity.
- Urethroscopy for any patients with suspected urethral warts
- Proctoscopy for patients at risk for anal condyloma

Condylomata Acuminata (Venereal Warts)

 Treatment

GENERAL MEASURES

- Diagnosis usually based on observation of characteristic lesions
- Current therapies have an equally low effectiveness in preventing wart recurrence and may not reduce disease transmission.

MEDICAL

- Trichloroacetic acid (Tri-Chlor): an 80% to 90% solution of TCA; apply directly to lesions; repeat weekly
- Podophyllin (Pod-Ben-25, Podocon, Podofin): applied to lesion (concentration 10%–25%) by health care worker once weekly for up to 6 weeks
- Podofilox (Condylox): Self-application of a 0.5% solution to warts twice daily for 3 days, followed by 4 days without treatment; can be repeated 4 to 6 times.
- 5-FU (Efudex, Fluoroplex): topical treatment with 5% cream 1 to 3 times per week for several weeks, as needed

SURGICAL

- Electrosurgery (electrodesiccation/loop electrosurgical excisional procedure): to destroy lesions; local anesthesia is usually sufficient.
- Surgical excision: often reserved for extensive disease; also effective for isolated warts
- CO_2 laser therapy: useful for lesions that have not responded to other therapies and for extensive disease. Magnification necessary to maximize efficacy; may produce less scarring
- Cryotherapy: application of liquid nitrogen on patients without extensive disease. This procedure can be repeated at 1- or 2-week intervals.

ALTERNATIVE THERAPIES

- Imiquimod (Aldara): potent inducer of interferon-alpha, which enhances cell-mediated cytolytic activity. Available as a 5% cream applied to external lesions 3 times per week up to a maximum of 16 weeks
- Interferon-alpha (IFN-α): provides immunomodulatory and antiproliferative effects as well as antiviral properties. Routes of delivery include intralesional, topical, and systemic administration.
- Vaccine: difficult to produce because of >20 different types of HPV that can cause genital lesions

PATIENT EDUCATION

- Genital condyloma is an STD, and counseling of the patient and sexual partner is advised.
- Women should undergo routine Pap smears.
- A patient may remain infective even after destruction of visible lesions.
- Treatment of lesions may not decrease recurrence rate.
- HPV Support Program: PO Box 13827, Research Triangle Park, NC 27709; (800)230-6039

 Follow-Up

MONITORING

- Patients should be examined shortly after therapy, to evaluate initial response rates.
- Yearly examinations to look for visible recurrences are optional.
- Educate the patient about self-examination.

PREVENTION

- Abstinence
- Condoms may reduce the risk of infection.

 Miscellaneous

SYNONYMS: N/A

ASSOCIATED CONDITIONS

- Cervical cancer is associated with HPV infection. HPV infection is not solely responsible for the malignant transformation of genital cells, but it may be a cofactor in development of malignancy.
- HPV-16 is found in approximately 40% to 60% of cervical cancers.
- HPV-18 is identified in 10% to 20%.
- PCR identifies HPV DNA in 93% of cervical cancers.
- HPV-6 and -11 are low-risk subtypes, and are seldom associated with malignancy.
- Anal carcinoma also associated with HPV infection.
- HPV DNA is detected in 80% of patients with anal carcinoma.
- HPV-16 is the most common type.
- Homosexuals are at 25 to 50 times greater risk for anal cancer.

NOTES

- See also Section I, "Penis—Lesion."

ABBREVIATIONS

- HPV, human papilloma virus; STD, sexually transmitted disease; DNA, deoxyribonucleic acid

REFERENCES

Beutner KR, Ferenczy A. Therapeutic approaches to genital warts. *Am J Med* 1997;102(5A):28.

Chuang T. Condyloma acuminata (genital warts). *J Am Acad Dermatol* 1987;16(22):376.

Mayman R, Shulman A, Maymon B. Penile condylomata: A gynecological epidemic disease: A review of the current approach and management aspects. *Obstet Gynecol Surv* 1994; 49(11):790.

Strauss MJ, Khanna V, Koenig JD, et al. The cost of treating genital warts. *Int J Dermatol* 1996;35:346.

Authors: Kenneth Ogan and Michael J. Manyak

Cushing Disease and Syndrome

 Basics

DESCRIPTION

• Cushing syndrome is a constellation of symptoms resulting from excessive amounts of glucocorticoids. The syndrome is multifactorial and includes patients with

—Cushing disease: pituitary hypersecretion of adrenocorticotropic hormone (ACTH)
—Adrenal hypersecretion: result of adrenal adenomas or carcinomas
—Ectopic secretion of ACTH or corticotropin-releasing hormone (CRH) from nonendocrine tumors

EPIDEMIOLOGY

• Rare; 3 to 4× more common in women than in men
• 20 to 60 years old; no racial predilection

GENETICS

• Unknown

STAGING: N/A

SIGNS AND SYMPTOMS

• Clinical appearance: "moon" facies; "buffalo" obesity in nuchal, truncal, and girdle regions; striae
• Hirsutism in women and feminization in men suggest adrenal cancer as cause of Cushing syndrome.
• Proximal muscle weakness due to protein wasting
• Depression or major psychoses
• Hypertension and edema due to increased mineralocorticoid activity
• Patients with Cushing's due to ectopic secretion of ACTH may present with cachexia from the underlying tumor.

PATHOPHYSIOLOGY

• Glucosteroids (including cortisol) are synthesized in the zona fasciculata of the adrenal gland. These regulate carbohydrate and protein metabolism.
• ACTH is a polypeptide that is secreted by the anterior pituitary and stimulates the secretion of cortisol by the adrenal glands.
• The release of ACTH is regulated by corticotropin-releasing factor (CRF), which is synthesized in the hypothalamus and reaches the pituitary via the portal–hypophyseal vessels.
• ACTH is most actively secreted in the morning, causing a diurnal variation in the resulting cortisol levels.
• The hypothalamic–pituitary axis is controlled by negative-feedback inhibition; cortisol inhibits the secretion of both CRF and ACTH.
• Evaluation of the hypothalamic--pituitary axis is essential in diagnosing the cause of Cushing syndrome (see below).

CAUSES/RISK FACTORS

• The etiology of increased glucocorticoids can be divided into four causes:

—Exogenous steroids: most common cause. N.B. creams and lotions contain steroids, which can have systemic effects.
—Hypersecretion of ACTH from pituitary (Cushing disease)
    —75% of patients with endogenous Cushing's
    —95% of patients have identifiable pituitary tumors (basophilic or chromophobic pituitary adenomas)
—Primary adrenal hypersecretion due to adrenal adenomas or carcinoma
    —Autonomous in their secretion of glucocorticoids; not limited by normal biofeedback mechanisms
    —Most unilateral; can be bilateral
    —In children <15 years old, adrenal carcinoma is the most common cause of Cushing syndrome.
—Ectopic ACTH secretion: Nonendocrine tumors can secrete polypeptides that biologically mimic ACTH or CRH. This is associated with hypokalemic acidosis, glucose intolerance, and hirsutism.
    —Causes of ectopic ACTH secretion in order of decreasing frequency: small cell (oat) bronchogenic carcinoma, tumors of the pancreas, thymomas, and ovarian tumors

• Risk factors: unknown

COMPLICATIONS

• Related to increased glucocorticoid activity

—Glucose intolerance and diabetes-related: poor wound healing and increased risk of cutaneous infections
—Health risk associated with obesity
—Decreased fertility in both sexes due to hormonal imbalances

DIFFERENTIAL DIAGNOSIS

• Some nonendocrine abnormalities can mimic both the clinical and biochemical manifestations of Cushing disease (pseudo-Cushing syndrome).

—Chronic alcoholism
—Major depression

• See also Section I, "Adrenal Mass."

 Database

HISTORY

• Change in physical appearance? Redistribution of fat?
• Weight gain or growth retardation? Most common presentation in children
• Difficulties with fertility? Change in menstruation? Impotence?
• Signs of glucose intolerance: diabetes, polyuria, polydipsia?
• Change in mental state or depression? Headaches?

• Signs/symptoms of underlying tumor to suggest ectopic secretion of ACTH?
• Cough, change in bowel habits, weight loss?

PHYSICAL EXAMINATION

• Appearance: central obesity, prominent supraclavicular fat pad, moon facies, hirsutism?
• Skin changes: acne, thin skin with poor wound healing, ecchymosis, and striae
• Musculoskeletal: osteoporosis and fractures, proximal muscle weakness and wasting, growth retardation in childhood
• Cardiovascular: hypertension, peripheral edema, congestive heart failure
• Renal: hypokalemic metabolic acidosis, urolithiasis

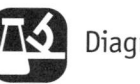 Diagnostic Studies

• Can be divided into two objectives:

—Determine if Cushing syndrome is present.
—Identify the cause of the syndrome.

LABORATORY TESTING

• To diagnose Cushing syndrome

—24-hour urinary cortisol
    —Obtain two or three consecutive 24-hour specimens.
    —Calculate as a function of creatinine excretion (measure cortisol and creatinine).
    —If elevated, it is due to either increased pituitary ACTH or ectopic location (corticotropin-dependent disease) or primary adrenal hypersecretion of cortisol (corticotropin-independent disease).
—AM/PM plasma cortisol level
    —Obtained if 24-hour urinary cortisol level is elevated
    —Determines presence/absence of normal circadian variations in cortisol
    —ACTH release in the morning results in an increased AM cortisol level.
    —Should be at least a 50% decrease (or to <5 ng/dL) in the PM cortisol
    —The diurnal variation is blunted in Cushing syndrome.
—Low-dose dexamethasone suppression test
    —Evaluates the pituitary biofeedback mechanism
    —Dexamethasone (synthetic glucocorticoid that suppresses secretion of ACTH and lowers endogenous glucocorticoids in normal controls)
    —Administer 0.5 mg po every 6 hours × 48 hours; then measure 24-hour urinary cortisol, 17-hydroxycorticosteroid, and creatinine and plasma cortisol. All of these levels should fall appropriately. Failure to suppress indicates disruption of the feedback mechanism, and rules out pseudo-Cushing syndrome.

—Single-dose dexamethasone test
    —Alternative to low-dose test
    —Less reliable, especially in obese patients, but easier to administer
    —1 mg of dexamethasone at midnight, with measurement of plasma cortisol at 8 AM.
    —Suppression to <5 μg/dL is normal.

- Labs to determine cause of Cushing syndrome

—Simultaneous plasma cortisol and corticotropin levels
    —Late PM or midnight sample
    —If cortisol >50 μg/dL and corticotropin <5 pg/mL, then cortisol is ACTH independent → primary adrenal disorder.
    —If corticotropin >50 pg/mL, then cortisol is ACTH dependent: pituitary disorder (Cushing disease); ectopic ACTH; CRH syndrome
—High-dose dexamethasone suppression test
    —Use if cortisol/corticotropin assay unavailable
    —Same protocol as low-dose study, with increased dose
    —2.0 mg po every 6 hours $\times$ 48 hours; then measure plasma cortisol and urinary free cortisol levels
    —Ectopic ACTH and adrenal tumors fail to suppress.
    —Cushing disease: Decrease to at least 50% of baseline.
—Metyrapone test
    —Metyrapone inhibits 11-beta-hydroxylase, preventing cortisol production.
    —This increases the secretion of ACTH (by lessening the negative feedback), and results in increased adrenal steroids, such as 11-deoxycortisol.
    —Cushing disease: exaggerated increase in 11-deoxycortisol levels
    —Ectopic ACTH production or adrenal tumors: no response
    —Not commonly used: risk of adrenal insufficiency and adrenal crisis
—Petrosal venous sinus catheterization
    —Measures ACTH levels in the petrosal venous sinus relative to peripheral plasma levels
    —Not commonly used: invasive nature with risks
—Catheterization of adrenal veins to localize active adrenal tumors
    —Measures cortisol and aldosterone levels (to ensure proper placement of catheter)
    —Difficult, especially catheterizing the shorter right adrenal vein
    —Potential for morbid complications

IMAGING

- CT fine cuts through the adrenal (3 mm)

—Localizes tumors and identifies adrenal hyperplasia
—Adrenal hyperplasia: thickening of adrenal rami and multinodularity bilaterally

—Most adrenal tumors are >2 cm and can be detected with CT.
    —Associated with contralateral atrophy
    —High-fat content manifests as low density on CT.
—Adrenal carcinomas: usually indistinguishable from adenomas on CT, except usually larger (>6 cm)
—Necrosis and calcification suggestive but not diagnostic for malignancy

- MRI: usually not necessary unless cancer suspected

—Evaluates contiguous organ and vascular involvement
—Generally, a higher signal intensity relative to the spleen indicates carcinoma.

SPECIAL STUDIES: N/A

 # Treatment

GENERAL MEASURES

- Treat the underlying cause.

MEDICAL

- Ectopic ACTH: Treat the primary tumor.

—Effects of hypersecretion of functional steroids can be diminished by agents that block steroid synthesis: metyrapone, cyproheptadine.

SURGICAL

- Cushing disease

—Transsphenoidal hypophysectomy: 70% to 95% success rate

- Bilateral adrenalectomy

—For patients who fail pituitary surgery
—10% to 20% develop pituitary tumors with hyperpigmentation (Nelson syndrome).
—Must follow with ACTH levels and evaluation of sella turcica
—Postoperatively: lifelong glucocorticoid and mineralocorticoid replacement

- Adrenal tumors

—The mainstay of therapy is surgical removal.
—Preoperative metyrapone blocks production of cortisol.
—Malignant adrenal tumors have a poor prognosis; 5-year survival is 50% with complete excision, and 35% overall.

ALTERNATIVE THERAPIES

- Cushing disease: pituitary irradiation

—4000 to 5000 cGy (cobalt)
—80% success rate in children; 20% cure rate in adults

PATIENT EDUCATION: N/A

 # Follow-Up

MONITORING

- Return for changes in symptoms.
- Periodic laboratory studies, including potassium and serum cortisol levels
- With bilateral adrenalectomies, require periodic ACTH levels and evaluation of the sella turcica

PREVENTION: N/A

 # Miscellaneous

SYNONYMS: N/A

ASSOCIATED CONDITIONS: N/A

NOTES: N/A

ABBREVIATIONS

- ACTH, adrenocorticotropic hormone; CRF, corticotropin-releasing factor

REFERENCES

Novick AC, Howards SS. The adrenals. In: Gillenwater JY, Grayhack JT, Howards SS, Duckett JW, eds. *Adult and Pediatric Urology*, 3rd ed. St Louis: Mosby–Year Book, 1996.

Orth DN. Cushing's syndrome. *N Engl J Med* 1995;332:791.

Vaughan ED Jr. Adrenal tumors. In: Richie JP, Oesterling JE, eds. *Urologic Oncology*. Philadelphia: WB Saunders, 1997.

Vaughan ED Jr. Diagnosis of surgical adrenal disorders. AUA Update Series (*in press*).

Author: Louis F. Plzak III

Cystitis—Emphysematous

 Basics

DESCRIPTION

• Emphysematous cystitis (EC) is an uncommon complication of cystitis that is characterized by the formation of air within the bladder lumen and wall.

EPIDEMIOLOGY

• Approximately 60% of patients are diabetic.
• 2:1 female predominance
• Middle-aged to elderly
• Patients with depressed immune status: hematologic malignancy, chemotherapy, immunosuppressive agents

GENETICS: N/A

STAGING: N/A

SIGNS AND SYMPTOMS

• Most commonly, the patient appears clinically well.
• Symptoms of mild cystitis are common.

—Frequent and urgent voiding
—Dysuria
—Foul-smelling urine
—Incontinence
—Gross hematuria
—Low abdominal or back pain

• Pneumaturia: The patient describes passing "bubbles" or "wind" per the urethra.
• The diagnosis of EC is usually made incidentally by characteristic findings on a fortuitously obtained radiograph.
• Patients may present acutely ill and febrile.

PATHOPHYSIOLOGY

• Impaired host responses to infection caused by local factors, such as urine stasis, or systemic factors, such as diabetes, lead to a complicated cystitis.
• The infecting organisms are postulated to ferment glucose to produce CO_2 that collects in the bladder lumen and soft tissues.
• Microbiology

—Most common organism: *Escherichia coli*
—Less common organisms: *Aerobacter/Klebsiella, Proteus, Staphylococcus, Streptococcus*
—Rare organisms: *Candida* and *Clostridium perfringens*
  —Suspect these when the urinalysis reveals bacteriuria and urine cultures are sterile.
  —Clinical presentation of these infections is more septic than in the usual patient with EC and is associated with a more guarded prognosis.

CAUSES/RISK FACTORS

• Diabetes
• Female sex
• Conditions of urine stasis: atonic diabetic bladder, prostate or urethral obstruction, bladder diverticulum

COMPLICATIONS: N/A

DIFFERENTIAL DIAGNOSIS

• Recent genitourinary tract instrumentation (e.g., Foley catheter insertion)
  —The most common cause for gas found within the bladder lumen

• Rectosigmoidal gas on a KUB mimicking a gas pattern consistent with EC
• Bladder fistulas

—Enterovesical fistulas associated with colonic diverticulitis, Crohn disease, rectosigmoidal cancer
—Vesicovaginal fistulas associated with vaginal surgery or traumatic vaginal delivery

 Database

HISTORY

• Identify patient factors that increase the likelihood of UTI complications: frequent past UTIs, diabetes, immunosuppressive agents, corticosteroids.
• Identify conditions associated with poor bladder emptying: neurogenic bladder, BPH, urethral stricture disease.
• Identify the history of above-cited conditions associated with bladder fistulas.
• Fevers, chills, nausea, vomiting?

—Symptoms suggest pyelonephritis.

• Flank pain or ureteral colic?

—Symptoms suggest ureteral obstruction, which must be investigated radiographically.

PHYSICAL EXAMINATION

• The patient usually appears clinically well and is afebrile. A septic-appearing and febrile patient indicates an infection with a more guarded prognosis.
• Costovertebral angle tenderness is absent.
• Mild lower back and abdominal tenderness without peritoneal signs
• Subcutaneous crepitus is not present.
• Feculent urine draining through the Foley catheter indicates an enterovesical fistula.

Diagnostic Studies

LABORATORY TESTING

- Urine chemistry: Hemoglobin, leukocyte esterase, nitrite, glucose, and ketone may all be positive.
- Urine microscopy: >5 WBCs/HPF and bacteriuria are present; hematuria may be present.
- Urine culture
- Complete blood count: WBC count may be normal or slightly elevated.
- Serum glucose and electrolytes: Identify perturbations of poor glucose control.

IMAGING

- KUB

—Gas–fluid level seen at the dome of the bladder on an upright film
—Submucosal gas vesicals give the internal diameter of the bladder a "bead necklace" contour.
—Thickened bladder wall
—A thin layer of gas defines the external diameter of the bladder.

- CT

—A thickened bladder wall with intramural gas is pathognomonic.
—Gas dissects into the soft tissues surrounding the bladder.
—Study of choice to evaluate for an enterovesical fistula

SPECIAL STUDIES

- Cystoscopy

—Not required for acute evaluation and management
—Classical appearance of EC
  —Submucosal gas bubbles (4 mm–1 cm)
  —An exaggerated light reflex gives submucosal bubbles a silver sheen.
  —Bubbles are easily ruptured with a cystoscope, liberating the gas into the bladder.

 ## Treatment

GENERAL MEASURES

- Urine drainage
- Hospital admission for prompt initial broad-spectrum intravenous antibiotics
- Strict management of diabetes
- Resolution of symptoms and radiographic findings usually in approximately 4 days
- Remove Foley catheter for voiding trial after symptoms resolve

—Check post-void residual urine volume.
—If residual urine is >150 cc, evaluate for neurogenic bladder or bladder obstruction.

MEDICAL

- Empiric parenteral agents

—Primary choice: ampicillin (1–2 g q6h) and gentamicin (1.7 mg/kg with interval adjusted for renal function)
—Alternative choices: ceftriaxone (2 g qd) or ciprofloxacin (400 mg bid)
—In immunocompromised patients, add metronidazole (500 mg q6h)

- Oral antifungal

—Fluconazole 200 mg on first day; thereafter, 100 mg

- Oral antibiotics

—Oral antibiotics are guided by urine culture and continued to achieve a total treatment period of 10 days.
—Primary choices: trimethoprim-sulfamethoxazole (DS tablet bid) or ciprofloxacin (500 mg bid)

SURGICAL

- Indicated in association with bladder outlet obstruction, bladder calculi, and anatomic abnormalities of the urinary tract
- Surgical debridement is rarely necessary and performed only when it is unavoidable.

ALTERNATIVE THERAPIES: N/A

PATIENT EDUCATION: N/A

 ## Follow-Up

MONITORING

- KUB: Persistence of gas indicates continued infection.
- Urine culture: posttreatment culture to document resolution of infection
- Urine microscopy: posttreatment evaluation to investigate for persistent hematuria, which warrants a formal evaluation

PREVENTION: N/A

 ## Miscellaneous

SYNONYMS: N/A

ASSOCIATED CONDITIONS: N/A

NOTES

- See also Section I, "Pneumaturia."
- Emphysematous pyelonephritis shares the epidemiology, microbiology, and pathophysiology of EC but is associated with a mortality rate of up to 40% and requires immediate percutaneous drainage or nephrectomy.
- EC is not usually associated with emphysematous pyelonephritis.
- Despite the alarming radiographic appearance of EC, the clinical presentation is otherwise not very impressive and the prognosis is excellent with prompt recognition and management.
- Outpatient treatment protocols for EC in the patient without other indications for admission to the hospital may be reasonable but are not yet currently evaluated.

ABBREVIATIONS

- BPH, benign prostatic hypertrophy; EC, emphysematous cystitis

REFERENCES

Bailey H. Cystitis emphysematous: 19 cases with intraluminal and interstitial collections of gas. *AJR* 1961;86:850.

Green MH. Emphysematous cystitis due to *Clostridium perfringens* and *Candida albicans* in patients with hematologic malignant conditions. *Cancer* 1992;70:2658.

Author: David L. Shepherd

Cystitis—Hemorrhagic (Infectious, Noninfectious)

 Basics

DESCRIPTION

- Acute or insidious diffuse bleeding from the luminal surface of the bladder

EPIDEMIOLOGY

- No age, sex, or race predilection
- Primarily seen in cancer patients treated with oxazaphosphorine alkylating agents (for lymphoproliferative disorders, solid tumors, collagen diseases, bone marrow transplant recipients) or pelvic radiation (prostate and cervical cancers)

—Incidence of cyclophosphamide-induced HC: 5% to 7%; mortality from hemorrhage: 4%
—Incidence of radiation-induced HC is about 10% in patients with history of pelvic radiation.

GENETICS

- Unknown

STAGING: N/A

SIGNS AND SYMPTOMS

- Gross hematuria (with or without pain)

—Mild: easily controlled, no acute hematocrit change
—Moderate: drops hematocrit, requiring <6 U PRBCs and local therapy
—Severe: refractory to simple therapies, requires >6 U PRBCs

- Frequency, urgency, dysuria
- Urinary retention from clots
- Occasional mucosal sloughing
- Signs and symptoms of hypovolemia, hemorrhagic shock, or anemia if severe

PATHOPHYSIOLOGY

- Urothelial damage: edema, necrosis, ulceration, hemorrhage, leukocyte infiltration, and neovascularization
- Direct contact by toxins to the bladder wall is believed to be the most common cause.
- Platelet-activating factor, nitric oxide, tumor necrosis factor-α, and interleukin-1 are key mediators in at least cyclophosphamide-induced HC.
- Radiation-induced cystitis may well result from a transmural angiitis.

CAUSES/RISK FACTORS

- Viral infection (adenovirus 11, influenza A, CMV, BK, and JC viruses)

—Outbreaks were seen in the mid-1970s, and now often after BMT.
—May present dramatically, but usually resolves spontaneously in <2 weeks

- Other infections: rarely cause severe HC

—Bacterial: *E. coli, Staphylococcus saprophyticus, Proteus, Klebsiella, Mycobacterium tuberculosis*
—Fungal: *Candida, Aspergillus, Cryptococcus, Torulopsis*

—Parasitic: *Schistosoma haematobium, Echinococcus granulosus*

- Systemic disease: rare, and often refractory to fulguration and irrigation

—Systemic amyloidosis associated with rheumatoid arthritis or Crohn's
—Carcinoma of the bladder

- Chemical toxins

—Anilines, toluidines, and chlordimeform are common industrial exposures (dyes, pesticides).
—Overdoses of methenamine mandelate; accidental urethral instillation of gentian violet douche or nonoxynol-9 contraceptive suppositories
—Thiotepa intravesical instillations and busulfan can cause delayed HC.

- Medications (penicillin, piperacillin, methicillin, carbenicillin, and danazol)

—Penicillin toxicity is likely immune mediated, while anabolic steroids cause damaging vascular changes.

- Radiation

—Induces an obliterative endarteritis that causes acute and chronic ischemia of the vesical wall
—Occurs as late as 15 to 20 years after exposure

- Oxazaphosphorine agents (cyclophosphamide and isophosphamide): most common cause of severe HC

—Acrolein, a liver metabolite of the agents, is the toxin that is believed to be directly implicated.
—Higher dosages, intravenous route of administration (vs. oral), and increased contact time between the bladder wall and the acrolein (because of dehydration and/or infrequent emptying) all worsen the HC.

COMPLICATIONS

- Small, fibrotic, noncompliant bladders are prone to UTIs and perforation.
- Vesicoureteral reflux resulting from bladder fibrosis
- Anemia, renal failure
- Bladder tumors/carcinoma

DIFFERENTIAL DIAGNOSIS

- Cancer anywhere in the urinary tract must first be ruled out.
- Stones, BPH, trauma

 Database

HISTORY

- Gross hematuria
- Receiving cyclophosphamide therapy, history of pelvic radiation or busulfan use
- Bone marrow transplant, possibly with a known viral infection or exposure
- Dysuria, frequency, fevers, chills, UTI

PHYSICAL EXAMINATION

- Hypotension, tachycardia, pallor: from acute or chronic anemia, hypovolemia
- Ocular infections: common with adenovirus infection
- Large hypertrophied tongue: amyloidosis
- Suprapubic pain/mass: distended bladder, infected and/or clot-filled bladder

 Diagnostic Studies

LABORATORY TESTING

- Urine for analysis, cytology, and cultures (including viral, if indicated)
- Coagulation factors and especially platelets (can be depleted)
- Serial hematocrits
- Serum creatinine

IMAGING

- Excretory urography, often done as work-up for hematuria, is usually not able to diagnose HC but may show clots in the lumen, a thickened irregular bladder wall, and/or small capacity.
- US, CT, and MRI will all show a thickened edematous bladder but are not necessary except to assess upper tracts.
- Cystogram to rule out vesicoureteral reflux; required before formalin instillations

SPECIAL STUDIES

- Cystoscopy, with or without biopsy

—May reveal amyloid deposits; eosinophilic inflammatory response of schistosomiasis; IgG, IgM, and C3 depositions; penicillin toxicity; whitish pseudomembranes or plaques of fungal infections
—Needed to distinguish the etiology from bladder cancer
—A biopsy may aggravate the problem, especially in systemic disease states.

- Blood tests for collagen disease markers, if appropriate

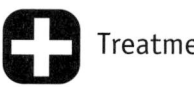 Treatment

GENERAL MEASURES

- Remove the offending toxin and treat the infectious agent.
- Once HC is diagnosed, the treatment for the acute condition is universal for all causes.
- Hydration and induction of diuresis
- Catheterization and clot evacuation
- Saline continuous bladder irrigation

MEDICAL

- Aminocaproic acid (Amicar): 1 to 5 g IV or po q6h

—Usually systemically dosed (IV or po), occasionally in bladder irrigation

—Adverse effects: formation and organization of bladder clots too large to pass, thrombosis, seizures

• Alum irrigation: run a 1% to 4% concentration at 300 to 1000 mL/h

—No need for anesthesia, low incidence of aluminum toxicity
—Adverse effects: spasms, precipitation and clogged catheters, cessation of bleeding rarely permanent

• Silver nitrate instillation: a 0.5% to 1.0% solution in bladder for 10 to 20 minutes, followed by saline flush

—Causes a chemical cauterization
—Adverse effects: painful, requiring anesthesia; crusty build-up can clog ureters; duration of response is often short

• Phenol instillation: 30 mL of 100% phenol in 30 mL of glycine for 1 minute, followed by ethanol and saline washes

—Destroys urothelium, not muscularis; less bladder fibrosis than with formalin
—Adverse effects: painful, requiring anesthesia; duration of response is often short

• Prostaglandin instillation: carboprost tromethamine, synthetic PGF2, 0.1 to 0.8 mg/dL solution. Dwell for 1 to 4 hours, four times a day for 5 to 7 days

—Stabilizes membranes, decreasing edema; causes vasoconstriction and platelet aggregation, decreasing hematuria
  —Low morbidity: no anesthesia required, no precipitate form, so there is no clogging of catheters
—Adverse effects: cost, requires intensive nursing care, moderate bladder spasms

• Formalin instillation: a 1% to 10% solution of no more than 50 mL for 5 to 30 minutes, with patient in reverse Trendelenburg to minimize vesicoureteral reflux (in OR with anesthesia)

—Check cystogram before instillation to rule out reflux; may need to occlude ureter with balloon to prevent potentially fatal renal absorption
—Hydrolyzes proteins, coagulating mucosa and submucosa; 80% effective
—Adverse effects: painful, requiring anesthesia; reflux could cause ureteral fibrosis and eventual renal obstruction, hydronephrosis, or papillary necrosis; extravasation could cause peritonitis and/or fistulas

• Hyperbaric oxygen

—Requires a hyperbaric chamber, which may not always be readily available
—Multiple treatments: helps acutely in most cases, but bleeding often recurs after treatment
—May require 30 to 60 daily treatments, possibly necessitating inpatient care

SURGICAL

• Usually only after all else has failed, and if the patient is unstable
• Bilateral percutaneous nephrostomy tubes with occlusive balloons; then allow bladder to self-tamponade or treat with prostaglandins
• Ligation occlusion of the hypogastric arteries
• Supravesical urinary diversion, cutaneous ureterostomy, ureterosigmoidostomy, cystectomy

ALTERNATIVE THERAPIES

• Selective embolization of the hypogastric arteries

—Can be done under local anesthesia on risky patients
—Complications range from gluteal claudication to bladder necrosis, lower limb paralysis, or impotence.

• Cystoscopic treatments

—With neodymium : YAG laser
—Application of formalin-soaked pledgets

PATIENT EDUCATION

• Rebleeding is common.
• Continue hydration for many days after bleeding ceases.
• Be aware of the long-term sequelae: rebleeding, vesical fibrosis, vesicoureteral reflux, upper tract injury.

Follow-Up

MONITORING

• Hematocrit, renal function, urine culture and sensitivities: repeatedly
• Maintain sterile urine.
• Increased risk for transitional cell carcinoma from cyclophosphamide and similar agents; may be years later
• After severe HC, the amount of bladder contracture and damage from the disease and treatment often necessitates urinary diversion or augmentation.

PREVENTION

• Before prophylaxis against HC was used with cyclophosphamide therapy, incidence of HC was almost 70%, and if it became "severe," mortality was quoted to be as high as 75%.
• Prior to cyclophosphamide administration, measures are taken to protect the urothelium.

—Intravenous hydration, frequent emptying, and sometimes indwelling catheters are used to reduce the time toxins are in contact with the bladder wall.
—Mesna and/or hyperbaric oxygenation treatments
—Avoid rapid decompression of an overdistended bladder due to neurogenic bladder dysfunction.

Miscellaneous

SYNONYMS: N/A

ASSOCIATED CONDITIONS

• Bone marrow transplantation, cyclophosphamide cystitis, radiation cystitis

NOTES: N/A

ABBREVIATIONS

• HC, hemorrhagic cystitis; mesna, 2-mercaptoethane sulfonate

REFERENCES

Del Pizzo JJ. Treatment of radiation induced hemorrhagic cystitis with hyperbaric oxygen: Long term follow up. *J Urol* 1998;160:731–733.

deVries CR, et al. Hemorrhagic cystitis: A review. *J Urol* 1990;143:1–9.

Etlik O, et al. Comparison of the uroprotective efficacy of mesna and HBO treatments in cyclophosphamide-induced hemorrhagic cystitis. *J Urol* 1997;158:2296–2299.

Souza-Fiho MV, et al. Involvement of nitric oxide in the pathogenesis of cyclophosphamide-induced hemorrhagic cystitis. *Am J Pathol* 1997;150:247–256.

West NJ. Prevention and treatment of hemorrhagic cystitis. *Pharmacotherapy* 1997;17:696–706.

Authors: Gregory J. Oleyourryk and Edward M. Messing

Cystitis—Radiation

 Basics

DESCRIPTION

• Acute (early) or delayed (late) inflammation of the urinary bladder during or following partial or total irradiation of the urinary bladder

EPIDEMIOLOGY

• Reactions are related to field size, radiation technique, dose, fractionation, and the status of the bladder prior to irradiation.

—Early reaction: transient irritative symptoms in 65% to 80% of patients undergoing external irradiation. Symptoms severe enough to require medical management between 0% and 10%. Modern radiation therapy technique with image-based planning may reduce the risk of acute sequelae.
—Late reaction: Severe late effects may occur in 5% of patients receiving 60 to 65 Gy to the entire bladder and in 50% receiving 70 to 75 Gy. With partial bladder irradiation, moderately severe effects may occur in 10% of patients and again depends on radiation dose. ≥75.6 Gy causing 13% late sequelae, whereas <70.2 Gy only 8%

GENETICS: N/A

STAGING: N/A

SIGNS AND SYMPTOMS

• Early reaction

—Early mucosal reactions usually produced at doses as low as 30 Gy are generally asymptomatic.
—Irritative symptoms generally occur 4 to 5 weeks after initiation of irradiation.
  —Subside 3 to 4 weeks after completion of irradiation
—Intense urinary frequency and urgency infrequently occur.
—Reduction in bladder capacity

• Late reaction

—May take years to develop
—Painless hematuria
—Urinary frequency and urgency from decreased bladder capacity
—Ulceration
—Fistulas
—Fibrosis

PATHOPHYSIOLOGY

• Mucosal and submucosal edema and hyperemia
• Submucosal blood vessels may appear tuftlike, dilated, or tortuous.
• Bullous edema, obliterative endarteritis, and telangiectasia
• Epithelium may appear atrophic or necrotic.

CAUSES/RISK FACTORS

• Systemic diseases
—Hypertension, diabetes, vascular disease, collagen vascular disease
• Prior pelvic surgery (multiple procedures increase risk)
—Open resections
—Transurethral resections
• Intravesical chemotherapy installations
—Methotrexate
—BCG
• Systemic chemotherapy
—Cyclophosphamide
• Other
—Infections
—Trauma

COMPLICATIONS: N/A

DIFFERENTIAL DIAGNOSIS

• Radiation prostatitis
• Urinary tract infection
• Tumor recurrence

 Database

HISTORY

• Symptoms

—Dysuria, urinary frequency and urgency, nocturia, and hematuria

• Characteristics of radiation therapy

—Timing, duration, radiation doses, technique, location, and volumes of irradiated tissues

• History of risk factors

PHYSICAL EXAMINATION

• Suprapubic fullness and tenderness

 Diagnostic Studies

LABORATORY TESTING

• Complete blood count
• Urinalyses
• Urine cultures

—Antibiotic and sensitivity tests if cultures are positive

IMAGING

• IVP

SPECIAL STUDIES

• Cystoscopy
• Urine cytology and/or biopsy if recurrent cancer is suspected

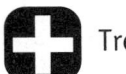 Treatment

GENERAL MEASURES

- Dietary restrictions

—Avoidance of
  —Alcohol
  —Caffeine
  —Tobacco

- Reduction in infection risk

—Drink at least 2 to 3 quarts of fluid daily.
—Ascorbic acid (vitamin C) to increase urine acidity

MEDICAL

- Topical analgesic

—Phenazopyridine (Pyridium) 200 mg tid or qid

- Urinary antispasmodic

—Urispas

- Potassium citrate and tincture of hyoscyamus
- Selective alpha-blockers
- Antibiotics

SURGICAL

- Cystoscopy with evacuation of clots and fulguration of bleeding sites
- Severe cases

—Cystectomy
—Supravesical urinary diversion by ileal conduit

ALTERNATIVE THERAPIES

- Hemorrhagic radiation cystitis

—Acidification of urine
—Bladder washout
  —Mercurochrome (1:200 dilution)
  —Potassium permanganate solution
  —1% to 2% formaldehyde solution
—Blood transfusion

PATIENT EDUCATION

- Radiation cystitis is generally self-limiting, so treatment is supportive in the majority of cases.

 Follow-Up

MONITORING

- Early reaction

—Weekly evaluations during radiation therapy and 4 to 6 weeks after completion of radiation therapy
  —Supportive care as indicated
  —Immediate urologic evaluation if urinary retention occurs

- Late reaction

—Every 3- to 6-month evaluation

PREVENTION

- Early reaction

—Minimize the volume of irradiated urinary bladder.

- Late reaction

—Avoidance of contractures may result from delayed micturition in an effort to "stretch" the bladder.

 Miscellaneous

SYNONYMS

- Bladder reaction

ASSOCIATED CONDITIONS

- Radiation prostatitis and urinary tract infections

NOTES

- See also Section II, "Cystitis—Hemorrhagic."

ABBREVIATIONS: N/A

REFERENCES

Hanks GE, Hanlon AL, Schulthesis TE, et al. Dose escalation with 3D conformal treatment: Five year outcomes, treatment optimization and future directions. *Int J Radiat Oncol Biol Phys* 1998;41(3):501–510.

Pearse HD. The urinary bladder. In: Moss WT, Cox JD, eds. *Radiation Oncology*, 6th ed. St Louis: Mosby, 1989:433–467.

Zelefsky MJ, Leibel SA, Gaudin PB, et al. Dose escalation with three-dimensional conformal radiation therapy affects the outcome in prostate cancer. *Int J Radiat Oncol Biol Phys* 1998;41(3): 491–500.

Authors: Richard K. Valicenti and Ben Corn

Cystocele and Enterocele

 Basics

DESCRIPTION

- Hernial protrusion of pelvic organs into the vagina and introitus is termed *pelvic prolapse*.
- Pelvic prolapse may contain bladder (cystocele), rectum (rectocele), peritoneum and its content (enterocele), or uterus (uterine prolapse).
- The site of prolapse determines the protruding structures and the treatment modalities.

—Anterior wall: cystocele
—Posterior wall: rectocele
—Apex: enterocele, vaginal vault or uterine prolapse

EPIDEMIOLOGY: N/A

GENETICS: N/A

STAGING

- Simple vs. complex prolapse (one structure vs. multiple structures)
- Degree of prolapse of the organ (bladder, small bowel, vaginal vault, uterus)

—Grade I: descent of the organ towards the introitus with straining
—Grade II: descent of the organ to the level of the introitus
—Grade III: descent of the organ outside of the introitus with straining
—Grade IV: descent of the organ outside of the introitus without straining

- Cystocele defect location

—Central: attenuation of endopelvic fascia in the midline under the bladder base
—Lateral: disruption of lateral attachments of endopelvic fascia or cardinal ligament
—Central and lateral combined is the most common.
—Nichols classification of enterocele (traction, pulsion, congenital, iatrogenic)

SIGNS AND SYMPTOMS

- Nonspecific symptoms
- Pelvic pressure; lower back pain; bulging sensation in the pelvis
- Symptoms and signs related to displaced organ

—Bladder (urgency and urge incontinence, obstructive voiding symptoms, recurrent cystitis)
—Urethra (anatomic stress incontinence, urgency and urge incontinence)
—Ureter (silent hydronephrosis, calculi, renal failure)
—Vagina (dyspareunia)
—Rectum (constipation)
—Small bowel (bowel obstruction)

- Other disturbances: emotional; psychosomatic; behavioral
- Manual reduction of the prolapsed organ facilitates its function (as in urinary obstruction, constipation)

PATHOPHYSIOLOGY

- Relevant anatomic fixation prevents extrusion of pelvic organs with increased abdominal pressure; with weakening of the suspending and supporting structures, prolapse occurs.
- Suspension

—Cardinal and uterosacral ligaments are most posterior condensation of levator fascia. Weakness or separation leads to cystocele, uterine prolapse, or enterocele in absence of the uterus.

- Support: levator ani (pubococcygeus, iliococcygeus, and ischiococcygeus)

—Anterior group (pubovisceral group) forms a hiatus for urethra, vagina, and rectum
—Posterior group (diaphragmatic group = levator plate) serves as horizontal support for upper third of the vagina and cervix and for maintenance of the axis of pelvic organs

- Other relevant structures

—Vesicopelvic fascia is a condensation of levator fascia that attaches the bladder base to the arcus tendinosis. Its weakening results in cystocele.
—Prerectal and pararectal fascia weakness and defect of the rectovaginal septum results in the rectocele.
—Sacrospinous ligament/coccygeus muscle serve as point of fixation of vaginal vault (beware of pudendal vessels, inferior gluteal vessels, and pudendal and sciatic nerve posteriorly).

CAUSES/RISK FACTORS

- Pregnancy (direct trauma, nerve damage, progesterone, and cortisol tissue softening)
- Menopause (estrogen withdrawal)
- Pelvic surgery

—Hysterectomy vaginal or abdominal retropubic urethropexy (enterocele formation results in 10% to 15%)
—Bladder neck suspension or colposuspension (enterocele in 3% to 17%)
—Radical pelvic surgery

- Neurogenic (multiple sclerosis, spinal dysraphism)
- Chronic increase in intraabdominal pressure (COPD, BOO, constipation, obesity, ascites, pelvic mass)
- Congenital (connective tissue disorders: Ehlers-Danlos syndrome)

COMPLICATIONS

- Venous congestion of chronically prolapsed vaginal mucosa

—Edema, serous seepage, ulceration, bleeding

DIFFERENTIAL DIAGNOSIS

- Discrimination between prolapsed organs difficult

—Vaginal examination (on withdrawal posterior speculum blade while patient is straining, a small furrow dividing enterocele and rectocele can be seen)

—Rectovaginal examination in standing position while straining (impulse of enterocele will be anterior to the tip of index finger in the rectum and thumb in the vagina)

 Database

HISTORY

- Symptoms
- Impact of prolapse onto vaginal, urinary, and bowel function
- Previous surgical procedures
- Hormonal status
- Obstetric history
- Conditions associated with increased intra-abdominal pressure

PHYSICAL EXAMINATION

- Grading of prolapse in standing and lithotomy (with and without straining)
- Inspection of prolapsed epithelium
- Q-tip test (assessment of rotational descent)
- Reduction of prolapsed organ (reduction of cystocele may reveal stress urinary incontinence)
- Inspection of anterior vaginal wall while posterior wall depressed with speculum with and without straining (diagnostic for cystocele)
- Inspection of posterior vaginal wall and apex with speculum blade anteriorly (diagnostic for enterocele and rectocele)
- Tongue depressor or half speculum can differentiate between

—Central defect (if reduction achieved while placed centrally)
—Lateral (if reduction while placed bilaterally)

- Rectal examination will differentiate rectocele from enterocele.

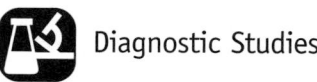 Diagnostic Studies

LABORATORY TESTING

- Urine analysis
- Urine culture as indicated
- BUN, creatinine: may indicate ureteral obstruction

IMAGING

- KUB: bowel gas in prolapsed enterocele or rectocele
- Voiding cystourethrogram while resting and straining in standing position

—Determines degree of hypermobility, presence of stress incontinence, and post-void residual measurement
—Differentiates central (urethra fixed) and lateral defect (urethra malpositioned with straining)

- Defecography (for rectocele assessment)
- Ultrasound or intravenous pyelogram (for suspected ureteral obstruction)

SPECIAL STUDIES

- Post-void residual urine
- Urodynamic studies according to the complexity of condition: mandatory if concomitant voiding dysfunction present

—Reduce cystocele prior to UDS.
—Components: urinary flow measurement, cystometrogram, pressure–flow studies, abdominal leak point pressure (if associated incontinence)

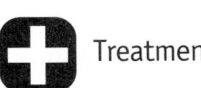 # Treatment

GENERAL MEASURES

- Kegel exercise
- Minimize straining on voiding and defecation.
- Pessary (donut, cube): cube specifically designed for vaginal vault prolapse

—Side effects: vaginal discharge and odor (especially with cube); inflammation, ulceration, erosion of the pessary; cervical or uterine incarceration; vesicovaginal fistula
—Uses: poor surgical candidate; temporary prior to surgery (if ulceration present) or in pregnancy (repair postpartum); temporary for diagnostic purposes (cystocele reduction prior to UDS may unmask SUI)

MEDICAL

- Stool softeners and bulk-forming agent
- Hormonal replacement: prior to surgery or poor surgical candidate

—Estrogen alone in postmenopausal women after hysterectomy
—Estrogen and progesterone if uterus present, even if postmenopausal

SURGICAL

- General measures

—Preoperative preparation
  —Hormonal replacement (same as above)
  —Bowel preparation optional (if bowel involved or for sacrospinous fixation)
  —DVT prophylaxis

- Perioperative 24 hours: antibiotic prophylaxis, suprapubic tube optional; vaginal packing impregnated with antimicrobials; indwelling urethral catheter for 24 hours

—Bladder drainage beyond 24 hours as required: suprapubic tube or intermittent catheterization

- Cystocele

—Transabdominal suspension suitable for lateral defect
  —Principle: apposition of vaginal wall and fascia to lateral pelvic wall by Burch colposuspension (to Cooper's ligament) or Richardson paravaginal repair (to obturator fascia)
—Transvaginal repair suitable for central defect
  —Principle: suture plication of vesicopelvic fascia and cardinal ligaments between vaginal cuff or cervix and mid-urethra by anterior colporrhaphy/Kelly plication with or without mash
—Transvaginal suspension suitable for lateral and central defect
  —Principle: suspension of cardinal and urethropelvic ligaments and vesicopelvic fascia toward the anterior abdominal wall
  —Six-corner suspension (for SUI and grade II or III cystocele with lateral defect)
  —Grade IV cystocele repair with goalpost incision (for SUI and combined lateral and central defect): combination of vaginal wall sling and anterior colporrhaphy
—Always consider concomitant bladder neck support if urethral or bladder neck malposition or hypermobility is present.
  —Vaginal vault prolapse (due to shortened vaginal vault anterior to levator plate)

- Enterocele and vaginal vault

—Transvaginal repair
  —Principle: mobilization, high ligation, and excision of entire peritoneal sac with approximation of cardinal/sacrouterine ligaments and vaginal cuff support
  —Simple enterocele repair: excision of hernia sac with high pursestring ligation and closure of McCall sutures (incorporating sacrouterine complex, prerectal fascia, and rectal wall)
  —As above, plus transvaginal suspension for cystocele if present
—Transvaginal sacrospinous fixation
  —Principle: Suture is placed through the sacrospinous ligament just above the ischial spine and through the vaginal cuff to fix the vaginal vault to the ligament.
  —Indicated for massive vaginal prolapse after hysterectomy; if cardinal/sacrouterine complex of limited strength; at the time of hysterectomy if vaginal suspension not intact; no concomitant cystocele present
  —Outcome: recurrence (0%–20%), enterocele (6%), rectocele (17%)
—Transabdominal repair
  —Moschcowitz's procedure: closure of the cul-de-sac with obliterating sutures (combined with Burch colposuspension)
  —Sacrocolpopexy: vaginal apex fixation to the presacral fascia at S3-S4, using dura mater or rectus fascia graft or synthetic material as a bridge

- Rectocele

—Transvaginal repair: plication of prerectal and pararectal fascia together with excised vaginal wall
  —Reconstruction of levator hiatus; repair of perineal body

- Uterine prolapse

—Transvaginal hysterectomy
  —Indication depends on degree, symptoms, and fertility
  —Contraindication: anatomic disproportion, pathologic conditions of internal genital organs

- Postoperative complications

—Intraoperative: bleeding; pelvic organ injury; neurologic damage; inadvertent cystotomy
—Postoperative early: pain, bladder dysfunction (urinary retention, de novo urgency, or stress incontinence), infection, bladder or ureteral fistula, ureteral obstruction (avoidable with good technique, cystoscopy, methylene blue)
—Postoperative late: vaginal shortening or narrowing, dyspareunia, recurrent pelvic organ prolapse, erosion of suture material

ALTERNATIVE THERAPIES

- Closure or removal of the vagina (colpocleisis or colpectomy)

—Disadvantage: no coital function, stress incontinence due to anatomic changes
—100% successful; older women only

PATIENT EDUCATION: N/A

 # Follow-Up

MONITORING

- Evaluation for recurrent incontinence, retention, or prolapse through history and examination

PREVENTION

- Culdoplasty at time of hysterectomy

 # Miscellaneous

SYNONYMS

- Pelvic organ prolapse

ASSOCIATED CONDITIONS

- Stress urinary incontinence, urgency–frequency syndrome, urinary retention

NOTES

- See also Section I, "Urinary Incontinence—Adult Female."

ABBREVIATIONS

- BOO, bladder outlet obstruction; UDS, urodynamic studies; SUI, stress urinary incontinence

REFERENCES

Klutke CG, Klutke JJ. Transvaginal sacrospinous fixation for the treatment of vaginal vault prolapse. *Adv Urol* 1996;9:275.

Raz S, Stothers L, Chopra A. Vaginal reconstructive surgery for incontinence and prolapse. In: Walsh PC, Retik AB, Vaughan ED, Wein AJ, eds. *Campbell's Urology,* 7th ed. Philadelphia: WB Saunders, 1998:1059–1093.

Richardson AC, Edmonds PB, Williams ML. Treatment of stress urinary incontinence due to paravaginal fascial defect. *Obstet Gynecol* 1981;57:357.

Authors: Peter Niemczyk and Carl G. Klutke

Deep Venous Thrombosis and Pulmonary Embolism

 Basics

DESCRIPTION

• Deep venous thrombosis (DVT): aggregation of platelets and fibrin within a deep vein (pelvis or lower extremity) that may lead to venous obstruction
• Pulmonary embolus (PE): propagation of a thrombus within the pulmonary artery or its branches that has arrived to its location by blood flow. Often arises from a DVT

EPIDEMIOLOGY

• DVT: more common in males

—2.5 million per year in United States, 0.5% to 2.7% in urologic procedures

• PE: 100,000 deaths per year and contribution to another 100,000

—1% to 3% in patients undergoing major urologic procedures

GENETICS

• Inherited deficiency/disorder
• Protein C deficiency
• Protein S deficiency
• Antithrombin III deficiency: can be decreased after surgery, congenitally, or through trauma
• Plasminogen deficiency: abnormal structure

STAGING: N/A

SIGNS AND SYMPTOMS

• DVT: pitting edema, blanching of skin, Homans' sign, increased girth of extremity
• PE: dyspnea, hemoptysis, tachycardia, tachypnea, pleuritic chest pain, cough, sudden death

PATHOPHYSIOLOGY

• Most PEs arise from DVT.
• DVT

—Initiating factors of Virchow's triad: stasis, intimal injury, and hypercoagulability
—Stasis: Stagnant hypoxemia causes endothelial injury.
—Injury: platelet accumulation and fibrin deposition
—Hypercoagulability: regional activation of coagulation cascade: obstruction, edema, pain

• Must differentiate from superficial thrombophlebitis/thrombosis that does not usually lead to DVT or PE
• PE: further thrombus propagation, leading to tails of debris floating within vessels that may dislodge and travel proximally

CAUSES/RISK FACTORS

• Age >40
• Major surgery: transurethral resection, prostatectomy, pelvic lymph node dissection, cystectomy
• Obesity, malignancy, prolonged immobilization
• Multiple trauma, prior thromboembolic event

COMPLICATIONS

• DVT

—Pulmonary embolus; recurrent venous thrombosis; pain
—Postphlebitic syndrome: caused by venous HTN that creates persistent obstruction, resulting in malfunction of contractile pump mechanism

• PE

—Death; pulmonary infarction; pain; dyspnea, shortness of breath

• PE and DVT

—Both of which require anticoagulation with its associated risk factors, create increased health care dollars, and prolonged or re-hospitalization

DIFFERENTIAL DIAGNOSIS

• DVT: cellulitis, thrombophlebitis, muscle sprain/strain, claudication, lymphedema
• PE: pneumonitis/pneumonia, pneumothorax, CHF, esophageal perforation, myocardial infarction

 Database

HISTORY

• DVT

—History of prolonged immobilization, postoperative stat, especially in patient with risk factors
—Complaint of pain with ambulation

• PE

—Must have high clinical suspicion with above history
—Acute onset of dyspnea, tachycardia

PHYSICAL EXAMINATION

• DVT: determined by level of obstruction

—Inspection: unilateral edema, discoloration below level of (occlusion), dilated superficial veins
—Palpation: tender cord or knot; Homans' sign (limitation of passive dorsiflexion of foot, 55% unreliable)

• PE

—Inspection: cyanotic, dyspneic, prominent jugular veins
—Auscultation: pleural rub, rales, S3-S4 heart sounds

Deep Venous Thrombosis and Pulmonary Embolism

 Diagnostic Studies

LABORATORY TESTING

- DVT: none initially for treatment, later evaluation for inherited deficiencies or disorders
- PE

—ABG: increased $P(A-a)O_2$
—PaO_2 below 80 mm Hg
—WBC <15,000 can rule out pulmonary infiltrate via pneumonitis.

IMAGING

- DVT

—Contrast venography (gold standard): invasive, expensive, not always available, time consuming, contrast risks
—Doppler ultrasound: 90% accurate above knee, versatile, noninvasive, painless
—Impedance plethysmography: highly sensitive and specific for proximal veins, less in calf veins, noninvasive
—Venous duplex scanning: more accurate than Doppler and plethysmography
—I-125 fibrinogen scan
  —No longer available secondary to hepatitis risks with human fibrinogen
  —Most sensitive for small clots below knee; results not readily available; expensive
  —High false-positive rate; leg pain following procedure in small percentage of patients

- PE

—Chest radiographs
  —Generally unremarkable; small unilateral effusion
  —Westermark sign (asymmetric vascular markings with segmental or lobar ischemia)
—Ventilation/perfusion scan
  —A perfusion defect ≥1 pulmonary segment and are all unmatched with ventilation defects supports a high probability of PE.
—Pulmonary angiogram (gold standard)
  —May be the appropriate first test in unstable patient. Should be performed when noninvasive tests are equivocal or contradictory

SPECIAL STUDIES: N/A

 Treatment

GENERAL MEASURES

- DVT: elevation, bed rest, pain relief
- PE: oxygen therapy, fluid resuscitation; maintain cardiac output with pressors as needed

MEDICAL

- DVT

—Proximal: anticoagulation with heparin for therapeutic PT for 5 days. Start Coumadin on day 1 and continue for 3 to 6 months, depending on risk.
—Distal: carries low risk of embolization but should be monitored noninvasively over next 2 weeks

- PE: systemic anticoagulation therapy with streptokinase, urokinase, or tissue plasminogen activator

SURGICAL

- DVT

—Thrombectomy: rarely needed
—IVC filter: used as prophylaxis in high-risk or multiple-trauma patient; useful if anticoagulation contraindicated

- PE

—Pulmonary embolectomy; considered rarely for patient who remains in shock despite medical therapy
—IVC interruption: recurrent emboli or contraindications to anticoagulation.

ALTERNATIVE THERAPIES: N/A

PATIENT EDUCATION

- The patient should be instructed to inform future health care providers of this diagnosis.
- Anticoagulated patients should avoid use of other medications (i.e., NSAIDs) that can alter the coagulation profile.

 Follow-Up

MONITORING

- Follow-up ultrasounds may be needed to assess propagation and/or resolution of the clot.
- Monitoring of PT/PTT/INR as needed based on usage

PREVENTION

- Physical: sequential compression hose in operating room and while patient bedridden: simple, inexpensive, can be combined with other modalities
- Ambulation: as soon pre- and postoperatively as feasible

- Medical

—Low-dose ultra-fractionated heparin: inhibits thrombin activity, decreases risk by 25% to 80%
—5000 U sq 2 hours preoperative, every 8 to 12 hours postoperative
—No increased risk of bleeding

- Low-molecular-weight heparin: inhibits factor Xa

—Better at preventing DVT; no difference in rates of bleeding
—Longer half-life; at least 5 formulations available; cost is 4× that of heparin

- Coumadin

—Highly effective in decreasing DVT
—Maintain at international rate 2 to 3; started 3 to 4 days preoperatively

- ASA: inhibits platelet aggregation; 28% reduction in DVT and 78% PE deaths
- Dextran: glucose polymer; decreases plasma viscosity, alters platelet function, and decreases fibrin polymerization

—Risk of allergic reactions, expensive, must monitor for volume overload

 Miscellaneous

SYNONYMS: N/A

ASSOCIATED CONDITIONS

- Malignancy, nephrotic syndrome, dysfibrinogenemia, lupus anticoagulant, drug abuse

NOTES: N/A

ABBREVIATIONS

- DVT, deep venous thrombosis; PE, pulmonary embolus; ASA, aspirin; CHF, congestive heart failure; HTN, hypertension; PT, prothrombin time

REFERENCES

Friedrichs P, et al. Facts and fallacies about DVT. *Contemp Urol* 1996;July:60–68.

Prevention of venous thrombosis and pulmonary embolism. NIH Consensus Development. *JAMA* 1986;256:744–749.

Authors: Natania Y. Piper and Ian M. Thompson

Detrusor Instability/Overactivity

 Basics

DESCRIPTION

• Symptomatic bladder overactivity is a condition with symptoms of urinary frequency, urgency, or urge incontinence, either singly or in combination, appearing in the absence of local pathologic factors explaining these symptoms.

EPIDEMIOLOGY

• The exact incidence of detrusor overactivity without incontinence is unknown. Thought to occur in 8% to 10% of the general population
• 10% to 22% of women with incontinence present with urge incontinence.
• Up to 75% of men with bladder outlet obstruction have associated detrusor overactivity.
• Female incidence > male

GENETICS

• Unknown

STAGING

• By voiding symptoms alone: frequency, urgency, urge incontinence
• By urodynamic testing

—Motor urgency: presence of uninhibited contractions during bladder filling. The term *detrusor instability* is used to denote the contractions with the sense of urgency.
—Sensory urgency: Urgency is present with filling, but no contractions are found.

SIGNS AND SYMPTOMS

• Urinary frequency
• Urinary urgency
• Urge incontinence
• Nocturia

PATHOPHYSIOLOGY

• Neurogenic theory

—Hyperreflexic detrusor in patients with a known neuropathy (spinal cord injury, multiple sclerosis, stroke) wherein loss of micturition reflex inhibition and bladder–sphincter coordination causes involuntary detrusor contractions
—Idiopathic detrusor overactivity: theory that a subclinical neurologic dysfunction affects the central and/or peripheral regulation of micturition

• Myogenic theory

—Detrusor instability or overactivity occurs when there is an alteration in the properties of the bladder smooth muscle cells such that they can spontaneously activate one another, bypassing neural regulation.

CAUSES/RISK FACTORS

• Neurologic lesion or disorder: *Detrusor hyperreflexia* is the term used to describe bladder overactivity.

—Spinal cord injury, stroke, Parkinson disease, multiple sclerosis, dementia

• Nonneurogenic: The terms *overactivity* and *instability* are used to describe bladder activity without a known neurologic deficit.

—Congenital (posterior urethral valves, obstruction)
—Bladder outlet obstruction (benign prostatic hyperplasia, urethral surgery)
—Urethral instability: sudden drop in urethral pressure triggering the bladder to contract
—Aging: common problem with advancing age, especially patients >80 years old
—Psychosomatic: children with Hinman-Allen syndrome
—Idiopathic: most common cause

COMPLICATIONS

• Social isolation from the constant urge to void and urinary frequency
• Urge incontinence with skin breakdown, candidiasis, recurrent urinary tract infections
• Detrusor hyperreflexia with obstruction (dyssynergia) can damage the bladder and kidneys.

DIFFERENTIAL DIAGNOSIS

• Urinary tract infection
• Carcinoma in situ of the bladder
• Urethral syndrome
• Interstitial cystitis
• Loss of detrusor compliance (radiation therapy, denervation)
• Foreign body in the bladder (stone, ureteral stent)

 Database

HISTORY

• Detail the daily frequency and urgency, with or without incontinence (voiding diary).
• Is there associated stress urinary incontinence?
• Is there a history of dysuria or hematuria?

—Suggests urinary tract infection, cancer, or stone

• Family, social, and environmental history
• Medical history

—Neurologic disorders
—Smoking (increased risk for bladder cancer)
—Medications (diuretics, psychoactive drugs)

• Surgical history

—Spine surgery, gynecologic procedures, pelvic procedures

PHYSICAL EXAMINATION

• Palpate the lower abdomen for a distended bladder.

—Suggests overflow incontinence or obstruction

• Pelvic examination to look for bladder prolapse or mass
• Digital rectal examination in men to assess the size, symmetry of the prostate

—Rule out the presence of a prostate nodule or induration (will need biopsy to rule out carcinoma).

• Focused neurologic examination to assess sensation and motor function

—Bulbocavernosus reflex, voluntary external anal sphincter contraction, perineal/perianal skin sensation

Diagnostic Studies

LABORATORY TESTING

• All patients

—Urinalysis: glucose, ketones, specific gravity, blood, nitrates, leukocyte esterase
—Urine cytology
—Post-void residual urine

• Selected patients

—Simple urodynamic testing: cystometrogram
  —When failing first-line drug and behavioral therapy
—Complex urodynamic testing: multiple channels, EMG, simultaneous fluoroscopy
  —Neurologic disease, failed incontinence surgery, obstructive uropathy

IMAGING

• Renal ultrasound

—When detrusor overactivity is associated with loss of bladder compliance or functional obstruction secondary to a neurologic lesion or disorder (spinal cord injury)

• Voiding cystourethrogram

—When the location of an obstructive process needs imaging for correction

SPECIAL STUDIES

• Cystourethroscopy

—Hematuria without infection; bladder stone; or suspicious cytology for cancer

 ## Treatment

GENERAL MEASURES

• Use a voiding diary to understand the actual daily frequency and urgency.

—Prescribe a timed voiding regimen (bladder drill) to slowly increase voiding intervals.
—Review the intake/output volumes to determine if oral intake is excessive.

MEDICAL

• Behavioral techniques in addition to timed voiding

—Pelvic floor exercises (Kegel): used to train the patient to effectively contract the pelvic floor, which will serve to reflexly inhibit the spontaneous bladder contraction causing the frequency and urgency
—Biofeedback: use of visual or auditory cues to reinforce the teaching of pelvic floor exercise

• Pharmacotherapy

—Anticholinergic and musculotropic relaxant medications: block the major neurotransmitter (acetylcholine) for detrusor contractions and/or directly relax the detrusor smooth muscle
  —Examples include oxybutynin chloride (Ditropan), propantheline bromide (Pro-Banthine), hyoscyamine (Cystospaz), hyoscyamine sulfate (Levsin), flavoxate hydrochloride (Urispas), and tolterodine (Detrol).
—Tricyclic antidepressants: have central and peripheral anticholinergic effects, block the reuptake of norepinephrine and serotonin, and are sedatives
  —Example is imipramine (Tofranil)
—All of these medications have bothersome side effects, including dry mouth, constipation, and blurred vision. Variable patient tolerance and compliance with the medications often requires titrating the medication to the desired result balanced with the side effects.

SURGICAL

• Reserved for medical therapy failures

• Augmentation cystoplasty

—Up to 90% effective for patients with neurogenic bladders and hyperreflexia
—The ability or means to perform intermittent catheterization is mandatory.

ALTERNATIVE THERAPIES

• Electrical stimulation

—Intravaginal or anal electrical stimulation has been used to augment the inhibitory reflex arc to the bladder, stopping the involuntary bladder overactivity.
—Percutaneous and extradural sacral nerve stimulation has been used successfully to modulate neural activity to the bladder and spinal cord, thereby suppressing the urinary urgency and frequency.

PATIENT EDUCATION

• Patients must understand the need to comply with medical regimens and behavioral techniques in order to get better.
• Medications often need adjustment in order to be both tolerable and effective.

 ## Follow-Up

MONITORING

• Periodic voiding diaries are helpful to objectify improvement.
• Periodically review compliance with the medications, timed voiding, and exercises.

PREVENTION: N/A

 ## Miscellaneous

SYNONYMS

• Hyperactive bladder, uninhibited bladder, spastic bladder, reflex bladder, hypertonic bladder

ASSOCIATED CONDITIONS

• BPH-mediated obstruction, detrusor–sphincter dyssynergia

NOTES

• See dosing of agents in Section V.

ABBREVIATIONS

• DI, detrusor instability; OAB, overactive bladder; DH, detrusor hyperreflexia

REFERENCES

Bates CP. The unstable bladder. *Clin Obstet Gynecol* 1978;5:109.

Cardoza LD, Abrams PD, Stanton SL, Finelly RCL. Idiopathic bladder instability treated by biofeedback. *Br J Urol* 1978;50:521.

Mark SD, Webster GD. Detrusor hyperactivity. In: Raz S, ed. *Female Urology*, 2nd ed. Philadelphia: WB Saunders, 1996.

Wein AJ. Drug treatment of voiding dysfunction. AUA Update Series, Vol 7, Lesson No. 15, AUA, Houston, 1988.

Author: Timothy B. Boone

Detrusor—Sphincter Dyssynergia

 Basics

DESCRIPTION

• Contraction of the sphincter mechanism occurring simultaneously with uninhibited involuntary contraction of the bladder detrusor muscle (detrusor hyperreflexia [DH]) in cases of neurogenic lower urinary tract dysfunction

EPIDEMIOLOGY

• Prevalent with spinal cord lesions; more prevalent at higher level (especially cervical) than lower (sacral) injury
• May affect those with multiple sclerosis, spinal cord tumor, traumatic spinal cord injury, arteriovenous malformation

GENETICS: N/A

STAGING: N/A

SIGNS AND SYMPTOMS

• Incontinence
• Risk for urinary tract infection; may present with urosepsis
• Poor bladder emptying, elevated residual urine, urinary retention
• May present with renal insufficiency; usually a late complication
• Urolithiasis

PATHOPHYSIOLOGY

• DSD causes a functional bladder outflow obstruction, resulting in dramatic elevation of intravesical pressure, which damages the urinary tracts directly with pressure and secondarily with infection and urolithiasis.
• DSD is always associated with DH, although DH may occur with synergic sphincter function (without DSD).
• Pontine mesencephalic reticular formation is responsible for coordinating sphincter relaxation with detrusor contraction.

—Spinal cord lesions impair the transmission of coordinating influences from the pons during reflex detrusor contraction.
—Uninhibited detrusor contraction stimulates a reflex sphincter contraction, resulting in bladder outflow obstruction.

• 10% to 20% of patients have internal (bladder neck) sphincter dyssynergia coexistent with external sphincter dyssynergia (DESD).
• Elevated intravesical pressure is responsible for the sequelae of DH-DSD, especially when sustained intravesical pressure exceeds 40 cm H_2O.

—Untreated DH-DSD may result in renal failure.

CAUSES/RISK FACTORS

• Suprasacral spinal cord lesions

—Tumor
—Trauma
—Arteriovenous malformation
—Plaques of multiple sclerosis
—Infarct
—Congenital malformation (myelodysplasia)

• Neurologic processes affecting the CNS below the level of the pons
• May be associated with autonomic hyperreflexia

COMPLICATIONS

• Bladder wall thickening, detrusor hypertrophy, diverticuli
• Recurrent urinary tract infection

—Males may be febrile with parenchymal involvement, potentially resulting in abscess formation.
  —Prostatitis
  —Epididymo-orchitis
  —Pyelonephritis: Recurrence results in scarring and decreased renal function.
—Febrile urinary tract infection is almost always indicative of pyelonephritis.

• Urolithiasis: results from urinary stasis but accelerated by chronic infection, especially with urea-splitting organisms

—Bladder
—Renal, ureteral: may complicate UTI with obstruction

• Urinary retention
• Hydroureteronephrosis

—Persistent elevation of intravesical pressure >40 cm H_2O impairs ureteral urine delivery to the bladder.
—Ureteral dilatation eventually impairs the ability of the ureterovesical junction to prevent backflow of urine (vesicoureteral reflux).
—Vesicoureteral reflux predisposes to chronic pyelonephritis.
—Chronic pyelonephritis may result in renal staghorn calculus formation.

• Renal insufficiency

—Results from pressure atrophy or chronic infection of the renal parenchyma

DIFFERENTIAL DIAGNOSIS

• In patients with DH, bladder outflow obstruction from other etiologies

—Benign prostatic hyperplasia
—Adenocarcinoma of the prostate
—Urethral stricture disease

• Bladder tumor

—Transitional cell carcinoma
—Adenocarcinoma
—Leiomyoma
—Squamous cell carcinoma

• Urethral tumor

—Transitional cell carcinoma
—Squamous cell carcinoma

• In patients with urinary retention/incomplete emptying and coexistent neurologic disease, consider impaired detrusor contractility/detrusor areflexia.

Database

HISTORY

- Neurologic disease: date of onset, duration of process
- Urinary voiding symptoms: frequency, urgency, urge incontinence
- Method of urinary management

—Condom catheter urinary collection
—Intermittent self-catheterization
—Indwelling urethral or suprapubic catheter

- Urinary tract infection

—Severity of infection
  —Response to antibiotics
  —Need for parenteral antibiotics
—Frequency of recurrence of infection

- Urolithiasis

—Episodes of lithiasis
—Surgical intervention
—Calculus composition

PHYSICAL EXAMINATION

- Fever

—Parenchymal urinary tract infection
  —Men: prostate, testes/epididymis/renal
  —Women: renal

- Hypertension

—During manipulation of the GI/GU systems, autonomic hyperreflexia may result.

- Generalized edema

—Severe renal insufficiency

- Palpable flank mass

—Secondary hydronephrosis

- Flank tenderness

—Ureteral obstruction
—Pyelonephritis

- Abdominal mass

—Distended bladder: urinary retention

- Incontinence of urine

—Spontaneously
—With stress maneuvers
—During abdominal/pelvic palpation

- Testicular mass

—Epididymo-orchitis/epididymitis
—Secondary abscess formation
—Hydrocele from recurrent infection

- Prostate mass/nodule

—Focal prostatitis

 Diagnostic Studies

LABORATORY TESTING

- Videourodynamic evaluation is essential to diagnose DH with DSD.

—Medium-fill cystometry at 50 cc/min
  —Uninhibited detrusor contraction
  —Intravesical pressure >40 cm H_2O during storage
  —Voiding pressure >60 cm H_2O during voiding
—Fluoroscopic monitoring
  —Bladder trabeculation, diverticulum formation
  —Dilated prostatic urethra
  —Narrow membranous urethra
  —Vesicoureteral reflux
  —Hydronephrosis
—Urethral pressure profile
  —Sustained or accentuated intraurethral pressure during involuntary uninhibited detrusor contraction
—Sphincter electromyography
  —Accentuated activity simultaneous with involuntary uninhibited detrusor contraction

- Blood studies

—Serum chemistry: Evaluate renal function, electrolyte levels.
—Complete blood count: Rule out secondary anemia due to decreased renal function or chronic infection.

- Urine studies

—Urine analysis
  —Proteinuria: renal dysfunction
  —Pyuria, nitrite, leukocyte esterase: acute or chronic infection
  —Hematuria: infection or lithiasis

IMAGING

- Renal ultrasound

—Effective in screening for upper urinary tracts
  —Calculus, hydronephrosis, masses

- Excretory urography

—Contraindicated in those with decreased renal function (serum creatinine <2.0)
—Delayed excretion of contrast with high urinary storage pressures
—Hydroureteronephrosis
  —Marked elevation of intravesical pressure
  —Usually in patients with longstanding DH-DESD
  —May be due to urinary calculi
—Bladder
  —Wall thickening, trabeculation, diverticulum formation, incomplete emptying

- Voiding cystourethrogram

—Bladder
  —Wall thickening, trabeculation, diverticulum formation, incomplete emptying
—Ureter
  —Vesicoureteral reflux
  —Hydroureter
  —Hydroureteronephrosis
—Urethra
  —Prostatic urethra dilated
  —Membranous urethra persistently narrow, stenotic, nonrelaxing
  —Distal urethra normal: Rule out stricture.
—Nuclear medicine renal scan
  —Objective quantification of glomerular filtration rate (GFR)
  —Sequential studies can detect deterioration of renal function prior to elevation of serum creatinine.
  —Determines whether obstruction exists with use of furosemide wash-out analysis

SPECIAL STUDIES

- Cystoscopy

—Normal penile urethra
—Spastic, nonrelaxing, stenotic membranous urethra
—Dilated prostatic urethra
—Bladder trabeculation/diverticuli
—Rule out calculus or bladder tumor.

(continued)

Detrusor—Sphincter Dyssynergia (continued)

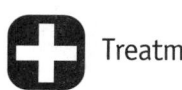 Treatment

GENERAL MEASURES

• Decrease intravesical pressure

—Decrease bladder contractility to allow low-pressure urinary storage.
—Defeat sphincter function to establish low-pressure urinary drainage per urethra.
   —This is an option only for males, as there is no effective external urinary collection device for females.

MEDICAL

• Anticholinergic therapy is effective in improving urinary storage under low pressure

—Oxybutynin 5 mg po tid-qid
—Propantheline bromide 15 mg po bid-tid
—Hyoscyamine 0.375 mg po bid-tid
—Tolterodine 2 to 4 mg po bid

• Alpha-adrenergic blockade may decrease internal sphincter function but is largely ineffective for DESD.

—Doxazosin 2 to 8 mg po qd
—Terazosin 2 to 5 mg po qd
—Prazosin 1 mg po tid
—Tamsulosin 0.4 mg po od
—Phenoxybenzamine 10 mg po bid (nonselective)

• Botulinum toxin injection into the external sphincter: efficacy short-lived; requires repeated injection

SURGICAL

• Endoscopic sphincter ablation (only in males): requires condom catheter urinary collection

—Electrosurgical or Nd:YAG laser sphincterotomy: Incise the external sphincter from the bulbous urethra to the mid-prostatic urethra.
   —Further incision through the prostate and bladder neck may be required if internal sphincter dyssynergia is present.
—Sphincter stent prosthesis placement: wire mesh stent placed endoscopically; bridges mid-prostatic to bulbous urethra
   —Maintains caliber of membranous urethra at 42Fr
   —Suprapubic tube cystostomy may be required in the perioperative period.
—Augmentation cystoplasty: bladder incised in clamshell fashion to disrupt detrusor contraction; gastrointestinal segment used to patch bladder; increasing storage with decreased pressure
   —Use large intestine, ileum, or gastric segment
   —Requires intermittent catheterization for urinary drainage
   —Limited dexterity may mandate creation of a continent catheterizable stoma for the urinary reservoir, especially in females.
—Ileal conduit cutaneous vesicostomy: conduit of ileum connecting dome of bladder to anterior abdominal wall
   —Continuous low-pressure drainage through an incontinent ileal conduit urostomy requires a stomal appliance urinary collection.
   —Useful if unable to perform self-catheterization (i.e., quadriplegia)

ALTERNATIVE THERAPIES

• Vanilloid agents: suppress uninhibited involuntary detrusor contraction in patients refractory to anticholinergic therapy

—Capsaicin, Resiniferotoxin: applied intravesically, requires repeated instillation

• Sacral deafferentation with sacral nerve root stimulation

—Deafferentation with dorsal rhizotomy abolishes spontaneous detrusor contraction, improving urinary storage.
—Nerve root stimulation allows control over detrusor contraction.
—Obstruction by the sphincter may require adjunctive sphincteric ablation.

PATIENT EDUCATION

• Patients must comprehend the potential dangers of untreated neurogenic lower urinary tract dysfunction, especially renal failure, infection, and urinary lithiasis.

Follow-Up

MONITORING

• Annual evaluation

—Videourodynamic testing to assure low intravesical pressure
—Upper tract imaging to rule out upper tract changes (calculi, hydronephrosis)
—Serum chemistry to confirm normal renal function and electrolyte balance

PREVENTION: N/A

 Miscellaneous

SYNONYMS

• Detrusor—external sphincter dyssynergia

ASSOCIATED CONDITIONS

• Neurogenic impotence, neurogenic bowel

NOTES

• See also Section I, "Neurogenic Bladder," and Section II, "Detrusor Instability/Overactivity" and "Spinal Cord Injury—Urologic Considerations."

ABBREVIATIONS

• DH, detrusor hyperreflexia; DSD, detrusor–sphincter dyssynergia; DESD, detrusor–external sphincter dyssynergia

REFERENCES

Blaivas JG. The neurophysiology of micturition: A clinical study of 550 patients. *J Urol* 1982;127: 958.

Kaplan SA, Chancellor MB, Blaivas JG. Bladder and sphincter behavior in patients with spinal cord lesions. *J Urol* 1991;146:113.

McGuire EJ, Woodside JR, Borden TA. Prognostic value of urodynamic evaluation in myelodysplastic patients. *J Urol* 1981;126:205.

Perkash I. Long-term urologic management of the patient with spinal cord injury. *Urol Clin North Am* 1993;20:423.

Watanabe T, Rivas DA, Chancellor MB. Urodynamics of spinal cord injury. *Urol Clin North Am* 1996;23:459.

Authors: David A. Rivas and Patrick J. Shenot

Diabetes Mellitus—Urologic Considerations

 Basics

DESCRIPTION

- Endocrin-based hyperglycemia with secondary metabolic abnormalities

EPIDEMIOLOGY

- 1% to 2% of general population

GENETICS

- Genetic predisposition permissive and not casual
- Possible chromosome 6 or 11 involvement

STAGING

- Primary

—Insulin-dependent diabetes mellitus (IDDM)
—Non–insulin-dependent diabetes mellitus (NIDDM)
—Non-obese NIDDM
—Obese NIDDM
—Maturity-onset NIDDM

- Secondary

—Pancreatic disease
—Hormonal based
—Chemical induced
—Pharmacologic
—Insulin receptor abnormalities
—Other

SIGNS AND SYMPTOMS

- Polyuria

—Secondary to osmotic diuresis

- Erectile dysfunction (ED)

—Approximate 40% incidence
—By age 60, double incidence in men with DM over general population
—By age 30, triple incidence in men with DM over general population
—May be presenting problem

- Ejaculatory failure

—Incidence up to 32% in men with DM

- Infertility
- Voiding dysfunction (VD)

—Classic lack of voiding sensation or urge
—Nocturia, urinary frequency

- Urinary tract infections (UTIs)

—Recurrent
—Rule out pyelonephritis

PATHOPHYSIOLOGY

- Polyuria

—Hyperglycemia causes secondary osmotic diuresis.

- ED

—Neurogenic factor: both autonomic and sensory component
—Arteriogenic: small vessel angiopathy

—Venogenic
—Psychologic

- Ejaculatory failure: secondary to AN
- Infertility

—Associated with ED, ejaculatory failure, as well as potentially poor semen quality and abnormal testes biopsy

- VD: Secondary to AN
- UTI

—Associated with glycosuria and VD
—Upper urinary tract associated with 80% of UTI in DM

CAUSES/RISK FACTORS

- Voiding dysfunction (VD)

—May be associated with BOO
—AN may be secondary to metabolic derangement of the Schwann cell that results in segmental demyelinization and impairment of nerve conduction.
—Polyuria may be secondary to poor control.

- ED

—2 to 5× higher incidence than in normal control subjects
—12% of impotent men have unrecognized DM.
—May be associated with autonomic/sensory neuropathy

- UTI

—Evaluate for glycosuria, upper and lower urinary tract obstruction, and VD.

COMPLICATIONS

- VD

—Atonic bladder with secondary urinary retention
—Recurrent UTI
—Hydroureteronephrosis with secondary renal insufficiency
—Urinary incontinence: SUI, urge, overflow

- UTI

—Cystitis
—Ascending infection with pyelonephritis, common with AN
—Obstruction with secondary pyelonephritis

DIFFERENTIAL DIAGNOSIS

- Polyuria: voluntary or psychogenic excessive fluid ingestion, diabetes insipidus, chronic renal failure
- Voiding dysfunction: BOO, HNP, tabes dorsalis, HZ, radical pelvic surgery
- Ejaculatory failure: ejaculatory duct obstruction, bladder neck surgery
- UTI: cystitis, pyelonephritis, emphysematous PNPS, bacterial nephritis, XGM, renal calculi, papillary necrosis, perinephric abscess, metastatic infection

 Database

HISTORY

- General

—Polyuria, polydipsia, polyphagia
—Weight loss, malaise
—Family history of DM
—ED in the younger man

- UTI

—History of recurrent UTI
—Flank pain, chills and fever, nausea and vomiting
—Hematuria
—History of urolithiasis

PHYSICAL EXAMINATION

- Flanks

—Evaluate for guarding, splinting, crepitation.

- Abdomen

—Check for distended bladder, incarcerated hernia.

- Genitals

—Phimosis, balanitis, diffuse yeast/bacterial dermatitis
—Testes atrophy

- Rectal

—Tone, perianal sensation
—BCR (sacral reflex arc)

- Prostate

—Symmetry, tone

Diagnostic Studies

LABORATORY TESTING

- General

—Fasting (overnight): venous plasma glucose concentration greater than 140 mg/dL on two different occasions
—Oral glucose tolerance test: may overdiagnose

- ED

—Testosterone: free/total
—Serum BUN, creatinine, FBS
—UA, glucose dipstick

- Ejaculatory dysfunction

—Postejaculatory UA

- UTI

—UA, C/S
—Serum BUN/creatinine
—FBS

- Polyuria

—Urine specific gravity: Dilute urine has a specific gravity of less than 1.007.
—FBS
—Urine glucose dipstick

IMAGING

- Voiding dysfunction

—Renal ultrasound is preferred over IVP. If IVP is done, check serum creatinine first.

- UTI

—Emphysematous pyelonephritis: See Section II, "Pyelonephritis—Emphysematous."

- Erectile dysfunction

—Penile duplex Doppler: Assess cavernosal arteries and response to ICRx.

SPECIAL STUDIES

- Voiding dysfunction: scan PVR (acceptable if less than 150 cc), voiding diary (polyuria associated with >2.5 L urine produced per day; quantify voided volume and fluid intake), uroflow (maximum uroflow may be altered by elevated PVR), CMG (evaluate sensation and bladder compliance)

 Treatment

GENERAL MEASURES

- Optimize serum blood glucose level, may require urgent measures

MEDICAL

- Erectile dysfunction

—Oral: yohimbine, sildenafil citrate (contraindicated with organic nitrates usage)
—ICRx: Prostaglandin E_1–Papaverine–Regitine mixture
—Intraurethral: MUSE
—Vacuum ErecAid device (VED)

- Ejaculatory failure

—Alpha-adrenergic therapy (beware with HTN, CAD)

- Voiding dysfunction

—Alpha blockade (Hytrin, Cardura, Flomax); check for secondary hypotension.
—Timed voiding
—Clean intermittent catheterization if residual urine markedly elevated

- UTI

—Antibiotics
—Fluid resuscitation
—If retention present, catheter drainage

SURGICAL

- ED: re-arterialization, venous ligation, penile prosthesis
- VD if able to document BOO; perform outlet procedure (TURP, TUIP, TUMT, etc.); then reestablish baseline.
- UTI

—If associated with obstruction, must unobstruct
—If emphysematous pyelonephritis: surgical emergency; must usually pursue nephrectomy

ALTERNATIVE THERAPIES: N/A

PATIENT EDUCATION

- Instruct on the urologic aspects of diabetes and stress control of hyperglycemia.

 Follow-Up

MONITORING

- ED: ICRx: serial phallus examination, liver function analysis
- VD: periodic renal ultrasound to rule out hydronephrosis, biannual physical examination, PVR, serum creatinine determination
- UTI: periodic UA, PVR, renal ultrasound

PREVENTION

- ED: tight diabetic control, active exercise, weight control, no smoking
- VD: timed voidings, Finasteride (may reduce serum PSA by 50%), alpha blockade
- UTI: timed voiding, optimal hydration, antimicrobial prophylaxis

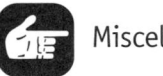 Miscellaneous

SYNONYMS: N/A

ASSOCIATED CONDITIONS: N/A

NOTES

- Diabetics are also prone to candidal infections of the external genitalia (see Section II topics).

ABBREVIATIONS

- Abx, antibiotic; AN, autonomic neuropathy; BCR, bulbocavernous reflex; BOO, bladder outlet obstruction; CAD, coronary artery disease; CMG, cystometrogram; DM, diabetes mellitus; ED, erectile dysfunction; FBS, fasting blood sugar; HNP, herniated nucleus pulposus; HTN, hypertension; HZ, herpes zoster; ICRx, intercavernosal therapy; IDDM, insulin-dependent diabetes mellitus; NIDDM, non–insulin-dependent diabetes mellitus; PVR, post-void residual; RPG, retrograde pyelogram; SUI, stress urinary incontinence; VD, voiding dysfunction; XGM, xanthogranulomatous pyelonephritis

REFERENCES

Dunsmuir WD, Holmes SAV. The etiology and management of erectile, ejaculatory, and fertility problems in men with diabetes mellitus. *Diabet Med* 1996;13:700–708.

Gillenwater JY, Grayhack JT, Howards SS, Duckett JW, eds. *Adult and Pediatric Urology*, 2nd ed. St Louis: Mosby, 1991.

Hackett GI. The treatment of patients with diabetes. *Int J STD AIDS* 1996;10[Suppl 3]:24–26.

Kaplan SA, et al. Urodynamic findings in patients with diabetic cystopathy. *J Urol* 1995;153:342–344.

Author: Steven P. Petrou

Endometriosis—Genitourinary

 Basics

DESCRIPTION

- Endometriosis externa is a condition in which endometrial tissue is found outside the uterus.

EPIDEMIOLOGY

- Occurs in 10% to 20% of premenopausal women
- Peak incidence age: 25 to 40 years
- No racial predilection

GENETICS

- A genetic predisposition is suggested but remains unproved.

STAGING

- Endometriosis is staged by intraoperative assessment. The pelvis is assessed using a point system that grades size, site, and scar sequelae of endometriosis. (*Fertil Steril* 1985;143:351).

—Stage I (minimal): 1 to 5 points
—Stage II (mild): 6 to 15 points
—Stage III (moderate): 16 to 40 points
—Stage IV (severe): >40 points

SIGNS AND SYMPTOMS

- Extremely variable
- May be totally asymptomatic
- May also present with dysmenorrhea and pelvic pain, infertility
- Urinary symptoms may include hematuria, dysuria, and frequency exacerbated at the time of menstruation
- The classic symptom of "cyclic hematuria," however, is uncommon.
- Ureteral involvement may cause flank pain, but silent obstruction may occur.

PATHOPHYSIOLOGY

- *Endometriosis externa* refers to any endometrial tissue outside the uterus.
- Three theories regarding the pathophysiology of endometriosis externa:

—Reflux menstruation with peritoneal implantation of endometrial tissue
—Metaplasia of peritoneal epithelium
—Hematogenous spread of endometrial tissue

- Ureteral obstruction due to endometriosis may be either intrinsic or extrinsic. Intrinsic lesions of the mucosa are due to direct invasion or embolization. Extrinsic lesions are due to external compression or scarring and fibrosis.
- The most common site of endometrial involvement of the urinary tract is the bladder. Endometriosis can present as a visible lesion in the bladder lumen or it can implant on the serosal surface of the bladder.
- Urethral and renal endometriosis are rare but have been reported.

CAUSES/RISK FACTORS

- The majority of cases of endometriosis occurs in menstruating females.
- Rare cases of endometriosis have been reported in postmenopausal women receiving estrogen therapy, and several cases of endometriosis of the bladder have been reported in male patients treated with oral estrogens for prostate cancer.

COMPLICATIONS

- Some cases of endometriosis of the urinary tract may cause silent ureteral obstruction. Loss of kidney function has been reported with untreated ureteral endometriosis.

DIFFERENTIAL DIAGNOSIS

- Endometriosis of the bladder

—Urinary tract infections
—Bladder cancer
—Radiation cystitis
—Bladder stone

- Endometriosis of the ureter

—Radiolucent stone
—Transitional cell carcinoma of the ureter
—Primary retroperitoneal malignancy
—Metastatic retroperitoneal malignancy
—Idiopathic retroperitoneal fibrosis

 Database

HISTORY

- Most commonly a young adult woman with a history of frequency and urgency with or without gross microhematuria.
- The urinary symptoms may or may not be exacerbated with menstruation.
- Non-urologic symptoms may include dysmenorrhea and pelvic pain. There may be infertility.

PHYSICAL EXAMINATION

- Pelvic examination: The ovaries may feel small, firm, indurated, or irregular. Tender nodularities may be palpable in the cul-de-sac or on the ureteral sacral ligaments.

Diagnostic Studies

LABORATORY TESTING

- Urinalysis
- Serum creatinine

IMAGING

- Renal ultrasound or IVP

Special Testing

- Laparoscopy

—The most common maneuver to provide a tissue diagnosis; gynecologic inspection of the pelvis under direct vision and to biopsy any areas suspicious for endometriosis

—A classic sign is the "chocolate cyst," which is an ovary filled with old blood.

 Treatment

GENERAL MEASURES

- The cornerstone of medical treatment is hormonal therapy of various forms.
- These may include suppression of ovulation with cyclic oral contraceptives, or induction of "pseudopregnancy" by continuous higher dose oral contraceptive administration.
- Danazol, a testosterone analogue, is also used to treat endometriosis, as are gonadotropin-releasing hormone agonists (e.g., Lupron).

MEDICAL: N/A

SURGICAL

- When medical treatment has not eliminated endometrial involvement of the ureter or bladder, surgery is often necessary.
- Bladder endometriosis can be successfully treated with a partial cystectomy; before a partial cystectomy is performed, a tissue diagnosis must be obtained.
- Ureteral involvement by endometriosis most commonly involves the distal 3 cm of the ureter and is most often, but not always, unilateral.

—Ureterolysis can be successful in mild cases, but usually a ureteral reimplant is required. Depending on the extent of the ureteral involvement, a psoas hitch or Boari flap may be necessary to complete a successful reimplant.

ALTERNATIVE THERAPIES

- With mild ureteral obstruction, a case can be made for placement of a ureteral stent while awaiting the outcome of hormonal therapy.

PATIENT EDUCATION: N/A

 Follow-Up

MONITORING

- A patient who has had ureteral involvement with endometriosis, regardless of the treatment chosen, should have serum creatinine levels and renal ultrasounds to monitor the status of the upper tracts.

PREVENTION

- None known

 Miscellaneous

SYNONYMS: N/A

ASSOCIATED CONDITIONS

- Infertility (female)

NOTES: N/A

ABBREVIATIONS: N/A

REFERENCES

Foster RS, Rink RC, Mulcahy JJ. Vesical endometriosis: Medical or surgical treatment. *Urology* 1987; 29(1):64.

Plous RH, Sunshine R, Goldman H, Schwartz IS. Ureteral endometriosis in post menopausal women. *Urology* 1985;26(4):408.

Ray J, Conger M, Ireland K. Ureteral obstruction in postmenopausal women with endometriosis. *Urology* 1985;26(6):577.

Author: Kevin R. Loughlin

Epididymis—Tumors and Cysts

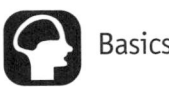 Basics

DESCRIPTION

- Dilatations of a ductus efferent may result in a common cystic lesion, called a spermatocele.
- Benign tumors of the epididymidis, predominantly adenomatoid tumors, are infrequently seen.
- Malignant tumors of the epididymidis are extremely rare.

EPIDEMIOLOGY

- Benign cystic lesions

—Spermatoceles: common; identified incidentally in up to 30% of men undergoing scrotal ultrasonography; usually small and may be multiple. Incidence increases with increasing age.
—Cysts, sperm granulomata

- Benign tumors: uncommon; adenomatoid tumors, leiomyoma, papillary cystadenoma, vascular lesions, cystic embryomas, fibromas, cholesteatomas, keratomas, lipomas, hamartomas, dermoid cysts, adrenal cortical adenomas

—Adenomatoid tumor: most common adnexal tumor of the scrotum; usually occur in men between 20 and 30 years of age.
—Pediatric population: Consider benign melanotic neuroectodermal tumor of infancy, as well as epididymal cystadenoma.
—Papillary cystadenoma: only known benign epididymal tumor of epithelial origin; when bilateral, suspect von Hippel-Lindau (VHL) disease.

- Malignant: rare; may be primary or metastatic

—Primary: adenocarcinoma, rhabdomyosarcoma, leiomyosarcoma, fibrosarcoma, liposarcoma
—Metastatic: GI tract, kidney, prostate

GENETICS: N/A

STAGING: N/A

SIGNS AND SYMPTOMS

- Most often present as a painless mass in the scrotum

PATHOPHYSIOLOGY

- The epididymis, which lies directly behind the testicle within the scrotum, is composed of a long, convoluted tubule measuring 3 to 4 m in length. Sperm enters this tubule at the head, or caput, via 8 to 12 ductuli efferentes extending from the rete testis. They move through the body or corpus to the cauda or tail, maturing along the way and exiting into the vas deferens.
- Benign

—Spermatocele
 —Appears to be continuous with the rete testis, either dilatations of efferent ducts or Haller's superior aberrant duct (vas aberrans of the rete testis)
 —Usually does not obstruct the epididymal tubule
 —Fluid often contains viable sperm

—Adenomatoid tumor: whitish, yellowish, or tan with a fibrous stroma that is often hyalinized. Smooth muscle is often present. Found in the epididymis more often than in the tunica or spermatic cord
—Papillary cystadenoma: cystic and pseudoencapsulated. Ducts may be dilated or microcystic. Glands are lined by glycogen-rich vacuolated or clear cells, which resemble renal cell carcinoma.

- Malignant: often larger and more irregular than benign masses

—Epididymal adenocarcinoma: usually tubular, tubulocystic, or tubulopapillary adenocarcinomas, often with an appreciable content of clear cells, which can usually be readily separated from other paratesticular malignant tumors, such as malignant mesothelioma and carcinomas of the mullerian type. Distinction from metastasis may be difficult and may depend largely on careful clinical evaluation.
—Rhabdomyosarcoma: spectrum from well to poorly differentiated areas within the same tumor
—Metastasis from GI, kidney, melanoma, and prostate

CAUSES/RISK FACTORS

- Von Hipple-Lindau syndrome

COMPLICATIONS

- Benign lesions: none
- Malignant: often aggressive (e.g., adenocarcinoma), requiring wide locoregional excision, adjuvant radiation, or chemotherapy; high mortality

DIFFERENTIAL DIAGNOSIS

- Essential to exclude intratesticular mass, which is likely to be a germ cell tumor
- See Section I, "Scrotum—Mass and/or Pain (Acute Scrotum)" and "Testicular Mass—Adult."
- Revised World Health Organization Classification of Tumors

—Tumors of collecting ducts, rete, epididymis, spermatic cord, capsule, supporting structures, and appendices
 —Adenomatoid tumor
 —Mesothelioma
 —Adenoma of epididymis
 —Carcinoma of epididymis
 —Adenoma of rete or collecting ducts or both
 —Carcinoma of rete or collecting ducts or both
 —Melanotic neuroectodermal tumor
 —Tumors of ovarian epithelial types
 —Soft-tissue tumors
—Unclassified tumors
—Tumor-like lesions
 —Epidermal (epidermoid cyst)
 —Nonspecific orchitis or epididymo-orchitis
 —Nonspecific orchitis
 —Nonspecific granulomatous orchitis
 —Specific orchitis
 —Malakoplakia
 —Fibromatous periorchitis
 —Sperm granuloma, lipogranuloma
 —Adrenal rests
 —Others

 Database

HISTORY

- Previous vasectomy associated with epididymal obstruction, inflammatory mass or cyst, sperm granuloma
- A family history of VHL disease suggests papillary cystadenoma.

—Tumors are bilateral in these patients.

PHYSICAL EXAMINATION

- Differentiation between hydrocele and spermatocele

—Hydrocele: variable sized mass anterior to and/or enveloping the testis
—A large hydrocele will make it difficult to palpate and examine the ipsilateral testis.
—Approximately 10% of benign lesions and a larger number of malignant tumors may be masked by hydroceles. May need to perform scrotal ultrasound to image the testis adequately
—Spermatocele: asymptomatic cystic mass of the epididymis, usually arising from the caput
 —Transillumination distinguishes them from a solid mass.
 —Can still palpate the testis, though it may be displaced by the spermatocele

- Benign and malignant tumors often present as a painless mass.

—Adenomatoid tumors are the most common benign tumors of the epididymis. Small and solid, they may be found anywhere on the epididymis.

Diagnostic Studies

LABORATORY TESTING

• Urinalysis should be performed to assure no evidence of infection.
• No other routine lab testing is usually necessary unless other testicular pathology is suspected.

IMAGING

• Scrotal ultrasonography

—Distinguish between intra- and extratesticular lesions, which determine the differential diagnosis.
—Distinguish between solid and cystic lesions.
—Tumors that may be obscured by a hydrocele can be identified.
—Cystadenomas in VHL patients
  —54% of male patients with VHL demonstrate either unilateral or bilateral solid abnormality in the head of the epididymis, suggestive of cystadenoma.
  —Sonographic appearances range from a solid mass with multiple tiny cysts to an almost completely solid mass.
  —Dilated efferent ductules may also be seen within the testicle, a result of chronic obstruction.

SPECIAL STUDIES: N/A

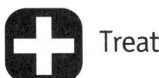 Treatment

GENERAL MEASURES

• Solid lesions less than 2.5 cm are more likely to be benign, while larger, irregular lesions are more suspicious for malignancy.

MEDICAL

• Antiinflammatory agents for occasional discomfort

SURGICAL

• Benign lesions can be observed unless the patient has significant discomfort.

—Transscrotal excision is the preferred route.

• Malignant or unknown diagnosis: inguinal exploration with orchiectomy high ligation of the cord.
• Rhabdomyosarcoma: adjuvant treatment: cobalt-60 teletherapy; chemotherapy with cyclophosphamide, vincristine, and dactinomycin

ALTERNATIVE THERAPIES

• Spermatocele

—Sclerotherapy is another nonsurgical option, but it has a higher failure rate.
—Spermatocele fluid often contains sperm that may be aspirated and utilized for in vitro fertilization methods in couples with infertility due to obstructive azoospermia.

PATIENT EDUCATION

• Stress the need for conservative management, unless malignancy or debilitating symptoms are present.
• Inform about no known impact on fertility.
• VHL patients may need genetic counseling.

 Follow-Up

MONITORING

• Benign: none needed, except for patients with cystadenoma and VHL syndrome

PREVENTION: N/A

 Miscellaneous

SYNONYMS: N/A

ASSOCIATED CONDITIONS

• Von Hippel-Lindau syndrome

NOTES

• See also Section I, "Scrotum—Mass and/or Pain (Acute Scrotum)," and Section II, "Von Hipple-Lindau Disease/Syndrome."

ABBREVIATIONS: N/A

REFERENCES

Goldstein M. Surgical management of male infertility and scrotal disorders. In: Walsh PC, Retik AB, Vaughan ED, Wein AJ, eds. *Campbell's Urology*, 7th ed. Philadelphia: WB Saunders, 1998.

Ritchie JP. Neoplasms of the testis. In: Walsh PC, Retik AB, Vaughan ED, Wein AJ, eds. *Campbell's Urology*, 7th ed. Philadelphia: WB Saunders, 1998.

Rowland RG, et al. Scrotum and testis. In: Gillenwater JY, Grayhack JT, Howards SS, Duckett JW, eds. *Adult and Pediatric Urology*, 3rd ed. St Louis: Mosby, 1996.

Authors: Kevin M. Slawin and Howard L. Adler

Epididymitis/Orchitis

 Basics

DESCRIPTION

- Clinical syndrome characterized by inflammation of the epididymis and/or testicles. Orchitis rarely exists in the absence of epididymitis.

EPIDEMIOLOGY

- Approximately 600,000 cases per year
- Highest prevalence: 19 to 35 years old
- 20% of military urologic admissions

GENETICS: N/A

STAGING: N/A

SIGNS AND SYMPTOMS

- Painful swelling in the scrotum
- Pain is usually severe and develops rapidly over 24 to 48 hours.
- Maximal tenderness is localized to the epididymis early in the disease process.
- The epididymis and testicle later may become one large inflammatory mass.
- Often associated with dysuria or irritative voiding symptoms
- May have a urethral discharge if urethritis present
- Prehn's sign: alleviation of pain with scrotal elevation
- A reactive hydrocele may be present.
- The patient may have a fever or elevated white blood cell count.

PATHOPHYSIOLOGY

- Epididymitis caused by spread of infections from the bladder or urethra

—Children: *E. coli* bacteriuria
—Heterosexual men less than 35 years old: *Neisseria gonorrhoeae* and *Chlamydia trachomatis* urethritis
—Homosexual men: *E. coli*
—Less common organisms: *Ureaplasma urealyticum, Staphylococcus* species, *Brucella, Blastomyces dermatitidis, Mycobacterium tuberculosis,* and *Coccidioides immitis*

- Tuberculous epididymitis

—Most common manifestation of genital tuberculosis
—Characteristic swelling of testis/epididymis, with "beadlike" irregularity of the vas deferens on occasion

- Bacterial orchitis

—Orchitis usually results from extension of infection or inflammation from neighboring epididymis.
—Rare as an isolated disease without associated epididymitis

- Mumps orchitis

—Rare today due to immunization for mumps
—Postpubertal boys (rare before 10 years of age)
—Usually begins 4 to 6 days after the onset of parotitis
—Occurs in 30% of patients with mumps
—One-third of boys with orchitis develop atrophy.
—Possible increased risk of infertility

CAUSES/RISK FACTORS

- Congenital anomalies of genitourinary tract
- Acquired lesions, such as a urethral stricture or enlarged prostate
- Three times greater risk in uncircumcised males
- Indwelling urethral catheters
- Recent urinary tract instrumentation
- Acute and chronic prostatitis
- Sexual abuse must be considered in children with epididymitis secondary to urethritis.

COMPLICATIONS

- Scrotal abscess
- Testicular infarction
- Cutaneous scrotal fistula
- Infertility
- Chronic epididymitis

DIFFERENTIAL DIAGNOSIS

- Testicular torsion
- Testicular tumors
- Torsion of appendix testes
- Scrotal hernias or hydroceles
- Trauma
- Henoch-Schönlein purpura
- Idiopathic scrotal edema

 Database

HISTORY

- Age of patient

—Epididymitis most common in adults (19–35 years old)

- Onset of symptoms

—Usually gradual onset over several days

- Fevers

—Occur in 14% to 28% of cases

- Complaints of dysuria or urethral discharge

—Seen with associated UTI or urethritis

- History of underlying urinary tract abnormality

—Epididymitis very uncommon in children without underlying abnormality

- Recent UTI or urologic instrumentation

—Increased risk in all age groups

PHYSICAL EXAMINATION

- Severe pain and swelling in epididymis and testicle upon palpation

—Inflammation often begins in the tail of the epididymis and may spread to the entire epididymis and testicle.

- Epididymis/testicle found in normal anatomic position
- Erythema in overlying scrotal skin is possible.
- Hydrocele

—A reactive hydrocele may occur from underlying inflammation.

- Urethral discharge

—Seen in men with associated urethritis

Diagnostic Studies

LABORATORY TESTING

- Gram stain of urethral smear for urethritis

—Intracellular gram-negative diplococci pathognomonic for *N. gonorrhoeae*
—White blood cells without bacteria are indicative of nongonococcal urethritis (two-thirds due to *C. trachomatis*)

- Gram stain and culture of midstream urine

—24% have pyuria.

IMAGING

- Nuclear medicine scan

—Study of choice to evaluate pediatric acute scrotal pain
—Sensitivity and specificity to detect torsion as high as 100% and 97%, respectively
—Increased perfusion of affected testicle and hemiscrotum on radionucleotide angiogram
—Disadvantages: Technology may not be available at all times.

- Color-flow Doppler ultrasound

—Sensitivity of 86% to 100% and specificity of approximately 100% in diagnosing torsion
—The affected testicle and epididymis appear hypoechoic.
—Increased flow is seen on the affected side due to inflammation.
—May identify associated complications such as scrotal abscesses
—Disadvantages: limited expertise and availability; efficacy not defined in younger age groups

SPECIAL STUDIES: N/A

 ## Treatment

GENERAL MEASURES

- Antibiotic therapy
- Bed rest
- Analgesics and/or antiinflammatory agents
- Scrotal elevation

MEDICAL

- *Always* treat the sexual partner if suspected secondary to sexual activity
- Gonococcal urethritis is associated with *C. trachomatis* in 30% to 50% of cases. Thus, treatment is indicated for both organisms when epididymitis is secondary to urethritis.
- Gonococcal urethritis

—Recommended regimen: ceftriaxone 125 to 250 mg IM once
—Alternative regimens: cefixime 400 mg orally once; cefotaxime 1g IM once; ciprofloxacin 500 mg orally once; ofloxacin 400 mg orally once; spectinomycin 2 mg IM once

- Nongonococcal urethritis

—Recommended regimens: doxycycline 100 mg orally twice a day for 7 days, or azithromycin 1 g orally once
—Alternative regimens: ofloxacin 300 mg orally twice a day for 7 days; erythromycin base 500 mg orally twice a day for 7 days; erythromycin ethylsuccinate 800 mg orally twice a day for 7 days

- Epididymitis secondary to bacteriuria should be treated with a 10- to 14-day course of a broad-spectrum antibiotic.
- Hospitalization and IV antibiotics for systemic manifestations of illness

SURGICAL

- May be necessary for treatment of an abscess or fistula

ALTERNATIVE THERAPIES

- Epididymectomy as a last resort for chronic epididymitis resistant to medical management

PATIENT EDUCATION

- Evaluation and treatment of sexual partners is mandatory in patients with epididymo-orchitis secondary to an STD.
- National STD Hotline: (800)227-8922

 ## Follow-Up

MONITORING

- Follow-up examinations are mandatory to monitor treatment and rule out *neoplasm.*
- Repeat cultures to document response to treatment

PREVENTION

- Sexual abstinence
- Condoms to reduce the risk of STDs

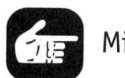 ## Miscellaneous

SYNONYMS: N/A

ASSOCIATED CONDITIONS

- See "Complications."

NOTES

- See Section I, "Urinary Tract Infection—Adult Male" and "Testicular Mass—Adult."

ABBREVIATIONS

- STD, sexually transmitted disease; UTI, urinary tract infection

REFERENCES

Barloon TJ, Weissman AM. Diagnostic imaging of patients with acute scrotal pain. *Am Fam Physician* 1996;53(5):1734.

Berger RE. Sexually transmitted diseases: The classic diseases. In: Walsh PC, Retik AB, Vaughan ED, Wein AJ, eds. *Campbell's Urology,* 7th ed. Philadelphia: WB Saunders, 1998:670–672.

Gilby RL. Infections of the urinary tract and male genitalia. In: Brillman JC, Quenzer RW, eds. *Infectious Disease in Emergency Medicine,* 2nd ed. Philadelphia: Lippincott-Raven, 1997:621–623.

Krieger JN. Prostatitis, epididymitis, and orchitis. In: Mandell GC, Dolin R, Bennett JE, eds. *Principles and Practice of Infectious Disease,* 4th ed. New York: Churchill Livingston, 1995:1098–1102.

Schul MW, Keating MA. The acute pediatric scrotum. *J Emerg Med* 1993;11:565.

Authors: Kenneth Ogan and Michael J. Manyak

Epispadias

 Basics

DESCRIPTION

- Developmental abnormality wherein the urethra opens on the dorsum of the penis. Often part of the exstrophy–epispadias complex, it can occur in the absence of exstrophy.

EPIDEMIOLOGY

- 1 in 117,000 newborn boys
- 1 in 484,000 newborn girls
- Male-to-female ratio: 5:1

GENETICS

- Rarity makes genetics difficult to obtain.

STAGING: N/A

SIGNS AND SYMPTOMS

- Usually low-set umbilicus
- Males

—Urethra opens anywhere from under pubic bone to tip of penis
   —Known as complete or penopubic epispadias, which is most common

- Females

—Urethra opens from bladder neck to tip of urethra
—Most severe and common type
—Labia may obscure the epispadias in females.

PATHOPHYSIOLOGY

- Embryologically, the cloacal membrane develops abnormally. Migration of mesenchyme from the lateral margins of the cloacal membrane medially is inhibited. The cloacal membrane fails to migrate caudally and so prevents the pubis from approximating. In extreme forms, exstrophy results.
- Wide pubic diastasis: usually not as wide as in bladder exstrophy
- Absence of urinary sphincters in complete type (penopubic) in males and type III in females
- Short, widened penis with dorsal chordee
- Urethra most commonly at base of penis under pubis; opening can be on shaft or also on glans
- Bifid clitoris, separated and rudimentary labia minora
- Vesicoureteral reflux: 30% to 75%

CAUSES/RISK FACTORS

- Unknown

COMPLICATIONS

- Urinary incontinence
- Upper tract damage
- Infertility

DIFFERENTIAL DIAGNOSIS

- Classic bladder exstrophy
- Lesser degrees of epispadias

 Database

HISTORY

- Family history of epispadias–exstrophy complex

PHYSICAL EXAMINATION

- Position of testis
- Pubic diastasis
- Presence of any degree of bladder prolapse or exstrophy

 Diagnostic Studies

LABORATORY TESTING

- CBC, serum electrolytes

IMAGING

- Plain x-ray of pelvis to determine pubic diastasis
- Renal ultrasound to assess presence of two kidneys and presence/absence of hydronephrosis

SPECIAL STUDIES: N/A

Epispadias

 Treatment

GENERAL MEASURES

- Careful, overall examination of infant

MEDICAL: N/A

SURGICAL

- Objectives

—Achievement of urinary continence
—Preservation of upper urinary tract
—Reconstruction of functional and cosmetically acceptable external genitalia

- Male

—Modified Cantwell-Ransley epispadias repair at 6 to 12 months of age after testosterone stimulation (3 mg/kg IM 2 weeks before surgery)
—Jeffs-Gearhart modification of Young-Dees-Leadbetter bladder neck repair at 4 to 5 years of age when bladder capacity is adequate and child is ready maturationally and motivationally to be continent and participate in postoperative voiding program

- Female

—Repair of urethra and genital reconstruction at around 12 months of age
—Bladder neck repair: same as male

ALTERNATIVE THERAPIES

- Males

—Combined repair of urethra and bladder neck reconstruction at the same time

- Females

—Same as above

PATIENT EDUCATION: N/A

 Follow-Up

MONITORING

- Follow-up after epispadias repair

—Urethral stent removed 10 to 12 days after surgery
—Renal and bladder ultrasound at 4 months after surgery
—Yearly cystoscopies and bladder capacity measurements under anesthesia until bladder capacity adequate for bladder neck repair
—Yearly ultrasound
—Urine cultures at three monthly intervals

- Follow-up after bladder neck repair

—Clamp the suprapubic tube at 3 weeks after surgery and begin the voiding trial.
—Cystoscopy and placement of small (8Fr) urethral catheter if child cannot void
—Removal of suprapubic tube when residuals are less than 15 cc and child is voiding well
—Urine culture before suprapubic tube is removed
—Renal and bladder ultrasound prior to removal of suprapubic tube and again at 3 months and 12 months after surgery
—Urinary prophylaxis until follow-up shows non-reflux and child is voiding well

PREVENTION: N/A

 Miscellaneous

SYNONYMS

- Subsymphyseal epispadias, complete epispadias, penopubic epispadias

ASSOCIATED CONDITIONS

- Exstrophy, bladder

NOTES

- See also Section II, "Exstrophy—Bladder."

ABBREVIATIONS: N/A

REFERENCES

Gearhart JP, Jeffs RD. Exstrophy–epispadias complex and bladder anomalies. In: Walsh PC, Retik AB, Vaughan ED, Wein AJ, eds. *Campbell's Urology,* 7th ed. Philadelphia: WB Saunders, 1997: 1939.

Gearhart JP, et al. The Cantwell Ransley epispadias repair: Lessons learned. *Urology* 1995;46(1): 92.

Gearhart JP, Jeffs RD. Bladder exstrophy: Increase in capacity following epispadias repair. *J Urol* 1989;142:525.

Author: John P. Gearhart

Exstrophy—Bladder (Classic)

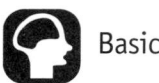 Basics

 Database

 Diagnostic Studies

DESCRIPTION

• The lower central abdomen is occupied by the posterior wall of the inner surface of the bladder.

EPIDEMIOLOGY

• 1 in 30,000 newborn infants
• Male-to-female ratio: 3:1

GENETICS

• Usually younger mother's first baby
• Multifactorial inheritance
• Risk of recurrence: 1 in 275
• Risk in offspring: 1 in 70 live births

STAGING: N/A

SIGNS AND SYMPTOMS

• Low-set umbilicus
• Bladder open from dome to tip of penile urethra (male)
• Bladder open from dome to tip of urethra (female)

PATHOPHYSIOLOGY

• Embryologically, there is a complete ventral defect of the urogenital sinus and overlying skeletal muscle.

—The typical migration of mesenchyme from the lateral margins of the cloacal membrane medially is inhibited. The cloacal membrane fails to migrate caudally and also prevents the pubis from approximating.

• Wide pubic diastasis
• 30% shortage of pubic bone
• External rotation of both anterior and posterior pelvis
• Absence of urinary sphincters
• High incidence of inguinal hernias in males
• Short, widened penis with dorsal chordee (exstrophy–epispadias complex)
• Bifid clitoris, separated labia, anterior vaginal opening
• Anterior anal opening
• Vesicoureteral reflux: nearly 100%

CAUSES/RISK FACTORS

• Unknown

COMPLICATIONS

• Urinary incontinence
• Upper tract damage
• Infertility
• Increased risk of uterine prolapse
• Increased risk of bladder cancer long term

DIFFERENTIAL DIAGNOSIS

• Superior vesical fissure
• Omphalocele
• Gastroschisis
• Cloacal exstrophy

HISTORY

• Family history of abdominal wall anomalies

PHYSICAL EXAMINATION

• Position of testes
• Size of bladder template
• Presence of omphalocele
• Position of anus
• Pubic diastasis
• Malleability of pelvis

—Only done under anesthesia at time of surgery to help determine whether pelvis can be brought together without pelvic osteotomy

LABORATORY TESTING

• CBC, serum electrolytes

IMAGING

• Plain x-ray of pelvis to determine actual pubic diastasis
• Renal ultrasound

—Assess presence of two renal units
—Presence or absence of hydronephrosis

SPECIAL STUDIES: N/A

Treatment

GENERAL MEASURES

• Careful, overall examination of infant and bladder template to determine suitability of newborn closure

MEDICAL: N/A

SURGICAL

• Closure of bladder, posterior urethra, abdominal wall, and creation of neoumbilicus
• Concomitant bilateral pelvic osteotomy if wide pubic diastasis or closure performed after 48 to 72 hours of age
• Epispadias repair after testosterone stimulation (3 mg/kg IM 2 weeks before surgery) at 6 to 12 months of age
• Jeffs-Gearhart modification of Young-Dees-Leadbetter bladder neck repair at 4 to 5 years of age when bladder capacity is adequate and child is ready maturationally and motivationally to be continent and participate in postoperative voiding program

ALTERNATIVE THERAPIES

• Combined bladder exstrophy and epispadias repair without bladder neck repair either in the newborn period (Mitchell) or in later infancy (Gearhart)

PATIENT EDUCATION

• Patients must be extensively educated in the serious nature of the exstrophy condition, the short- and long-term consequences of therapy, and the long term outcomes in this condition.
• ABC (Association of Bladder Exstrophy Children) parent support group based in North Carolina
• Johns Hopkins Exstrophy Center web page: www.med.jhu.edu/pediurol/web2.htm

 Follow-Up

MONITORING

• Follow-up after primary closure

—After initial bladder exstrophy closure, the ureteral stents are removed at 2 to 3 weeks after surgery
—The suprapubic tube is clamped after 4 weeks, and residuals are checked to ensure adequate outlet drainage.
—Urine culture prior to removal of suprapubic tube
—Renal ultrasound just prior to removal of suprapubic tube
—Renal and bladder ultrasound at 3 to 4 months after surgery to ensure absence of hydronephrosis and lack of residual urine; repeat at 6 months and 1 year after surgery.
—Urine cultures at three monthly intervals for first year of life
—Urinary prophylaxis with antibiotics on daily basis

• Follow-up after epispadias repair

—Yearly cystoscopies and bladder capacity measurements under anesthesia until bladder capacity is adequate for bladder neck repair
—Yearly ultrasounds
—Urine cultures at three monthly intervals

• Follow-up after bladder neck repair

—Clamp the suprapubic tube 3 weeks after surgery and begin a voiding trial.
—Cystoscopy and placement of a small (8Fr) urethral catheter if child cannot void
—Removal of suprapubic tube when residuals are less than 15 to 20 cc and child is voiding well
—Urine culture before suprapubic tube removal
—Renal and bladder ultrasound prior to removal of suprapubic tube and again at 3 months and 12 months after surgery
—Urinary prophylaxis until follow-up shows no reflux and child is voiding well

PREVENTION: N/A

 Miscellaneous

SYNONYMS

• Ectopic vesicae

ASSOCIATED CONDITIONS

• Normal fertility in females, increased risk of uterine prolapse, and impaired fertility in males (will likely require assisted reproductive techniques)

NOTES

• See also Section II, "Exstrophy—Cloacal" and "Epispadias."

ABBREVIATIONS: N/A

REFERENCES

Ben-Chaim J, et al. The outcome of adult exstrophy patients. *J Urol* 1996;155:1251.

Gearhart JP, Jeffs RD. Exstrophy–epispadias complex and bladder anomalies. In: Walsh PC, Retik AB, Vaughan ED, Wein AJ, eds. *Campbell's Urology*, 7th ed. Philadelphia: WB Saunders, 1997: 1939.

Gearhart JP, et al. Combined vertical and horizontal pelvic osteotomy approach for the initial and secondary repair of bladder exstrophy. *J Urol* 1996;155:689.

Author: John P. Gearhart

Exstrophy—Cloacal

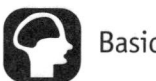 Basics

DESCRIPTION
- Most severe form of exstrophy wherein both the anterior bladder and anterior rectal wall fail to develop

EPIDEMIOLOGY
- Incidence: 0.5 per population 400,000
- Male-to-female ratio: 2:1

GENETICS
- Unknown inheritance, no recorded cases of fertility

STAGING: N/A

SIGNS AND SYMPTOMS
- Exstrophy of foreshortened hindgut or cecum, prolapsed ilium, blind-ending tailgut
- Single or paired appendix on exstrophied cecum
- Exstrophy of two hemi-bladders either side of hindgut hemi
- Ureteric orifices on each exstrophied hemi-bladder
- Small, divided penis (small corporal bodies) or bifid clitoris
- Undescended testis
- Omphalocele (85%)

PATHOPHYSIOLOGY
- Embryology: persistence or overgrowth of the cloacal membrane on the lower anterior abdominal area; prevents normal mesenchymal ingrowth

—This causes divergence of the lower abdominal muscular structures and forces the genital ridges to fuse caudal to the cloacal membrane.
—The stage of ingrowth of the urorectal septum at the time of rupture determines whether one will produce an exstrophic urinary tract alone (classic bladder exstrophy or epispadias) or cloacal exstrophy with the hindgut interposed between the hemi-bladders.

- Skeletal and central nervous system anomalies

—Pelvic abnormalities and asymmetry
  —Extremely wide pubic diastasis
  —External rotation of posterior pelvis (45-degree iliac wing)
  —37% shortage and external rotation of anterior pelvic segment
  —Sacroiliac malformations
—Hip external rotation, abduction, and sometimes malformations
—Vertebral anomalies (in up to 80%)
—Spina bifida (29%–86%)
  —Meningocele
  —Meningomyelocele
  —Lipomeningocele
—Congenital hip dislocation
—Lower limb abnormalities (12%–65%)
  —Clubfoot and other deformities
  —Agenesis

- Genital tract anomalies
—Partial or complete duplication of uterus (in up to 95%)
—Duplication of vagina (43%–65%) or vaginal agenesis (25%–43%)
- Upper urinary tract anomalies
—Pelvic kidney
—Renal agenesis
—Hydronephrosis/hydroureter
—Ureteric ectopia (to vas deferens, fallopian tubes, vagina, or uterus)
- Gastrointestinal anomalies
—Malrotation
—Duplication
—Duodenal atresia
—Meckel's diverticulum
—Short-gut syndrome/absorptive dysfunction (25%–50%)
- Cardiovascular and pulmonary anomalies rare

CAUSES/RISK FACTORS
- Unknown

COMPLICATIONS
- Urinary incontinence
- Vesicoureteric reflux (after bladder closure, in 100%)
- Fecal incontinence
- Upper urinary tract damage
- Infertility

—?Need for male gender reassignment, depending on phallic size and adequacy for reconstruction

DIFFERENTIAL DIAGNOSIS
- Omphalocele
- Gastroschisis
- Classic exstrophy
- Superior vesical fissure

 Database

HISTORY
- Family history of abdominal wall defects

PHYSICAL EXAMINATION
- Evaluate exstrophy–espadias complex

—Assessment of hindgut exstrophy
—Assessment of hemi-bladder templates
—Presence of omphalocele
—Pubic diastasis and malleability of pelvis
—Position of testes
—Formation of phallus
—Presence of imperforate anus

- Evaluate associated anomalies.

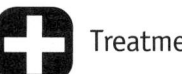 Diagnostic Studies

LABORATORY TESTING
- CBC, creatinine, electrolytes

IMAGING
- Prenatal ultrasound

—Cystic mass from infraumbilical anterior abdominal wall
—Splaying of pubic rami
—Meningomyelocele (in 50%)
—Rocker-bottom feet
- Neonatal

—Hematology and serum biochemistry assessment
—Plain abdominal radiograph, including bony pelvis
—Ultrasound examination of kidneys

SPECIAL STUDIES: N/A

✚ Treatment

GENERAL MEASURES
- Supportive care in collaboration with neonatologist

MEDICAL: N/A

SURGICAL
- Functional bladder closure ± gender reassignment in males
- One-stage repair (robust infant with few associated anomalies)

—Neonatal period
  —Bilateral pelvic osteotomy with external fixator
  —Omphalocele excision
  —Cecal plate and hemi-bladder separation
  —Bladder rejoining and closure
  —Gonadectomy in males with very diminutive or absent penis
  —Genital revision if required
  —Epispadias repair (for those few males to be raised as male)
  —Terminal ileostomy/colostomy

- Two-stage repair (frail or premature infant or multiple associated anomalies)

—Neonatal period
  —Omphalocele excision
  —Cecal plate and hemi-bladder separation
  —Bladder rejoining
  —Gonadectomy in males with duplicated or absent penis
  —Terminal ileostomy/colostomy

—At 4 to 6 months or later
  —Bilateral pelvic osteotomy
  —Bladder closure
  —Genital revision if required

- Antiincontinence/reflux procedure

—Orthotopic reconstruction for capable and motivated child

- Young-Dees-Leadbetter bladder neck reconstruction (only rarely applicable)
- Bilateral Cohen ureteral reimplantation
- Bladder augmentation (with bowel or stomach)

—Diversion

- Continent diversion with abdominal/perineal stoma for clean intermittent self-catheterization

- Vaginal reconstruction

—Vaginal construction or augmentation after puberty

- Restoration of bowel continuity (small, select minority of patients without spinal anomalies)

—Parenteral nutrition
—Correction of imperforate anus
—Pull-through procedure (anorectoplasty), depending on ability to achieve continence

ALTERNATIVE THERAPIES: N/A

PATIENT EDUCATION

- Prenatal counseling and planning for perinatal management
- Parent education in serious nature of cloacal exstrophy and associated anomalies, short- and long-term consequences of therapy, and long-term outcome
- Early pediatric psychiatric involvement for all patients and families, and especially long-term counseling of patients who undergo gender reassignment

 Follow-Up

MONITORING

- Follow-up after primary closure

—Ureteral stents are removed 2 to 3 weeks after initial bladder closure.
—The suprapubic tube is clamped at 4 weeks and residual is checked to ensure adequate outlet drainage.
—Urine culture prior to suprapubic tube removal
—Renal ultrasound just prior to removal of suprapubic tube
—Renal and bladder ultrasound at 3 to 4 months to ensure absence of hydronephrosis and lack of residual urine; repeated at 6 months and 1 year
—Urine culture at three monthly intervals for first year
—Urinary prophylaxis with antibiotics on daily basis
—Cystoscopy at 2 years of age to measure bladder capacity and yearly to check growth of bladder

- Follow-up after epispadias repair (rare)

—Annual cystoscopy and bladder capacity measurement, until adequate for bladder neck reconstruction
—Annual renal ultrasound
—Urine culture every 3 months

- Follow-up after bladder neck repair

—The suprapubic tube is clamped at 3 weeks and a trial voiding is begun.
—If child cannot void, cystoscopy and placement of small (8Fr) urethral catheter
—Urine culture prior to suprapubic tube removal
—Removal of suprapubic tube when residuals less than 15 to 20 cc and child is voiding well
—Renal and bladder ultrasound just prior to removal of suprapubic tube, at 3 and 12 months from surgery
—Urinary prophylaxis with antibiotics on daily basis until no reflux and child is voiding well

PREVENTION: N/A

 Miscellaneous

SYNONYMS

- Vesicointestinal fissure, extrophia splanchnia

ASSOCIATED CONDITIONS: N/A

NOTES

- See also Section II, "Exstrophy—Bladder."

ABBREVIATIONS: N/A

REFERENCES

Gearhart JP, Jeffs RD. Techniques to create urinary continence in cloacal exstrophy. *J Urol* 1991;146:616.

Gearhart JP, Jeffs RD. Exstrophy–epispadias complex and bladder anomalies. In: Walsh PC, Retik AB, Vaughan ED, Wein AJ, eds. *Campbell's Urology*, 7th ed. Philadelphia: WB Saunders, 1998: 1971.

Authors: Mark R. Feneley and John P. Gearhart

Fournier's Gangrene

 Basics

DESCRIPTION

- Fournier's gangrene is a rare, progressive, necrotizing fasciitis of the genitalia or perineum.

EPIDEMIOLOGY

- More common in older individuals but has been reported in all age groups
- Mean age: 54 years
- Male predominance

GENETICS: N/A

STAGING: N/A

SIGNS AND SYMPTOMS

- Prodromal period of genital discomfort or pruritus
- Progression to painful or edematous genitalia with cellulitic changes, eschar, necrosis, or crepitus

—May extend to abdominal wall, axilla, thighs, or buttocks
—Cutaneous findings may underestimate the extent of disease.
—Foul odor often present

- Fever, chills, nausea, vomiting, malaise, or mental status changes may reflect sepsis.
- A delay in diagnosis is common (mean: 5–7 days).

PATHOPHYSIOLOGY

- Aerobic and anaerobic organisms act synergistically to produce a progressive, obliterative endarteritis leading to vascular thrombosis and gangrene.
- Resultant ischemia allows further proliferation of pathogenic organisms.
- Microbiology
- Most common organisms are *E. coli*, *Bacteroides*, streptococci, and staphylococci

—*Clostridium*, *Pseudomonas*, *Proteus*, and *Klebsiella* are isolated less frequently.
—Streptococci and staphylococci predominate in the pediatric population.

CAUSES/RISK FACTORS

- Source identifiable in nearly all cases

—Genitourinary: extension of urinary tract infection with dissection along fascial planes to involve the penis and scrotum (i.e., urethral stricture with extravasation)
—Rectal: extension of infection in perianal area along fascial planes to the penis and scrotum (i.e., perianal abscess)
—Dermal: Trauma to skin provides access of organisms to subcutaneous tissues.

- In children, trauma, insect bites, circumcision, burns, perirectal disease, perineal skin infections, and systemic infection are potential etiologies.

- Risk factors

—Immunosuppressed conditions: diabetes, advanced age, malnutrition, alcoholism, intravenous drug use, cortisone therapy, malignancy, chemotherapy, radiation therapy, renal failure, hemodialysis, cirrhosis, vasculitis, and HIV infection
—Recent procedures or operations: herniorrhaphy, orchiectomy, hydrocelectomy, penile prosthesis, vasectomy, hemorrhoidectomy, circumcision, prostate biopsy, hypospadias repair, coital injury, colonoscopy

COMPLICATIONS

- Morbidity: 25% to 30%
- Frequent complications

—Acute renal failure
—ARDS
—Multiorgan system dysfunction
—Infertility
—Urethral stricture

DIFFERENTIAL DIAGNOSIS

- Balanitis
- Cellulitis
- Epididymitis
- Orchitis
- Hydrocele
- Testicular torsion
- Strangulated inguinal hernia
- Meleney's gangrene
- Hidradenitis suppurativa
- Pyoderma gangrenosum

 Database

HISTORY

- Urinary frequency, urgency, dysuria, cloudy urine, urethral discharge, decreased force of stream, or straining to void suggests a urinary source.
- Rectal pain or bleeding, a history of anal fissures, fistulas, or hemorrhoids suggest a rectal source.
- A history of acute and chronic infections of the scrotum (recurrent hidradenitis suppurativa, balanitis, genital skin drug injection) suggests a dermal source.
- Medical history

—Diabetes, alcoholism, malignancy, immunosuppression

- Surgical history

—A recent surgery or procedure is a risk factor.

PHYSICAL EXAMINATION

- Genitalia and perineum

—Assess for pain, inflammation, or crepitus.
—Note the presence and extent of erythema or eschar.
—Cutaneous findings may vary and often underestimate the degree of involvement.

- Abdomen

—Note abdominal pain or signs of abdominal wall involvement.

- Rectal examination

—Assess for perirectal abscess or anal sphincteric involvement.

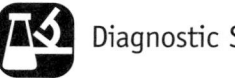 Diagnostic Studies

LABORATORY TESTING

- Complete blood profile: leukocytosis, anemia, or thrombocytopenia
- Serum electrolytes: hyponatremia, hyperkalemia, or hypokalemia
- Hyperglycemia common
- Renal function tests: Elevated BUN and creatinine are associated with worse outcome.
- Coagulopathy may be present.
- Other blood tests: hypoalbuminemia, hypocalcemia, or hypocholesterolemia
- Urinalysis: glucosuria or pyuria
- Microbiology

—Wound cultures may demonstrate four or more organisms.
—Blood cultures are occasionally positive.
—Urine culture may be positive if there is a urinary source.

IMAGING

- Plain radiographs

—Help to assess the presence and extent of subcutaneous gas
—Absence of subcutaneous gas does not rule out disease.
—May help to assess intraabdominal involvement

- Retrograde urethrography

—May reveal urethral stricture, disruption, or urinary extravasation

- Ultrasonography

—Allows examination of the scrotal contents, perineum, and abdomen
—May demonstrate soft-tissue gas before evident on physical examination

- CT of abdomen, pelvis, and perineum may help to reveal underlying pathology and demonstrate the extent of inflammation and subcutaneous emphysema.

—May be particularly helpful if there is an intraabdominal or retroperitoneal process

SPECIAL STUDIES

- MRI has been reported as helpful in assessing extent of inflammation and fascial involvement.

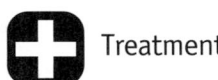

Treatment

GENERAL MEASURES

• Fournier's gangrene is a true urologic emergency and demands early recognition and prompt medical and surgical treatment.
• Metabolic stabilization: Correct electrolyte disturbances, hyperglycemia, or acidosis.
• Hemodynamic stabilization: Aggressive fluid resuscitation, correction of coagulopathy, invasive monitoring; inotropic support is often necessary prior to early surgical intervention.

MEDICAL

• Initiation of prompt broad-spectrum intravenous antibiotic therapy is important.
• Empiric triple therapy

—Penicillin G is bactericidal and offers good coverage against gram positives (3–5 million IU q6h)
　—Covers streptococci, clostridia, and some anaerobes
　—Does not cover *Bacteroides* or gram-negative rods
—Aminoglycosides: gentamicin or tobramycin (3–5 mg/kg/d)
　—Offers excellent gram-negative rod coverage
—Clindamycin (600–1200 mg/d in divided doses)
　—Covers *Bacteroides* and other anaerobes

• Alternative regimens

—Third-generation cephalosporin and an aminoglycoside
　—May offer better gram-negative coverage with less nephrotoxicity
　—Gram-positive coverage is not as good.
—Other frequently used agents: Ampicillin (2 g q4h), ticarcillin with clavulanic acid (3.1 g q6h), and metronidazole (500 mg q6h) may be used in conjunction with one or more of the above agents

• Consider tetanus toxoid administration.

SURGICAL

• Prompt and aggressive surgical debridement minimizes progression of necrosis.
• The dorsal lithotomy position provides optimal access.
• If perirectal disease is suspected, examination under anesthesia and proctoscopy should be performed.
• Consider a diverting colostomy if the sphincter is grossly infected or if there is colonic or rectal perforation.
• Cystoscopy can help assess urethral involvement.
• Consider proximal urinary diversion (cystotomy) in cases of urinary extravasation, significant urethral disease, or extensive penile involvement or edema.
• Extent of debridement should include all affected tissues.

—Deep fascia and muscle are often not involved and usually do not require debridement.

—Areas with questionable viability may be managed with drainage by surgical incision, placement of drains, and close observation.
—Testes have their own separate vascular supply and usually are viable.
　—Orchiectomy is indicated if there is gross disease of the testicles or spermatic cord.
　—Placement of the testes in a subcutaneous abdominal or thigh pouch may be necessary.

• Intraoperative irrigation with bactericidal solution: Dakin's solution (25%), bacitracin, kanamycin, or hydrogen peroxide
• Wound should be packed with fine-mesh gauze soaked in Dakin's solution (25%), Clorpactin, or saline.
• Treatment in children is similar to that in adults, with fluid resuscitation, systemic antibiotics, and a more conservative approach to debridement.

ALTERNATIVE THERAPIES

• Hyperbaric oxygen

—Reportedly successful in promoting wound healing and improving survival
—Increased oxygen concentration is bactericidal, enhances phagocytic activity, and promotes epithelialization.
—Should be considered adjunctive therapy and should not delay appropriate surgical intervention

PATIENT EDUCATION: N/A

Follow-Up

MONITORING

• Follow volume status closely and adjust accordingly.
• Extended critical care support may be required postoperatively.
• Wound culture results and sensitivities may guide antibiotic therapy.
• Postoperative wound care

—Wet-to-dry dressing changes 3 times per day
—Silvadene cream may be added to dressing changes.
—Routine careful inspection
—Daily whirlpool therapy
—Repeat debridement in the operating room is often necessary.

• Nutritional support

—Important in wound healing
—Patients are catabolic and in a negative nitrogen balance and require early nutritional support.
—Early enteral feeding vs. intravenous hyperalimentation

• Reconstructive techniques: delayed primary closure, split-thickness skin grafts, or skin flaps

PREVENTION

• Appropriate intraoperative antibiotics and postoperative care for urethral/scrotal/perineal surgery

Miscellaneous

SYNONYMS

• Fournier's disease, necrotizing fasciitis, genitourinary gangrene

ASSOCIATED CONDITIONS

• Diabetes mellitus, malignancy, alcoholism, intravenous drug abuse

NOTES

• See Section I, "Perineal Pain."

ABBREVIATIONS

• ARDS, adult respiratory distress syndrome; CT, computed tomography; MRI, magnetic resonance imaging

REFERENCES

Kane CJ, Nash P, McAninch JW. Ultrasonographic appearance of necrotizing gangrene: Aid in early diagnosis. *Urology* 1996;48:142.

Laucks SS. Fournier's gangrene. *Surg Clin North Am* 1994;74:1339.

Lowe FC. Gangrene of the male genitalia. In: Marshall FF, ed. *Operative Urology*. Philadelphia: WB Saunders, 1996.

Paty R, Smith AD. Gangrene and Fournier's gangrene. *Urol Clin North Am* 1992;19:149.

Weiner DM, Lowe FC. Gangrene of the male genitalia. AUA Update Series, Lesson 6, Volume XVII, 1998.

Authors: Jeffrey F. Williams and J. Stuart Wolf, Jr.

Glomerulonephritis—Acute

 Basics

DESCRIPTION

• Acute glomerulonephritis (AGN) is characterized by intraglomerular inflammation and cellular proliferation associated with hematuria.
• In some of these conditions, the glomerulus is the affected site, and in other conditions, the kidney is the manifestation of a systemic disease.
• The hallmarks of glomerulonephritis (GN) are abrupt onset of proteinuria, hematuria, and RBC casts.
• AGN can be divided into acute onset (postinfectious) and rapidly progressive glomerulonephritis (subacute glomerulonephritis).
• Chronic glomerulonephritis (CGN) is discussed in Section II, "Glomerulonephritis—Chronic."

EPIDEMIOLOGY

• Etiology
—Poststreptococcal GN: streptococcal infection of upper respiratory tract or of the skin.
  —Specific serotypes: Group A beta-hemolytic streptococci wit M and T antigens: "nephritogenic" strains (M-serotypes: pharyngitis: #12, 1, 3, 4; skin: #49, 2, 55, 57; T-antigens: T-14).
  —GN-rate poststreptococcal pharyngitis or impetigo: 15%
  —More common in children (ages 2–10 years), but can occur at any age. Rare in children younger than 2 years
—Postpharyngitis GN
  —Latent period between pharyngitis and development of GN: 9 to 11 days
  —More common in cold climates, with peak seasonal incidence during winter and springs.
  —Boys:girls ratio: >2:1
—Postimpetigo GN
  —Latent period: 3 weeks or longer
  —More common in hot or tropical climates
  —Boys:girls ratio: equal
—Rapidly progressive GN
  —Probably secondary to autoimmune disorder
  —Seen in systemic lupus, periarteritis nodosa. When associated with pulmonary disease, it is referred to as Goodpasture syndrome.

GENETICS: N/A

STAGING: N/A

SIGNS AND SYMPTOMS

• Streptococcal pharyngitis or impetigo, which is followed by a latent period, and then the abrupt onset of nephritis
• Patients develop edema (periorbital), oliguria, dark urine ("tea-colored" urine), gross hematuria, hypertension, headaches, visual disturbances.
• Edema probably occurs secondary to sodium retention due to diminished GFR.

PATHOPHYSIOLOGY

• Immune-complex disease in which streptococcal antigens provoke an antibody response.
• The antigen–antibody complexes are deposited in the glomerular capillary wall.
• The complexes activate the complement pathway, leading to damage to the capillary wall and glomerular basement membrane.
• Depression of serum complement activity. Cultures are negative for streptococcal infection during the nephritic state. Other infections and viruses can produce a similar clinical picture.
• Pathology: limited to glomeruli. Enlarged and hypercellular glomeruli. Large number of neutrophils, and later, mononuclear cells. Proliferation of endothelial and mesangial cells. Discrete nodular deposits along the epithelial aspects of the glomerular basement membrane (deposits of IgG and C3). All of these changes tend to resolve by 2 months after the onset of the condition.

CAUSES/RISK FACTORS

• Streptococcal pharyngitis or skin infection with specified nephritogenic serotypes. AGN-proven biopsy has also been associated with pneumococcal, staphylococcal, and viral infections.

COMPLICATIONS

• For most, the course is mild to moderate in severity, with complete resolution in 2 to 3 months.
• Rarely, fulminant course, with hypertension, seizure disorders, anuria, hyperkalemia, possibly death

DIFFERENTIAL DIAGNOSIS

• Membranoproliferative GN
• Systemic lupus erythematosus
• Schönlein-Henoch purpura
• Berger disease
• Malaria nephropathy
• Focal sclerosing GN
• Goodpasture syndrome
• Polyarteritis nodosa
• Chronic pyelonephritis
• Renal trauma
• Acute tubular injury and necrosis
• Acute hemorrhagic cystitis

 Database

HISTORY

• Hematuria, edema, and fatigability following pharyngitis or skin infection
• Any other relatives with similar symptoms?
• A history of hematuria during the acute streptococcal infection increases the likelihood of subsequent GN.

PHYSICAL EXAMINATION

• Hallmarks include periorbital edema, dependent edema, and hypertension.
• Oliguria is common. Evidence of vascular congestion

Diagnostic Studies

LABORATORY TESTING

- Urinalysis: hematuria and proteinuria. Urine may be scanty, brown, or smoky. The urinary sediment contains RBCs, WBCs, and renal tubular cells. RBC casts in the urinary sediment are characteristic and pathognomonic of poststreptococcal GN in patients with previous symptoms of pharyngitis.
- Dysmorphic RBCs due to glomerular bleeding
- Proteinuria is mild, with levels of 1 g/24 h.
- Elevated ASO and ASH titers, diminished complement titers (particularly C3)
- Mild normochromic anemia is common.
- Elevated ESR, BUN, and serum creatinine
- Hyponatremia may occur secondary to fluid overload.
- Negative throat cultures at the time of onset of GN

IMAGING

- Renal ultrasound is likely to be normal in its appearance. Not necessary for diagnosis. Chest x-ray may show increased pulmonary markings consistent with fluid overload.

SPECIAL STUDIES

- Serum complement levels (C1, C2, C3, C4). ASO, ASH titers
- Immunofluorescence microscopy typically reveals coarse granular pattern of deposits of C3 and IgG.
- Renal biopsy is not routinely necessary.

 ## Treatment

GENERAL MEASURES

- Systemic support for fluid overload and possible acute renal insufficiency
- Bed rest until the hematuria clears; subsequent physical activity should be limited as long as abnormalities in the urinary sediment persist.
- Dietary protein intake should be restricted if azotemia is present.
- Likewise, sodium restriction is recommended for cases of fluid overload, edema, or severe hypertension. Diuretics (furosemide) may be of value in this situation.
- Hypertensive treatment with drugs such as hydralazine may be necessary in some patients.

MEDICAL

- All patients should receive penicillin (600,000 U/d for 8 days).
- Exposed members of the family should receive prophylactic penicillin for a similar period.

SURGICAL: N/A

ALTERNATIVE THERAPIES: N/A

PATIENT EDUCATION

- With AGN, family members should receive penicillin prophylaxis.

 ## Follow-Up

MONITORING

- Spontaneous resolution usually occurs in 2 to 3 weeks.
- Serial monitoring of blood pressure and urine output and assessment of urinary sediments
- Complete recovery is expected in the majority of patients.
- Hypertension, proteinuria, and chronic renal insufficiency can occur in up to 20% of patients.

PREVENTION

- Penicillin therapy of culture-proven streptococcal pharyngitis

 ## Miscellaneous

SYNONYMS

- Poststreptococcal GN, postinfectious GN, lupus nephritis

ASSOCIATED CONDITIONS

- Renal insufficiency, systemic lupus erythematosus, streptococcal pharyngitis

NOTES

- See also Section II, "Glomerulonephritis—Chronic."

ABBREVIATIONS

- ASO, antistreptolysin-O; AGN, acute glomerulonephritis; CGN, chronic glomerulonephritis; BUN, blood urea nitrogen; GFR, glomerular filtration rate

REFERENCES

Couser WG. Pathogenesis of glomerulonephritis. *Kidney Int* 1993;42[Suppl]:S19–S26.

Hricik DE, et al. Glomerulonephritis. *N Engl J Med* 1998;339(13):888–899.

Johnson RJ. The glomerular response to injury: Progression or resolution? *Kidney Int* 1994;45:1769–1782.

Noe HN. Hematuria in children. AUA Update Series XVI (34):266, 1997.

Author: T. Ernesto Figueroa

Glomerulonephritis—Chronic

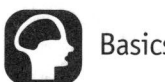 Basics

DESCRIPTION

• Chronic glomerulonephritis (CGN) is also referred to as slowly progressing GN, a condition of chronic and progressive diffuse sclerosis of glomeruli and clinical proteinuria and loss of renal function.
• A syndrome characterized by progressive renal insufficiency in patients with glomerular inflammation, hematuria, and hypertension
• Characterized by intraglomerular inflammation and cellular proliferation associated with hematuria. In some of these conditions, the glomerulus is the affected site, and in other conditions, the kidney is the manifestation of a systemic disease.
• The hallmarks of glomerulonephritis (GN) are proteinuria, hematuria, and RBC casts.

EPIDEMIOLOGY

• Diverse causes, and often the exact etiology, of the condition are uncertain and cannot be demonstrated.
• Patients may be asymptomatic for many years before the disease becomes clinically evident.
• Incidence at autopsy is 0.5% to 1%; no good estimates of incidence in general population
• Lupus nephritis is one of the common causes of CGN.

GENETICS: N/A

STAGING: N/A

SIGNS AND SYMPTOMS

• Various presentations, depending on the severity of the disease
• Patients may be asymptomatic, with the exception of proteinuria or hematuria.
• May present with advanced disease with uremic symptoms (nausea, vomiting, pruritus, dyspnea, edema)
• Hypertension is common.

PATHOPHYSIOLOGY

• Multiple pathophysiologic processes, usually uncertain
—Pathology: diffuse, progressive glomerular sclerosis
—Organized glomerular synechiae are seen in 50% of the cases.
—Infiltration and sclerosis of the interstitium
—Tubular atrophy. Increase in extracellular matrix

CAUSES/RISK FACTORS

• Systemic lupus; most others unknown

COMPLICATIONS

• Chronic renal failure, hypertension, uremia, death

DIFFERENTIAL DIAGNOSIS

• Membranoproliferative GN
• Systemic lupus erythematosus
• Schönlein-Henoch purpura
• Berger disease
• Malaria nephropathy
• Focal sclerosing GN
• Goodpasture syndrome
• Polyarteritis nodosa
• Chronic pyelonephritis
• Renal trauma
• Acute tubular injury and necrosis
• Acute hemorrhagic cystitis

 Database

HISTORY

• Elicit drug use, previous infections, previous episodes of pharyngitis or skin infections, history of cardiac valvular disease and subacute bacterial endocarditis
• May have intermittent episodes of hematuria
• Shortness of breath and chronic fatigability are also common. Nausea and vomiting may be elicited.

PHYSICAL EXAMINATION

• Dependent edema, hypertension
• Heart murmurs may be apparent.

Diagnostic Studies

LABORATORY TESTING

- Hematuria and moderate-to-severe proteinuria
- RBC casts may be absent, whereas finely and coarsely granular tubular cell and hyaline casts are uniformly present in the urinary sediment.
- BUN and serum creatinine may be elevated.

IMAGING

- Renal ultrasound may show small kidneys with poor corticomedullary differentiation.

SPECIAL STUDIES

- A renal biopsy is needed to confirm the diagnosis.

—A biopsy may help in distinguishing between benign recurrent hematuria, tubulointerstitial disease, or other forms of glomerular disease.
—Particularly important in the early phases of the disease
—Biopsy indicated in patients with systemic lupus erythematosus and proteinuria, to exclude lupus nephritis
—If the kidneys are shrunken and scarred, as in the latter stages of the disease, little can be learned from the biopsy.

 ## Treatment

GENERAL MEASURES

- Hypertensive treatment may be necessary in some patients.
- Protein restriction based on the degree of azotemia. Similarly, sodium restriction is recommended.

MEDICAL

- Antihypertensive agents are used if hypertension is a significant factor (furosemide 2–7 mg/kg divided into 2 or 3 daily doses).
- Alkali therapy: if $CO_2 < 15$ mmol/L (sodium bicarbonate 1 g tid, or sodium citrate 10% solution, 1 tsp tid)
- Lupus nephritis: Systemic steroids should be considered.

—Cytotoxic immunosuppressive drugs (cyclophosphamide) in addition to prednisone has been used in the management of rapidly progressive renal failure secondary to lupus.
—Plasmapheresis does not improve the outcome of patients with severe lupus nephritis.

SURGICAL: N/A

ALTERNATIVE THERAPIES: N/A

PATIENT EDUCATION

- Counseling on the possibility of dialysis

 ## Follow-Up

MONITORING

- Chronic monitoring of renal function, level of proteinuria, and blood pressure

PREVENTION

- None known

 ## Miscellaneous

SYNONYMS

- Lupus nephritis, slowly progressive GN

ASSOCIATED CONDITIONS

- Renal insufficiency, systemic lupus erythematosus

NOTES

- See also Section II, "Glomerulonephritis—Acute."

ABBREVIATIONS

- ASO, antistreptolysin-O; AGN, acute glomerulonephritis; CGN, chronic glomerulonephritis; GFR, glomerular filtration rate

REFERENCES

Couser WG. Pathogenesis of glomerulonephritis. *Kidney Int* 1993;42[Suppl]:S19–S26.

Hricik DE, et al. Glomerulonephritis. *N Engl J Med* 1998;339(13):888–899.

Johnson RJ. The glomerular response to injury: Progression or resolution? *Kidney Int* 1994;45:1769–1782.

Noe HN. Hematuria in children. AUA Update Series XVI (34):266,1997.

Author: T. Ernesto Figueroa

Gonadal Dysgenesis (Mixed and Pure)

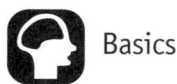 Basics

DESCRIPTION

• A group of disorders with abnormal gonadal development. Gonadal dysgenesis may involve either ovaries or testes.

EPIDEMIOLOGY

• Pure gonadal dysgenesis (PGD) is a rare condition causing delayed puberty.

—Patients usually present as phenotypic females.
—62% of females have delayed puberty, and Turner syndrome (45XO PGD) is the most common cause.
—Turner syndrome (45XO PGD) occurs in 1 in 2000 to 3000 female births.

• Mixed gonadal dysgenesis (MGD) is rare condition causing ambiguous genitalia.

—Patients may be raised as males or females, depending on androgen exposure during development.
—MGD is the second most frequent cause of ambiguous genitalia.

GENETICS

• PGDs have one of three karyotypes: 45XO, 46XX, and 46XY.
• MGD: usually 46XY/45XO mosaic karyotype; 47XXY, 45XO, and 46XY have been reported.
• 46XX PGD: some autosomal recessive inheritance
• 46XY PGD: some X-linked recessive or autosomal dominant inheritance

STAGING: N/A

SIGNS AND SYMPTOMS

• Presentation

—PGD: often present as adolescent phenotypic females with delayed puberty
　—Turner syndrome patients (45XO PGD): short stature
　—46XX and 46XY PGD: normal or tall stature
　—46XY PGD: may develop rapid breast or clitoral enlargement due to hormonally active gonadoblastomas within the streak gonads
　—Infants with 45XO PGD: usually signs of Turner syndrome (webbed neck, shield-shaped chest, and low posterior hairline)
—MGD: usually present as neonates with ambiguous genitalia
　—Genitals vary from phenotypic males to phenotypic females.
　—Most common: partially virilized female
　—Some have features similar to Turner syndrome.

PATHOPHYSIOLOGY

• Patients with PGD have two dysplastic streak gonads.

—Streak gonads: excessive fibrous stromal tissue, few or no germinal cells, found within the abdomen
—45XO and 46XX PGD have bilateral streak ovaries.
　—Usually found in the broad ligament; little malignant potential
—46XY PGD (Swyer syndrome) has bilateral streak testis.
　—Gonads in the abdomen; high malignant potential
　—Histology of testis: fibrous stroma and disorganized tubules
　—Tumors may develop at any age and may be bilateral.
　—Tumor types: gonadoblastomas (most common and benign), dysgerminoma, teratoma, and choriocarcinoma
—Hypoplastic mullerian internal ductal structures present

• MGD: testis on one side, streak gonad on the other

—Bilateral streaked gonads or bilateral dysgenetic testis has been reported.

• Intrascrotal or intraabdominal testis
—Sertoli and Leydig cells, but no germinal cells
—Often fail to produce adequate testosterone
—Undescended testicle: embryonal cell carcinoma or seminoma
—Streak gonad: 25% to 30% risk of tumor
　—Tumor types: gonadoblastoma, dysgerminoma, teratoma, and choriocarcinoma
　—MGD with 46XY: highest risk of tumor
—Internal duct development is usually mixed and may vary.
　—Usually a vas and epididymis on the testis side
　—A fallopian tube and unicorn uterus usually develop on the streak side.
　—Vagina: opens into the urethra

CAUSES/RISK FACTORS

• Positive family history

COMPLICATIONS

• Malignant degeneration of dysplastic gonads in 46XY PGD and MGD
• Infertility, failure of sexual maturity
• Turner syndrome has increased risk of

—Skeletal, cardiac, and renal abnormalities
—Osteoporosis and inflammatory bowel disease
—Lymphedema in infants

DIFFERENTIAL DIAGNOSIS

• Other causes of ambiguous genitalia in addition to MGD include

—Congenital adrenal hyperplasia (CAH)
—Partial androgen insensitivity
—True hermaphrodites
—Hypospadias

• Other causes of delayed puberty in addition to PGD include

—Hypothalamic–pituitary defects (Kallmann, Prader-Willi, etc.)
—Chronic illness (anorexia, inflammatory bowel disease, diabetes, etc.)
—Complete androgen insensitivity
—Imperforate hymen and Mayer-Rokitansky syndrome
—Ovarian injury (irradiation, surgery, torsion, sickle cell disease)
—Tumors
—MGD

 Database

HISTORY

• A family history of ambiguous genitalia, genital reconstructive surgery, unexplained infant deaths, and infertility may identify an inherited condition. Maternal exposure to drugs or androgens during pregnancy may be important in the causation of ambiguous genitalia.

PHYSICAL EXAMINATION

• In evaluating the newborn with ambiguous genitalia and possible MGD, the degree of virilization is important.

—Phallus: size, shape, and position
—Labioscrotal folds: rugation, color, size, and fusion
—Gonads: If palpated in the scrotum or groin, then the patient does not have PGD.
—Increased pigmentation of the labioscrotal folds or the areola
　—Caused by overproduction of melanocyte-stimulating hormone
　—Associated with CAH
—Infant uterus
　—May be detected in the first days of life due to effect of maternal hormones
　—Palpate on rectal examination as a midline mass.

• Evaluating adolescents for delayed puberty and PGD

—Signs of sexual development: breast development, pubic hair
—Turner syndrome (45XO PGD): short stature, webbed neck, cubis valgus, and sexual infantilism (sparse pubic and axillary hair, no breast development)
—46XX and 46XY PGD: normal or tall stature

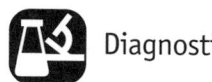 Diagnostic Studies

LABORATORY TESTING

- If suspicion of PGD or MGD: karyotype analysis immediately
- If ambiguous genitalia

—Urine 17-ketosteroid, serum 17-hydroxyprogesterone, and electrolytes to rule out CAH

- If delayed puberty

—LH and FSH: Evaluate the level of stimulation of the ovaries by the pituitary.
—Estrogen levels indicate ovarian function.

IMAGING

- Infants with ambiguous genitalia: should have genitograms to delineate the lower urinary tract and the genital tract

—A pelvic ultrasound may help identify the uterus and ovaries.

- Patients with delayed puberty: pelvic ultrasound

SPECIAL STUDIES

- Cystoscopy, vaginoscopy, and laparoscopy may be necessary to accurately diagnose the condition.

 Treatment

GENERAL MEASURES

- Family counseling and education are of utmost importance.

—Intersex states are often handled best by a team of urologists, endocrinologists, pediatricians, and counselors.

MEDICAL

- Replacement hormones not provided by the dysgenetic gonads can be given after the age of puberty.

SURGICAL

- As a rule, the gonads in MGD and in 46XY PGD should be excised at diagnosis.
- The sex of rearing in MGD is determined by the external genitalia, and once a sex has been decided, the genitalia should be reconstructed appropriately.

—Reconstructive genital surgery between 3 and 12 months
—Since infants with MGD are poorly virilized, the most common surgical procedure is a feminizing genitoplasty.
　　—An enlarged clitoris is surgically reduced, while the glans and nerves are preserved for sensation.
　　—Phallic skin can be made into a clitoral hood and labia minora.
　　—Fused labioscrotal folds are split to create labia majora.
　　—The urogenital sinus is reconstructed to separate the urinary tract from the reproductive system.
—Gender assignment and reassignment are controversial and should be discussed openly with the family and the team of physicians.

ALTERNATIVE THERAPIES: N/A

PATIENT EDUCATION

- Patients and families must be educated about problems of infertility, the need for hormone replacement, and potential malignancies in retained gonads.

 Follow-Up

MONITORING

- If the patient has retained gonads, they must be monitored for malignant degeneration.
- Patients with Turner syndrome should be monitored for osteoporosis and adequate skeletal growth.

PREVENTION: N/A

 Miscellaneous

SYNONYMS: N/A

ASSOCIATED CONDITIONS: N/A

NOTES

- See also Section I, "Ambiguous Genitalia," and Section II, "Intersex Disorders."

ABBREVIATIONS

- PGD, pure gonadal dysgenesis; MGD, mixed gonadal dysgenesis; CAH, congenital adrenal hyperplasia

REFERENCES

Berkovitz GD, et al. Clinical and pathologic spectrum of 46, XY gonadal dysgenesis: Its relevance to the understanding of sex differentiation. *Medicine* 1990;70:375.

Muller J, et al. Gonadal malignancy in individuals with sex chromosome anomalies. *Birth Defects* 1991;26:247.

Siegel SF, et al. Abnormal sexual differentiation and hypogonadism: Management and therapy. In: Sanfilippo JS, et al., eds. *Pediatric and Adolescent Gynecology*. Philadelphia: WB Saunders, 1994.

Author: Anthony J. Casale

Gonorrhea

Basics

DESCRIPTION

• Gonorrhea is a highly infectious, sexually transmitted disease caused by *Neisseria gonorrhoeae,* a gram-negative intracellular diplococcus.

EPIDEMIOLOGY

• 1400 in 100,000 people in the United States
• More common in males than in females (symptomatic disease)
• Very common in teenagers and racial and ethnic minorities
• Higher prevalence in heterosexual Black men then heterosexual White men
• 15% to 30% risk of contracting disease when men have intercourse with an infected woman
• 60% to 90% risk of contracting disease when women have intercourse with an infected man
• Risk increases with amount of sexual intercourse.
• Up to 35% will have concomitant chlamydial infection.
• Pharyngeal (25%) and rectal infections (40%) are more common in the homosexual than in the heterosexual male population.

GENETICS

• Individuals with congenital absence of the late components of the complement cascade (C7, 8, 9) are more prone to the development of local gonococcal infections.

STAGING: N/A

SIGNS AND SYMPTOMS

• Asymptomatic in 40% to 60% of the contacts of partners with gonorrhea. Lack of symptoms is more common in women than in men. Without treatment, even symptomatic gonorrhea will improve, but the host may remain a carrier and be potentially infectious.
• Men

—Urethral discharge, yellowish or gray-brown, profuse and purulent, associated with itching, in up to 75% of the cases. In other cases, urethral discharge can be scant or absent.
—Dysuria (slight discomfort to extreme pain)
—Frequency
—Testicular or epididymal tenderness
—Proportion of asymptomatic cases: 5% to 10%

• Women

—Cervicovaginal discharge
—Dyspareunia
—Abdominal pain
—Cervical erythema, edema, friability
—Bartholinitis
—Cervical motion or adnexal tenderness (early pelvic inflammatory disease)
—Proportion of asymptomatic cases: 50% dysuria or pelvic pain

PATHOPHYSIOLOGY

• The bacteria cause a purulent inflammation of mucus membrane surfaces. Virtually any mucus membrane may be infected.
• The male urethra and the endocervical canal in women are the usual sites of infection.
• Significant inflammatory response with resultant tissue damage

CAUSES/RISK FACTORS

• *Neisseria gonorrhoeae* is the pathogen.
• Sexual exposure to an infected partner without the use of barrier contraceptive methods
• Multiple sexual partners
• Autoinoculation (finger to eye)
• Use of intrauterine devices (pelvic inflammatory disease)
• Infant: through the infected birth canal of the mother
• Children: sexual abuse by infected individual

COMPLICATIONS

• Periurethritis is a common complication that may lead to abscess formation, urethral fibrosis, and urethral stricture (leading to obstructive urinary symptoms).
• Infertility in women (tubal scarring due to pelvic inflammatory disease)
• Disseminated infection (0.5% of untreated cases): fever; small, tender papules; or petechiae may appear on the arms and legs and may turn into hemorrhagic or necrotic pustules.
• Tenosynovitis and arthritis may occur, involving most commonly the knees.
• Hematogenous dissemination may rarely lead to endocarditis and meningitis.
• Corneal scarring after eye infections
• Destruction of articular surfaces
• Death from congestive heart failure or meningitis

DIFFERENTIAL DIAGNOSIS

• Nongonococcal urethritis

—Chlamydial infections: 50% to 60%
—*Ureaplasma urealyticum, Trichomonas vaginalis, Gardnerella vaginalis, Candida albicans,* viral warts, herpes virus: 5% to 10%
—Unknown: 30% to 45%

• Urinary tract infections
• Other infectious vaginitides (yeast, *Trichomonas,* bacterial vaginosis)

Database

HISTORY

• Detailed history of sexual activity and partners. Usually teenagers and young adults, sexually active, multiple partners, no protection during intercourse
• Onset of symptoms in relation to suspected sexual intercourse
• The incubation period is 3 to 10 days. May range from 12 hours to 3 months before manifestation
• "Bon jour spot": drop of urethral exudate, commonly seen on arising and before urination

PHYSICAL EXAMINATION

• Routine genitourinary examination (should be performed at least 1 hour after last voiding, preferably 4 hours)
• Aspects of discharge (urethral or vaginal): watery, thick, mucoid or purulent, whitish or yellowish
• Signs of proctitis in anoscopy (friable, purulent rectal mucosa)
• Signs of pharyngeal infection: sore throat, exudative pharyngitis
• Other signs of mucous inflammation in relation to the surface affected, as well as other signs of disseminated disease

Diagnostic Studies

LABORATORY TESTING

- Urethral smear (preferably 4 hours after last voiding, but at least 1 hour): The specimen must be collected within the urethra (2 cm proximal to the meatal opening) and not simply from a drop of discharge. In women, a cervical specimen is collected by rotating the swab for 20 to 30 seconds within the endocervical canal, after the cleansing of the external cervical area with a large swab (procto swab).

—A finding of gram-negative diplococci within polymorphonuclear leukocytes is diagnostic.
—Finding only extracellular diplococci is equivocal and will depend on the results of the culture.
—No gram-negative diplococci seen, negative for gonorrhea

- Culture (Thayer-Martin agar in CO_2 incubator)
- Pharyngeal and rectal smears should be done if the history is positive for contact.

IMAGING

- A pelvic ultrasound or CT scan may demonstrate thick, dilated tubes or abscess formation in pelvic inflammatory disease due to gonococcal infection.
- Retrograde urethrogram if male urethral disease suspected

SPECIAL STUDIES

- Genetic probe techniques and polymerase chain reaction are new tools in detecting gonococci. Useful in places where cultures are not reliable (isolated rural areas or locales with severe climate conditions). Sensitivity and specificity are lower than culture.
- Strain typing: autotyping and serovar identification
- Antibiotic sensitivity tests, if suitable

 ## Treatment

GENERAL MEASURES

- Avoid sexual intercourse until cure has been established and partners evaluated and treated.
- Investigation of another sexually transmitted disease must be considered.

MEDICAL

- Always remember to treat concomitant chlamydial infection (up to 35% of the cases) when treating gonococcal urethritis.
- Persistence of symptoms after treatment calls for investigation for nongonococcal urethritis.

—Uncomplicated urethral, endocervical, or rectal infection
   —Recommended: ceftriaxone 125 mg IM plus doxycycline 100 mg 2 times daily for 7 days
   —Alternative regimens: cefixime 400 mg orally once; ciprofloxacin 500 mg orally once; ofloxacin 400 mg orally once; spectinomycin 2 g IM (recommended in cases of allergy to cephalosporins and quinolones)
—Epididymitis
   —Recommended: ceftriaxone 250 mg IM once, plus doxycycline 100 mg bid for 10 days
   —Alternative regimens: ofloxacin 300 mg orally twice daily for 10 days
—Pregnancy
   —Ceftriaxone 125 mg IM
   —Spectinomycin 2 g IM
   —Cefixime 400 mg orally, single dose
—Neonates
   —Ophthalmia neonatorum: ceftriaxone 25 to 50 mg/kg/d IV or IM, not to exceed 125 mg, single dose
   —Disseminated gonococcal infections: ceftriaxone 25 to 50 mg/kg/d IV or IM, single daily dose for 7 days; 10 to 14 days if meningitis is documented
—Disseminated disease
   —Ceftriaxone 1 g IV once daily for 7 days, followed by ciprofloxacin 750 mg/d po bid for 5 days
—Pelvic inflammatory disease
   —Ceftriaxone 500 mg IM on day 1 and on day 5, plus doxycycline 100 mg po bid for 14 days

SURGICAL: N/A

ALTERNATIVE THERAPIES: N/A

PATIENT EDUCATION

- Education of persons at risk about modes of disease transmission and the means of reducing that risk

 ## Follow-Up

MONITORING

- Repeat cultures and reexamination 3 to 7 days after therapy is begun. A negative culture must always be obtained after treatment.
- Persistence of symptoms: The patient is still infected or presenting a postgonococcal urethritis.

PREVENTION

- Initial prevention

—Use of condoms (offers partial protection)
—Nonoxynol-9, a spermaticide, has been shown to kill the gonococcus.
—Postcontact antibiotics

- Recurrence: no sexual intercourse until culture results are known and partner(s) have been tested and treated

 ## Miscellaneous

SYNONYMS

- "Clap," "the drip"

ASSOCIATED CONDITIONS

- Concurrent infection due to *Chlamydia trachomatis* in 10% to 35% of patients
- Other sexually transmitted diseases, such as syphilis, HIV, hepatitis B, and herpes

NOTES: N/A

ABBREVIATIONS: N/A

REFERENCES

Berger RE. Sexually transmitted diseases: The classic diseases. In: Walsh PC, Retik AB, Vaughan ED, Wein AJ, eds. *Campbell's Urology*, 7th ed. Philadelphia: WB Saunders, 1997:663–681.

Sherrard J. Modern diagnosis and management of gonorrhoea. *Br J Hosp Med* 1996;55(7):394–397.

Zenilman JM. Gonorrhea: Clinical and public health issues. *Hosp Pract (Off Ed)* 1993;28(2A):29–35, 39–40, 43–45.

Authors: David M. Albala and Fernando C. Koleski

Granuloma Inguinale

 Basics

DESCRIPTION

• Asexually transmitted, chronic infection ("dono-vanosis") affecting the genital and anorectal mucosal membranes, inguinal regions, and neighboring subcutaneous tissues

EPIDEMIOLOGY

• Causative agent: *Calymmatobacterium granulomatis*, a nonmotile, gram-negative rod related to *Klebsiella pneumoniae*.
• Incubation period: typically 1 to 4 weeks, but may be as long as 6 months
• United States incidence is low; higher in Third World nations

GENETICS: N/A

STAGING: N/A

SIGNS AND SYMPTOMS

• A small, painless, elevated papule with irregular edges is the first sign.
• No inguinal lymphadenopathy
• A subcutaneous granulomatous process referred to as a "pseudobubo" is present.
• Base of ulcer is nontender, indurated, and firm

PATHOPHYSIOLOGY

• Commonly occurs in people who have unprotected sexual activity

CAUSES/RISK FACTORS

• *Calymmatobacterium granulomatis*
• History of sexual partner with known granuloma inguinale
• History of other sexually transmitted diseases
• High-risk (unprotected) sexual activity

COMPLICATIONS: N/A

DIFFERENTIAL DIAGNOSIS

• Syphilis: painless ulcer with sharply demarcated edges; dark-field examination and serologic testing are diagnostic.
• Herpes: grouped, tiny, painful vesicles associated with tender lymphadenopathy; viral cultures are positive.
• Chancroid: multiple, very painful papules with irregular edges
• Lymphogranuloma venereum: painless vesicle, papule, or ulcer
• Traumatic ulcer: consistent with history
• Fixed drug reaction: consistent with history

 Database

HISTORY

• Important to take a thorough sexual history

—Past and current sexual contacts
—Sexual preferences
—Sexual behaviors
—History of HIV or other immunocompromised state

• Consider in any patient (or partner) with recent (1 to 3 months) foreign travel
• Consider recent drug usage
• Consider recent trauma (e.g., sexual activity, zipper, human or insect bite, scratch)

PHYSICAL EXAMINATION

• Typically young, sexually active, generally healthy person
• Examine the genitalia.

—Type of lesion: papule, pustule, vesicle
—Characteristics of lesion(s)
—Number
  —One (syphilis, lymphogranuloma venereum)
  —Multiple (herpes, chancroid, donovanosis)
—Edges
  —Sharply demarcated (syphilis)
  —Irregular (chancroid, donovanosis)
—Base (smooth, purulent)
—Size (in millimeters)

• Examine inguinal nodal areas.

—Painless (donovanosis, syphilis)
—Painful (herpes, chancroid, lymphogranuloma venereum)
—"Matted" pseudobubos (donovanosis)

• Examine the anus for lesions.
• Type of lesion: papule, pustule, vesicles

Diagnostic Studies

LABORATORY TESTING

• Routine laboratory testing is not informative.

IMAGING: N/A

SPECIAL STUDIES

• Preferred study: cytologic examination (crushed preparation)

—Retrieval of small piece of tissue from ulcer base, crushing it between two slides
—Stain with Leishman, Giemsa, or Wright stain.

• "Donovan bodies" seen on cytologic examination

—Pathognomonic lesion
—Reproduces itself inside of lysosomes of infected cells that contain 20 to 30 nonmobile, gram-negative rods
—Found at base of ulcer

• Ancillary tests include a histologic examination.
• Microbiologic cultures are impractical.
• No serologic tests are available.

Treatment

GENERAL MEASURES

- Rule out other sexually transmitted diseases.

MEDICAL

- Tetracycline 500 mg po qid for 20 days

SURGICAL: N/A

ALTERNATIVE THERAPIES

- Bactrim one DS tablet po bid for 20 days
- Erythromycin 500 mg po qid for 20 days

PATIENT EDUCATION

- Sexual education about modes of transmission and the use of protective devices and behaviors is essential for all patients and their partners.

 Follow-Up

MONITORING

- Reevaluate those patients who have been appropriately treated but have persistent lesions.
- Clarify that the diagnosis is correct.

PREVENTION

- Patient education
- Sexual abstinence
- Use of condoms

Miscellaneous

SYNONYMS

- Donovanosis, granuloma donovani, granuloma pudenda tropicum, *Calymmatobacterium,* and granuloma venereum

ASSOCIATED CONDITIONS

- Other sexually transmitted diseases

NOTES

- See also Section I, "Penis—Lesion" and "Inguinal Lymphadenopathy."

ABBREVIATIONS: N/A

REFERENCES

Berger RE, Rothman I. Sexually transmitted diseases in males. In: Tanagho EA, McAninch JW, eds. *Smith's General Urology,* 14th ed. Norwalk, CT: Appleton & Lange, 1995:262–275.

Berger RE. Sexually transmitted diseases: The classic diseases. In: Walsh PC, Retik AB, Vaughan ED, Wein AJ, eds. *Campbell's Urology.* Philadelphia: WB Saunders, 1998:663–683.

Krieger JN. Biology of sexually transmitted diseases. *Urol Clin North Am* 1984;11(1):15–25.

Authors: Byron D. Joyner and J. Brantley Thrasher

Herpes Simplex—Genital

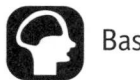 Basics

DESCRIPTION

• Genital herpes is a sexually transmitted viral infection causing painful lesions of the genitalia of men and women, as well as constitutional symptoms and lymphadenopathy.

EPIDEMIOLOGY

• Affects approximately 55 million people in the United States
• Incidence is rising, but only 20% to 25% are ever clinically detected.

GENETICS: N/A

STAGING: N/A

SIGNS AND SYMPTOMS

• First episode

—Severe illness lasting several weeks
—Malaise, flu-like constitutional symptoms
—Tender inguinal lymphadenopathy
—Crops of fluid-filled painful vesicles surrounded by erythema
—Ruptured vesicles leave painful ulcers, which often coalesce and eventually crust.
—Symptoms more severe in women; urinary retention may result.

• Recurrences

—Less severe, last 5 to 10 days, fewer constitutional symptoms or lymphadenopathy
—Prodromal symptoms: pain, burning, or tingling at future site of vesicles 12 to 72 hours before
—Women have more severe symptoms, but symptoms last longer in men.

PATHOPHYSIOLOGY

• Sexually transmitted by infected individual to partner
• Infectious sites can be the mouth or genitals.
• Symptoms or lesions need not be present for transmission to occur.
• Latency from acquisition to onset of symptoms may be short or long.
• Herpes simplex virus type 2 (HSV-2) is more common than type 1 (HSV-1).

CAUSES/RISK FACTORS

• Sexual contact with infected individual
• Other sexually transmitted diseases increase likelihood.
• Risk factors for recurrences: stress, fatigue, trauma, immunocompromised state, pregnancy, menstruation

COMPLICATIONS

• Difficulty voiding or urinary retention

—Secondary to reflex inhibition of voiding secondary to fear of pain
—Some instances may be secondary to sacral radiculopathy.
—Suprapubic catheter placement may be preferable to urethral catheterization to prevent intravesical spread.

• Headaches in 20%
• Aseptic or herpetic meningitis

—Lumbar puncture may be necessary to exclude bacterial meningitis.
—Aseptic meningitis usually has a benign course; herpetic meningitis may cause confusion or cerebellar symptoms and has a worse prognosis.

• Extragenital lesions may occur in moist mucocutaneous areas or in locations where a breach in the epidermis has occurred (nail, finger).
• Herpetic keratoconjunctivitis from ocular inoculation can cause eye pain, blurry vision, and excessive tearing.

DIFFERENTIAL DIAGNOSIS

• Syphilis
• Chancroid
• Behçet disease
• Traumatic lesions of genitalia

 Database

HISTORY

• Sexually active?

—Number of partners, infected partners

• History of prior sexually transmitted diseases
• Recent stressors, presence of immunocompromised state

PHYSICAL EXAMINATION

• Examine the genitalia for lesions, ulcerations, encrusted areas, and vesicles.

—Painful? Surrounding erythema?

• Examine for inguinal lymphadenopathy.

—Tender?

Diagnostic Studies

LABORATORY TESTING

- Collect vesicular fluid or ulcer exudate on a swab and send it in appropriate media (check with laboratory for available testing media).
- Viral culture (via cell lines), typing using antiserum, or antigen detection (ELISA or direct immunofluorescence) can be done.

IMAGING: N/A

SPECIAL STUDIES: N/A

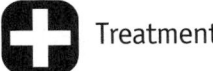 ## Treatment

GENERAL MEASURES

- Oral analgesics suffice for most patients.
- Warm soaks may be helpful in women, especially if they have difficulty voiding.
- Anesthetic jelly applied locally may be helpful.

MEDICAL

- First episodes: Oral antiviral agents may ease local and constitutional symptoms.

—Acyclovir (200 mg 5 times daily) for 5 to 10 days is safe and effective.
—Valacyclovir is the prodrug for acyclovir and needs less frequent dosing because of better bioavailability (500 mg twice daily).
—Famciclovir (250 mg tid) has the best oral bioavailability (77%) and is the prodrug for the active compound penciclovir.

- Recurrences: may be reduced in severity and frequency by using continuous antiviral suppressive therapy with the agents above.

—Therapy should be reserved for individuals with frequent, painful recurrences.
—Famciclovir is especially useful in these patients due to its long persistence in infected cells (250 mg twice daily).

- Baseline CBC, chemistry panel, and BUN/creatinine should be performed prior to initiating therapy.
- Women should be advised to avoid pregnancy while on therapy.

SURGICAL: N/A

ALTERNATIVE THERAPIES: N/A

PATIENT EDUCATION

- Educating the general population about the risks of orogenital and genitogenital transmission may reduce incidence.
- All partners should be identified and examined.
- Patients should be counseled regarding the prompt diagnosis and treatment of recurrent lesions.

 ## Follow-Up

MONITORING

- Patients should be monitored until the disappearance of the primary lesion and should be asked to report any recurrences.
- The pattern of recurrences should be monitored and antiviral therapy initiated if indicated.

PREVENTION

- Patient education is the best method of prevention.
- Preventing transmission by using condoms and spermicidal sponges and creams is effective but incomplete.

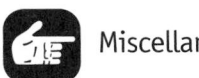 ## Miscellaneous

SYNONYMS: N/A

ASSOCIATED CONDITIONS: N/A

NOTES

- See also Section I, "Penis—Lesions."

ABBREVIATIONS: N/A

REFERENCES

Sacks SL, Aoki FY, Diaz-Mitoma F, Sellors J, Shafran SD. Patient-initiated, twice daily oral famciclovir for early recurrent genital herpes. *JAMA* 1996;276:44–49.

Thackray AM, Field HJ. Comparison of effects of famciclovir and valaciclovir on pathogenesis of herpes simplex virus type 2 in a murine infection model. *Antimicrob Agents Chemother* 1996;40: 846–851.

Woolley P. Update on genital herpes. *Infect Urol* 1998;11:42–46.

Author: Mantu Gupta

HIV Infection—Urologic Considerations

 Basics

DESCRIPTION

- Urologic manifestations of HIV include atypical and nonbacterial infections, unusual malignancies, impaired renal function, and voiding dysfunction.

EPIDEMIOLOGY

- Over 22 million people worldwide are living with HIV/AIDS.
- As of December 1997, 84% of AIDS cases reported to the CDC were males, and nearly one-fifth were at least 50 years old.
- For most current data: CDC National AIDS Clearinghouse: www.cdcnac.org

GENETICS

- 25% perinatal transmission from HIV-positive mother (decreased with zidovudine therapy)

STAGING

- Current AIDS definition

—CD4 $< 200/\mu$L
—AIDS-defining illnesses: updated periodically in the *HIV/AIDS Surveillance Report,* published by the CDC

SIGNS AND SYMPTOMS

- Acute retroviral syndrome

—Fever, malaise, lymphadenopathy, skin rash
 —Occurs in first few weeks after HIV infection

- Infection

—Typical: dysuria, frequency, urgency, fever, or lumbar pain
—Atypical: gross hematuria, asymptomatic bacteriuria, refractory UTI Sx despite antimicrobial therapy

- Neoplasms

—Lymphoma may have upper tract obstruction symptoms secondary to retroperitoneal involvement or testicular mass.
—Kaposi's sarcoma (KS)
 —Reddish-purple, macular lesions; in darker pigmented individuals, lesions may be brown or black.
 —Visible oral or cutaneous lesions are present in 95% of AIDS patients with KS.
 —Lesions involve the genitalia in 20% of KS patients.

- HIV-associated nephropathy: mild hypertension
- Indinavir nephropathy

—Asymptomatic crystalluria (20%)
—Renal colic secondary to urolithiasis (3.6%)
—Dysuria or urgency

- Neurologic infections or tumors

—Wide range of voiding-dysfunction symptoms

PATHOPHYSIOLOGY

- Genitourinary infections

—UTI incidence as high as 50% in HIV-infected patients, frequently asymptomatic
—Incidence increases with degree of immunosuppression
 —Bacteriuria more common with CD4 counts less than $200/\mu$L
—Ascending routes of transmission have been described.
—Bacterial pathogens
 —Common: *E. coli, Enterobacter, Proteus*
 —Less common: *Staphylococcus, Serratia, Salmonella*
—Nonbacterial infections: usually associated with severe immunodeficiency (CD4 $< 100/\mu$L)
 —Viruses: CMV, adenovirus
 —Fungi and yeast: *Candida, Aspergillus, Blastomyces, Cryptococcus, Histoplasma, Pneumocystis*
 —Parasites: *Cryptosporidium, Toxoplasma*
—Infection not limited to urinary tract, e.g., CMV prostatitis, *Candida epididymitis, Toxoplasma orchitis*
—Miscellaneous infectious sequelae: CMV-induced ATN, enterovesical fistula with *Cryptosporidium* cystitis

- Malignancies

—Lymphoma
 —Usually undifferentiated B-cell, but large-cell and T-cell have been reported.
 —May involve kidneys in 6% to 12% of AIDS patients (commonly bilateral)
 —Retroperitoneal adenopathy may cause ureteral obstruction
 —May present as primary testicular lymphoma
—Kaposi's sarcoma
 —Strong evidence that KS-associated herpesvirus (KSHV, or HHV-8) is etiologic pathogen
 —Usually affects skin, but may involve other organs, including urinary tract

- Intrinsic renal disease

—HIV-associated nephropathy
 —May occur at any stage of HIV infection; more common in Black males
 —Unique histopathology: focal and segmental glomerulosclerosis; segmental deposition of IgM and C3. Other observations: tubules with microcystic dilation, tubular necrosis, interstitial edema, glomerular capillary collapse associated with hyalin deposition and edema
 —May be reversible as viral load decreases
 —Although most patients will require dialysis, mortality is low.
—Acute tubular necrosis
 —Up to 13% of HIV patients will experience ATN during the course of their disease.
 —Usually the result of hemodynamic changes (not HIV-nephropathy)

- Drug-associated renal disease

—Nephrotoxic antivirals
 —Cidofovir (CMV agent); dose-dependent nephrotoxicity (80% have proteinuria, 29% have serum creatine elevations); should not be given if baseline Scr > 1.5
 —Acyclovir (varicella or herpes agent); nearly 50% have rise in Scr with bolus infusion; bolus is associated with crystal precipitation in renal tubules and ATN
 —Foscarnet sodium (CMV and HIV agent); as many as one-third have progressive renal insufficiency secondary to direct tubular toxicity; rare dose-dependent hypocalcemia

—Indinavir nephropathy (protease inhibitor for HIV)

  —Urine pH > 5.5 promotes indinavir crystal formation in the urine, and can progress to symptomatic stones.

  —Composition is usually pure indinavir, but other components may be present.

  —Stones may occur more frequently with doses >2.4 g/d.

  —Stones may be associated with hypocitraturia.

  —Intratubular crystal formation my lead to renal injury.

  —Crystals may become soluble in vitro upon acidification less than 4.5.

• Voiding dysfunction

—As many as 10% with HIV or AIDS report moderate subjective problems.

—Neurologic lesions associated with AIDS

  —Inflammatory: arachnoiditis

  —Infectious: cerebral toxoplasmosis, herpes radiculitis, herpes transverse myelitis, HIV encephalitis, HIV myelopathy, tuberculous meningitis, CMV infection

  —Malignancy: lymphoma, disseminated KS

CAUSES/RISK FACTORS

• For HIV

—Unprotected intercourse, anal or oral sex

—IV drug abuse/needle sharing

—Concomitant STDs

—Multiple blood product transfusions

• For atypical GU infections

—Immunosuppression

  —Bacterial: CD4 < 200/μL

  —Nonbacterial: CD4 < 100/μL

—Prophylactic antibiotics, e.g., co-trimoxazole for PCP prophylaxis

  —May suppress urine culture growth

  —May select out more resistant organism

• For malignancy: immunosuppression

• For HIV nephropathy: progressive clinical stage of disease

• For indinavir nephropathy: dose >2.4 g/d; daily fluid intake of <1.5 L/d while taking drug

COMPLICATIONS

• See drug-associated renal disease

DIFFERENTIAL DIAGNOSIS: N/A

 Database

HISTORY

• General HIV screening: known exposure to HIV, unprotected intercourse, multiple partners, anal or unprotected oral sex, history of STDs, IV drug abuse, needle sharing, weight loss, constitutional symptoms, rashes, multiple blood product infusions

• In patient with known HIV or AIDS

—Dysuria, frequency, urgency, flank pain, hematuria

  —GU infection, including STDs

  —Indinavir stones

  —Lymphoma-induced ureteral compression

—Incontinence, urinary retention

  —Suggests possible neurologic lesion

—Lethargy, confusion, urticaria

  —Suggests possible renal failure

—Adenopathy, skin lesions

  —Suggests possible malignancy

PHYSICAL EXAMINATION

• General

—Skin lesions, adenopathy, abnormal neurologic examination

• GU examination in HIV or AIDS patient

—Tenderness to palpation of prostate, epididymis, testis

  —Suggests possible infection

—Testicular mass

  —Possible lymphoma

—Penile skin lesions

  —Penile infection, KS, HSV

—Inguinal adenopathy, diffuse adenopathy

  —Infection, malignancy, acute retroviral syndrome

 Diagnostic Studies

LABORATORY TESTING

• HIV testing

—A screening HIV-1 antibody test should be performed first (enzyme immunoassay [EIA])

—Supplemental test required for confirmation of diagnosis

  —Western blot (WB); immunofluorescence assay (IFA)

• Tests if HIV-positive: CD4 cell count; plasma HIV RNA level; PPD; baseline toxoplasma IgG, VDRL, hepatitis B and C serology, CMV IgG

• Urine culture if infection suspected

—Selective cultures if on antibiotics

—Viral and fungal cultures if immunosuppressed (CD4 < 100/μL)

• Urinalysis

—Hematuria suggests stone, infection, invasive malignancy.

—Leukocytes suggest stone, infection.

—Crystalluria with indinavir crystals

  —Tapered or flat rectangular plates

  —Circular or symmetrical fan-shaped and starburst forms

  —Birefringence with straight extinction

—Proteinuria

  —Heavy proteinuria with nephrotic syndrome associated with HIV-nephropathy

• Complete blood count with differential WBC

—Anemia, leukopenia suggestive of immunosuppression, malignancy

—Lymphopenia may suggest AIDS, lymphoma.

(continued)

HIV Infection—Urologic Considerations (continued)

IMAGING

- Chest radiograph

—In all HIV-positive patients, to screen for pneumonia, tuberculosis

- Ultrasound

—TRUS for prostatic abscesses
—A renal ultrasound may diagnose renal abscesses and indinavir stones, or suggest intrinsic renal disease.
  —HIV nephropathy: bilateral, echogenic, large kidneys without hydronephrosis

- KUB

—Indinavir stones with a calcium component may be radiopaque.

- IVU

—Filling defects are suggestive of indinavir stones and fungal masses.
—Obstruction is suggestive of retroperitoneal lymphoma, tuberculosis, and indinavir stones.
—Parenchymal defects are suggestive of abscesses, fungal infection, and parenchymal disease.

- Abdomen and pelvis CT

—Renal abscesses, parenchymal disease, fungal masses, retroperitoneal adenopathy (lymphoma), indinavir stones in some, tumor metastasis

SPECIAL STUDIES

- Renal biopsy

—Diagnosis of HIV nephropathy

- Prostate or bladder biopsy (in case of culture-negative infective symptoms or negative hematuria work-up)

—CMV infection with diagnostic inclusion bodies in prostate or bladder tissue
—Tissue for viral cultures, AFB and fungal cultures, diagnosis of parasites

- Resistant infective symptoms: Viral cultures, isolator cultures, or tissue culture may be necessary to make a diagnosis.

 Treatment

GENERAL MEASURES

- HIV treatment with antiretroviral drugs must be maximized to augment treatments for specific urologic manifestations.

MEDICAL

- Genitourinary infections

—Treatment of infections must be culture-specific.
—Broad-spectrum antibiotics should be avoided if possible.

- Malignancy

—NHL: treated with combination systemic chemotherapy
—KS: if focal, local radiation; if disseminated, multidrug chemotherapy, interleukin, interferon

- HIV nephropathy may require dialysis.
- Indinavir nephropathy

—Temporarily stop drug if renal failure or symptomatic stones
  —Consider surgery for symptomatic stones (see below).
  —Reduce indinavir doses to <2.4 g/d in less severe cases.
—H_2O consumption >1.5 L/d
—Potassium citrate or sodium citrate supplementation may be helpful.
—Acidification of urine not reasonable or practical (pH < 4.5)

- Voiding dysfunction

—Treat the underlying neurologic disorder.
—Patients may achieve symptomatic improvement with appropriate pharmacotherapy.

SURGICAL

- Genitourinary infections: Prostatic abscesses may require surgical drainage.
- Malignancy

—Lymphoma
  —Testis: surgical excision if diagnosis not already made
  —Retroperitoneal involvement: may require ureteral stenting to relieve obstruction
—KS
  —Focal lesions of external genitalia: respond well to laser ablation
  —Urethral strictures resulting from local radiation may require dilation, incision, or reconstruction.

- Indinavir stones

—Ureteral stenting for symptomatic relief
—Ureteroscopic stone extraction
—Ureteroscopic lithotripsy: no studies to determine comparative effectiveness (electrohydraulic lithotripsy, laser, etc.)
—ESWL

ALTERNATIVE THERAPIES: N/A

PATIENT EDUCATION

- All patients with HIV should be referred to health centers with comprehensive HIV treatment and counseling programs.
- Encourage increased water intake if the patient is taking indinavir.

Follow-Up

MONITORING

- CD4 and plasma HIV RNA level should be checked regularly (every 6 months or more frequently).
- HIV-positive patients should be screened regularly for STDs: gonorrhea, chlamydial infection, syphilis.

PREVENTION

- Preventative measures are the same for all sexual and blood-transmissible diseases.

—Male latex condoms only preventable for anal, oral, or vaginal transmission of HIV (sheepskin condoms ineffective)
—Female latex condoms not thoroughly tested for HIV prevention of transmission
—Needle sharing should be strongly discouraged.

 Miscellaneous

SYNONYMS: N/A

ASSOCIATED CONDITIONS

- Sexually transmitted diseases

NOTES: N/A

ABBREVIATIONS

- CDC, Centers for Disease Control and Prevention; HIV, human immunodeficiency virus; AIDS, acquired immunodeficiency syndrome; STD, sexually transmitted disease; KS, Kaposi's sarcoma; NHL, non-Hodgkin's lymphoma; PCP, *Pneumocystis carinii* pneumonia; CMV, cytomegalovirus; AFB, acid-fast bacteria

REFERENCES

Sable CA, Wispelwey B. Genitourinary manifestations of HIV infection. In: Resnick MI, Older RA, eds. *Diagnosis of Genitourinary Disease.* New York: Thieme, 1997.

Sharifi R, Lee M. Urinary tract infections in HIV-infected men. *Infect Urol* 1997;10(1):24.

Steele BW, Carson CC. Recognizing the urologic manifestations of HIV and AIDS. *Contemp Urol* 1997;9(9):39.

Authors: Bradley W. Steele and Culley C. Carson III

Hot Flushes (Vasomotor Instability)

 Basics

DESCRIPTION

• Vasomotor instability, characterized by flushing and profuse sweating, is a common, bothersome side effect of androgen deprivation therapy in men with advanced adenocarcinoma of the prostate.

EPIDEMIOLOGY

• Occurs in 55% to 75% of patients treated with androgen deprivation
• No relationship to race or disease stage
• Symptomatic patients tend to be younger than asymptomatic patients.
• Rarely severe enough to discontinue therapy
• 20% of men will actively seek medical attention.

GENETICS

• Unknown

STAGING: N/A

SIGNS AND SYMPTOMS

• Sensation of overall increased body temperature, mainly upper arms, face, and thorax
• Profuse sweating follows increased temperature sensation in most patients.
• Cutaneous erythema of affected body parts often visible
• Occasional sense of suffocation, mild dyspnea, or anxiety
• Rarely, patients may experience sleep disturbances or irritability.

PATHOPHYSIOLOGY

• Occurs in response to the precipitous and persistent drop in serum testosterone levels following androgen ablation therapy (i.e., LH-RH analogue, orchiectomy, etc.)
• Gonadotropin levels may be high or low; no correlation to symptoms
• The main physiologic defect is altered hypothalamic thermoregulation.
• Mechanism unknown; increased hypothalamic catecholamine release may contribute
• Sex steroids normally stimulate hypothalamic release of opioid peptides, which inhibit catecholamine release.
• An abrupt decrease in circulating testosterone leads to a rapid increase in local catecholamine release.
• A catecholamine neurotransmitter is released in close proximity to the hypothalamic thermoregulatory neurons, which leads to peripheral vasodilatation.

CAUSES/RISK FACTORS

• Development of hot flushes

—Age: men with hot flushes tend to be slightly younger than asymptomatic men.
—Pre-androgen ablation testosterone levels are not predictive of development of symptoms.
—Stage of disease does not correlate with a likelihood of hot flushes.

• Hot flush stimuli

—Shifting to reclining position, particularly at bedtime
—Drinking hot fluids, alcohol ingestion
—Warm environment, cigarette smoking
—Exercise, caffeine

COMPLICATIONS

• Bothersome hot flushes will decrease the overall quality of life in men with advanced prostate cancer.
• Cessation of therapy rarely occurs secondary to bothersome hot flushes.
• Sleep disturbance, leading to fatigue, irritability, and anxiety
• Social withdrawal may occur secondary to profuse sweating episodes.
• No long-term adverse cardiopulmonary sequelae

DIFFERENTIAL DIAGNOSIS

• Pertinent in the absence of medical or surgical castration
• Systemic illness

—Carcinoid syndrome
—Pheochromocytoma
—Mastocytosis
—Carcinoma
—Medullary thyroid
—Renal cell
—Pancreas: VIP-secreting tumors

• Medications

—Any vasodilatory agent
—Calcium channel blockers
—Opiates
—Tamoxifen
—Cephalosporins

• Neurologic etiology

—Autonomic hyperreflexia
—Parkinson disease
—Anxiety
—Migraine headaches
—Multiple sclerosis
—CNS malignancy

• Dietary

—Ethanol, sulfite ingestion, monosodium glutamate

 Database

HISTORY

• Typically, men complain of the abrupt, paroxysmal onset of warmth, frequently followed by profuse, body-wide sweating
• Sensation of warmth most prominent in the face, upper extremities, neck, and upper chest
• Patients may complain of dyspnea and anxiety.
• Occasionally, sweating is so severe that clothing and/or bedding requires changing.
• Episodes typically last 1 to 5 minutes and require no acute intervention for resolution.
• Nighttime episodes common (40%)
• Majority of patients (two-thirds) have daily episodes; of these, over half experience more than six episodes per day.
• Nearly one-half of men characterize hot flush episodes as "extremely bothersome."
• The onset of hot flushes is typically within 1 year of therapy (90%); one-third will develop symptoms within 1 month.
• Hot flushes will spontaneously resolve in up to half of men within 2 years.

PHYSICAL EXAMINATION

• Unremarkable when hot flushing quiescent
• During an acute episode, visible erythema is noted on the upper chest, throat, and face.
• Mild increased temperature of the involved skin
• Sweating variably present
• Mild tachycardia secondary to effect of peripheral vasodilatation and/or anxiety and dyspnea

Diagnostic Studies

LABORATORY TESTING

• No pattern of characteristic changes in serum testosterone, FSH, LH, or prolactin
• Men who experience flushing have normal urine catecholamine studies.
• No routine laboratory evaluation is indicated for hot flushes.

IMAGING: N/A

SPECIAL STUDIES: N/A

Treatment

GENERAL MEASURES

• Reassurance: if symptoms mild, no treatment necessary
• Avoidance of inciting stimuli
• Eliminate hot beverages, particularly if caffeine-containing
• Stop cigarette smoking
• Minimize alcohol use
• Keep environment cool
• Watchful waiting: Up to 50% of symptomatic patients will experience resolution within 2 years.

MEDICAL

• Testosterone replacement strictly contraindicated in men with advanced prostate cancer
• Sex steroid replacement: restores feedback inhibition on hypothalamus, decreasing catecholamine release

—Megestrol acetate (Megace): 20 mg po daily or bid
  —Progesterone derivative
  —Complete resolution rate of 70%, partial response in 20%
  —Side effects minimal and include weight gain (appetite stimulation), diarrhea, nausea/vomiting, dyspepsia
  —Onset of action is delayed for 2 to 3 months.
  —Response rate durable and well tolerated long-term
  —Safest and most effective first-line therapy
—Diethylstilbestrol (DES): 0.30 to 1.0 mg po daily
  —Complete resolution rate of 70%, partial resolution rate of 20%
  —Painful gynecomastia occurs in a majority of patients, leading to discontinuance of therapy.
  —Additional side effects are severe: thromboembolism, myocardial infarction, and subarachnoid hemorrhage.
  —No longer available in the United States; custom pharmacy service compounding available

—Cyproterone acetate (Androcur): 50 mg po bid to tid
  —Progestational and antiandrogen effects
  —Modestly effective, but not available in the United States
• Nonendocrine therapy
—Clonidine (Catapres): 0.1 to 1.0 mg daily (oral or patch formulation)
  —Central inhibition of CNS norepinephrine outflow
  —It will rarely completely eliminate hot flushes, but one-third of men will report a partial response.
  —Side effects prevalent and include constipation, dry mouth, orthostatic hypotension, fatigue
  —May be used as a second-line agent
—Phenobarbital/ergotamine preparations: (1 tablet po bid)
  —Ergot alkaloids stabilize peripheral vasculature by a vasoconstrictive effect.
  —The barbiturate component eliminates anxiety.
  —It rarely eliminates hot flushes, but nearly half of patients report a reduction in severity and frequency of symptoms.
  —May be used as a second-line agent

SURGICAL: N/A

ALTERNATIVE THERAPIES

• Behavioral therapy: Slow, deep breathing may reduce the frequency of hot flushes.
• Vitamin and mineral therapy: There are anecdotal reports that vitamins C, E, and B-complex may be helpful, but no scientific evidence exists to support these claims.
• Bee pollen and ginseng are marketed as useful, but no scientific data exist.
• Muscle relaxation techniques are shown to have no clinical benefit.

PATIENT EDUCATION

• Prior to the initiation of therapy, all patients should be informed about the potential development of hot flushes.
• Patients should be counseled as to the benign nature of their condition.
• When treating with sex steroid replacement, patients should be made aware of the 2- to 3-month delay in drug activity.
• Patients should be taught to avoid external factors that can stimulate hot flushes.
• Each patient should be carefully instructed to continue androgen therapy despite the development or persistence of bothersome hot flushes.

Follow-up

MONITORING

• Specific questioning with regard to the presence and severity of vasomotor instability should be a part of all clinical evaluations of patients treated for advanced carcinoma of the prostate with androgen ablation.
• Response to therapy for hot flushes and the bother of side effects should be ascertained.
• Intermittent cessation of treatment for hot flushes is reasonable, as flushing is usually self-limited.

PREVENTION

• Directed clinical intervention will prevent the development of hot flushes in a majority of patients.

Miscellaneous

SYNONYMS

• Vasomotor instability, hot flushes, hot flashes, flushing, vasomotor flushing

ASSOCIATED CONDITIONS

• Adenocarcinoma of the prostate

NOTES: N/A

ABBREVIATIONS: N/A

REFERENCES

Bucholz NP, et al. Post-orchiectomy hot flushes. *Eur Urol* 1994;26:120–122.

Charig CR, et al. Long-term side effect of orchiectomy in treatment of prostatic carcinoma. *Urology* 1989;33:175–178.

McGuffey EC. Treating hot flashes. *Am Pharm* 1995;35:14, 17.

Mohyi D, et al. Differential diagnosis of hot flushes. *Maturitas* 1997;27:203–214.

Smith JA. A prospective comparison of treatments for symptomatic hot flushes following endocrine therapy for carcinoma of the prostate. *J Urol* 1994;152:132–134.

Authors: Christopher G. Schrepferman and William A. See

Hydrocele (Adult and Pediatric)

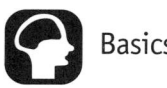 Basics

DESCRIPTION

- A hydrocele is a collection of serous fluid in some part of the processus vaginalis, usually in the tunica. Can be congenital or acquired

EPIDEMIOLOGY

- More common in childhood
- 1% of adult males; prevalence: 1000 in 100,000
- No racial predilection

GENETICS

- Unknown

STAGING: N/A

SIGNS AND SYMPTOMS

- Translucent swelling in the scrotum or inguinal canal or both
- Apart from congenital hydrocele, it is possible to get examining fingers above the swelling.
- Demonstrated fluctuation in size in congenital hydrocele
- Usually not painful
- Sensation of heaviness or discomfort in the scrotum
- Positive pinch test in a secondary hydrocele (ability to pinch the tunica)

PATHOPHYSIOLOGY

- Congenital: The processus vaginalis (PV) does not close after testicular descent. Four anatomic variants: vaginal (PV around the testis), infantile (PV around testis and cord), congenital communicating (PV communicates with the peritoneal cavity), hydrocele of the cord (PV patent with obliteration above and below)
- Acquired: can be primary (idiopathic) or secondary to disease of the testis. Secondary hydroceles may present acutely or chronically.
- The hydrocele of the canal of Nuck is comparable in females. The cyst is in relationship with the round ligament and located in the inguinal canal.
- Hydrocele fluid characteristics

—Amber colored; specific gravity of 1.022 to 1.024
—Components: water, inorganic salts, 6% albumin, and fibrinogen
—Nonclotting, unless a drop of blood added
—Chronic hydrocele: cholesterol-rich
—Occasionally, tyrosine crystals are present.

CAUSES/RISK FACTORS

- The hydrocele is produced by

—Connection with the peritoneal cavity (PPV); AKA congenital hydrocele
—Defective absorption of fluid by tunica vaginalis, e.g., primary hydrocele (common in adults)
—Excessive production of fluid within the sac, e.g., secondary hydrocele (epididymitis, bleeding, etc.)
—Lymphatic obstruction, e.g., filariasis, scrotal surgery (varicocele), renal transplantation, pelvic radiation, malignancy
—Migration of ventriculoperitoneal shunt

- Prematurity, low birth weight: risk factors

COMPLICATIONS

- Rupture: usually traumatic
- Hernia of the hydrocele sac: Tension causes herniation through the dartos muscle.
- Calcification of the wall: may occur with long-standing cases
- Hematocele: following trauma or aspiration, or presents chronically simulating a neoplasm

DIFFERENTIAL DIAGNOSIS

- Inguinal hernia
- Epididymo-orchitis
- Spermatocele
- Traumatic injury to the testis (hematocele)
- Varicocele (large)
- Torsion (testis or appendix testis)
- Testicular or paratesticular tumors
- Lymphedema of the external genitalia

 Database

HISTORY

- Symptoms of epididymitis, urinary tract infection, or acute pain?

—Secondary hydrocele with infection, torsion, and trauma usually painful

- Is there change in size of the swelling (i.e., size varies throughout day)?

—Suggests congenital communicating hydrocele

- Birth history

—Hydrocele more common in premature and low-birth-weight infants

- Medical or surgical history

—Varicocelectomy, renal transplant, VP shunt, trauma to the genitalia can be causes

PHYSICAL EXAMINATION

- Transilluminate mass

—If transilluminates, favors simple hydrocele, but is *not* diagnostic

- Palpation of testes bilaterally

—Especially in children, need to rule out undescended testicle. Adults, attempt to feel for testicular mass

- Examine the groin for inguinal hernia.
- Lymphedema of external genitalia or lower extremities

—Tissue edema can be mistaken for the hydrocele.

Diagnostic Studies

LABORATORY TESTING

• Urinalysis and urine culture if epididymo-orchitis suspected
• Tumor markers (bhCG, AFP) if tumor suspected

IMAGING

• Transscrotal ultrasound in adults with hydrocele to detect underlying testicular abnormality (i.e., tumor)
• Nuclear scan or Doppler ultrasound examination in cases of torsion

SPECIAL STUDIES: N/A

 Treatment

GENERAL MEASURES

• Adults: No treatment is necessary unless the hydrocele causes discomfort or cosmetic concerns or there is a significant underlying cause, patent such as a tumor.
• Children: Most will resolve in first year of life. Persistence suggests the presence of a patent indirect hernia sac that should be repaired.

MEDICAL: N/A

SURGICAL

• Children: inguinal incision between internal and external rings. High ligation of the processus vaginalis and excision of the sac. In hydrocele of the cord, the sac can be completely removed.
• Adults: scrotal approach with drainage of the hydrocele and resection of the tunica vaginalis; drain for 24 to 48 hours
• "Bottle procedure": (thin hydrocele sac) incise anteriorly, wrap sac back around testicle
• Jaboulay-Winkelman procedure (thick hydrocele sac): hydrocele sac resected and edge wrapped posteriorly around cord structures (resected edges can also simply be oversewn)
• Lord procedure (thin hydrocele sac): radial sutures used to gather sac posterior to testis

ALTERNATIVE THERAPIES

• Aspiration of the hydrocele, with or without the injection of sclerosing agents, should be discouraged.
• Aspiration may have a role in postoperative hydroceles.

PATIENT EDUCATION

• Parents of a newborn with a hydrocele should be instructed in the natural history of the condition in children.

 Follow-Up

MONITORING

• Periodic follow-up (baseline ultrasound) suggested if managed by observation; return for any acute changes in symptoms

PREVENTION: N/A

Miscellaneous

SYNONYMS: N/A

ASSOCIATED CONDITIONS

• Ehlers-Danlos syndrome
• Exstrophy of the bladder
• Indirect inguinal hernia
• Hydrocephalus (with ventriculoperitoneal shunt)
• Peritoneal dialysis
• Testicular tumors or epididymo-orchitis in secondary hydrocele
• Undescended testicle with PPV

NOTES

• Most authors consider transscrotal ultrasound essential in adults with a hydrocele.
See also Section I, "Scrotum—Mass and/or Pain (Acute Scrotum)."

ABBREVIATIONS

• PPV, patent processus vaginalis

REFERENCES

Lord PH. A bloodless operation for the radical cure of idiopathic hydrocele. *Br J Surg* 1964;51:914.

Skoog SJ, Conlin, MJ. Pediatric hernias and hydroceles: The urologist's perspective. *Urol Clin North Am* 1995;22:119.

Szabo R, Kessler R. Hydrocoele following internal spermatic vein ligation: A retrospective study and review of the literature. *J Urol* 1984;132:924.

Authors: Mohammed T. Ismail and Leonard G. Gomella

Hyperaldosteronism—Primary (Conn Syndrome)

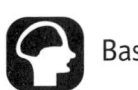 Basics

DESCRIPTION

• Characterized by hypertension, hypokalemia, hypernatremia, and alkalosis due to excess production of aldosterone

EPIDEMIOLOGY

• 1% of hypertensive population
• Adrenal adenoma more common in women
• Peak incidence during fourth and fifth decades

GENETICS

• A rare form of autosomal dominant primary hyperaldosteronism is glucocorticoid remediable aldosteronism (GRA).
• Hereditary pattern for more common aldosterone-producing adenomas unclear

STAGING: N/A

SIGNS AND SYMPTOMS

• Nocturia, urinary frequency, muscular weakness, cramp, and paresthesias
• Headaches, tetany
• Hypertension with K < 3.0 strongly suggests hyperaldosteronism.

—If normokalemic, symptoms milder

PATHOPHYSIOLOGY

• Excess aldosterone leads to inappropriate Na reabsorption.

—Extracellular fluid volume is increased until renal escape occurs, leading to mild hypertension.

• Renal escape occurs after approximately 1.5 kg of extracellular fluid is absorbed; then a decrease in Na retention occurs, limiting hypertension and preventing significant edema.
• Excess aldosterone leads to K loss and hydrogen ion secretion in urine, leading to hypokalemia and alkalosis.
• The biochemical hallmark of the disease is increased aldosterone after Na loading and low plasma renin activity during Na depletion.

CAUSES/RISK FACTORS

• Four subtypes

—Unilateral aldosterone-producing adrenal adenoma, most common
—Bilateral adrenal hyperplasia
—Glucocorticoid remediable aldosteronism due to aldosterone-producing, renin-responsive adenoma
—Adrenal cancer producing aldosterone: extremely rare

COMPLICATIONS

• Those due to hypertension
• Those due to low potassium (tetany, headache, etc.)

DIFFERENTIAL DIAGNOSIS

• Other causes of hypertension
• Other causes of hypertension and hypokalemia, such as

—Overingestion of licorice

• Use of chewing tobacco
• Hyperdeoxycorticosteronism

 Database

HISTORY

• Symptoms of polyuria, muscle weakness, cramps, headaches, temporary paralysis, visual disturbances

—Symptoms better with low-salt diet in some patients

• Family history of hypertension *not* important.

PHYSICAL EXAMINATION

• Mild-to-moderate hypertension
• Not usually distinguishable from essential hypertension
• Malignant hypertension rare

Diagnostic Studies

LABORATORY TESTING

• Serum potassium

—Hypertension with K < 3.0 usually has an aldosterone-producing adenoma.
—If present, can generally proceed to studies designed to localize adenoma
—Normal serum K in 20% of patients with hyperaldosteronism, usually in adrenal hyperplasia

• Serum aldosterone levels

—If restricted Na diet, severe hypokalemia often absent; only test patients if adequately salt loaded
—Salt loading suppresses aldosterone in essential hypertension vs. aldosterone levels >14 μg/d in primary hyperaldosteronism.

• Plasma renin activity low in primary hyperaldosteronism; if plasma renin >1, diagnosis unlikely
• An elevated ratio of plasma aldosterone to renin indicates hyperaldosteronism and may be a useful screening test; it also may be helpful if serum K levels are normal.

IMAGING

• A CT scan with thin cuts through the adrenals is the preferred noninvasive test; MRI may not be as accurate.
• Adrenal scintigraphy using ^{131}I-6-iodomethyl-19-nor-cholesterol is available, but it is inaccurate in many cases; it may have role if CT and vein sampling are inconclusive.

SPECIAL STUDIES

• Postural test useful to distinguish adenoma from bilateral hyperplasia

—Adrenal adenoma: suppressed plasma renin activity and low aldosterone after 2 hours of recumbency
—Adrenal hyperplasia: no suppression of renin and continued elevated aldosterone

• Adrenal vein sampling for aldosterone is the gold standard in localizing the site of excess production.

—Adenoma: high levels on involved side and suppressed from contralateral adrenal gland

 ## Treatment

GENERAL MEASURES

• Treatment selected based on etiology of hyperaldosteronism
• Control hypertension.

MEDICAL

• Hyperaldosteronism due to bilateral adrenal hyperplasia is treated by spironolactone.

—Amiloride may also be used, especially if gynecomastia or other side effects of spironolactone occur.

• Other antihypertensives, such as calcium channel blockers, angiotensin-converting enzyme inhibitors, and alpha-blockers, may also be effective in some cases.

SURGICAL

• Unilateral adrenalectomy is indicated in patients with hyperaldosteronism due to an adenoma.

—Hypertension is cured or improved significantly in more than 90% of such cases.
—Adequate control of blood pressure for several weeks and correction of metabolic abnormalities should be done before surgery.

• Some patients with hyperaldosteronism and a normal CT or hyperplasia can be cured by surgery.

—Tests suggestive of potential for cure include the positive postural stimulation test, elevated plasma 18-methyloxygenated cortisol metabolites, and increased aldosterone secretion from one adrenal compared with the opposite adrenal.

ALTERNATIVE THERAPIES: N/A

PATIENT EDUCATION: N/A

 ## Follow-Up

MONITORING

• Blood pressure and serum electrolytes should be evaluated postoperatively and following medical therapy.

PREVENTION: N/A

 ## Miscellaneous

SYNONYMS

• Conn syndrome, aldosteronism

ASSOCIATED CONDITIONS

• Adrenal cancer (rare), essential hypertension

NOTES

• Diagnosis may be difficult in those with normal serum K levels and those being treated with antihypertensives or diuretics.

ABBREVIATIONS

• GRA, glucocorticoid remediable aldosteronism

REFERENCES

Conn JW. Primary aldosteronism: A new clinical syndrome. *J Lab Clin Med* 1989;16:481.

Noth RH, Biglieri EG. Primary aldosteronism. *Med Clin North Am* 1988;72:1117.

Author: Glenn S. Gerber

Hyperprolactinemia

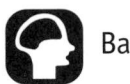 Basics

DESCRIPTION
- Hypersecretion of prolactin by the pituitary

EPIDEMIOLOGY
- Rare finding in men during evaluation of impotence or infertility

GENETICS: N/A

STAGING: N/A

SIGNS AND SYMPTOMS
- Decreased libido
- Erectile dysfunction
- Infertility
- Gynecomastia
- Galactorrhea

PATHOPHYSIOLOGY
- Regulation of prolactin is inhibited by dopamine.
—Any CNS disturbance of dopamine may affect prolactin.
- Prolactinomas in the pituitary can cause a direct hypersecretion of prolactin.
—Prolactin can interfere with peripheral conversion of testosterone to dihydrotestosterone.

CAUSES/RISK FACTORS
- Four most common causes
—Central nervous system dopamine disturbances
—Prolactinomas
—Compensated hypothyroidism
—Medications (e.g., chlorpromazine, perphenazine, fluphenazine, imipramine, amitriptyline, haloperidol)
- Other causes
—Granuloma formation, infiltrative disorders (e.g., histiocytosis X, temporal arteritis, cavernous sinus thrombosis, pituitary stalk trauma, meningitis, herpes zoster, chest-wall trauma, breast biopsy or augmentation, renal failure, bronchial carcinoma, renal cell carcinoma (paraneoplastic)
—Chronic renal failure and dialysis

COMPLICATIONS
- Infertility
- Erectile dysfunction
—Thought to be mediated via a hormonal effect

DIFFERENTIAL DIAGNOSIS
- Prolactinoma
- Hypothyroidism
- Hypothalamic dysfunction
- CNS tumor
- Hypogonadism

 Database

HISTORY
- Decreased libido, erectile dysfunction
—Present in 80% to 90% of men with hyperprolactinemia
- Infertility
- Gynecomastia, galactorrhea (rare)
- Headaches, visual disturbances (if large pituitary tumor)
- Symptoms of hypothyroidism (if cause is thyroid)

PHYSICAL EXAMINATION
- May have soft testes of decreased volume, but most will have normal testes
- Visual field examination
—Sensitive method for detection of compression of optic nerves
—Usually associated with larger lesions
- Breast examination
—If indicated by history

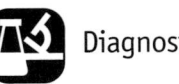 Diagnostic Studies

LABORATORY TESTING
- Serum prolactin
—Three measurements should be obtained from either morning specimens on different days or specimens on the same day q2h.
—Two elevated prolactin measurements confirm hyperprolactinemia.
- Serum TSH if history consistent with hypothyroidism
- Semen analysis (if patient presenting with infertility)
—May have oligospermia secondary to inhibitory effect on LH-RH and testosterone
—May have motility defects

IMAGING
- X-ray of sella
—Will detect if large macroadenoma
- CT scan pituitary
—Sensitive test
—Will not detect all microadenomas
- MRI scan, pituitary
—The future standard
—Will not detect all microadenomas

SPECIAL STUDIES: N/A

Treatment

GENERAL MEASURES

- Treat the underlying cause.
- Aim to reduce prolactin levels surgically or medically.
- 80% to 90% success overall in treatment. A majority will regain potency if hyperprolactinemia is the sole cause of erectile dysfunction.

MEDICAL

- Bromocriptine 2.5 mg po bid or tid
- Testosterone replacement (if hypogonadal and low serum testosterone)

SURGICAL

- Pituitary adenomectomy

ALTERNATIVE THERAPIES: N/A

PATIENT EDUCATION: N/A

 Follow-Up

MONITORING

- Serial serum prolactin
- The patient may require repeat imaging of the pituitary if prolactin remains elevated despite pituitary surgery.

PREVENTION: N/A

 Miscellaneous

SYNONYMS: N/A

ASSOCIATED CONDITIONS: N/A

NOTES

- See also Section I, "Erectile Dysfunction."

ABBREVIATIONS: N/A

REFERENCES

Blackwell RE. Hyperprolactinemia: Evaluation and management. *Endocrinol Metab Clin North Am* 1992;21(1):105–124.

Hermanns U, Hafez ESE. Prolactin and male reproduction. *Arch Androl* 1981;6:95–125.

Authors: Jay Lee and Jeremy P.W. Heaton

Hypospadias

 Basics

DESCRIPTION

• Common urogenital malformation in males, characterized by incompletely formed urethra wherein the misplaced meatus variably opens on the ventral aspect of the penis, scrotum, or perineum

—Malformation varies greatly in severity, ranging from the extreme form of perineal hypospadias with genital ambiguity to mild distal glans hypospadias.
—Commonly associated with chordee (abnormal ventral curvature of the penis) in 50% of cases and/or meatal stenosis 30% of cases

EPIDEMIOLOGY

• Incidence: 1 in 300 of live male births
• More common in Whites than in Blacks; and in Italians and Jews than in other ethnic groups

GENETICS

• Familial tendency: 8% of fathers of affected children have hypospadias; 14% of male siblings affected

STAGING

• Classification

—Based on location of meatus: glans, subcoronal, penile, penoscrotal, scrotal, or perineal
—Distal hypospadias (subcoronal or penile) comprises 62% of cases.

SIGNS AND SYMPTOMS

• Associated anomalies

—Undescended testicles: 9%
—Inguinal hernias: 9%
—Clinically significant upper tract anomalies: rare

• Chordee

—Generally caused by superficial tethering of the skin and dartos fascia, not by the urethral plate
—Chordee can occur without hypospadias, but is rare (0.6%).
—The more proximal the meatus, the greater the chordee.
—The more distal the meatus, the greater the incidence of meatal stenosis.

PATHOPSYSIOLOGY

• Unknown, but several factors involved
• Normal penile development

—The genital tubercle fuses by the sixth week; the lateral mesoderm forms the urethral and genital folds.
—The external genital structures develop the male configuration due to testosterone.
—As the phallus elongates, urethral folds coalesce in the midline, closing the urethra and forming the median raphe of the scrotum and penis.

• Alterations of the urethral fold closure result in hypospadias.
• Testosterone biosynthetic defects occur in half of proximal hypospadiacs.
• Exposure to synthetic "endocrine disrupters" that block the effect of testosterone is critical from 9 to 12 weeks' gestation.
• Related to low birth rate in discordant monozygotic twins

CAUSES/RISK FACTORS

• Unknown; some suggestion of familial risk

COMPLICATIONS

• Infertility
• Cosmetic psychological trauma
• See surgical complications in "Treatment" section, below.

DIFFERENTIAL DIAGNOSIS

• Glandular
• Subcoronal
• Penile
• Penoscrotal
• Scrotal
• Perineal

 Database

HISTORY

• Any family history?

PHYSICAL EXAMINATION

• The urethral opening may be anywhere along the shaft of the penis or into the perineum.

—62% of the openings subcoronal or penile, 22% penoscrotal angle, and 16% scrotum or perineum

• Severe hypospadias (proximal) may be confused with intersex disorders.
• The more proximal the meatus, the more the ventral curvature (chordee) will be seen.
• Undescended testes and inguinal hernia

Diagnostic Studies

LABORATORY TESTING: N/A

IMAGING

• Incidence of upper urinary tract abnormalities is rare. With more severe (proximal) cases of hypospadias, some recommend screening the upper tracts.

SPECIAL STUDIES: N/A

Treatment

GENERAL MEASURES

• With any suspicion of hypospadias, neonatal circumcision should *not* be performed
• Many consider severe hypospadias to be a type of intersex disorder.

MEDICAL: N/A

SURGICAL

• Timing of repair

—Best between 6 and 18 months
—Factors favoring early repair
  —Anesthetic risks optimal after 4 months of age
  —Penile growth modest during the first few years of life
  —Operative amnesia before age 3
  —Modern-day surgical and optical refinements facilitate repairs on infant genitalia.
  —Younger patients, still in diapers, make management of stents and catheters easier.
  —Genital awareness begins after 18 months of age.

• Technique selection for distal repairs

—Depends on the new location of the meatus after chordee is corrected
—Broadly, three types of distal repairs: mobilizations, tubulizations, and extensions
—Mobilizations: native urethra left intact, but must mobilize penile urethra to the scrotum (long run for short slide)
—Tubularizations: require deeply clefted glans and wide urethral plate or surgical steps to create comparable anatomy, e.g., tubularized, incised plate repair (Snodgrass).
—Extensions: The MAGPI (meatal advancement and glanduloplasty) is ideally suited for distal (glanular and coronal) hypospadias without chordee (Duckett). Perimeatal-based flaps (Mathieu) are also popular. A more reliable repair is the onlay island flap (Hollowell) from the inner prepuce. Not suitable if chordee persists after shaft skin is mobilized

• Technique selection for proximal hypospadias (midshaft and posterior)

—If no chordee is present, the first choice is the onlay island flap (Hollowell).
—If chordee persists, the best option is the transverse preputial island flap (Duckett).

• Complications

—Urethral cutaneous fistulas: Most occur near the coronal sulcus.
—Meatal regression
—Meatal stenosis: Fix with meatoplasty.
—Buccal or bladder mucosa: Tissue for secondary urethral reconstruction following breakdown of initial repairs if there is a deficiency of well-vascularized skin for flap procedures

ALTERNATIVE THERAPIES

• Psychosocial support as part of overall care

PATIENT EDUCATION

• Primarily involves education of the parents

Follow-Up

MONITORING

• Short-term follow-up examinations for development of fistulas and stricture
• Current techniques are superior to older techniques.

PREVENTION: N/A

Miscellaneous

SYNONYMS: N/A

ASSOCIATED CONDITIONS

• Hernia, undescended testicles, adrenogenital syndrome, Reifenstein syndrome, true hermaphroditism, mixed gonadal dysgenesis

NOTES

• See also Section I, "Ambiguous Genitalia," and Section II, "Intersex Disorders."

ABBREVIATIONS: N/A

REFERENCES

Culp OS, McRoberts JW. Hypospadias. In: Alken CE, Dix V, Goodwin WE, et al., eds. *Encyclopedia of Urology.* New York: Springer-Verlag, 1968: 11307–11344.

Duckett JW, Snyder HM III. Meatal advancement and glanduloplasty hypospadias repair after 1,000 cases: Avoidance of meatal stenosis and regression. *J Urol* 1992;147:665–668.

Duckett JW. Transverse prepubital island flap technique for repair of severe hypospadias. *Urol Clin North Am* 1980;7:423–431.

Author: J. William McRoberts

Inflammatory Bowel Disease—Urologic Considerations

 Basics

DESCRIPTION

• Inflammatory bowel disease (IBD) encompasses Crohn disease (CD) and ulcerative colitis (UC) and can involve the urinary tract in 2% to 10%.

EPIDEMIOLOGY

• CD (regional enteritis) prevalence: 20 to 40 per 100,000 U.S. population
• UC prevalence: 70 to 150 per 100,000 U.S. population
• Peak occurrence: ages 15 to 35 years for all IBD
• Males and females equally affected

GENETICS

• IBD is more common in Whites than in Blacks; Jews have three- to sixfold higher incidence of CD.
• Familial involvement in 2% to 5% of persons with CD or UC
• Increased incidence of CD in monozygotic twins

STAGING: N/A

SIGNS AND SYMPTOMS

• CD: fever, anorexia, abdominal pain, diarrhea, malaise, weight loss, and right lower quadrant mass or fullness

—Commonly causes fistulas; typically produces ileovesical fistulas, usually right sided

• UC: bloody diarrhea, abdominal pain, fever, and, in severe cases, weight loss

—Extracolonic involvement: arthritis, skin changes, or evidence of liver disease

PATHOPHYSIOLOGY

• CD: transmural inflammation involving all layers of intestine, mesentery, and regional lymph nodes; small bowel more frequently affected; terminal ileum most commonly affected; frequent infection with *Yersinia enterocolitica;* skip lesions; rectum spared in 50%; and granuloma formation
• UC: inflammation involving colonic mucosa, hyperemic areas with ulceration, uniform and continuous involvement, rectum involvement in 95%, and pseudopolyp formation

CAUSES/RISK FACTORS

• The causes of CD and UC remain unknown.

—Possible factors include the infectious, familial, and immunologic.

• The primary risk factor for urinary tract involvement is the chronicity of IBD.

—Mean duration of CD at first symptoms of enterovesical (EV) fistula: 10 years

COMPLICATIONS

• Higher incidence of urolithiasis in IBD (2%–3%), with 10% occurring in patients with ileal resection

—Predominantly calcium oxalate stones caused by loss of calcium in feces, promoting increase colonic oxalate absorption
—Chronic dehydration is a significant risk factor, predisposing IBD patients to urolithiasis.
—Higher incidence of uric acid urolithiasis in IBD
—IBD often leads to hypomagnesuria and hypocitraturia (urinary magnesium and citrate are stone inhibitors).

• Fistula formation with any organ, including the urinary tract, is one of the pathognomonic features of CD.

—EV fistula: colovesical (most commonly associated with diverticulitis), rectovesical, ileovesical (most common in CD), and appendicovesical
  —The clinical hallmark of EV fistula is Gouverneur syndrome: suprapubic pain, frequency, dysuria, and tenesmus.
  —Patients with enterovesical fistula present with recurrent UTI, multiorganism etiology, pneumaturia, and fecaluria.

• Ureteral obstruction in CD (5%–20%) is from periureteral fibrosis, almost exclusively involving the right distal ureter.

—Average age at presentation: mid-20s.

DIFFERENTIAL DIAGNOSIS

• Infectious colitis: bacterial, fungal, and protozoan
• Radiation enteritis, ischemic colitis, irritable bowel disease, appendicitis, diverticulitis, sprue, sarcoidosis, and Behçet syndrome
• Lymphoma, colonic adenocarcinoma, polyposis syndromes

 Database

HISTORY

• Symptoms of bowel-to-urinary tract fistula: pneumaturia (60%), fecaluria (pathognomonic occurs in 40%), recurrent urinary tract infection, and hematuria
• Ureteral obstruction from CD rarely causes symptoms referable to the urinary tract, and it is usually found incidentally.
• Recurrent urolithiasis, especially calcium oxalate and uric acid

PHYSICAL EXAMINATION

• Physical examination findings in IBD are often nonspecific.
• Abdominal examination for masses, right lower quadrant fullness/mass (CD), abdominal distention, and colonic area tenderness (UC)

Diagnostic Studies

LABORATORY TESTING

- Findings are often nonspecific.
- Urinalysis may reveal fecal material in the enterovesical fistula.
- Hypoalbuminemia, elevated alkaline phosphatase may indicate hepatobiliary disease (UC).
- Mild anemia, leukocytosis, and elevated ESR (CD)

IMAGING

- In suspected fistula, IVP or retrograde pyelogram to rule out ureteral involvement
- Noncontrast CT of pelvis, demonstrating air in noninstrumented bladder: 92% sensitive for fistula
- Cystogram may demonstrate "herald" sign, a crescentic defect on upper bladder margin
- A barium enema (BE) rarely defines a fistula, but may show underlying bowel pathology, particularly diverticular disease.

—Radiography of urinary sediment after BE may enhance sensitivity in an enterovesical fistula.

- IVP and renal ultrasound for cases of suspected ureteral obstruction, with Lasix renal scan for confirmation of obstruction

SPECIAL STUDIES

- Cystoscopy provides a definitive diagnosis of EV fistula in 35% to 46% of cases.
- Oral activated charcoal with antacid slurry and examination of voided urine over 3 days is very sensitive in diagnosis of EV fistula.

 ## Treatment

GENERAL MEASURES

- Medical therapy for both CD and UC is the mainstay.
- Surgery is reserved for specific complications, such as urinary fistula, abscess, and intractable disease.

MEDICAL

- Sulfasalazine and glucocorticoids are most effective in both CD and UC.

—Metronidazole for CD patients with chronic perineal fistulas

- Primary treatment of ureteral obstruction in CD is bowel treatment with medical and/or surgical excision of the involved bowel. Subsequently, ureteral obstruction resolves without primary ureteral surgery. Nephrectomy for nonfunctional renal units
- Azathioprine and/or cyclosporine for steroid-sparing high-risk cases

SURGICAL

- An EV fistula in CD should be surgically repaired only after adequate medical therapy.

—Surgical excision of an associated abscess and involved bowel segment is the key step with multilayer bladder closure. Interposition of omentum is desirable, but may not be possible in many cases of CD.

—A staged approach may be necessary, especially in cases involving abscess.

ALTERNATIVE THERAPIES: N/A

PATIENT EDUCATION

- Dietary control with a high-residue diet and close monitoring by a gastroenterologist are key to avoid complications

 ## Follow-Up

MONITORING

- Yearly serum creatinine in all patients with IBD
- Renal ultrasound for high-risk patients

PREVENTION

- None known

 ## Miscellaneous

SYNONYMS

- CD: regional enteritis, granulomatous colitis

ASSOCIATED CONDITIONS: N/A

NOTES

- See also Section I, "Fistula—Enterovesical."

ABBREVIATIONS

- IBD, inflammatory bowel disease; CD, Crohn disease; UC, ulcerative colitis

REFERENCES

Glickman RM. Inflammatory bowel disease: Ulcerative colitis and Crohn's disease. In: Fauci AS, et al., eds. *Harrison's Principles of Internal Medicine,* 14th ed. New York: McGraw-Hill, 1997.

Resnick MI, Kursh ED. Extrinsic obstruction of the ureter. In: Walsh PC, Retik AB, Vaughan ED, Wein AJ, eds. *Campbell's Urology,* 7th ed. Philadelphia: WB Saunders, 1998.

Velagapudi SRC, Pollack HM, Weiss JP. Acquired fistula of the urinary tract. AUA Update Series 12:18, 1993.

Authors: Raymond S. Lance and J. Brantley Thrasher

Intersex Disorders

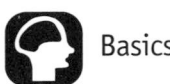 Basics

DESCRIPTION

• Developmental anomalies of sexual differentiation characterized by genital ambiguity that are classified into four main groups:

—Overandrogenization of a genetic female: female pseudohermaphrodite
—Underadrogenization of a genetic male: male pseudohermaphrodite
—Disorders of chromosomal sex
  —Mixed gonadal dysgenesis (one dysgenetic testicle, one streak gonad)
  —Anomalies of sex chromosomes without genital ambiguity: Klinefelter syndrome, Turner syndrome, XX male
—Disorders of gonadal sex
  —True hermaphrodite (both testicular and ovarian tissue represented)
  —Pure gonadal dysgenesis (no genital ambiguity)

EPIDEMIOLOGY

• Female pseudohermaphroditism incidence: 1 in 5000 to 15,000
• Male pseudohermaphroditism due to androgen insensitivity: 1 in 20,000 to 64,000
• True hermaphrodites are relatively common among the Bantu population (300 cases reported).
• Incidence of other conditions is unknown.

GENETICS

• Female pseudohermaphrodites: 46XX
• Male pseudohermaphrodites: 46XY
• Mixed gonadal dysgenesis: 45X0/46XY mosaic (60%), 40% 46XY, complex mosaics occasionally found.
• True hermaphrodites are 46XX (90%); remainders have either a mosaic 46XY/46XX or 46XY.
• Other genes involved in sex determination are located on autosomes or chromosome X.

—The defective SOX-9 gene is located on 17q, and defects in 9p and 10q are associated with sex reversal.
—21-hydroxylase is encoded by a gene located on 6p, and the 5-alpha-reductase gene is on chromosome 19.
—The receptor for dihydrotestosterone is encoded by a gene located on the X chromosome.

STAGING: N/A

SIGNS AND SYMPTOMS

• Female pseudohermaphroditism

—Clitoral enlargement of various degree, from trivial to an almost normal looking male phallus, with the opening of the urogenital sinus at its tip
—Not palpable, gonad hyperpigmented, and enlarged labia majora to form labioscrotal folds, sometimes fused in the midline
—Usually no vaginal opening visible in the perineum. Urogenital sinus anomaly
—Severe 21-hydroxylase and 3-beta-hydroxysteroid dehydrogenase defects cause the salt-wasting syndrome: low Na, high K, possible hypotension, and life-threatening adrenogenital crisis 5 to 7 days after birth due to lack of corticosteroids
—11-hydroxylase defects cause severe hypertension and water-salt retention.

• Male pseudohermaphroditism

—Pseudohermaphroditism type I (testicular feminization syndrome)
—Complete androgen insensitivity (X-linked): normal female phenotype with small infertile testes retained in the groin. Usually short vagina. At puberty: primary amenorrhea, breast development, but scanty pubic and axillary hair
—Incomplete androgen insensitivity: phenotypes from normal female with minor clitoral enlargement to hypospadias with one or two descended testes
—Pseudohermaphroditism type II (5-alpha-reductase defect): severe penoscrotal hypospadias, prepenile scrotum, undescended testes. Progressive virilization at puberty
—Congenital defects of testosterone biosynthesis
  —Defect of: 20,22-desmolase and 3-beta-hydroxysteroid dehydrogenase: hypospadiac small penis and undescended testes, severe salt-wasting syndrome
  —17-alpha-hydroxylase: ambiguous genitalia and hypertension, hypokalemic alkalosis
  —17-KS-reductase and 17-OH-dehydrogenase: ambiguous genitalia, virilization at puberty
—Mixed gonadal dysgenesis
  —Small hypospadiac penis, asymmetric labioscrotal folds, one gonad often palpable, occasionally fully descended in the better developed side. Urogenital sinus
—True hermaphroditism
—Phenotype varies from the hypospadiac male to the female with mild clitoral enlargement. Most patients severely virilized. Asymmetric labioscrotal folds, one gonad (testis or ovotestis) often palpable in the better developed side

PATHOPHYSIOLOGY

• Female pseudohermaphroditism

—Enzyme defect in the biosynthesis of glucocorticoids and mineralocorticoids: Increased ACTH causes fetal androgen overproduction in the adrenals (congenital adrenal hyperplasia [CAH]), and occasionally salt wasting due to a lack of mineralocorticoids (21-hydroxylase and 3-beta-dehydrogenase).
—11-beta hydroxylase defect: CAH with increased deoxycorticosterone synthesis (virilization, salt retention, and hypertension)
—Absent Müllerian inhibitory substance (MIS)
—Normal ovaries and uterus. Urogenital sinus due to a high or low confluence of vagina and urethra

• Male pseudohermaphroditism

—Hypoandrogenization of a genetic male may be caused by
  —Defects in testosterone synthesis or in its reduction to dihydrotestosterone
  —Block of androgen receptors
  —Normal MIS production: absent mullerian derivatives
  —Several enzymes are required in testosterone biosynthesis (20,22-desmolase, 17-hydroxylase, 3-beta hydroxysteroid dehydrogenase, 17-ketosteroid reductase). A defect causes deficiency in both androgen and adrenal steroids: External genitalia are ambiguous, testes may be small or undescended or both, and internal genitalia are wolffian derivatives.
—Na/K metabolism may be affected.

• Dihydrotestosterone is the biologically active androgen; its deficiency, due to the 5-alpha-reductase defect, causes

—Severe feminization
—Undescended testes with spermatogenesis
—Short vagina or urogenital sinus
—Internal genitalia are wolffian.
—Receptor deficiency
  —Complete or partial
  —Female phenotype with short vagina
  —Infertile testes
  —Rudimentary Wolffian or absent internal genitalia
  —Increased risk of germ cell cancer

—Mixed gonadal dysgenesis
  —Pathogenesis and etiology are obscure.
  —Asymmetrical gonads: a small, dysgenetic, and undescended testis on one side and an intraabdominal streak gonad on the other
  —Low MIS: Mullerian derivatives present on the side of the streak gonad.
  —Low testosterone: wolffian derivatives on the testicular side, ambiguous external genitalia with urogenital sinus anomaly and clitoral enlargement
  —Increased gonadal cancer risk: gonadoblastoma in the streak gonad, germ cell tumor in the testis
—True hermaphroditism
  —The reasons for gonadal asymmetry are unclear.
  —Coexistence of well-developed ovary and testis, separated on both sides or combined as an ovotestis. In ovotestis, testicular tissue is central and the ovary is peripheral.
  —Mullerian derivatives on the ovarian side, wolffian on the testicular side, both duct systems in case of an ovotestis. Rudimentary uterus and often large vagina opening in a urogenital sinus
  —External genitalia frequently masculinized
  —Low incidence of gonadal tumors

CAUSES/RISK FACTORS

• Female pseudohermaphroditism

—Excess maternal androgens
—Adrenal steroid synthesis enzymes deficiency (90% involves a mutation of 21-hydroxylase gene, located on 6p within the autosomal HLA class III of major histocompatibility complex)

• Male pseudohermaphroditism

—Testicular androgen synthesis enzymes deficiency
—Peripheral 5-alpha-reductase deficiency (gene located on chromosome 19)
—Receptor deficiency in target organs (deletion or point mutation of the receptor gene located on chromosome X)

• Mixed gonadal dysgenesis

—Chromosomal abnormalities (most common mosaic 45XO/46XY)
—Other factors are unknown.

• True hermaphroditism: unknown

COMPLICATIONS

• Female pseudohermaphroditism due to CAH

—Salt-wasting syndrome
—Life-threatening adrenogenital crisis 5 to 7 days after birth: severe vomiting, dehydration, and hypotension
—Hypertension in 11-hydroxylase defects

• Male pseudohermaphroditism

—Germ cell cancer in androgen receptors defects

• Mixed gonadal dysgenesis

—Gonadal tumors (30% of untreated cases): gonadoblastoma, seminoma, and embryonal cell cancer
—Wilms' tumor and glomerulonephritis (Denys-Drash syndrome)

• True hermaphroditism

—Gonadoblastoma and dysgerminoma

DIFFERENTIAL DIAGNOSIS

• Gender assignment must be rapid and correct at birth.
• Fluorescence to detect Yq may rapidly define genotypic sex.

—Y-positive subjects are divided according to gonadal symmetry.
  —Gonads symmetrically located above or distal to inguinal ring: male pseudohermaphrodite
  —Asymmetrically located gonads: mixed gonadal dysgenesis

—Y negatives are accordingly subdivided.
  —Symmetrically nonpalpable gonads: CAH
  —Asymmetrically located gonads: true hermaphroditism
—Karyotype is more accurate in ascertaining the chromosomal pattern and in detecting mosaicism (multiple tissues must be sampled).

• Further identification of involved metabolic pathways is obtained by biochemical evaluation (see Laboratory Testing in "Diagnostic Studies" section):

—hCG stimulation test in XY subjects: 2000 IU/d for 4 days
  —Testosterone rises more than 2 ng/mL from baseline: androgen resistance
  —Testosterone rises less than 2 ng/mL: testosterone synthesis defect
  —If testosterone/DHT ratio is >30: 5-alpha-reductase deficiency

 Database

HISTORY

• Family history

—True hermaphroditism and the XX male syndrome are hereditary.
—Other relevant information about members of the family
—Sudden deaths in infancy

• Hirsutism, primary amenorrhea, and infertility
• Virilizing tumors
• Drugs during pregnancy
• Personal history

—Vomiting and failure to thrive in infants
—Impaired or inappropriate pubertal development in adolescents
—Primary amenorrhea
—Unexplained pseudohematuria (menstruation in virilized hermaphrodites)

PHYSICAL EXAMINATION

• Vomiting and dehydration or hypertension in the newborn
• Rectal examination: In a newborn, the uterus is easily detected.
• Development of secondary sexual characters in adolescents
• Gynecomastia
• Hirsutism, development and distribution of body hair
• Genital examination

—Pigmentation of genitalia (CAH)
—Presence and position of gonads: If a gonad is palpable in the groin or in a labioscrotal fold, it is a testis or contains testicular tissue (e.g., an ovotestis).
—Size and aspect of phallus
—Position of urethral or urogenital sinus meatus
—Location of a vaginal introitus, if any

(continued)

Intersex Disorders (continued)

 Diagnostic Studies

LABORATORY TESTING

- Genetic analysis

—Amniocentesis and PCR analysis of involved genes may allow for prenatal diagnosis of CAH.
—Rapid analysis at birth
  —Barr bodies (inactivated second X chromosome): unreliable
  —Fluorescence to detect Yq
  —PCR analysis to detect SRY zone of Yp
—Karyotype
—PCR analysis of single genes involved in sex determination
—Biochemical testing: Specific enzyme defects are identified based on the type of steroid excreted in the urine.
  —3-beta-hydroxysteroid DH: dehydroepiandrosterone (DHEA)
  —21-hydroxylase: 17-hydroxyprogesterone
  —11-hydroxylase: 11-deoxycorticosterone (DCS), 11-deoxycortisol (DOC)
  —17-KS-reductase: androstenedione (ADS)
  —hCG stimulation test: See Differential Diagnosis in "Basics" section above.

IMAGING

- Abdominal ultrasound
- Genitography

SPECIAL STUDIES

- Laparoscopy with gonadal biopsy
- Laparotomy and biopsy

 Treatment

GENERAL MEASURES

- Intersex treatment requires a team approach, including a pediatric endocrinologist, a urologist, a geneticist, and a psychologist.

MEDICAL

- Female pseudohermaphroditism due to CAH

—Prenatal diagnosis: dexamethasone starting by fifth or sixth week of gestation; treatment is discontinued in males, but continued to term in affected females.
—Postnatal treatment: oral hydrocortisone 8 to 10 mg/m^2/d, or cortisone acetate 25 mg/IV plus fluorocortisone 0.05 mg to 0.2 mg/d in salt-wasting syndromes
—Adrenogenital crisis: Hydrate with half-strength saline in 5% to 10% dextrose plus hydrocortisone Na succinate (25 mg/IV in newborn; 50–100 mg in older patients).

- Male pseudohermaphrodites

—Reared as males: (after diagnosis) testosterone 10 to 25 mg IM once a month per 3 months to observe penile growth; then testosterone replacement at puberty
—Reared as females: estrogen replacement at adolescence
—Enzyme deficiency: Replace minerals and glucocorticoids (see above).
—True hermaphrodites and mixed gonadal dysgenesis: hormonal replacement at adolescence according to sex of rearing

SURGICAL

- All female pseudohermaphrodites and patients with complete androgen receptor deficiency must be reared as females.
- All other intersex patients may be reared as male or female according to the size of the phallus and the degree of masculinization of external genitalia. Most patients are assigned to the female gender.
- Feminizing genitoplasty

—Clitoral reduction
—Exteriorization of vagina and vulvovaginoplasty, possibly as a single-stage procedure in infancy
—Remove dysgenetic gonads.

- Male reconstruction

—Pretreatment with testosterone to make the repair easier
—Staged hypospadias repair
—Remove Müllerian remnants and dysgenetic gonads.
—Pex the testes in the scrotum.
—Correct the prepenile scrotum.

ALTERNATIVE THERAPIES: N/A

PATIENT EDUCATION

- After feminizing genitoplasty, patients of appropriate age are taught to self-dilate the vaginal introitus to avoid stenosis.
- Situations requiring increase in hormonal supplementation: fever and infectious diseases, surgery, exposure to a hot environment

Follow-Up

MONITORING

- Electrolytes, growth chart, urinary steroids

PREVENTION

- Gonadoblastoma and germ cell cancer in retained dysgenetic gonads
- Seminoma in testes
- Osteomalacia due to lack in estrogens (start replacement early!)

 Miscellaneous

SYNONYMS

- Ambiguous genitalia

ASSOCIATED CONDITIONS: N/A

NOTES

- See also Section I, "Ambiguous Genitalia."

ABBREVIATIONS

- CAH, congenital adrenal hyperplasia; MIS, Müllerian inhibitory substance; hCG, human chorionic gonadotropin; DHT, dihydrotestosterone; PCR, polymerase chain reaction

REFERENCES

Aaronson IA. Sexual differentiation and intersexuality. In: Kelalis P, King L, Belman B, eds. *Clinical Pediatric Urology*, 3rd ed. Philadelphia: WB Saunders, 1992:977–1014.

Donahoe PK, Schnitzer JJ. Ambiguous genitalia in the newborn. In: O'Neill T, et al. eds. *Pediatric Surgery*, 5th ed. St. Louis: Mosby, 1998:1797–1818.

Hensle TW, Kennedy WA II. Surgical management of intersexuality. In: Walsh PC, Retik AB, Vaughan ED, Wein AJ, eds. *Campbell's Urology*, 7th ed. Philadelphia: WB Saunders, 1998:2155–2171.

Mandell J. Sexual differentiation: Normal and abnormal. In: Walsh PC, Retik AB, Vaughan ED, Wein AJ, eds. *Campbell's Urology*, 7th ed. Philadelphia: WB Saunders, 1998:2145–2154.

Authors: Douglas A. Canning and Emilio Merlini

Interstitial Cystitis

 Basics

DESCRIPTION

- Interstitial cystitis (IC) is a chronic inflammatory condition of the bladder, characterized by irritative voiding symptoms with bladder and/or pelvic pain. The etiology is unknown, and the diagnosis of IC is one of exclusion.

EPIDEMIOLOGY

- Prevalence estimates of 10.8 to 30 cases/100,000 population
- Female-to-male ratio: 10:1
- More common among Jewish women (14%), compared with the general population (3%)
- Rarely found in African Americans
- Average age of onset: third to fourth decade
- Up to 50% of patients experience spontaneous regression.

GENETICS

- The HLA-DR6 allele may be associated with a specific gene for IC.

STAGING

- The National Institute of Arthritis, Diabetes, Digestive, and Kidney Diseases (NIADDK) in 1987 (revised a year later) established a research criteria as a guide to homogenize the IC patients under study. This has become a defacto definition of the disease.
- Exclusion criteria

—Frequency of urination; while awake, <8 times/d
—Duration of symptoms <9 months
—Radiation cystitis
—Cyclophosphamide or any chemical cystitis
—TB cystitis
—Absence of nocturia
—Symptoms relieved by antibiotics, anticholinergics, or antispasmodics
—Vaginitis
—Age <18 years old
—Active genital herpes
—Uterine, cervical, vaginal, or urethral cancer
—Urethral diverticulum
—Bacterial cystitis or prostatitis within a 3-month period
—Benign or malignant bladder tumors
—Bladder capacity of >350 mL on awake cystometry
—Absence of intense urge to void with bladder filled to 100 to 150 mL during cystometry
—Phasic involuntary bladder contractions on cystometry using fill rate of 30 to 100 mL/min
—Bladder or ureteral calculi in cystoscopy

- Inclusion criteria

—Pain associated with bladder or urinary urgency
—Glomerulations or Hunner's ulcer after cystoscopy and hydrodistention

SIGNS AND SYMPTOMS

- Disease onset is usually subacute, with symptoms including

—Intense frequency, nocturia, urgency
—Bladder and/or pelvic pain

- Less common symptoms

—Dyspareunia
—Hematuria

PATHOPHYSIOLOGY

- Currently, there are no pathognomonic histologic characteristics of IC.

—Suburothelial edema and telangiectasia are the only consistently observed histopathologic features in classic and nonulcer IC.

- Grossly: On cystoscopic evaluation, in about <10% of cases one may see chronic inflammatory cell infiltrate, and the "Hunner's ulcer" described by Hunner in 1915, considered classic IC.
- A recent detailed ultrastructural study of bladder biopsies of IC patients posthydrodistention has revealed distinctive features in nonulcer IC.

—Discohesive urothelium with disrupted permeability barrier and accelerated turnover; querciphylloid profiles of detrusor muscles cells; damage of intrinsic nerves and blood vessel walls.

CAUSES/RISK FACTORS

- Unknown etiology. Suggested theories include

—Infectious agents: Few studies suggest an infectious cause: No specific bacterial agent has been isolated; however, secondary infection is a common feature.
—Increase in mast cells, with release of histamine
—Defect in epithelial permeability of bladder surface glycosaminoglycan (GAG) layer
—Neurogenic inflammation: Neuropeptides can exert direct effects on vascular smooth muscle endothelium and initiate inflammatory changes.
—Autoimmunity
—Reflex sympathetic dystrophy (RDS): a neurovascular pain syndrome with abnormalities in sympathetic outflow leading to constriction of blood vessels and tissue ischemia; no conclusive studies
—Inherent urine toxin

COMPLICATIONS: N/A

DIFFERENTIAL DIAGNOSIS

- UTI
- Neurogenic bladder
- Vaginitis or urethritis
- CIS
- Radiation, chemical or TB cystitis

 Database

HISTORY

- The patient may have associated systemic disease, including fibromyalgia, systemic lupus erythematous, and Sjögren syndrome.
- Need to rule out other causes of cystitis

—Chemotherapy drugs, radiation, TB, or infection

- Patients are likely to report a history of childhood bladder problems.
- Duration of symptoms prior to presentation usually 3 to 5 years
- Patients usually can remember the exact day or week symptoms began.
- Disease onset is subacute rather than insidious.
- Pattern of voiding

—Frequency >8 times per day
—Patients usually do not respond to anticholinergics or antispasmodics.

PHYSICAL EXAMINATION

- Typically unremarkable
- Pelvic examination

—Rule out herpetic lesions, GU malignancy, or urethral diverticulum.

Diagnostic Studies

LABORATORY TESTING

- Urine analysis and culture

—A positive urine culture is indicative of UTI and precludes a diagnosis of IC.
—>5 RBCs is significant and should warrant the usual hematuria work-up.

- Urine cytology

—Helpful to exclude diagnosis of TCC of bladder, particularly CIS

IMAGING

- Routinely, no imaging tools are necessary in the diagnosis of IC.

SPECIAL STUDIES

- Cysto and bladder biopsy
- Urodynamics/VUD

—Sensory urgency, characteristic finding
—A >350-cc bladder capacity excludes diagnosis.
—Absence of urgency to void with filling excludes diagnosis.

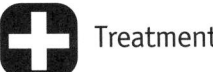 Treatment

GENERAL MEASURES

- Cystoscopy with hydrodistention of the bladder under GA for 1 to 2 minutes at 80 to 100 cm of water pressure is the first therapeutic modality and is often part of the diagnostic evaluation.
- Assess symptoms after hydrodistention.
- Start with the least invasive therapy, which may include watchful waiting.

MEDICAL

- Amitriptyline 25 mg qhs; may increase up to 75 mg per dose
- Hydroxyzine 25 to 50 mg qhs; plus 25 mg qd
- Nifedipine (calcium channel antagonist)
- Sodium pentosan polysulfate/Elmiron (PPS) 500 mg tid
- Nalmefene (opiate antagonist)
- Long-term opioid therapy in selected patients
- Intravesical therapy

—DMSO, heparin, Clorpactin WCS 90, capsaicin, lidocaine
—Doxorubicin, GAG, BCG, cromolyn (in trial studies)

SURGICAL

- Last resort after conservative methods have failed

—Transurethral resection of Hunner's ulcer
—Supratrigonal cystectomy with enterovesical anastomosis
—Total cystectomy and urinary diversion

ALTERNATIVE THERAPIES

- Pain diversion by transcutaneous electric nerve stimulation
- Acupuncture

PATIENT EDUCATION

- The patient should understand that there is no cure for this disease at this time and that treatment is directed at controlling symptoms.
- Up to 50% of patients may have spontaneous resolution of symptoms.
- The Interstitial Cystitis Association is an important resource for information and support for patients
- Altering diet and abstaining from caffeine, alcohol, and acidic beverages have improved symptoms in some patients.
- Stress reduction and exercise may be helpful.

 Follow-Up

MONITORING

- prn basis, depending on symptomatology

PREVENTION: N/A

 Miscellaneous

SYNONYMS

- Painful bladder syndrome

ASSOCIATED CONDITIONS

- Allergies (44%), irritable bowel syndrome (30%), SLE, inflammatory bowel disease (7%), vulvar vestibulitis syndrome, Sjögren syndrome

NOTES: N/A

ABBREVIATIONS

- CIS, carcinoma in situ; DMSO, dimethyl sulfoxide; GA, general anesthesia; GAG, glycosaminoglycan; IC, interstitial cystitis; TCC, transitional cell carcinoma; VUD, video urodynamics

REFERENCES

Batra AK, Wein AJ, Hanno PM. Interstitial cystitis. AUA Update Series, Vol XII, Lesson 8: 63, 1993.

Elbadawi A. Interstitial cystitis: A critique of current concepts with a new proposal for pathologic diagnosis and pathogenesis. *Urology* 1997; 49[Suppl 5A]:14.

Jones CA, Nyberg L. Epidemiology of interstitial cystitis. *Urology* 1997;49[Suppl 5A]:2.

Pontari MA, Hanno PM, Wein AJ. Logical and systematic approach to the evaluation and management of patients suspected of having interstitial cystitis. *Urology* 1997;49[Suppl 5A]:114.

Thompson AC, Christmas TJ. Interstitial cystitis—An update. *Br J Urol* 1996;78:813.

Authors: Corlis L. Archer and Ashok K. Batra

Interstitial Nephritis

 Basics

DESCRIPTION

• Syndrome characterized by sudden onset of renal insufficiency. Divided into three categories: drug induced, infectious, autoimmune

EPIDEMIOLOGY

• Infectious is most commonly seen in children
• Adults more likely drug induced

GENETICS: N/A

STAGING: N/A

SIGNS AND SYMPTOMS

• Sudden decrease in renal function
• May present with rash, fevers, and/or flank pain
• Patients usually asymptotic and have recently started new medications

PATHOPHYSIOLOGY

• Infiltration of inflammatory cells into interstitial compartment with sparing of glomeruli

—Edema and infiltration cause disruption of the basement membrane.

• Granuloma formation may occur.

—Deposition of immune complexes are seen in autoimmune-induced nephritis.

CAUSES/RISK FACTORS

• Usually drug induced

—Beta-lactam antibiotics, NSAIDs, sulfa drugs

• Infection

—Systemic infection usually caused by streptococcal infection

• Autoimmune

—Not associated with systemic rash
—Known underlying autoimmune disorder
—Tubulointestinal nephritis and uveitis syndrome: AIN and uveitis usually seen in young girls

COMPLICATIONS

• Acute renal failure
• Interstitial fibrosis
• End-stage renal disease

DIFFERENTIAL DIAGNOSIS

• Pyelonephritis
• Bilateral renal obstruction/obstructive uropathy
• Glomerulonephritis
• Lupus
• IgA nephropathy
• Risk factors

—Analgesic abuse
—Recent addition of new medication, especially antibiotic

 Database

HISTORY

• Any new medications?
• Have there been any recent infections, such as strep?
• Complaints of fever, flank pain, and hematuria?

PHYSICAL EXAMINATION

• Fever or macular, papular rash and unilateral flank pain
• Facial and peripheral edema

 Diagnostic Studies

LABORATORY TESTING

• Elevated serum creatinine
• Peripheral blood eosinophilia
• Urinalysis: gross or microscopic hematuria

—WBC and RBC casts
—Proteinuria

• 24-hour urine for creatine clearance and protein determination

IMAGING

• Renal ultrasound

—Rule out other causes of renal insufficiency.
—Interstitial nephritis: increased cortical echogenicity

• A gallium scan shows increased renal uptake.

SPECIAL STUDIES

• Renal biopsy is the gold standard.

Treatment

GENERAL MEASURES

- Discontinue offending medications.
- Ultrasound-directed renal biopsy often necessary

MEDICAL

- Acute dialysis may be necessary.
- High-dose steroids

—Cyclophosphamide if corticosteroids are not helpful

SURGICAL

- Usually no role, unless open/laparoscopic biopsy needed

ALTERNATIVE THERAPIES: N/A

PATIENT EDUCATION

- Avoidance of offending medications

 Follow-Up

MONITORING

- Periodic creatinine to monitor renal function
- Renal function usually resolves, but may take months.

PREVENTION: N/A

 Miscellaneous

SYNONYMS: N/A

ASSOCIATED CONDITIONS: N/A

NOTES

- See also Section I, "Renal Failure—Acute."

ABBREVIATIONS

- AIN, acute interstitial nephritis; TINU, tubulointerstitial nephritis and uveitis

REFERENCES

Bennett CJ, Plum F. *Cecil Textbook of Medicine.* Philadelphia: WB Saunders, 1996.

Michel DM, Kelly CJ. Acute interstitial nephritis. *J Am Soc Nephrol* 1998;9(3):506–515.

Authors: Gabriel P. Haas and Satbir Singh

Latex Allergy

 Basics

DESCRIPTION

• Individuals with certain medical conditions or occupations that are heavily exposed to products containing natural rubber latex (NRL) may became sensitized to NRL and develop allergic reactions.

EPIDEMIOLOGY

• 7% of health care workers have allergic reactions; patients with spina bifida have an 18% to 40% incidence; no sex or race variations

GENETICS

• No evidence

STAGING: N/A

SIGNS AND SYMPTOMS

• Local reactions: erythema, swelling, papules, and edema at the site of mechanical irritation
• Allergic reaction: from local erythema and swelling to systemic life-threatening anaphylactoid reactions

—Generalized itching, urticaria, angioedema involving skin and gastrointestinal tract
—Respiratory tract: bronchial asthma, rhinoconjunctivitis, dyspnea
—Cardiovascular system: hypotension, tachycardia, shock

PATHOPHYSIOLOGY

• Three types of humoral and cellular reactions to NRL

—Irritant reactions occur when dermal cells are actually damaged by agents such as processing chemicals or donning agents through a process of mechanical irritation. Made worse by
    —Macerating conditions within a moist, confined, occlusive environment; preexisting eczema; mechanical trauma (i.e., scrubbing)
—Type IV delayed hypersensitivity. Clinical signs similar to irritant reactions but different underlying mechanism: acquired immune reaction mediated by T cells and macrophages
—Type I immediate hypersensitivity to protein antigens (Ag)
    —Mediated by B cells and IgE antibodies (Ab)
    —Depends on the allergic potential of the individual
    —The Ag-Ab complex results in the degranulation of the mast cells and basophils with release of histamine, kinins, leukotrienes, and prostaglandins.

CAUSES/RISK FACTORS

• General population risk to become sensitized to latex: 1%
• Certain occupations and medical conditions have a 5% to 60% higher risk.

—Occupations: health care providers, workers in rubber industries, food industries, sanitation and electronic industry
—Medical conditions frequently associated with latex hypersensitivity (also frequently treated by urologists)
    —Congenital: spina bifida and urogenital malformation
    —Acquired: spinal cord injury and cerebral palsy
    —Any group of patients frequently and intensely exposed to latex: repeated surgical procedures and treatments, such as intermittent catheterization, Texas catheters, manual bowel evacuation, etc. (see list of products containing latex in "Miscellaneous" section)

• History of atopy or hand eczema has increased risk for type I reactions to NRL (example: two-thirds of a group of physicians and nurses with latex allergy, where also atopic)

COMPLICATIONS

• Range from local irritation, inconvenience, to fatal anaphylaxis
• Professional career changes to minimize/eliminate exposure

DIFFERENTIAL DIAGNOSIS

• Contact dermatis, eczema other dermatologic conditions
• Allergic reaction to other agents, environmental factors

 Database

HISTORY

• Patients are usually in the high-risk categories, being either institutionalized or unaware of their condition (physicians, nurses, sanitation workers, etc.).
• A detailed history of past reaction to latex should be obtained from the patient, care taker, or medical charts. The severity of the reactions and the level of precaution have to be assessed before any examination or procedure.

PHYSICAL EXAMINATION

• Depends on type of reaction and severity (see Signs and Symptoms in "Basics" section)
• Vinyl latex-free gloves for patient contact

Diagnostic Studies

LABORATORY TESTING

• Routine testing uninformative

IMAGING: N/A

SPECIAL STUDIES

• Skin-prick test

—Frequently used in Europe; reports of anaphylactic reactions deemed the test unsafe in United States

—Most convenient and sensitive method of diagnosis of type I and IV reactions

—Antigen diluted in saline is dropped on the forearm and gently pricked with a lancet

—Determine wheal-and-flare response time.

   —10 to 60 minutes suggests a type I reaction.
   —4 to 6 hours suggests a type IV reaction.

• The radioallergosorbent test (RAST) is a noninvasive screening assay, and is commercially available.

—Currently the most specific test for IgE antibody

—Unfortunately, low sensitivity (40%–70%) limits its clinical utility.

—Diagnosis of a patient with a known history of anaphylaxis should first start with RAST. If this is negative, proceeding with the skin-prick test should be done cautiously by a trained specialist with standby emergency drugs and resuscitative equipment.

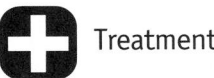 Treatment

GENERAL MEASURES

• The mainstay of the treatment of patients with latex allergy is prevention.

MEDICAL: N/A

SURGICAL

• See Prevention in the "Follow-Up" section below.
• The OR should have a protocol in place for latex allergy precautions.
• Surgical, anesthesia, and OR staff should maintain vigilance for intraoperative/perioperative manifestations of potentially life-threatening latex allergy in high-risk patients.

ALTERNATIVE THERAPIES: N/A

PATIENT EDUCATION: N/A

 Follow-Up

MONITORING: N/A

PREVENTION

• Patients and families need ongoing education to understand the potential for catastrophic reaction.
• Patients should query manufacturers about the content of products about which they are uncertain and should avoid using any products about which they are unsure.
• Enforce regulations for proper labeling of products and discourage use of the term *hypoallergenic,* which is inconsistent and misleading.
• Patients should wear Medic-Alert bracelets and carry an emergency epinephrine kit at all times.
• Protect patients by prominent flagging of charts, rooms, and beds.
• Perioperative management

—Patients, especially those in high-risk groups, should be routinely and carefully questioned about a history of reaction to exposure to products containing latex.

—Review latex allergy protocols with the OR staff before scheduling any procedures.

   —The OR and hospitals should maintain an inventory of latex-free products.

—Prophylaxis by premedication with antiinflammatory agents (steroids) and H1 and H2 blockers has not proved to prevent an anaphylactic reaction.

 Miscellaneous

SYNONYMS: N/A

ASSOCIATED CONDITIONS

• See Causes/Risk Factors in "Basics" section.

NOTES

• Some common products containing latex (this list is not comprehensive; contact manufacturer, if necessary, for a specific product)

—Medical devices: anesthesia masks, catheters, cervical caps, condoms, diaphragms, douche bulbs, endotracheal tubes, esophageal dilators, eyedropper bulbs, hemodialysis machine components, gastric tubes, gloves, Penrose drains, pessaries, tourniquets, surgical implants, syringes, vascular grafts

—Consumer products: balloons, galoshes, household rubber gloves, Koosh balls, rubber bands, scuba diving equipment, shower caps, swimming goggles, swimsuits, tennis shoes, underwear

ABBREVIATIONS

NRL, natural rubber latex

REFERENCES

Hamann CP, Kick SA. What the practicing urologist should know about latex allergy today. AUA Update Series Vol. 13, Lesson 14, 1994.

Hamon CB, Connolly SM, Larson TR. Condom-related allergic contact dermatitis. *J Urol* 1995; 153(4):1227–1228.

Jones JM, Sussman GL, Beezhold DH. Latex allergen levels of injectable collagen stored in syringes with rubber plungers. *Urology* 1996;47(6): 898–902.

Maguerian PA, Klein RB, Graven MA, et al. Intraoperative anaphylactic reaction due to latex hypersensitivity. *Urology* 1991;38:301–304.

Nguyen DH, Burns MW, Shapiro GG, et al. Intraoperative cardiovascular collapse secondary to latex allergy. *J Urol* 1991;146:571–574.

Authors: Mihai Alexianu and Gary H. Weiss

Lyme Disease—Urologic Considerations

 Basics

DESCRIPTION

• Lyme disease, first described in Lyme, Connecticut, in 1975, is a multisystem infection by *Borrelia burgdorferi,* begins with a characteristic skin lesion, erythema migrans (EM), which may be followed by neurologic, cardiac, and joint involvement.

EPIDEMIOLOGY

• Most prevalent vector-born disease in the United States
• In 1994, 13,083 cases were reported in the United States, which is 58% more than in 1993.
• National incidence: 5.2 per 100,000 population in 1994
• Affects both sexes and all ages
• Most likely infected in spring and summer
• The rate of transmission after tick bite: as low as 3%

GENETICS: N/A

STAGING

• See below.

SIGNS AND SYMPTOMS

• Clinical manifestation

—Stage 1 (early localized infection): erythema chronicum migrans, an annular skin lesion
—Stage 2 (acute disseminated infection): cardiac and acute neurologic manifestations
—Stage 3 (chronic disseminated infection): arthritis and chronic neurologic dysfunction

• Erythema migrans (EM): classic early symptom

—Most common and distinctive
—Characterized as an expanding annular erythematous skin lesion that clears centrally
—Occurs in 50% to 70% of patients
—Develops 2 days to 2 weeks after tick bite
—Multiple EM lesions: indicators of hematogenous spread
—Systemic Sx: fever, malaise, headache, stiff neck, fatigue, transient hepatitis, and lymphadenopathy

• Myocarditis or pericarditis: up to 8% of adult patients
• Atrioventricular block: reversible; congestive heart failure
• Acute neurologic disease: acute meningitis, acute encephalitis, cranial neuritis, radiculoneuropathy
• Chronic neurologic diseases: chronic encephalopathy, polyneuropathy
• Arthritis: median period 4 weeks after onset of EM

—In large joints such as the knee; chronic arthritis develops in 10%.

• Urologic manifestation
—Involved in two different ways
  —Secondary to neuroborreliosis
  —Direct invasion of the urinary tract by the spirochete (Lyme cystitis)
—Transient microscopic hematuria and mild proteinuria lasting for 1 to 2 weeks
—Urinary retention
—Urinary urgency, frequency, nocturia, and urge incontinence

PATHOPHYSIOLOGY

• At present, Lyme disease is principally a clinical diagnosis based on the medical history and physical examination, with laboratory studies used for support and confirmation.
• Etiologic agent: *B. burgdorferi*; family Spirochaetaceae, genus *Borrelia*
• Vector: species of *Ixodes* ticks ("deer tick")

—Three-stage ticks (larval, nymphal, and adult)
—Nymphal form
  —Most frequent vehicle for transmission of the infection to humans
  —Cannot be transmitted from one animal to another or from one person to another

• Reservoirs: the white-footed mouse and the wood rat
• Commonly infected along river valleys, lakeshores, and coastal areas because of 85% surface humidity of tick
• Spirochetes readily visible by phase-contrast or dark-field microscope
• Acridine orange, Giemsa stain, silver stains (Dieterle and Warthin-Starry)

—Difficult to demonstrate the spirochete in chronic disease

CAUSES/RISK FACTORS

• Exposure to endemic areas of United States (i.e., coastal northeastern United States)

COMPLICATIONS

• Heart, nervous system, migratory polyarthritis, urinary tract (rare)

DIFFERENTIAL DIAGNOSIS

• Multiple sclerosis
• Alzheimer syndrome
• Pseudotumor cerebri
• Polyneuritis multiplex
• Acute facial palsy
• Psychiatric disorder
• Rheumatoid arthritis

 Database

HISTORY

• Deer tick exposure, history of annular rash or arthritis

PHYSICAL EXAMINATION

• Skin lesion: EM
• Neurologic findings

—Quadriparesis or paraparesis of the lower extremities
—Hyperreflexia and spastic gait
—Cognitive dysfunction and memory loss

Diagnostic Studies

- The diagnosis of Lyme disease is clinical, not serologic.

—Diagnostic criteria from the CDC: (1) a person with EM or (2) a person with at least one late manifestation and (3) laboratory confirmation of infection

LABORATORY TESTING

- Urine analysis: normal
- Culture from punch skin biopsy specimens of EM lesions: proved as high as 85%
- Serologic test: A two-test approach (ELISA or IFA followed by Western immunoblot) is recommended.

—ELISA (enzyme-linked immunosorbent assay): 13% to 73% sensitivity
—IFA (indirect immunofluorescent assay)
—Western immunoblot: specificity (>95%), sensitivity (30%–40%)

- Polymerase chain reaction with primers specific for the outer surface protein A genes (ospA) in the CSF: specific but not sensitive (25%–66%)

IMAGING: N/A

SPECIAL STUDIES

- Bladder biopsy: spirochetal forms consistent with *B. burgdorferi* in the bladder wall
- Urodynamic evaluation: detrusor hyperreflexia or detrusor areflexia

—Detrusor–external sphincter dyssynergia was not noted on electromyography in any patient.

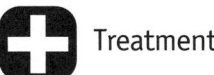 ## Treatment

GENERAL MEASURES

- No evidence to recommend prophylactic antibiotic therapy after a tick bite, even in endemic area
- Treatment based only on laboratory tests and routine testing in the absence of symptoms is not recommended.
- Not appropriate to prescribe a lengthy course of antibiotics for persistent nonspecific symptoms
- Maintain continence and preserve the upper urinary tracts.

—Detrusor areflexia: intermittent catheterization
—Detrusor hyperreflexia: anticholinergics

MEDICAL

- Milder forms

—Doxycycline 100 mg orally twice daily or amoxicillin 500 mg orally three times daily for 10 to 21 days

- Severe forms: central nervous system Lyme disease

—Ceftriaxone 2 g IV or IM daily for 14 days
—Doxycycline 100 mg twice daily for 30 days
—Combination of amoxicillin and probenecid, each 500 mg four times daily for 30 days

SURGICAL: N/A

ALTERNATIVE THERAPIES: N/A

PATIENT EDUCATION: N/A

 ## Follow-Up

MONITORING: N/A

PREVENTION

- Don't sleep with dogs and cats.
- Wear white or light colors and tightly woven fabrics.
- Avoid tall grass and low brush.
- Proper removal of ticks (by tweezers) from the skin
- Permethrin
- Repellents: DEET (diethyltoluamide), indoline, dimethyl carbate, dimethyl phthalate, benzyl benzoate
- Acaricides to gardens, lawns, and the edge of woodland near homes
- Recombinant vaccine; not yet approved in children

 ## Miscellaneous

SYNONYMS

- "New Great Imitator"

ASSOCIATED CONDITIONS: N/A

NOTES: N/A

ABBREVIATIONS

- EM, erythema migrans; ELISA, enzyme-linked immunosorbent assay; IFA, indirect immunofluorescent assay; DEET, *N,N*-diethyl-m-toluamide

REFERENCES

Burgdorfer W, et al. Lyme disease—A tick-borne spirochetosis? *Science* 1982;216:1317.

Chancellor MB, et al. Urinary dysfunction in Lyme disease. *J Urol* 1993;149:26.

Nagi KS, et al. Cardiac manifestations of Lyme disease: A review. *Can J Cardiol* 1996;12:503.

Warshafsky S, et al. Efficacy of antibiotic prophylaxis for prevention of Lyme disease. *J Gen Intern Med* 1996;11:329.

Authors: Suk Young Jung and Michael B. Chancellor

Lymphocele—Pelvic

 Basics

DESCRIPTION

- A collection of lymph fluid in a cavity that is not lined by epithelium. Generally occurs following extraperitoneal surgery

EPIDEMIOLOGY

- Incidence: 0.6% to 18% after renal transplant
- Incidence: 0.7% to 15% after pelvic lymphadenectomy (up to 27% if all patients are imaged with US)
- May also occur after retroperitoneal lymphadenectomy or radical gynecologic surgery

GENETICS: N/A

STAGING: N/A

SIGNS AND SYMPTOMS

- Lower extremity and/or genital edema
- Low abdominal pain or mass
- Deep vein (venous) thrombosis (DVT) (in lower extremities)
- Renal insufficiency (in transplant patients)
- Hydronephrosis (if ureter obstructed)
- Urinary frequency (if compressing bladder)
- Constipation

PATHOPHYSIOLOGY

- Lymph fluid leaks from transected lymphatic vessels following extraperitoneal pelvic surgery.
- The lymph accumulates in the extraperitoneal space and is poorly reabsorbed (intraperitoneal fluid is efficiently reabsorbed).
- Most lymphoceles are asymptomatic, but size and location may result in significant mechanical compression of adjacent structures.

CAUSES/RISK FACTORS

- Inadequate intraoperative lymphostasis
- Additional risk factors

—Prior radiation and/or chemotherapy
—Anticoagulation: Mini-dose heparin is a controversial risk factor.
—Rejection of renal allograft (results in 20-fold increase of lymph flow)

COMPLICATIONS

- Deep venous thrombosis (and pulmonary embolus) from compression of iliac vein
- Lower extremity/genital edema
- Compromised function of renal allograft
- Obstructive/irritative voiding dysfunction

DIFFERENTIAL DIAGNOSIS

- Lymphocele
- Urinoma
- Hematoma
- Abscess

 Database

HISTORY

- Recent pelvic surgery, i.e., PLND, renal transplant, RPLND
- Prior chemotherapy or pelvic radiation
- Timing of onset of symptoms: Abscess, hematoma, and urinoma tend to occur earlier in the postoperative period.

PHYSICAL EXAMINATION

- Palpable abdominal mass
- Lower extremity/genital edema (painful leg swelling suggests DVT)

 Diagnostic Studies

LABORATORY TESTING

- Serum creatinine, BUN (especially to follow renal function in transplant patient)
- Aspirated fluid creatinine and BUN (to distinguish between lymphocele and urinoma), Gram stain and culture (to determine infection)

—Urinoma, markedly elevated creatinine; lymphocele creatinine usually equal to serum creatinine

IMAGING

- Key to diagnosis, but cannot distinguish between lymphocele and urinoma
- Ultrasound

—Pelvic: to identify fluid collection that is separate from bladder, adjacent to renal allograft
—Retroperitoneal: to evaluate hydronephrosis, if suspected
—Duplex study of lower extremities: to evaluate for DVT

- Pelvic CT: best definition of size and location of lymphocele. Can demonstrate relationship to bladder and renal allograft. The allograft ureter must be identified by contrast or by a previously placed ureteral stent (if elevated creatinine prohibits use of IV contrast).
- IVP: may show displacement of ureter and compression of bladder, but is seldom necessary

SPECIAL STUDIES

- Lymphangiography/lymphoscintigraphy: if other studies unclear, may aid diagnosis

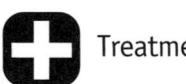 ## Treatment

GENERAL MEASURES

- Treat DVT if present.
- Foley catheter in bladder if patient has significant voiding dysfunction

MEDICAL

- Systemic antibiotics (with percutaneous drainage) if lymphocele is infected

SURGICAL

- Open marsupialization (internal drainage) into the peritoneum is the historic gold standard.

—A window of peritoneum is excised, allowing the lymph to be reabsorbed by the peritoneum.
—Omentoplasty may decrease recurrence by keeping the window patent. Success: 75% to 100%

- Laparoscopic marsupialization is equally effective and less invasive.

—Three transperitoneal ports provide access for excision of the peritoneal window and optional omentoplasty. Success: 77% to 100%

- Open external drainage is an historic procedure, with prolonged drainage and high infection rates (25%).

ALTERNATIVE THERAPIES

- Needle aspiration: good for differentiating between lymph and urine, but high recurrence rate (80%–100%)
- Percutaneous drainage: minimally invasive but requires prolonged treatment (up to 4 months), with risk of infection, especially in immunocompromised (transplant) patients. Success: 70%
- Sclerotherapy (povidone–iodine, 95% ethanol, tetracycline 0.5–2 g in 50-mL NS, bleomycin 1 U/mL): Cavity is aspirated, then filled gently with a sclerosing agent.

—Requires prolonged treatment (3–5 weeks), and may need to be repeated. The intense inflammatory response may be worrisome around the renal allograft. Successful in 70% to 90%

PATIENT EDUCATION: N/A

 ## Follow-Up

MONITORING

- Repeat imaging 2 to 4 months after treatment to detect recurrence
- Late recurrence is uncommon.

PREVENTION

- Meticulous intraoperative lymphostasis is critical, especially in patients with risk factors.

 ## Miscellaneous

SYNONYMS

- Lymphocyst (gynecology)

ASSOCIATED CONDITIONS

- Deep venous thrombosis

NOTES

- Subclinical lymphoceles are common after lymphadenectomy for radical prostatectomy and usually resolve spontaneously.

ABBREVIATIONS

- PLND, pelvic lymph node dissection; RPLND, retroperitoneal lymph node dissection; NS, normal saline; DVT, deep venous thrombosis

REFERENCES

Glass GL, Cockett ATK. Lymphoceles: Diagnosis and management in urologic patients. *Urology* 1998;51[Suppl 5A]:135.

Hamilton BD, Winfield HN. Laparoscopic marsupialization of pelvic lymphoceles. *Technol Urol* 1997; 2(4):220.

Kay R, Fuchs E, Barry JM. Management of postoperative pelvic lymphoceles. *Urology* 1980;15:345.

Authors: Blake D. Hamilton and Howard N. Winfield

Lymphogranuloma Venereum

 Basics

DESCRIPTION

• Aggressive ulcerative venereal disease caused by three of 15 immunotypes (L1, L2, L3) of *Chlamydia trachomatis*

EPIDEMIOLOGY

• Common in tropical and semitropical climates (especially Africa and the Far East)
• Approximately 500 cases per year in the United States, usually among the population that has traveled

GENETICS: N/A

STAGING: N/A

SIGNS AND SYMPTOMS

• Primary lesion

—Painless ulcerations, papules, and vesicles commonly on glans and vaginal wall
　—50% of initial lesions asymptomatic, often go unnoticed
—Urethritis
—Anorectal infections with proctitis: purulent or bloody diarrhea, tenesmus, ulcerations/granulomatous inflammation similar to Crohn disease

• Secondary lesion

—Painful, suppurative inguinal lymphadenopathy
—Tender fluctuant, unilateral buboes in groin (appear 2–6 weeks after exposure)
　—Bubo: tender, firm lymph node collection
—"Groove sign": inguinal and femoral nodes enlarged and separated by inguinal ligament

• Tertiary lesion

—Fistula and stricture formation
—Chronic ulceration
—Lymphatic obstruction leading to elephantiasis

• Constitutional symptoms

—Fever, malaise, myalgias, arthralgias, anorexia

PATHOPHYSIOLOGY

• Sexually transmitted through unprotected intercourse with infected partner
• Incubation period: 5 to 7 days
• Three known LGV strains of *C. trachomatis* virulent and invasive

—Penetrates host cell, replicates, and spreads to contiguous host cells

CAUSES/RISK FACTORS

• Unprotected intercourse
• Multiple partners
• Travel to endemic area

COMPLICATIONS

• Perineal fistula
• Rectal stricture
• Chronic ulceration, chronic sinus formation
• Abscess of supralevator muscle
• Lymphatic obstruction

DIFFERENTIAL DIAGNOSIS

• Syphilis
• Chancroid
• Granuloma inguinale
• Herpes simplex
• Associated HIV

 Database

HISTORY

• Inquire about protected intercourse.

—Any travel to endemic areas?

• History of other STDs
• Painless ulcerations, papules, or vesicles on glans or vulva
• Painful, suppurative inguinal nodes/mass
• Fever, malaise, myalgias, anorexia

PHYSICAL EXAMINATION

• Primary lesion

—Nontender vesicles, papules, or ulcers on glans or labia
—Pelvic examination: lesions on cervix and/or vaginal wall

• Secondary lesion

—Tender groin lymphadenopathy, fluctuant
—Groove sign

• Tertiary lesion

—Groin fistula, chronic ulceration

Diagnostic Studies

LABORATORY TESTING

- Culture for *C. trachomatis* most specific lab test

—Cervical/urethral swabs
—Swabs of material aspirated from buboes

- Complement fixation titers (titers >1:64 strongly suggestive of infection with LGV strains)

IMAGING: N/A

SPECIAL STUDIES

- Direct fluorescent antibody staining for *C. trachomatis*

 ## Treatment

GENERAL MEASURES

- Treat partners who have been exposed.
- Counsel regarding HIV risks/testing
- Test for concomitant STDs.
- Protected intercourse with barrier (e.g., condom, female condom)

MEDICAL

- Doxycycline 100 mg po bid × 21 days

SURGICAL

- For secondary and tertiary lesions

—Aspiration of buboes
—Excision of fistula
—Repair of rectal or vaginal strictures/fistulas

ALTERNATIVE THERAPIES

- Tetracycline 500 mg po qid × 21 days
- Erythromycin 500 mg po qid × 21 days
- Sulfasoxazole 1 g po qid × 21 days

PATIENT EDUCATION

- Safe-sex guidelines
- HIV-risk counseling; increased risk of infections with ulcers (portal of entry)

 ## Follow-Up

MONITORING

- After treatment of primary, groin examination
- Follow-up of tertiary lesions: rectal examination, radiologic investigations if warranted

PREVENTION

- Protected intercourse with barrier

 ## Miscellaneous

SYNONYMS: N/A

ASSOCIATED CONDITIONS

- HIV, other STDs (e.g., chlamydia, gonorrhea, syphilis)

NOTES: N/A

ABBREVIATIONS

- LGV, lymphogranuloma venereum

REFERENCES

Burgoyne R. Lymphogranuloma venereum. *Prim Care* 1990;17(1):153–157.

Faro S. Lymphogranuloma venereum, chancroid, and granuloma inguinale. *Obstet Gynecol Clin North Am* 1989;16(3):517–529.

Goens JL, Schwartz RA, De Wolf K. Mucocutaneous manifestations of chancroid, lymphogranuloma venereum and granuloma inguinale. *Am Fam Physician* 1994;49(2):415–425.

Authors: Jay Lee and Jeremy P.W. Heaton

Medullary Sponge Kidney

Basics

DESCRIPTION

• Medullary sponge kidney (MSK) is characterized by dilated collecting duct tubules in one or more papillae as demonstrated by intravenous urography.

EPIDEMIOLOGY

• Present in roughly 1 in 200 unselected intravenous urograms
• No definitive male:female ratio
• Bimodal pattern: first in adolescence, second in third and fourth decades
• Has been associated with Ehlers-Danlos syndrome, congenital pyloric stenosis, and hyperparathyroidism

GENETICS

• Most cases are sporadic.
• Autosomal dominant inheritance has been described.

STAGING: N/A

SIGNS AND SYMPTOMS

• Flank pain and renal colic from associated renal calculi

—Pain may be related to passage of ureteral calculi, but not necessarily.

• Urinary tract infection
• Hematuria

PATHOPHYSIOLOGY

• Terminal collecting ducts (ducts of Bellini) are dilated.

—Confined to papillary portions of pyramids
—Frequently contain calculi

• Kidneys may be asymmetric, the more involved kidney generally the larger.

—Most cases are bilateral, but may involve only one papilla.

• Cystic spaces found in tip of affected papillae

—Calculi form in cysts, in part due to stasis.
—Medullary nephrocalcinosis is common.

• No cysts in other organs; liver normal

CAUSES/RISK FACTORS

• Cause is unknown.
• Rarely congenital

—Incidence in autopsies of newborns is 2 in 12,000.

COMPLICATIONS

• Uncomplicated MSK: neither symptoms nor abnormal renal function
• Calculi in 60% of patients
• Urinary tract infections in 35%; instrumentation should be avoided to reduce risk of infection, which can be difficult to eradicate.
• Hematuria in 30%
• Papillary nephrocalcinosis common
• Renal failure uncommon

DIFFERENTIAL DIAGNOSIS

• Papillary blush

—Results from normal concentration of contrast in nondilated collecting ducts

• Papillary necrosis

—Not associated with nephrocalcinosis
—One or two irregular cavities in papillary necrosis vs. multiple striations in MSK
—Cavities fill on retrograde ureteropyelography

• Tuberculosis

—Associated with strictures, caseous necrosis

• Calyceal diverticulum

Database

HISTORY

• Often an incidental finding on IVU
• Renal colic may be related to passage of ureteral calculi.
• Chronic flank pain in severe cases
• Urinary tract infection
• Hematuria
• History of recurrent stones

PHYSICAL EXAMINATION

• Usually unremarkable

—Hypertension no more common than in general population

• Costovertebral angle tenderness uncommon

Diagnostic Studies

LABORATORY TESTING

• Urinalysis may show RBCs, WBCs, bacteria, and crystals.
• Urine culture may reveal infection.
• Electrolytes generally normal, but may show decreased bicarbonate consistent with renal tubular acidosis
• Serum calcium and phosphate hyperparathyroidism
• 24-hour urine collection indicated for recurrent stone-formers

—May show hypercalciuria, hypocitraturia, impaired concentration, and/or acidification of urine

IMAGING

• *Diagnosis of MSK is made by intravenous urography,* which reflects the severity of pathologic changes.

—Plain film may be normal or show medullary nephrocalcinosis and/or nephrolithiasis. The pattern of nephrocalcinosis is characteristic of MSK.
—Minimal disease: discrete linear densities in one or more papilla
—Moderate disease: cystic dilatation of collecting ducts in clusters; calculi seen on plain film surrounded by contrast
—Advanced disease: Papillae and calyces are distorted from large cavities; calcifications are large and diffuse. May have associated renal and ureteral calculi

• CT, ultrasound not helpful
• Retrograde usually does not fill many cavities unless performed forcefully; in unusual circumstances, it may help differentiate MSK from papillary necrosis or tuberculosis. It is not generally indicated, since any instrumentation may lead to infection, which can be difficult to eradicate.

SPECIAL STUDIES: N/A

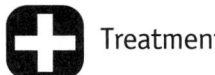 Treatment

GENERAL MEASURES

• Asymptomatic patients require no specific treatment except to maintain a reasonable fluid intake.

MEDICAL

• Recurrent stone-formers should undergo testing to determine the cause.

—Treatment is no different than in other stone-forming patients.

SURGICAL

• ESWL or ureteroscopy may be necessary to treat ureteral stones.
• ESWL has been used to treat nephrocalcinosis in several reported series

—Benefit is uncertain, since few, if any, patients become stone-free.
—Some authors report improvement in frequency of episodes of renal colic.

ALTERNATIVE THERAPIES: N/A

PATIENT EDUCATION

• If a specific metabolic abnormality is identified, nutritional advice may help to reduce the risk of recurrent stones.

 Follow-Up

MONITORING

• Plain abdominal films at 6- to 12-month intervals are indicated to assess progression of disease.
• If medical treatment is undertaken, regular serum and 24-hour urine testing is indicated to assess response.

PREVENTION: N/A

 Miscellaneous

SYNONYMS

• Renal tubular ectasia, cystic disease of renal pyramids, precalyceal canalicular ectasia, Cacchi-Ricci disease, cystic dilatation of renal tubules

ASSOCIATED CONDITIONS

• Nephrocalcinosis, renal tubular acidosis, hyperparathyroidism

NOTES

• MSK is not to be confused with medullary nephrocalcinosis, which can be associated with MSK.

ABBREVIATIONS

• MSK, medullary sponge kidney

REFERENCES

Ginalski JM, Portmann L, Jaeger P. Does medullary sponge kidney cause nephrolithiasis? *AJR* 1990;155:299–302.

Goldman SM, Hartman DS. Medullary sponge kidney. In: Pollack HM, ed. *Clinical Urography*. Philadelphia: WB Saunders, 1990:1167–1177.

Pyrah LN. Medullary sponge kidney. *J Urol* 1996;95:274.

Vandeursen H, Baert L. Prophylactic role of extracorporeal shock wave lithotripsy in the management of nephrocalcinosis. *Br J Urol* 1993;71:392–395.

Author: Francis X. Keeley, Jr.

Megacystis

 Basics

DESCRIPTION

- Megacystis, or an abnormally large bladder, includes congenital megacystis (CM), megacystis–megaureter syndrome (MMS), microcolon–hypoperistalsis–megacystis syndrome (MHMS), and acquired megacystis (AM).

EPIDEMIOLOGY

- CM: variable age of presentation, rare
- MMS: may be seen on antenatal sonogram
- MHMS: rare, more common in females and usually detected early
- AM: variable age of presentation, depending on mechanism

GENETICS

- Unknown

STAGING: N/A

SIGNS AND SYMPTOMS

- Distended lower abdomen/suprapubic area, with or without pain
- Flank pain
- Incontinence (dribbling)
- Foul urine (infection)

PATHOPHYSIOLOGY

- CM: large bladder and large post-void residual (PVR), without obstruction or reflux, normal upper tracts
- MMS: large bladder secondary to massive reflux that leads to refilling (cycling) of the bladder, large post-void residual, with eventual bladder decompensation
- MHMS: unknown mechanism results in functional obstruction to the bladder and small bowel, resulting in extremely large PVR, reflux, hydronephrosis, and dilated small intestine, with hypoperistalsis and malrotation
- AM: secondary to functional obstruction, variable degree of severity

CAUSES/RISK FACTORS

- CM: unknown cause, risk of infection
- MMS: cause related to inadequate intramural ureteral position (inadequate submucosal tunnel), allowing massive reflux. Infection and upper tract deterioration are risks.
- MHMS: unknown cause, may be fatal in first year
- AM: may be due to posterior urethral valves, urethral stricture, voiding dysfunction (sphincter dyssynergy)

COMPLICATIONS

- All: failure to thrive, infection, incontinence (overflow)
- MMS: bladder decompensation (inability to contract), upper tract deterioration
- MHMS: death
- AH: bladder decompensation, diverticula, upper tract deterioration

DIFFERENTIAL DIAGNOSIS

- Constipation
- Tumor
- Pelvic mass: hydrocolpos, torsed ovary
- Prune-belly syndrome (Eagle-Barrett syndrome)

 Database

HISTORY

- Day and/or nighttime wetting
- Symptoms of urinary tract infection
- Poor urinary stream or dribbling (overflow incontinence)
- Difficulty toilet training
- Poor appetite
- Constipation/bloating

PHYSICAL EXAMINATION

- Visible/palpable suprapubic mass
- CVA (flank) tenderness on palpation
- Palpable flank mass(es)
- Dribbling from meatus
- Moist introitus, vaginal pooling

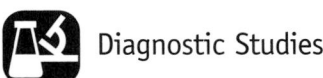 ## Diagnostic Studies

LABORATORY TESTING

- Urinalysis and urine culture
- Serum chemistries (BUN, creatinine, electrolytes) if upper tract injury suspected

IMAGING

- Renal/bladder ultrasound, pre- and post-void views if possible
- Voiding cystourethrogram
- If upper tract injury suspected, renal scan

SPECIAL STUDIES

- Urodynamics: cystometrogram (CMG), electromyography (EMG), urethral pressure profile (UPP)
- Urinary flow study

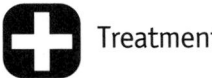 ## Treatment

GENERAL MEASURES

- Treat all acute infections, followed by antibiotic suppression or prophylaxis.

MEDICAL

- As above, and assess renal function; if impaired, nephrology consultation
- Timed voids, with double voids, if inadequate emptying, intermittent catheterization

SURGICAL

- CM: none
- MMS: Repair reflux; initial vesicostomy may be necessary.
- MMHS: parenteral alimentation, bowel plication to improve peristalsis, urinary diversion (vesicostomy)
- AM: Relieve obstruction: resection of posterior urethral valves, incision of urethral stricture.

ALTERNATIVE THERAPIES

- Biofeedback for sphincter dyssynergy

PATIENT EDUCATION

- Patients must be aware of the need for close monitoring of the urinary tract and the long-term potential for renal deterioration.

 ## Follow-Up

MONITORING

- Periodic follow-up with appropriate ultrasound/x-ray/renal scan
- Periodic monitoring of renal function (serum chemistries)
- Monitoring of urinalysis, urine culture

PREVENTION

- Antibiotic prophylaxis for reflux

 ## Miscellaneous

SYNONYMS

- Neurogenic bladder

ASSOCIATED CONDITIONS

- Prune-belly syndrome

NOTES

- See also Section I, "Neurogenic Bladder."

ABBREVIATIONS

- CM, congenital megacystis; MMS, megacystis–megaureter syndrome; MMHS, megacystis–microcolon–hypoperistalsis syndrome; AH, acquired megacystis

REFERENCES

Berdon WE, Baker DH, Blane WA, et al. Megacystis-microcolon-intestinal hypoperistalsis syndrome: A new cause of intestinal obstruction in the newborn. Report of radiologic findings in five newborn girls. *AJR* 1976;126:957.

Inamdar S, Mallouh C, Ganguly R. Vesical gigantism or congenital megacystis. *Urology* 1984;24:601.

Williams DI. Congenital bladder neck obstruction and megaureter. *Br J Urol* 1957;29:389.

Authors: Michael G. Packer and Mark Zaontz

Megalourethra

 Basics

DESCRIPTION

• Megalourethra is a congenital dilatation of the penile urethra.

EPIDEMIOLOGY

• Congenital

GENETICS

• Unknown

STAGING: N/A

SIGNS AND SYMPTOMS

• Gross ballooning of urethra (ventral and/or dorsal) with voiding

—May appear incontinent or experience post-void dribbling from retention of urine in capacious urethra

• Erectile dysfunction

—Complete (deficiency of erectile tissue of corpus spongiosum and corpora cavernosa)
—Partial (deficiency of only the corpus spongiosum)
   —Erections with dorsal curvature

PATHOPHYSIOLOGY

• Maldevelopment/arrest in embryogenesis of corporal erectile tissue

—There are two anatomic variants; however, megalourethra is probably a spectrum with an arbitrary division.
   —Scaphoid (most common variant, deficiency of only the corpus spongiosum, seen with prune-belly syndrome, may be associated with dilatation of prostatic urethra and vesicoureteral reflux)
   —Fusiform (least common, deficiency of erectile tissue of both corpora cavernosa and spongiosum)

CAUSES/RISK FACTORS

• It is theorized that embryologic arrest early in development results in absence or atresia of corporal bodies.
• No identifiable anatomic obstruction

COMPLICATIONS

• Associated nongenitourinary abnormalities may be life threatening.
• Urinary tract infections
• Erectile dysfunction
• Abnormal cosmetic appearance

DIFFERENTIAL DIAGNOSIS

• Congenital urethral diverticulum

—With or without anterior urethral valves

• Urethral diverticulum secondary to hypospadias repair

 Database

HISTORY

• Previous hypospadias surgery suggests acquired diverticulum.
• History of prune-belly syndrome?

PHYSICAL EXAMINATION

• Witnessed voiding

—Urethral ballooning (ventral or dorsal) suggests megalourethra.
—Post-void dribbling suggests retention of urine in the capacious urethra.

• Witnessed erections

—Dorsal curvature implies the presence of corpora cavernosa and absence/atresia of corpus spongiosum.
—Lack of any erection suggests atresia of all corporal bodies.

• Palpation of phallus

—Not a congenital megalourethra if all corporal bodies present and palpably normal
—Excess urethral mucosa and penile skin
—Urethral massage may express pooled urine.

• Associated congenital anomalies, such as prune-belly syndrome

 Diagnostic Studies

LABORATORY TESTING

• Urinalysis to rule out infection; hematuria can be seen.

IMAGING

• Voiding cystourethrogram

—May distinguish from a congenital urethral diverticulum
—May identify concomitant genitourinary pathology

• Renal ultrasound

—May detect upper tract abnormalities

SPECIAL STUDIES: N/A

Treatment

GENERAL MEASURES

• Ensure adequate drainage of the upper tracts.

MEDICAL

• Prevent urinary tract infections.

SURGICAL

• Reduction urethroplasty

—Excision of redundant urethral mucosa and penile skin with reconstruction

ALTERNATIVE THERAPIES: N/A

PATIENT EDUCATION: N/A

 Follow-Up

MONITORING

• Periodic follow-up, including voiding history and voiding cystourethrogram

PREVENTION: N/A

 Miscellaneous

SYNONYMS: N/A

ASSOCIATED CONDITIONS

• Prune-belly syndrome (triad syndrome, Eagle-Barrett syndrome)

NOTES: N/A

ABBREVIATIONS: N/A

REFERENCES

Appel R, Kaplan G, Brock W, Streit D. Megalourethra. *J Urol* 1986;135:747.

Mortensen P, Johnson H, Coleman G, Lirenman D, Taylor G, McLoughlin M. Megalourethra. *J Urol* 1985;134:358.

Stephens FD, Fortune DW. Pathogenesis of megalourethra. *J Urol* 1993;149:1512.

Authors: Mark E. Kolligian and Israel Franco

Megaureter—Congenital

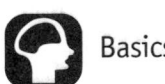

Basics

DESCRIPTION
• This is a collective, generic term describing a dilated ureter. Numerous types and causes; L.R. King classification recommended

EPIDEMIOLOGY
• Most commonly diagnosed by antenatal ultrasound
• The megaureter comprises 20% of antenatally diagnosed urologic anomalies.
• No sex or racial predilection
• Prevalence depends on type of megaureter; cf specific types for these data.

GENETICS
• Unknown, overall
• Certain specific diseases have recognized inheritance, e.g., vesicoureteric reflux.

STAGING
• A grading system proposed by Pfister and Hendren; unlike that for vesicoureteral reflux, may not correlate with prognosis.
• L.R. King classification

—Refluxing
—Obstructed
—Both refluxing and obstructed
—Nonrefluxing and nonobstructed
—Each of the above types can be further subdivided into primary and secondary.

SIGNS AND SYMPTOMS
• Asymptomatic; common

—Incidental detection on antenatal ultrasound
—Unable to determine the cause of megaureter on antenatal ultrasound

• Symptomatic; uncommon

—Urinary infection
—Hematuria
—Abdominal, flank pain
—Abdominal mass

• Features of certain specific disease states

—Prune-belly syndrome
—Posterior urethral valves
—Diabetes insipidus

PATHOPHYSIOLOGY
• Depends on specific type of megaureter

—Primary and secondary refluxing megaureter
  —Primary: deficient longitudinal muscle of intravesical ureter, short submucosal tunnel
  —Secondary: to bladder outlet obstruction and consequent elevated bladder pressure

—Primary obstructive megaureter
  —Aperistaltic juxtavesical ureteral segment 3 to 4 cm long
  —Unable to propagate urine at acceptable flow

—Variety of histologic and ultrastructural abnormalities
—These abnormalities include disorientation of muscle, muscular hypoplasia, muscular hypertrophy, mural fibrosis, and excessive collagen deposition.

—Secondary obstructive megaureter
  —Seen in neurogenic and nonneurogenic voiding dysfunction, infravesical obstruction
  —Other causes: ureteroceles, post-reimplant fibrosis

—Secondary nonobstructive, nonrefluxing megaureter
  —Not discussed in this chapter; noncongenital in nature
  —More common than realized
—Primary nonobstructive, nonrefluxing megaureter
  —Most megaureters in newborns are in this category.
  —Possible causes: "physiological"–transitory; persistent ureteral folds; delays in development of ureteral patency; immaturity of ureteral peristalsis

CAUSES/RISK FACTORS
• See above.

COMPLICATIONS
• Urinary tract infection; stasis of urine probable cause
• Urolithiasis; stasis of urine probable cause
• Progressive renal damage/failure

—Higher risk in primary and secondary refluxing megaureter; secondary obstructive megaureter
• Urinary extravasation/urinary ascites: rare

DIFFERENTIAL DIAGNOSIS
• Entails differentiation between the various types of megaureter and their cause by diagnostic studies mentioned below

Database

HISTORY
• Antenatal presentation

—What is the sex of the fetus?
—Is the megaureter unilateral or bilateral?
—What is the appearance of the ipsilateral kidney?
  —Hypoplastic, dysplastic, or hydronephrotic?
—Is the bladder normal or distended?
—Does the megaureter appearance vary with the state of bladder filling?
—What is the amount of amniotic fluid?
—Any other abnormalities of the urinary tract?

• Postnatal presentation

—Symptoms and signs of urinary infection
—Symptoms and signs of hematuria
—Abdominal/flank pain
—Difficulty with urination
—Polyuria/polydipsia

PHYSICAL EXAMINATION
• Abdominal

—Palpable flank/abdominal mass
—Tenderness
—Signs of prune-belly syndrome

• External genitalia

—No specific abnormality to detect in patient with megaureter

• Spine

—Evidence of a myelomeningocele

Diagnostic Studies

LABORATORY TESTING
• Urinalysis, urine culture and sensitivity to assess for urine concentration, hematuria, and urinary infection
• Serum electrolytes, BUN, and creatinine to assess renal function

IMAGING
• Renal and bladder ultrasound to detect

—Degree of ureteric dilation
—Degree of hydronephrosis
—Quality of renal parenchyma
—Evidence of duplex kidney
—Presence of a ureterocele

• Voiding cystourethrogram to detect

—Vesicoureteral reflux
—Neurogenic bladder
—Posterior urethral valve
—Features of prune-belly syndrome

• Excretory urography (IVP)

—Rarely done
—Useful if level of obstruction cannot be defined or if determination of anatomic detail is complex

• Diuretic renogram (DTPA or MAG3)

—Has limitations; no standardized technique
—Subjective estimates of regions of interest
—An immature neonatal kidney affects the quality of the result.
—Best done after neonate is more than 2 months of age

SPECIAL STUDIES
• Pressure perfusion study (Whitaker test)

—Invasive test/general anesthesia often needed
—Infusion rate of 10 mL/min excessive for young children
—Parameters of obstruction are empirically defined.

• Urodynamic tests

—Especially used for those patients with a neurogenic bladder or nonneurogenic voiding dysfunction

• Retrograde pyelogram

—Rarely indicated unless anatomic detail of ureter cannot be determined by other tests

Treatment

GENERAL MEASURES: N/A

MEDICAL

• Antibiotics

—Short term; to treat acute urinary infection
—Long term (prophylactic), especially for neonate/infant
 —Neonate: amoxicillin drops (50 mg/mL) 25 mg/kg once a day
 —>3 months of age: trimethoprim-sulfamethoxazole suspension (40 mg/5 mL) 2 mg/kg once a day or nitrofurantoin suspension (25 mg/5 mL) 1 to 2 mg/kg once a day
—Prolonged usage in children with megaureter in association with reflux and/or prune-belly syndrome

• Nonoperative treatment with monitoring by repeat laboratory and organ imaging studies

—Particularly in primary nonobstructive, nonrefluxing megaureter
—Many patients with primary nonrefluxing, obstructive megaureter
—Patient selection for reconstructive ureteral surgery in patients with prune-belly syndrome and primary obstructive, nonrefluxing megaureter is controversial.

SURGICAL

• Patient selection for surgery is influenced by the specific type of megaureter.
• Indications for surgery

—Recurrent urinary infection with or without breakthrough on prophylactic antibiotic treatment
—Urolithiasis
—Deterioration of renal function

• Details of surgery for the ureter

—Depends on the type of megaureter
—Ureteroneocystostomy (reimplantation of ureter) without any tapering of the distal ureter is uncommon.
—Type of taper of ureter
 —Excision: Hendren
 —Infolding: Starr plication
 —Overlap: Kaliscinski plication
—Careful preservation of the ureteral blood supply is essential.
—Delicate handling of tissues
—Total tapering of megaureter controversial and done, uncommonly
—Type of reimplantation of ureter into bladder
 —Politano-Leadbetter
 —Cross-trigonal
—Excision tapering almost always stented for 5 to 7 days; plicated tapering not always stented

• Complications of surgery

—Vesicoureteral reflux
—Stricture of the distal ureter
—Fistula between reimplanted ureter and bladder lumen: uncommon

ALTERNATIVE THERAPIES

• Temporary cutaneous vesicostomy

—Uncommon
—Useful in some patients with the prune-belly syndrome, neurogenic bladder, or posterior urethral valves

• Temporary end cutaneous ureterostomy

—Rarely necessary
—Primary reconstruction of the ureter, if necessary, is preferable.

PATIENT EDUCATION: N/A

 ## Follow-Up

MONITORING

• Type and frequency of, is case dependent
• Nonoperative group

—Urinalysis, urine culture and sensitivity about every 3 months or at times of suspected urinary infection
—Serum electrolytes, BUN, and creatinine about every year
—Renal and bladder ultrasound about every year
—Voiding cystogram, depends on the initial type of megaureter
—Nuclear imaging every 1 to 2 years, depending on the type of megaureter

• Operative group

—Monitor urine and serum as for the nonoperative group.
—Renal and bladder ultrasound 1 month after operation and then at 6 months; other ultrasounds depends on the particular patient and type of operation done
—Voiding cystourethrogram 6 months after the operation; thereafter depends on particular patient
—Nuclear imaging; case dependent

PREVENTION: N/A

 ## Miscellaneous

SYNONYMS

• "Wide" ureter, megaloureter, hydroureter, big ureter, dilated ureter

ASSOCIATED CONDITIONS

• Posterior urethral valves
• Prune-belly syndrome
• Neurogenic bladder
• Voiding dysfunction
• Diabetes insipidus

NOTES

• Differentiation between obstructive and non-obstructive megaureters and indications for surgery are controversial.

ABBREVIATIONS

• MGU, megaureter

REFERENCES

Atala A, et al. Vesicoureteral reflux and megaureter. In: Walsh PC, Retik AB, Vaughan ED, Wein AJ, eds. *Campbell's Urology,* 7th ed. Philadelphia: WB Saunders, 1998.

Kass EJ. Megaureter. In: Kelalis PP, et al., eds. *Clinical Pediatric Urology.* Philadelphia: WB Saunders, 1992.

King LR. Megaloureter: Definition, diagnosis and management. *J Urol* 1980;123:222.

Noe HN. The wide ureter. In: Gillenwater JY, Grayhack JT, Howards SS, Duckett JW, eds. *Adult and Pediatric Urology,* 3rd ed. St Louis: Mosby, 1996.

Author: R. Bruce Filmer

Mesoblastic Nephroma—Congenital

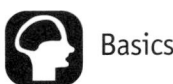 Basics

DESCRIPTION

- A solid renal neoplasm seen in early infancy that carries a remarkably good prognosis

EPIDEMIOLOGY

- The most common renal solid tumor of early infancy, particularly from birth to 3 months of age
- The incidence occurs at a younger age than the peak occurrence for Wilms' tumors.

GENETICS

- None known

STAGING: N/A

SIGNS AND SYMPTOMS

- A palpable, smooth abdominal mass
- Has been associated with polyhydramnios

PATHOPHYSIOLOGY

- Grossly, a solid tumor that resembles a uterine fibroid or leiomyoma on cut surface
- Microscopically, interlacing bundles of spindle-shaped cells with indistinct borders
- Variant with increased cellularity and more mitotic activity, represents a more aggressive tumor

—Some have referred to this more aggressive cellular type as "clear cell sarcoma."

- Almost uniformly benign, with 20% demonstrating a tendency for local recurrence in the more aggressive cellular variant
- Metastases rarely, if ever, are seen with this type of renal tumor.

CAUSES/RISK FACTORS

- None known

COMPLICATIONS

- May be locally aggressive, tendency for local recurrence; rarely, metastases

DIFFERENTIAL DIAGNOSIS

- Wilms' tumor (primary differential)
- See also Section I, "Abdominal Mass—Newborn/Child."

 Database

HISTORY

- A newborn or young infant, usually male, with a palpable abdominal mass
- History of polyhydramnios during pregnancy

PHYSICAL EXAMINATION

- Patients appear healthy.
- Large, palpable, smooth abdominal mass that crosses the midline
- No palpable nodes

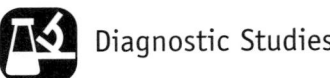 Diagnostic Studies

LABORATORY TESTING

- Serum electrolytes, serum creatinine
- Urinalysis

IMAGING

- Abdominal ultrasound or CT scan

—Solid, smooth, noncalcified renal mass creating distortion of the pelvicalyceal system

- Chest x-ray

SPECIAL STUDIES: N/A

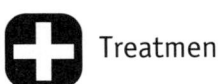 Treatment

GENERAL MEASURES

• Assessment of renal function and contralateral renal appearance

MEDICAL

• No medical treatment or radiation is indicated.

SURGICAL

• Transperitoneal radical nephrectomy with clear margins of uninvolved perirenal margins
• Surgery is both diagnostic and curative.

ALTERNATIVE THERAPIES: N/A

PATIENT EDUCATION: N/A

 Follow-Up

MONITORING

• Serial abdominal sonography every 6 to 12 months for 5 years

PREVENTION: N/A

 Miscellaneous

SYNONYMS

• Fetal renal hamartoma, mesenchymal or leiomyomatous hamartoma of infancy, Bolande disease

ASSOCIATED CONDITIONS

• Polyhydramnios

NOTES

• See also Section I, "Renal Masses—Benign and Malignant."

ABBREVIATIONS

• CMN, congenital mesoblastic nephroma

REFERENCES

Kelalis P, et al. Tumors of the upper urinary tract. In: Kelalis P, et al., eds. *Clinical Pediatric Urology*. Philadelphia: WB Saunders, 1992.

Retik A. Congenital mesoblastic nephroma. In: Siedmon J, Hanno P, eds. *Current Urologic Therapy*. Philadelphia: WB Saunders, 1994.

Snyder HM, et al. Pediatric oncology. In: Walsh PC, Retik AB, Vaughan ED, Wein AJ, eds. *Campbell's Urology*. Philadelphia: WB Saunders, 1992.

Author: T. Ernesto Figueroa

Microphallus (Micropenis)

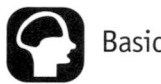 Basics

DESCRIPTION

- Penile length <2.5 standard deviations below mean for age and race, but otherwise normal

EPIDEMIOLOGY

- Statistical definition based on stretched penile length
- Incidence: statistically, occurs in 0.6% of population
- The normal newborn penis is at least 1.9 cm long.
- The term *micropenis* should not be used with other abnormalities of the penis, e.g., hypospadias
- Environmental factors: none

GENETICS

- There is no genetic determinant for micropenis, but some genetic syndromes are associated with it.
- Chromosomes: abnormal number, e.g., Klinefelter and Down syndromes
- Genes: genetic mutation, e.g., androgen insensitivity ("testicular feminization")

STAGING: N/A

SIGNS AND SYMPTOMS

- Signs
—Small penis
- Symptoms
—None, unless part of a syndrome

PATHOPHYSIOLOGY

- Penile development includes androgen-dependent and -independent growth.
- Majority of development depends on secretion of androgens
- First 3 months of gestation
—Maternal hCG causes fetal testis Leydig cells to produce testosterone.
—Testosterone is converted to dihydrotestosterone in the genital tubercle by 5α-reductase type 2.
—The penis and urethra become completely formed during the first trimester.
- Fourth month of gestation onward
—The fetal hypothalamus and pituitary drive testosterone production by the testis.
- Micropenis is generally due to inadequate testosterone stimulation during the second and third trimesters of gestation.
- Additional growth at puberty, ages 11 to 18, due to increase in serum testosterone to adult levels
- Cessation of penile growth appears related to downregulation of AR in the penis.
—Androgen therapy after puberty does not cause growth of the penis.
- Non–androgen-dependent growth: The penis also grows in a relative absence of androgens, indicating biochemical signal amplification or androgen-independent growth factors.

CAUSES/RISK FACTORS

- CNS abnormalities: hypogonadotropic hypogonadism
—Hypothalamus: inadequate GnRH secretion
  —Most common cause of micropenis
—Anterior pituitary: inadequate gonadotropin release; inadequate hypothalamic-releasing factors or pituitary response
- Testes: hypergonadotropic hypogonadism, inadequate synthesis of testosterone
- Androgen insensitivity: AR mutations
- Chromosomal defects: abnormalities of number or genetic mutations
- Rare syndromes
- Idiopathic: no definable cause; diagnosis of exclusion
- Antiandrogen medications taken during pregnancy
- Family history
  —Genetic or familial syndromes
- Advanced maternal age
—Nondisjunction during meiosis, e.g., Klinefelter and Down syndromes

COMPLICATIONS

- Medical
—Related to underlying endocrine abnormalities
—Related to treatment: complications of testosterone therapy (see below)
- Psychological
—Most with persistent micropenis, even after treatment, adjust well to the male sexual role and develop stable heterosexual relationships; however, some refuse sexual intimacy and elect sexual abstinence.

DIFFERENTIAL DIAGNOSIS

- Concealed penis
—Suprapubic fat
—Phimosis due to circumcision
- Webbed penis
- Hypospadias with chordee
- Female pseudohermaphroditism
- Male pseudohermaphroditism
- Hypothalamic—pituitary dysfunction
—Hypogonadotropic hypogonadism syndromes; insufficient GnRH or LH secretion (most common cause: 50% of cases)
  —Kallmann syndrome: most common; low GnRH; anosmia
  —Prader-Willi syndrome: poor muscle tone, short stature, obesity, mental retardation, diabetes, behavioral problems
  —Lawrence-Moon-Biedl syndrome: obesity, mental retardation, pigmented retinopathy (blindness), polydactyly
  —Rud syndrome: mental retardation, epilepsy, ichthyosis
—Isolated hormone deficiencies (hypopituitarism)
  —GnRH deficiency: may occur without Kallmann syndrome
  —LH deficiency: fertile eunuch syndrome; small penis, normal-sized testes
  —Growth hormone deficiency: both deficiency of hormone and effect (Laron dwarfism)
  —Thyroid hormone deficiency
  —ACTH deficiency: leads to cortisol deficiency and circulatory collapse
  —Panhypopituitarism

Microphallus (Micropenis)

- Testosterone underproduction (primary testicular failure)

—Hypergonadotropic hypogonadism (25% of cases)

  —Testicular dysgenesis: hCG stimulation test and radiographic imaging may not detect; requires exploration to remove dysgenetic testes to prevent malignant degeneration; sporadic or familial

  —Klinefelter syndrome: testicular dysgenesis

  —Laurence-Moon-Biedl syndrome (see above): can also be associated with hypergonadotropic hypogonadism

  —Multiple X syndromes

  —Vanishing testis syndrome: intrauterine torsion; bilateral loss results in micropenis

  —Robinow syndrome: mesomelic dwarfism, dental anomalies

  —LH receptor defect/mutation

- 5α-reductase type 2 deficiency

—Usually associated with hypospadias or genital ambiguity

- Androgen insensitivity

—Due to an AR mutation

—Usually associated with ambiguous genitalia

- CNS abnormalities

—Structural brain defects

  —Anencephaly, congenital pituitary aplasia, agenesis of corpus callosum, septo-optic dysplasia, occipital encephalocele, Dandy-Walker cystic malformation of fourth ventricle, cerebellar malformations with ataxia

- Chromosome defects

—Klinefelter syndrome and variants of polysomy

—Down syndrome

—Translocations, deletions, trisomy involving chromosomes 8, 13, and 18

—69, XXY triploidy

- Rare syndromes

—Rud, Martsolf, Gorlin's multiple lentigines, Robinow, Fanconi's anemia, Smith-Lemli-Opitz, Boucher-Neuhauser, Möbius

- Idiopathic: diagnosis of exclusion (10% of cases)

—Endocrine studies show normal HPT axis

—May result from abnormal timing of fetal gonadotropin secretion

—Virilize normally at puberty

 Database

HISTORY

- May suggest a transmitted genetic defect
- Maternal history

—Medications during pregnancy

—Fetal ultrasounds

—Previous stillbirth

—Decreased fetal movements or floppiness at birth: Consider Prader-Willi syndrome.

- Family history

—GU: hypospadias, cryptorchidism, infertility

—Anosmia, deafness, vision impairment

—Major congenital anomalies

PHYSICAL EXAMINATION

- Face: stigmata of chromosomal or midline brain defect

—Microcephaly, hypertelorism (widely spaced eyes), low-set ears, small mouth, high arched palate

- Hands and feet: small size, syndactyly, polydactyly
- Height, weight, body habitus: growth hormone abnormalities, Prader-Willi syndrome
- Skin: nevi or ichthyosis
- Hearing: central brain defects
- Smell: Anosmia suggests Kallmann syndrome.
- Fundoscopic retina examination: pigment changes
- Penis

—General appearance: prepuce, urethral meatus

—Stretched penile length

  —Correlates with length of penis in erect state

  —Measured with a rigid ruler from the base of the penis at the pubic symphysis to the tip of the glans

  —Compare with standards for penile length (nomogram).

  —Measure according to physiologic age, not chronologic age.

—Penile girth: usually normal in relation to length

- Scrotum appearance: development in terms of size, symmetry, rugae
- Palpation of gonads: size, shape, consistency, position

(continued)

Microphallus (Micropenis) (continued)

 Diagnostic Studies

LABORATORY TESTING

- Need to determine central (brain) or gonadal hormone deficiency
- All patients

—Karyotype: Exclude Klinefelter syndrome or a major chromosomal defect.
—Genetic testing: Prader-Willi, Kallmann syndromes (done only at research centers)
—Anterior pituitary screening: ACTH, GH, TSH; measure directly and indirectly (stimulation products).
—Gonadotropin studies: LH, FSH, and T; procedure varies according to age
  —0 to 6 months: Elevated levels of LH, FSH, and T are normal; low T suggests testis failure; confirm with hCG stimulation test.
  —6 months to 14 years: Low LH, FSH, and T levels are normal; check testis function with the hCG stimulation test.
  —Older than 14 years: Increasing LH, FSH, and T levels are normal; baseline LH, FSH, and T levels in micropenis are usually low; diagnosis is usually constitutional delay or hypothalamic dysfunction; do the hCG stimulation test or treat with testosterone injections; if the penis grows, repeat hormone studies in 1 year; pubertal delay may resolve in response to T injections.
  —At puberty, check testis size, which should be increasing at this time, with a Prader orchidometer.
  —When testicular function is proven intact, CNS function is evaluated.
—Diagnosis of androgen insensitivity
  —Increased LH, FSH, and T after puberty
  —Suspect in infant unresponsive to T stimulation, after hCG test negative
  —Confirm with receptor studies on cultured genital fibroblasts or DNA analysis of AR gene

IMAGING

- All patients
—MRI of the head
  —Evaluate the hypothalamus, pituitary, and midbrain.
  —Craniofacial anomalies: Check the optic chiasm, fourth ventricle, and corpus callosum.
  —Kallmann syndrome: Check the size of olfactory sulci.

- Renal imaging

—Should be done in all cases of hypogonadotropic hypogonadism because of association with unilateral renal agenesis
—Initial study: renal ultrasound; DMSA renal scan if ultrasound suggests renal agenesis to detect dysplastic or ectopic renal tissue

- Optional

—MRI of the pelvis to assess corpora cavernosa

SPECIAL STUDIES

- Laparoscopy

—Used for cases of hypergonadotropic hypogonadism (testicular failure) when testes are nonpalpable
—Excludes vanishing testis syndrome and Müllerian duct structures
—Used for hypogonadotropic hypogonadism with nonpalpable testes to determine testicular position before orchidopexy
—Abnormal-appearing testes are biopsied to exclude dysgenesis; abnormal testes are removed.

- Genitogram

—Not generally indicated unless laparoscopy reveals dysgenetic gonads, an ovotestis, or mullerian duct structures or if androgen insensitivity suspected

 Treatment

GENERAL MEASURES

- Correction of metabolic disturbances

—Hypoglycemia: dextrose
—Adrenal insufficiency: hydrocortisone and saline
—Long-term replacement of cortisol, growth hormone, and thyroxine if hypopituitarism present

- Stimulation of penile growth: hCG stimulation or testosterone
- Management of cryptorchidism: orchidopexy or orchiectomy (for dysgenetic gonads)
- Induction of puberty

—Gonadal deficiency: testosterone injections or transdermal patches
—Central deficiency
  —hCG injections: includes benefits of testis growth and spermatogenesis induction
  —GnRH therapy: most physiologic but very inconvenient because requires frequent administration

- Testosterone therapy

—Stimulation of penile growth
—Replacement therapy for hypogonadism
—Long-term use may decrease fertility.

MEDICAL

- Testosterone therapy

—25 to 50 mg testosterone enanthate in oil IM injection for infants/children: diagnostic and therapeutic

- Potential complications

—Closure of epiphyseal plate (limits long-bone growth), behavioral changes (aggression), CNS (unknown)
—Early stimulation of penile growth does not appear to limit ultimate penile length, based on studies of males with CAH.

Microphallus (Micropenis)

SURGICAL

- Penile reconstruction

—Lengthening procedures are generally disreputable and ineffective.
—Penile prosthesis generally not used
—Radial forearm flap reconstruction rarely used

- Orchidopexy for undescended testes

ALTERNATIVE THERAPIES

- Sex reassignment/gender conversion

—Rarely indicated; best done when less than 18 months of age
—Must first demonstrate failure of penile growth with androgen stimulation
—Considered for severe androgen insensitivity/testicular feminization or severe penile maldevelopment

PATIENT EDUCATION

- Psychotherapy

—Address behavioral and psychosocial problems.
—Reassure for concerns about penis size, masculinity, potency, and sex appeal.
—Educate that penis size is unimportant for sexual satisfaction.
—Help establish sexual identity.

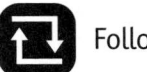 Follow-Up

MONITORING

- Biochemical

—Pituitary and gonadal hormone replacement
—Follow growth, vital signs, electrolytes, glucose, renin, ACTH, GH, TFTs, gonadotropins, and serum testosterone.

- Physical

—Serial penile length measurements and correlation with body growth and established nomograms

PREVENTION

- Family screening and genetic counseling

—Kallmann, Prader-Willi, Laurence-Moon-Biedl, X-linked, and familial syndromes

- Prenatal care

—Amniocentesis or CVS to determine sex and detect chromosome abnormalities
—Fetal ultrasound to detect CNS abnormalities

 Miscellaneous

SYNONYMS

- As above

ASSOCIATED CONDITIONS

- As above

NOTES

- See also Section I, "Ambiguous Genitalia."

ABBREVIATIONS

- ACTH, adrenocorticotropic hormone; AR, androgen receptor; CAH, congenital adrenal hyperplasia; CVS, chorionic villi sampling; GH, growth hormone; GnRH, gonadotropin-releasing hormone; HPT, hypothalamus—pituitary–testis; LH, luteinizing hormone; T, testosterone; T4, thyroxine; TBG, thyroid-binding globulin; TFTs, thyroid function tests

REFERENCES

Aaronson IA. Micropenis: Medical and surgical implications. *J Urol* 1994;152:4–14.

Husmann DA, et al. Micropenis: Current concepts and controversies. AUA Update Series, Vol. XVII, Lesson No. 10, pp. 74–79, 1998.

Lee PA, O'Dea LSL. Testes and variants of male sexual development. In: Hung W, ed. *Clinical Pediatric Endocrinology*. St Louis: Mosby–Year Book, 1992:268–312.

Author: Richard I. Silver

Molluscum Contagiosum

 Basics

DESCRIPTION

• Mildly contagious viral infection confined to the skin

EPIDEMIOLOGY

• Worldwide prevalence: 1% to 8%
• U.S. prevalence: 1%
• More prevalent in children
• Children: boys > girls
• Adults: men same as women
• Prevalence increased in immunosuppressive state

—10% to 20% of AIDS patients have molluscum contagiosum.

• Adult (genital form) increasing in the United States

GENETICS: N/A

STAGING: N/A

SIGNS AND SYMPTOMS

• 2- to 4-mm flesh-colored papules with central depression (umbilicated)

—Usually in groups, but can be single
—Can occur anywhere on body, except palms and soles
—Children: lesions usually on face, trunk, extremities
—Adults: lesions usually on lower abdomen, upper thighs, skin of genitalia
—Usually asymptomatic, but can itch
—Extensive lesions outside genital area in adults rare unless immunocompromised (AIDS, sarcoidosis, leukemia, therapy with immunosuppressive agents)
—Giant lesions (>1 cm) also suggest an immunocompromised state.

PATHOPHYSIOLOGY

• Viral infection

—Caused by unclassified poxvirus (double-stranded DNA virus)
—Occurs only in humans
—Cannot be cultured in vitro

• Disease seen in two different forms: one in adults, other in children

—Adults: spread by sexual contact (lesion in genital area)
—Children: spread by skin-to-skin contact during play (lesions on trunk, limbs, face)
—Can also be spread by autoinoculation or fomites

• Molluscum contagiosum virus infects follicular epithelium
• Viral replication in cytoplasm of epidermal cells
• Hyperplasia and hypertrophy of epidermal cells occur.
• Large oval or brick-shaped intracytoplasmic inclusion bodies (molluscum body or Henderson-Patterson body) seen in epidermal cells microscopically

—Compress nuclei of infected cells peripherally
—Contain viral particles
—Infected keratinocytes discharge into the center of the lesion (pilar canal of infected follicle).
—No neural involvement or nerve root dormancy has been demonstrated.

CAUSES/RISK FACTORS

• Sexual contact in adults
• Immunocompromised patients at increased risk

COMPLICATIONS: N/A

DIFFERENTIAL DIAGNOSIS

• Warts, keratoacanthomas, syringomas, pyodermas
• Large lesions can be confused with furuncles, epidermal inclusion cysts, basal cell carcinoma, or squamous cell carcinoma.
• In AIDS patients, deep fungal infections (cryptococcosis, histoplasmosis, or coccidioidomycosis) may look like molluscum contagiosum.

 Database

HISTORY

• In adults: characteristic lesions in sexually active patient

—Incubation period: 2 weeks to 3 months
—Lesions start as grouped, flesh-colored or pearly papules at point of contact (asymptomatic).
—Lesions progress to develop a distinct central depression.
—Usually 3 to 30 lesions
—A given lesion usually persists for about 2 months.
—New crops of lesions can appear for 6 months to 3 years (autoinoculation).
—In immunocompetent patients, the process resolves spontaneously in 6 to 12 months (as host immunologic response starts to work).

PHYSICAL EXAMINATION

• Adults: 3 to 10 lesions, 2 to 3 mm (rarely can be up to 10 cm), with characteristic umbilicated lesions on lower abdomen, upper thighs, and skin of genitalia, grouped at points of contact
• Children: characteristic lesions on trunk, limbs, face

Diagnostic Studies

LABORATORY TESTING

• Diagnosis often easy clinically: characteristic lesions in expected distribution
• Biopsy if diagnosis unclear, large lesions, or atypical appearance

—H&E prep shows basophilic cytoplasmic inclusion bodies (molluscum bodies) in the stratum granulosum and stratum corneum.

• A crush prep of expressed comedonal plug or curdlike material will show molluscum bodies in cellular elements with PMS or Giemsa stain.

IMAGING: N/A

SPECIAL STUDIES: N/A

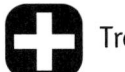 ## Treatment

GENERAL MEASURES

• No specific therapy required

—Self-limited
—Lesions heal without scars unless secondarily infected.

MEDICAL

• If desired, can be treated
• Destruction with liquid nitrogen most efficacious

—May require several sessions

• Simple painting with tincture of iodine may be helpful.
• Electrodesiccation or curettage with a local is an alternative.
• Chemical eradication possible

—Cantharidin in collodion base
—5% salicylic acid plus 5% lactic acid in collodion base
—Phenol
—Retin A cream
—Silver nitrate
—Trichloroacetic acid

SURGICAL: N/A

ALTERNATIVE THERAPIES: N/A

PATIENT EDUCATION

• Adult patients need to understand the sexually transmitted nature of the disease and the self-limiting nature of the disease.

 ## Follow-Up

MONITORING

• Not necessary unless lesions persist

PREVENTION

• Educate patients about modes of transmission.

 ## Miscellaneous

SYNONYMS

• "A nuisance sexually transmitted disease"

ASSOCIATED CONDITIONS: N/A

NOTES: N/A

ABBREVIATIONS

• MCV, molluscum contagiosum virus

REFERENCES

Billstein SR, Mattaliano VJ. The "nuisance" sexually transmitted diseases: Molluscum contagiosum, scabies, and crab lice. *Med Clin North Am* 1990;74:1487.

Epstein WL. Molluscum contagiosum. *Semin Dermatol* 1992;11:184.

Gellis SE. Warts and molluscum contagiosum in children. *Pediatr Ann* 1987;16:89.

Schwartz JJ, Myskowski PL. Molluscum contagiosum in patients with human immunodeficiency virus infection: A review of twenty-seven patients. *J Am Acad Dermatol* 1992;199:583.

Author: Paul R. Young

Multicystic Dysplastic Kidney

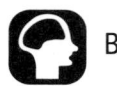 Basics

DESCRIPTION
• Nonfunctioning kidney replaced by multiple cysts of varying size

EPIDEMIOLOGY
• Second most common cause (after UPJO) of abdominal mass in the neonate
• 1 in 4300 live births
• Male:female ratio: 3:2
• Left > right (56% vs. 44%)
• Contralateral kidney abnormal in 10% to 20%, i.e., UPJO, UVJO, renal dysplasia
• Bilateral (Potter syndrome): 20% of cases are incompatible with life.

GENETICS
• Unknown

STAGING: N/A

SIGNS AND SYMPTOMS
• Typically none; most picked up on antenatal US
• Abdominal mass in 13%

PATHOPHYSIOLOGY
• Results from early and complete obstruction of the fetal ureter
• No intercommunication between cysts; associated with ipsilateral ureteral atresia or hypoplasia

CAUSES/RISK FACTORS
• Failed coordination of development of the metanephros and the branching ureteric bud

COMPLICATIONS
• Hypertension: risk extremely low
• Pain: rare
• Infection: rare
• Neoplasia: only 10 cases reported in 25 years

DIFFERENTIAL DIAGNOSIS
• Hydronephrosis due to UPJO
• Cystic Wilms' tumor
• Multilocular cyst (cystic nephroma)
• Cystic mesoblastic nephroma

 Database

HISTORY
• Typically detected in the antenatal period on ultrasounds

PHYSICAL EXAMINATION
• Negative in most
• Abdominal mass: 13% of cases

 Diagnostic Studies

LABORATORY TESTING: N/A

IMAGING
• Ultrasound multiple noncommunicating cysts of variable size. No identifiable renal parenchyma.
• Renal scan (DTPA or MAG3): no function or rarely, minimal function on delayed images
• VCUG: 15% have vesicoureteral reflux to contralateral kidney

SPECIAL STUDIES: N/A

Treatment

GENERAL MEASURES: N/A

MEDICAL

• Nonoperative: 13% disappear by age 3 years, and 23% by 5 years.
• 50% are unchanged at 5 years (but relatively smaller).

SURGICAL

• Nephrectomy: for large size, hypertension, malignancy

ALTERNATIVE THERAPIES: N/A

PATIENT EDUCATION

• Solitary kidney precautions, i.e., avoidance of contact sports

 ## Follow-Up

MONITORING

• US of the abdomen every 3 to 4 months in first year of life; every 6 to 12 months between 1 and 5 years; every 12 years thereafter
• The follow-up schedule may be modified as increased knowledge of the natural history of the condition is acquired.
• Annual BP

PREVENTION: N/A

 ## Miscellaneous

SYNONYMS

• Multicystic dysplasia

ASSOCIATED CONDITIONS

• Potter syndrome

NOTES

• See also Section II, "Renal Dysplasia, Hypodysplasia, and Hypoplasia."

ABBREVIATIONS: N/A

REFERENCES

Kelalis P, King L, Belman B, eds. *Clinical Pediatric Urology,* Vol 2. Philadelphia: WB Saunders. 1992:772–781, 1154–1166.

Minevich E, et al. The importance of accurate diagnosis and early close followup in patients with suspected multicystic dysplastic kidney. *J Urol* 1997;158[3 Part 2]:1301–1304.

Author: Hyman H. Rabinovitch

Multilocular Cystic Nephroma

 Basics

DESCRIPTION

- Multilocular cystic nephroma is an uncommon benign renal tumor.

EPIDEMIOLOGY

- Bimodal incidence: 0 to 4 years in males, >4 years in females (to adult)

GENETICS: N/A

STAGING: N/A

SIGNS AND SYMPTOMS

- Children: asymptomatic flank mass most common
- Adults: abdominal pain and hematuria

PATHOPHYSIOLOGY

- Lesions are bulky and circumscribed by a thick capsule.
- Loculi range from a few millimeters to centimeters and do not intercommunicate.
- Lined by cuboidal or low columnar epithelium
- Must distinguish between those cysts containing foci of Wilms' tumor
- Essential diagnostic criterion

—Lesion must be multilocular
—Cysts mostly lined by epithelium
—Cysts do not communicate with the renal pelvis.
—Mature nephronic elements must be absent from septa.

CAUSES/RISK FACTORS: N/A

COMPLICATIONS: N/A

DIFFERENTIAL DIAGNOSIS

- Multilocular cyst
- Multilocular cyst with foci of Wilms' tumor
- Mesoblastic nephroma
- Cystic Wilms' tumor
- Clear cell sarcoma
- Cystic renal cell carcinoma

 Database

HISTORY

- Flank or abdominal mass in children
- Abdominal pain or hematuria in adults

PHYSICAL EXAMINATION

- Flank or abdominal mass is the hallmark of large lesions.

 Diagnostic Studies

LABORATORY TESTING

- Usually not helpful

IMAGING

- CT and/or US are the diagnostic studies of choice.
- Angiography may be useful if planning a partial nephrectomy.

SPECIAL STUDIES

- Cyst aspiration yields clear to yellow fluid, but is usually not helpful.

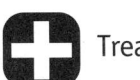 Treatment

GENERAL MEASURES

- Evaluate the contralateral kidney based on imaging studies.
- If there a possibility of Wilms' tumor, the approach is modified.

MEDICAL: N/A

SURGICAL

- The treatment of choice for multilocular cyst is nephrectomy.

ALTERNATIVE THERAPIES

- Partial nephrectomy or enucleation for lesions <2 cm

PATIENT EDUCATION: N/A

 Follow-Up

MONITORING

- If Wilms' tumor treated with local excision, must be followed with US and/or CT scan
- A benign histology requires no long-term follow-up.

PREVENTION: N/A

 Miscellaneous

SYNONYMS

- Mulilocular cyst, cystic nephroma

ASSOCIATED CONDITIONS: N/A

NOTES: N/A

ABBREVIATIONS: N/A

REFERENCES

Eble JN, Bonsib SM. Extensively cystic renal neoplasms. *Semin Diagn Pathol* 1998:Feb. 15:2–20.

Glassberg KI. Renal dysplasia and cystic disease of the kidney. In: Walsh PC, Retik AB, Vaughan ED, Wein AJ, eds. *Campbell's Urology,* 6th ed. Philadelphia: WB Saunders, 1992:1469–1472.

Minevich E. The importance of accurate diagnosis and early close follow-up in patients with suspected multicystic dysplastic kidney. *J Urol* 1997;158[3 Pt 2]:1301–1304.

Authors: Michael Cram and Robert R. Bahnson

Multiple Sclerosis—Urologic Considerations

 Basics

DESCRIPTION

• Multiple sclerosis (MS): a neurologic disease causing focal demyelination of white matter, resulting in mild-to-severe neurologic impairment

EPIDEMIOLOGY

• Most commonly affects ages 20 to 45
• Females with 2× greater incidence than males
• Caucasians highest ethnicity affected; rare in Japanese and Black Africans
• 1 in 1000 people per year in the United States

GENETICS

• Increased risk if MS is present in a first-degree relative
• Identical twin: 300× increased risk if other twin develops MS
• Unknown pattern of inheritance

STAGING: N/A

SIGNS AND SYMPTOMS

• Most common: weakness, visual disturbances, ataxia, diplopia, and sensory disturbances
• Urologic manifestations: presenting complaint in 2.0% to 2.5% of MS patients

—In patients with MS >10 years, 90% will have urologic symptoms.
—Detrusor hyperreflexia with urge incontinence is the most common GU symptom present in 78% of patients with voiding dysfunction.
—Impotence: up to 80% of males
—Detrusor hypocontractility and poor emptying are seen in some patients.
—Detrusor-sphincter dyssynergia (DSD) present in 30% to 65%: leads to poor emptying and possible upper tract damage

PATHOPHYSIOLOGY

• Autoimmune attack of the CNS myelin

—Focal demyelination with relative axon sparing
—Histopathology shows perivenular lymphocytic infiltrates, macrophages within the white matter, gliosis, and scarring.

• GU pathophysiology

—MS affects the cervical spinal cord in the pyramidal and reticulospinal tracts, affecting innervation of the bladder and external urethral sphincter, causing detrusor hyperreflexia and DSD.
—MS can affect the sacral cord: may lead to bladder areflexia and large post-void residuals

CAUSES/RISK FACTORS

• Autoimmune cause

—T cells invade the CNS and attack antigens expressed on the myelin by release of cytokines.

• Risk factors are heritable.

COMPLICATIONS

• The course can be rapid and severely debilitating or mild, with episodes of exacerbation.
• Urologic complications

—Hydronephrosis due to elevated voiding pressures
—Renal insufficiency due to elevated voiding pressures, recurrent infections, and poor emptying (more common in men)
—Recurrent urinary tract infections (UTIs) and pyelonephritis
—Urethral erosion for indwelling catheters left in for long periods of time

DIFFERENTIAL DIAGNOSIS

• With respect to urologic diseases

—Bladder instability due to infection, inflammatory conditions, CIS
—Detrusor hyperreflexia due to other neurologic causes, i.e., CVA, tethered cord, herniated disc
—Sexual dysfunction due to medications or coexisting disease
—Detrusor areflexia due to diabetes, medications, or obstruction

 Database

HISTORY

• Presence of neurologic symptoms:

—Blurry vision, balance problems, numbness, or tingling?
—Lhermitte's sign: an "electric shock" in the arms, back, or legs intermittently associated with stretching of neck or back
—Uhthoff's sign: heat intolerance

• Urinary history

—Stress incontinence or urge incontinence? Note exacerbating and alleviating factors.
—Hematuria or recurrent infections
—Current medications
—Previous pelvic surgery

PHYSICAL EXAMINATION

• Genitourinary examination

—Testicular and prostate examination in male to rule out neoplasm or infection
—Pelvic examination in female to assess pelvic support, rule out urethral or vaginal pathology
—Bulbocavernosus reflex to asses function of sacral nerves (although absent in up to 30%)

• Focused neurologic examination

—Deep tendon reflexes, proprioception, Babinski reflex, and cranial nerve examination

Multiple Sclerosis—Urologic Considerations

 Diagnostic Studies

LABORATORY TESTING

- Urinalysis: concomitant infection or hematuria
- Cerebrospinal fluid

—May see increases in monocyte count or elevated protein levels but oftentimes normal

IMAGING

- MRI

—The most useful tool for diagnosing MS; diagnostic in 70% to 95% of cases
—Increased signal intensity on T2-weighted images in areas of demyelination

- Upper tract imaging

—Rule out presence of hydronephrosis; US a good screening test
—Important in patients with known DSD or in patients with indwelling catheters

- Lower tract imaging

—Lateral voiding cystourethrogram in female helps exclude reflux and calculi as well as assess anatomic support of the bladder and urethra

SPECIAL STUDIES

- Urodynamics

—Absolutely necessary to characterize voiding dysfunction to allow for proper management
—Predicts patients at risk for upper tract deterioration (elevated storage and voiding pressures)
—Demonstrate presence of DSD
—May suggest diagnosis of MS in patient with few other neurologic symptoms
—Need follow-up urodynamics, as patterns of voiding dysfunction may change

 Treatment

GENERAL MEASURES

- Physical therapy and exercise

—Helps prevent muscle atrophy, loss of postural tone, osteoporosis, and deep venous thrombosis

- Avoidance of known stressors

MEDICAL

- Steroids for exacerbations

—Reduces severity of the exacerbation

- Interferon-beta IA: decreases exacerbations by 33%
- Urologic treatment

—Ditropan: 67% to 80% of patients respond for symptoms of detrusor hyperreflexia; however, there is a high attrition rate due to side effects.
—Levsin (hyoscyamine) may add the extra benefit of smooth muscle relaxation and perhaps fewer anticholinergic side effects.
—Clean intermittent catheterization: cornerstone of treatment for patients with hypocontractility or DSD and poor emptying; protects upper tracts
—Avoid indwelling Foley catheters
—Appropriate treatment of UTIs, as MS patients at risk for recurrent UTIs and pyelonephritis

SURGICAL

- Suprapubic cystotomy

—If unable to perform self–intermittent catheterization; avoids urethral erosion; allows for better hygiene; reduces incidence of epididymitis and prostatitis
—Drawbacks include risk of bladder calculi and development of squamous cell carcinoma.

- Sphincterotomy for the male patient with DSD and inability to catheterize
- Augmentation cystoplasty: when conservative management has failed
- Urinary diversion either through ileal conduit or ileovesicostomy

ALTERNATIVE THERAPIES

- Artificial urinary sphincter for the selected patient
- Injection of bulking agents such as collagen or fat for urethral incompetence

PATIENT EDUCATION

- The urologic consequences of MS should be explained to the patient.

 Follow-Up

MONITORING

- Patients with bladder dysfunction secondary to MS can be stratified into low risk and high risk.

—High-risk patients: DSD, elevated storage pressures >40 cm H_2O, indwelling catheters
　—Follow closely for upper tract deterioration, development of squamous cell carcinoma of the bladder, and other problems associated with long-term indwelling catheters.
—Low-risk patients: These patients do not require frequent upper tract imaging.

- All patients should undergo periodic urodynamic testing, especially if there is a change in symptoms, an increase in infections, or an overall worsening of the MS.

PREVENTION

- Upper tract deterioration and renal insufficiency prevention through urologic monitoring, as above

 Miscellaneous

SYNONYMS: N/A

ASSOCIATED CONDITIONS

- Detrusor sphincter dyssynergia

NOTES: N/A

ABBREVIATIONS

- DSD, detrusor sphincter dyssynergia; MS, multiple sclerosis

REFERENCES

Blavas JG, Kaplan SA. Urologic dysfunction in the patient with multiple sclerosis. *Semin Urol* 1988; 8:159.

Mayo ME, Chetner MP. Lower urinary tract dysfunction in multiple sclerosis. *Urology* 1992;39:67.

Walsh PC, Retik AB, Vaughan ED, Wein AJ, eds. *Campbell's Urology*, 7th ed. Philadelphia: WB Saunders, 1998.

Authors: Jeffrey M. Holzbeierlein and Douglas F. Milam

Myasthenia Gravis—Urologic Considerations

 Basics

DESCRIPTION

• Myasthenia gravis is a rare autoimmune disorder in which impaired neuromuscular transmission due to the presence of antibodies against nicotinic acetylcholine (ACH) receptors causes early fatigability and weakness in striated muscle.

EPIDEMIOLOGY

• More common in younger women and older men
• Prevalence rate of 14.2 in 100,000

GENETICS

• Moderate association with HLA-B8 and -DRw3

STAGING

• Focal disease involving ocular muscles only
• Generalized mild-to-moderate muscle weakness
• Generalized severe weakness
• Myasthenic crisis (respiratory depression)

SIGNS AND SYMPTOMS

• Weakness/fatigability of skeletal muscle, increasing with repeated activity

—Ptosis/diplopia common and early; involvement of eye muscles only occurs in 15%.
—Generalized weakness (85%), proximal limb muscles, neck, and diaphragm most commonly affected

• No loss of reflexes, sensation, or coordination
• GU manifestations are uncommon but may include detrusor areflexia or incontinence after TURP in males.

PATHOPHYSIOLOGY

• Antibody-mediated loss of ACH receptors at neuromuscular junctions

—80% to 90% have demonstrable antibody levels by radioimmunoassay (RIA).
—Widening of synaptic gap and flattening of postsynaptic membrane

CAUSES/RISK FACTORS

• Exact cause unknown

—75% of patients have an associated abnormality of the thymus.
—? Immune response to infection

COMPLICATIONS

• Myasthenic crises: rare but life threatening

—Exacerbation of symptoms with commonly used drugs: anesthetic agents, aminoglycosides, corticosteroids, contrast media, and overuse of anticholinesterases

• Urologic complications

—Marked increase in incidence of incontinence post-TURP
—Primary detrusor failure

DIFFERENTIAL DIAGNOSIS

• Drug-induced myasthenia
• Hyperthyroidism, Graves disease
• Lambert-Eaton syndrome
• Botulism
• Progressive external ophthalmoplegia, intracranial mass lesions

 Database

HISTORY

• Classical symptoms of diplopia, ptosis, dysarthria, dysphagia, and peripheral muscle weakness exacerbated by repeated action

PHYSICAL EXAMINATION

• Above symptoms easily elicited

—No loss of sensation, reflexes, or coordination
—Positive Tensilon test

Diagnostic Studies

LABORATORY TESTING: N/A

- Consider screening for thyroid disease with the thyroid function test.

IMAGING

- CT brain, if signs limited to ocular or cranial muscles
- CT thorax to exclude thymoma

SPECIAL STUDIES

- Diagnostic tests

—Anticholinergic (Tensilon) test
—ACH receptor antibody titer (RIA)
  —Repetitive nerve stimulation
  —Single-fiber electromyography

- If urologic symptoms, full urodynamic evaluation, including EMG

 Treatment

GENERAL MEASURES

- Avoidance of known aggravating factors, antimuscarinic agents contraindicated

MEDICAL

- Anticholinesterases (e.g., Pyridostigmine)

—Improvement is usually incomplete and temporary.

- Immunosuppressants

—Response is generally good in conjunction with thymectomy; however, treatment usually needs to be prolonged.

SURGICAL

- Thymectomy

—Complete remission or improvement in 85% of patients

ALTERNATIVE THERAPIES

- Plasma exchange and immune globulin

—Short-term effect but very useful in myasthenic crisis

PATIENT EDUCATION: N/A

 Follow-Up

MONITORING: N/A

PREVENTION: N/A

 Miscellaneous

SYNONYMS: N/A

ASSOCIATED CONDITIONS

- Thymic tumors, hyperthyroidism, other autoimmune disorders

NOTES: N/A

ABBREVIATIONS

- ACH, acetylcholine; RIA, radioimmunoassay

REFERENCES

Christmas TJ. Detrusor failure in myasthenia gravis. *Br J Urol* 1990;65:442.

Drachman DB. Myasthenia gravis. *N Engl J Med* 1994;330:1797–1810.

Khan Z. Urinary incontinence after TURP in myasthenia gravis patients. *Urology* 1989;34:168–169.

Phillips LH. The epidemiology of myasthenia gravis. *Neurol Clin North Am* 1994;12:263–271.

Sandler PM. Detrusor areflexia in a patient with myasthenia gravis. *Int J Urol* 1998;5:188–190.

Authors: Seamus J. Teahan, John P. Lavelle, and Michael Chancellor

Myelodysplasia (Myelomeningocele) — Urologic Considerations

 Basics

DESCRIPTION

• *Myelodysplasia* is a term used to describe a wide range of vertebral column defects, including meningocele, lipomyelomeningocele, and myelomeningocele. Children affected by this disorder often have neurogenic bladder dysfunction.

EPIDEMIOLOGY

• Incidence is 1 per 1000 births in the United States, but has been steadily decreasing over the past 10 years.

GENETICS

• Familial association has been observed.
• When a sibling has spina bifida, a second sibling has a 2% to 5% incidence of myelodysplasia
• Incidence doubles when two or more children are already affected in one family.

STAGING: N/A

SIGNS AND SYMPTOMS

• A neurologic lesion is unpredictable.
• Bony vertebral level of defect can be unrelated to the neurologic level of involvement.

—20% of children have a bony or intraspinal abnormality further cephalad in relation to the vertebral defect and coexisting myelodysplasia.
—Children with thoracic and upper lumbar dysraphias can have a normal sacral spine with intact sacral reflex arcs.

• Consequently, the degree of lower urinary tract dysfunction cannot be predicted according to the spinal or vertebral defect.

PATHOPHYSIOLOGY

• Normal development of spinal cord begins on day 18 of gestation.

—The canal closes in a cephalocaudal direction, with complete closure by day 35 of gestation.
—Mechanism of dysraphism remains undefined

• Myelodysplastic states can be subdivided.

—Meningocele: The meninges or dural sac extends beyond the confines of the vertebral canal. No neural elements are contained in the sac.
—Myelomeningocele: Neural tissue (nerve roots or spinal cord) has evaginated with the meningocele.
—Lipomyelomeningocele: Fatty tissue along with cord structures extrude into the sac.

• Myelomeningocele: 90% of spinal dysraphism

—85% of children have an associated Arnold-Chiari malformation.
   —Cerebellar tonsils herniate through the foramen magnum.
   —The fourth ventricle is obstructed, and ventricular—peritoneal shunting is needed to prevent hydrocephalus.

CAUSES/RISK FACTORS

• Exact cause of dysraphism unknown
• Various environmental and genetic factors have been implicated.
• Folate supplementation prior to conception and during pregnancy has led to a significant reduction of incidence.

COMPLICATIONS

• Usually urologic (UTI, incontinence, neurogenic bladder)

DIFFERENTIAL DIAGNOSIS

• Other causes of neurogenic bladder (see Section I, "Neurogenic Bladder")

 Database

HISTORY

• Developmental and medical histories must be reviewed when neurovesical dysfunction is suspected.

—Acute vs. chronic, stable vs. progressive, and primary vs. secondary to a period of normal continence
—Other neurologic symptoms are present, such as change in bowel habits or gait, onset of leg or back pain, or onset of seizures or other neurologic symptoms.

• Incontinence is a common presenting complaint.

—A detailed characterization of incontinence is important.
—Is it primary or secondary? Stress or urge? Nocturnal vs. diurnal? Strength of stream must be assessed.

PHYSICAL EXAMINATION

• Assessment of gait, balance, muscular development, and general neurologic state
• Reflexes
• Back examination: skin tags, dimples, hemangiomas, hair patches, or any signs of spinal dysraphism
• An attempt to empty the bladder by the Credé maneuver should be performed.
• Genitalia: evidence of excoriation, hypospadias, cryptorchidism, or labiovulvar abnormalities
• Rectal examination: perianal sensation and tone, along with evidence of fecal impaction
• The presence or absence of bulbocavernosal reflex should be documented.

Diagnostic Studies

LABORATORY TESTING

• Urinalysis and culture, along with serum electrolytes/creatinine, should be performed.
• If an elevated serum creatinine is present or any evidence of renal scarring, then a 24-hour creatinine clearance should be performed.

IMAGING

• Plain abdominal x-rays

—Bony abnormalities such as sacral agenesis or widened interpedicular distance
—Rule out severe constipation and calculus disease.

• Ultrasound: good general screening study

—If the ultrasound is abnormal, IVP or nuclear studies are needed.

• VCUG should be obtained if evidence of hydronephrosis, renal scarring, or pyelonephritis

Myelodysplasia (Myelomeningocele) — Urologic Considerations

SPECIAL STUDIES

- Any child with proven or suspected spinal dysraphism should have urodynamics performed.

—The newborn should only have the study performed when the patient can be safely transported to the urodynamics suite.
—It is important to counsel the child and family in order to build an atmosphere of trust.
—Proper patient cooperation is indispensable to obtaining a good study.

- An accurate urodynamic evaluation is essential in the development of treatment guidelines for patients with neurovesical dysfunction.
- Three categories of lower urinary tract dynamics can be defined according to the relationship between the sphincter and bladder contractility.

—Dyssynergy occurs when the external sphincter increases activity during detrusor contraction.
—Synergy occurs when the sphincter completely relaxes during detrusor contractions.
—Complete denervation is observed when a complete lack of bioelectric potentials is seen during micturition or Credé.

- Outlet pressures greater than 40 cm H_2O are the major factors in upper tract deterioration.

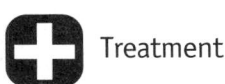 ## Treatment

GENERAL MEASURES

- Children with outlet obstruction and detrusor-sphincter dyssynergia are at the greatest risk for upper tract damage

—Clean intermittent catheterization (CIC) and anticholinergic treatment are instituted in these children.
—These measures limit upper tract deterioration to an 8% to 10% incidence in the setting of high filling pressures or high voiding pressures.

- The neurologic deficits of myelodysplasia can change during periods of growth acceleration, such as puberty.

—Any such change can reveal central nervous system lesions, such as tethered cord, syrinx or hydromelia of the cord, increased cranial pressure, or herniation of the brainstem or cerebellum.
—Due to this phenomena, yearly urodynamics is recommended from the newborn period until 5 years of age.

MEDICAL

- Management of associated reflux

—Occurs in 3% to 5% of neonates with myelodysplasia
—Generally associated with dyssynergia and detrusor hypertonicity
—With no treatment, 40% of children develop reflux by 5 years of age.

- Grades 1–3 reflux can be managed conservatively.

—These children must void spontaneously, have very little outlet resistance, and be able to completely empty their bladders.

—Management here is with antibiotic prophylaxis only.

- Grades 4–5 reflux are managed with intermittent catheterization to ensure complete bladder emptying.
- Any child who is incapable of complete bladder emptying is managed with CIC regardless of grade of reflux.

—This technique of nonsterile intermittent catheterization is used to manage reflux uropathy, upper tract deterioration, urinary tract infection, and incontinence in children with spinal dysraphias.
—Children with detrusor hypertonicity are also treated with oxybutynin in order to achieve lower detrusor pressures.
—The Credé maneuver should be avoided in children with high outlet resistance, detrusor-sphincter dyssynergy, and high intravesical pressures.

SURGICAL

- Antireflux surgery is performed for standard indications.

—Recurrent urinary infections while on appropriate antibiotics and catheterization schedule
—Evidence of persistent upper tract dilation despite adequate bladder emptying

- Achieving continence

—Initial attempts at continence are nonsurgical and involve CIC and anticholinergic therapy.
—At times, a multidrug regimen may have to be employed, including anticholinergics and sympathomimetic drugs.

- Surgical intervention is carried out to treat incontinence when conservative measures fail.

—Usually wait until the child is 5 years old
—Several bladder neck reconstructions have been used, such as Young-Dees, Leadbetter, Kropp, and the Pippi-Salle modification.
—Fascial sling operations and artificial urinary sphincters have been employed to maintain continence.
—Continent urinary diversion is another reliable option utilized to achieve urinary continence.

- Bladder augmentation

—Children may have a persistence of hydronephrotis, reflux, or continued incontinence despite CIC and pharmacotherapy.
—Such children are candidates for bladder augmentations with or without continent diversions, bladder neck revisions, and ureteral reimplants.
—In order to be an augmentation candidate, urodynamic studies must reveal diminished capacity and/or compliance. An adequate bladder outlet must be demonstrated, an adequate length of bowel must be present, and the patient must be able to follow a strict regimen of CIC.

ALTERNATIVE THERAPIES: N/A

PATIENT EDUCATION: N/A

 ## Follow-Up

MONITORING

- A follow-up regimen should be designed in infancy.
- If sonography, urine culture, and urodynamics are normal in a child who is able to spontaneously void, a yearly sonogram is acceptable monitoring, along with close urologic follow-up.
- Long-term monitoring of children with varying degrees of bladder and sphincter dysfunction usually entails yearly sonograms and urodynamic studies.

PREVENTION

- Adequate folic acid intake during pregnancy may decrease risk.

 ## Miscellaneous

SYNONYMS

- Spina bifida, spinal dysraphism, myelomeningocele

ASSOCIATED CONDITIONS: N/A

NOTES

- See also Section I, "Neurogenic Bladder," and Section III, "Tethered Cord Syndrome."

ABBREVIATIONS

- CIC, clean intermittent catheterization

REFERENCES

Bauer S. Neurogenic dysfunction of the lower urinary tract in children. In: Walsh PC, Retik AB, Vaughan ED, Wein AJ, eds. *Campbell's Urology*, 7th ed. Philadelphia: WB Saunders, 1997.

Bellinger MF. Myelomeningocele and neuropathic bladder. In: Gillenwater JY, Grayhack JT, Howards SS, Duckett JW, eds. *Adult and Pediatric Urology*, 3rd ed. St Louis: Mosby, 1996.

Poppas DP, Bauer SB. Urologic evaluation of the myelodysplastic child. AUA update Series, Vol. XVI, Lesson 36, 1997.

Authors: G. Bino Rucker and Dix P. Poppas

Nephrocalcinosis

 Basics

DESCRIPTION

- Radiographically detectable diffuse parenchymal calcification in living patients
- First used by Albright et al. 1934 in patients with hyperparathyroidism
- Some authors define *nephrocalcinosis* as histologically demonstrable renal calcification.
- Calcium salts deposited in renal parenchyma in postmortem examination in 5% to 25% of all kidneys
- Not a single entity but associated with multiple renal diseases
- Not nephrolithiasis (calcifications are located within the pyelocalyceal lumina)

EPIDEMIOLOGY

- Histologic classification

—Dystrophic: Calcification occurs in diseased tissue.
　—Serum calcium and phosphorus levels are normal.
　—Calcium oxalate and phosphate salts are deposited in the renal tubules and interstitium in devitalized tissues.
　—Secondary to ischemia, necrosis
　—Associated with renal infections, neoplasia, or vascular disease
　—Metastatic: Calcification occurs in normal tissue.
　—Secondary hypercalcemia, hypercalciuria, hyperoxaluria, and increased tissue alkalinity or structural abnormality
　—Associated with hyperparathyroidism, renal tubular acidosis, medullary sponge kidney, milk–alkali syndrome, or renal failure

- Radiographic classification by location

—Cortical nephrocalcinosis: Calcification is predominately located in the renal cortex.
　—Acute cortical necrosis: methoxyflurane (Penthrane) anesthesia, chronic glomerulonephritis, ethylene glycol poisoning, Alport syndrome, sickle cell disease, rejected renal transplant
—Medullary nephrocalcinosis: calcification in medullary interstitium or renal tubular lumina
　—Hyperparathyroidism, chronic pyelonephritis, medullary sponge kidney, idiopathic hypercalciuria, renal tubular acidosis(RTA), sarcoidosis, milk–alkali syndrome, vitamin D excess, primary hyperoxaluria, structural abnormalities
—Nephrolithiasis: calcification in the pyelocalyceal lumina
　—Associated with many of the same causes of medullary calcifications

GENETICS: N/A

STAGING: N/A

SIGNS AND SYMPTOMS

- Varies based on etiology of nephrocalcinosis

—A specific disorder can be recognized in most cases, unlike renal lithiasis, in which a cause may not be known.
—Age may correlate with the cause of nephrocalcinosis.
　—It may occur at any age, but elderly patients are more likely to have hyperparathyroidism and children are more likely to have hyperchloremic acidosis (RTA).
　—Sex, familial, and racial factors were not found to be a predisposition in most series.

- Nephrocalcinosis is a radiologic diagnosis, and there may not be specific signs or symptoms.

—Cortical nephrocalcinosis
　—Distinguished radiographically from medullary by peripheral location of calcium deposits
　—Hematuria, proteinuria, urinary tract infection, renal insufficiency, or renal failure
　—Most common causes: acute cortical necrosis, chronic glomerulonephritis
—Medullary nephrocalcinosis
　—Most common causes: hyperparathyroidism (40%) and RTA (20%)
　—Commonly associated with hypercalciuria and often hypercalcemia
　—Radiographic appearance: bilateral clusters of stippled calcifications involving renal pyramids
　—May be difficult to distinguish parenchymal from intraluminal calcifications
　—Both cortical and medullary calcifications may be associated with hematuria, persistent urinary tract infections, renal insufficiency, and renal failure with uremia

- Stones that extrude into the collecting system can cause flank pain and urinary obstruction.

PATHOPHYSIOLOGY

- Cortical nephrocalcinosis
- Acute cortical necrosis: any condition producing prolonged shock
　—Hemorrhage, burns, snake bite, sickle cell, fever, dehydration, sepsis from any cause
　—Fever or dehydration
　—All these conditions lead to ischemia and tissue death in the renal cortex.
　—Ischemia due to vasospasm of small vessels with primary intravascular thrombosis following excessive release of thromboplastin
　—Calcium deposits occur in devitalized tissue.
—Chronic glomerulonephritis
　—Multiple etiology
　—No apparent history of preceding renal disease (85%–90%)
　—Late manifestation of acute poststreptococcal infection (10%)
　—Inflammation of glomeruli that progresses to sclerosis and scarring with deposition of intercellular material, leading to collapse and compression of the capillaries and vascular sclerosis
　—Ischemia leads to progressive atrophy and calcium deposition.
　—Differs from chronic pyelonephritis, which shows changes predominantly in tubules and interstitial tissue, while glomeruli remain intact
—Alport syndrome
　—Nephritis is accompanied by nerve deafness.
　—Late tubular atrophy and interstitial infiltrate and fibrosis with generalized shrinkage of the kidney and nephrocalcinosis
—Rejected renal transplants
　—Interstitial cellular infiltration with edema and tubular necrosis, destruction of glomerulus by fibrous tissue
　—Nephrocalcinosis is more likely seen in slowly progressive rejection than in an acute process.
—Severe primary hyperoxaluria
　—Deposition of calcium oxalate crystals in many organs of the body, including the kidneys
　—Calcium oxalate crystals are deposited in proximal and distal convoluted tubules.
　—Impart a diffuse stippled or subtle homogeneous opacity to the kidneys
—Methoxyflurane anesthesia or ethylene glycol poisoning
　—Intranephronic deposition of calcium oxalate

—Medullary nephrocalcinosis
  —Usually associated with hypercalciuria and often with hypercalcemia
  —Most common cause: primary hyperparathyroidism (40%)
  —Second most common cause: RTA (20%)
  —Most conditions that cause medullary nephrocalcinosis can also cause nephrolithiasis.
  —Metabolic conditions that result in increased filtration of calcium and decreased reabsorption of calcium, resulting in increased calcium excretion
  —Most conditions that cause nephrocalcinosis produce either cortical or medullary calcifications; oxalosis produces both.
  —Any structural abnormality of the urinary tract that allows for stasis of urine predisposes to stone formation based on the principle of increased particle retention time; small stone particles or gravel that would normally pass spontaneously may be retained long enough to allow crystal growth and stone formation.
  —Medullary sponge kidney, dilatation of terminal nephron (distal collecting ducts)
  —Stasis leads to calculi formation in 50% of patients.
  —Calcifications develop in the medullary area rather than in the pyelocalyceal lumen.

CAUSES/RISK FACTORS

• Hypercalcemia: structural abnormality; hypercalciuria: shock, sepsis, ischemia

COMPLICATIONS

• Vary depending on the etiology of nephrocalcinosis

—Renal insufficiency and renal failure: bone demineralization, spontaneous
—Hypertension, fracture in PHP, hematuria, muscle weakness, and coma
—Flank pain or renal colic, hypokalemia of RTA
—Obstructive uropathy, persistent UTI, or urosepsis

DIFFERENTIAL DIAGNOSIS

• In renal nephrolithiasis, we cannot, in most cases, diagnosis cause from radiographic appearance.
• In nephrocalcinosis, the clinical presentation and x-ray characteristics allow identification of underlying disease in most cases.
• Multiple diffuse recumbence calculi associated with spinal injury
• Dystrophic calcifications of renal tuberculosis may be seen in renal pyramids and may mimic nephrocalcinosis.
• Dystrophic calcific foci found in congenital cystic kidney
• Renal artery calcifications
• Milk of calcium
• Calcified "rim" sign in chronic UPJ obstruction, or ureterocele with both hydronephrotic or pyonephrotic changes

—Calcifications with hypernephroma
—Calcification of renal infarction

 Database

HISTORY

• Nephrocalcinosis, clinically, is often a surprise, identified on abdominal x-ray or sonogram. Patients most often have no presenting symptoms to suggest the condition.

—Symptoms, when present, may include blood in urine, flank pain, nausea or vomiting, frothy or foaming urine, weakness, muscle aches, weight loss, headaches, stomach pain or ulcer pain, painful urination, fever, fluid retention, swelling of extremities, mental status change, sleep disturbance, and seizures.
—History of excessive intake of vitamin D, milk, alkalis
—History of bone pain or bone fractures
—History of stone or gravel passage

PHYSICAL EXAMINATION

• More than half of patients who present with nephrocalcinosis will have an entirely normal examination.

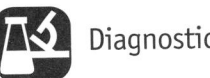 Diagnostic Studies

LABORATORY TESTING

• Diagnosis is made on roentgenographic studies; other clinical laboratory testing to identify nephrocalcinosis may not be necessary.
• Testing to identify a causative disorder may include BUN, creatinine, calcium, phosphorous, uric acid, electrolytes, alkaline phosphate, and albumin.
• 24-Hour urine for calcium, oxalate, uric acid, phosphate, creatinine, protein, citrate, magnesium, sodium
• Urinary pH testing: Have the patient use Nitrazine test paper and record pH over 48 hours.

—Routine urinalysis and urine culture when indicated

IMAGING

• In nephrolithiasis, the radiographic appearance of stones does not allow for a diagnosis.
• In nephrocalcinosis, most often the correlation between the radiologic appearance and clinical features will suggest a causative disease.
• Radiographic extent or degree of renal calcium deposition is not a reliable indication of the degree of impairment of renal function and is not a satisfactory guide to prognosis.
• The prognosis is significantly poorer for patients who have advanced renal insufficiency at the time nephrocalcinosis is recognized.
• Conditions causing hypercalcemia (PHP, sarcoidosis, Cushing disease) tend to produce slight-to-moderate calcinosis with normal or small kidneys.
• Conditions causing hypercalciuria without hypercalcemia (RTA, idiopathic hypercalciuria) produce moderate-to-marked calcinosis with normal or large kidneys.
• The renal damage caused by hypercalcemia has a tendency to produce renal shrinkage. The presence of small kidneys is a poor prognostic sign. A rise in BUN with normal renal size that the impairment of renal function can be temporary or reversible.

(continued)

Nephrocalcinosis (continued)

- *Cortical nephrocalcinosis*

—Acute cortical necrosis: Three patterns of calcifications are seen:
  —Thin peripheral band, often with perpendicular extension into the necrotic Bertin's septa
  —Two thin parallel calcific tracts at the interface of necrotic cortex with viable subcapsular cortex on one side and juxtamedullary cortex on the other
  —Diffuse punctate calcific densities

—Similar patterns of cortical nephrocalcinosis are seen in chronic glomerulonephritis, rejected renal transplant, Alport syndrome, and severe forms of primary hyperoxaluria.

—Diffuse stippled or subtle homogenous opacity to kidney
  —Methoxyflurane anesthesia or ethylene glycol poisoning
  —Diffuse mottled or speckled cortical nephrocalcinosis

—Medullary nephrocalcinosis
  —Hyperparathyroidism (PHP) renal lithiasis more common than renal calcinosis.
  —Nephrocalcinosis appears as millet seed densities confined to medulla.
  —Fine streaks along the line of the ducts of Bellini
  —Medullary nephrocalcific deposits are not confined to the lumen of the nephron, but occur in medullary interstitium.
  —In sponge kidney, the tubular concretions will be engulfed by contrast, but in PHP, the interstitial nephrocalcific deposits will not be engulfed.
  —Contrast-filled ectatic tubules, the hallmark of sponge kidney, will not be seen in PHP.
  —Medullary sponge: round or oval deposits with clear-cut margins situated in the papillary portion of the pyramids, unilateral or bilateral; kidneys usually enlarged

—RTA/idiopathic hypercalciuria
  —Larger calcifications or staghorn calculi are common.
  —Similar radiographic appearance to PHP

—Chronic pyelonephritis: large calcifications of unequal distribution

—Oxalosis: may produce both cortical and medullary calcifications

SPECIAL STUDIES: N/A

 Treatment

GENERAL MEASURES

- Treatment must be tailored to the specific etiology of nephrocalcinosis.

MEDICAL

- Cortical nephrocalcinosis

—Acute cortical necrosis
  —Correct conditions producing shock, fever, dehydration
  —IV fluids
  —Broad-spectrum antibiotics, blood products as needed

- Chronic glomerulonephritis

—Long-term support for renal insufficiency
—Dialysis for renal failure
—Low-protein diet
—Treat hypertension to slow progression of vascular disease.
—Steroids to decrease proteinuria in nephrotic syndrome

- Alport syndrome

—Supportive measures to stabilize and reduce uremia
—Monitor and treat UTI or hypertension as indicated.

- Medullary nephrocalcinosis

—Hyperparathyroidism
—Best treated with surgery to remove parathyroid adenoma
—If the patient is not a candidate for surgery, correct the hypercalciuria with thiazide therapy.
—Monitor the serum calcium level when using thiazides.

- Renal tubular acidosis

—High fluid intake to produce >2 L urine per day
—Potassium citrate (20 mEq bid)

- Medullary sponge kidney

—Maintain aggressive hydration to produce >2 L of urine per day.
—Monitor urine cultures to rule out UTI.
—Rule out possible hypercalcemia/hypercalciuria.

- Hypervitaminosis D: Alter diet.
- Sarcoidosis: Reduce dietary calcium.

—Sodium cellulose phosphate to reduce calcium absorption
—Thiazide therapy to reduce hypercalciuria

SURGICAL

- Prophylactic ESWL for precalyceal calcifications in patients with medullary nephrocalcinosis is disappointing; most studies demonstrate poor fragmentation and poor evacuation.
- Upper tract ureterorenoscopy helps to assess location of calcification and determine which ones are intracalyceal and will respond to ESWL or laser lithotripsy and which ones are in the papillae and will not respond

ALTERNATIVE THERAPIES: N/A

PATIENT EDUCATION: N/A

Follow-Up

MONITORING: N/A
- Perioptic renal function testing
Perioptic renal ultrasound

PREVENTION: N/A

 Miscellaneous

SYNONYMS: N/A

ASSOCIATED CONDITIONS
- See above

NOTES: N/A

ABBREVIATIONS: N/A

REFERENCES

Banner M. Nephrocalcinosis. In: Pollack HM, et al., eds. *Clinical Urography.* Philadelphia: WB Saunders, 1990.

Engel WJ. Urinary calculi associated with nephrocalcinosis. *J Urol* 1952;68:105.

Kreel LN. Radiological aspects of nephrocalcinosis. *Clin Radiol* 1962;13:218.

Mortensen JD, Emmett JL. Nephrocalcinosis: A collective and clinicopathological study. *J Urol* 1954;71:398.

Pyrah LN, Hodgkinson A. Nephrocalcinosis. *Br J Urol* 1960;32:361.

Author: John J. Pahira

Nephrolithiasis/Renal Calculi

 Basics

DESCRIPTION

• Renal stone disease is a major cause of morbidity. Approximately 12% of the American population will form a kidney stone at some time. Prompt diagnosis and therapy are required to prevent complications such as infection, obstructive uropathy, and bleeding. After an initial episode, the incidence of recurrence is about 50% over the next 10 years, increasing up to 75% by 25 years.

EPIDEMIOLOGY

• Peak incidence: third to fifth decade
• Males affected 3 times more often than females
• Infected stones are more common in women than in men (3:2).
• Renal calculi are especially common in Europe, North America, and Japan (high intake of refined carbohydrate with a low intake of crude fiber).
• Prevalence is believed to be higher in those who live in mountainous, desert, and tropical areas.
• Types of urolithiasis

—Pure calcium oxalate stones: 36% to 70%
—Pure calcium phosphate stones: 6% to 20%
—Mixed calcium oxalate and phosphate: 11% to 31%
—Struvite: 6% to 20%
—Uric acid: 6% to 17%
—Cystine: 0.5% to 3.0%
—Miscellaneous: 1% to 4%

GENETICS

• Cystine stones are due to an inborn error in amino acid transport, producing cystinuria.
• A small number of leading gene loci (3–4) are probably the principal contributors to the observed heritability of calcium oxalate disease.

STAGING: N/A

SIGNS AND SYMPTOMS

• Wide variations in symptoms, depending on location of the stone; may also be asymptomatic
• Usually agonizing back pain, abrupt onset
• Radiation of pain to groin, testicles, suprapubic area, or labia
• Hematuria, varying from microscopic to grossly bloody
• Frequency, dysuria, urgency, strangury
• Symptoms related to concomitant urinary infection, as well as fever and chills
• Gastrointestinal symptoms: nausea, vomiting, abdominal distension with associated reflex ileus
• Tachycardia, tachypnea (in the presence of renal colic)
• Costovertebral angle tenderness
• While in acute pain, the patient is usually restless and pale and has cold perspiration.

PATHOPHYSIOLOGY

• Remains poorly understood. A prerequisite for urinary stone formation is urinary crystal formation.
• Some chemical and physical factors are known to play a role.

—Supersaturated urine (overabundance of solute in a solution). Depends on the amount of solute presented to the kidney, urine pH, and temperature). Stones will be formed when the concentration of urinary constituents exceeds their solubility.
—Lack of sufficient urinary inhibitors (pyrophosphates, citrates, magnesium, zinc, and macromolecules)
—Presence of matrix (a noncrystalline mucoprotein often associated with urinary calculi)

CAUSES/RISK FACTORS

• Calcium oxalate stones

—Idiopathic hypercalciuria
　—Absorptive hypercalciuria with an increased calcium absorption
　—Renal hypercalciuria: renal leak of calcium
　—Resorptive hypercalciuria secondary to increased bone demineralization
　—Hypercalciuric conditions
　　—Primary hyperparathyroidism
　　—Hypercalcemia of nonparathyroid origin: malignancy (most common), granulomatous diseases, pheochromocytoma, immobilization, thiazides, exogenous
—Hyperoxaluria
　—80% endogenous in origin, 20% dietary intake
　—Hyperuricosuria: excessive dietary intake of purines
　—Low urinary citrate
—Magnesium ammonium phosphate (struvite, usually mixed with some calcium phosphate)
　—Persistently alkaline urine (usually associated with infection; *Proteus mirabilis* is the most frequent organism associated)
—Calcium phosphate (as apatite or apatite plus brushite)
　—Persistently alkaline urine (renal tubular acidosis, oral antacids, carbonic anhydrase inhibitors)
　—Primary hyperparathyroidism
—Uric acid
　—Persistently acid urine (inability to excrete NH_3 buffer)
　　—Gout
　　—Hyperuricosuria
—Cystine
　—Cystinuria, an autosomal recessive disorder (defective renal tubular absorption)

• Risk factors

—Metabolic state
—Hormonal imbalances
—Environmental factors
—Dietary excesses
—Medications: acetazolamide, antacids, protein supplements, triamterene, vitamins C and D, indinavir

—Anatomic abnormalities leading to chronic infection or stasis (ureteropelvic obstruction, calyx diverticulum, tubular ectasia, ureteral stricture, ureterocele, horseshoe kidney)

COMPLICATIONS

- Infection and sepsis
- Hydronephrosis, loss of kidney function in several degrees
- Pain and disability

DIFFERENTIAL DIAGNOSIS

- Muscular back pain
- Acute appendicitis
- Acute peritonitis
- Salpingitis
- Cholecystitis
- Gastroenteritis
- Colitis
- Diverticulitis
- Peptic ulcer disease
- Pancreatitis
- Ruptured aortic aneurysm
- Pyelonephritis

 Database

HISTORY

- A detailed history must be obtained in all patients: number of urinary infections, calcium and fluid intake, occupation, symptoms of hypercalcemia, hypertension, or renal failure.
- 25% of patients have a positive family history (first-degree relatives), and higher in conditions such as cystinuria and hyperoxaluria
- History of previous calculi (age of onset; type of calculi if available; number of events; most recent event; interval between events)
- Use of medications, previous surgeries

PHYSICAL EXAMINATION

- Special attention to temperature or signs of generalized infection
- Careful genitourinary examination
- Abdominal examination: subcostal and loin tenderness

 Diagnostic Studies

- A simplified evaluation may be used in a single-stone episode. Further, extensive evaluation is required for recurrent stones or patients at high risk

LABORATORY TESTING

- Urinalysis

—Gross or microscopic hematuria (80%–100%)
—Pyuria (culture if infection or fever/chills)
—Crystalluria
—Cystine crystals
—Urinary pH: <5.5, uric acid stone; >7.5, struvite

- Serum chemistries

—Calcium, phosphorus, electrolytes, uric acid, creatinine

- Parathyroid hormone if serum calcium high

IMAGING

- Plain abdominal x-ray

—Radiopaque stones (85% of all stones)
—May miss radiolucent uric acid stones

- Intravenous pyelography

—Can determine if opacity seen on plain x-ray is within the kidney
—May disclose radiolucent stones
—Gives details about collecting system anatomy and kidney conditions
—Shows options for further management of the stones

- Ultrasonography: shows the size of the stone, localization in the kidney or ureter, degree of obstruction, quality of renal parenchyma

—Retrograde ureteropyelogram: useful in special situations
—Computed tomography: shows the size of the stone, localization in the kidney or ureter, degree of obstruction, quality of renal parenchyma
—Spiral computed tomography: very useful in acute renal colic, as a substitute for IVP.

SPECIAL STUDIES

- In high-risk patients

—Serum concentrations of calcium, uric acid, and phosphate
—24-hour urine pH and concentrations of oxalate, phosphate uric acid, and calcium
—Spot urine test for cystine

- Stone analysis

(continued)

Nephrolithiasis/Renal Calculi (continued)

 Treatment

GENERAL MEASURES

- 90% of stones <4 mm pass spontaneously. 50% of stones between 4 and 6 mm pass spontaneously.
- 10% of stones >6 mm pass spontaneously.
- Acute therapy

—Narcotic analgesics for pain relief (IM meperidine, morphine, or buprenorphine)
—Intravenous fluids are necessary in dehydrated patients and to increase urinary flow (facilitates stone migration).
—Ask patients to strain urine up to 3 or 4 days after symptoms cease. It is usual to pass small stones without even noticing it.

- Indications for hospitalization

—Intractable pain and vomiting
—Severe urinary tract infection or sepsis
—Complete ureteral obstruction
—Partial obstruction of a solitary kidney

- Conservative observation

—Depends on stone size, shape, location, and associated ureteral edema

- Dissolution agents

—Depends on stone surface area, stone type, volume of irrigant, mode of delivery
—Oral alkalinizing agents include sodium or potassium bicarbonate and potassium citrate.
—Intrarenal alkalinization must be done under a low-pressure system (<25 cm water). Agents include sodium bicarbonate, 2 to 4 ampules in 1 L of normal saline, producing a urinary pH between 7.5 and 9.0.
—Cystine calculi can be dissolved with D-penicillamine (0.5% solution), *N*-acetylcysteine (2%–5% solution), and alpha-mercapto-propionylglycine (Thiola) (5% solution).

- Relief of obstruction

—Obstructive urinary calculi with fever and infected urine require emergent drainage. This can be accomplished by the placement of a double-J ureteral stent or a percutaneous nephrostomy tube.

MEDICAL

- Hypercalciuric patient

—Thiazide diuretics (e.g., hydrochlorothiazide 25–50 mg twice a day). Dietary sodium must be restricted. K-citrate must also be given to prevent thiazide-induced hypocitraturia. Very effective in renal hypercalciuria and mild absorptive hypercalciuria (type 2)
—Cellulose sodium phosphate (5 g three times a day with meals). Useful in the treatment of absorptive hypercalciuria. Dietary oxalate restriction is often needed, since hyperoxaluria and hypomagnesuria can occur.
—Neutral sodium phosphate (500 mg four times a day) increases pyrophosphate excretion, corrects hypophosphaturia, and decreases calcium excretion in absorptive hypercalciuria.
—Allopurinol is useful in patients with hyperuricosuria (inhibits uric acid production).

- Hypocitraturia

—Citrate as the K salt, since oral Na loads increase urinary Ca excretion

- Struvite stones

—Appropriate antimicrobial agent for at least 6 weeks
  —Eliminate any metabolic predisposition to stone formation.
  —Sandwich therapy: PCNL followed by ESWL followed by PCNL.

- Uric acid stones

—Alkalinize urine to decrease uric acid precipitation (NaHCO$_3$, K-citrate, or Shohl solution, 1–3 mEq/kg/d in 4 doses)
—Avoid purine-rich foods.
—Allopurinol when hyperuricosuria is present (>1000 mg/d)

- Cystine stones

—A large fluid output of up to 4 L/d is required.
—Alkalization of the urine up to pH >7.5 can be tried. However, alkali administration to achieve this degree of alkalosis is difficult and requires 15 to 25 g/d of NaHCO$_3$.
—Dietary restriction of methionine will decrease cystine excretion.
—D-penicillamine forms soluble mixed disulfide bonds with cystine. Used when other measures fail

SURGICAL

- Indications for surgical treatment are persistent pain, intractable with medication, recurrent UTIs, persistent bleeding, damage to the kidney, and/or signs of loss of renal function.
- The best method is still quite controversial. It will depend on localization, size and composition of the stone, patient preferences, surgeon preference, and availability of urologic equipment.
- Options for surgical treatment are mentioned briefly below.

—ESWL: for stones in the renal pelvis, upper or distal ureter, size <1.5 cm. Pregnancy is currently the only absolute contraindication for this procedure. Success rates up to 90% have been reported, according to the size and location of the stones.
—Ureteroscopy with or without intracorporeal lithotripsy: feasible in all portions of the ureter up to the renal pelvis and calyces. Best results are reported in the lower third of the ureter. The higher the stone, the greater the risk of ureteric damage.
—PCNL with or without intracorporeal lithotripsy: stones located in the renal collecting system or in the upper third of the ureter, greater than 1.5 cm, cystine or uric acid stones, struvite, infection, obesity
—Open surgery (very few indications nowadays): large, complex staghorn calculi; stone that is impossible to remove by other means; patient whose health precludes other procedures

ALTERNATIVE THERAPIES: N/A

PATIENT EDUCATION

- Recurrence in untreated patients is 50% to 100%. In treated patients, recurrence is 10% to 15%, depending on stone composition.
- Achieve adequate fluid intake to produce at least 2 L of urine per day (distributed over the day).
- Dietary restrictions will depend on the type of stone.
- Reduce dietary intake of calcium if excessive. Avoid calcium restriction to prevent a negative calcium balance, bone mineral loss, and increased intestinal absorption of oxalate. There is no evidence that calcium restriction is beneficial. The dietary intake of calcium must be at least 800 mg/d.
- Limit the intake of animal protein and foods with a high purine content.
- If hyperoxaluria is present, avoid foods high in oxalate (spinach, cranberries, tea, cocoa, and nuts) and increase intake of potassium-rich foods.
- In the presence of hypercalciuria, restrict NaCl to 6 g/d; intake of vitamin C must be done in moderate amounts.

 Follow-Up

MONITORING

- Assess the effect of medical therapy by measurement of urinary and plasma chemistries 1 to 2 months after initiating treatment, and then yearly.
- KUB x-ray at 3 and 6 months and at 1 year (or less, depending on each case) to identify new stones and assess effectiveness of therapy.

PREVENTION

- See Patient Education in "Treatment" section.

 Miscellaneous

SYNONYMS

- Urinary lithiasis, nephrolithiasis, kidney stones

ASSOCIATED CONDITIONS

- Infections, gout, hyperuricemia, hyperparathyroidism, sarcoidosis, cystinuria, prolonged immobilization

NOTES

- See Section II, "Pregnancy—Urolithiasis" and specific stone topics in Sections II and III.

ABBREVIATIONS

- PCNL, percutaneous nephrolithotomy; ESWL, extracorporeal shock wave lithotripsy

REFERENCES

Babayan RK. Urinary calculi and endourology. In: *Manual of Urology: Diagnosis and Therapy,* 1st ed. Boston: Little, Brown, 1990:123–131.

Curhan GC, et al. Dietary factors and kidney stone formation. *Compr Ther* 1994;20(9): 485–489.

McDonald MW, et al. Urinary stone disease: A practical guide to metabolic evaluation. *Geriatrics* 1997;52(5):38–56.

Stoller ML, et al. Urinary stone disease. In: Tanagho EA, McAninch JW, eds. *Smith's General Urology,* 14th ed. Norwalk, CT: Appleton and Lange, 1995:27–304.

Authors: David M. Albala and Fernando C. Koleski

Nephroptosis

 Basics

DESCRIPTION

- Renal descent of more than two vertebral bodies (>5 cm) when the patient moves from a supine to an erect position

EPIDEMIOLOGY

- More common in thin women, with the right kidney affected more often. Overall, a very rare disease entity

—The radiologic diagnosis far exceeds the occurrence of symptomatic nephroptosis.

GENETICS

- Unknown

STAGING: N/A

SIGNS AND SYMPTOMS

- May be totally asymptomatic, but nephroptosis is noted by radiologic studies
- Symptomatic patients

—Report pain in the abdomen, ipsilateral flank, or pelvic regions when moving from the supine to the erect position.
—Exacerbated by sitting or standing for long periods, increased physical activity, or shaking movements
—Discomfort may be partially or totally relieved when returning to the supine position.

- Microhematuria (>80% cases)
- Rarely have associated recurrent UTIs, pyelonephritis, renal calculi, or findings of hypertension

PATHOPHYSIOLOGY

- Insufficiency of perirenal fat and fascial support in very thin patients, usually females. In addition, there may be anomalous development of the renal vascular pedicle being longer than usual. These factors lead to downward displacement of the kidney in the frontal and sagittal axis.
- Ptosis of kidney may result in proximal ureteric angulation or kinking, with temporary hydronephrosis and pain. Stretching of the renal vessels may cause partial narrowing of the lumen, with associated renal ischemia.

CAUSES/RISK FACTORS

- Severe weight loss
- Long-distance running, jogging, or other vigorous physical activities
- Females

COMPLICATIONS

- Pyelonephritis, renal calculi, hematuria, hypertension, renal ischemia
- Incapacitating severe flank and abdominal pain

DIFFERENTIAL DIAGNOSIS

- Renal colic associated with urolithiasis
- Cholecystitis (on right side)
- Spastic bowel disorder
- Intermittent bowel obstruction
- Hematuria–loin pain syndrome
- Pyelonephritis
- Ovarian vein syndrome
- Nutcracker syndrome (compression of left renal vein between SMA and aorta)

 Database

HISTORY

- Typical pain patterns associated with symptomatic nephroptosis

—Does the pain increase when moving from the supine to the upright position?
—Does it become worse with vigorous physical activities, such as long-distance running or jogging?
—Does the pain diminish when returning to the supine position?

- Has there been a large weight loss or marked thinness throughout the adult lifetime?

—Marked slenderness, usually in females

- Has there been history of hematuria, recurrent UTIs, renal calculi, or hypertension?

—Occasionally associated with symptomatic nephroptosis

PHYSICAL EXAMINATION

- Usually very thin, female
- Rarely febrile unless associated pyelonephritis
- The kidney may be palpated in the ipsilateral lower abdomen when the patient moves into the upright position. In some cases, an indenting of the anterior abdominal wall may be seen.
- Costovertebral pain may be present during a symptomatic attack.

 Diagnostic Studies

LABORATORY TESTING

- Urinalysis: may show microhematuria
- Urine culture usually normal
- BUN, creatinine, electrolytes usually normal

IMAGING

- IVP

—Shows renal descent of two or more vertebral bodies when moving from the supine to the upright position
—Hydronephrosis may also develop in the erect position, with delayed images.

- Diuretic furosemide renogram from supine to upright position: may demonstrate hydronephrosis and/or decreased split renal function
- Retrograde pyelogram: usually normal with patient supine
- CT scan and ultrasound: usually normal in supine state

SPECIAL STUDIES: N/A

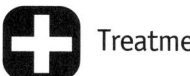 ## Treatment

GENERAL MEASURES

• Treatment is reserved only for the rare patient who presents with the full array of symptoms and signs of nephroptosis.
• Analgesics, antibiotics, and antihypertensive drugs, if needed

MEDICAL: N/A

SURGICAL

• Renal fixation by performing a nephropexy: securing the kidney high in the retroperitoneum by open surgery or laparoscopic surgery

—Securing the renal capsule to the psoas or quadratus lumborum muscles by the use of nonabsorbable sutures, fascial or muscle bands, polyglactin mesh

• Percutaneous nephrostomy tube insertion through an upper pole or mid-calyceal posterior calyx and then allowing the nephrostomy tract to mature × 3 weeks. This may create sufficient retroperitoneal scarring to fixate the kidney.

ALTERNATIVE THERAPIES

• Insertion of double-J catheter. Requires changing every 3 to 4 months. May sometimes be used as a "diagnostic" test

PATIENT EDUCATION

• Comprehension that nephroptosis is a rare clinical entity, which is diagnosed only after all other more common differential diagnostic diseases have been ruled out

 ## Follow-Up

MONITORING

• Postoperative IVP or diuretic renal scan 6 to 8 weeks postoperative
• Return for any recurrence of symptoms

PREVENTION

• Avoid excessive weight loss.
• If symptoms develop during vigorous athletic or physical activities, these may need to be curtailed if definitive surgical intervention is not undertaken.

 ## Miscellaneous

SYNONYMS

• Floating kidney, ptotic kidney

ASSOCIATED CONDITIONS

• UTI, renal calculi, hypertension, hematuria

NOTES

• Symptomatic nephroptosis is often a diagnosis of exclusion after more common urinary tract etiologies have been ruled out.

ABBREVIATIONS

• SMA, superior mesenteric artery

REFERENCES

deZeeuw D, Donker AJM, Burema J, van der Hem GK, Mandema E. Nephroptosis and hypertension. *Lancet* 1977;1:213.

Fornara P, Doehn C, Jocham D. Laparoscopic nephropexy: 3-year experience. *J Urol* 1997; 158:1679–1683.

O'Reilly PH, Pollard AJ. Nephroptosis: A cause of renal pain and a potential cause of inaccurate split renal function determination. *Br J Urol* 1988;61:284–288.

Author: Howard N. Winfield

Nephrotic Syndrome

 Basics

DESCRIPTION

- Nephrotic syndrome (NS) involves the tetrad of proteinuria (>3 g/d/1.73 m²), hypoproteinemia, edema, and hyperlipidemia. Can be secondary (associated with systemic disease) or primary (idiopathic). Presentation of nephrotic syndrome in adults may signal a serious underlying disease.

EPIDEMIOLOGY

- Uncommon disease
- Incidence varies, depending on age, race, prevalence of infections (malaria, hepatitis B, schistosomiasis)
- 80% in children are primary NS, usually minimal change disease (incidence 2–7/100,000). More common in males
- Only 25% of adult patients have primary NS.
- The most common cause in the United States is diabetes mellitus.

GENETICS

- Some etiologies have association with HLA types.
- Heredofamilial syndromes are rare.

STAGING: N/A

SIGNS AND SYMPTOMS

- The most common manifestations are related to fluid overload.

—Edema, especially face, lower extremities, sacrum
—Dyspnea/orthopnea secondary to pleural effusion
—Ascites, hypertension

- Signs/symptoms may be related to systemic disease causing nephrotic syndrome

PATHOPHYSIOLOGY

- All forms of NS feature severe proteinuria.

—NS is primary, or secondary to systemic disease affecting the glomerulus
—Signs/symptoms of NS worsen as serum albumin falls below 2.5 g/dL

- Various pathologic patterns can be differentiated on kidney biopsy.

—Minimal change glomerulopathy
—Membranous glomerulopathy
—Focal segmental glomerulosclerosis (FSGS)
—Mesangioproliferative glomerulonephritis
—Membranoproliferative glomerulonephritis
—Diabetic glomerulosclerosis
—Amyloidosis
—Fibrillary glomerulonephritis
—Light-chain deposition disease
—Rarer other lesions

- Pathophysiology: abnormal leakage of proteins across glomerular basement membrane (GBM). GBM normally restricts passage of proteins >70 kd.

—Minimal change nephropathy: Loss of charge selectivity results in selective proteinuria.
—Membranous nephropathy: Abnormal pore size results in nonselective proteinuria.
—FSGS, a plasma factor produced by lymphocytes, increases albumin excretion.
—Renal ablation syndromes: Hyperfiltration can result in proteinuria.

CAUSES/RISK FACTORS

- Idiopathic: See Pathophysiology in the "Basics" section.
- Medications: NSAID agents, captopril, gold, penicillamine, heroin
- Infectious

—Bacterial: syphilis, endocarditis, poststreptococcal glomerulonephritis (PSGN)
—Viral: HIV, hepatitis B, hepatitis C
—Protozoal: malaria
—Helminthic: schistosomiasis, trypanosomiasis, filariasis

- Neoplastic: tumors (lung, colon, stomach, breast); leukemia, lymphoma, multiple myeloma
- Toxins and allergens: bee stings, pollens
- Systemic disease: systemic lupus, sarcoid, amyloidosis, vasculitis, rheumatoid arthritis
- Metabolic diseases: diabetes mellitus, myxedema
- Heredofamilial disease: sickle cell anemia, Alport syndrome, Fabry disease
- Miscellaneous: preeclampsia, renal artery stenosis, reflux nephropathy, morbid obesity

COMPLICATIONS

- Sodium retention: NS is characterized by increased tubular resorption of sodium.
- Hyperlipoproteinemia

—Both cholesterol and triglyceride levels elevated; high-density lipoprotein (HDL) usually normal
—Caused by overproduction and impaired catabolism of lipoproteins

- Thromboembolism

—Hypercoagulable state due to abnormalities in coagulation factors and platelet function
—Renal vein thrombosis in 20% to 30% of patients with membranous glomerulopathy
—Risk of deep vein thrombosis and pulmonary embolus
—Arterial thrombosis much rarer

- Infections: susceptibility due to low levels of both IgG and components of alternative complement pathway

DIFFERENTIAL DIAGNOSIS

- Any edema-forming state (congestive heart failure, cirrhosis, malnutrition, protein-losing enteropathy); however, these conditions usually do not cause heavy proteinuria.

 Database

HISTORY

- Symptoms of fluid/sodium retention?

—Periorbital edema, especially on awakening
—Peripheral edema, especially at end of day

- History of systemic disease causing NS?

—See Causes/Risk Factors in "Basics" section.
—History of infection: HIV disease, hepatitis B or C
—Medication or illicit drug use
—History of cancer or signs of malignancy (weight loss, bowel changes, bleeding)
—Travel history (especially to endemic areas for malaria)
—Evidence of other systemic disease: rash, arthralgias, nightsweats
—Other medical illnesses: diabetes, hypertension
—Family history: deafness, renal disease, sickle cell

PHYSICAL EXAMINATION

- Vital signs: blood pressure, temperature, weight
- Skin examination: rash (e.g., butterfly rash of SLE), pallor, edema, lymphadenopathy
- Ophthalmic examination: uveitis in sarcoid, diabetic retinopathy
- Heart/lung examination: endocarditis, pleural effusion
- Abdominal examination: masses, ascites
- Pelvic/rectal examination
- Neurologic examination: diabetic neuropathy, CNS lesion, mononeuritis multiplex in vasculitis

Diagnostic Studies

LABORATORY TESTING

- Urine analysis

—Marked proteinuria causes urine to "foam."
—Albuminuria detected by dipstick; all proteinuria detected by sulfosalicylic acid (SSA)
—Positive SSA and negative dipstick: non-albumin proteinuria (multiple myeloma)
—Characteristic dipstick reading of 3+ to 4+ in NS patients
—Glycosuria: suggests diabetes mellitus as possible cause of NS
—Hematuria common (usually microscopic)
—Microscopic: "Maltese crosses," oval fat bodies, fatty casts, hematuria. Cellular casts suggest NS.

- 24-hour urine protein: NS characterized by massive proteinuria (mostly albumin)
- Complete blood count

—Cause of anemia should be evaluated.
—Leukocytosis suggests infection or leukemia.
—Leukopenia or thrombocytopenia may be seen in SLE, lymphoma, etc.

- Renal function/electrolytes: Abnormal renal function suggests long-standing NS or a nephritic syndrome.
- Albumin level: Clinical features of NS worsen as serum albumin falls below 2 g/dL.
- Serology

—Liver function enzymes
—VDRL test, HIV, hepatitis panel may be appropriate.
—Other screening tests: antinuclear antibody (ANA), complements, rheumatoid factor

- Urine and serum protein electrophoresis if multiple myeloma suspected
- Coagulation profile
- Lipid profile: cholesterol, triglycerides

IMAGING

- Renal ultrasound

—Increased echogenicity of renal parenchyma suggests advanced glomerular disease.
—A solitary kidney (unilateral renal agenesis, previous nephrectomy) can result in FSGS.
—Doppler ultrasound: renal artery stenosis

- Chest x-ray: Sarcoidosis or malignancy is suspected. Other studies (CT, endoscopy, etc.), as needed, to rule out malignancy

SPECIAL STUDIES

- Renal biopsy

—In children, due to high prevalence of minimal change disease, biopsy not necessary and treatment usually empiric
—If cause of NS not identified in an adult, kidney biopsy indicated
—Contraindications to biopsy: coagulopathy, uncooperative patient, uncontrolled hypertension, pyelonephritis, severe anemia. Solitary kidney: relative contraindication

 ## Treatment

GENERAL MEASURES

- Secondary NS: Treat the underlying cause.
- Sodium restriction (2–3 g/d)
- Low-protein, low-lipid/cholesterol diet
- Patients being considered for steroid treatment should have a PPD skin test.

MEDICAL

- Diuretics to treat edema
- Angiotensin converting enzyme (ACE) inhibitors: reduce proteinuria, hyperlipidemia

—Indicated even in normotensive patients
—Side effects include hyperkalemia and potential worsening of renal function.

- NSAIDs: also reduce proteinuria but significant GI side effects
- Cholesterol-lowering agents
- Prophylactic anticoagulation therapy in high-risk patients (serum albumin <2.5 g/dL, protein­uria >10 g/d)

—Low-dose aspirin may be of benefit.
—Chronic anticoagulation: indicated if a thrombo-embolic complication has occurred

- Pneumococcal, influenza vaccination recommended
- Specific therapy for primary NS depends on the pathologic lesion.

—Minimal change disease: steroids alone in children; alkylating agents or cyclosporine for nonresponse to steroids alone
—FSGS: responds less well to steroids; may also require alkylating agents
—Membranous glomerulonephritis: no response to steroids alone; requires an alkylating agent. Cyclosporine also used

SURGICAL: N/A

ALTERNATIVE THERAPIES: N/A

PATIENT EDUCATION

- Prognosis depends on age, race, pathology, presence of hypertension, underlying systemic disease, degree of renal dysfunction, and degree of proteinuria.

—Minimal change disease in children has an excellent prognosis.
—Prognosis of the other glomerulopathies much more variable

 ## Follow-Up

MONITORING

- 24-Hour urine for protein to judge response to therapy
- Monitor for treatment toxicity.

—Leukopenia: alkylating agents
—Infections: steroids, alkylating agents, cyclosporine
—Steroid-induced hyperglycemia, osteoporosis

- Attention to sodium retention, hyperlipidemia, thromboembolic complications

PREVENTION

- None for primary NS
- Secondary NS: treatment or prevention of systemic disease (e.g., tight control of diabetes, prevention of STD)

 ## Miscellaneous

SYNONYMS: N/A

ASSOCIATED CONDITIONS: N/A

NOTES: N/A

ABBREVIATIONS

- ACE, angiotensin converting enzyme; FSGS, focal segmental glomerulosclerosis; GBM, glomerular basement membrane; NS, nephrotic syndrome; PSGN, poststreptococcal glomerulonephritis; SSA, sulfosalicylic acid

REFERENCES

Glassock RJ, Cohen AH, Adler SG. Primary glomerular disease. In: Brenner BM, ed. *The Kidney*, 5th ed. Philadelphia: WB Saunders, 1996:1392–1497.

Orth SR, Ritz E. The nephrotic syndrome. *N Engl J Med* 1998;338:1202.

Schnaper HW, Robson AM. Nephrotic syndrome: Minimal change disease, focal glomerulosclerosis, and related disorders. In: Schrier RW, Gottschalk CW, eds. *Diseases of the Kidney*, 6th ed. Boston: Little, Brown, 1997:1725–1780.

Authors: Joel D. Glickman and Joseph F. Harryhill

Neuroblastoma

Basics

DESCRIPTION

- Solid tumor of childhood, arising from cells of neural crest that form the sympathetic nervous system

EPIDEMIOLOGY

- 1 in 100,000 live births
- 7% to 8% of all childhood malignancies
- No sex predilection
- Most common malignancy of infants
- Second most common solid malignancy of childhood
- 50% in children <2 years of age
- Peak age: 1.5 years
- Site of primary tumor in decreasing order: abdomen (adrenal the most common), chest, neck, pelvis, and neck
- Incidental autopsy finding 400-fold higher than clinical incidence

GENETICS

- The risk of NB in a sibling or offspring is <6%.
- 20% familial autosomal dominant
- 70% to 80% chromosome 1p deletion
- 30% N-myc oncogene amplification

STAGING

- 70% have metastasis at the time of diagnosis.
- Marrow involvement in 50%, even in absence of bony metastasis
- TNM classification based on anatomic location of tumor determined by surgery, adopted by the Pediatric Oncology Group (POG)
- Evan's classification (1971) adopted by the Children's Cancer Group (CCG)
- The Shimada classification (1984), based on histopathology, describes degree of cellular differentiation, stromal content, mitosis–karyorrhexis index, and age at diagnosis.
- Worldwide consensus on staging: International Neuroblastoma Staging System (INSS) in 1986

—Stage 1: localized tumor with complete excision, bilateral nodes negative
—Stage 2A: localized tumor with incomplete excision, bilateral nodes negative
—Stage 2B: localized tumor with incomplete excision, ipsilateral nodes positive
—Stage 3: unresectable midline tumor, or unresectable unilateral tumor infiltrating across the midline, or localized unilateral tumor with contralateral nodes positive
—Stage 4: any primary tumor with metastasis to distant nodes, bone, bone marrow, liver, skin
—Stage 4S: localized primary (1, 2A, 2B) age <1 year, with metastasis limited to skin, liver, or bone marrow

SIGNS AND SYMPTOMS

- Depend on site of primary, existence of metastasis, and secretion of biochemical products

—Site of primary: abdominal mass, urinary retention, constipation, extremity paresis, or Horner syndrome
—Presence of metastasis: fever, lethargy, weight loss, bony pain, and pallor
—Active biochemical products (catecholamines): paroxysmal hypertension, headache, palpitation, flushing, and diarrhea

PATHOPHYSIOLOGY

- Gross: vascular, purple mass usually solid but may be cystic, hemorrhagic, poorly encapsulated
- Histology: classified as small round cell tumor of childhood, with lobular growth, and cells forming psuedorosettes

—Microscopically resembles lymphoma, rhabdomyosarcoma, Ewing's sarcoma

- Neuron-specific enolase stains for intracellular catecholamines: highly specific for NB
- Forms that neuroblastoma (carcinoma in situ) undergo spontaneous regression within first year of life; explains the high rate of NB found incidentally in infant autopsies (1/100) vs. its low clinical rate (1/100,000)
- Metastasis to bone more common in older children; liver more common in younger children
- Biochemical products

—90% of tumors produce catecholamines in excess. Hypertension, flushing, and headaches occur only in 5% because catecholamines are sequestered within intracellular vacuoles.
—HVA is the primary by-product in less differentiated tumors.
—VMA is the primary by-product in more differentiated tumors.
—VIP secreted by some NBs; causes diarrhea

CAUSES/RISK FACTORS

• NB, ganglioneuroma, and ganglioneuroblastoma appear to form a spectrum of diseases resulting from an incorrect maturation process.
• Commonly used histopathologic markers for NB include *N-myc,* DNA ploidy, Shimada histopathology, NSE, and, recently, Trk neurotrophin receptors and the multidrug resistance protein (MRP).
• Favorable prognostic factors include nonadrenal primary; stages I, II, IV-S; age at diagnosis <1; serum ferritin <150 ng/mL; mature and "stroma-rich" (tumor with high volume of connective tissue rather than NB cells) histology; and low mitosis to karyorrhexis index (MKI) in "stroma-poor" types of tumors.
• Poor prognostic factors include adrenal origin; age >1; stages III and IV; diploid DNA content; N-*myc* amplification; serum ferritin >150 ng/mL; neuron-specific enolase >100 ng/mL; chromosome 1p deletion; and increased vascularity.

COMPLICATIONS

• Acute myoclonic encephalopathy occurs in 2%.
• Spinal cord compression with paravertebral tumor growing into an intervertebral foramen (dumbbell tumor); more common with ganglioneuroblastoma
• Retinal hemorrhage, extraocular muscle paresis, optic atrophy
• Spontaneous remission in 1% to 2% diagnosed tumors
• No association with any congenital malformations

DIFFERENTIAL DIAGNOSIS

• Related conditions
—Ganglioneuroma: benign counterpart of NB
—Ganglioneuroblastoma: intermediate differentiation between NB and ganglioneuroma

• Intraabdominal mass in childhood

—Wilms' tumor, teratomas, rare primary neoplasms of liver and pancreas
—Lymphoma, rhabdomyosarcoma, Ewing's sarcoma: Periodic-acid Schiff (PAS) staining can distinguish sarcomas; neuron-specific enolase staining is specific for NB.

 Database

HISTORY

• Early satiety, poor appetite, vomiting?

—A large intraabdominal mass may cause partial intestinal tract obstruction.

• Unexplained fever, weight loss, anorexia, pallor, irritability?

—Constitutional symptoms usually indicate metastatic disease from neuroblastoma.

• Urinary frequency, urinary retention, or constipation?

—A mass in the presacral region may cause extrinsic compression of pelvic organs, leading to obstructive symptoms.

• Poor truncal balance, jerky muscle movements, or uncontrolled eye movement?

—Acute myoclonic encephalopathy occurs in 2%, probably due to toxic effects of biochemical products or an autoimmune phenomenon.

• Pain in skull and long bones?

—Metastasis to the bones indicates a poor prognosis, and usually involves the long bones.
—Metastasis to bone from NB should be differentiated from bone tumors and infection.

• Pallor and anemia?

—Bone marrow involvement leads to anemia, and is present in 50% of children with neuroblastoma.

• Bleeding diathesis, easy bruising?

—Extensive metastasis to the liver may cause coagulopathy.

• Lower or upper extremity weakness, sensory symptoms?

—Paravertebral sympathetic ganglia NB may compress the spinal cord.

• Paroxysmal hypertension, sweating, headaches, palpitations?

—Rarely, NB releases catecholamines.

• Watery diarrhea?

—Some NBs secrete vasoactive intestinal peptide (VIP).

• Family history of NB?

—20% are familial.

(continued)

Neuroblastoma (continued)

PHYSICAL EXAMINATION

- Hypertension

—Rare; may be due to catecholamine release

- Abdominal mass

—55% NB within the abdomen; adrenal gland most common site

- Bluish/erythematous subcutaneous nodules

—Metastatic spread is to the skin; origin of monomer "blueberry muffin baby"

- Ataxia, myoclonus, multidirectional eye movement

—Toxic effects of catecholamine by-products or autoimmune phenomenon

- Ptosis, loss of pupillary dilation, unilateral anhydrosis

—Unilateral Horner syndrome: tumor compressing sympathetic ganglia or spinal cord

- Ocular proptosis and upper eyelid ecchymosis

—Periorbital metastasis

- Extremity paresis, sensory deficits

—Paravertebral lesion growing into and compressing spinal cord

 Diagnostic Studies

LABORATORY TESTING

- CBC: Anemia indicates bone marrow replacement.
- PT/PTT: Elevated levels indicate liver involvement.
- 24-Hour urine for VMA and HVA

—Elevated in 95% of patients with NB

- Serum ferritin

—Elevated in 40% to 50% with advanced disease
—Must be elevated >3 standard deviations above the mean per milligram for age

IMAGING

- IVP: displacement of kidney by suprarenal mass
- KUB: Speckled calcification in 50% of abdominal NB
- CT: Solid vs. cystic nature and location of mass; examine presence of possible metastatic lesions
- Ultrasound of abdomen/pelvis: tumor/mass localization
- MRI: evaluation of intraspinal extension. Paravertebral tumors may grow through the intervertebral foramen into the spinal canal, forming a dumbbell-shaped tumor.
- Skeletal survey/bone scan: routine; rule out skeletal metastasis
- Chest x-ray: obtained to evaluate posterior mediastinum

SPECIAL STUDIES

- Iodine-125 MIBG scan: images primary as well as metastatic sites

—MIBG structurally similar to norepinephrine: taken up by NB cells
—Used in place of technetium-99m bone scan for metastatic bone survey

- Bone marrow aspiration: performed in all cases of NB

—Tumor cells forming pseudorosettes

 Treatment

GENERAL MEASURES

- Common modalities: surgery, chemotherapy, and bone or stem cell transplantation
- Various combinations of these four modalities are employed in different treatment protocols.
- Generally, the more advanced the disease, the more complex and radical the protocol needed to induce remission.
- International collaboration has led to a risk assignment schema based on INSS stage, age, N-myc, amplification, DNA ploidy, and Shimada histopathology.
- Current POG/CCG intergroup studies use this risk-based stratification in evaluating new treatment protocols.
- Low-risk (stages 1, 2A, 2B, 4S with age <1 year, or age >1 year with favorable pathology) treatment is primarily surgical. Five-year survival: 85% to 98%
- Intermediate-risk (stage 3 with age <1 year, or >1 year with favorable pathology, or stages 4, 4S with age <1 year) treatment multiagent chemotherapy and surgery. Five-year survival: 55% to 90%
- High-risk (stages 2A, 2B with age >1 year with unfavorable histopathology, or stages 3, 4, 4S with amplification of N-myc regardless of age) treatment is intensive chemotherapy, with or without bone marrow ablation, with repeated surgery, relapses common. Five-year survival: 10% to 30%

MEDICAL

- Low risk: low-dose cycles of cyclophosphamide/Adriamycin and cisplatin/NV-26 if surgery fails
- Intermediate risk

—Induction with cyclophosphamide/Adriamycin cycles with or without radiotherapy. Maintenance with cisplatin/VM-26 or others after complete response

- High risk

—Common agents: cyclophosphamide, Adriamycin, VM-26, doxorubicin, cisplatin, etoposide in various combination for 8 to 12 months
—Myeloablation with autologous PBSCR or BMT

- Radiation therapy: indications

—Cytoreduction in anticipation of second-look surgical excision
—Adjunct to chemotherapy
—Palliation/treatment of pain
—Part of bone marrow transplant protocol
—Symptomatic liver enlargement from metastasis

- Dumbbell NB with spinal cord compression is best treated with chemotherapy. Neurosurgical intervention is reserved for emergent decompression.

SURGICAL

- Low risk

—Surgery is the primary treatment of choice.
—Resection of a primary tumor in stage 4S may prevent recurrence.

- Intermediate risk

—Primary surgery followed by induction chemotherapy
—Second-look surgery and maintenance chemotherapy are often required.

- High risk

—Medical reduction followed by surgery and often repetitive cycles of surgery and chemotherapy with or without radiotherapy for recurrence

- Second-look surgery

—Stage 3: Post chemotherapy/radiation therapy, excision of resectable mass may increase survival by 30%.
—Stage 4: Second-look: no increased survival; may be part of experimental protocol

ALTERNATIVE THERAPIES

- Iodine-131 MIBG for refractory NB
- Monoclonal antibody 3F8 directed to GD2 ganglioside-positive tumors and metastatic lesions
- Prolonged isotretinoin maintenance following intensive chemotherapy
- Interferon-alpha plus tretinoin for refractory NB
- Cyclophosphamide plus topotecan for refractory NB
- Temozolomide for recurrent CNS NB
- Docetaxel for recurrent solid tumor

PATIENT EDUCATION

- NCI Cancer Information Service: (800)422-6237; www.graylab.ac.uk/cancernet
- The Neuroblastoma Children's Cancer Society: (800)532-5162; www.granitewebworks.com/nccs.htm
- Children's Cancer Web: www.ncl.ac.uk/~nchwww/guides/guide2n.htm

 Follow-Up

MONITORING

- First year: examination every month, with imaging and bone marrow biopsy every 3 months
- Second year: examination every 2 months, with imaging and bone marrow biopsy every 6 months
- Third year: examination every 3 months, with imaging and bone marrow biopsy if indicated clinically
- HVA or VMA may be followed if the pretreatment work-up showed elevated levels.

PREVENTION

- Screening initiatives (Japan and Quebec) using urinary catecholamines are not effective.

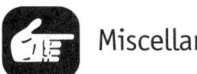 Miscellaneous

SYNONYMS: N/A

ASSOCIATED CONDITIONS: N/A

NOTES

- See also Section II, "Adrenal Medullary Neuroblastoma."
- Young adults and adults

—Tumor growth slower, similar site distribution; more resistant to chemotherapy

ABBREVIATIONS

- BMT, bone marrow transplantation; CCG, Children's Cancer Group; HVA, homovanillic acid; INSS, International Neuroblastoma Staging System; MIBG, metaiodobenzylguanidine; NB, neuroblastoma; NSE, neuron-specific enolase; POG, Pediatric Oncology Group; PBSCR, peripheral stem cell rescue; VIP, vasoactive intestinal peptide; VMA, vanillylmandelic acid

REFERENCES

Coplen DE, Evans AE. Neuroblastoma update. AUA Update Series XII:35, 1993.

Katzenstein HM, Cohn SL. Advances in the diagnosis and treatment of neuroblastoma. *Curr Opin Oncol* 1998;10:43–51.

Ritchey ML, Andrassy RJ, Kelalis PP. Pediatric urologic oncology. In: Gillenwater JY, Grayhack JT, Howards SS, Duckett JW, eds. *Adult and Pediatric Urology*, 3rd ed. St Louis: Mosby, 1996.

Authors: S. Adam Ramin, Mark Thompson, and Herbert C. Ruckle

Paraphimosis

 Basics

DESCRIPTION

• Painful swelling of the foreskin distal to a phimotic ring after retraction of the foreskin for a prolonged period

EPIDEMIOLOGY: N/A

GENETICS: N/A

STAGING: N/A

SIGNS AND SYMPTOMS: N/A

PATHOPHYSIOLOGY

• In children

—A congenitally narrowed preputial opening is present.
—The foreskin is retracted behind the glans penis and not promptly reduced.
—Entrapment in the coronal sulcus occurs secondary to swelling of the glans.
—This leads to venous congestion, edema, and enlargement of the glans, followed by arterial occlusion and necrosis of the glans.

• In adults

—Typically occurs in elderly men and may be associated with poor hygiene and/or chronic balanoposthitis
—This inflammation leads to a contraction of the opening of the prepuce and forms a fibrotic ring of tissue.
—This in turn leads to constriction when the foreskin is retracted behind the glans.
—Results in venous congestion with edema
—Failure to promptly reduce the paraphimosis can result in arterial occlusion and necrosis of the glans penis. This constitutes a urologic emergency.

CAUSES/RISK FACTORS

• Chronic balanoposthitis
• Chronic indwelling Foley catheterization and catheter changes
• Patients requiring clean intermittent catheterization
• Phimosis

COMPLICATIONS

• Necrosis of glans and distal urethra

DIFFERENTIAL DIAGNOSIS

• Balanitis
• Balanoposthitis
• Angioneurotic edema
• Anasarca

 Database

HISTORY

• Has the patient been circumcised?
• Recurrent bouts of chronic balanitis?
• Chronic indwelling Foley catheterization?
• Clean intermittent catheterization?
• Diabetes mellitus: may be risk factor for phimosis
• Phimosis

PHYSICAL EXAMINATION

• Edema and swelling of penile shaft proximal to glans and corona
• Tight phimotic ring proximal to corona
• Late finding: swelling of the glans, venous congestion, necrosis of the glans penis

 Diagnostic Studies

LABORATORY TESTING

• Not usually necessary
• If surgery planned, preoperative lab studies, including coagulation factors

IMAGING: N/A

SPECIAL STUDIES: N/A

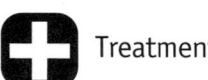 Treatment

GENERAL MEASURES

- Considered a urologic emergency
- Delay in reducing paraphimosis can result in necrosis of the glans.

MEDICAL

- Gentle steady pressure to foreskin to decrease swelling

—May use elastic wrap or Kerlix bandage

- Push against the glans with thumbs, pulling the foreskin forward over the glans with the fingers.

—Use a gauze pad to facilitate traction on the foreskin.

- As an adjunct to simple reduction, a 25-gauge needle is used to make multiple stab wounds in the edematous foreskin to help remove edema fluid.

—May use 2% lidocaine gel or EMLA cream (2.5% prilocaine and 2.5% lidocaine)

- Hyaluronidase 1 cc (150 U/cc Wydase)

—Injected into one or more sites in the edematous prepuce (spreading agent)
—Modifies permeability of the intracellular ground substance (limited utility)

SURGICAL

- Dorsal or ventral slit using 1% lidocaine penile block
- Convert to formal circumcision

ALTERNATIVE THERAPIES

- Penile block, then tourniquet to base of penis, then 20-gauge needle to aspirate blood from glans penis
- Parallel to the urethra, then constricting ring gently reduced over shrunken glans

PATIENT EDUCATION: N/A

 Follow-Up

MONITORING

- Circumcision should be performed when the edema/inflammation resolves.
- If there is no definitive treatment, paraphimosis tends to recur.
- Debridement of necrotic tissue is rarely indicated.

PREVENTION

- Emphasize to caregivers, when inserting or changing Foley catheters or performing clean intermittent catheterization: Reduce the foreskin after the procedure is completed.

 Miscellaneous

SYNONYMS: N/A

ASSOCIATED CONDITIONS: N/A

NOTES

- See also Section II, "Phimosis."

ABBREVIATIONS: N/A

REFERENCES

Brown MR, et al. Common office problems in pediatric urology and gynecology. *Pediatr Clin North Am* 1997;44(5):1091–1115.

DeVries CR, et al. Reduction of paraphimosis with hyaluronidase. *Urology* 1996;48(3):464–465.

Raveenthiran V. Reduction of paraphimosis. *Br J Surg* 1996;83(9):1247–1248.

Williams JC, et al. Paraphimosis in elderly men. *Am J Emerg Med* 1995;13(3):351–353.

Authors: Phillip C. Ginsberg and Richard C. Harkaway

Paratesticular Tumors

 Basics

DESCRIPTION

• Intrascrotal tumors involving the testicular tunic, epididymis, or cord structures. The most common paratesticular tumor of significance is rhabdomyosarcoma.

EPIDEMIOLOGY

• Rhabdomyosarcoma

—Occurs predominantly in children and adolescents
—White-to-Black ratio: 3:1

GENETICS: N/A

STAGING: N/A

SIGNS AND SYMPTOMS

• Slowly enlarging scrotal or inguinal mass that is distinct from the testicle

—Usually painless, unless associated with trauma or epididymitis

PATHOPHYSIOLOGY

• Rhabdomyosarcoma

—97% belong to the favorable histology group of embryonal cell tumors.
—Electron microscopy may be helpful in identifying cytoplasmic myofilaments when the diagnosis is in doubt.

• Cystadenoma of the epididymidis histologically corresponds to benign prostatic hyperplasia.

CAUSES/RISK FACTORS

• Marijuana and cocaine use in the parents has been associated with rhabdomyosarcoma in general.
• Patients with von Hippel-Lindau syndrome may have epididymal cystadenomas.

COMPLICATIONS

• Disease-associated complications include death in approximately 10%.
• Treatment-associated complications

—Retrograde ejaculation and intestinal obstruction secondary to retroperitoneal surgery
—Growth abnormalities secondary to radiation therapy
—Hypogonadism of contralateral testis and hemorrhagic cystitis secondary to chemotherapy

DIFFERENTIAL DIAGNOSIS

• Adenomatoid tumors: the most common benign paratesticular tumor
• Cystadenoma of the epididymis
• Leiomyosarcoma
• Liposarcoma
• Fibrosarcoma
• Malignant fibrous histiocytoma
• Malignant mesothelioma of the tunica vaginalis: associated with asbestos exposure
• Testicular torsion
• Epididymitis
• Hydrocele
• Inguinal hernia
• Traumatic injury
• Spermatocele
• Varicocele
• Tunica albuginea lesions (cysts, fibrous pseudotumor)
• Postoperative changes (sperm granuloma after vasectomy, etc.)

 Database

HISTORY

• Lower urinary tract symptoms

—Suggests epididymitis

• Acute pain

—Suggests torsion

• History of trauma or previous scrotal surgery

PHYSICAL EXAMINATION

• Palpation of the testes, epididymis, and cord structures bilaterally

—Rhabdomyosarcoma reveals a firm mass that is usually distinct from the testis.
—Transillumination suggests a fluid-filled lesion such as a hydrocele.

• Careful examination of the groin is necessary to rule out hernia.

Diagnostic Studies

LABORATORY TESTING

- Urinalysis and culture if epididymitis is suspected

IMAGING

- A scrotal ultrasound is crucial.

—Rules out an intratesticular lesion
—Solid lesions almost always require exploration.
—Simple cystic lesions are almost always benign.

- CT scan of the abdomen with and without contrast when diagnosis is made

—Clinical staging of retroperitoneal lymph nodes

SPECIAL STUDIES

- Percutaneous biopsies are contraindicated.
- Bone marrow aspirate

—Routine part of staging at time of diagnosis

- Radioisotope bone scan

—Especially for elevated alkaline phosphatase or symptoms with rhabdomyosarcoma

 Treatment

GENERAL MEASURES

- Ultrasound suggests initial management.
- Lesions suggestive of a benign process can be observed with serial examinations.
- If there is any concern about the malignant potential, the scrotum should be explored through an inguinal incision.
- Transscrotal manipulation or biopsy is contraindicated.

MEDICAL

- Usually necessary only for malignant tumors
- For rhabdomyosarcoma, always secondary to surgical treatment of the primary lesion

—Vincristine and actinomycin D–based chemotherapy
—Cyclophosphamide or ifosfamide reserved for higher stage disease

- Radiation therapy for stage II rhabdomyosarcoma and higher

—Some use radiation as salvage for chemotherapeutic and surgical failures.

SURGICAL

- Suspicious lesions are explored through an inguinal incision.

—Therapy for the primary lesions is always radical orchiectomy.

- For rhabdomyosarcoma

—Consider hemiscrotectomy for any degree of scrotal wall involvement.
—Routine retroperitoneal lymphadenectomy is controversial.
—A recent report suggests significant understaging and relapse when only CT scan is used.

ALTERNATIVE THERAPIES: N/A

PATIENT EDUCATION

- Discuss serial testicular self-examination.

 Follow-Up

MONITORING

- Serial ultrasounds for equivocal lesions, especially in the epididymis
- Routine guidelines are not established for rhabdomyosarcoma.

—A suggested schedule is a physical examination, chest x-ray, and CT every 2 to 3 months for the first year and every 3 to 4 months the next.
—In subsequent years, the examinations can be spread out to every 6 months and then annually.
—Patients who present with metastases require much closer monitoring.
—Recurrence after 2 years is unusual.

PREVENTION: N/A

 Miscellaneous

SYNONYMS: N/A

ASSOCIATED CONDITIONS: N/A

NOTES

- See also Section I, "Scrotum—Mass and/or Pain (Acute Scrotum)."

ABBREVIATIONS: N/A

REFERENCES

Crist W, et al. The Third Intergroup Rhabdomyosarcoma Study. *J Clin Oncol* 1995;13:610.

deVries JDM. Paratesticular rhabdomyosarcoma. *World J Urol* 1995;13:219.

Ferrari A, et al. The management of paratesticular rhabdomyosarcoma: A single institutional experience with 44 consecutive children. *J Urol* 1998; 159:1031.

Wiener E, et al. Changing pattern of relapse with localized paratesticular rhabdomyosarcoma in the Intergroup Rhabdomyosarcoma Study (IRS) Group trials. *Proc Am Soc Clin Oncol* 1997;16:519a.

Author: B. Mayer Grob

Parkinson Disease—Urologic Considerations

 Basics

DESCRIPTION

• A common neurologic disease causing voiding dysfunction, classically resulting in detrusor overactivity and sphincter bradykinesia, an impairment of relaxation of the striated external urinary sphincter

EPIDEMIOLOGY

• Prevalence of 100 to 150 per 100,000, chiefly in the sixth and seventh decades
• Men and women equally affected

GENETICS

• Genetic component long hypothesized; probably accounts for small proportion of cases
• Evidence for linkage to polymorphic markers on chromosome 4

STAGING: N/A

SIGNS AND SYMPTOMS

• Voiding dysfunction in up to 75% of patients

—Irritative symptoms (frequency, urgency, and urge incontinence) are seen in 57%, obstructive symptoms (hesitancy, incomplete emptying, and retention) in 23%, and mixed symptoms in 20% of patients with urologic symptoms.
—Symptomatology may be affected by preexisting detrusor or bladder outlet abnormalities.

• Cardinal neurologic signs are hypokinesia, rigidity, and tremor.
• Characteristic masked facies, festinating gait, and "pill-rolling" tremor of fingers and wrist

PATHOPHYSIOLOGY

• Degeneration of pigmented neurons in the extrapyramidal system (substantia nigra and locus ceruleus) results in characteristic cytoplasmic inclusions (Lewy bodies).
• Focal dopamine deficiency in neurons projecting from substantia nigra to the striatum results in an imbalance between dopaminergic and cholinergic activity.

—Results in extrapyramidal signs of bradykinesia, skeletal rigidity, and tremor
—The extrapyramidal system is inhibitory of the pontine micturition center; detrusor hyperreflexia may result.
—Skeletal muscle of the external urinary sphincter is subject to bradykinesia, resulting in urinary hesitancy from delayed sphincteric relaxation with the onset of detrusor activity.

CAUSES/RISK FACTORS

• Many theories about causes of idiopathic Parkinson disease

—Environmental toxins, causing selective destruction of dopaminergic neurons
—Genetic cause
—Free radicals cause oxidative damage to neuronal tissue.
—Accelerated aging, resulting in loss of dopaminergic neurons

• Many causes of secondary parkinsonism are known.

—Postencephalitic parkinsonism
—Drug-induced parkinsonism: chlorpromazine, haloperidol, reserpine, metoclopramide
—Toxin-induced parkinsonism: MPTP, a contaminant of illicit heroin-like street drug in 1980s

COMPLICATIONS

• Urinary tract infection
• Hydronephrosis is relatively uncommon.

DIFFERENTIAL DIAGNOSIS

• BPH in men
• Anatomic stress urinary incontinence in women
• Shy-Drager syndrome: autonomic dysfunction consisting of postural hypotension and extrapyramidal symptoms

 Database

HISTORY

• Assess for concurrent urologic conditions.

—BPH in men and stress urinary incontinence in women

• Careful review of medications

—Trihexyphenidyl hydrochloride (Artane) and benztropine mesylate (Cogentin) may impair detrusor contractility, resulting in urinary retention.

PHYSICAL EXAMINATION

• Geared toward recognizing subtle and gross neurologic signs

—Observation of mental status, coordination, and motor movements is important, as many patients are best managed by intermittent self-catheterization.

• A neurourologic examination permits direct assessment of sacral spinal cord segments.

—Should focus on perianal sensation, anal tone and control, and bulbocavernosal reflex

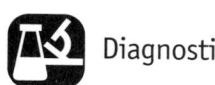 ## Diagnostic Studies

LABORATORY TESTING

- Serum creatinine
- No specific tests for Parkinson disease

IMAGING

- Renal ultrasound (hydronephrosis)

SPECIAL STUDIES

- Urodynamic investigation with close attention to sphincter electromyography (EMG) forms the basis for rational treatment.

—Detrusor hyperreflexia is present in up to 90%.
—Sphincter bradykinesia, or delayed relaxation of the external sphincter at the onset of voluntary micturition, is common.
—Bladder outlet obstruction: BPH vs. neuropathic external sphincter activity
—Impaired contractility less common; may coexist with detrusor hyperreflexia
—Detrusor areflexia is uncommon.

 ## Treatment

GENERAL MEASURES

- Begin with least invasive treatments.
- Must assess patient's cognitive and physical limitations

MEDICAL

- L-dopa may significantly improve symptoms. Alpha$_1$ antagonists (doxazosin, terazosin, tamsulosin) or finasteride for outflow obstruction
- Anticholinergics (oxybutynin, tolterodine) to control uninhibited bladder contractions

—Increased sensitivity to anticholinergics: Start at a low dose and titrate up.

SURGICAL

- Treatment is aimed at concomitant outlet obstruction from BPH.

—Transurethral prostatectomy (TURP or TUIP)
—Transurethral microwave thermotherapy (TUMT)

- Risk of postprostatectomy incontinence is approximately 20%.

ALTERNATIVE THERAPIES

- Intermittent catheterization with or without anticholinergics
- Behavioral therapies: timed voiding
- Intraprostatic stent prosthesis; potentially reversible if incontinence worsens

PATIENT EDUCATION

- National Parkinson Foundation Inc.: www.parkinson.org
- Parkinson's Support Groups of America, 11376 Cherry Hill Road, #204, Beltsville, MD 20705; (301)937-1545

 ## Follow-Up

MONITORING

- Voiding diary to assess response to therapy
- Post-void residual determination before and 1 to 2 weeks after starting medical therapy, especially if anticholinergics used
- Renal ultrasound if urodynamics suggest high risk of upper tract compromise

PREVENTION: N/A

 ## Miscellaneous

SYNONYMS

- Paralysis agitans

ASSOCIATED CONDITIONS

- Depression and insomnia are common.

NOTES: N/A

ABBREVIATIONS

- TURP, transurethral resection of prostate; TUIP, transurethral incision of prostate; TUMT, transurethral microwave thermotherapy; BPH, benign prostatic hyperplasia

REFERENCES

Berger Y, et al. Urodynamic findings on Parkinson's disease. *J Urol* 1987;138:836.

Blaivas JG, Chancellor MB. Parkinson's disease. In: Chancellor MB, Blaivas JG, eds. *Practical Neurourology: Genitourinary Complications of Neurologic Disease.* Boston: Butterworth-Heinemann, 1995.

Author: Patrick J. Shenot

Penis Cancer—General

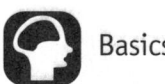 Basics

DESCRIPTION

• Penile cancer is almost always a squamous carcinoma of the penile skin, which may involve the prepuce, the glans, the shaft, or the base of the penis. It may metastasize to inguinal and pelvic lymph nodes, and thence to other organs.

EPIDEMIOLOGY

• Rare in the United States (prevalence: 0.2/100,000); may constitute 10% to 20% of male cancers in parts of Africa and South America
• In the United States, Blacks are affected about twice as often as Whites.
• Rare before age 40; peak incidence around age 75; mean age: 58
• Circumcision appears to protect against development; chronic irritative effect of smegma may be a factor; history of condyloma acuminata, balanitis xerotica obliterans, and leukoplakia may predispose

GENETICS

• Unknown

STAGING

• TNM staging: see the Appendix
• Jackson System

—Stage I: tumor confined to glans or prepuce
—Stage II: invasion into shaft or corpora; no nodal or regional metastases
—Stage III: tumor confined to penis; operable inguinal nodal metastases
—Stage IV: tumor involves adjacent structures; inoperable inguinal nodes and/or distant metastases

SIGNS AND SYMPTOMS

• Widely variable: The presenting lesion may range from patchy erythema, induration, or verrucoid growth to extensive destruction of penile tissue.
• The lesion may be flat or papillary.
• May present as itching or burning under foreskin, which may progress to ulceration
• Usually long history of inability to retract foreskin; tumor may be concealed by prepuce
• Usually not painful; often secondarily infected

PATHOPHYSIOLOGY

• Most (95%) of penile cancers are squamous cell carcinomas. Less common are sarcoma (including Kaposi's sarcoma), melanoma, basal cell carcinomas, and lymphomas.
• The Buschke-Lowenstein tumor (giant condyloma, verrucous carcinoma) is a histologically benign tumor that is characterized by aggressive local extension, which may destroy the penis if not treated.
• Tumors are graded as well differentiated (grade I), moderately well differentiated (grade II–III), and poorly differentiated (grade IV) (Broders classification system)

• Biopsy of the lesion makes the diagnosis; special stains are not usually required.
• Tumors that metastasize usually spread first to superficial inguinal nodes, then deep inguinal nodes, then pelvic nodes. Both groins may be involved.

CAUSES/RISK FACTORS

• Circumcision appears to protect against development; disease is rare where infant circumcision is widely practiced.
• Poor hygiene: The chronic irritative effect of smegma may be a factor.
• History of condyloma acuminata, balanitis xerotica obliterans, and leukoplakia may predispose

—HPV-16 and HPV-18 human papilloma virus strains identified in >50% of squamous carcinomas of the penis

COMPLICATIONS

• Biopsy has never been associated with tumor spread.
• Development of metastasis

DIFFERENTIAL DIAGNOSIS

• Erythroplasia of Queyrat (Bowen disease of penis)
• Mycotic skin infections
• Balanitis xerotica obliterans
• Sarcoma
• See also Section I, "Penis—Lesion."

 Database

HISTORY

• Duration of lesion
• History of condyloma or other inflammatory conditions

PHYSICAL EXAMINATION

• Lesion on penis: glans most common (50%), prepuce (21%), both prepuce and glans (9%), coronal sulcus (6%), shaft (2%)

—Palpate shaft to assess for corporal involvement; rectal examination for urethral/prostatic involvement

• Palpate groins for lymphadenopathy

—Most productive if done under anesthesia
—Examination repeated after 4 to 8 weeks of antibiotic therapy to rule out lymphatic enlargement from infection
—Persistently enlarged nodes require lymphadenectomy.

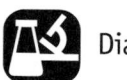 ## Diagnostic Studies

LABORATORY TESTING

• Biopsy of lesion to include some normal adjacent penile skin
• Serology, cultures, and skin tests may be required.
• Rarely, hypercalcemia (without evidence of bone metastases) may occur.

IMAGING

• Ultrasound and CT scan may be helpful in staging or identifying inguinal nodal involvement in some patients.

—CT-guided biopsy of abnormal inguinal or pelvic nodes may guide the planning of surgical therapy or chemotherapy.

• MRI may be helpful in delineating corporal and adjacent tissue involvement.
• Lymphangiography and cavernosography may be helpful in selected cases.

SPECIAL STUDIES: N/A

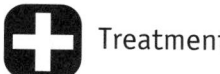 ## Treatment

GENERAL MEASURES

• Spontaneous regression of tumor has never been reported in penile cancer.
• Treatment of the primary tumor is followed by 4 to 8 weeks of therapy with broad-spectrum antibiotics to reduce inguinal nodal inflammation.
• Additional surgical therapy of the groin and pelvic nodes is required where nodal enlargement persists.

MEDICAL

• Four to 8 weeks of antibiotic therapy (e.g., cephalosporin) to reduce infection/inflammation in the groin nodes is administered before proceeding with inguinal lymphadenectomy. About 50% of enlarged nodes will regress.

SURGICAL

• Primary excision: Depending on the size and location of the lesion, this may involve

—Wide excision, circumcision, partial penectomy, total penectomy

• A 2-cm margin is essential. In patients in whom partial penectomy does not leave sufficient penile length to allow voiding while standing, total penectomy with perineal urethrostomy may be preferable.
• For persistent lymphadenopathy or suspected groin node metastases, inguinal node dissection is indicated.

—Modified superficial inguinal lymphadenectomy (after Catalona)
—Classical superficial and deep lymphadenectomy (after Daseler)
—Pelvic lymphadenectomy (unilateral or bilateral)

• With palpably negative nodes and stage To, Ta, or TI, grade I–II tumor, careful follow-up may be used.
• With palpably negative nodes and tumor ≥T2, or any grade III–IV histology, bilateral modified superficial lymphadenectomy is performed, proceeding to complete lymphadenectomy and pelvic lymphadenectomy if positive nodes are found.
• Because of lymphatic crossover at the base of the penis, bilateral superficial inguinal lymphadenectomies are performed, with deep inguinal and pelvic dissections done on the involved side if nodal metastases are confirmed.

ALTERNATIVE THERAPIES

• Radiotherapy: may be an effective treatment in small primary lesions, but complicated by severe edema and skin problems. May be a useful palliative measure in poor surgical candidates or in unresectable disease
• Laser surgery of the primary lesion may be effective in small tumors, but does not provide tissue for histologic evaluation and staging.

• Combination chemotherapy has demonstrated effectiveness in selected cases and is being further evaluated.

PATIENT EDUCATION

• Patients should be instructed to examine groins and report any adenopathy.

 ## Follow-Up

MONITORING

• In patients being followed expectantly, groin examinations should be conducted at least every 2 months for the first 2 years after diagnosis, then every 6 months for 2 years, then annually. A periodic groin ultrasound, CT, or MRI may be indicated.

—Poorly compliant patients may be better managed with inguinal lymphadenectomy.

• Patients who have undergone lymphadenectomy should be followed every 3 months for 2 years, then every 6 months for 2 years, then annually.

PREVENTION

• Circumcision may have a role in prevention. Hygiene should be stressed in uncircumcised boys and men.

 ## Miscellaneous

SYNONYMS: N/A

ASSOCIATED CONDITIONS: N/A

NOTES

• Debate on the indications for and timing of lymphadenectomy persists. Recent literature suggests that higher grade tumors appear to behave more aggressively.
• See also Section I, "Penis—Lesion."

ABBREVIATIONS: N/A

REFERENCES

Burgers JK, Badalament RA, Drago JR. Penile cancer: Clinical presentation, diagnosis, and staging. *Urol Clin North Am* 1992;19:247.

Catalona WJ. Modified inguinal lymphadenectomy for carcinoma of the penis with preservation of the saphenous vein: Technique and preliminary results. *J Urol* 1988;140:306.

Lynch DF, Schellhammer PF. Tumors of the penis. In: Walsh PC, Retik AB, Vaughan ED, Wein AJ, eds. *Campbell's Urology,* 7th ed. Philadelphia: WB Saunders, 1998.

Author: Donald F. Lynch, Jr.

Peyronie Disease

Basics

DESCRIPTION

• Peyronie disease (PD) is an idiopathic, sexually disabling penile condition caused by fibrotic scarring of the tunica albuginea surrounding the corpus cavernosa, resulting in curvature of the erect penis.

EPIDEMIOLOGY

• Usually occurs in fifth or sixth decades; mean age: 53 years
• Estimated prevalence: 388 in 100,000 men

GENETICS

• Few families identified with autosomal dominant trait

—Increased association with Dupuytren's contracture
—Association with HLA B27 antigen cross-reactivity

• HLA testing in a PD population vs. a control group revealed no significant difference of HLA antigen distribution.

STAGING: N/A

SIGNS AND SYMPTOMS

• Painful, progressive penile curvature with erection; usually becomes less painful over time
• New-onset erectile dysfunction associated with curvature
• Decreased penile sensation associated with curvature

PATHOPHYSIOLOGY

• Idiopathic
• Described by François de la Peyronie in 1743
• Natural history varies widely

—Spontaneous regression reported in 6% to 50%
—Results of study following 97 men as long as 8 years after diagnosis
    —40% with no difference in sexual function, pain, or curvature
    —40% with worsening sexual function or curvature
—6% with worsening pain

• Curvature characteristics

—Dorsal or dorsolateral curvature in vast majority
—Ventral curvature in only 6%

• Microscopic changes

—Early in course of disease
    —Abundance of lymphocytes and plasmocytes in areolar connective tissue between corpus cavernosum and tunica albuginea
—Later in course of disease
    —Thick fibrous plaques separating corpus cavernosum and tunica albuginea, replacing smooth muscle bundles in intercavernous septum

• Peyronie's plaque composition

—Collagen in plaque with increased type III collagen
—Ratio of α-1 to α-2 collagen chains increased above normal ratio
—Decreased glycine and alanine content of collagen, implicating increased non-collagen proteins

• Associated conditions

—Dupuytren's contractures
    —10% of patients with PD
    —As many as 78% of patients with familial PD
—Paget disease of the bone
—Dermatomyositis

CAUSES/RISK FACTORS

• Inherent tendency to abnormal production of fibrous tissue
• Mechanical stresses implicated in etiology, mainly during intercourse

—History of sexual trauma likely unimportant

• Reports of impotence treatments resulting in PD

—Prostaglandin intracorporeal injection
—Phentolamine/papaverine intracorporeal injection
—Vacuum erection device use

• Case reports of association with β-blocker use (metoprolol and propranolol)

COMPLICATIONS

• Complications of PD plaque formation

—Significant pain, or inability to achieve penetration
—Significant penile vascular abnormalities
—Decreased sensation associated with dorsal nerve involvement by plaques

• Complications of surgical treatment

—Penile shortening
    —Especially with all operations involving corporeal plication
—Erectile dysfunction
    —Veno-occlusive more common
—Numbness or loss of sensation
    —More common with plaque excision
—Infection
    —Higher in operations involving synthetic grafts or penile prosthesis
—Hematoma
    —Especially concerning under patch grafts
—Urethral injury
—Phimosis
—Suture granuloma

DIFFERENTIAL DIAGNOSIS

• See Section I, "Penis—Curvature and/or Pain."

Database

HISTORY

• Timing of curvature, duration of curvature
• Association with penile trauma

• Association of pain with intercourse
• Assess changes in penile sensation
• Quality of erection both currently and before the development of curvature must be assessed to treat appropriately.

—If on treatment for erections, did treatment precede development of curvature?

• Ability to penetrate with erection

PHYSICAL EXAMINATION

• Palpation of plaque; assess size of plaque
• Polaroid photograph of erect penis very helpful
• Examine for associated Dupuytren's contractures

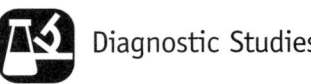

Diagnostic Studies

LABORATORY TESTING

• Alkaline phosphatase if Paget disease suspected

IMAGING

• Ultrasound

—In one study, a three-dimensional demonstration of plaques was possible in 75%.
—Color Doppler ultrasonography to assess significant vascular abnormalities

• Dynamic infusion cavernosography/cavernosometry

—Helpful to evaluate veno-occlusive dysfunction prior to treatment

SPECIAL STUDIES

• Nocturnal penile tumescence studies

—Helpful when there is a question of potency prior to treatment

• Prostaglandin E1 intracorporeal injection to assess curvature in an office setting or intraoperatively

Treatment

GENERAL MEASURES

• Spontaneous regression of curvature/pain may occur in 8% to 50%.
• Nonoperative treatment has best results in younger patients treated early in the course of their disease.
• Patients with curvature or pain preventing intercourse are unlikely to respond to medical therapy.

MEDICAL

• All therapies reported in small series, rarely placebo-controlled, and have yet a defined role in treatment
• All therapies have reported a decrease in pain, angulation of erection, and plaque size.
• Vitamin E

—Theoretic augmentation of connective tissue repair
—Dose: 400 IU tid for 3 months; then reevaluate

- Para-aminobenzoate (POTABA)

—Inhibitor of collagen cross-linkage
—Dose: 12 g daily in four divided doses for at least 3 months

- Colchicine

—Induces collagenase activity and decreases collagen synthesis

- Tamoxifen

—Dose: 20 mg bid for 3 months; then reevaluate

SURGICAL

- Definitive treatment for severe, disabling, stable PD
- Operation should not be considered until approximately 12 months after the onset of disease (when curvature progression has ceased).
- Choose the most conservative procedure to produce the desired result of penile straightening.
- Corporeal plication

—Should be used in patients with mild curvature, good erection, and adequate penile length
—Plication sutures (nonabsorbable) placed opposite of plaque, straightening convex side of curvature
  —Intraoperative artificial erection should be used to determine the point of maximal curvature.
—Complications include penile shortening, numbness, suture granuloma, and hematoma.
—The most problematic complication is unacceptable penile shortening.

- Nesbit procedure (corporeal excision opposite plaque)

—Same indications and complications as for corporeal plication
—One or more ellipses of corporeal tissue excised opposite point of maximal curvature and closed with running suture
—When compared with plication procedures, overall results appear somewhat better.
—Nesbit modifications that do not involve excision of tunica albuginea
  —Partially shaving an ellipse of tunica albuginea at convexity, followed by plication
  —Longitudinal incision of tunica albuginea with horizontal closure of incision

- Plaque incision/excision with grafting

—Should be used in patients with severe curvature and good erections
—Involves incising plaque or excising plaque to straighten convex portion of curvature, followed by corporeal grafting to allow erection without penile shortening
—Plaque incision technique
  —Usually transverse incisions at point of maximal curvature as determined by artificial erection
  —CO_2 laser has been used to evaporate the plaque substance and incise the corpora.
—Horton-Devine technique
  —Excision of plaque with dermal grafting of resultant corporeal defect
  —Excellent, durable results supported well in urologic literature

—May be used in conjunction with laser plaque management
—Alternative graft materials
  —Deep dorsal vein or saphenous vein; lympholized human dura mater; temporalis fascia; arterial patch
  —Dacron, Dexon mesh, Silastic sheets, Gore-Tex
—Complications include loss of sensitivity, infection (especially with artificial graft material), hematoma under graft, urethral injury, and veno-occlusive erectile dysfunction.

- Penile prosthesis with or without penile straightening

—For patients with significant erectile dysfunction, or if other procedures have been unsuccessful
—Inflatable prostheses have better reported results than semirigid prostheses.
—Penile straightening
  —Plaque incision with or without graft placement to fill the resultant defect
  —Plaque excision rarely necessary
  —Penile remodeling by implantation and inflation of prosthesis, followed by manual bending opposite of curvature to "fracture" penile plaque
  —All straightening techniques have reported excellent results.
—Complications same as for inflatable penile prosthesis placement

ALTERNATIVE THERAPIES

- Data supporting long-term results are lacking.
- Injection techniques

—Verapamil
  —Calcium channel blockers alter metabolic pathways of fibroblasts, promoting remodeling of extracellular matrix.
  —Intralesional injection weekly or biweekly for 6 months
  —Single-blind, controlled study in 14 patients with significant improvement in pain, angulation, plaque size, and erection quality
—Collagenase
  —Intralesional injection with purified clostridial collagenase
  —Patients with a lesser deformity responded more favorably in a placebo-controlled double-blind study.
—Orgotein
  —Antiinflammatory metalloprotein with superoxide dismutase activity is used mainly in Europe.
  —Injected monthly into indurated areas of penis
  —Best effect on pain control

- Focal ultrasound

—Used in conjunction with topical hydrocortisone
—Daily treatments for 2 weeks
—Best effect on reducing plaque size in patients with shorter duration of symptoms

- Radiation therapy

—Best results with focused linear accelerator
—Most effective in relieving pain associated with PD
—Not effective in treating penile curvature

PATIENT EDUCATION

- Patients with new onset and mild curvature or pain should be reassured of the benign nature of the disease and reevaluated regularly to monitor symptoms.

 Follow-Up

MONITORING

- Patients should be reexamined every 3 months after the onset of their symptoms to assess plaque size, pain, degree and progression of curvature, sexual function, and response to medical therapies.

PREVENTION: N/A

 Miscellaneous

SYNONYMS

- Acquired penile curvature, penile induration

ASSOCIATED CONDITIONS

- Dupuytren's contractures, Paget disease of the bone, dermatomyositis

NOTES

- See also Section I, "Penis—Curvature and/or Pain."

ABBREVIATIONS

- PD, Peyronie disease

REFERENCES

Carson CC. Peyronie's disease: Newer diagnostic studies and surgical alternatives. *Curr Opin Urol* 1994;4:180.

Carson CC. Peyronie's disease. In: Kirby RS, Carson CC, Webster GD, eds. *Impotence: Diagnosis and Management of Male Erectile Dysfunction*. London: Butterworth, 1991:248.

Jordan GH, Angermeier KW. Preoperative evaluation of erectile function with dynamic infusion cavernosometry/cavernosography in patients undergoing surgery for Peyronie's disease. *J Urol* 1993;150:1138.

Poulsen J, Kirkeby HJ. Treatment of penile curvature—A retrospective study of 175 patients operated with plication of the tunica albuginea or with the Nesbit procedure. *Br J Urol* 1995;75:370.

Authors: Bradley W. Steele and Culley C. Carson III

Pheochromocytoma

 Basics

DESCRIPTION

- Neoplastic growth derived from neuroectodermal cell line that produces excess catecholamines

EPIDEMIOLOGY

- No sex predilection
- Accounts for <1% of cases of hypertension (HTN)
- Average age: 50 to 60

GENETICS

- 90% sporadic
- 10% familial, autosomal dominant, with locus on chromosome 10

STAGING: N/A

SIGNS AND SYMPTOMS

- Hypertension: most common sign, three patterns, only 10% normotensive

—Sustained HTN: most common in children (90%), and MEA 2 syndrome
—Paroxysmal HTN: dramatic attacks of HTN, females > males, occur 3 to 4 times a week
—Sustained HTN with superimposed paroxysms: 50% incidence

- Hypertensive attacks may be initiated by a variety of stimuli.

—Compression of tumor: physical activity, trauma, increase abdominal pressure with Valsalva, micturition, etc.
—Foods rich in tyramine: beer, wine, cheese, etc.
—Drugs: tyramine, histamine, nicotine, glucagon, etc.

PATHOPHYSIOLOGY

- Tumors arise form chromaffin cells of neural crest origin in the sympathetic nervous system.
- In sporadic cases, the Rule of Nines holds true.

—90% are sporadic.
—90% of sporadic tumors occur in the adrenal gland.
—9% found elsewhere in the abdomen (organ of Zuckerkandl, abdominal sympathetic ganglia)
—1% found elsewhere in the body (posterior mediastinum, carotid body)
—10% of sporadic tumors bilateral, 50% of familial tumors bilateral

- Sporadic tumors are solitary, well circumscribed, and encapsulated.
- Average weight: 100 g
- 2.5% to 10.0% malignant

—Histologic determination of malignancy not possible; diagnosed based on metastases
—Extraadrenal tumors have a higher incidence of malignancy.

- Tumors contain enzymes necessary to convert tyrosine to catecholamines.
- Clinical manifestations secondary to the release

of these catecholamines, norepinephrine (NE), and epinephrine (EPI)

- Bladder pheochromocytomas account for <1% of bladder tumors and <1% of pheochromocytomas.

—Can present with micturition syncope
—Partial cystectomy with complete excision of tumor is the treatment of choice. Transurethral excision is contraindicated because it may precipitate a hypertensive crisis.

CAUSES/RISK FACTORS

- Familial tumors associated with multiple endocrine neoplasia (MEN) syndrome

—MEN IIA (Sipple syndrome): pheochromocytoma (<50%), medullary carcinoma of the thyroid (50%), and parathyroid adenoma (25%). Autosomal dominant, chromosome 10, secrete mostly EPI, with paroxysmal HTN
—MEN IIB (MEN III): pheochromocytoma, medullary carcinoma of the thyroid, ganglioneuromatosis, multiple mucosal neuromas of eyelids, lips, tongue

- Neuroectodermal syndromes

—Von Recklinghausen syndrome: 1% have pheochromocytoma; 5% of patients with pheochromocytoma have neurofibromatosis.
—Von Hippel-Lindau disease (retinal cerebellar hemangioblastomatosis): 10% with pheochromocytoma

COMPLICATIONS

- Persistent HTN can result in retinopathy and nephropathy.
- Catecholamine-induced cardiomyopathy

—Injected catecholamines can cause foci of myocardial necrosis, with inflammation and fibrosis.
—Can see hypotension secondary to global reduction of myocardial pump due to downregulation of β-receptors and decrease in effective myofibril contraction
—Cardiomyopathy reversible with α-blockade and β-methylparatyrosine
—All patients should have cardiac evaluation, including echocardiogram.

- Cholelithiasis: 30% with paroxysmal HTN, 10% with persistent HTN; cause unknown
- Cerebral vascular accident
- Unexplained shock
- Renal insufficiency
- Hemorrhagic necrosis of pheochromocytoma
- Dissecting aneurysm
- Ischemic enterocolitis

DIFFERENTIAL DIAGNOSIS

- Essential hypertension
- Renovascular disease
- Anxiety, tension states, psychoneurosis
- Hyperthyroidism
- Paroxysmal tachycardia
- Menopause
- Vasodilating headaches (migraine and cluster)
- Acute hypertensive encephalopathy
- Nephrologic diseases
- Cocaine, amphetamines

 Database

HISTORY

- Most patients are symptomatic, presenting with paroxysms of HTN with severe headache, drenching perspiration, and palpitations.
- Other symptoms include nervousness, tremor, pallor, and pain in the chest and abdomen.
- Symptomatic attacks may be induced (see Signs and Symptoms in the "Basics" section).
- HTN and accompanying symptoms are paroxysmal in half of patients.

—Paroxysmal attacks occur 3 to 4 times per week, lasting 15 to 30 minutes per attack.

PHYSICAL EXAMINATION

- Can be unremarkable if patient not symptomatic at time of examination
- Occurs in thin and obese patients
- Signs include fine tremors, pallor, and perspiration.
- Rarely have palpable tumor
- Accelerated hypertensive retinopathy: papilledema, exudate, A-V knicking
- Raynaud's phenomenon or livedo reticularis
- Hyperhidrosis

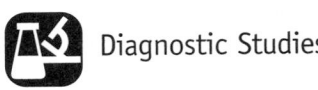 Diagnostic Studies

LABORATORY TESTING

- Diagnosis rests on the demonstration of elevated levels of catecholamines and/or their metabolites in the blood or urine.
- Urine test: 24-hour urine for NE/EPI, metanephrine (MN), normetanephrine (NMN), and vanillylmandelic acid (VMA)

—First test in work-up: The patient should be hypertensive during the test, and off of all medication if possible.
—Normal values: NE < 100 μg/24 h; EPI < 25 μg/24 h; VMA < 6.5 mg/24 h; NMN + MN < 1.3 mg/24 h
—If urinary values are >3× normal, then proceed to localize the tumor.
—If urinary values are <3× normal and suspicious, then repeat the test and proceed to pharmacologic testing.

- Plasma catecholamine testing

—Measure NE, EPI with the patient fasting and supine, with the needle in place in the vein for at least 20 minutes prior to drawing the sample.
—Test positive if plasma NE + EPI > 950 pg/mL (sensitivity: 88%–100%)

- Pharmacologic testing

—Stimulation and suppression tests are generally not utilized.
—Useful in patients with essential HTN but borderline elevated catecholamines
—Provocative tests dangerous, with several reported deaths

- Clonidine suppression test

—Most often used suppression test

—Centrally acting α_2-agonist that suppresses sympathetic outflow

—Normally results in decrease blood pressure and lower levels of plasma catecholamines

—Draw blood for NE/EPI before and 3 hours after administering clonidine (0.3 mg/70 kg)

—Plasma catecholamines remain the same or elevated in patients with pheochromocytoma.

IMAGING

- CT scan most widely used (sensitivity: 98%)

—Detects tumors >1 cm (most are >2 cm)

- MRI: several advantages over CT

—The bright "light bulb" appearance of the tumor on T2-weighted images distinguishes it from other tumors.

—No radiation exposure: procedure of choice for pregnant women

—Can provide excellent anatomic information concerning tumor and surrounding vasculature

—Procedure of choice (sensitivity: 100%)

- MIBG: scintigraphic localization with ^{131}I-metaiodobenzylguanidine

—Provides both anatomic and functional characterization of the tumor

—Concentrated in sympathomedullary tissue through the catecholamine pump

—Useful to evaluate for residual or multiple tumors, and MEA syndromes

SPECIAL STUDIES: N/A

 Treatment

GENERAL MEASURES

- Surgical removal of the tumor is the only definitive method of treatment.

MEDICAL

- Appropriate antihypertensive drugs are used to manage HTN, control symptoms, and prepare for surgery.

—α-Adrenergic blocking agents are most commonly used.
  —Phenoxybenzamine 10 to 40 mg bid or tid
  —Prazosin 1 to 10 mg bid

—β-Blocking agents are contraindicated in the absence of established α-blockade.
  —Use only for concomitant cardiac arrhythmias or persistent tachycardia.

SURGICAL

- Close hemodynamic monitoring and anesthetic management are essential.
- Recommend induction with agent such as thiopental, followed by isoflurane as inhalation agent
- Surgical approach

—Posterior or flank approach for small, localized tumors

—Thoracoabdominal or transabdominal for large or multiple tumors

—Initial dissection aimed toward early control and division of the main adrenal vein

- Pheochromocytoma in pregnancy

—Simultaneous cesarean section and removal of tumor is indicated if fetal maturity is compatible with extrauterine survival at the time of diagnosis; if not, treat with α-blockers.

- Malignant pheochromocytoma

—Usually slow growing; attempt complete resection

—Large masses can be debulked surgically to relieve symptoms.

ALTERNATIVE THERAPIES

- Malignant pheochromocytoma

—Some are radiosensitive using ^{131}I-MIBG.

—Combination chemotherapy with cyclophosphamide, vincristine, and dacarbazine: 50% to 60% partial response

—Local radiation or chronic blockade with metyrosine for symptomatic disease

PATIENT EDUCATION: N/A

 Follow-Up

MONITORING

- 10-year survival for nonmalignant tumors: >80%

—Because of uncertainties about which tumors are malignant, measure urinary or plasma catecholamines 1 to 2 weeks postoperatively and annually for 5 years.

—Blood pressure should be monitored every month for the first 6 months, then every 6 months thereafter.

—25% of patients have persistent HTN after surgery.

PREVENTION: N/A

 Miscellaneous

SYNONYMS: N/A

ASSOCIATED CONDITIONS

- MEN IIa, MEN IIb: See Section III, "Multiple Endocrine Neoplasia (MEN I, MEN II, and MEN III)."

NOTES

- See also Section I, "Adrenal Mass."

ABBREVIATIONS

- NE, norepinephrine; EPI, epinephrine; MN, metanephrine; NMN, normetanephrine; VMA, vanillylmandelic acid

REFERENCES

Bravo EL, Gifford RW, Manger WM. Adrenal medullary tumors: Pheochromocytoma. In: Mazzaferri EL, Samaan NA, eds. *Endocrine Tumors*. Blackwell Scientific, 1993:426–444.

Keiser HR. Pheochromocytoma and related tumors. In: DeGroot LJ, ed. *Endocrinology*. Philadelphia: WB Saunders, 1995:1853–1877.

Vaughan ED. Diagnosis of surgical adrenal disorders. AUA Update Series, Lesson 39, Vol. 16, 1997.

Authors: Stephen D.W. Beck and Michael O. Koch

Phimosis

 Basics

DESCRIPTION

• Inability to retract the foreskin

—Physiologic phimosis: first few years of life. Most foreskins can be retracted by age 3 to 5 years.
—Pathologic phimosis: The foreskin cannot be retracted after it has previously been retractable.

EPIDEMIOLOGY

• 10% of boys have nonretractile foreskin; 1% at puberty

GENETICS: N/A

STAGING: N/A

SIGNS AND SYMPTOMS

• Progressive inability to retract foreskin
• Discharge, soiling of undergarment
• Irritation, cracking and bleeding from foreskin

PATHOPHYSIOLOGY

• Physiologic phimosis

—The glans penis is adherent to the prepuce in infants.
—Glandular secretions and epithelial debris (smegma) facilitate separation.

• Pathologic phimosis

—Cicatricial preputial ring from irritation results in inflammation and scarring, caused by
  —Poor local hygiene
  —Early forceful retraction of foreskin
  —Chronic balanitis, especially in diabetics
—May balloon during voiding

CAUSES/RISK FACTORS

• Pathologic phimosis

—Chronic balanoposthitis
—Poor hygiene
—Diabetes mellitus

COMPLICATIONS

• Infection
• Possibility of increased risk of penile cancer

DIFFERENTIAL DIAGNOSIS

• Physiologic phimosis in the neonate
• Pathologic phimosis
• Postcircumcision phimosis

 Database

HISTORY

• Pathologic phimosis

—Could the foreskin be previously retracted?
—Has there been a prior circumcision?
—Hygiene problems?
—Ballooning of foreskin when voiding?
—Post-void dribbling?
—History of diabetes mellitus?
—Prior episodes of balanoposthitis?

PHYSICAL EXAMINATION

• Classification of retractability of the foreskin

—0: full retraction
—1: full retraction, tight behind glans
—2: partial exposure of the glans
—3: partial retraction, meatus just visible
—4: slight retraction, unable to visualize meatus
—5: no retraction

• Appearance of the foreskin

—0: normal
—1: crack in prepuce and skin splitting on gentle retraction
—2: small, partially circumferential white scar
—3: balanitis xerotica obliterans or severe scarring

• Frenular lacerations
• Preputial fissures
• Cicatricial band
• "Foreskin pearls" (smegma collection)
• Inflammation or active infection?
• Evidence of malignancy?

—Increased risk of penile cancer if uncircumcised

 Diagnostic Studies

LABORATORY TESTING

• Consider surface culture and sensitivity of the subpreputial space.
• Consider serum glucose to evaluate for diabetes.

IMAGING: N/A

SPECIAL STUDIES: N/A

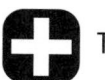 Treatment

GENERAL MEASURES

• Physiologic phimosis

—Note: Never circumcise a newborn with evidence of hypospadias or other anomaly of the external genitalia.
  —Prepuce may be needed for reconstruction.
—Encourage good hygiene.
—Instruct parents in gentle and gradual retraction of newborn foreskin.
—Gentle cleaning of smegma

• Pathologic phimosis

—Good hygiene
—Systemic or topical antibiotics to treat infection if present
—Steroid ointment

MEDICAL

• Nonsurgical treatment

—Local steroid application (topical vs. injectable has been studied)
—Nonsteroidal drug application has been used: EMLA cream (lidocaine and prilocaine).

SURGICAL

• Physiologic phimosis

—Circumcision, although not absolutely indicated
—Surgical correction of phimosis with preservation of the foreskin

• Pathologic phimosis

—Circumcision generally considered standard of care
—Preputial dilation
—Dorsal/ventral slit
—Y-V or V flap repairs
—Surgical correction of phimosis with preservation of foreskin

ALTERNATIVE THERAPIES: N/A

PATIENT EDUCATION: N/A

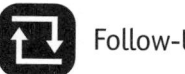 Follow-Up

MONITORING

• Postcircumcision phimosis

—May occur with Plastibell, Gomco clamp, or Guillotine techniques
—May be due to inadequate primary procedure or postprocedure scarring
—Usually requires formal surgical revision

• Glandular hyperesthesias may take several months to resolve after circumcision.

—Epithelium develops a squamous keratinized layer.

• Complications of circumcision are low (0.2%–0.6%).

—Meatal stenosis
—Fibrous bridges
—Infection
—Urethrocutaneous fistula
—Hemorrhage
—Cysts of the glans
—Avascular necrosis
—Preputial cysts
—Concealed penis
—Lymphedema of penile shaft
—Penile denudation

PREVENTION: N/A

 Miscellaneous

SYNONYMS: N/A

ASSOCIATED CONDITIONS

• Diabetes

NOTES

• See also Section II, "Paraphimosis."

ABBREVIATIONS: N/A

REFERENCES

Atilla MK, et al. A non-surgical approach to the treatment of phimosis. *J Urol* 1997;158(1): 196–197.

Brown MR, et al. Common office problems in pediatric urology and gynecology. *Pediatr Clin North Am* 1997;44(5):1091–1115.

Golubovic Z, et al. The conservative treatment of phimosis in boys. *Br J Urol* 1996;78(5):786–788.

Kikiros CS, et al. The response of phimosis to local steroid application. *Pediatr Surg Int* 1993; 8:329.

Authors: Phillip C. Ginsberg and Richard C. Harkaway

Polycystic Kidney Disease—Autosomal Dominant

 Basics

DESCRIPTION

• Characterized by renal and extrarenal cysts with hypertension and variable progression to end-stage renal disease (ESRD), requiring either dialysis or transplantation
• Autosomal dominant disease; usually presents in adulthood

EPIDEMIOLOGY

• Most frequent autosomal dominant fatal disease (1:500–1:1,000 incidence)

—10× greater than Huntington disease; 2× greater than cystic fibrosis

• >500,000 persons in United States; >5 million at risk worldwide
• Multisystem disease; can lead to ESRD
• Contributes 10% of all patients on chronic hemodialysis

GENETICS

• Autosomal dominant inheritance with 100% penetrance
• At least three genes are responsible.

—PKD1 (chromosome 16p13.3) (85%–90%) encodes polycystin. Expression regulated during renal development. May regulate cell-to-cell and/or cell-to-extracellular matrix interaction in the maintenance of renal epithelial differentiation and organization
—PKD2 on chromosome 4q.21-23 encodes a 968 amino acid protein. Both PKD1 and PKD2 encoded proteins are postulated to function as a voltage-gated ionic channel.
—No assignment of genomic locus for the third gene

STAGING: N/A

SIGNS AND SYMPTOMS

• Renal manifestations

—Usually bilateral renal cysts in an enlarged kidney
—Four to 5× the risk of renal adenomas, but renal cell carcinoma (RCC) risk is not elevated.
  —If RCC is present, it is more often bilateral, multicentric, and sarcomatoid.
—Can have decreased urinary concentrating ability, decreased citrate excretion, increased renin production

• Extrarenal manifestations

—Hepatic and pancreatic cysts, colonic diverticula, cardiac valvular abnormalities (mitral valve prolapse, aortic incompetence, and tricuspid prolapse), intracranial aneurysms, and rare miscellaneous cysts (arachnoid, pineal, splenic, testicular, seminal vesicle, and ovarian)

• Usual presentation: 30 to 50 years old with hypertension (60%–80%), flank pain (50%–70%), microscopic or gross hematuria (50%) without anemia, gastrointestinal symptoms, and intracerebral (from hypertension) or subarachnoid bleeding (from berry aneurysms)
• Hypertension most common symptom; is renin mediated through ischemia caused by the stretching of intrarenal vessels around the cyst. Patients not anemic due to adequate erythropoietin production
• Anemia may be present in ESRD due to cystic hemorrhage and/or uremic hematopoietic depression.
• 70% of intracranial bleeds are intracerebral due to hypertension; 10% to 40% have berry aneurysms, but only 10% die of subarachnoid hemorrhage.
• Renal cysts are found in utero in 2% of ADPKD patients, with a high recurrence (45%) of early polycystic kidney presentation in subsequent siblings.
• Neonates present with renomegaly and respiratory distress. Children (<1 year old) present with hypertension and renomegaly.
• Men tend to develop hypertension and renal insufficiency earlier, while women have a high incidence of liver cysts, urinary tract infections, and flank pain.

PATHOPHYSIOLOGY

• Gross pathology

—Enlarged kidneys with renal cysts ranging from millimeters to centimeters in diameter, creating a cobblestone-like surface with either a normal or distorted kidney morphology. Cyst fluid can be straw-yellow, hemorrhagic, or gelatinous.

• Histopathology

—Cysts can involve all portions of the nephron, and the wall epithelium can resemble the nephron segment from which it arose. Also, epithelial hyperplasia, arteriosclerosis, and interstitial fibrosis are present.

Polycystic Kidney Disease—Autosomal Dominant

CAUSES/RISK FACTORS

- Etiology theories

—Epithelial hyperplasia: epidermal growth factor and receptor found in cyst fluid and wall. Hyperplasia causes tubular obstruction with weakening and outpouching.

—Defect in extracellular connective tissue matrix: similar manifestations with other multiorgan diseases (Ehlers-Danlos and Marfan syndromes)

—Abnormal cell polarity: Na^+-K^+ ATPase and epidermal growth factor receptor found apically as well as its normal basolateral position; may reverse sodium transport and allow fluid accumulation within cysts

- Risk factors: parents or close relatives with the disease
- Progression of symptoms

—Increased severity of manifestations in males, patients with PKD1, age of diagnosis before 30, age of hypertension diagnosis before 35, gross hematuria before age 30, and three or more pregnancies

—Severity of manifestations may be directly related to maternal imprinting (receiving the defective gene from the mother) and anticipation (disease more severe and earlier onset in the next generation).

—Diet is not shown to affect progression to ESRD.

COMPLICATIONS

- Death from ESRD, intracerebral or subarachnoid hemorrhage
- Chronic pain, nephrolithiasis, renal cyst hemorrhage, and infection are common.
- Liver cysts rarely lead to portal hypertension, while congenital hepatic fibrosis and cholangiocarcinoma are also rare.

DIFFERENTIAL DIAGNOSIS

- Autosomal recessive PKD (autosomal recessive disease that presents in childhood with hepatic fibrosis), medullary dysplastic kidney (dysplastic renal parenchyma without a reniform configuration and increased risk of contralateral UPJ obstruction [3%–12%] or VUR [18%–43%])
- Simple renal cysts
- Von Hippel-Lindau syndrome: autosomal dominant disease with cerebellar hemangioblastomas, retinal angiomatosis, pheochromocytoma, pancreatic and epididymal cysts, with 35%–38% incidence of RCC
- Tuberous sclerosis: hamartomas in brain, skin, and kidneys; CNS abnormalities such as mental retardation and seizure activity; renal angiomyolipomas; <5% also present with polycystic kidneys; 2% incidence of RCC; and associated PKD contiguous gene syndrome (see Associated Conditions in "Miscellaneous" section)
- Sporadic glomerulocystic kidney disease: nonheritable condition diagnosed in neonates with bilateral enlarged kidneys, glomerular cysts, and no extrarenal abnormalities
- Contrast nephropathy and renal vein thrombosis must be considered in a neonate with bilateral renomegaly and homogenous hyperechogenic kidneys.

 Database

HISTORY

- Family: at least three generations of renal disease, hypertension, and strokes
- Patient history of renal disease, hypertension, stroke, hematuria, stones, urinary tract infections

PHYSICAL EXAMINATION

- Blood pressure, hypertensive changes of the retina
- Heart murmur, signs of uremia, cysts within the seminal vesicles
- Enlarged kidneys on abdominal palpation

(continued)

Polycystic Kidney Disease—Autosomal Dominant (continued)

 Diagnostic Studies

LABORATORY TESTING

• Electrolytes, blood urea nitrogen, serum creatinine, urine analysis

IMAGING

• Ultrasound of abdomen, CT scan of abdomen or head, MRI of head. Bilateral renal cysts and two of the following: bilateral renal enlargement; >3 hepatic cysts; cysts of spleen, pancreas, or pineal gland; cerebral artery aneurysm
• IVP: bilateral renal enlargement with calyceal distortion and the "bubble/Swiss cheese nephrogram." This reflects the nonfunctional cysts within the normal renal tissue.

SPECIAL STUDIES

• Cytogenetics: Due to genetic heterogeneity of ADPKD mutations, linkage analysis is still needed to confirm diagnosis at the molecular level.

—Phenotypic heterogeneity between family members with the same genomic genetic mutation may be explained by somatic "second-hit" loss of heterozygosity.

 Treatment

GENERAL MEASURES

• Control of symptoms and preservation of renal function

MEDICAL

• Hypertension (ACE inhibitors in patients with *early* disease)
• Pain (caution in using NSAIDs because of their nephrotoxic potential) can be caused by intracystic hemorrhage, cyst pressure, obstruction by blood clot or stone, and infection.
• Hematuria/cyst hemorrhage usually resolves spontaneously. Treat conservatively, but uncontrolled bleeding may need embolization.
• Infections: most commonly in females and occurs in cysts (87%) and in parenchyma (91%). Treat cystic infection with lipid-soluble antibiotics (trimethoprim-sulfamethoxazole, chloramphenicol, ciprofloxacin, vancomycin, clindamycin, and erythromycin).
• Stones: with normal renal function, can treat stones with same standard of care as given to non-ADPKD patients
• Dialysis for ESRD

SURGICAL

• Cyst pressure relief: Aspirate percutaneously or perform "Rovsing's procedure" (unroofing cyst) via the open or laparoscopic method.

—Two approaches: Treat as many cysts as possible or treat only the largest cyst(s).
—Results: 90% pain-free 6 months after procedure; 77% pain-free at 5 years

• Transplantation: success same between ADPKD and non-ADPKD recipients
• Removal of native kidney(s) indicated only if (1) recurrent pyelonephritis poorly controlled by medical therapy, (2) hematuria requiring transfusion, (3) bulky kidneys that pose an obstacle to caval flow or to transplanted kidney

ALTERNATIVE THERAPIES: N/A

PATIENT EDUCATION

• Renalnet: http://www.renalnet.org
• National Institute of Diabetes and Digestive and Kidney Diseases of the NIH: http://www.niddk.nih.gov
• American Association of Kidney Patients: (800)749-2257; http://www.aakp.org
• Prognosis

—Life expectancy is 4 to 13 years after clinical presentation. Death is usually due to uremia, heart failure, or cerebral hemorrhage.
—ADPKD will cause ESRD in 2% at age 40, 23% at age 50, and 48% at age 73 years. ADPKD diagnosed in utero has a poor prognosis; 43% died before the age of 1 year, and 67% of survivors developed hypertension.

Follow-Up

Monitoring

- Presymptomatic patients: Follow blood pressure and creatinine.
- For marriage, prenatal diagnosis and the search for potential kidney donors in the family
- Issue of early diagnosis of disease

—In favor: Early diagnosis allows early medical management and a chance to rule out the disease early.
—Against: emotions of anxiety, grief, and fear of being a burden with early diagnosis. Also, exclusion from career opportunities and health/life insurance

PREVENTION

- Genetic counseling; in utero ultrasound and genetic testing, with termination of pregnancy if disease is found

 Miscellaneous

SYNONYMS

- Adult-onset polycystic kidney disease

ASSOCIATED CONDITIONS

- TSC2 (tuberous sclerosis)/PKD1 contiguous gene syndrome: characteristics of both ADPKD and TSC, but ESRD earlier (second decade)

NOTES

- Apoptosis may play a role in renal cell destruction, leading to ESRD.

ABBREVIATIONS

- ACE, angiotensin converting enzyme; ADPKD, autosomal dominant polycystic kidney disease; ESRD, end-stage renal disease; PKD, polycystic kidney disease; RCC, renal cell carcinoma; TSC, tuberous sclerosis; UPJ, ureteropelvic junction; VUR, vesicoureteral reflux

REFERENCES

Gabow PA. Autosomal dominant polycystic kidney disease. *N Engl J Med* 1993;329:322–342.

Glassberg KI. Renal dysplasia and cystic disease of the kidney. In: Walsh PC, Retik AB, Vaughan ED, Wein AJ, eds. *Campbell's Urology*, 7th ed. Philadelphia: WB Saunders, 1998:1757–1813.

Grantham JJ. The etiology, pathogenesis, and treatment of autosomal dominant polycystic kidney disease: Recent advances. *Am J Kidney Dis* 1996;28(6):788–803.

Sessa A, et al., eds. *Contributions to Nephrology: Hereditary Kidney Diseases.* Basel: Karger, 1997:122.

Tsiokas L, et al. Homo- and heterodimeric interactions between gene products of PKD1 and PKD2. *Proc Natl Acad Sci U S A* 1997;94:6965–6970.

Authors: Louis S. Liou and Eric A. Klein

Polycystic Kidney Disease—Autosomal Recessive

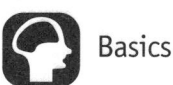 Basics

DESCRIPTION

- A group of inherited disorders involving cystic dilatation of the renal collecting ducts and varying degrees of biliary dysgenesis and periportal fibrosis

EPIDEMIOLOGY

- Commonly discovered in perinatal period, can present early in childhood or adolescence
- Incidence: 1 to 2 in 10,000 live births
- Males and females involved equally
- Severely affected neonates usually die hours after birth; overall survival is much improved if they live beyond the neonatal period.
- Survival: for patients living to 1 month: 86% alive at 1 year, 67% alive at 15 years

GENETICS

- Autosomal recessive, heterozygotes unaffected, gene locus at chromosome 6p21
- Multiple allelism is likely responsible for variable phenotypic presentation.
- Offspring of heterozygotes: 25% risk of disease, 50% carriers

STAGING

- An overlap in the spectrum of renal and liver involvement precludes use of the Blyth and Orkenden classification (perinatal, neonatal, infantile, and juvenile subtypes).
- Best grouped as polycystic disease of newborn and young infant, polycystic disease of childhood, and congenital hepatic fibrosis

SIGNS AND SYMPTOMS

- Prenatal: abnormal prenatal ultrasound (oligohydramnios, enlarged reniform kidneys, absent urine in bladder, seen after 30 weeks' gestation)
- Neonates: palpable flank masses, difficult vaginal delivery, respiratory distress (most common cause of death in neonates), poor urine output, edema, feeding intolerance, Potter's phenotype (deep-set eyes, beaked nose, micrognathia, low-set ears, extremity contractures)
- Infants: palpable flank masses, abdominal mass, respiratory distress, hypertension, polydipsia, polyuria, edema, feeding intolerance, Potter's phenotype, nonspecific GI complaints, failure to thrive, growth retardation, infection
- Older children: palpable flank mass, abdominal mass, Potter's phenotype, GI bleed, hematuria, pyuria, polydipsia, polyuria, hypertension, nonspecific GI complaints, edema, growth retardation, fatigue, infection

PATHOPHYSIOLOGY

- Renal
—Bilateral enlarged kidneys with reniform shape
—Pinpoint opalescent dots on capsule (cortical collecting duct cysts)
—Cut surface with spongelike quality due to linear distention of nephrons in radial pattern
—Normal pelvicalyceal system and renal vessels
—In neonates, kidneys at least 10% of body weight
—Older children: Macrocyst development can give the appearance of autosomal dominant polycystic kidney disease (ADPKD).
—Microscopic pathology: fusiform cysts ($<$2 mm + diameter) lined by low columnar or cuboid epithelium
—Decreased number of glomeruli secondary to collecting duct ectasia and interstitial edema
—No obstruction shown by microdissection studies or electron microscopy
—No normal parenchyma

- Clinical course (renal)
—Severely affected neonates commonly die of pulmonary complications hours after birth.
—Patients surviving the neonatal period have a better prognosis; they can have some renal maturation.
—Progressive renal cyst enlargement, fibrosis, and renal insufficiency
—Eventually, most develop renal failure.
—Later presentation: less severe renal component

- Hepatobiliary
—Can have hepatosplenomegaly at presentation; frequently normal
—Elongated, hyperplastic biliary ducts with ectasia
—Periportal fibrosis with normal hepatocellular histology

- Clinical course (hepatobiliary)
—Development of hepatosplenomegaly, portal hypertension, extrahepatic bile duct dilation, gall bladder enlargement, occasional choledochal cyst formation, and hepatic dysfunction
—Liver failure ultimately develops later in childhood.

CAUSES/RISK FACTORS

- The cause of ARPKD remains poorly understood.
- Genetic and/or epigenetic factors may promote aberrant epithelial hyperplasia.
- Causing cystic expansion of the collecting ducts and fluid accumulation. Less is known about hepatobiliary changes; however, epithelial hyperplasia may have role.
- Risk factors: heterozygous parents

COMPLICATIONS

- Renal: renal failure (concentrating defect with polydipsia and polyuria), HTN, anemia, occasional metabolic acidosis, hyponatremia, osteodystrophy, growth failure
- Hepatobiliary: hepatosplenomegaly, bleeding esophageal varices, portal thrombosis, hypersplenism, choledochal cysts, bacterial cholangitis
- Pulmonary: respiratory failure, pulmonary hypoplasia, pneumothorax, atelectasis, poor diaphragmatic excursion
- Gastrointestinal: feeding intolerance, failure to thrive

DIFFERENTIAL DIAGNOSIS

- ADPKD, juvenile nephronophthisis, renal dysplasia, Meckel-Gruber syndrome, Jeune syndrome, Zellweger syndrome, Ivemark syndrome, Bardet-Biedl syndrome, chondrodysplasia syndrome, Trisomy 9 and 13, glutaric aciduria type II, Caroli disease, congenital hypernephronic nephromegaly with tubular dysgenesis

 Database

HISTORY

- Age of the patient?
—Other cystic renal disorders rarely present in the pediatric population: younger, more respiratory and renal issues; older, more hepatobiliary issues.
- Did the mother have prenatal care?
—Characteristic changes on prenatal US after week 30, abnormal uterine growth measurements, maternal α-fetoprotein levels, amniocentesis results, history of stillbirth
- Birth history
—Difficult delivery suggests possible flank or abdominal mass.
- Family history
—Normal parents with a normal renal US suggests recessive disease.
- Medical history
—For older patient, may suggest clues to evolution of disease
- Present illness: polydipsia, polyuria, fatigue, unexplained fever, hematuria, pyuria, edema, difficult feeding, recent GI bleed or vague GI symptoms

PHYSICAL EXAMINATION

- Hypertension, respiratory rate, temperature
- General appearance
—Potter's phenotype, pallor
- Palpable kidneys: hepatosplenomegaly
- Extremities: joint contractures, edema

Polycystic Kidney Disease—Autosomal Recessive

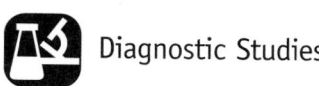 Diagnostic Studies

LABORATORY TESTING

- Electrolytes, blood chemistry, UA, urine culture
- CBC (exclude anemia, hypersplenism), coagulation profile (access liver disease), liver function tests (usually normal), high maternal α-fetoprotein (associated with ARPKD), high amniotic fluid release (possible correlation)

IMAGING

- Ultrasound (best test): prenatal-enlarged kidneys, oligohydramnios, normal liver, no bladder filling (more reliable after 30 weeks' gestation); infancy-enlarged reniform kidneys, cortical echogenicity, loss of corticomedullary differentiation, hypoechoic subcapsular rim; older macrocysts (<2-cm diameter), decreased size, medullary echogenicity, hepatosplenomegaly
- IVP (rarely obtained now) and CT: provide similar information

SPECIAL STUDIES

- Renal biopsy
- Liver biopsy

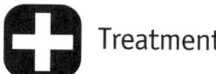 Treatment

GENERAL MEASURES

- No specific therapy for ARPKD. Treatments are supportive.
- Pulmonary issues first priority initially; survival better with advances in perinatology
- Goals: Delay progression to renal failure, liver failure, and portal hypertension.
- Social support and respite care

MEDICAL

- Advanced pulmonary support as required
- Correct acid-base and electrolyte abnormalities.
- Thiazides to help urine concentrating defect
- Aggressive HTN control
- Treatment of renal osteodystrophy with vitamin D phosphate binders
- Recombinant human erythropoietin
- Growth hormone treatment
- Peritoneal dialysis
- Enteral feedings
- Adequate hydration

SURGICAL

- Preemptive bilateral nephrectomy and peritoneal dialysis catheter (significant pulmonary distress)
- Unilateral nephrectomy (improve feedings, help with breathing)
- Gastrostomy tube placement (improve feedings)
- Splenorenal shunt or portocaval shunt procedures (portal hypertension)
- Renal transplantation (ESRD)
- Liver transplantation (hepatic failure)

ALTERNATIVE THERAPIES: N/A

PATIENT EDUCATION

- Genetic counseling

—Thorough understanding of the pathogenesis and progression of disease
—Emphasis on team approach; pediatric subspecialists and support staff

 Follow-Up

MONITORING

- Close monitoring of renal and liver function. Prevent associated complications of renal and hepatobiliary disease.

PREVENTION

- Genetic counseling for families with proven ARPKD (linkage studies with polymorphic DNA markers)

 Miscellaneous

SYNONYMS

- Infantile polycystic kidney disease; Potter type I polycystic kidneys

ASSOCIATED CONDITIONS

- Ehlers-Danlos syndrome

NOTES

- See also Section II, "Polycystic Kidney Disease—Autosomal Dominant."

ABBREVIATIONS: N/A

REFERENCES

Levine E, Hartman DS, Mellstrup JW, Van Slyke MA, Edgar KA, Barth JC. Current concepts and controversies in imaging of renal cystic disease. *Urol Clin North Am* 1997;24:523.

Roy S, Dillon MJ, Trompeter RS, Barratt TM. Autosomal recessive polycystic kidney disease: Long-term outcome of neonatal survivors. *Pediatr Nephrol* 1997;11:302.

Zerres K, Mucher G, Becker J, et al. Prenatal diagnosis of autosomal recessive polycystic kidney disease: Molecular genetics, clinical experience, and fetal morphology. *Am J Med Genet* 1998;76:137.

Zerres K, Rudnik-Schoneborn S, Steinkamm C, Becker J, Mucher G. Autosomal recessive polycystic kidney disease. *J Mol Med* 1998;76:303.

Authors: Matthew T. Gettman and Michael J. Erhard

Posterior Urethral Valves

 Basics

DESCRIPTION

• Congenital valvular obstruction of the posterior urethra that can cause variable degrees of dysfunction of all segments of the urinary tract, including the bladder, ureters, and kidney

EPIDEMIOLOGY

• Congenital only
• Prevalence: 1 in 5000 to 1 in 8000 male births
• No racial predilection
• Most common cause of lower urinary tract obstruction in males

GENETICS

• Unknown

STAGING: N/A

SIGNS AND SYMPTOMS

• The use of antenatal ultrasonography has changed the presentation and timing of diagnosis of this disease.

—Antenatal features
—Bilateral hydroureteronephrosis
—Distended bladder
—Distended proximal, posterior urethra: "keyhole" sign
—Oligohydramnios
—Urinary ascites
—Postnatal presentation
—Abdominal mass(es): bladder, kidneys
—Failure to thrive
—Urosepsis
—Poor urinary stream
—Urinary ascites

PATHOPHYSIOLOGY

• Congenital mucosal membrane (fold/valve) in the posterior urethra
• Hugh H. Young Classification, 1919

—Type I
—Obstructing mucosal membrane attached proximally to the verumontanum and distally, extending to the membranous urethra: most common type (95%)
—Type II
—Mucosal fold extending from the verumontanum to the bladder neck, superiorly: regarded as nonobstructive and secondary to the type I or type III valve
—Type III
—Transverse membrane in the posterior urethra; has a central aperture; no attachment to the verumontanum and located distal to the verumontanum: uncommon (5%)

• Secondary effects of the valve

—Dilation of the urethra proximal to the valve
—Dilation of the bladder
—Trabeculation of the bladder wall with increased deposition of fibrous tissue

—Vesicoureteric reflux noted in about 50% of the patients
—Hydroureteronephrosis
—Possible renal dysplasia/hypoplasia
—Leakage of urine from the fornix of the kidney, causing perirenal urinoma or urinary ascites
—Oligohydramnios: range of severity from mild to severe; the severe type can be associated with pulmonary hypoplasia and Potter's facies.

CAUSES/RISK FACTORS

• Type I valve: embryology not completely understood. Possibly the end result of anomalous insertion of the mesonephric ducts into the primitive fetal cloaca
• Type II valve thought to be hypertrophy of superficial muscle that extends from the ureteral orifice to the verumontanum
• Type III valve could be the result of incomplete dissolution of the urogenital membrane; this valve is not attached to the verumontanum and can have bizarre configurations at times (e.g., the "windsock" valve).

COMPLICATIONS

• Early

—Urinary infection
—Fluid and electrolyte imbalance
—Urinary ascites
—Respiratory distress syndrome; more common in those patients with significant oligohydramnios

• Later

—Poor renal function in about one-third
—End-stage renal failure in about 15%
—Death from renal failure in about 10%

• Other

—Persistence of vesicoureteral reflux; after treatment of the valve, reflux persists in about one-third to one-half of the patients.
—A unilateral nonfunctional kidney is associated with unilateral reflux and renal dysplasia.
—Bladder dysfunction is associated with a poorly compliant or fibrotic bladder.
—Urinary incontinence is rarely due to damage to the external sphincter; it is usually secondary to the poorly compliant bladder and high-output renal impairment.
—Potential for sterility secondary to retrograde ejaculation

DIFFERENTIAL DIAGNOSIS

• Antenatally and postnatally

—Anterior urethral valve
—Prune-belly syndrome
—Severe bilateral vesicoureteric reflux (megacystis/megaureter syndrome)
—Congenital urethral stricture
—Neurogenic bladder
—Megacystis/microcolon syndrome
—Bilateral prolapsing ureteroceles
—Bladder neck obstruction: It is regarded that this condition was overdiagnosed previously; this condition is rare.

 Database

HISTORY

• Antenatally

—There are no specific questions in the maternal or family history to aid in the diagnosis.

• Postnatally

—Since the diagnosis is either suspected antenatally on ultrasound examination or in the neonatal period for the reasons mentioned above, no history can be obtained from the patient.
—Questioning the mother or nursing staff about the nature of the urinary stream or noticing if the child strains to void is most unreliable method to make the diagnosis of PUVs.
—Failure to thrive
—Symptoms indicative of sepsis in a neonate/infant
—Delayed presentation of PUVs in childhood is rare these days; They are to be considered in any male with a chronic history of day and night urinary incontinence; urinary tract infection; chronic polydipsia/polyuria.

PHYSICAL EXAMINATION

• Neonatal presentation

—General: Potter's facies, limb deformities (rare; in patients with severe obstruction and oligohydramnios); clinical features of the prune-belly syndrome: wrinkled abdominal wall, undescended testes, palpable bladder
—Pulmonary: respiratory distress syndrome, pulmonary hypoplasia
—Abdominal: palpable bladder, kidneys; abdominal distention secondary to ascites
—Genitalia: Observing a bulge in the penoscrotal junction during urination is indicative of an anterior urethral valve.
—Spine: Examine for evidence of a myelomeningocele.

• Childhood presentation

—Urinary incontinence with or without a palpable bladder

Diagnostic Studies

LABORATORY TESTING

• Urinalysis and urine culture. Check for urinary infection.
• Serum electrolytes, BUN, and creatinine. Check for salt wasting, acidosis, and elevated BUN and creatinine.
• CBC: Check for signs of sepsis, anemia.
• Blood culture/spinal tap if there are signs of sepsis

IMAGING

• Renal and bladder ultrasound to assess for degree of hydroureteronephrosis, quality of renal parenchyma (corticomedullary differentiation, echogenicity feature of renal dysplasia, thickness of renal parenchyma, thickness of the bladder wall)
• Contrast (fluoroscopic) voiding cystourethrogram: This is the only study that can diagnose the urethral valve accurately. Check for vesicoureteral reflux.
• A radionuclide renal scan (DMSA) is usually delayed until the neonate is a few weeks old, so that better imaging can be obtained of the differential function of the kidneys.

SPECIAL STUDIES: N/A

 ## Treatment

GENERAL MEASURES

• Insertion of a 5Fr to 8Fr feeding tube into the bladder and left indwelling. Passage of the catheter into the bladder is not difficult, as a rule.
• Daily weights
• Accurate input and output fluid-balance record
• Routine vital signs
• Establishing an intravenous line in order to give fluids and electrolytes, and antibiotics

MEDICAL

• Correction of any fluid and electrolyte imbalance
• Administration of broad-spectrum antibiotics. If gentamicin is used, careful monitoring of the gentamicin levels in the blood is mandatory

SURGICAL

• Transurethral incision/destruction of the valve possible in more than 80% of neonates. Miniaturization of cystoscopes/resectoscopes has made this possible.
• Cutaneous vesicostomy in patients whose urethra is too small to accept the urethral instruments

—Transurethral destruction of the valve and closure of the vesicostomy is done, simultaneously, at a later age (2–4 months of age).
—Bilateral cutaneous ureterostomies as immediate treatment; rare today, but popular 20 years ago
—Nephroureterectomy of a nonfunctional upper tract is done at a later stage.
—Reimplantation of a persistently refluxing, functioning upper tract might be necessary.
—Bladder augmentation is rarely needed for patients with PUVs.

ALTERNATIVE THERAPIES

• Suprapubic endoscopic ablation of the valve is described but rarely done.
• Ablation of the valve by an insulated "crotchet hook" through the urethra has been described but rarely used.

PATIENT EDUCATION

• Instruct parents to watch for signs of urinary infection.
• Explain that additional fluid replacement by mouth might be a lifelong need.
• Explain the patient's limited tolerance of dehydration.
• Stress that long-term follow-up is essential.
• Inform parents of the long-term complications of this disease and its treatment.

 ## Follow-Up

MONITORING

• Frequent follow-up is necessary. Frequency of visitation is determined by the severity of the disease.

—Urinalyses and urine culture and sensitivity
—Serum electrolyte, BUN, and creatinine assessment to observe renal function
—Renal and bladder ultrasounds to follow upper tract dilation
—Voiding cystourethrograms to assess ablation of valve, bladder size, progress of vesicoureteral reflux
—Radionuclide scans to assess for individual renal function

PREVENTION

• Prophylactic antimicrobials if vesicoureteral reflux is present

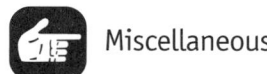 ## Miscellaneous

SYNONYMS

• Urethral valves

ASSOCIATED CONDITIONS: N/A

NOTES

• It is hoped that the earlier diagnosis of children with PUVs could result in some reduction in the incidence of renal failure.

ABBREVIATIONS

• PUVs, posterior urethral valves

REFERENCES

Cendron M, et al. Perinatal urology. In: Gillenwater JY, Grayhack JT, Howards SS, Duckett JW, eds. *Adult and Pediatric Urology*, 3rd ed. St Louis: Mosby, 1996.

Gonzales ET. Posterior urethral valves and other anomalies. In: Walsh PC, Retik AB, Vaughan ED, Wein AJ, eds. *Campbell's Urology*, 7th ed. Philadelphia: WB Saunders, 1998.

Hulbert WC, et al. Posterior urethral valve obstruction. AUA Update Series, Lesson 29, Volume XI, 1992.

Kaplan GW, et al. Infravesical obstruction. In: Kelalis PP, et al., eds. *Clinical Pediatric Urology*, 3rd ed. Philadelphia: WB Saunders, 1992.

Author: R. Bruce Filmer

Postobstructive Diuresis

 Basics

DESCRIPTION

• Polyuria resulting from the relief of bilateral ureteral obstruction or obstruction of a solitary kidney

EPIDEMIOLOGY

• Peak incidence in men 70 to 90 years old, due to increased obstruction from benign prostatic hyperplasia (BPH) and prostatic cancer
• Peak incidence in women 40 to 60 years old, due to obstruction from pregnancy and carcinoma of the cervix and uterus

GENETICS: N/A

STAGING: N/A

SIGNS AND SYMPTOMS

• Obstruction

—Asymptotic but is often associated with flank pain radiating to groin and/or ipsilateral thigh, nausea, vomiting, fevers, chills
—Resulting uremia may cause mental status changes, tremors, and GI bleeding.

• Diuresis

—Increase in urine output out of proportion to fluid intake, usually >200 cc/h

PATHOPHYSIOLOGY

• Retained urea, sodium, and water; impaired sodium reabsorption and concentrating ability of the renal tubule; and circulating hormones all contribute.

—Increased sodium, potassium, and magnesium losses result in increased water excretion.
—Accumulated urea acts as an osmotic agent, bringing fluid with it as it is cleared, thereby increasing diuresis.
—Impaired concentrating ability of the renal tubule leads to continuing fluid losses and hypovolemia.

• Atrial natriuretic peptide (ANP), which causes vasodilation, natriuresis, and diuresis, has been found to be elevated in patients with ureteral obstruction.

CAUSES/RISK FACTORS

• Urinary tract obstruction is caused by a number of processes, grouped into extrinsic and intrinsic causes.

—Intrinsic: nephrolithiasis, blood clot, ureteral strictures, urethral strictures, neurogenic bladder, anticholinergic agents, levodopa
—Extrinsic: BPH, prostate cancer, tubo-ovarian abscess, ovarian tumor or cyst, endometriosis, arterial aneurysms, tumors of the kidney, ureter, bladder, and urethra and their corresponding lymphatic and metastatic spread

• Obstructed patients most likely to have POD are those with chronic obstruction, edema, congestive heart failure, hypertension, weight gain, azotemia, and uremic encephalopathy.

COMPLICATIONS

• Uremic death
• Hypovolemic circulatory collapse
• Bladder mucosal bleeding secondary to vein rupture resulting from rapid bladder decompression
• Arrhythmia secondary to electrolyte abnormalities

DIFFERENTIAL DIAGNOSIS

• Causes of polyuria

—Medications
  —Lithium carbonate, methoxyflurane, demethylchlortetracycline, amphotericin B, mannitol, glycerol, diuretics, ethanol, opiate antagonist, phenytoin
—Diabetes insipidus, diabetes mellitus
—Renal disease: diuretic phase of ATN

• Physiologic diuresis from fluid excess

 Database

HISTORY

• Chronic obstruction

—Weight gain, malaise, fatigue, shortness of breath

• Acute obstruction

—Flank pain associated with forced diuresis (consumption of coffee, tea, or alcohol), nausea, vomiting, hematuria, anuria

PHYSICAL EXAMINATION

• Chronic obstruction

—Pulmonary congestion, pitting edema of lower extremities, hypertension

• Acute obstruction

—Abdominal mass, suprapubic tenderness, flank tenderness

Diagnostic Studies

LABORATORY TESTING

• CBC, urine culture and sensitivity

—Infection in the setting of obstruction requires emergent evaluation and treatment.

• SMA-7

—BUN and creatinine are typically elevated and are monitored after relief of obstruction.
—POD may cause profound hypokalemia.

• Urine osmolality

—Evaluate the kidney's ability to concentrate urine; typically impaired concentrating ability

IMAGING

• Ultrasound is the screening test of choice to evaluate obstruction.

—Avoids risk of contrast agents
—Without hydronephrosis, diagnosis of POD should be questioned.

SPECIAL STUDIES

• Monitor urine output.

—After relief of obstruction, >3 L over 24 hours or more than 200 cc/h over each of 2 consecutive hours is diagnostic of polyuria found with POD.

 ## Treatment

GENERAL MEASURES

• After the obstruction is relieved, admit the patient to the hospital to closely monitor hemodynamic status and electrolytes.
• Monitor urine output q2h and replace with intravenous fluids (0.5–1.0 cc of one-half NS per cubic centimeter of urine output) in addition to po fluids.
• Check serum sodium and potassium every 6 to 12 hours and replace as needed.
• Follow BUN and creatinine values to normal.

—If they remain elevated, obtain a follow-up renal ultrasound to rule out hydronephrosis.
—If there is persistent hydronephrosis, consider persistent obstruction of ureter(s) above the level of the bladder or a nonfunctioning stent/percutaneous tube.

MEDICAL: N/A

SURGICAL: N/A

ALTERNATIVE THERAPIES: N/A

PATIENT EDUCATION: N/A

 ## Follow-Up

MONITORING

• Serial renal function testing, using blood work and imaging as indicated

PREVENTION

• Treat and repair the cause of obstruction, to prevent recurrence.

 ## Miscellaneous

SYNONYMS

• Postobstructive uropathy

ASSOCIATED CONDITIONS

• Benign prostatic hyperplasia

NOTES

• In a male with long-standing BPH and retention, monitor for POD after Foley catheter insertion in the emergency setting.

ABBREVIATIONS

• POD, postobstructive diuresis

REFERENCES

Gulmi FA, Felsen D, Vaughan ED. Management of post-obstructive diuresis. AUA Update Series 17:177–183.

Gulmi FA, Mooppan UMM, Chou S, et al. Atrial natriuretic peptide in patients with obstructive uropathy. J Urol 1989;142:268–272.

Authors: Jerome Zink and Leonard G. Gomella

Pregnancy—Urolithiasis

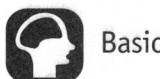 Basics

DESCRIPTION: N/A

EPIDEMIOLOGY

- Incidence: 0.03% to 0.53%
- Usually presents in second or third trimester
- Incidence of symptomatic stones equal, right side vs. left side
- Multiparous women are more commonly affected than are primiparous women.

—May be due to increasing incidence of stones with aging overall

GENETICS: N/A

STAGING: N/A

SIGNS AND SYMPTOMS

- Flank pain
- Abdominal pain

—Renal colic is the most common source of non-obstetric abdominal pain in pregnancy.

- Urgency
- Dysuria, hematuria
- Nausea/emesis
- Fever

PATHOPHYSIOLOGY

- Associated with a higher incidence of maternal urinary tract infections (10%–20%)
- Premature passage can precipitate premature labor and/or interfere with normal labor.
- May cause a higher rate of spontaneous abortions (controversial)
- Physiologic dilation of calyces, ureters, and renal pelves begins in the first trimester and persists into the postpartum period.
- Dilation of right upper tract greater than of left upper tract
- Decreased ureteral peristaltic activity due to hormonal and mechanical factors
- Dilation and decreased peristalsis allow urinary stasis and infection.
- Increased urinary calcium excretion in pregnancy

—Increases 2 to 3 times
—Increased levels of 1,25-dihydroxy vitamin D (Calcitrol)
—Increase in calcium salt excretion
—Glomerular filtration rate (GFR) increases 25% to 50% in pregnancy.

- Urine is more alkaline in pregnancy.

—Protective against uric acid stones

- Increase in excretion of stone inhibitors: citrate and magnesium
- Overall, with all factors considered, pregnancy has no adverse affect on stone disease.

CAUSES/RISK FACTORS

- Dehydration
- Genetic predisposition
- Immobility (relative)
- Voluntary dietary modification (increased calcium)

COMPLICATIONS

- Premature labor, fetal loss
- Urosepsis, renal insufficiency

DIFFERENTIAL DIAGNOSIS

- Hydronephrosis of pregnancy
- Acute pyelonephritis
- Renal vein thrombosis
- Gastroenteritis
- Appendicitis
- Cholecystitis
- Neurologic/musculoskeletal pathology
- Obstetric etiology of pain

 Database

HISTORY

- Pregnancy history
- History of previous stones
- Medications
- Dietary modifications

PHYSICAL EXAMINATION

- Costovertebral angle tenderness
- Abdominal tenderness

 Diagnostic Studies

LABORATORY TESTING

- Serum creatinine

—Adjust for baseline lower values, given the increased GFR (25%–50%) in pregnancy.

- Urinalysis

—Accept some degree of microscopic hematuria secondary to the gravid state.
—Pyuria suggests infection.

- Urine culture

—UTIs are more common in pregnancy associated with stone disease (10%–20%).
—A UTI can induce premature labor.

IMAGING

- KUB, "one-shot" IVP

—Timing of IVP (30, 60, 120 minutes) not standardized
—No adverse affect of contrast material on the fetus has been reported.
—A greater concern is radiation exposure to the fetus.
 —A typical urogram gives <1.5 rads of exposure.
 —5 to 15 rads to the maternal pelvis in the first trimester increases the risk of congenital anomalies by 1% to 3%.
 —However, fetal exposure to as little as 0.4 to 1.0 rads can increase the risk of childhood malignancy 2.4 times.

- Renal ultrasound

—Hydronephrosis
—Renal stones/proximal ureteral stones
—Extravasation/perirenal urinoma
—Resistive index >0.70 in intrarenal arteries supportive of acute obstruction
—Abscess
—Poor assessment of pyelonephritis
—No radiation exposure to fetus

- Transvaginal ultrasound

—Useful for visualizing distal ureteral stones
—May visualize ureteral jets, verifying lack of a complete obstruction
—Document the diameters of distal ureters.

- Noncontrast helical/spiral CT

—Increasing utilization in nonpregnant patients
—Unlikely to be utilized much, due to relatively high radiation exposure

- MRI urography

—Effect on fetal development unknown
—Unlikely to prove useful in this setting

- Percutaneous nephrostogram

—Presumably can be performed at time of placement of percutaneous nephrostomy tube

—Radiation exposure with fluoroscopy is time dependent.

—Unlikely to be used as a diagnostic tool until obstruction is proven by another modality

SPECIAL STUDIES: N/A

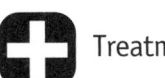 ## Treatment

GENERAL MEASURES

- Observation/hydration/analgesia

—Passage of at least 50% of symptomatic stones

- Intervention required in up to one-third of patients

MEDICAL: N/A

SURGICAL

- Cystoscopy/stent placement

—With or without USS guidance

—With or without ureteroscopy

- Percutaneous nephrostomy tube

—USS can be used for guidance to minimize radiation exposure.

—The stone/obstruction can then be addressed postpartum.

- Nephrolithotomy/ureterolithotomy

—Extremely rare during gestation, given the other temporizing options available

- ESWL

—Not enough data to prove safety during pregnancy

ALTERNATIVE THERAPIES: N/A

PATIENT EDUCATION: N/A

 # Follow-Up

MONITORING

- During gestation

—Conservative management with hydration
  —Indications for intervention
  —Worsening renal function associated with persistent obstruction
  —Intractable pain
  —Obstruction of a solitary kidney
  —Persistent infection associated with an obstruction
  —Renal colic, precipitating premature labor that is refractory to tocolysis

—Preventive medications have unacceptable side effects during pregnancy.
  —Thiazides: can cause fetal thrombocytopenia, hypoglycemia, and hyponatremia
  —Xanthine oxidase inhibitors: no adverse effects on fetal animals; effects on human fetus unknown
  —Penicillamine: teratogenic in rats; fetal defects have been found in infants of mothers who took this during gestation.

- Postpartum

—Metabolic screening should be delayed until postdelivery and lactation.
  —Calcium and urate metabolism is not at baseline during these times.

PREVENTION: N/A

 # Miscellaneous

SYNONYMS: N/A

ASSOCIATED CONDITIONS: N/A

NOTES

- See also Section II, "Pregnancy—Urologic Considerations."

ABBREVIATIONS: N/A

REFERENCES

Hendricks SK, Russ SO, Krieger JN. An algorithm for diagnosis and therapy of management and complications of urolithiasis during pregnancy. *Surg Gynecol Obstet* 1991;172:49–54.

Loughlin KR. Management of urologic problems during pregnancy. *Urology* 1994;44(2):159–169.

Loughlin KR, Bailey RB Jr. Internal ureteral stents for conservative management of ureteral calculi during pregnancy. *N Engl J Med* 1986;315:1647–1649.

Maikranz P, Coe FL, Parks J, Lindheimer MD. Nephrolithiasis in pregnancy. *Am J Kidney Dis* 1987; 9(4):354–358.

Murthy LNS. Urinary tract obstruction during pregnancy: Recent developments in imaging. *Br J Urol* 1997;80[Suppl]:1–3.

Swanson SK, Heilman RL, Eversman WG. Urinary tract stones in pregnancy. *Surg Clin North Am* 1995;75(1):123–142.

Authors: Matthew S. Tobin and Kevin R. Loughlin

Prostate—Benign Hyperplasia

 Basics

DESCRIPTION

• BPH is a noncancerous enlargement of the prostate gland.

EPIDEMIOLOGY

• An estimated 25% of males >50 years old have symptomatic BPH.
• Increased age and normal androgen status are risk factors.
• No racial differences

GENETICS

• First-degree relatives of patients with early onset BPH have 4× the risk for development of BPH.

STAGING: N/A

SIGNS AND SYMPTOMS

• Obstructive symptoms

—Hesitancy, weak stream, straining to void, incomplete bladder emptying, prolonged micturition, acute or recurrent urinary retention

• Irritative symptoms

—Urgency, frequency, nocturia, urge incontinence

PATHOPHYSIOLOGY

• BPH develops in the periurethral transition zone of the prostate. Histologic changes occur as the result of hyperplasia of the stromal nodules. Stimulation of the prostatic smooth muscle leads to increased resistance of the prostatic urethra.
• Prostate growth is under the control of testosterone and its active metabolic dihydrotestosterone. BPH develops when growth factor production is increased from DHT. Increased resistance leads to detrusor instability and ultimately detrusor decompensation with larger residual urine volumes, decreased micturition, and urinary hesitancy.

CAUSES/RISK FACTORS

• Increasing age and normal hormonal states are the only known risk factors.
• Cellular proliferation leading to hyperplasia occurs as the result of an imbalance between growth factors inducing excessive cell division and decreased growth factors with reduced apoptosis.

COMPLICATIONS

• Urinary retention, urinary tract infection, bladder calculus, bladder decompensation, bladder diverticulum, chronic renal insufficiency, acute renal failure, hematuria, upper urinary tract obstruction

DIFFERENTIAL DIAGNOSIS

• Prostate cancer, urinary tract infection, bladder cancer
• Bladder calculus, nonspecific cystitis, uninhibited bladder contractions following CVA, urethral stricture, spinal cord injury
• Parkinson disease, multiple sclerosis, prostatitis, interstitial cystitis, bladder neck dyssynergia, external sphincter dyssynergia

 Database

HISTORY

• Symptoms of voiding dysfunction

—Sensation of incomplete bladder emptying after voiding, urinary frequency, urinary intermittency, urinary urgency, decreased urinary stream, hesitancy in initiation urination, nocturia
—Medical or surgical history, current prescription and over-the-counter medications

• AUA Symptom Score (see Section III) to determine degree of prostatic obstructive symptoms

—Mild (score ≤7); moderate (score 8–19); severe (score 20–35)

PHYSICAL EXAMINATION

• Abdomen

—Palpable bladder secondary to retained urine (usually must be >150 mL to be palpable in adults)

• Digital rectal examination

—To determine size, consistency, palpable nodules, and anatomic limit of prostate and to assess anal sphincter tone

Diagnostic Studies

LABORATORY TESTING

- Urinalysis by dipstick on microscopic examination of spun specimen to rule out urinary tract infection or hematuria; serum creatinine to determine presence or absence of renal insufficiency
- Serum prostate-specific antigen in combination with digital rectal examination to detect possible carcinoma of the prostate

IMAGING

- Transrectal ultrasound of the prostate for accurate assessment of prostate size in patients with large prostates
- Renal ultrasonography if serum creatinine elevated, to determine the presence of hydronephrosis

SPECIAL STUDIES

- Cystoscopy: Evaluate for another pathology that may cause voiding symptoms (i.e., stricture disease, bladder calculus).
- Uroflowmetry to measure peak urinary flow rate, post-void residual urine volume
- Pressure–flow study to determine if low peak flow rate secondary to obstruction or a decompensated neurogenic bladder

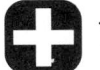 ## Treatment

GENERAL MEASURES

- Treatment primarily based on patient's symptoms

—Mild symptoms: watchful waiting; moderate and severe symptoms: medical therapy or surgical therapy

- Refractory urinary retention, recurrent gross hematuria, a bladder calculus, and renal insufficiency secondary to BPH require surgical therapy.

MEDICAL

- Finasteride (Proscar) 5 mg qd; may be more effective in larger prostate glands (i.e., >40 g)
- Doxazosin (Cardura) 1 to 8 mg qd
- Terazosin (Hytrin) 1 to 8 mg qd
- Tamsulosin (Flomax) 0.4 to 0.8 mg qd

SURGICAL

- Surgical therapy: transurethral incision of the prostate, transurethral resection of the prostate, open prostatectomy

—Minimally invasive treatment: prostatic stents, electrovaporization of the prostate, laser ablation of the prostate (contact, noncontact, interstitial), transurethral needle ablation (TUNA), transurethral microwave thermotherapy (TUMT)

ALTERNATIVE THERAPIES

- Phytotherapy: utilization of extracts from plant compound for relief of BPH symptoms

—Saw palmetto, pumpkin seed, *Pygeum africanum*, alfalfa, forage crops, South African star grass, stinging nettle, aspen, purple cone flower, garlic, rye pollen

PATIENT EDUCATION

- Patients should be educated in regard to symptoms, effect on the quality of life, and risks and implications of different therapeutic options.

 ## Follow-Up

MONITORING

- Periodic follow-up of patients on watchful waiting or medical therapy, with yearly visits or return if any increase in symptoms. Should include assessment of symptoms, periodic uroflow, and determination of residual urine

PREVENTION

- None known

 ## Miscellaneous

SYNONYMS

- Prostatism, lower urinary tract symptoms (LUTS), bladder outlet obstruction (BOO)

ASSOCIATED CONDITIONS: N/A

NOTES

- See also Section II, "Bladder Outlet Obstruction."

ABBREVIATIONS

- BPH, benign prostatic hyperplasia

REFERENCES

Buck AC. Phytotherapy for the prostate. *Br J Urol* 1996;78:325.

Gee WF, Holtgrewe HL, Albertson PC, et al. Practice trends in the diagnosis and management of benign prostatic hyperplasia in the United States. *J Urol* 1995;154:205.

Kirby RS, McConnell JD. *Benign Prostatic Hyperplasia.* Oxford: Health Press, 1997.

McConnell J. Epidemiology, etiology, pathophysiology and diagnosis of benign prostatic hyperplasia. In: Walsh PC, Retik AB, Vaughan ED, Wein AJ, eds. *Campbell's Urology,* 7th ed. Philadelphia: WB Saunders, 1998.

McConnell J, et al. Benign prostatic hyperplasia diagnosis and treatment. Clinical practice guideline. U.S. Dept. of Health and Human Services, Agency for Health Care Policy and Research, 1994.

Author: W. Bruce Shingleton

Prostate Cancer—General

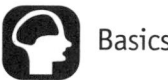 Basics

DESCRIPTION

• Adenocarcinoma of the prostate (CaP)

EPIDEMIOLOGY

• Most common solid tumor in U.S. males; 179,500 cases in 1999; over 37,000 deaths
• With PSA blood test in mid-1980s, rate of CaP skyrocketed 69% between 1989 and 1992, and peaked in 1992 for White Americans at 186 in 100,000 and in 1993 for Black Americans at 265 in 100,000
• In 1994, rate declined 27% for Whites and 11% for Blacks; decrease continues over time
• Mean age at diagnosis: 65 years, rare <50
• Higher risk in African Americans, Africans, and in the Caribbean; lower in Asians; Caucasians: intermediate risk
• Unknown if racial differences are environmental or genetic or a combination
• High rate of clinically unimportant cancer in men over 70
• Familial: approximately 15%. Suspect if diagnosis young, <60 years, or 5 or more family members affected

GENETICS

• Unknown, but human prostate cancer-1 (HPC-1) on chromosome 1 linked to some familial CaP
• HPC-1 or other undiscovered gene(s) could account for 10% to 15% of CaP in men <60 years with family history.
• Familial not more aggressive than sporadic cases
• Other genes: *p53* tumor suppressor gene, *bcl-2* oncogene, E-cadherin, *c-erbB-2*, PTEN1, androgen receptor (AR) implicated. *p53* and *bcl-2* appear to be prognostic biomarkers.
• Multifocality and heterogeneity of CaP makes genetic studies difficult, especially on needle biopsy.

STAGING

• CaP spreads from the prostate gland to local periprostatic tissue to pelvic lymph nodes and/or to distant nodes and frank metastases. CaP metastasizes to skeletal system (bones), less likely to lungs and in end-stage to liver and other organs, such as CNS. Staging studies dictated by prediagnosis level of serum prostate-specific antigen (PSA). Patients with PSA <10 ng/mL have a low likelihood of metastases, and radiographic studies (i.e., bone scan, computed tomography) are not necessary. A bone scan is usually obtained for PSA > 10 ng/mL, and CT of the pelvis and abdomen may be obtained when initial PSA is >25 ng/mL. Endorectal coil magnetic resonance imaging (MRI) is not proven to be of significant value for local tumor staging.
• See TNM classification in Section VII.
• Traditional staging system: A, B, C, D; preferred staging is TNM (see also Section VII)

—T1 (A): nonpalpable, clinically confined to gland
—T2 (B): palpable, clinically confined to gland
—T3 (C): palpable, local extension of tumor outside of gland
—T4 (C): palpable fixed local extension
—Tany N1-3 (D1): pelvic lymph node metastases
—Tany Nany M1 (D2): distant metastatic disease: bone, lung, liver, CNS

SIGNS AND SYMPTOMS

• No symptoms in early stage; most cases detected by PSA and/or digital rectal examination (DRE)
• Symptoms of local growth: urinary obstructive or irritative voiding symptoms, occasional impotence, hematuria, hematospermia
• Late stage: symptoms of metastases: bone pain, low back pain, weight loss, malaise. Very late: spinal cord compression from vertebral metastases

PATHOPHYSIOLOGY

• Normal prostate: 20 to 25 g, base of bladder surrounding urethra; normal function: produces 30% ejaculate
• Main diseases: prostatitis; benign prostatic hyperplasia (BPH), and prostate cancer
• CaP is adenocarcinoma majority; rarely small cell carcinoma, sarcoma
• Precursor of CaP is prostatic intraepithelial neoplasia (PIN); 50% with PIN are subsequently found to have CaP.
• Prostate produces PSA, a protein secreted into ejaculate, a protease that liquefies seminal fluid; small amount of PSA in serum normally; prostate diseases increase PSA in serum.

CAUSES/RISK FACTORS

• Cause unknown; genetics and environment implicated
• Genetics: Progression of genetic alterations transforms prostate cell to PIN through early and late stage disease (see above).
• Environmental: diet implicated: saturated fat, higher protein "Western" diet. Selenium, vitamin E, lycopene (cooked tomatoes) implicated to be protective
• Hormonal: testosterone/androgens stimulate CaP growth; a known risk factor is elevated testosterone.
• Risk factors: increased age, family history

COMPLICATIONS

- Complications of disease: early stage: urinary symptoms; late stage: bone pain, vertebral Mets, spinal cord compression, ureteral obstruction, bladder outlet obstruction
- Complications of treatment: early stage (i.e., surgery, radiation): impotence, incontinence; late stage (i.e., androgen deprivation therapy): hot flashes, loss of libido, impotence, malaise, loss of muscle mass, possible osteoporosis

DIFFERENTIAL DIAGNOSIS

- Key differential: prostate cancer vs. benign prostatic hyperplasia (BPH)
- Early stage: no symptoms or urinary symptoms; perform DRE and PSA test; if either is abnormal, referral to a urologist is essential.
- Late stage: low back pain, bone pain in older male; consider possibility of CaP; perform PSA and DRE as above.
- Adenocarcinoma of unknown primary: consider CaP; perform special pathology stains for PSA, prostatic acid phosphatase (PAP); consider prostate biopsy.

 Database

HISTORY

- Typical case in 1990s: middle-aged male with elevated PSA on screening; referral to urologist for transrectal ultrasound of prostate (TRUS-prostate) and prostate needle biopsy. Rare scenario: man with symptoms of metastases, such as bone pain

PHYSICAL EXAMINATION

- Key examination: digital rectal examination (DRE), prefer standing in bent-over position with elbows on knees. Careful palpitation for nodules or internal induration. Any abnormality: referral to urologist
- Late stage: palpable bladder on abdominal examination, rare: supraclavicular adenopathy

 Diagnostic Studies

LABORATORY TESTING

- Mainstay for screening and staging

—Traditional normal value: 0 to 4 ng/mL
—Age- and race-adjusted normal ranges now commonly used

AGE RANGE	ASIANS	BLACKS	WHITES
40–49	0–2.0	0–2.0	0–2.5
50–59	0–3.0	0–4.0	0–3.5
60–69	0–4.0	0–4.5	0–4.5
70–79	0–5.0	0–5.5	0–6.5

—Traditional "normal" up to 4.0 ng/mL too high for young men; many now use 0 to 2.5 ng/mL as normal cut-off.

- Free PSA: "total" PSA (as noted above) is the traditional test; "free" PSA is the proportion of total PSA that is not bound to other proteins in the serum (i.e., free).

—Lower free PSA: higher risk of CaP

- Probability of cancer: based on PSA and %FPSA results

—Men with nonsuspicious DRE results, any age
—%FPSA can stratify risk for men with PSA between 4 and 10 ng/mL

PSA	CANCER RATE	%FPSA	PROBABILITY OF CANCER
0–2 ng/mL	1%	0%–10%	56%
2–4 ng/mL	15%	10%–15%	28%
4–10 ng/mL	25%	15%–20%	20%
>10 ng/mL	>50%	20%–25%	16%
		>25%	8%

- Prostatic acid phosphatase (PAP): no role in screening; ? prognostic in predicting recurrence in early stage CaP
- Alkaline phosphatase: if elevated, may signify bone metastases; higher level: poorer survival in metastatic CaP
- Creatinine: primary or nodes may obstruct ureter
- Hematocrit: prognostic factor in metastatic CaP

(continued)

Prostate Cancer—General (continued)

IMAGING

- Transrectal ultrasound of the prostate (TRUS-P) is mainstay of imaging prostate gland to direct systematic prostate needle biopsies; not a stand-alone screening test but indicated to evaluate abnormal DRE or PSA
- Magnetic resonance imaging (MRI) with endorectal coil: used in selected cases to determine local staging, sensitivity, and specificity for extra-prostatic disease extension; is suboptimal
- Bone scan: to evaluate for metastasis; should be used with PSA > 10 ng/mL
- CT pelvis and abdomen: to evaluate for lymph node and soft-tissue metastases; limited value unless significantly elevated PSA (i.e., >25–50 ng/mL)
- ProstaScint (indium-III-labeled monoclonal antibody scan): nuclear medicine scan to detect occult metastases via monoclonal antibody directed against prostate-specific membrane antigen (PSMA). Has some ability to differentiate local vs. distant recurrence; studies are ongoing.

SPECIAL STUDIES

- Unknown adenocarcinoma primary metastases: stained for PSA, PSMA, and/or PAP to identify prostatic primary
- Prognostic biomarkers: *p53, bcl-2* promising but investigational
- DNA ploidy flow cytometry or image analysis: debated whether DNA ploidy adds unique prognostic value
- Reverse-transcriptase polymerase chain reaction (RT-PCR) of PSA-expressing potential occult metastatic cells in blood/marrow/nodes strictly investigational

 Treatment

GENERAL MEASURES

- Depends on stage and general health of individual
- Many diagnosed in older men (>70 years); some men may die of other causes, even with untreated CaP.
- Early stage: radical prostatectomy, external beam radiotherapy, brachytherapy (seed implant radiation), with or without neoadjuvant or adjuvant hormonal therapy, and watchful waiting (observation without treatment)
- Late stage: mainstay is hormonal therapy (i.e., any treatment to lower androgens), with or without radiation

MEDICAL

- Hormonal therapies

—LH-RH agonists (medical castration): leuprolide acetate injection every 1, 3, or 4 months (Lupron). Goserelin acetate injection every 1 or 3 months (Zoladex)

—Antiandrogens: flutamide (Eulexin) 250 mg tid po; bicalutamide (Casodex) 50 mg qd po; nilutamide (Nilandron) 300 mg qd po first month, then 150 mg qd po

—LH-RH injections may be administered alone or along with daily antiandrogens (orally). Called "combination hormonal therapy"

- Chemotherapy: indicated for hormone refractory prostate cancer (HRPC). No single agent or combination has been proven to prolong survival, but significant palliation can be achieved.

—Two FDA-approved chemotherapies: estramustine phosphate (Emcyt) and mitoxantrone (Novantrone), along with steroids

—Commonly used chemotherapies: vinblastine, etoposide, paclitaxel, and many clinical trials

SURGICAL

- Radical prostatectomy

—Complete surgical removal of prostate and seminal vesicles with reanastomosis of bladder to urethra; used since early 1900s

—Can be curative if organ confined; most commonly used local treatment for curative intent

—Side effects: impotence in 25% to 100%, depending on nerve sparing and age/health of patient. Incontinence: total 1% to 3%; stress incontinence: 10% to 30%

- Brachytherapy (radiation seed implants): TRUS-P guided placement of radioactive I^{125} or Pd^{103} into prostate. Current technique used since early 1990s; short-term results comparable to radical prostatectomy for early-stage patients; long-term cure rate unknown; lower rate of incontinence; suspected lower rate of impotence than prostatectomy
- Orchiectomy (castration): removal of testicles in late-stage prostate cancer as method of hormonal therapy; very effective, inexpensive; few men choose this treatment in era of medical (LH-RH) injections

ALTERNATIVE THERAPIES

- External beam radiation therapy: a standard treatment, can be combined with hormones to increase effectiveness in bulky tumors; comparable 10-year control rates compared with prostatectomy for low-stage disease. Three-dimensional conformal improves delivery, minimizes side effects.
- Cryosurgery: computer-controlled liquid nitrogen–cooled perineal probes placed via TRUS-P guidance to freeze prostate gland

—Investigational with long-term results is unknown; high rate of impotence. Salvage after radiation: high rate of incontinence

- Proton and neutron radiation therapy: investigational; deliver higher doses of radiation with fewer effects to surrounding normal tissue. No long-term data

PATIENT EDUCATION

- Support groups

—US TOO, International: (800)80-USTOO; www.ustoo.com
—American Cancer Society Man-to-Man support groups; contact local ACS chapter.
—American Foundation for Urologic Disease (AFUD): (800)82USTOO
—National Cancer Institute (NCI): (800)4CANCER

 Follow-Up

MONITORING

- PSA gold standard

—Radical prostatectomy: should decline to undetectable (<0.1 ng/mL)
—Radiation or hormones should decline to very low nadir level (i.e., <0.2–0.5 ng/mL)
—Rising PSA indicates disease recurrence. *Recurrence* is defined as two or three documented increased PSA values after the posttreatment nadir.

- Typical follow-up: every 3 months during the first year, every 6 months for years 2 to 4, annually year 5 and beyond
- Follow-up tests: PSA, DRE; other tests are individualized.

PREVENTION

- No proven preventative strategy
- Ongoing studies with diet (low-fat, saturated-fat), finasteride, lycopene (tomato-based foods), vitamin E, and selenium

 Miscellaneous

SYNONYMS

- Prostate cancer, adenocarcinoma of the prostate, prostate carcinoma

ASSOCIATED CONDITIONS

- Benign prostatic hyperplasia (BPH): Noncancerous enlargement of the prostate may elevate PSA and cause similar symptoms, but this is *not* a precancerous condition.

NOTES

- See other topics on PSA, prostate nodules, and specific stages of prostate cancer

ABBREVIATIONS

- CaP, prostate cancer

REFERENCES

Moul JW. Treatment options for prostate cancer. Part I: Stage, grade, PSA, and changes in the 1990s. *Am J Managed Care* 1998;4:1031–1036.

Moul JW. Treatment options for prostate cancer. Part II: Early and late stage and hormone refractory disease. *Am J Managed Care* 1998;4:1171–1180.

Author: Judd W. Moul

Prostate Cancer—Hormone Refractory (D3)

 Basics

DESCRIPTION

- Clinical or biochemical progression of prostate cancer disease after a period of hormonal ablation

EPIDEMIOLOGY

- Historically, the median duration to biochemical failure is 16 to 18 months.
- 50% mortality 24 months after progression
- Occurs after periods of androgen deprivation for prostate cancer

GENETICS

- Clonal selection of androgen-independent cancer cells and/or adaptation to new hormonal environment

STAGING

- T×N×M1 in the TNM staging system
- D3 in the ABCD staging system

SIGNS AND SYMPTOMS

- Weight loss, anorexia, lethargy, hematuria, urinary retention, ureteral obstruction, rectal obstruction, bone pain, neurologic deficits, visual impairment, altered mental status

PATHOPHYSIOLOGY: N/A

CAUSES/RISK FACTORS

- Not understood

COMPLICATIONS

- Anemia from hematuria
- Uremia from urinary retention or ureteral obstruction
- Cord compression syndrome from collapse of spinal column
- Ambulatory difficulty from fracture of weight-bearing bones
- Visual impairment or mental status alteration from brain metastasis

DIFFERENTIAL DIAGNOSIS

- Bone pain
—Degenerative joint disease
—Paget disease

 Database

HISTORY

- Initial Gleason score, stage, serum PSA
- Past treatment(s)
- PSA nadir level posttreatment
- Time and level of PSA relapse
- Duration of androgen deprivation
- Sensory and motor functions
- Visual/mental status alteration
- Voiding function
- Overall physical health and psychological well-being

PHYSICAL EXAMINATION

- Chest examination to rule out gynecomastia
- Genitourinary examination
- Neurologic examination

 Diagnostic Studies

LABORATORY TESTING

- PSA every 3 to 4 minutes
- Electrolytes, BUN, and creatinine every 6 months

IMAGING

- Bone scan performed every 6 to 12 months
- X-rays, MRI to rule out cord compression
- Renal ultrasonography to rule out hydronephrosis
- Post-void residual to assess urinary retention

SPECIAL STUDIES: N/A

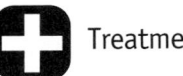 Treatment

GENERAL MEASURES

- No effective treatment
- 70% of these patients will die of prostate cancer.
- Continue androgen deprivation
- Radiation treatment for symptomatic bony metastasis
- If available, enroll the patient in clinical trials.

MEDICAL

- Withdraw antiandrogens if on maximal androgen blockade (MAB)
- Medications to suppress the adrenal testosterone (5% of all testosterone)
—Corticosteroid
—Suppressing the pituitary production of ACTH
—Hydrocortisone 50 mg/d, or dexamethasone 0.75 mg bid
—20% to 80% response rate
—Ketoconazole
—Inhibiting the cytochrome P-450 in the synthesis of steroid. Additionally, some cytotoxic effects
—200 to 400 mg tid
—As high as 30% response rate
—Side effects: nausea, vomiting, skin rash, hepatitis
—Aminoglutethimide
—Inhibiting the cytochrome P-450 in the steroidogenesis
—1000 to 1750 mg/d
—Highly variable response rate, ranging from 0% to 40%
—Side effects: lethargy, nausea, skin rash, hypothyroidism, hepatitis
—Antiandrogens
—Steroidal antiandrogen: cyproterone
—Nonsteroidal antiandrogens: flutamide (Eulexin), bicalutamide (Casodex), nilutamide (Nilandron)
—Monotherapy agent or a component of MAB

- Bone pain palliation by analgesics, diphosphonate, or radiation treatment
—Analgesics
  —Aspirin or other NSAIDs
  —Opiates: codeine or oxycodone
  —Long-acting opiate: fentanyl patch
—Diphosphate
  —Effective if given intravenously
  —Suppresses one resorption by directly inhibiting osteoclasts
—Local radiation
  —Pain palliation for a single site of the metastasis
  —Given in divided doses (30 Gy, total) over 2 to 3 weeks
—Wide-field irradiation
  —Hemibody irradiation reserved for widespread metastasis
  —Alleviation of pain is immediate and significant.
  —Gastroenterologic and hematologic side effects
—Strontium-89 (Metastron)
  —Deposit in areas of bony metastasis
  —Provides comparable pain relief as the external beam radiation
  —Delays disease progression and incidences of new sites of pain
  —Hematologic side effects
  —Criteria for strontium-89 treatment: presence of multiple metastases and diffuse bony pain; WBCs >3000, and platelets >60,000; life expectancy >3 months; refractory to the hormonal or chemotherapy treatment

SURGICAL

- Bilateral orchiectomy considered, if not yet done

ALTERNATIVE THERAPIES

- Working through direct cytotoxic effects or regulation of cellular receptors
- A combination therapy of these agents may prove to be beneficial in the future.
- Cytotoxic agents: estrogens, progestins, and their derivatives
- Estrogens

—Diethylstilbestrol (DES): suppression of the steroidogenesis; direct cytotoxic effect by inhibiting DNA polymerase; cardiovascular and thromboembolytic complications
—Estramustine phosphate (EMP)
  —Metabolized to estradiol and estrone
  —Accumulates in the prostate and binds to microtubule-associated proteins to cause microtubule disintegration
  —60% response rate; significant hematologic side effects

- Progestins
—Medroxyprogesterone
  —Direct cytotoxic effects
  —Downregulation of the gonadotropin secretion
  —Limited use other than relief of bone pain
—Megestrol
  —Most common progestin used for prostate cancer
  —Low response rate
  —Primarily used as an appetite stimulant
- Receptor-regulating agents: somatostatin, suramin, calcitriol, Taxol, Retinoid, Liarozole
—Somatostatin
  —Blocks the growth hormone action
  —Prevents secretion of insulin-like growth factors (IGFs)
  —Moderate response rate
  —Minimal side effects
  —Further investigation underway
—Suramin
  —A growth factor inhibitor
  —Significant neuromuscular toxicity and adrenal insufficiency
—Calcitriol
  —Inhibits growth of prostate cancer in vitro
  —Minimal response rate in current trial
  —May cause hypercalcemia
—Taxol
  —High affinity for polymerized microtubules
  —Moderate response rate
  —Report of leukopenia as the only significant side effect
  —Undergoing further trials
—Retinoid
  —A transcription regulator that inhibits angiogenesis and tubule formation
  —Its role in chemoprevention is currently under investigation
—Liarozole
  —Inhibits the metabolism of retinoic acid and thus increases the retinoic acid level. Not well-documented efficacy and side effects

PATIENT EDUCATION

- Teach patients the signs and symptoms of advanced prostate cancer.
—Cord compression syndrome
—Urinary retention
—Bone pain
—Hematuria
- Support groups
—USTOO International: www.ustoo.com
—Man to Man (American Cancer Society): (800)ACS-2345; www.cancer.org
—American Cancer Society: (800)ACS-2345; www.cancer.org
—National Cancer Institute: (800)4-CANCER; www.nci.nih.gov
—National Prostate Cancer Coalition: (202)463-9455; www.4npcc.org

 Follow-Up

MONITORING

- Regular follow-up for bone scan, physical examination, laboratory tests, and ultrasonography for kidneys; post-void residuals should be instituted.
- In addition to the physical health, the patient's as well as the family's psychological well-being should be monitored. A multidisciplinary approach, involving a team of a urologist, a geriatrician, a psychiatrist, and nurses, provides the best possible care for the patient and family.

PREVENTION: N/A

 Miscellaneous

SYNONYMS

- Androgen (hormone)-resistant, -independent, -insensitive, -escaped, and -refractory

ASSOCIATED CONDITIONS

- Hematuria, urinary retention, ureteral obstruction, renal failure, bone fractures, visual impairment, altered mental status, impotence, infertility

NOTES: N/A

ABBREVIATIONS

- LH-RH agonist, luteinizing hormone–releasing hormone agonist; NSAID, nonsteroidal anti-inflammatory drug

REFERENCES

Kelly WK, Scher HL. Prostate-specific antigen decline after antiandrogen withdrawal: The flutamide withdrawal syndrome. *J Urol* 1993;149:607.

Vorreuther R. Biphosphonates as an adjunct to palliative therapy of bone metastases from prostatic carcinoma. A pilot study on clondonate. *Br J Urol* 1993;72:792.

Authors: David Wei and Arnon Kongrad

Prostate Cancer—Localized (T1, T2)

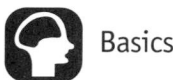 Basics

DESCRIPTION

- Prostate adenocarcinoma that has not clinically spread beyond the prostate capsule. T1a and b diagnosed on TURP; T1c diagnosed because of elevated PSA. T2 is organ confined based on rectal examination.

EPIDEMIOLOGY

- Early detection has increased due to PSA, DRE, and prostate needle biopsy with TRUS (200,000 men/year).
- Age at diagnosis: 70 to 72 years
- Incidence rates: low in Asian men; higher in Scandinavian and African-American men
- Median age at death: all Americans, 77 years; African Americans, 75 years
- Mortality: African-American men have the highest mortality; ≥39,000 men die per year due to PCa.

GENETICS

- Cancer susceptibility gene: autosomal dominant allele, long arm of chromosome 1
- Oncogenes: A mutation of *Ras* occurs in 25% of PCa in Japanese men.
- Tumor suppressor genes: chromosomes *8p, 10q, 13q* (retinoblastoma gene), *16q, 17p (p53)*, and *18q*. Chromosome *17q; p53*: occurs in 53% of high-grade, metastatic tumors. Deletions of chromosomes: *8p22* (70% of cases in localized PCa); *13q* (retinoblastoma gene); *16q* (suppressor gene E-cadherin). Correlates with increased invasiveness and poor survival

STAGING

- See the Appendix for TNM.

SIGNS AND SYMPTOMS

- Symptoms are typically absent in early, localized disease.

PATHOPHYSIOLOGY

- Etiology

—Origin: epithelial, germ, or mesenchymal cells. Pathologic types: epithelial neoplasms (adenocarcinoma: the most common); carcinosarcoma; nonepithelial neoplasms; and germ cell tumors. PIN grade III (severe atypical hyperplasia or hyperplasia with anaplasia) is neoplastic by cytologic patterns and associated with coincidental PCa.

- PCa spread

—Via local extension, lymphatic and hematogenous spread (bones, lung, liver, or brain)

- Gleason grading: low-power microscopy. Grades 1 to 5 (highest grade) assigned for primary (most prevalent pattern) and secondary patterns. Gleason sum (primary + secondary) ranges from 2 to 10.

—Predictive values for organ-confined disease: 70%, Gleason 2 to 6; and 35%, Gleason 7 to 10

—A Partin nomogram (T stage, serum PSA level, and biopsy Gleason score) represents a specific pathologic stage combining all parameters (see Section III).

CAUSES/RISK FACTORS

- Etiology: unknown
- Definitive risk factors

—Age >50 years: exponential increase in incidence and mortality
—Family history: autosomal dominant fashion. Incidence is 6× higher in men with a first- and second-degree relative with PCa.

- Probable/potential risk factors

—Dietary fat: high soy protein diet may lower mortality; higher mortality in countries with high-fat diets
—Vasectomy and cadmium: may increase risk (controversial)
—Hormones: undefined role

COMPLICATIONS

- Localized disease: none before tumor grows larger (i.e., >T3)
- Therapy related

—Hormonal: gynecomastia, decreased size of testis, mood swings, decreased libido
—Radiation: rectal bleeding, hematuria, and pain
—Surgery: 25% require blood transfusion; rectal injury (<1% of cases), myocardial infarction, wound problems will occur in <2% of cases. Bladder neck contracture (5%–12%), urinary incontinence (10%), sexual dysfunction (improved due to better surgical techniques)

DIFFERENTIAL DIAGNOSIS

- Increased PSA

—BPH
—Prostatitis
—Prostatic biopsy/massage, TRUS, TURP

 Database

HISTORY

- Family history (PCa and malignancies) and risk factors

PHYSICAL EXAMINATION

- DRE

—DRE misses 23% to 45% of cases detected by elevated PSA or TRUS abnormalities. Organ-confined disease occurs in ≤50% of cases of PCa found by DRE alone, and >50% of patients diagnosed by an abnormal DRE have advanced disease. Prostate biopsy is recommended in abnormal DRE.

 Diagnostic Studies

LABORATORY TESTING

- PSA: serine protease from prostatic epithelium and periurethral glands. Half-life is 2 to 3 days. 25% of men with PCa have normal DRE and serum PSA level <4 ng/mL.

—PSA level without DRE is *not* recommended. PSA is the single test with the highest predictive (30%) value for PCa. If >4 ng/mL, sensitivity is 72%; specificity, 49%; and positive predictive value, 30% to 40%.
—PSA density, PSA velocity, age-specific PSA, and free and total PSA (see Special Studies below)

IMAGING

- TRUS lesions

—Hypoechoic: the most common prostatic lesion
—Hypoechoic: overall accuracy of 43%
—Isoechoic: 20% to 40% of all cases of PCa
—The overall staging accuracy of TRUS is 58%.

- TRUS-guided prostate biopsy

—Biopsy a suspicious lesion detected by TRUS, and perform systematic sextant biopsies in nonhypoechoic areas (i.e., three biopsies from each side of the prostate; one from the base, middle, and apex of the gland). More sampling may increase detection of PCa.
—Indications: abnormal DRE, elevated serum PSA level

- MRI

—Overall staging accuracy from 55% to 69%. Detects only 9.6% of positive nodes

- Endorectal coil MRI

—Better resolution than conventional MRI. Staging accuracy is 54%.

- Pelvic computed tomography (CT) scan

—Evaluates nodal metastases (normal size: <1 cm). Indications: PSA >20 ng/mL, percutaneous aspiration of enlarged nodes, Gleason score ≥8 and/or high-stage, bulky local disease, and patients unlikely to undergo traditional staging

- Radionuclide bone scan

—Accurate to assess bony metastases. False-negative rate: <1%; sensitivity: >99%
—Indication: PSA level ≥10 ng/mL

- CYT-356 antibody

—Monoclonal antibody against prostate-specific membrane. Useful for imaging sites of disease spread and recurrence. Further studies are necessary.

SPECIAL STUDIES

- PSA

—Density: serum PSA level/the prostate volume (TRUS). PSA density ≥0.15 is significant when the PSA level is 4 to 10 ng/mL. Sensitivity is 75% and specificity is 40%.

—Velocity: rate of change of PSA levels over time. Minimal length of time is 18 months to 2 years and 3 repeat measurements. An increase ≥0.75 ng/mL/yr is a specific marker for PCa (sensitivity: 55%; specificity: 96%).

- Age-specific: Ranges are 40 to 50 years: 0 to 2.5 ng/mL; 50 to 60: 0 to 3.5 ng/mL; 60 to 70: 0 to 4.5 ng/mL; 70 to 80: 0 to 6.5 ng/mL.
- Total and free PSA: A free/total PSA cutoff ≥0.25 improves detection of PCa compared with PSA level alone.
- For PSA levels 4 and 10 ng/mL: Free PSA may provide predictive information for PCa.
- RT-PCR: highly variable but sensitive; detects 1 prostate cell in 106 lymphocytes. May give prognostic information
- *bcl-2* (apoptosis-suppressing oncogene)

—Related to development of androgen-resistant PCa, acts as independent prognostic indicator of PCa (independent of Gleason grade and clinical stage), and is correlated with poor survival

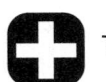

Treatment

GENERAL MEASURES

- Evaluation of comorbid diseases

—Diabetes mellitus, cardiovascular and pulmonary diseases

- Objective discussion of risk/benefit for an individual patient
- Watchful waiting

—The Scandinavian Prostatic Cancer Group and the Prostate Cancer Intervention Versus Observation Trial (PIVOT) are the studies in progress to compare expectant management and radical prostatectomy.

—Rationale for observation: no decline in the last 30 years in disease-specific mortality rate despite advances in therapy; prevalence of PCa exceeds clinical incidence of disease, and retrospective, uncontrolled studies suggested that low-grade untreated lesions have limited progression and high survival rates (5–10 years' follow-up).

- Radical prostatectomy (retropubic or perineal)

—Nonprogression rates of PCa are reported to be 69% to 89% at 5 years and 47% to 79% at 10 years.

—Mortality: <0.5%

- PLND

—Gold standard for detecting nodal metastases. It may be done as an isolated procedure if the risk of metastases is high, prior to perineal prostatectomy or radiation, or at the time of radical prostatectomy.

- Radiation

—External beam radiation 60 to 70 Gy over 6 weeks; neoadjuvant hormonal therapy for bulky disease, studies pending for early disease PLND may be helpful for staging high risk prior to radiation. Improved technology optimizes radiation delivery, decreasing side effects.

—Brachytherapy or interstitial radiation: beads or pellets of isotope material. Early data promising for low-risk disease

- Cryotherapy

—Use of liquid nitrogen into the tumor. High-resolution TRUS and better percutaneous instruments improved this modality of treatment for localized PCa.

- Hormonal treatment

—Neoadjuvant hormonal treatment decreases PSA levels by 95% to 98% and gland volume by 25% to 30%. Decreased margin positivity in 3-month studies, but no benefit on PSA progression; 8-month studies underway

- Orchiectomy

—Alternative hormonal treatment decreasing levels of testosterone. Recommended to patients with severe comorbid disease(s), advanced age, or to patients refusing other type of treatment

MEDICAL: N/A

SURGICAL: N/A

ALTERNATIVE THERAPIES

- No clear scientific evidence

PATIENT EDUCATION

- Counsel patients about treatment.

—Consider risks and benefits of all the current treatments, including watchful waiting.

—Reinforce the importance of rigorous follow-up.

Follow-Up

MONITORING

- DRE and serum PSA levels

—Every 3 months for 1 year after treatment, then every 6 months for 1 year, and yearly thereafter

- Abnormal DRE and/or increase in PSA levels

—Evaluation for recurrence

PREVENTION

- No scientific data

Miscellaneous

SYNONYMS: N/A

ASSOCIATED CONDITIONS

- Diabetes mellitus, cardiovascular and pulmonary diseases

NOTES

- See Section II for other prostate cancer topics.

ABBREVIATIONS

- PLND, pelvic lymph node dissection; PCa, prostate cancer; PIN, prostatic intraepithelial neoplasia; PSA, prostate-specific antigen; RT-PCR, reverse-transcription polymerase chain reaction; TRUS, transrectal ultrasonography

REFERENCES

Crawford D, Oesterling J, Richie J, Waters B, Lindgreen B. In: *Urologic Oncology*, Ch. 26–31. 1997: 378–453.

Kim E, Grayhack J, Narayan P, et al. *Comprehensive Textbook of Genitourinary Oncology*. 1996: 557–920, 1996.

Pienta K, Epstein J, Partin A, et al.. In: Walsh PC, Retik AB, Vaughan ED, Wein AJ, eds. *Campbell's Urology*, 7th ed., Ch. 80–90. Philadelphia: WB Saunders, 1998:2487–2658.

Authors: Robert C. Flanigan and Fernando J. Kim

Prostate Cancer—Locally Advanced (T3)

 Basics

DESCRIPTION

• Stage of PCa where the cancer cells have locally invaded beyond the capsule of the prostate, but have not yet metastasized. Traditionally, T3 disease has been digital rectal examination (DRE) staged and defined as locally advanced with extracapsular extension. DRE-based or DRE-influenced staging of T3 disease has most recently prompted a rather empiric definition: a positive biopsy of (a) seminal vesicles or (b) transrectal ultrasound biopsy (TRUS)–demonstrated sites of extracapsular extension.

EPIDEMIOLOGY

• T3: most commonly diagnosed form of PCa.
• 20% to 50% of radical prostatectomy for clinically localized disease is pathologically T3 (p T3).
• 37% of T1c tumors (elevated PSA only), will be T3. Patients undergoing RT are likely to have similar rates of extraprostatic disease.
• T3 disease (c T3 and p T3) accounts for over 150,000 cases annually.

GENETICS

• See Section II, "Prostate Cancer—General."

STAGING

• See the Appendix, "TNM Classification."

SIGNS AND SYMPTOMS

• Often asymptomatic
• Occasionally obstructive or irritative symptoms
• Stage T3 can present clinically in a variety of ways:

—Bulky disease: bladder obstruction and voiding symptoms. Bulky disease is decreasing in prevalence, but this presentation was common when DRE was the sole diagnostic method used for clinical staging.
—Apparent, which includes apical lesions palpated on DRE, capsular violations seen on magnetic resonance imaging (MRI), a biopsy core that happens to catch the capsule edge, and/or PSA >30 ng/mL
—Predicted: (i.e., Partin tables) from prognostic methods including PSA and its indices, biopsy Gleason grade, radiographic studies, and newer molecular markers

PATHOPHYSIOLOGY

• Gleason grade is predictive of whether extracapsular disease exists, but only at the extreme ends of the grading scale.
• Most cases of T3 are intermediate Gleason grades of 5 to 7.
• Capsular violation (p T3) will include capsular penetration; either positive surgical margins exist or the lesion is specimen-confined after prostatectomy.

CAUSES/RISK FACTORS

• Family history and being African American are general risk factors for PCa.

COMPLICATIONS

• Local obstruction, bleeding, renal insufficiency, development of metastasis
• Recurrence after radical prostatectomy

—Most important predictor of local recurrence: positive surgical margins with high tumor grade
—Tumors involving surgical margins without extraprostatic extension experience biochemical failure rates (i.e., rising PSA) higher than those of patients with confined tumors and less than those with extraprostatic disease. PSA failure is related to the degree of the surgical margin positivity.

DIFFERENTIAL DIAGNOSIS

• No single diagnostic modality can diagnose, confirm, or rule out cancer confinement within the prostate except biopsy evidence.
• Digital rectal examinations (DREs) have been the traditional method of staging prostate cancer, although its poor sensitivity characteristically understages the extent of disease.

—Of clinically staged T1/T2 tumors, only 58% are organ-confined.
—If judged to be T2/T3, it is more likely to be T3.

• Can only differentiate "probably organ-confined" (i.e., normal DRE, PSA of <10 ng/mL, and Gleason grade of <6) from the "probably extracapsular" (i.e., suspicious DRE, PSA >10 ng/mL, and Gleason grade of >6) when DRE, PSA, and Gleason score are combined.
• Partin et al. devised nomograms that combine PSA, Gleason grading, and DRE to predict the pathologic stage in men with localized prostate cancer (see Section VII, "Partin Tables")

 Database

HISTORY

• Family history of PCa
• Voiding symptomatology

PHYSICAL EXAMINATION

• Palpable induration may extend into the lateral sulcus on one (T3a) or both sides (T3b) or cephalad into the seminal vesicles (T3c).

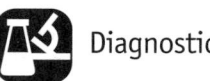 Diagnostic Studies

LABORATORY TESTING

• PSA: high sensitivity for detecting cancer, but little predictive value alone in determining stage. A linear correlation exists between tumor volume and PSA levels, but an inverse relationship between PSA and Gleason score has been suggested.
• In the bulky T3 category, the contribution of (BPH) PSA elevation must be considered.

—PSA density (PSAD) is a volume-based quotient that accounts for PSA per gram of prostate and can nullify any contribution of BPH to elevated PSA levels. In one study, a PSAD cutoff value above 0.35 was associated with 66% extraprostatic extension.

IMAGING

• TRUS and TRUS-guided biopsy have consistently proven effective. The TRUS-guided biopsy staging together with preoperative PSA and biopsy Gleason score can establish probabilities of extraprostatic disease.

—With PSA >20 ng/mL, 70% of patients had extraprostatic disease; but at Gleason scores of 8 to 10, only 23% had seminal vesicle (SV) involvement.
—With logistic regression, however, it was the combination of these three factors that provided the greatest predictive value of extracapsular extension with or without positive margins.
—Other diagnostic imaging modalities currently available are not reliable in detecting extracapsular involvement.
—AUA guidelines: Bone scans should only be done with PSA >10 ng/mL, whereas a CT scan or MRI should only be ordered with PSA levels greater than 20 ng/mL.

SPECIAL STUDIES

• ProstaScint cannot distinguish T3.
• Investigational: molecular and genetic markers that may signify the extent of disease: RT-PCR PSA, ploidy, morphometry/nuclear roundness, *p53*, *bcl-2*, tumor vascularity

Treatment

GENERAL MEASURES

- Management of PCa is controversial; dependent on many factors (age, life expectancy, co-morbidities, extent of disease, quality-of-life issues, preferences of patient and family)
- Variety of treatment options: watchful waiting, surgery, external radiation, and hormonal therapy
- Existence of extracapsular disease may influence treatment expectations more than choice of treatment.
- Bulky T3 disease is not as prevalent as it was a decade ago. Historically, TURP or hormonal therapy was used to relieve obstructive symptoms, with RT or hormones for palliation.

MEDICAL

- External RT: mainstay for apparent T3 disease. PSA survival is poor with radiotherapy alone for T3, with progression-free rates being only 30% to 40% at 5 and 10 years.
- Combined hormonal therapy and RT: Local progression and overall survival may be enhanced with hormones combined with radiation.
- Recent advances with techniques and equipment (three-dimensional conformal) are designed to deliver a higher dosage and limit the side effects associated with radiation.

SURGICAL

- Radical prostatectomy for c T3 disease is often contraindicated. The benefits of prostatectomy may outweigh the risks associated with predicted T3 prostate cancer.
- Neoadjuvant hormonal therapy might improve surgical outcomes; and adjuvant hormonal therapy or RT could minimize the risk of immediate post-surgery biochemical failure.
- Some support for radical prostatectomy uncertain T2/T3 tumors, but the ambiguous results of patients with and without adjuvant therapy after RP preclude conclusive answers.

ALTERNATIVE THERAPIES

- Adjuvant RT and/or androgen deprivation are available for patients thought to have clinical, organ-confined disease but who demonstrate p T3.
- The lower the PSA (as well as the delay of PSA rise), the more likely that patients would benefit from radiation therapy.
- Adjuvant hormonal therapy with positive margins or seminal vesicle involvement can prolong time to progression, but there is no evidence of a survival advantage.

PATIENT EDUCATION: N/A

 Follow-Up

MONITORING

- Follow-up PSA provides a lead time of years before the appearance of metastatic disease, but the timing of treatment and the mode of therapy are still controversial.

—Survival advantages for patients with metastatic disease treated with early hormonal therapy in contrast to deferred treatment waiting for development of symptoms.
—Single-agent antiandrogens have recently been utilized and are an appealing treatment option. Studies of flutamide and finasteride are ongoing. Intermittent androgen deprivation is utilized in many patients as a compromising treatment option.
—"Watchful waiting" is not acceptable for many men.
—Additionally, the side effects of combined androgen blockade are not easily tolerated. The disadvantage of controlling prostate cancer disease by androgen deprivation is the development of cancer cells resistant to hormonal manipulations.

PREVENTION: N/A

 Miscellaneous

SYNONYMS

- T3, locally advanced prostate cancer

ASSOCIATED CONDITIONS: N/A

NOTES: N/A

ABBREVIATIONS

- c T3, clinical T3; p T3, pathologic T3; PCa, prostate cancer; RT, radiation therapy

REFERENCES

Boges GE, McNeal JE, Redwine EA, Freiha FS, Stamey TA. Morphologic analysis of surgical margins with positive findings in prostatectomy for adenocarcinoma of the prostate. *Cancer* 1992;69: 520–526.

Bolla M, Gonzalez D, Warde P, et al. Improved survival in patients with locally advanced prostate cancer treated with radiotherapy and goserelin. *N Engl J Med* 1997;337:295–300.

Fallon B, Williams RD. Current options in the management of clinical stage C prostatic carcinoma. *Urol Clin North Am* 1990;17:853–866.

Middleton RG, Thompson IM, Austenfeld MS, et al. Prostate Cancer Clinical Guidelines Panel Summary report on the management of clinically localized prostate cancer. The American Urologic Association. *J Urol* 1995;154:2144–2148.

Morgan WR, Bergstralh EJ, Zinke H. Long-term evaluation of radical prostatectomy as treatment for clinical stage C (T3) prostate cancer. *Urology* 1993;41:113–120.

Authors: Ali M. Ziada and E. David Crawford

Prostate Cancer—Metastatic (N+, M+)

 Basics

DESCRIPTION

- Prostate cancer (PCa) that has spread from the prostate gland to nodes or distant tissue

EPIDEMIOLOGY

- 30% of patients with PCa present with regional or distant metastasis.
- Slightly higher incidence and lower 5-year survival rates with metastatic PCa in African-American males

GENETICS

- No known genetic predisposition to develop metastatic PCa
- 9% of PCa is hereditary.
- Several genetic aberrations (*p53, H-ras, KAI-1*) and growth factors have some association with metastatic PCa.

STAGING

- See TNM table in the Appendix.

SIGNS AND SYMPTOMS

- Signs of metastatic disease are nonspecific.

—Weight loss in advanced cases
—Symptoms relate to the organ system involved.
—Most common sites of metastasis (in decreasing order of occurrence): pelvic LN, bone, abdominal LN, lung, liver, adrenals, other

- Bone pain: most common with M+

—Persistent, often severe in back or hip
—Pathologic fractures
—Degree of bone pain prognostic for survival

- Neurologic manifestations

—20% to 37% of patients with M+
—Acute spinal cord compression from epidural metastases is an emergency.
—CNS symptoms present with brain metastases.

- LN metastases may cause lower extremity edema (uncommon).
- Urinary tract symptoms related to local PCa growth into bladder
- Other symptoms (rare)

—Paraneoplastic syndrome (ectopic ACTH, SIADH, or hypercalcemia)
  —Hematologic: disseminated intravascular coagulation, anemia, DVT

PATHOPHYSIOLOGY

- Metastasis occurs through lymphatic or hematogenous routes.
- LN metastasis is usually sequential from regional to distant LN; skip lesions are noted in up to 17%.

—Medial branch of internal iliac LN chain is most common site; often called obturator LN because of proximity to obturator nerve
—Extensive LN involvement may occur with little or no bony involvement and vice versa.

- Bone metastasis in 65% to 85% at autopsy, though often not symptomatic until extensive

—Most common sites are spine, ribs, pelvis, femur, and shoulder (in decreasing order).

- Metastasis to other visceral organs is a late manifestation.

CAUSES/RISK FACTORS

- High Gleason grade of primary tumor
- Increased incidence of metastasis with increasing serum PSA value
- Local disease extension on histopathologic evaluation of surgical specimen
- Rising serum PSA value after definitive therapy

COMPLICATIONS

- Acute spinal cord compression
- Renal failure secondary to lymphatic obstruction of ureters
- Bladder outlet obstruction
- Severe bone pain
- Pathologic fractures
- Deep vein thrombosis
- Priapism
- Paraneoplastic syndromes
- Severe weight loss

DIFFERENTIAL DIAGNOSIS

- Depends on the organ systems involved

 Database

HISTORY

- Personal

—Age
—Family history of cancer in first-degree relative
—Previous diagnosis and treatment (if applicable)
—Medications

- Review of systems

—Urinary tract function
—Neurologic deficits
—Weight loss
—Flank or back pain
—Lower extremity edema (especially unilateral)

PHYSICAL EXAMINATION

- Digital rectal examination (DRE) to determine local extent of disease

—Higher incidence of metastasis with locally extensive PCa

- LN palpation: inguinal, abdominal, supraclavicular, cervical

—Presence of palpable LN suggests high volume, advanced disease

- Neurologic examination if history suggests neurologic involvement

—Emergency CT or MRI if cord compression suspected

Diagnostic Studies

LABORATORY TESTING

• PSA most sensitive test for PCa

—Failure of PSA to return to undetectable levels after radical prostatectomy suggests
—Progressive PSA rise within 1 year of definitive treatment suggests metastasis.
—2% of patients with distant metastases do not express PSA.

• PAP is less sensitive than PSA but occasionally useful.
• Alkaline phosphatase may be elevated with metastatic disease.
• Creatinine is elevated with ureteral or bladder outlet obstruction.
• Anemia is a late manifestation of extensive bone marrow involvement.

IMAGING

• Cannot detect microscopic disease
• Bone scan (scintigraphy) most sensitive test for skeletal metastasis

—Very low yield with PSA less than 20 ng/mL
—8% false negative due to no osteoblastic activity or to diffuse disease throughout bones

• Bone radiographs

—Used to confirm equivocal findings on bone scan
—Osteoblastic lesions: 50%; osteolytic lesions: 10%; mixed: 33%
—50% of bone involvement necessary before radiographic findings apparent

• CT

—Not very sensitive for LN or bone metastasis
—Threshold for LN detection: 1.0 to 1.5 cm

• MRI

—Slightly better sensitivity than CT
—May be best study for local extension (endorectal coil)
—May detect bone lesions in case of equivocal bone scan

• Ultrasound

—Not useful for soft-tissue or bony disease but will detect hydronephrosis
—May identify locally advanced disease

• Lymphangiography is labor intensive, difficult to interpret, and rarely used.
• Monoclonal antibody nuclear scan (radioimmunoscintigraphy)

—More sensitive than CT or MRI for soft-tissue disease
—Not recommended to detect bone lesions
—Early studies suggest this may be the best test for local recurrence.

SPECIAL STUDIES

• Used in patients at relatively high risk for metastatic disease at diagnosis or to obtain tissue confirmation of abnormal imaging studies
• Soft tissue

—Pelvic LN dissection (open, minilaparotomy, laparoscopic)
—CT- or MRI-guided biopsy
—TRUS biopsy of the prostatectomy surgical site has low yield.

• Bone biopsy to confirm metastasis

(continued)

Prostate Cancer—Metastatic (N+, M+) (continued)

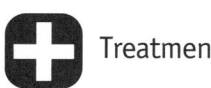 Treatment

GENERAL MEASURES

• There is no cure for metastatic PCa. It is important to establish the goal of any planned therapy.

—Control of disease progression
—Palliation of symptoms

MEDICAL

• Control of disease progression

—Endocrine therapy through androgen ablation
—75% with metastatic PCa have a serum PSA decrease to androgen deprivation.
—Testes produce 95% of androgen (testosterone), and adrenals produce 5% (DHEA, androstenedione).
—Controversial whether combined androgen blockade to block all androgens offers any advantage over monotherapy to block testosterone alone

• Medical ablation of primary gonadal function

—Aminoglutethimide: requires steroid supplement; used in patients refractory to hormone therapy
—Spironolactone: significant side effects; not often used
—Ketoconazole: inhibits cytochrome P-450; used in patients refractory to hormone therapy
—LH-RH agonist or antagonist given monthly or every 3 to 4 months (depot formulation)
   —Indirect gonadal suppression. Most common therapy used for androgen suppression. Expensive; associated with hot flashes, gynecomastia, liver function abnormalities. Leuprolide (Lupron), goserelin acetate (Zoladex), triptorelin pamoate (Decapeptyl), buserelin acetate

—Estramustine phosphate (Emcyt): oral medication used in hormone-refractive patients
—Estrogens: indirect gonadal suppression
   —Diethylstilbestrol (DES): inexpensive oral medication with CV side effects
   —Diethylstilbestrol diphosphate (Stilphostrol): intravenous estrogen
   —Conjugated estrogens and progesterone used rarely
—Antiandrogens: often used in conjunction with LH-RH antagonist or orchiectomy for complete androgen blockade. May have transient and occasional long-term PSA decrease on withdrawal of antiandrogen therapy. Patients on antiandrogens with increasing PSA should have a trial of medication withdrawal before use of other combination therapy.
   —Flutamide (Eulexin): tid dosage, associated with diarrhea (15%), gynecomastia (20%)
   —Bicalutamide (Casodex): single daily dosage, generally fewer side effects
   —Nilutamide (Nilandron): tid dosage, associated with night vision problems
   —Cyproterone acetate: nonsteroidal agent that also blocks LH release (not available in United States)
—Chemotherapy: multiple agents have been used alone or in combination with modest, relatively short-term effect from several agents, though often associated with significant toxicity. Used in patients refractory to hormone therapy. Most promising results from
   —Estramustine phosphate plus vinblastine
   —Paclitaxel (Taxol) alone or with other agents

• Palliation of symptoms

—Narcotic analgesics for bone or visceral pain
—Endocrine therapy alone or in combination with radiotherapy has often been used to decrease tumor volume to relieve neurologic symptoms and urinary obstruction.
—Mitoxantrone chemotherapy for palliation

SURGICAL

• Control of disease progression. Surgical approaches instead of medical therapies may be used for androgen ablation.

—Orchiectomy: inexpensive, outpatient procedure
—Hypophysectomy, adrenalectomy: no longer done

• Palliation of symptoms

—Transurethral resection of prostate for relief of urinary obstruction
—Ureteral stent or nephrostomy placement for relief of ureteral obstruction

ALTERNATIVE THERAPIES

• External beam radiation therapy

—Effective for palliation of bone pain from specific site
—May decrease tumor volume of primary tumor to relieve urinary obstructive symptoms
—Treatment of choice for impending cord compression

• Radiopharmaceutical treatment: bone pain relief in 60% to 90% of patients. Toxicity is hematologic. Not recommended for cord compression

—Strontium-89 has a longer half-life, longer duration of response, and higher toxicity.
—Samarium-153

• Investigational

—Agents for differentiation, antiangiogenesis, signal transduction inhibition, metalloprotease inhibition; bisphosphate therapy, vitamin D analogs
—Dietary agents or supplements
—Gene therapy/immunotherapy

- USTOO International: www.ustoo.com
- Man to Man (American Cancer Society): (800)ACS-2345; www.cancer.org
- American Cancer Society: (800)ACS-2345; www.cancer.org
- National Cancer Institute: (800)4-CANCER; www.nci.nih.gov
- National Prostate Cancer Coalition: (202)463-9455; www.4npcc.org

 Follow-Up

MONITORING

- Serology

—PSA: most sensitive test for PCa detection, progression, and response to treatment. Usually obtained every 3 to 6 months, depending on disease status

—Creatinine as necessary in patient with progressive disease

—Liver function tests every 6 months for patients on LH-RH agonist or antiandrogens

- Imaging: Stable patients rarely need further imaging studies.

—CT, MRI, monoclonal antibody scan, bone scan, or sonography may be indicated for disease progression.

- Physical examination: brief examination every 3 to 6 months unless progression warrants a different schedule.

PREVENTION: N/A

 Miscellaneous

SYNONYMS: N/A

ASSOCIATED CONDITIONS

- See above.

NOTES

- See other Section II prostate cancer topics.

ABBREVIATIONS

- ACTH, adrenocorticotropic hormone; DES, diethylstilbestrol; DHEA, dehydroepiandrosterone; LH-RH, luteinizing hormone–releasing hormone; LN, lymph node; PAP, prostatic acid phosphatase; SIADH, syndrome of inappropriate antidiuretic hormone secretion; TRUS, transrectal ultrasound

REFERENCES

Landis SH, Murray T, Bolden S, Wingo PA. Cancer statistics, 1998. *CA Cancer J Clin* 1998;48:6–29.

Manyak MJ, Javitt MC. The role of computerized tomography, magnetic resonance imaging, bone scan, and monoclonal antibody nuclear scan for prognosis prediction in PC. *Semin Urol Oncol* 1998;16:145–152.

Moul JW. Contemporary hormonal management of advanced PC. *Oncology* 1998;12:499–508.

Roth BJ. New therapeutic agents for hormone-refractory PC. *Semin Oncol* 1996;23[Suppl 14]: 49–55.

Saitoh H, Yoshida K-I, Uchijima Y, et al. Two different lymph node metastatic patterns of a prostatic cancer. *Cancer* 1990;65:1843–1846.

Author: Michael J. Manyak

Prostate Sarcoma

 Basics

DESCRIPTION

- Neoplasm arising from the stromal cells of the prostate, generally associated with early local spread and poor prognosis. Leiomyosarcoma, rhabdomyosarcoma, and fibrosarcoma the most common types.

EPIDEMIOLOGY

- <0.1% of prostate malignancies
—136 cases reported in the past 50 years
- Child and young adult predominance
—30% in first and second decades of life (primarily rhabdomyosarcoma)
—45% in ages 20 to 40
—30% after age 40 (primarily leiomyosarcoma)
- Mean age at diagnosis: 48 years

GENETICS: N/A

STAGING

- No standardized staging system

SIGNS AND SYMPTOMS

- Obstructive voiding symptoms
—Early invasion of the prostatic and perivesical tissues, causing compression of the prostatic urethra
—Onset of symptoms prior to diagnosis: 1 month
- Bowel symptoms (constipation, sense of fullness, bloody stools, inability to defecate)
—Compression and direct involvement
—Bowel symptoms in conjunction with obstructive urinary symptoms are strongly suggestive of prostatic sarcoma.
- Palpable perineal or suprapubic mass
—Rapid enlargement
—Early lymphatic and vascular spread
- Hematuria
—Gross or microscopic
—Later occurrence, compared with bladder sarcoma
- Enlarged prostate by digital rectal examination (symmetrically or asymmetrically)
—Hard/soft/rubbery or cystic (sometimes mistaken for an abscess)
- Deep pelvic pain
- Edema of scrotum, perineum, lower extremities
—Advanced disease

PATHOPHYSIOLOGY

- Mesodermal in origin
—Variable degrees of differentiation into striated muscle (rhabdomyosarcoma), smooth muscle (leiomyosarcoma), and connective tissue (fibrosarcoma)

- Histologic subtypes in order of frequency
—Leiomyosarcoma
——More common in older patients
——Slow growth rate
——Gross: smooth, encapsulated, friable
——Microscopic: actin and myosin without cross-striations (stain red with trichrome stain)
—Rhabdomyosarcoma
——Most occur in children.
——Most rapid growth rate
——Gross: varies; often pearly "grapelike" clusters (sarcoma botryoides) with necrotic areas
——Microscopic: actin and myosin cross-striations visible in some cells (seen better with phosphotungstic stain)
—Fibrosarcoma
——More common in older patients
——Slow growth rate
——Spindle/fusiform cells arranged in whirls or bundles
—Less common: reticulum cell lymphosarcoma, angiosarcoma, malignant fibrous histiocytoma
- Natural history
—Rapid growth/early compression of the urethra
—Local extension
——75% of cases associated with extension to bladder/abdominal wall anteriorly and rectum/perineum posteriorly
—Early lymphatic and vascular invasion
—Metastases to liver, lungs, and bones (osteolytic)
——20% of patients have metastases at the time of diagnosis.
—Very poor prognosis
——Worse prognosis in children

CAUSES/RISK FACTORS

- Radiation
—Rhabdomyosarcoma reported after radiotherapy for other malignancy

COMPLICATIONS

- Local morbidity
—Bladder/bowel obstruction, edema, pelvic pain
- Metastatic disease
- Death
—5-year survival: 10% to 28% in adults (less in children)
—No improvement in survival over the past 50 years

DIFFERENTIAL DIAGNOSIS

- Chronic prostatitis/prostatic abscess
- Benign prostatic hyperplasia
- Postoperative spindle cell nodule (overgrowth of benign-appearing stromal cells after transurethral resection of the prostate (TURP))
- Prostatic lymphoma
- Prostatic adenocarcinoma
- Carcinosarcoma of the prostate (both epithelial and mesodermal neoplastic components)

 Database

HISTORY

- Age of the patient?
—Histology and potential differential diagnoses disparate between young and old
- Voiding pattern?
—New onset of obstruction or complete urinary retention common
- Change in bowel habits?
—Constipation, fullness characteristic (historically thought to be pathognomonic when seen in conjunction with urinary obstruction)
- History of hematuria?
—Common with prostatic sarcoma, but numerous other potential causes
- New-onset bone pain or fracture?
—Osteolytic bone metastases
- History of prostatic adenocarcinoma treated with radiation?
—Increased risk of carcinosarcoma and rhabdomyosarcoma
- Surgical history?
—Postoperative spindle cell nodule after TURP
- History of lymphoma?
—Secondary involvement of the prostate

PHYSICAL EXAMINATION

- Abdominal examination
—Visible or palpable suprapubic mass
- Digital rectal examination
—Prostate size/consistency/nodularity
—Evidence of local spread
- Scrotum/perineum/lower extremities
—Evidence of edema, indicating advanced disease
- Bimanual examination under anesthesia
—To further evaluate evidence of local spread

Prostate Sarcoma

 ## Diagnostic Studies

LABORATORY TESTING

- Urinalysis and culture
—Pyuria and positive culture suggestive of prostatitis
—Leukocyte esterase or nitrite positive suggestive of infection
- Serum electrolytes
- Liver function studies
—Suggestive of metastatic disease if elevated
—Evaluate with CT.
- Complete blood count
—Leukocytosis with prostatitis or abscess
- Prostate-specific antigen
—Elevation secondary to sarcoma not reported
—Elevated in carcinosarcoma

IMAGING

- Abdominopelvic CT or MRI with or without contrast
—Local staging
- Chest x-ray
—CT scan for suspicious findings or high clinical suspicion
- Bone radiographs/nuclear bone scan
—Indicated for elevated alkaline phosphatase/bone pain

SPECIAL STUDIES

- Transrectal prostate biopsy
—Usual method of diagnosis
- Cystoscopy
—To check for bladder-base involvement

 ## Treatment

GENERAL MEASURES

- If clinically localized, aggressive local surgical excision optimal
- Bilateral staging pelvic lymphadenectomy and radical prostatectomy or cystoprostatectomy appropriate in the absence of obvious metastases
- Metastatic disease: palliative chemo/radiotherapy

MEDICAL

- Doxorubicin-based combination chemotherapy for metastatic disease most current recommendation
- Actinomycin D, vincristine, and cyclophosphamide historically used
—Several protocols with varying dosages
—Some remissions reported
—Durable remissions unusual
—Adjuvant chemotherapy suggested in patients with high-grade leiomyosarcomas or rhabdomyosarcomas and in patients with positive nodes
- Radiotherapy
—Leiomyosarcoma may be more radiosensitive.
—Adjuvant radiotherapy suggested in patients with low-grade leiomyosarcomas with positive resection margins
—40 to 60 Gy to the pelvis and lymphatic areas
—Some case reports suggest conventional radiotherapy or brachytherapy as a primary modality.

SURGICAL

- Radical prostatectomy for small localized disease
- Radical cystoprostatectomy for large tumors or tumors involving the bladder
—Nerve-sparing radical prostatectomy and hemicystectomy with good outcome in a patient with fibrosarcoma invading the bladder has been described (Walsh).
- Total pelvic exenteration for disease involving the rectum

ALTERNATIVE THERAPIES: N/A

PATIENT EDUCATION

- Poor prognosis
—Overall 5-year survival: 10% to 28%
—Leiomyosarcoma has a better prognosis (42% 5-year survival in one series).
—Rhabdomyosarcoma has a worse prognosis (13% 5-year survival in one series).

 ## Follow-Up

MONITORING

- Periodic monitoring for metastases is reasonable.
—Chest x-ray, liver function studies

PREVENTION: N/A

 ## Miscellaneous

SYNONYMS: N/A

ASSOCIATED CONDITIONS: N/A

NOTES

- See also Section II, "Prostate Cancer—General."

ABBREVIATIONS

- CT, computed tomography; MRI, magnetic resonance imaging; TURP, transurethral resection of the prostate

REFERENCES

Mostofi FK, Price EB Jr. Tumors of the male genital system. In: Atlas of Tumor Pathology. Washington, D.C.: Armed Forces Institute of Pathology, 2nd series, fascicle 8, 1973.

Narayana AS, Loening S, Weimar GW, Culp DA. Sarcoma of the bladder and prostate. J Urol 1978;119:72–76.

Quinlan DM, Stutzman RE, Peters CA, Walsh PC. Unilateral nerve-sparing radical prostatectomy and hemicystectomy in management of prostate sarcoma. Urology 1993;41(4):308–310.

Takahashi S, Tsukamoto T, Lieber MM. Genitourinary sarcomas in adults. In: Vogelzang NJ, Scardino PT, Shipley WU, Coffey DS, eds. Comprehensive Textbook of Genitourinary Oncology. Baltimore: Williams & Wilkins, 1996:1124–1139.

Tannenbaum M. Sarcomas of the prostate gland. Urology 1975;5(6):810–814.

Authors: Robert R. Byrne and Cary N. Robertson

Prostate—Transitional Cell Carcinoma

 ## Basics

DESCRIPTION

• Transitional cell carcinoma (TCC) arising from the prostate either as an isolated entity or associated (either synchronous or metachronous) with TCC occurring elsewhere in the urinary tract

EPIDEMIOLOGY

• TCC of the prostate (TCC-P) accounts for 4% to 5% of prostate cancers.
• With TCC of the bladder, the incidence of prostatic involvement of TCC increases to 12% to 45%.
• 75% associated with either concurrent or history of TCC
• 25% of cases occur as isolated entities.
• Smoking is a risk factor for TCC of the urothelium.
• Two types: Secondary direct extension of urinary bladder TCC into the prostate is more common than primary TCC of the prostate.
• Prostatic urethral involvement is an ominous risk factor associated with urethral recurrence. Prostatic stromal invasion is the strongest single predictor for subsequent recurrence in the anterior urethra.
• Cystoprostatectomy specimens for bladder cancer: 43% of prostates contained TCC; 8% to 45% of prostates removed for bladder cancer also had prostatic adenocarcinoma.
• Significant association between carcinoma in situ (CIS) of bladder neck and trigone and increased incidence of TCC-P

GENETICS

• Unknown, but bladder TCC associated with inactivation or deletions of tumor suppressor genes (p53, Rb genes)

STAGING

• No universally accepted system
• If associated with bladder TCC: pT4a disease
• Currently staged according to Jewett-Strong (stage D1) and TNM (T4) systems for urinary bladder. These imply that prostatic TCC-P is a high-stage neoplasm with a poor prognosis, which is not always accurate.
• Prostatic urethral or ductal TCC does not alter the survival determined by the primary bladder cancer stage.
• Prostatic stromal invasion arising intraurethrally significantly decreases survival across primary bladder cancer stages.
• Patients with primary bladder cancers that invade through detrusor muscle into the prostate have a lower survival compared with patients with primary bladder cancers of lower stage associated with urethral cancers that arise in the prostate.
• P4a (primary bladder tumor extended full thickness through bladder wall to invade prostate) has a 5-year recurrence rate of 75% and an overall survival rate of 21%. In contrast, prostatic involvement arising from within prostatic urethra has a 5-year recurrence rate of 36% (30% rate without

stromal invasion and 70% rate with stromal invasion.) The overall survival rate is 55%.
• Patients with a P1 bladder tumor with prostatic stromal invasion arising intraurethrally have a survival rate of 45%, and it has been suggested that it should be called "P1str," as it clearly has a prognosis different than P4a bladder cancer (survival of only 21%).
• Conclusion: Prostatic urethral or ductal TCC does not alter survival determined by bladder stage alone, and it should not be classified as P4a.

SIGNS AND SYMPTOMS

• Gross or microscopic hematuria in those with intact urinary tracts
• Bloody urethral discharge, a palpable perineal/urethral mass, and less commonly, inguinal adenopathy in those who have undergone cystectomy without urethrectomy
• Deep transurethral biopsy of prostate is necessary in anyone with a suspected invasive bladder cancer.
• Signs and symptoms of urethral recurrence after cystectomy

—10% risk of urethral recurrence after cystectomy for bladder cancer
—Screening cytologies for urethral recurrence. Urethroscopy and biopsy are not indicated following a positive cytology; total urethrectomy is indicated.
—Recurrences tend to be high grade and invasive.

PATHOPHYSIOLOGY

• Composed of pleomorphic cells arranged in sheets, with frequent mitoses
• Fails to stain with antibodies to PSA and PAP, may stain with antibodies to CEA
• Occurs in five patterns

—CIS of the prostatic urethra and periurethral glands
—TCC of the prostatic ducts and acini
—TCC with submucosal or prostatic stromal invasion
—Extraprostatic extension to seminal vesicles or other periprostatic tissues
—Metastases to regional lymph nodes or more distantly

• Cancers confined to the periurethral glands and ducts are associated with a high survival rate; it drops to 42% for those with stromal invasion and less than 15% for those with extraprostatic extension or regional disease.
• 10% of patients with TCC of the bladder and prostate will develop anterior urethral recurrence following radical cystectomy alone.
• Anterior urethral recurrence occurs in 10% to 25% of those with mucosal or ductal involvement and in 30% to 64% of those with prostatic stromal invasion.
• TCC is biologically different than prostatic adenocarcinoma. (TCC is hormonally resistant and frequently has distant metastasis, including osteolytic bone Mets.) Therefore, an accurate diagnosis is paramount.

CAUSES/RISK FACTORS

• Transitional cells line the prostatic urethra and ducts, making these structures susceptible to malignant transformation in response to the same factors that cause bladder tumors.
• The anatomic barrier to tumor spread in prostatic TCC is the basement membrane of the prostatic urethra, periurethral glands, and prostatic ducts and acini.
• CIS and intraductal involvement are associated with a significantly lower risk of urethral recurrence (10%–25%) as compared with stromal invasion (30%–64%).

COMPLICATIONS

• Hematuria, obstructive voiding, or signs and symptoms of metastatic disease
• Complications of urethrectomy: local abscesses, perineal sinuses, rectoperineal fistulas

DIFFERENTIAL DIAGNOSIS

• TCC-P and adenocarcinoma of the prostate may occur concurrently.
• Must be differentiated from adenocarcinoma of the prostate, which occurs in glands and stains positive with antibodies for PSA and PAP.

 ## Database

HISTORY

• Gross or microscopic hematuria, obstructive voiding symptoms in those with intact lower urinary tracts
• Urethral discharge or periurethral mass in those who have undergone urethrectomy
• Constitutional symptoms of weight loss, fatigue, anorexia, or bone pain

PHYSICAL EXAMINATION

• Periurethral mass, regional lymphadenopathy, bloody urethral discharge
• Digital rectal examination: nodularity, fixation

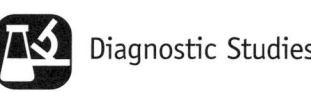 ## Diagnostic Studies

LABORATORY TESTING

• PSA of limited value

IMAGING

• Cross-sectional imaging (CT or MRI) to exclude regional extension
• Radionuclide bone scan indicated in those at risk of metastases based on grade and/or extent

SPECIAL STUDIES

- Cystoscopy

—Most often flat lesion in prostatic urethra seen on cystoscopy
—Papillary, flat, or sessile cancers within the bladder seen on cystoscopy

- Biopsy

—Transurethral resection most accurate and is associated with at least a 90% sensitivity for detection

- Transrectal fine- or core-needle biopsy is less accurate and associated with low sensitivities for detection (20%–40%).

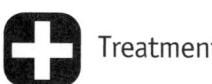 ## Treatment

GENERAL MEASURES

- Treatment is almost always indicated and is based on extent of disease: urethral/ductal vs. stromal vs. disease beyond the prostate.
- Treatment based on depth of involvement: all Ta, T1, Tis diseases are candidates for bacille Calmette-Guérin (BCG).

—Tumor limited to mucosa or superficial ducts? BCG with 70% response at 5 years
—Tumor invades deeper ducts or with stromal invasion? Radical cystectomy with urethrectomy

MEDICAL

- Intravesical administration of BCG is appropriate in those with disease confined to the urethra or prostatic ducts.

—Approximately 50% response
—Complete resection of the bladder neck may not be necessary, as BCG may bind to fibronectin receptors.
—BCG (120 mg in 50 cc NS) given after resolution of bleeding
—BCG given weekly for 6 weeks
—Repeat endoscopy, cytology, and biopsy performed 6 weeks after cessation of BCG induction. If disease has resolved, BCG given weekly for 3 weeks and maintenance regimen considered
—If recurrent/persistent disease is noted after BCG, consider repeat induction for 6 weeks.
—If the patient fails BCG, proceed to surgery or systemic therapy.

- Systemic chemotherapy for metastasis or in neoadjuvant setting

—Neoadjuvant: Downstaging of the primary tumor occurs, and less extensive treatment is needed (i.e., a partial instead of radical cystectomy can be done).
—Adjuvant: based on adverse pathologic findings at surgery (nodal or extravesical tumor extension is documented or when evidence of vascular or lymphatic invasion)
—No specific therapies studied only for TCC-P; bladder regimens used
  —MVAC
  —Preliminary three-drug regimen of ITP (ifosfamide, paclitaxel, and cisplatin). Median survival of ITP: 18.3 months vs. MVAC's 12.5 months

- Medical–systemic chemotherapy followed by selective surgery or radiation

—Platinum-based chemotherapy alone has a low complete response rate for patients with stromal and extraprostatic extension.
—Platinum-based chemotherapy may be followed by concurrent platinum and external beam radiotherapy.
—Combined modality treatment has been associated with an initial response rate.
—Patients who receive combined modality treatment are at risk for both invasive and superficial recurrence.

SURGICAL

- Radical cystectomy, rarely radical prostatectomy alone, is indicated for patients with invasive transitional cell cancers of the urethra.
- Urethrectomy is indicated in those with any TCC involving the distal aspect of the prostatic urethra and should be considered in those with stromal invasion, even when it does not reach the apical portions of the prostate.
- Orthotopic urinary diversion may be performed cautiously in those with proximal prostatic urethral involvement and no evidence of distal prostatic involvement.
- Radical cystectomy is associated with a 30% to 64% 5-year survival, depending on the extent of the bladder primary (if any) and depth of urethral involvement.

ALTERNATIVE THERAPIES: N/A

PATIENT EDUCATION: N/A

 ## Follow-Up

MONITORING

- Urethral cytologies in those patients with bladder TCC and/or prostatic urethra who have undergone either intravesical therapy or cystectomy
- Cystoscopy should complement cytology in those with an intact lower urinary tract.

PREVENTION: N/A

 ## Miscellaneous

SYNONYMS: N/A

ASSOCIATED CONDITIONS: N/A

NOTES

- See also Section II, "Bladder Cancer—TCC, Superficial (CIS, Ta, T1)" and "Bladder Cancer—TCC, Invasive (T2/3/4)."

ABBREVIATIONS

- TCC, transitional cell carcinoma

REFERENCES

Bajorin D. Treatment of patients with transitional-cell carcinoma of the urothelial tract with ifosfamide, paclitaxel, and cisplatin: A phase II trial. *J Clin Oncol* 1998;16(8):2722.

Cheville JC. Transitional cell carcinoma of the prostate. *Am Cancer Soc* 1998;82(4):703.

Esrig D. Transitional cell carcinoma involving the prostate with a proposed staging classification for stromal invasion. *J Urol* 1996;156: 1071.

Iselin CE. Does prostate transitional cell carcinoma preclude orthotopic bladder reconstruction after radical cystoprostatectomy for bladder cancer? *J Urol* 1997;158:2123.

Scgekkgannerm OF. Intravesical bacillus Calmette-Guerin for treatment of superficial transitional cell carcinoma of the prostatic urethra in association with carcinoma of the bladder. *J Urol* 1995;153(53):53.

Authors: Nathalie M. Barnes and Peter R. Carroll

Prostatic Intraepithelial Neoplasia

 Basics

DESCRIPTION

• Prostatic intraepithelial neoplasia (PIN) is characterized by cellular proliferation in prostatic ducts and acini, which can mimic cancer. It is subdivided into low- and high-grade PIN.

EPIDEMIOLOGY

• Present in 15% of prostatic needle core biopsies
• Coexists in 85% of prostates with adenocarcinoma

GENETICS

• 30% to 68% of high-grade PIN are aneuploid.
• Gain of chromosome 8 and allelic loss of 8p, 10q, and 16q in some cases of PIN and carcinoma

STAGING: N/A

SIGNS AND SYMPTOMS: N/A

PATHOPHYSIOLOGY

• Strong association between high-grade PIN and prostatic adenocarcinoma
• Cellular proliferation within preexisting ducts and acini with

—Cytologic atypia
—Nuclear and nucleolar enlargement

CAUSES/RISK FACTORS

• Unknown

COMPLICATIONS

• Possible association with carcinoma, although no cause-and-effect relationship has yet been proven

• Risk factors

—Most likely similar to prostatic carcinoma, such as age, race, and geography

DIFFERENTIAL DIAGNOSIS

• Lobular atrophy and postatrophic hyperplasia
• Atypical basal cell hyperplasia
• Cribriform hyperplasia
• Metaplastic changes after infarction, irradiation, or prostatitis
• Cribriform, ductal endometrioid and urothelial adenocarcinoma

 Database

HISTORY

• Is there a family history of prostate cancer?

PHYSICAL EXAMINATION

• The rectal examination is often usually normal in PIN.

 Diagnostic Studies

LABORATORY TESTING

• PSA levels are variable in PIN.

IMAGING

• May show as hypoechoic foci on transrectal ultrasound, probably due to a background of coexistent carcinoma

SPECIAL STUDIES

• Transrectal ultrasound-guided prostatic needle biopsy to evaluate for prostate cancer
• Recent data suggest that sextant biopsied directed more laterally or increasing the number of biopsies to 12 or more, including laterally directed and transitional zone, may increase cancer detection rates
• Immunostaining of histologic sections with high-molecular-weight cytokeratin (HMW-CK) to document presence of intact basal layer and thus absence of carcinoma

Treatment

GENERAL MEASURES

• No treatment is advocated now, as a direct cause-and-effect relationship with carcinoma has not been established.

—See below for repeat biopsy recommendations.

MEDICAL: N/A

SURGICAL: N/A

ALTERNATIVE THERAPIES: N/A

PATIENT EDUCATION

• Information on probability of coexistent carcinoma

 Follow-Up

MONITORING

• Repeat biopsy and follow-up (suggested by some authors) within 6 to 12 months of the biopsy of high-grade PIN

—Clinical follow-up every 3 months for 2 years, and then yearly for life (recommended by some authors)

—Low-grade PIN, in and of itself, does not require any specific follow-up.

PREVENTION

• Unknown. Long-term studies are underway to evaluate chemoprevention strategies (i.e., finasteride, others).

 Miscellaneous

SYNONYMS

• Intraductal dysplasia, large acinar atypical hyperplasia

ASSOCIATED CONDITIONS

• Prostatic adenocarcinoma

NOTES: N/A

ABBREVIATIONS

• PIN, prostatic intraepithelial neoplasia

REFERENCES

Bostwick D, Eble J, eds. Neuroplasms of the prostate. *Urologic Surgical Pathology* 1997;343–422.

Authors: Shahandeh Haghir and Gabriel P. Haas

Prostatitis—Acute Bacterial

 ## Basics

DESCRIPTION

- A serious illness requiring aggressive treatment with parenteral antibiotics. It is generally associated with infection of both the prostate and bladder.

EPIDEMIOLOGY

- Rarely affects pubertal or prepubertal boys. Adult men are most commonly affected.

GENETICS

- Unknown

STAGING: N/A

SIGNS AND SYMPTOMS

- Acute onset of lower back pain, perineal pain, fever, chills, dysuria, hematuria, and general malaise. Later arthralgias and myalgias may develop.
- Prostate examination usually reveals a warm, tender, and indurated gland.

PATHOPHYSIOLOGY

- Mechanisms are unknown. Possible routes of infection include ascending urethral infection, reflux of urine into prostatic ducts, lymphatic spread, and hematogenous spread.
- The agents that cause acute bacterial prostatitis are similar to those that cause urinary tract infections.

—Nonhospitalized patients: Aerobic gram-negative bacilli predominate (*Escherichia coli, Klebsiella pneumonia, Proteus mirabilis, Pseudomonas aeruginosa*); gram-positive organisms include *Staphylococcus aureus, Enterococcus*; also *Neisseria gonorrhoeae, Chlamydia trachomatis*
—Hospitalized patients: more resistant forms of *Enterococcus, Pseudomonas, S. aureus*

CAUSES/RISK FACTORS

- Bladder outlet obstruction, recent prostate biopsy, cystoscopy, catheterization

COMPLICATIONS

- Rectal examinations in acutely ill patients can produce a bacteremia and thus should be carefully performed.
- Urosepsis, urinary retention
- Pyelonephritis, epididymitis, or prostatic abscess

DIFFERENTIAL DIAGNOSIS

- Distinct entity from other forms of prostatitis such as chronic bacterial prostatitis, wherein there may be evidence of a UTI, but the patient is not toxic
- Urethritis, cystitis, prostatic abscess, seminal vesiculitis
- See also Section I, "Urinary Tract Infection—Adult Male."

 ## Database

HISTORY

- Typically acute onset of signs/symptoms

—Fever, chills, dysuria, perineal or suprapubic pain

- Any recent instrumentation, i.e., cystoscopy, prostate biopsy?

PHYSICAL EXAMINATION

- Signs of sepsis: fever, tachycardia, hypotension
- Evidence of lower abdominal fullness may suggest retention.
- Perineal tenderness is common.
- The rectal examination should be performed cautiously. (Some suggest deferring the examination if the diagnosis is apparent.)

 ## Diagnostic Studies

LABORATORY TESTING

- CBC typically demonstrates signs of systemic infection.
- Urinalysis and cultures are consistent with a UTI.

—Segmented urinalysis: usually not necessary in cases of acute prostatitis

IMAGING

- Ultrasound to confirm bladder emptying to evaluate upper tracts for obstruction if clinically indicated

SPECIAL STUDIES: N/A

Treatment

GENERAL MEASURES

• The diagnosis of acute bacterial prostatitis is often made based on the patient's history and symptoms.
• Bed rest, analgesics, antipyretics, and stool softeners are recommended.
• For acute urinary retention secondary to acute bacterial prostatitis, a suprapubic catheter is recommended.
• Transurethral instrumentation should be avoided.
• Acutely ill patients should be hospitalized for IV antibiotic therapy.
—When afebrile, switch to appropriate oral therapy.
• Urine culture and sensitivity and blood cultures should be performed.

MEDICAL

• Treatment should be started prior to culture and sensitivity results.
• When the organism and its sensitivity are known, treat for 30 days to prevent chronic bacterial prostatitis.
• Severe
—Empiric therapy with IV ampicillin and gentamicin for broad-based urinary coverage
—Fluoroquinolones
  —Ciprofloxacin (Cipro) 400 mg IV q12h
  —Ofloxacin (Floxin) 400 mg IV q12h
• Mild forms: fluoroquinolones or trimethoprim-sulfamethoxazole

—Norfloxacin (Noroxin) 400 mg po q12h
—Ciprofloxacin (Cipro) 500 mg po q12h
—Ofloxacin (Floxin) 400 mg po q12h
—Trimethoprim-sulfamethoxazole (Bactrim) 160 mg trimethoprim/800 mg sulfamethoxazole bid

SURGICAL

• Suprapubic drainage if patient is in retention
• Drainage of prostatic abscess if present

ALTERNATIVE THERAPIES: N/A

PATIENT EDUCATION

• Parents of newborn with a hydrocele should be instructed in the natural history of the condition in children.

 Follow-Up

MONITORING

• Follow-Up cultures off antibiotics
• Evaluate for bladder outlet obstruction.
• Failure of therapy to alleviate symptoms may indicate that an abscess has formed. Transrectal ultrasound can be used to detect a prostatic abscess.

PREVENTION: N/A

 Miscellaneous

SYNONYMS: N/A

ASSOCIATED CONDITIONS: N/A

NOTES

• See recommended changes in the classification of prostatitis, Section III, "Prostatitis—NIH Classification System."
• Must treat for at least 1 month with oral antibiotics to minimize development of chronic bacterial prostatitis
• Never check a PSA in the setting of an acute prostatitis until all symptoms are resolved (falsely elevated).

ABBREVIATIONS: N/A

REFERENCES

Dalhoff A, et al. Diffusion of ciprofloxacin into prostatic fluid. *Eur J Clin Microbiol* 1984;3:360.

Mears EM Jr. Prostatitis. *Med Clin North Am* 1991;75:405.

Mears EM Jr, Stamey TA. Bacteriologic localization patterns in bacterial prostatitis and urethritis. *Invest Urol* 1968;5:492.

Sanford JP. *Guide to Antimicrobial Therapy 1990*. West Bethesda, MD: Antimicrobial Therapy Inc., 1990:3–32.

Schwager EJ. Treatment of bacterial prostatitis. *Am J Fam Physician* 1991;44:2137.

Authors: John B. Maggioncalda and Leonard G. Gomella

Prostatitis—Chronic Bacterial

 Basics

DESCRIPTION

- Prostatitis associated with positive urine culture, but no signs of systemic infection

EPIDEMIOLOGY

- Prostatitis is the most common urologic diagnosis in men <50 years old and the third most common diagnosis in men >50 years old.
- Prostatitis results in over 2 million office visits per year in the United States.
- 25% of all genitourinary office visits are for prostatitis.
- 5% to 40% of patients with prostatitis syndrome have chronic bacterial prostatitis.

GENETICS

- No known genetic predisposition

STAGING: N/A

SIGNS AND SYMPTOMS

- Pain

—Perineal, suprapubic, groin, penile, scrotal, rectal

- Voiding

—Dysuria, poor stream, frequency, urgency, nocturia

- Sexual

—Pain on ejaculation, decreased libido

PATHOPHYSIOLOGY

- Etiologic organism

—Uropathogenic bacteria (i.e., E. coli)
—Presumed uropathogenic bacteria (i.e., enterococci)
—Possible uropathogenic bacteria (i.e., coagulase-negative staphylococci)
—Noncultured organisms (i.e., chlamydia, mycoplasma, etc.)
—Cryptic unculturable organisms

- Etiologic mechanisms

—Obstructive, turbulent and/or high-pressure voiding combined with intraprostatic ductal reflux
—Begins as acute or subacute intraductal inflammation
—Progresses to chronic intraductal inflammation
—Bacteria present in inflamed ducts in protected bacterial aggregates or bacterial biofilms
—Ductal epithelium and basement membranes break down, with inflammation spilling over into stroma.
—End-stage: fibrosis (scarring) of interstitium with obliteration of normal ductal architecture

CAUSES/RISK FACTORS

- Causes

—High-pressure turbulent voiding associated with intraductal prostatic reflux of infected urine from bladder or urethra

- Risk factors

—Acute bacterial prostatitis
—Obstructive, turbulent, or high-pressure voiding
—Urinary tract infection
—Urethritis
—Foley catheterization
—Bladder neck hypertrophy
—Detrusor/sphincter dyssynergia
—Urethral stricture
—Urethral meatal stenosis
—Balanitis

COMPLICATIONS

- Recurrent infections

—Recurrent cystitis
—Epidiymo-orchitis
—Urethritis

- Chronic pelvic pain syndrome

—Patients cured of chronic bacterial prostatitis sometimes continue to suffer from nonbacterial prostatitis or chronic pelvic pain syndrome long after bacteria have been eradicated.

DIFFERENTIAL DIAGNOSIS

- Cystitis
- Urethritis
- Acute bacterial prostatitis
- Chronic nonbacterial prostatitis (NIH chronic pelvic pain syndrome or category IIIA prostatitis)
- Prostatodynia/pelvic floor myalgia (NIH chronic pelvic pain syndrome or category IIIB prostatitis)

 Database

HISTORY

- History

—Prostatitis (acute or chronic)
—Urinary tract infections
—Sexually transmitted diseases
—Sexual history (partners, sexual orientation, condoms, etc.)
—Catheterizations
—Lower genitourinary surgery

- Pain

—Location
—Description
—Nature
—Duration
—Voiding
  —Obstructive symptoms
  —Irritative symptoms

- Quality of life

—How do they feel about their problem?
—Bother
—Effect on employment

PHYSICAL EXAMINATION

- Abdominal examination

—Tenderness, bladder distension, hernias

- External genitalia

—Testes, epididymis, penis, scrotum
—Focused neurologic examination
  —Anal tone, sensation, bulbocavernosal reflex
—Digital rectal examination
  —Size, consistency, tenderness
  —Concurrent with collection of urine specimens before and after massage, as well as collection of expressed prostatic secretions (see Laboratory Testing below)

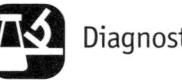 Diagnostic Studies

LABORATORY TESTING

- Traditional

—Culture of VB1 (first voided urine), VB3 (second voided urine or midstream urine), EPS (expressed prostatic secretion) and VB3 (third voided urine after prostate massage)
—Microscopy of VB2 and VB3 or EPS wet-mount specimen
  —Chronic bacterial prostatitis diagnosed when there is excessive leukocytosis (>tenfold) compared with VB1 and VB2 or >10 white blood cells in EPS and culture of VB3 and/or EPS quantitatively grows more (>tenfold) uropathogens than VB1 and/or VB2

- Pre- and postmassage test (PPMT)

—Culture of urine and microscopy of sediment of urine before (pre-M) and after (post-M) prostate massage
  —Chronic bacterial prostatitis diagnosed when there is excessive leukocytosis and uropathogens (as described in traditional method above) in post-M specimen compared with pre-M specimen

IMAGING

- Transrectal ultrasound, abdominal/pelvic ultrasound, intravenous pyelogram, retrograde urethrogram, and videourodynamics very occasionally will be required to rule out pathology other than simple chronic bacterial prostatitis.

SPECIAL STUDIES

- A cystoscopy will occasionally be required to rule out a urethral or bladder outlet abnormality.

 ## Treatment

GENERAL MEASURES

- Avoid stress, alcohol, acidic drinks, spicy foods, and high-impact sports and activities.
- Drink lots of fluids, continue low-impact activities, and do not avoid sex.

MEDICAL

- Blood–prostate barrier

—There is a "blood–prostate barrier" based on differential pH gradients between the prostatic interstitium and the prostatic ducts and acini. Only drugs with a unique pKa can penetrate this barrier in bacteriocidal concentrations.

- Antimicrobials

—Antimicrobials indicated in chronic prostatitis secondary to proven uropathogens include
  —Trimethoprim (or trimethoprim combinations such as trimethoprim-sulfamethoxazole)
  —Fluoroquinolones (i.e., norfloxacin, ciprofloxacin, ofloxacin)
—Antimicrobials indicated in chronic prostatitis if chlamydia or mycoplasma suspected
  —Tetracyclines (including Vibramycin), ofloxacin, and erythromycin may be considered.
—Duration of antimicrobial therapy
  —Antimicrobials should be prescribed for a minimum of 6 weeks for the initial episode.
  —For symptoms that are improving, 12 weeks of therapy is recommended.
  —For relapsing cases (same organism), low-dose long-term suppressive therapy is recommended.
  —For recurrent cases (different organisms), low-dose long-term prophylactic therapy is recommended.

SURGICAL

- Surgery is to be avoided unless a strong definite indication is noted.

—Internal urethrotomy: for urethral strictures
—Bladder neck surgery: for documented bladder neck hypertrophy and obstruction
—Radical TURP: may be of benefit in refractory cases with infected prostatic calculi and/or obstructed prostate
—Total prostatectomy: may be of benefit in very selected cases of refractory bacterial prostatitis in which it can be documented that antimicrobials do not clear bacterial infection originating in the prostate

ALTERNATIVE THERAPIES

- Prostate massage

—Repetitive prostate massage is an historic therapy for chronic prostatitis, and appears to be of benefit when combined with antibiotics in some cases.
  —Hypothesized to work by stimulating "hibernating" bacterial biofilms (making them more susceptible to antimicrobials), draining the obstructed inflamed ducts (allowing for better antimicrobial penetration), and stimulating the blood supply to the area

- Phytotherapy

—Plant extracts and herbal medications are becoming very popular and appear to be as effective as placebo.

PATIENT EDUCATION

- See General Measures above

—Patients must understand the difficulties in obtaining complete amelioration of symptoms and that the disease has a tendency to recur.

 ## Follow-Up

MONITORING

- Symptoms

—If improved or cured: midstream urine collection for culture
—If symptoms continue: repeat EPS and/or VB3 (post-M) culture

- Cultures

—See above

PREVENTION

- No known method to prevent recurrent prostatitis, except for protected intercourse (i.e., condom)

 ## Miscellaneous

SYNONYMS

- NIH (National Institutes of Health) category II prostatitis

ASSOCIATED CONDITIONS

- Recurrent cystitis, urethritis, epididymo-orchitis

NOTES

- See recommended changes in classification of prostatitis, Section III, "Prostatitis—NIH Classification System."
- See other prostatitis topics in Section II.

ABBREVIATIONS

- EPS, expressed prostatic secretion; VB1, voided bladder 1 (urethral specimen); VB2, voided bladder 2 (bladder specimen); VB3, voided bladder 3 (urine specimen collected after prostatic massage); Pre-M, urine before prostate massage (i.e., VB2); Post-M, urine after prostate massage (i.e., VB3)

REFERENCES

Nickel JC. Prostatitis: Myths and realities. *Urology* 1998;51:362–366.

Nickel JC. Prostatitis. In: Mulholland SG, ed. *Antibiotic Therapy in Urology*. Philadelphia: Lippincott-Raven, 1996:57–70.

Nickel JC. A practical approach to the management of prostatitis. *Techniques Urol* 1995;1:162–167.

Nickel JC. New concepts in the pathogenesis and treatment of prostatitis. *Curr Opin Urol* 1992;2:37–43.

Author: J. Curtis Nickel

Prostatitis—Chronic, Nonbacterial, Inflammatory

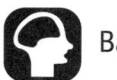 Basics

DESCRIPTION

• Inflammatory condition of unknown etiology, rarely associated with infectious organism, and with similar symptomatology to chronic bacterial prostatitis

EPIDEMIOLOGY

• In general, 50% of men will experience an episode of some form of prostatitis; approximately 25% of men evaluated for urologic problems have prostatitis symptoms, nonbacterial type, estimated to be 8 times more frequent than bacterial prostatitis.

GENETICS: N/A

STAGING: N/A

SIGNS AND SYMPTOMS

• Voiding symptoms: dysuria, frequency; urgency, nocturia, postvoid dribbling
• Pain symptoms: suprapubic, perineal, back, scrotal, penile, and with ejaculation
• Possible hematospermia; symptoms may be intermittent.

PATHOPHYSIOLOGY

• Reflux of urine into prostatic ducts may play a role; possible chemical inflammatory response

CAUSES/RISK FACTORS

• Unsure etiology; possible agents such as gram-positive organisms, *Ureaplasma urealyticum* and *Chlamydia* species have been unproved as causative factors; other hypotheses include unidentified infectious agent, chemical agent, an autoimmune response, or viral agent. Possible risk factors include a history of GU infections and possible estrogens.

COMPLICATIONS

• Fertility is uncommonly affected, as sperm quality may be adversely affected.
• Quality of life is significantly impacted, with a significant sickness impact profile; up to one-half of patients may meet the criteria for major depression.

DIFFERENTIAL DIAGNOSIS

• Any cause of lower urinary tract symptoms

—Chronic bacterial prostatitis
—Acute bacterial prostatitis
—Prostatodynia
—Bladder neck dysfunction
—Prostate cancer
—Granulomatous prostatitis
—Urethral stricture
—Bladder disorders, including cancer

 Database

HISTORY

• Bladder or prostate infections/fever?
• History of hematuria?
• History of GU surgery?
• STDs may suggest stricture disease.
• Urologic Symptom Score (IPSS, AUA-SS)

—Provides baseline assessment to gauge interventions (see Section III)

PHYSICAL EXAMINATION

• Digital rectal examination

—Usually nonspecific findings; may have tenderness, bogginess, firmness, or nodularity

 Diagnostic Studies

LABORATORY TESTING

• UA should be normal; urine culture sterile
• Urine cytology should be negative.
• EPS has excessive WBCs (>10/HPF) and lipid-laden macrophages; no organisms should be identified; found to have increased urate and creatinine
• PSA not useful unless ruling out prostate cancer

IMAGING

• Ultrasound rarely helpful

SPECIAL STUDIES

• Stamey localization technique (VB-1, 2, 3; see Section III) for prostatic fluid examination
• Occasional patients presenting with lower urinary tract symptoms, even of young age (20s–40s), may have bladder outlet obstruction due to bladder neck dysfunction. Pressure–flow urodynamic testing is necessary to exclude this diagnosis.

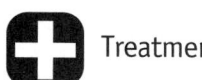 Treatment

GENERAL MEASURES

• A definitive treatment is difficult because of the uncertain etiology.
• Conservative measures include sitz baths, non-steroidal antiinflammatory agents (e.g., ibuprofen 600–800 mg tid-qid), and prostatic massage for those men who have infrequent ejaculation.

MEDICAL

• Antibiotic use is controversial.
• Empiric trial of antibiotics (e.g., Bactrim or Septra DS bid, or a fluoroquinolone for 2–4 weeks)

—If improvement is noted, continue for 6 weeks minimum.

• Many believe in a 2-week trial of tetracycline 500 mg qid, or doxycycline 100 mg bid, or erythromycin 250 mg tid to treat *Chlamydia* and *Ureaplasma.*

—If no response, should terminate antibiotics

SURGERY

• Should attempt medical management first
• TUIP, single incision, may be helpful in the case of bladder outlet obstruction.
• TUMT has also shown improvement in small patient studies.

ALTERNATIVE THERAPIES

• Allopurinal 600 mg/d initially for short period, decreasing to 300 mg/d, has improved discomfort.
• Pollen extract (Cernilton RN one tab tid for 6 months) has decreased WBCs in EPS and caused a favorable subjective response in the majority of patients.
• Alpha-blockers may improve symptoms, as in patients with prostatodynia.

PATIENT EDUCATION: N/A

 Follow-Up

MONITORING: N/A

PREVENTION: N/A

 Miscellaneous

SYNONYMS

• Chronic pelvic pain syndrome: inflammatory, idiopathic prostatitis, abacterial prostatitis

ASSOCIATED CONDITIONS: N/A

NOTES

• See recommended changes in the classification of prostatitis, Section III, "Prostatitis—NIH Classification System."
• See other prostatitis topics in Section II.

ABBREVIATIONS

• EPS, expressed prostatic secretions; TUIP, transurethral incision of prostate; TUMT, transurethral microwave therapy

REFERENCES

Berger RE, Krieger JN, Kessler D, et al. Case-control study of men with suspected chronic idiopathic prostatitis. *J Urol* 1989;141(2):328–331.

Doble A. Chronic prostatitis. *Br J Urol* 1994;74(5): 537–541.

Moul JW. Prostatitis: Sorting out the different causes. *Postgrad Med* 1993;94(5):191–194.

Persson BE, Ronquist G. Evidence for a mechanistic association between nonbacterial prostatitis and levels of urate and creatinine in expressed prostatic secretion. *J Urol* 1996;155(3):958–960.

Pewitt EB, Schaeffer AJ. Urinary tract infection in urology, including acute and chronic prostatitis. *Infect Dis Clin North Am* 1997;11(3):623–646.

Authors: Sam S. Chang and Douglas F. Milam

Prostatitis—Granulomatous

 Basics

DESCRIPTION

• Inflammation of the prostate associated with granuloma formation. Often confused with carcinoma of the prostate

EPIDEMIOLOGY

• Very rare type of prostatitis
• 0.8% of benign inflammatory prostatic specimens

GENETICS

• Unknown

STAGING: N/A

SIGNS AND SYMPTOMS

• Often asymptomatic
• Symptoms similar to other forms of prostatitis

—Irritative voiding symptoms, including urgency, frequency, dysuria
—Obstructive voiding symptoms, including acute urinary retention

• Signs on physical examination may mimic prostate cancer.

—Hard gland with global induration and/or nodule

• If associated with systemic vasculitis or granulomatous disease, may have constitutional symptoms or signs
• Often associated with UTI 2 to 3 months prior to onset of symptoms

PATHOPHYSIOLOGY

• Due to infectious, iatrogenic, systemic granulomatous disease; allergic, idiopathic etiology; or malakoplakia
• Intense localized foreign body inflammatory response caused by blockage of prostatic ducts

—Tissue necrosis occurs, and with destruction of the gland structures, secretions, cellular debris, or infectious agents spill.
—Spilled materials are recognized as foreign in the interstitium, and foreign-body reaction formation occurs.

• Eosinophilic and noneosinophilic histologic subtypes

CAUSES/RISK FACTORS

• Infectious: bacterial, viral, fungal, parasitic, including *Mycobacterium*
• Iatrogenic causes: TURP, BCG instillation therapy for bladder cancer
• Systemic granulomatous diseases: Wegener's granulomatosis, Churg-Strauss syndrome, sarcoidosis, rheumatoid arthritis, polyarteritis nodosa, malakoplakia
• UTI or STD

COMPLICATIONS

• Undetected prostate cancer
• Acute urinary retention
• If infectious in etiology, may pass organism to sexual partner

DIFFERENTIAL DIAGNOSIS

• Carcinoma of the prostate
• Acute prostatitis
• Chronic prostatitis
• BPH with calcifications

 Database

HISTORY

• Previous UTI or STD?

—Syphilis, TB, or other infectious agent

• History of LUTS?

—Voiding symptoms are often associated.

• Systemic granulomatous disease?

—Secondary involvement of the prostate

• History of prostate surgery or bladder cancer?

—BCG or TURP can cause granulamatous prostatitis.

• Fever, chills, or other constitutional signs?

—Suggest infectious, systemic etiology

PHYSICAL EXAMINATION

• Rectal examination: hard, indurated gland with/without nodule

—Tender vs. painless

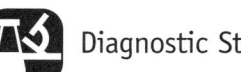 Diagnostic Studies

LABORATORY TESTING

• Urinalysis

—Leukocytosis may occur during UTI.

• Urine cultures are often sterile.
• Blood sampling may reveal elevated sedimentation rate, acid phosphatase, or eosinophilia; PSA findings variable
• If evidence of TB or mycotic disease, appropriate tests should be ordered of AFB, etc.

IMAGING

• The transrectal ultrasound has limited utility.

SPECIAL STUDIES

• Prostate biopsy is the definitive test.

—Histopathology typically shows noncaseating granuloma formation with multiple types of inflammatory cells.
—Fibrotic tissue replaces parenchyma.

Treatment

GENERAL MEASURES

- Spontaneous resolution of symptoms usually occurs, but rectal examination findings may persist.
- Symptomatic treatment may be given.

—Sitz baths, fluids, antiinflammatory and other symptomatic medications

MEDICAL

- Treat the underlying cause if one is known.

—Antibiotics, antituberculous agents

- Some advocate corticosteroids and antihistamines.
- Temporary transurethral urinary catheterization if symptoms severe/retention of urine

SURGICAL

- Prostatectomy is rarely advocated.

ALTERNATIVE THERAPIES: N/A

PATIENT EDUCATION

- Most will spontaneously resolve; physical examination findings may persist for years.

 Follow-Up

MONITORING

- Despite a previous history of granulomatous prostatitis on biopsy, abnormal glands may need to be re-biopsied so as not to miss a concomitant cancer.

PREVENTION: N/A

 Miscellaneous

SYNONYMS: N/A

ASSOCIATED CONDITIONS

- Wegener's granulomatosis, Churg-Strauss syndrome, bladder cancer

NOTES: N/A

ABBREVIATIONS

- BCG, bacillus Calmette-Guérin; BPH, benign prostatic hyperplasia; STD, sexually transmitted disease; LUTS, lower urinary tract symptoms

REFERENCES

Bryan RL. Granulomatous prostatitis: A clinicopathologic study. *Histopathology* 1991;19:453.

Mears EM. Prostatitis and related disorders. In: Walsh PC, Retik AB, Vaughan ED, Wein AJ, eds. *Campbell's Urology,* 7th ed. Philadelphia: WB Saunders, 1998.

Roberts RA. Review of clinical and pathological prostatitis syndromes. *Urology* 1997;49(6):809.

Stillwell TJ. The clinical spectrum of granulomatous prostatitis: A report of 200 cases. *J Urol* 1987;138:320.

Authors: Deborah Glassman and Richard B. Alexander

Prostatitis—Nonbacterial, Noninflammatory (Prostatodynia)

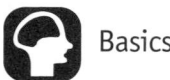 Basics

DESCRIPTION

• Nonbacterial, noninflammatory prostatitis, also referred to by some as prostatodynia, is a clinical diagnosis made in patients with voiding symptoms and pain similar to that of prostatitis, with a negative urine culture, noninflammatory expressed prostatic secretions, and a normal prostate examination.

EPIDEMIOLOGY

• The typical patient is 20 to 45 years old.

GENETICS: N/A

STAGING: N/A

SIGNS AND SYMPTOMS

• Urinary symptoms

—May have irritative or obstructive urinary symptoms

• Pelvic pain

—Complaints of perineal, scrotal, suprapubic, urethral pain

PATHOPHYSIOLOGY

• The exact cause of prostatodynia is not known.
• The most commonly held theory is that there is intraprostatic urinary reflux, which is responsible for this form of prostatitis.
• Many patients will have evidence of "spastic" bladder neck on urodynamic studies. The elevated prostatic urethral pressures cause the intraprostatic reflux and a chemical prostatitis.
• Stress may also be a factor; it may cause tension myalgia of pelvic musculature.

CAUSES/RISK FACTORS

• Stress
• Anxiety

COMPLICATIONS

• Sexual dysfunction
• Quality-of-life issues

DIFFERENTIAL DIAGNOSIS

• Acute bacterial prostatitis
• Chronic bacterial prostatitis
• Nonbacterial prostatitis
• Parasitic prostatitis
• Mycotic prostatitis
• Tuberculous prostatitis
• Gonococcal prostatitis

 Database

HISTORY

• Age of patient?

—Typically occurs in younger males 20 to 50 years old

• Urinary symptoms?

—May have irritative or obstructive voiding symptoms; hesitancy and intermittency common

• Pain?

—Often complain of perineal, urethral, or suprapubic pain

• History of urinary tract infection?

—Urinary tract infection is more often associated with acute/chronic bacterial prostatitis.

• History of sexually transmitted disease?

—May be associated with other forms of prostatitis

• Social history?

—Prostatodynia can be associated with "high stress" and anxiety.

PHYSICAL EXAMINATION

• No specific abnormalities either neurologically or on physical examination
• Rectal examination

—May have increased sphincter tone
—May have tender paraprostatic tissue, but prostate is usually nontender

• The remaining genitourinary examination is typically normal.

 Diagnostic Studies

LABORATORY TESTING

• Urinalysis and urine culture

—Rule out urinary tract infection.
—Prostatodynia is not associated with urinary tract infection.

• Expressed prostatic secretions (EPS)

—Examination of fluid determines whether inflammation is present.
—10 WBCs/HPF indicates inflammation.
—Prostatodynia is not associated with inflammation or infection of the EPS.

IMAGING

• A transrectal ultrasound of the prostate to determine inflammatory changes within the prostate has not been shown to be clinically useful.

SPECIAL STUDIES

• Videourodynamics

—May demonstrate incomplete relaxation of bladder neck and prostatic urethra with decreased peak and average flow rates

• Cystoscopy

—May reveal signs of bladder outlet obstruction

Prostatitis—Nonbacterial, Noninflammatory (Prostatodynia)

 Treatment

GENERAL MEASURES

• Supportive care
• Warm sitz baths may provide symptomatic relief.
• Dietary irritants should be avoided if identified as problematic (i.e., caffeine, spicy foods).
• Prostatic massage remains controversial; it may assist patients with a "congested prostate" from infrequent ejaculation.

MEDICAL

• Alpha-blockers are a mainstay of treatment.

—These relax the bladder neck, therefore improving urinary symptoms, and may decrease urinary reflux into the ejaculatory ducts.

• Diazepam (Valium)

—Can be used in conjunction with alpha-blockers to relieve perineal tension

• Nonsteroidal antiinflammatory medications

—Can be helpful for pain and discomfort (i.e., ibuprofen)

• Anticholinergics

—May eliminate irritative voiding symptoms

SURGICAL

• Various surgical options have been tried, including transurethral resection; laser ablation with medical therapy is considered the mainstay of therapy.
• Recently, microwave hyperthermia has shown some activity.

ALTERNATIVE THERAPIES

• Psychiatric/psychological counseling regarding stress management may be necessary in those who do not respond well to medical treatment.
• Biofeedback

PATIENT EDUCATION

• Some patients may benefit from stress management.

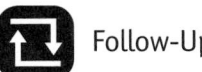 Follow-Up

MONITORING: N/A

PREVENTION: N/A

 Miscellaneous

SYNONYMS

• Stress prostatitis, chronic pelvic pain syndrome, prostatodynia, NIH category III β prostatitis

ASSOCIATED CONDITIONS: N/A

NOTES

• Patients who fail therapy should be evaluated for possible interstitial prostatitis.
• See recommended changes in classification of prostatitis, Section III, "Prostatitis—NIH Classification System."
• See other prostatitis topics in Section II.

ABBREVIATIONS

• EPS, expressed prostatic secretions

REFERENCES

Meares EM. Prostatitis. *Med Clin North Am* 1991; 75(2):405–424.

Nickel JC. Effective management of chronic prostatitis. *Urol Clin North Am* 1998;25:4.

Nickel JC, Sorensen R. Transurethral microwave therapy for nonbacterial prostatitis and prostatodynia: Initial experience. *Urology* 1994;44(3): 458–460.

Authors: M. Louis Moy and Leonard G. Gomella

Prune-Belly (Triad) Syndrome

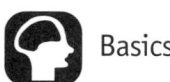 Basics

DESCRIPTION

• Triad necessary for diagnosis

—1: deficiency of abdominal musculature
—2: bilateral undescended testicles, usually abdominal
—3: dilated prostatic urethra, bladder, and lower ureters

• Incomplete variant where two parts of triad exist

EPIDEMIOLOGY

• 1 per 35,000 to 50,000 live births
• Predominantly male; females are incomplete variants.

GENETICS

• Possibly two-step autosomal dominant with sex-limited inheritance

STAGING

• I: oligohydramnios, pulmonary hypoplasia, or pneumothorax
• II: typical features but no immediate problem with survival; may have mild or unilateral renal dysplasia
• III: mild external features and uropathy; renal function is stable.

SIGNS AND SYMPTOMS

• Urologic

—Cryptorchidism
  —Generally nonpalpable
—Urinary tract infection and dysfunctional voiding
—Renal insufficiency
—Megalourethra
  —Fusiform type, associated with stillbirth
  —Scaphoid type, less severe

• Pulmonary

—Bronchitis and respiratory distress
—Pectus excavatum

• Abdomen
—Wrinkled lower abdomen as neonate
  —Becomes "pot-bellied" with standing
  —Infants have difficulty sitting from a supine position.

• Musculoskeletal
—Elbow and knee dimples, clubfoot, congenital hip dislocation

• Gastrointestinal
—Intestinal obstruction
—Constipation

• Cardiac problems

PATHOPHYSIOLOGY

• Abdomen
—Muscle is diffusely deficient lateral and inferior

• Testicles are undescended
—Generally nonpalpable, usually found at level of iliac vessels
—Reports of decreased spermatogonia
—Risk of malignancy undefined, but rare

• The prostatic urethra is dilated.
—Wide-open bladder neck on voiding
  —Contrast to posterior urethral valve patients with bladder neck hypertrophy.
—Dilation tapers down to the membranous urethra.
—Reports of urethral stenosis, atresia, and valves in autopsy series
  —Rare occurrence in living patients
—Paucity of prostatic tubules (epithelium)

• The bladder is enlarged.
—No trabeculation
  —No muscle hypertrophy
—Pseudodiverticulum of dome
  —Occasional patent urachus
—Incomplete emptying
  —Recurrent bacterial colonization

• Vesicoureteral reflux in three-fourths of patients
• Ureteral dilation
—Bilateral
—Distal significantly more involved than proximal
  —Deficiency of smooth muscle

• Renal hypodysplasia
—Variable severity of renal insufficiency
—Calyceal and pelvic dilation considerably less than distal ureteral dilation

• Fertility: no reported cases
—Testicular dysfunction
—Prostatic dysfunction
  —Normal erection and orgasm
  —Probable retrograde ejaculation

• Pulmonary hypoplasia secondary to oligohydramnios
—Bronchitis and respiratory distress
  —Poor pulmonary toilet secondary to hypoplastic abdominal musculature

• Gastrointestinal
—Intestinal malrotation
—Constipation common

• Cardiac
—Atrial and ventricular septal defects
—Tetralogy of Fallot

CAUSES/RISK FACTORS

• Etiologic theories of triad syndrome
—Lateral plate mesodermal arrest
—In utero transient urethral obstruction

COMPLICATIONS

• Death
—Renal failure and/or pulmonary hypoplasia

• Urosepsis
• Renal failure (30%)

DIFFERENTIAL DIAGNOSIS

• Megacystis microcolon—intestinal hypoperistalsis syndrome

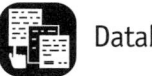 Database

HISTORY: N/A

• Diagnose as neonate

PHYSICAL EXAMINATION

• Lung auscultation for pneumothorax
• Cardiac auscultation for murmurs
• Abdominal palpation for dilation of upper collecting system, megacystis, and location of testicles
• Observe the urinary stream if possible.
• Examine extremities for clubbing, dimples, hip dislocation.

Diagnostic Studies

LABORATORY TESTING

- Serum electrolytes, creatinine, and urea nitrogen

—Creatinine should stabilize below 1 mg/dL.

- Urinalysis and urine culture

IMAGING

- Chest x-ray for pneumothorax and pulmonary hypoplasia
- Renal and bladder ultrasound before and after voiding

—Dilation of entire urinary tract
    —Distal ureters worse
—Bladder wall thickened, usual post-void residual
—Renal parenchymal changes are variable.

- Voiding cystourethrogram with antibiotic prophylaxis

—Vesicoureteral reflux in 75%
    —Reflux may demonstrate the entire collecting system.
—Large, irregular-shaped bladder with pseudodiverticulum
    —No trabeculation
—Wide-open bladder neck
—Dilated, triangular prostatic urethra tapering down to membranous urethra

- Radioisotope renal scan for differential function

—If possible, wait until 1 month of age

SPECIAL STUDIES: N/A

 Treatment

GENERAL MEASURES

- Parent reassurance
- Ensure urine sterility.

MEDICAL

- Monitor serum creatinine and pulmonary function.
- Bladder massage in infants to promote emptying
- Antibiotic prophylaxis

—Neonate: amoxicillin drops (50 mg/mL) 25 mg/kg once a day
—3 months of age: trimethoprim-sulfamethoxazole suspension (40 mg/5 mL) 2 mg/kg once a day, or nitrofurantoin suspension (25 mg/5 mL) 1 to 2 mg/kg once a day

- Urine culture every 3 months

SURGICAL

- Neonatal drainage indications: worsening function or dilation, recurrent urinary infections, or urosepsis

—Cutaneous vesicostomy affords the easiest drainage.
    —If present, remove the pseudodiverticulum at the same time.
—Bilateral pyelostomies if ureters are redundant and stagnant
    —Avoid upper ureterostomies.

- Orchiopexy relative indications: allows palpation for tumor, is cosmetic, fertility never reported

—Best achieved transabdominally
—Often done in conjunction with other procedure, always before 1 year of age

- Extensive surgical remodeling: indications and timing extremely controversial; no controlled studies to show whether surgery is superior to conservative management

—Reduction cystoplasty
—Distal ureterectomy
—Upper ureteral reimplantation and tapering if necessary

- Urethrotomy indications: valves, uncommon, but reported; outflow obstruction, difficult to document due to impaired detrusor function
- Abdominoplasty

—May facilitate bladder emptying

- Nephrectomy
- Renal transplantation

ALTERNATIVE THERAPIES: N/A

PATIENT EDUCATION

- National Prune Belly Syndrome Association, 30 Salem Blvd., Naugatuck, CT 06770; (203)729-6054; http://prunebelly.org

 Follow-Up

MONITORING

- Urine culture every 3 months
- Serum creatinine at least annually
- Imaging is individualized.

PREVENTION: N/A

 Miscellaneous

SYNONYMS

- Eagle-Barrett syndrome, triad syndrome

ASSOCIATED CONDITIONS

- Megalourethra, intestinal malrotation, pulmonary hypoplasia, atrial and ventricular septal defects

NOTES: N/A

ABBREVIATIONS: N/A

REFERENCES

Coplen DE, Snow BW, Duckett JW. Prune belly syndrome. In: Gillenwater JY, Grayhack JT, Howards SS, Duckett JW, eds. *Adult and Pediatric Urology.* St Louis: Mosby–Year Book, 1996:2297.

Greskovich FJ, Nyberg LM. The prune belly syndrome: A review of its etiology, defects, treatment and prognosis. *J Urol* 1988;140:707.

Woodard JR, Smith EA. Prune belly syndrome. In: Walsh PC, Retik AB, Vaughan ED, Wein AJ, eds. *Campbell's Urology*, 7th ed. Philadelphia: WB Saunders, 1998:1917.

Woodard JR, Zucker I. Current management of the dilated urinary tract in prune belly syndrome. *Urol Clin North Am* 1990;17(2):407.

Authors: Eric A. Kurzrock and Laurence S. Baskin

Pseudohermaphroditism—Male and Female

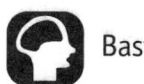 Basics

DESCRIPTION

Female Pseudohermaphrodite

- Karyotype 46XX
- Gonads: histologically normal ovaries
- External genitalia: varying degrees of masculinization
- Classification

—Congenital adrenal hyperplasia
—Most common cause in females
—Results from block in cortisol synthesis pathway
—Exogenous virilization
—Progestational agents administered in the first trimester
—Virilizing tumors
—Maternal ovarian/adrenal tumors

Male Pseudohermaphrodite

- Karyotype: 46XY
- Gonads: histologically normal testes
- External genitalia: incomplete masculinization
- Classification

—Androgen insensitivity
—5α-Reductase deficiency
—Disordered steroidogenesis (testosterone)

CAUSES/RISK FACTORS

- Maternal progestational agents
- Family history

COMPLICATIONS

- Infertility
- Psychological trauma

DIFFERENTIAL DIAGNOSIS

- See Section I, "Ambiguous Genitalia."

FEMALE PSEUDOHERMAPHRODITE (CONGENITAL ADRENAL HYPERPLASIA)

EPIDEMIOLOGY

- 21-Hydroxylase deficiency

—90% of CAH
—1 in 15,000 births

- 11β-Hydroxylase deficiency

—5% to 8% of CAH

- 3β-Hydroxysteroid dehydrogenase deficiency

—Rare

GENETICS

- Recessively inherited
- 21-Hydroxylase deficiency

—Locus on short arm of chromosome 6

- 11β-Hydroxylase deficiency
—Locus on long arm of chromosome 8
- 3β-Hydroxysteroid dehydrogenase deficiency
—Locus on chromosome 1

STAGING: N/A

SIGNS AND SYMPTOMS

- Genitals

—Clitoral hypertrophy with chordee
—Single urogenital sinus emptying at base of clitoris
—Rugose and pigmented labial scrotal folds

- Somatic (untreated)

—Advanced bone age with early epiphyseal closure and short stature
—Precocious pubic and axillary hair
—Acne, amenorrhea, failure of breast development

- Electrolytes

—One-half to one-third with salt-wasting form (21-hydroxylase and 3β-hydroxylase deficiency)
—Hypotension, hyponatremia, hyperkalemia, elevated renin
—Increased severity of hypotension with 3β-hydroxylase deficiency
—11-hydroxylase deficiency: salt retention
—Hypertension, hypernatremia

PATHOPHYSIOLOGY

- CAH: Disruption in cortisol synthetic pathway. Cortisol unable to provide negative feedback control of ACTH release

—21-Hydroxylase deficiency
— ↓ 11-deoxycortisol and cortisol
—Resultant increase in ACTH production: ↑ 17-hydroxyprogesterone and 17-hydroxypregnenolone: metabolized to dehydroepiandrosterone and androstenedione (converted to testosterone peripherally)
—11β-Hydroxylase deficiency
—Occurs later in cortisol synthetic pathway
—Accumulation of precursors including deoxycorticosterone (DOC), and 17-hydroxyprogesterone
— ↑ DOC: hypertension in two-thirds
—3β-Hydroxysteroid dehydrogenase deficiency
—Early block in cortisol synthetic pathway
—Accumulation of dehydroepiandrosterone (not converted to testosterone)
—Less virilization than with other forms of adrenogenital syndrome

- Exogenous progestational agents

—Ethisterone and Norlutin administered to prevent miscarriage
—Structure homologous to testosterone
—Virilization when administered in first trimester

- Virilizing maternal tumors

—Luteoma
—Arrhenoblastoma

MALE PSEUDOHERMAPHRODITE

EPIDEMIOLOGY

- Androgen insensitivity

—1 in 20,000 to 1 in 64,000 incidence with complete testicular feminization
—Complete form 10× more common than incomplete form

- 5α-Reductase deficiency: rare
- Disordered steroidogenesis (testosterone): rare

GENETICS

- Androgen insensitivity: X-linked
- 5α-Reductase deficiency: autosomal recessive
- Disordered steroidogenesis (testosterone)

—Autosomal or X-linked recessive

STAGING: N/A

SIGNS AND SYMPTOMS

- Genitals

—Androgen insensitivity
—Complete form: complete feminization; undescended testes/absent wolffian duct remnants; vagina short or rudimentary
—Incomplete form: Some virilization of external genitalia (labial fusion, clitoromegaly, vagina short or rudimentary, wolffian duct remnants) may be present.
—5α-Reductase deficiency
—Severe hypospadias
—Blind vaginal pouch
—Testes with wolffian duct development
—No Müllerian structures
—Enlargement of phallus at puberty
—Disordered steroidogenesis (testosterone)
—Wide range from mild hypospadias to full feminization

- Somatic

—Androgen insensitivity
—Breast development
—Scant pubic hair with complete form
—5α-Reductase deficiency
—Female habitus but without breast development
—Muscle development at puberty
—Disordered steroidogenesis (testosterone)
—With or without gynecomastia

- Electrolytes

—Androgen insensitivity: normal
—5α-Reductase deficiency: normal
—Disordered steroidogenesis
—Congenital adrenal hyperplasia: 20,22-desmolase deficiency: salt wasting; 3β-hydroxysteroid dehydrogenase deficiency: salt wasting; 17α-hydroxylase deficiency: hypokalemic alkalosis, hypertension; 17,20-desmolase deficiency: normal adrenocortical function; 17β-hydroxysteroid dehydrogenase deficiency: normal adrenocortical function

PATHOPHYSIOLOGY

- Androgen insensitivity

—Faulty androgen receptor with elevation of LH and testosterone

- 5α-Reductase deficiency

—Failure of conversion of testosterone to dihydrotestosterone
—Resultant failure of virilization of genital tubercle and urogenital sinus
—LH levels normal or slightly elevated, testosterone levels normal

- Disordered steroidogenesis

—Congenital adrenal hyperplasia: disruption in cortisol synthetic pathway
 —20,22-Desmolase deficiency; deficiency prior to synthesis of pregnenolone; cholesterol major secreted steroid; impaired testosterone synthesis
 —3β-Hydroxysteroid dehydrogenase deficiency; early block in cortisol synthetic pathway; accumulation of dehydroepiandrosterone (not converted to testosterone); impaired testosterone synthesis
 —17α-Hydroxylase deficiency; accumulation of corticosterone and 11-deoxycorticosterone
 —17,20-Desmolase deficiency; normal adrenocortical function; failure of conversion of 17-hydroxyprogesterone to androstenedione
 —17β-Hydroxysteroid dehydrogenase deficiency; normal adrenocortical function; failure of conversion of androstenedione to testosterone

 ## Database

HISTORY

- Maternal progestational agents
- Family history

—Ambiguous genitalia, unexplained infant mortality, hirsutism, infertility, amenorrhea

PHYSICAL EXAMINATION

- In the infant

—Suspicious genital examination
 —Clitoromegaly
 —Bilateral undescended testes
 —Hypospadias with unilateral or bilateral cryptorchidism
—Presence of a palpable gonad: excludes diagnosis of pseudohermaphrodite
—Rectal examination with palpable uterus: excludes diagnosis of male pseudohermaphrodite
—Increased pigmentation of labioscrotal folds/areola: consistent with CAH
—Hypotension/dehydration: consistent with CAH

- In the adolescent

—Gynecomastia/female habitus in the male
—Amenorrhea in the female

 ## Diagnostic Studies

LABORATORY TESTING

- Karyotype: Peripheral blood leukocyte analysis has replaced the buccal smear.
- Plasma 17-hydroxyprogesterone: elevated with 21-hydroxylase deficiency
- Urinary 17-ketosteroids and pregnanetriol: elevated with 21-hydroxylase deficiency
- Plasma testosterone

—Pre- and post-hCG administration (in the male pseudohermaphrodite)
 —Level of post-stimulation testosterone/dihydrotestosterone (if suspicious of 5α-reductase deficiency)

- Fibroblast skin cultures (if suspicious of androgen insensitivity)

IMAGING

- Genitogram

—Configuration of urogenital sinus
—Cervical impression/fallopian tubes excludes diagnosis of male pseudohermaphrodite

- Abdominal/pelvic USG

—Müllerian structures may be detected.

SPECIAL STUDIES

- Endoscopy

—Configuration of urogenital sinus
—Visualized cervix excludes diagnosis of male pseudohermaphrodite

- Exploratory laparotomy

—Consider if other studies inconclusive
—Gonadal biopsy to rule out dysgenesis or true hermaphrodite

 ## Treatment

GENERAL MEASURES

- Sex assignment based on ability to construct functioning genitalia
- Fertility secondary consideration
- Sex assignment completed prior to discharge from nursery

MEDICAL

- CAH

—Fluid/salt repletion for salt-wasting variant
—Glucocorticoid/Florinef replacement
—Monitoring of BP and electrolytes

SURGICAL

- Female pseudohermaphrodite (CAH)

—Reduction clitoroplasty
—Vaginoplasty

- Male pseudohermaphrodite

—Androgen insensitivity (complete)
 —Orchiectomy: timing controversial
 —Raised as female
—Disordered steroidogenesis and 5α-reductase deficiency
 —Sex assignment based on ability to reconstruct phallus/testosterone response

ALTERNATIVE THERAPIES: N/A

PATIENT EDUCATION

- Family counseling critical during evaluation

—Sensitivity essential
—Explain that genital formation is incomplete and that reconstructive efforts will complete normal development.

 ## Follow-Up

MONITORING: NA

PREVENTION: N/A

Miscellaneous

SYNONYMS

- Intersex

ASSOCIATED CONDITIONS

- Hypospadias, cryptorchidism

NOTES

- See also Section I, "Ambiguous Genitalia," and Section II, "Intersex Disorders."

ABBREVIATIONS

- CAH, congenital adrenal hyperplasia; DHEA, dehydroepiandrosterone; LH, luteinizing hormone; FSH, follicle-stimulating hormone; DOC, deoxycorticosterone acetate; hCG, human chorionic gonadotropin

REFERENCES

Allen T. Disorders of sexual differentiation. In: Kelalis PP, King LR, Belman AB, eds. *Clinical Pediatric Urology,* 2nd ed. Philadelphia: WB Saunders, 1992:904–921.

Figueroa TE. Congenital adrenal hyperplasia. In: Seidmon EJ, Hanno PM, eds. *Current Urologic Therapy,* 3rd ed. WB Saunders, 1994:2–6.

Griffin JE, Griffin JD. Disorders of sexual differentiation. In: Walsh PC, Retik AB, Stamey TA, Vaughan ED Jr, eds. *Campbell's Urology,* 6th ed. Philadelphia: WB Saunders, 1992:1509–1532.

Author: Gregory E. Dean

Pyelonephritis—Acute

 Basics

DESCRIPTION

• An inflammatory process involving the renal pelvis and renal parenchyma. It is most often a result of bacterial infection, but fungi, parasites, and viruses may be involved.

EPIDEMIOLOGY

• >250,000 episodes annually in the United States

GENETICS

• Related to vesicoureteral reflux

STAGING: N/A

SIGNS AND SYMPTOMS

• Onset is usually sudden, with manifestations ranging from mild illness to life-threatening sepsis.

—Fever and chills (80%–90%)
—Flank pain (85%–100%)
—Costovertebral angle tenderness
—Ileus with nausea and vomiting (35%–70%)
—Abdominal pain and tenderness (60%–85%)
—Frequency, urgency, and dysuria (50%–60%)
—Gross hematuria is uncommon.

PATHOPHYSIOLOGY

• Most common organisms are gram-negative rods, with *E. coli* accounting for 80% of cases
• Bacteria enter urinary the tract.

—Ascending infection: urethra and bladder
—Lymphatic and hematogenous dissemination to the kidneys is uncommon.

• Bacteria adhere to the urothelium, with subsequent invasion and inflammatory response.

—Bacterial virulence factors
  —Adhesins and fimbriae: allow bacteria to adhere to urothelium
  —Lipopolysaccharides: have toxic and inflammatory effects
  —Hemolysins: allow for bacterial invasion by damaging cells
  —Aerobactin: enables bacteria to compete for iron, which is necessary for aerobic metabolism and reproduction

CAUSES/RISK FACTORS

• Anatomic or functional abnormalities: incomplete emptying of the bladder; urine is more easily infected.

—Vesicoureteral reflux
—Neurogenic bladder
—Bladder outlet obstruction

• Foreign body: Bacterial colonization occurs, and the foreign body acts as a nidus for infection.

—Calculous disease
—Indwelling catheters

• Medical conditions
—Diabetes mellitus
—Immunosuppression
—Alcoholism

• Women are at increased risk because the female urethra is shorter and in close proximity to the anus, allowing gram-negative organisms to more easily colonize the urinary tract.

COMPLICATIONS

• Short-term
—Septic shock
—Abscess formation

• Long-term
—Renal scarring (20%)

• Children with developing kidneys are at significant risk of scarring from even one episode of acute pyelonephritis.
• Diabetics are at significant risk of developing emphysematous pyelonephritis, a more fulminant process with a high mortality.

—Characterized by renal intraparenchymal gas and detectable on KUB

• Patients with calculi or urinary tract obstruction who have recurrent episodes of pyelonephritis may develop xanthogranulomatous pyelonephritis.

—Characterized by large nonfunctioning renal mass
—Stones are present in 80% of cases.

• Pregnant patients are at high risk because of the physiologic changes of pregnancy to the urinary tract.

—Sepsis
—Adult respiratory distress syndrome
—Preterm delivery with low-birth-weight infants

DIFFERENTIAL DIAGNOSIS

• Any intraabdominal inflammatory process
—Appendicitis, cholecystitis, diverticulitis, pancreatitis

• Gynecologic conditions
—Pelvic inflammatory disease, ectopic pregnancy, ruptured ovarian cysts

• Urologic conditions
—Renal colic with fever
—Renal and perinephric abscesses

• Lower lobe pneumonia

 Database

HISTORY

• Fevers, chills, malaise, nausea or vomiting
• Flank or abdominal pain
• Dysuria, urgency or frequency, gross hematuria
• Prior episodes of urinary tract infections
• History of renal calculi or urinary tract abnormalities
• History of diabetes, immunosuppression, or alcoholism
• Children may present with failure to thrive.

PHYSICAL EXAMINATION

• Vital signs for signs of sepsis
• Costovertebral angle tenderness
• Abdominal distension with decreased bowel sounds may be present.

Diagnostic Studies

LABORATORY TESTING

- Complete blood count (CBC): leukocytosis with neutrophil predominance (90%)
- Serum chemistry: renal failure uncommon unless obstruction or sepsis present
- Blood culture: 12% of hospitalized pyelonephritis patients will have bacteremia.
- Urinalysis: pyuria (>5–10 WBCs/HPF), WBC casts, red blood cells, bacteria
- Urine culture: positive with >100,000 bacteria/mL and identifies the causative organism

IMAGING

- In uncomplicated acute pyelonephritis, imaging studies are unnecessary.
- Failure to respond to appropriate therapy within 72 hours requires further evaluation to rule out obstruction, abscess, or other abnormalities.
- Pediatric patients are at risk of scarring and should undergo radiologic evaluation.
- Abdominal x-ray (KUB)

—Evaluate for renal or ureteral calculi, if suspected.
—Intraparenchymal gas: emphysematous pyelonephritis
—Renal shadow may be enlarged and poorly defined secondary to parenchymal edema.

- Intravenous pyelogram (IVP)

—75% of patients with uncomplicated acute pyelonephritis will have a normal IVP.
—IVP shows an enlarged kidney (>15 cm in length or 1.5 cm greater than the unaffected side with decreased nephrogram and delayed excretion)
—Cortical striations may be seen.
—Focal enlargement of the kidney is consistent with focal bacterial nephritis, or acute lobar nephronia may be confused with tumor or abscess.
—Nonobstructive dilation of the renal pelvis and ureter may be present (endotoxins impair ureteral peristalsis).

- Ultrasonography

—Renal enlargement with hypoechoic parenchyma and loss of corticomedullary differentiation
—Noninvasive and does not use ionizing radiation

- CT scan

—Noncontrast CT of the abdomen reveals an enlarged kidney with decreased attenuation parenchyma, and perinephric fat streaking.
—Contrast administration shows delayed enhancement with delayed excretion.

- Radionuclide scan

—Cortical agents (e.g., DMSA) reveal decreased activity in the affected kidney.
—Useful to identify areas of scarring

SPECIAL STUDIES: N/A

 ## Treatment

GENERAL MEASURES

- Supportive care consists of hydration, antipyretics, and analgesics.
- Antibiotics that are active against the possible causative organisms, and achieve adequate levels in the renal parenchyma and urine, are used.

MEDICAL

- Outpatient therapy

—Uncomplicated acute pyelonephritis, those who are reliable, tolerate oral intake, and do not have signs of sepsis do not require hospitalization.
—Oral fluoroquinolones (ciprofloxacin 500 mg po bid, or levofloxacin 250 mg po qd); empiric agents until urine culture results available
—An alternative antibiotic is trimethoprim-sulfamethoxazole (TMP-SMZ).
—Therapy is continued for 14 days.

- Inpatient therapy

—If signs of sepsis, bacteremia, or cannot tolerate oral medications: hospitalize
—Also recommended for children, the elderly, pregnant patients, diabetics, and the immunocompromised
—Parenteral antibiotic therapy
  —Ampicillin (2 g IV q6h) and gentamicin (1.5 mg/kg IV q8h) is traditional treatment; or
  —Ceftriaxone (1 g IV qd) empirically; or
—Intravenous fluoroquinolones
—Most patients continue to have fever or flank pain for several days after appropriate therapy has been started.
—IV therapy continued until the patient is afebrile, or cultures indicate another appropriate antibiotic
—When able to tolerate oral intake, the patient is switched to an oral antibiotic for a 14-day course.
—Pregnant patients: Place on suppression therapy (e.g., nitrofurantoin 100 mg po qd, cephalexin 250 mg po qd) after treatment until delivery, due to a relapse rate of up to 60% in nonsuppressed patients.

SURGICAL

- Diversion (stent/nephrostomy) if obstructed

ALTERNATIVE THERAPIES: N/A

PATIENT EDUCATION: N/A

 ## Follow-Up

MONITORING

- Urine cultures 4 to 6 weeks after completion of antibiotics to ensure infection cleared
- 10% to 30% suffer a relapse and may be treated with a second 14-day course of antibiotics.
- Occasionally, a 6-week course is necessary for cure.

PREVENTION

- Anatomic or functional abnormalities must be eliminated (See Causes/Risk Factors in "Basics" section).
- Patients with recurrent infections may require low-dose prophylactic antibiotics.

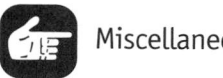 ## Miscellaneous

SYNONYMS: N/A

ASSOCIATED CONDITIONS: N/A

NOTES

- See also Section I, "Urinary Tract Infection—Adult Male," "Urinary Tract Infection—Adult Female," and "Urinary Tract Infection—Pediatric."

ABBREVIATIONS: N/A

REFERENCES

Donovan MP, Carson CC. Urinary tract infections. In: Resnick MI, Older RA, eds. *Diagnosis of Genitourinary Disease,* 2nd ed. New York: Thieme Medical Publishers, 1997.

Hooton TM, Stamm WE. Diagnosis and treatment of uncomplicated urinary tract infection. *Infect Dis Clin North Am* 1997;11:551.

Sant GR. Pyelonephritis. In: Seidmon EJ, Hanno PM, eds. *Current Urologic Therapy,* 3rd ed. Philadelphia: WB Saunders, 1994.

Schaffer AJ. Infections of the urinary tract. In: Walsh PC, Retik AB, Vaughan ED, Wein AJ, eds. *Campbell's Urology,* 7th ed. Philadelphia: WB Saunders, 1997.

Authors: David Hom and Robert M. Moldwin

Pyelonephritis—Chronic

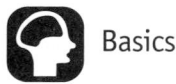 Basics

DESCRIPTION

• Chronic pyelonephritis (CP) is a number of renal lesions that result from recent or remote bacterial infection. This produces a coarsely scarred or contracted atrophic kidney. CP is a diagnosis based on pathologic and radiologic evidence.

EPIDEMIOLOGY

• No known association with race, sex, or age
• Predominantly originates in childhood

GENETICS: N/A

STAGING: N/A

SIGNS AND SYMPTOMS

• Patients are frequently asymptomatic.
• No typical symptoms associated with the condition
• Condition discovered incidentally with episodes of acute infections

—More common in children than in adults

• Nonspecific signs of chronic infection

—Azotemia
—Anemia
—Fever

• Pregnant women

—Chronic azotemia (i.e., hypertension, visual impairment, headaches, fatigue, etc.)
—May present as UTI

• Hypertension

—Bilateral chronic pyelonephritis
—Advanced chronic pyelonephritis

PATHOPHYSIOLOGY

• The pathologic changes of chronic pyelonephritis are comparable to many types of noninfectious interstitial nephritis; therefore, the diagnosis cannot be made on a histologic basis alone.
• Most of the changes of chronic pyelonephritis occur during early childhood.

—Growing kidney most susceptible to scarring
—Theory that nonviable bacterial antigens and autoimmune reactions may account for scarring

• Portions of parenchyma may be replaced by fibrosis.
• Histologic changes reveal accumulations of lymphocyte, plasma cells, and occasional polymorphonuclear cells.
• The kidney is most susceptible to scarring during early childhood.
• Atrophy of kidney
• Thickening of the arteries and arterioles
• Diffuse infiltration of the parenchyma with plasma cells and lymphocytes
• Renal damage is rare in nonobstructed UTIs in adults.
• Inflammation and fibrosis of renal parenchyma
• The capsule is pale and strips poorly.

• The renal surface is pitted and depressed in areas of scarring.

CAUSES/RISK FACTORS

• Vesicoureteral reflux
• Recurrent urinary tract infections
• Severe reflux in children
• Urinary tract obstruction
• Neurogenic bladders
• Congenital urinary tract anomalies
• End-stage renal disease
• Reflux nephropathy

COMPLICATIONS

• Perinephric abscess

—Surgical drainage required
—May dissect further within retroperitoneal space

• Urosepsis

—Life-threatening
—Fever, chills, mental status changes, multiorgan system failure

• Hypertension
• Infected renal stones

DIFFERENTIAL DIAGNOSIS

• Lower urinary tract infection
• Analgesic nephropathy
• Renal tuberculosis
• Renal tumors (hypernephroma)
• Xanthogranulomatous pyelonephritis
• Gouty nephritis
• Hypertensive renal disease
• Renal artery stenosis
• Diabetic nephropathy
• Interstitial nephritis
• Psoas and subdiaphragmatic abscess
• Renal stones

 Database

HISTORY

• Recurrent episodes of acute pyelonephritis
• Severe suppurative disease

—Diabetes mellitus
—Renal transplant patients

• Fever of unknown origin
• Association with vesicoureteral reflux
• Frequently asymptomatic and discovered incidentally

PHYSICAL EXAMINATION

• Nonspecific, usually associated with acute pyelonephritis

—Flank pain
—Peritoneal signs
—Abdominal distention
—Costovertebral angle pain

Diagnostic Studies

LABORATORY TESTING

- Urine analysis

—Pyuria and bacteriuria in presence of active disease
—Findings vary with severity of disease.
—Excessive proteinuria indicates advanced disease with glomerular involvement.
—May see elevated creatinine with advanced disease
—Medullary defect in pyelonephritic kidney causes loss of filtered water and sodium

- Erythrocyte sedimentation rates

—May be elevated with active infection

- CBC

—May show anemia of chronic infection

IMAGING

- Intravenous urogram

—Best technique for diagnosis
—Small atrophic kidney overlying dilated calyces
—Focal coarse renal scarring with clubbing of the underlying calyx
—Compensatory hypertrophy of contralateral kidney
—Dilation of the ipsilateral ureter may indicate vesicoureteral reflux or obstruction.

- Voiding cystourethrography

—Useful in evaluation of children who frequently have vesicoureteral reflux

- CAT scan/renal ultrasound

—Differentiates renal tumors from changes of chronic pyelonephritis
—A renal abscess may be visualized.

- Renal scan to evaluate function

SPECIAL STUDIES

- Cystoscopy

—Cystitis with active infection
—Investigate the possibility of vesicoureteral reflux.

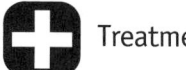 ## Treatment

GENERAL MEASURES

- Close supervision of renal function and timely treatment of acute infection in patients with CP are important in order to minimize the sequelae.

MEDICAL

- Prompt identification and treatment of UTIs, especially in children (young kidney), is important in avoiding the renal damage and resultant scarring that accompanies CP.
- Long-term use of prophylactic antibiotics may be required, especially in children, to prevent recurrent infections.

SURGICAL

- Nephrectomy

—Anatomic defects, perinephric abscess, infected stones

- Repair of high-grade vesicoureteral reflux

ALTERNATIVE THERAPIES: N/A

PATIENT EDUCATION

- Need for follow-up for recurrent UTI or hypertension, if present

 ## Follow-Up

MONITORING

- Sequential studies of renal structure and function should be performed (ultrasound, renal scan) on a 1- to 2-year basis.
- Repeat urine cultures during and after therapy for acute infection for a follow-up period of 6 months to 1 year.

PREVENTION

- Early detection of childhood UTIs, with prompt treatment
- Prompt detection and repair of obstructive uropathy

 ## Miscellaneous

SYNONYMS

- Chronic tubulointerstitial renal disease, interstitial nephritis, reflux nephropathy, chronic atrophic pyelonephritis, focal-course renal scarring

ASSOCIATED CONDITIONS: N/A

NOTES: N/A

ABBREVIATIONS

- CP, chronic pyelonephritis

REFERENCES

Kunin C. Pyelonephritis and other infections of the kidney. In: Kunin C, ed. *Urinary Tract Infections: Detection, Prevention, and Management,* 5th ed. Baltimore: Williams & Wilkins, 1997:189–225.

Schaeffer AJ. Infection of the urinary tract. In: Walsh PC, Retik AB, Vaughan ED, Wein AJ, eds. *Campbell's Urology,* 7th ed. Philadelphia: WB Saunders, 1998:570–573.

Tanagho E. Chronic pyelonephritis. In: Tanagho EA, McAninch JW, eds. *Smith's General Urology,* 14th ed. Norwalk, CT: Appleton and Lange, 1995:210–212.

Authors: C.B. Threatt and C.N. Robertson

Pyelonephritis—Emphysematous

Basics

DESCRIPTION

• A serious, acute necrotizing renal parenchymal and perirenal infection associated with the presence of gas formation

EPIDEMIOLOGY

• Adults most frequently
• Women > men

GENETICS: N/A

STAGING: N/A

SIGNS AND SYMPTOMS

• Severe, acute pyelonephritis that fails to resolve within 3 days of commencing antimicrobial treatment

—Fever, vomiting, flank pain

• Acutely ill or septic presentation
• Urologic problems are often complicated by medical abnormalities.

—Electrolyte imbalances
—Dehydration
—Metabolic acidosis
—Hyperglycemia

• Average duration of symptoms before diagnosis: 12 to 18 days

PATHOPHYSIOLOGY

• Impaired host response allows enhanced proliferation of microorganisms.

—Hyperglycemia and ketoacidosis impair cellular defenses with protection of bacteria from the bactericidal activity of lactic acid.

• Presence of gram-negative facultative anaerobes

—Ferment glucose within necrotic tissue.

• Decreased elimination of gas due to impaired tissue perfusion
• Pathology reveals multiple abscesses with an empty central region.
• Glomerulosclerosis, arteriosclerosis, intrarenal vascular thrombi, or papillary necrosis may be present.

CAUSES/RISK FACTORS

• Diabetes mellitus

—80% to 90% of cases

• Obstruction is almost always present in absence of diabetes.
• *E. coli* is the most common organism.

—*Klebsiella* and *Proteus* are less frequently isolated.

COMPLICATIONS

• Overall mortality is approximately 43%, associated with delay in diagnosis.
• Nephrectomy may be required in many cases with resultant renal failure.

DIFFERENTIAL DIAGNOSIS

• Perirenal abscess
• Xanthogranulomatous pyelonephritis
• Necrotic renal neoplasm
• Upper urinary tract obstruction with pyelonephritis
• Emphysematous pyelitis

Database

HISTORY

• Acute onset of fevers, chills, nausea or vomiting
• Dysuria and frequency
• Pneumaturia is not present unless the collecting system is also involved.

PHYSICAL EXAMINATION

• Marked pyrexia
• Flank or abdominal tenderness, nonspecific
• Findings may be consistent with sepsis—tachycardia and hypotension.

Diagnostic Studies

LABORATORY TESTING

• Urine cultures should be positive.

—Blood cultures are almost always positive for the same organism as in the urine.

• Serum creatinine is commonly elevated >2.0 mg/dL.

IMAGING

• Establishes the diagnosis
• Plain-film radiography (KUB)

—Hallmark finding: gas in the region of the kidney
—Should not be confused with cases of pyelonephritis with air in the collecting system. This is termed *emphysematous pyelitis* and is less severe. Frequently found in nondiabetics

• Excretory urography (IVP): rarely of value

—The affected kidney is usually nonfunctioning or significantly impaired.

• Ultrasound

—Strong focal echoes, suggesting presence of intraparenchymal gas
—Will show obstruction in 25%

• CT: ideal study to localize gas and determine extent of infection

—Single or multiloculated, ill-defined abscesses with air and fluid
—Confirms diagnosis in 100% of cases
—Contrast not necessary

SPECIAL STUDIES: N/A

Treatment

GENERAL MEASURES

• Rapid supportive measures with fluid resuscitation and correction of electrolyte imbalances
• Surgical emergency

MEDICAL

• Appropriate antimicrobial agents

—Broad-spectrum initially, then tailor to culture sensitivities
  —Cefazolin 1 g IV q8h, gentamicin 120 mg IV q12h, metronidazole 500 mg IV q8h

• Management of diabetes

—Correction of hyperglycemia

• Determine function of contralateral kidney
• Medical treatment alone often inadequate (approximate 71% mortality rate)

SURGICAL

• Almost always requires wide surgical drainage or nephrectomy

—Should have low threshold for intervention if not improved after several days of conservative therapy

• Eliminate the obstruction of the affected kidney, if present.

—Perform percutaneous catheter drainage of the affected renal unit.
—If the patient's condition improves, it is possible to avoid or defer nephrectomy.

ALTERNATIVE THERAPIES

• Percutaneous drainage with CT guidance in combination with medical therapy

—Select patients that are extremely poor operative risks, or choose minimally invasive therapy
—Recommend a follow-up CT scan in 4 to 7 days.
—Remove the drain when gas has resolved, which may be weeks.

PATIENT EDUCATION: N/A

 Follow-Up

MONITORING

• Follow-up CT scans, especially if managed conservatively

—Gas may often take much longer to resolve than the clinical picture.

• Follow up with radionuclide functional studies if conservative management is chosen.

PREVENTION

• Long-term antibiotic prophylaxis

—Ciprofloxacin 500 mg po qd for 6 months

• Improved medical control of diabetes mellitus

 Miscellaneous

SYNONYMS

• Gas-forming renal infection

ASSOCIATED CONDITIONS

• Poor renal function, diabetes, immunocompromised status

NOTES: N/A

ABBREVIATIONS: N/A

REFERENCES

Chen MT, et al. Percutaneous drainage in the treatment of emphysematous pyelonephritis: 10-year experience. *J Urol* 1997;157:1569–1573.

Patel NP, et al. Gas-forming infections in genito-urinary tract. *Urology* 1992;39:341–345.

Schaeffer AJ. Infections of the urinary tract. In: Walsh PC, Retik AB, Vaughan ED, Wein AJ, eds. *Campbell's Urology*, 7th ed. Philadelphia: WB Saunders, 1998:573–574.

Shokeir AA, et al. Emphysematous pyelonephritis: A 15 year experience with 20 cases. *Urology* 1997;49:343–346.

Authors: Charles Best and Howard N. Winfield

Pyelonephritis—Xanthogranulomatous

 Basics

DESCRIPTION

• Xanthogranulomatous pyelonephritis (XGP) is a rare and severe form of chronic renal infection. The infection results in a chronic granulomatous inflammatory disease characterized by parenchymal destruction and replacement by lipid-laden macrophages (foamy or xanthoma cells). Most cases are unilateral and result in a nonfunctioning, enlarged kidney associated with obstructive uropathy secondary to nephrolithiasis.

EPIDEMIOLOGY

• Rare disease: 0.6% to 1.4% of all patients with renal inflammation
• Female-to-male ratio of 3:1
• Peak age: 40 to 60; can occur in children and elderly
• Almost always unilateral
• 15% of patients with XGP are diabetic.

GENETICS

• No known genetic predisposition

STAGING: N/A

SIGNS AND SYMPTOMS

• Usually nonspecific signs

—Fever, flank pain, chills, anorexia, malaise

• Hematuria usually *absent*
• Persistent bacteriuria common despite antibiotic treatment

PATHOPHYSIOLOGY

• Chronic severe infection that may involve kidney only, kidney and perinephric fat, or kidney, perinephric fat, and retroperitoneum
• Gross examination

—Pyonephrosis (renal pelvis filled with pus)
—Orange-yellow nodules covering the exterior of the kidney, next to areas of necrosis

• Microscopic examination

—"Xanthoma cells": lipid-laden macrophages arranged in sheets around parenchymal abscesses
—Necrosis and inflammation with infiltrating plasma cells, neutrophils, and hemosiderin-laden macrophages
—Granulomas in the renal pelvis and calyces

CAUSES/RISK FACTORS

• Exact pathogenesis unknown
• Primary factors for development are obstruction and infection.

—Obstruction most commonly from a stone, but may be from UPJ or stricture
—Infection is a UTI most commonly due to *Proteus mirabilis* or *E. coli.*
—Immunosuppressive conditions
  —Seen more frequently in diabetics

COMPLICATIONS

• Due to extensive nature and diffuse process of XGP, usually necessitates removal of the kidney
• Perinephric abscesses not uncommon
• Squamous metaplasia of the urothelium and transitional cell carcinoma of the renal pelvis due to chronic inflammation have been reported.
• Pyelocutaneous fistula reported
• Sepsis

DIFFERENTIAL DIAGNOSIS

• XGP has been called the "great imitator" due to its propensity to mimic renal cell carcinoma.
• Transitional cell carcinoma of the renal pelvis
• Renal abscess
• Tuberculosis of the kidney
• Renal neoplasms
• Inflammatory renal parenchymal diseases

 Database

HISTORY

• History of fever, chills, malaise, anorexia, flank pain, weight loss

—Symptoms often present for weeks to months
—Recurrent UTIs, despite antibiotic treatment, may be present, although urinary symptoms are usually minimal.

• Medical history

—35% with history of stone disease
—Obstructive uropathy
—Diabetes mellitus

PHYSICAL EXAMINATION

• Tender palpable flank mass (62% of patients)
• Elevated temperature
• Hypertension in 20%

Diagnostic Studies

LABORATORY TESTING

- Urinalysis shows leukocytes, protein, and bacteria.
- Urine culture may be mixed-growth, *Proteus,* or *E. coli,* but one-third of patients will have no growth on urine culture due to previous antibiotic treatment.
- Tissue culture at surgery demonstrates *Proteus* or *E. coli* most commonly.
- Serum chemistries

—67% microcytic anemia
—46% with leukocytosis
—17% with Stauffer syndrome (hypoalbuminemia, elevated bilirubin, alkaline phosphatase, elevated SGOT and SGPT) that return to normal after nephrectomy
—BUN/creatinine usually normal due to unaffected contralateral kidney

- Urine cytologic examination reveals xanthoma cells in 80% of cases (nonspecific).

IMAGING

- CT scan

—Accurate in making diagnosis in 90% of cases; best study to demonstrate extent of involvement
—Demonstrates large reniform mass with a renal pelvis filled with low attenuating material
—May see calcification in pelvis, representing a stone
—"Bear paw sign": multiple rounded, low-density areas with enhancing rings in a hydronephrotic pattern

- IVP

—30% to 80% show nonvisualization of the kidney.
—30% to 80% will have a stone demonstrated on IVP.
—75% demonstrate a renal mass with a calyceal deformity that cannot be differentiated from a neoplasm.

- Retrograde pyelogram demonstrates an abnormal pelvocalyceal system.
- Ultrasound shows an enlarged kidney with an echogenic central area and an anechoic parenchymal pattern.
- MRI of no additional value

SPECIAL STUDIES: N/A

 Treatment

GENERAL MEASURES

- Patients have often been on inadequate courses of antibiotics and need broad-spectrum IV antibiotics with good gram-negative and anaerobic coverage.

MEDICAL

- Antibiotics

—Broad-spectrum

SURGICAL

- Mainstay of treatment for XGP
- Usually requires nephrectomy
- Partial nephrectomy may be appropriate if infection is localized.
- Nephrectomy is often done because the diagnosis is in question and the mass is worrisome for renal cell carcinoma.
- If the retroperitoneum or perinephric tissue are involved, then extensive removal of this tissue is recommended, as this tissue is also usually infected.
- The flank approach is usually used, unless wide debridement of the retroperitoneum is also needed.
- The patient should receive mechanical and antibiotic bowel prep prior to surgery in case the colon is involved and requires resection.

—The area should be well drained with multiple drains postoperatively.

ALTERNATIVE THERAPIES: N/A

PATIENT EDUCATION: N/A

 Follow-Up

MONITORING

- Follow-up laboratory

—Anemia and hepatic dysfunction resolve after nephrectomy.
—Repeat urine culture should be negative.
—BUN and creatinine remain normal throughout the illness.

- If any neoplastic elements are found (i.e., renal cell or transitional cell carcinoma), appropriate follow-up is necessary.

PREVENTION: N/A

 Miscellaneous

SYNONYMS: N/A

ASSOCIATED CONDITIONS

- Urolithiasis

NOTES

- See also Section II, "Pyelonephritis—Acute."

ABBREVIATIONS

- XGP, xanthogranulomatous pyelonephritis

REFERENCES

Donovan MP, Carson CC. Urinary tract infections. In: Resnick MI, Older RA, eds. *Diagnosis of Genitourinary Disease,* 2nd ed. New York: Thieme Medical Publishers, 1997:278–281.

Meares EM Jr. Nonspecific infections of the genitourinary tract. In: Tanagho EA, McAninch JW, eds. *Smith's General Urology,* 14th ed. Norwalk, CT: Appleton & Lange, 1995:213–218.

Schaeffer AJ. Infections of the urinary tract. In: Walsh PC, Retik AB, Vaughan ED, Wein AJ, eds. *Campbell's Urology,* 7th ed. Philadelphia: WB Saunders, 1998:579–580.

Authors: Jeff M. Holzbeierlein and Michael S. Cookson

Renal and Perirenal Abscess

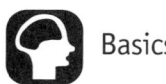 Basics

DESCRIPTION

• Renal abscess/carbuncle: collection of purulent material confined to the renal parenchyma
• A perirenal abscess often results from extension of an acute cortical abscess into the perinephric space, confined by Gerota's fascia.
• When a perinephric abscess ruptures through Gerota's fascia into the pararenal space, the abscess is classified as a paranephric or pararenal abscess.

EPIDEMIOLOGY

• See below.

GENETICS

• No genetic predisposition

STAGING: N/A

SIGNS AND SYMPTOMS

• Symptoms are often present for several days.

—Fever, chills
—Abdominal or flank pain
—Malaise
—Weight loss

PATHOPHYSIOLOGY

• *E. coli, Proteus mirabilis,* and *Staphylococcus aureus* (in descending order of occurrence) account for the majority of infections.
• Gram-negative organisms isolated in majority of adults with abscess
• Infected hydronephrosis associated with destruction of parenchyma, leading to abscess formation
• Obstruction from urolithiasis common
• Hematogenous spread from extragenitourinary site

CAUSES/RISK FACTORS

• Two-thirds of gram-negative abscesses associated with renal calculi or kidney with poor function

—Polycystic kidney diseases
—Hemodialysis
—Diabetes mellitus

• Ascending infection

—Distal urinary obstruction most common causative factor
—Vesicoureteral reflux second most common

• Neuropathic bladder
• Pregnancy

—Untreated bacteriuria associated with higher incidence of pyelonephritis
—Hematogenous spread
—Skin infection with gram-positive organisms
—IV drug abuse
—Immunocompromised status
—Tuberculosis: Renal infection is among the most common sites for extrapulmonary disease.

COMPLICATIONS

• Perinephric abscess is historically associated with mortality as high as 56%.

—Delay in diagnosis associated with higher mortality

• Loss of renal function (kidney destruction or nephrectomy)
• Delay in diagnosis still associated with higher mortality
• Rupture of abscess may lead to

—Psoas abscess
—Nephrobronchial fistula
—Pyelocutaneous fistula
—Nephrocolonic fistula

DIFFERENTIAL DIAGNOSIS

• Decreasing order of occurrence

—Pyelonephritis
—Infected hydronephrosis (pyonephrosis)
—Xanthogranulomatous pyelonephritis
—Emphysematous pyelonephritis
—Renal tuberculosis
—Bowel perforation with retroperitoneal spread of infection

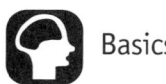 Database

HISTORY

• Significant chronic or acute illnesses

—Diabetes
  —Neuropathic bladder
—Chronic renal failure

• Renal calculi
• IV drug abuse
• Recent skin infections
• Persistent fever after 48 to 72 hours of appropriate antibiotics
• Flank pain

PHYSICAL EXAMINATION

• Elevated temperature
• Abdominal and/or flank mass

—Hydronephrosis
—Abscess
—Distended bladder

• Skin carbuncles or dermatologic evidence of IV drug abuse
• Costovertebral or flank tenderness
• Heart murmurs

—Bacterial endocarditis

Diagnostic Studies

LABORATORY TESTING

• Urine analysis: includes urine dipstick, microscopic analysis, and culture

—Pyuria and bacteria often present
—Pyuria may be absent if there is no communication with the collecting system or with obstruction.
—Gram-positive organisms not routinely cultured from urine with hematogenous source
—Gram-negative organisms often the same as cultured from abscess
—Sterile pyuria seen with tuberculosis

• Complete blood count

—Leukocytosis

• Blood cultures

—Gram-negative organisms most commonly cultured

IMAGING

• Differentiation between early renal abscess and acute pyelonephritis is difficult at times, due to the small size of the abscesses.
• Intravenous urography (IVP)

—Abnormal in up to 80% of patients
—Generalized enlargement of involved renal unit
—Distortion of renal contour and collecting system
—Psoas shadow obscured on affected side
—Mimics renal mass

• Abdominal ultrasonography

—Quickest and least expensive method to demonstrate abscess
—Abscess
——Rounded, focal, hypoechoic, space-occupying lesion
——Poorly marginated in early phases of infection
——Well-defined mass in later stages
——Surrounding renal parenchyma often edematous

• Abdominal CT scan

—Diagnostic procedure of choice
—The abscess is well defined before and after contrast enhancement.
—Destruction of adjacent parenchyma common
—Excellent to determine if confined to perinephric space
—The "ring sign" results from increased vascularity in the wall of a chronic abscess.
—Renal tuberculosis associated with calcified thick-walled abscess

SPECIAL STUDIES: N/A

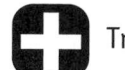 ## Treatment

GENERAL MEASURES

• Suspected pyelonephritis treated with antibiotics for 48 to 72 hours without significant improvement requires radiographic evaluation to rule out obstruction and/or abscess formation.
• Obstruction, if present, must be relieved.
• Hospitalization with initiation of IV antibiotics and hydration

MEDICAL

• Antibiotic therapy: may prevent surgical intervention unless abscess involves perinephric space

—Initiate empirical treatment
—IV third-generation cephalosporins, aminoglycosides, or antipseudomonal penicillins
—Adjust antibiotic coverage according to culture/sensitivity results.
—Adjust dose for renal function.
—Suspected hematogenous source of infection
——Penicillin-resistant *Staphylococcus* most likely organism
——Ampicillin/sulbactam (UNASYN) 1.5 to 3.0 g IM or IV q6h
——Penicillin allergy: ceftriaxone (Rocephin); adults, 1 to 2 g IM/IV q24h
——Vancomycin: adults, 500 mg to 2 g daily in 3 to 4 divided doses IV

SURGICAL

• Standard treatment of renal abscess has been rapid incision and drainage.
• Relief of coexisting obstruction is mandatory.
• Primary treatment remains drainage for all perinephric abscesses.
• Nephrectomy may be required for adequate treatment if medical therapy fails.

ALTERNATIVE THERAPIES

• Percutaneous nephrostomy tube placement

—Rapid relief of obstruction with urosepsis

• Percutaneous drainage may not be effective for large, loculated abscesses.

PATIENT EDUCATION: N/A

 ## Follow-Up

MONITORING

• Address the underlying medical conditions to prevent recurrent infections.
• Repeat radiographic studies to confirm complete resolution.
• Extended antibiotic therapy is often required.

PREVENTION

• Prompt recognition and treatment of infection, especially in face of obstruction

 ## Miscellaneous

SYNONYMS

• Renal carbuncle (renal abscess), perinephric abscess (perirenal abscess)

ASSOCIATED CONDITIONS

• See above.

NOTES

• See also Section II, "Pyelonephritis—Acute," "Pyelonephritis—Emphysematous," and "Pyelonephritis—Xanthogranulomatous."

ABBREVIATIONS: N/A

REFERENCES

Angulo JC, et al. Successful conservative management of emphysematous pyelonephritis, bilateral or in a solitary kidney. *Scand J Urol Nephrol* 1997;31(2):193–197.

Dunnick NR, Sandler CM, Amis ES Jr, Newhouse JH. Renal inflammatory disease. In: Dunnick NR, et al, eds. *Textbook of Uroradiology*, 2nd ed. Baltimore: Williams & Wilkins, 1997:163–189.

Lowe LH, et al. Role of imaging and intervention in complex infections of the urinary tract. *AJR* 1994;163:363–367.

Siegel JF, Smith A, Moldwin R. Minimally invasive treatment of renal abscess. *J Urol* 1996;155:52–55.

Authors: K. Shane Geib and Michael J. Manyak

Renal Angiomyolipoma

 Basics

DESCRIPTION

- Renal angiomyolipoma (AML) is a benign kidney tumor (hamartoma); it may occur sporadically or may be associated with the tuberous sclerosis complex (TSC).

EPIDEMIOLOGY

- AML: uncommon neoplasm: 2% to 5% of all renal tumors
- 80% of patients with renal AML do not have TSC.

—TSC: autosomal dominant inherited disorder: mental retardation, epilepsy, adenoma sebaceum, and hamartomas of the brain, eye, heart, lung, bone, and kidney

- 80% with tuberous sclerosis develop AML (usually multiple and bilateral).
- Female predominance (male:female ratio: 1:4)
- Mean age: 50 years without TSC; 30 years with TSC
- Renal AML associated with pulmonary lymphangiomyomatosis (LAM), a progressive and fatal lung disease
- LAM occurs in a subset of patients with TSC.
- 40% with LAM have renal AMLs.

GENETICS

- Tuberous sclerosis complex

—Autosomal dominant; two-thirds of cases sporadic, representing new dominant mutations
—Genetically heterogeneous, with half of familial cases linked to a locus (TSC1) on chromosome 9q34 and the other to (TSC2) on chromosome 16p13.3

STAGING: NA

SIGNS AND SYMPTOMS

- Depends on tumor size, number, bilaterality, and associated TSC

—TSC present at a younger age, have tumors (usually multiple and bilateral) that tend to grow and are more likely to require treatment
—AML: often incidental in patients imaged for unrelated complaints or with known TSC
—Tumors <4 cm are rarely symptomatic.
—Tumors >4 cm are symptomatic in 46% to 82% of cases.
  —Most common: abdominal/flank pain, palpable mass, hemorrhage, hematuria, hypertension, and anemia
—Can present as hemorrhagic shock: spontaneous rupture of AML into the kidney or retroperitoneum

PATHOPHYSIOLOGY

- Grossly: yellow to pink-tan, depending on proportion of smooth muscle and fat
- Microscopically: AML named for the three primary components

—Mature fat cells; abnormal, tortuous, thick-walled blood vessels; and sheets of smooth muscle
—Pleomorphism is common; sometimes one predominant cell type
—Lymph node and extrarenal disease: reflects multicentricity and not metastatic disease
—Epithelioid angiomyolipoma: variant with malignant potential
—Multiple renal cysts: common with TSC and AML
—RCC occasionally associated with AML

CAUSES/RISK FACTORS

- Family history or other characteristics of TSC
- Tuberous sclerosis (80% develop renal AML)
- Isolated lymphangiomyomatosis (40% develop renal AML)

COMPLICATIONS

- Most significant is hemorrhage

—Sudden pain and/or hypotension secondary to massive hemorrhage
—Pregnancy and pseudoaneurysms associated with hemorrhage
—Flank/abdominal pain and gastrointestinal symptoms: tumor compression on adjacent organs
—Renal failure in 15% with TSC, a result of multiple bilateral AMLs and cysts that replace the kidneys

DIFFERENTIAL DIAGNOSIS

- Solid renal/perirenal neoplasms

—RCC, renal pelvic urothelial tumors, oncocytoma, rare benign and malignant connective-tissue tumors (lipoma, fibroma, sarcomas)

- Spontaneous renal/retroperitoneal hemorrhage

—AML and RCC; systemic vasculitides affecting the kidneys (e.g., polyarteritis nodosa); vascular disease (aneurysms, AV malformations)

 Database

HISTORY

- Family history of TSC
- History of mental retardation, seizure disorder, adenoma sebaceum, pulmonary disease (spontaneous pneumothorax, LAM)
- Symptoms of abdominal/flank pain, gastrointestinal complaints (nausea, vomiting, early satiety)
- History of anemia, hypertension, renal failure

PHYSICAL EXAMINATION

- Signs

—Of tuberous sclerosis (adenoma sebaceum, mental retardation, ungual fibromas, pulmonary disease)
—Abdominal/flank tenderness or palpable mass
—Hypertension, anemia, or hypotension

Diagnostic Studies

LABORATORY TESTING

- Generally not helpful in the diagnosis
—Anemia is common.
—Baseline renal function
—Microscopic or gross hematuria may be present.

IMAGING

- Today, virtually all AMLs are diagnosed before treatment on the basis of fat density.
—IVP cannot differentiate AML from other neoplasms.
—Angiography: similar to RCC (vascular tumor with abnormal vessels)
—Ultrasound: AMLs are the most echogenic renal masses because of the multiple fat–nonfat interfaces (a small proportion of RCCs are also echogenic).
—CT scan detects fat densities (>-30 Hounsfield units) that are characteristic of AML and is the preferred imaging modality for these tumors in most situations (ultrasound can be used to follow lesions after the diagnosis is firmly established).
—MRI can also reliably detect fat densities because of the characteristic high signal intensity on T1-weighted images.
—Diagnostic problems may arise because, rarely, RCCs may exhibit fat densities and occasionally AMLs may have very little fat density detectable on imaging studies.

SPECIAL STUDIES

- Fine-needle aspiration (biopsy) may be useful when the diagnosis is not firmly established by imaging studies.
- Special stains are occasionally useful: AML stains negative for epithelial cell markers (e.g., cytokeratin) and positive for melanosome-associated protein (HMB-45)

 Treatment

GENERAL MEASURES

- Management controversial and depends on presence and degree of symptoms, size and bilaterality of the tumor, and accuracy of diagnosis
- Isolated AML <4 cm and asymptomatic
—Observe with serial imaging (yearly CT or ultrasound)
—Rarely grow on follow-up. With growth or symptoms, consider selective arterial embolization or renal-sparing surgery.
- Isolated renal AML >4 cm and asymptomatic
—May follow conservatively with more frequent imaging (CT or ultrasound every 6 months). If growth is observed (even in the absence of symptoms), consider embolization or renal-sparing surgery.
- Isolated renal AML >4 cm and symptomatic
—Symptomatic or bleeding: requires either selective arterial embolization or renal-sparing surgery
- Acute hemorrhage: selective arterial embolization initial management
- Multiple tumors: RCC can exist with AML; renal-sparing surgery preferred when all are not unequivocally AMLs or have other complicating features (e.g., calcifications)
- Patient with tuberous sclerosis: greater likelihood for tumor growth and treatment; closer follow-up and reasonable to treat earlier (before tumors are large) with to embolization or renal-sparing surgery

MEDICAL: N/A

SURGICAL: N/A

ALTERNATIVE THERAPIES

- Cryoablation investigational at present

PATIENT EDUCATION

- TSC: Counsel patients and families on the importance of screening and follow-up for renal tumors.
- AML: Inform of the risks and potential complications of AML and to promptly report any symptoms as noted.

 Follow-Up

MONITORING

- Conservative follow-up: serial imaging with CT or ultrasound at intervals dictated by the clinical situation (discussed above)
- Local recurrence unusual following excision; has been reported with large tumors
- Following embolization: serial imaging, progressively longer intervals

PREVENTION: N/A

 Miscellaneous

SYNONYMS

- Renal angiomyolipoma (renal hamartoma), tuberous sclerosis (Bourneville disease)

ASSOCIATED CONDITIONS

- Tuberous sclerosis, lymphangiomyomatosis

NOTES

- See also Section I, "Renal Masses—Benign and Malignant."

ABBREVIATIONS

- AML, angiomyolipoma; TSC, tuberous sclerosis complex; LAM, lymphangiomyomatosis; RCC, renal cell carcinoma

REFERENCES

Eble JN. Angiomyolipoma of kidney. *Semin Diagn Pathol* 1998;15:21.

Kennelly MJ, et al. Outcome analysis of 42 cases of renal angiomyolipoma. *J Urol* 1994;152:1988.

Lemaitre L, et al. Renal angiomyolipoma: Growth followed up with CT and/or ultrasound. *Radiology* 1995;197:598.

Oesterling JE, et al. The management of renal angiomyolipoma. *J Urol* 1986;135:1121.

Steiner MS, et al. The natural history of renal angiomyolipoma. *J Urol* 1993;150:1782.

Author: M. Craig Hall

Renal Capsular Neoplasms

 Basics

DESCRIPTION

- Mesenchymal neoplasms arising from components of renal capsule

EPIDEMIOLOGY

- Extremely rare
- Most are benign.
- Typically present after age 40 years
- No known racial or gender preferences

GENETICS

- Unknown

STAGING: N/A

SIGNS AND SYMPTOMS

- Benign lesions typically remain asymptomatic.
- Local symptoms may occur, especially for larger lesions.

—Persistent pain or fullness in upper abdomen
—Abdominal/flank mass
—Hematuria rarely occurs.

- Constitutional symptoms

—Weight loss
—Fevers, leukocytosis

PATHOPHYSIOLOGY

- Benign

—Lipoma, fibroma, leiomyoma, hemangioma, mixed (neurofibroma, angiomyolipomas)

- Malignant

—Liposarcoma, fibrosarcoma, leiomyosarcoma, malignant fibrous histiocytoma, hemangiopericytoma

CAUSES/RISK FACTORS

- None known

COMPLICATIONS

- Local invasion and metastases
- Hemorrhage

DIFFERENTIAL DIAGNOSIS

- Primary renal parenchymal neoplasms
- Metastatic lesions
- Retroperitoneal neoplasms
- The diagnosis is often difficult to make on clinical or radiologic grounds. Pathologic examination is often necessary to make a correct diagnosis.

 Database

HISTORY

- Identify comorbidities that may mandate more conservative surgical management.

—Diabetes mellitus, hypertension, other renal pathology that compromise renal function

- Clinical evidence of disease

—Intractable bleeding and/or pain may occur from advanced local disease.
—Anorexia, weight loss, malaise, fevers, and bone pain may signify metastatic disease.

PHYSICAL EXAMINATION

- Hemodynamic lability

—Hypotension and tachycardia may suggest significant bleeding.

- Physical signs of advanced disease

—Upper abdominal/flank mass
—Adenopathy and cachexia

 Diagnostic Studies

LABORATORY TESTING

- Urinalysis

—Hematuria is less prominent than with parenchymal lesions.

- Serum chemistries and complete blood count

—Creatinine for estimation of renal function; liver enzymes to evaluate for possible metastases
—Anemia may indicate a bleeding lesion.

IMAGING

- Chest x-ray to rule out metastatic disease
- Intravenous pyelography, CT, and MRI

—May show mass arising in periphery of renal contour but cannot accurately differentiate capsular vs. parenchymal lesions
—CT scan or MRI preferable

SPECIAL STUDIES

- Angiography

—Not routinely necessary
—Benign lesions lack neovascularity and show sharp borders.
—May show predominant arterial masses in renal fossa to be supplied by capsular vessels

Treatment

GENERAL MEASURES

• Due to the rarity and heterogeneity of these lesions, there is no consensus for management or follow-up. However, malignant lesions are typically aggressive, and surgical excision appears to offer best hope of cure.
• Symptomatic treatment

—Analgesia for pain, transfuse for symptomatic anemia, nutritional support if malnourished.

MEDICAL

• Consider chemotherapy for metastatic and/or locally invasive malignant lesions.

—Cyclophosphamide, vincristine, doxorubicin, and actinomycin D or cisplatinum
—Questionable benefit

SURGICAL

• Radical nephrectomy
• Consider partial nephrectomy, especially when preoperative evaluation suggests a capsular origin of the lesion.

ALTERNATIVE THERAPIES

• Radiotherapy of no proven benefit for most sarcomas
• Angioinfarction

—May palliate symptomatic lesions

PATIENT EDUCATION

• Generally poor prognosis for malignant lesions

 ## Follow-Up

MONITORING

• Benign disease

—No follow-up if pathology is clearly benign. Otherwise, serial CT scans to monitor for change in radiologic appearance, size, and impingement on other structures

• Malignant disease

—Serial CT scans, chest x-ray, bone scans, liver enzymes, history, and physical

PREVENTION: N/A

 ## Miscellaneous

SYNONYMS: N/A

ASSOCIATED CONDITIONS

• None proven

NOTES

• See also Section I, "Renal Masses—Benign and Malignant."

ABBREVIATIONS: N/A

REFERENCES

Belldegrun A, deKernion JB. Renal tumors. In: Walsh PC, Retik AB, Vaughn ED Jr, Wein AJ, eds. *Campbell's Urology,* 7th ed. Philadelphia: WB Saunders, 1998:2283.

Gelb AB, Simons ML, Weidner N. Solitary fibrous tumor involving the renal capsule. *Am J Surg Pathol* 1996;20(10):1288–1295.

Joseph TJ, Becker DI, Turton AF. Renal malignant fibrous histiocytoma. *Urology* 1990;37(5): 483–489.

Lopez JI, Angulo JC, Flores N, Toledo JD. Malignant fibrous histiocytoma of the renal capsule and synchronous transitional cell carcinoma of the bladder. *Pathol Res Pract* 1996;192:468–471.

Rifai GH. Renal and perirenal hemangiopericytoma. *Urology* 1973;1(2):148–150.

Authors: Marvin Young and Arnon Kongrad

Renal Cell Carcinoma—General

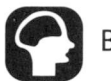 Basics

DESCRIPTION

• Renal cell carcinoma (RCC) is the most common malignant neoplasm of the renal parenchyma.

EPIDEMIOLOGY

• 3% of all malignancies. U.S. 1999 incidence: 30,000; RCC-related deaths: 11,900
• Male:female ratio: 2:1
• Typical, fifth to seventh decade; racial expression equal

GENETICS

• Most sporadic; familial clusters identified
• Associated with von Hippel-Lindau syndrome (VHL)
• VHL gene on 3p25-26 (transcription factor). Altered or absent in sporadic and VHL cases

STAGING

• See Section VII for TNM staging.

SIGNS AND SYMPTOMS

• Usually none; often discovered incidentally discovered
• Occasionally hypochromic anemia hematuria, weight loss, fever, flank mass, pain
• "Classic" triad of pain, flank mass, and hematuria only 11%

PATHOPHYSIOLOGY

• The proximal tubule cell is the principle site of lesion.
• VHL gene: principal tumor suppressor gene responsible for abnormalities and downstream events
• Growth factor alterations evident (VEGF, TGF-alpha), multiple drug resistance exhibited (MDR1)
• Paraneoplastic syndromes: hypercalcemia (PTHrp), Stauffer syndrome, neuropathy, or amyloidosis
• Fuhrmann classification system for nuclear grading I–IV (see Section III)
• Adenocarcinoma; broad histologic categorization

—Clear cell carcinoma (glycogen content)
—Granular cell (distinguish from oncocytoma)
—Papillary type (genetically and pathologically distinct from VHL)

CAUSES/RISK FACTORS

• Increased risk: tobacco use (including pipe and cigar use)
• Weak association with heavy metal exposure
• Acquired renal cystic disease from dialysis and possibly polycystic disease

COMPLICATIONS

• Metastases to lung, liver, bone, or multiple other sites
• Paraneoplastic syndromes; cachexia, bleeding (hematuria, internal)
• Vascular extension (tumor thrombus)
• Mass effect of lesion (GI pulmonary effects)

DIFFERENTIAL DIAGNOSIS

• See also Section I, "Renal Masses—Benign and Malignant."
• Oncocytoma: benign lesion, highly differentiated eosinophilic cells
• Angiomyolipoma: benign hamartoma; fat content on CT can define the lesion.
• Transitional cell carcinoma of collecting system
• Lymphoma
• Complicated cyst: best demonstrated on thin-cut CT or MRI
• Abscess: usually associated with symptoms
• Tumor metastasis (lung or breast most common)
• Rare tumors: hemangiopericytoma, collecting-duct tumors

 Database

HISTORY

• Smoking history, heavy-metal exposure
• Dialysis
• Family history of RCC, polycystic kidney disease

PHYSICAL EXAMINATION

• Hypertension, flank mass, adenopathy, new onset of left varicocele (persistent when recumbent), lower extremity edema, Caput medusa, neuropathy

 Diagnostic Studies

LABORATORY TESTING

• Urinalysis: gross or microscopic hematuria, often negative
• CBC hypochromatic anemia, normal hematocrit, or erythrocytosis (4%)
• Normal or elevated WBC
• Chemistry panel: elevated liver function tests (Stauffer syndrome), hypercalcemia (PTH-related protein)

IMAGING

• CT scan (with and without contrast) demonstrates renal mass with attenuated contrast enhancement (best test). Helical CT permits better definition and three-dimensional reconstruction.
• MRI (with and without gadolinium contrast); also MRI multicoil array

—Similar to CT (advantage of multiplanar imaging: useful if contrast allergy or poor renal function present)

• Ultrasound demonstrates the solid or cystic nature of the renal mass.
• Intravenous urography can demonstrate a renal mass.
• Angiography: Abnormal vasculature is practically a tissue signature for RCC. Most useful in planning complex surgery on solitary renal units
• Venacavagram: to define any tumor thrombus; generally replaced by Doppler ultrasound and MRI
• A radionuclide scan can distinguish normal parenchyma (column of Bertin) from other renal mass.

SPECIAL STUDIES

• Needle biopsy of renal mass rarely employed unless suspicion of metastasis or lymphoma

Treatment

GENERAL MEASURES

- After initial diagnosis, a metastatic evaluation is performed: imaging of chest abdomen and skeletal system.
- RCC is essentially a surgical disease, other modalities being adjunctive.

MEDICAL

- Cytoreductive chemotherapy: limited in effectiveness; used in advanced disease
- Vinblastine and CCNU (a nitrosourea) are classic agents, with a response rate of 15%. Pooled studies: 5% to 6% response
- Floxuridine: up to 57% response; pooled studies, 16% response

SURGICAL

- Radical nephrostomy

—Classically consists of removal of the entire kidney, and a portion of the ureter and the ipsilateral adrenal within Gerota's fascia.
—Multiple approaches: thoracoabdominal, extrapleural interspace flank, transabdominal, and subcostal
—Surgical mortality <1%; complications: blood loss; bowel, splenic, or pancreatic injury; chronic incisional pain; or flank laxity

- Partial nephrectomy

—Partial nephrectomy: option in 4 cm or less in size
—Partial nephrectomy generally required in case of solitary renal unit, bilateral poor renal function, or bilateral lesions
—"Enucleation" with lesions <2 to 3 cm

- Tumors with vena caval thrombus: venacavotomy, use of cardiopulmonary bypass for thrombus above diaphragm in absence of metastases
- Resection of one to two isolated metastases (especially pulmonary) an option for treating primary or recurrent disease

ALTERNATIVE THERAPIES

- External beam radiation: poor response for primary tumor; may palliate painful metastasis

—No data to support adjuvant therapy in locally advanced disease

- Biologic response modifier therapy

—This is presently protocol in nature.
—Lymphokine-activated killer (LAK) cells or tumor-infiltrating lymphocyte (TIL) cells with interleukin-2 (IL-2). Initial responses of up to 30%. This process is cumbersome, with significant toxicity.
—IL-2 alone: 15% response rate, with 4% complete response. Median response: 23 months

- Interferons (usually alpha): response rate of 15% to 20%, with a short duration of 8 to 10 months
- Interferons are also studied in combination with 13 cis-retinoic acid.
- Tumor vaccine approach in progress. Autologous vaccine with granulocyte-macrophage colony–stimulating factor to enhance T-cell response
- Expectant management suggested in elderly or medically compromised with small lesions. The natural history and true risk of such follow-up is indeterminate.

PATIENT EDUCATION

- Oncolink: http://www.oncolink.upenn.edu
- American Cancer Society: (800)ACS-2345; www.cancer.org
- Kidney Cancer Association: (800)850-9132; www.nkca.org
- National Cancer Institute: (800)4-CANCER; www.nci.nih.gov

 Follow-Up

MONITORING

- Postoperative follow-up: physical examination, chest x-ray, chemistry panel, CBC and urinalysis every 6 months for at least 3 years
- Yearly follow-up for at least 5 years
- CT on a yearly basis for at least 5 years
- Beyond 5 years, no guidelines exist. Late recurrences at any site are reported.

—Yearly: PE chest x-ray, and laboratory studies and every-other-year CT reasonable

- Partial nephrectomy patients: more intensive CT imaging on an every-6-month schedule for 5 years

PREVENTION

- Smoking cessation
- Ultrasound "screening" if familial history of RCC or VHL, and if on dialysis

 Miscellaneous

SYNONYMS

- Hypernephroma, Grawitz tumor, kidney cancer

ASSOCIATED CONDITIONS

- Von Hippel-Lindau disease, hypertension, renal insufficiency, paraneoplastic syndromes (e.g., hypercalcemia, fever of unknown origin)

NOTES

- See also Section I, "Renal Masses—Benign and Malignant," and Section II, "Renal Cell Carcinoma—Localized (T1–T4)" and "Renal Cell Carcinoma—Metastatic (N+, M+)."

ABBREVIATIONS

- RCC, renal cell carcinoma; VHL, von Hippel-Lindau syndrome; VEGF, vascular endothelial growth factor; MDR, multiple drug resistance; PTHrp, parathyroid hormone–related polypeptide

REFERENCES

Belldegrun A, deKernion JB. Renal tumors. In: Walsh PC, Retik A, Vaughan ED, Wein AJ, eds. *Campbell's Urology*, 7th ed. Philadelphia: WB Saunders, 1998:2283.

Malkowicz SB. Clinical aspects of renal tumors. *Semin Roentgenol* 1995;30:102.

Montie JE. Follow-up after partial or total nephrectomy for renal cell carcinoma. *Urol Clin North Am* 1994;21:589.

Author: S. Bruce Malkowicz

Renal Cell Carcinoma—Localized (T1–T4)

 Basics

DESCRIPTION

• A localized or locally advanced tumor of the kidney without metastases to nodes or other sites

EPIDEMIOLOGY

• 30,000 new cases in 1999
• Male:female ratio is 2:1.
• Peak incidence in sixth decade
• 25% of patients with kidney cancer present with metastases.

GENETICS

• Clear cell type, von Hippel-Lindau disease (VHL) gene (tumor suppressor gene on chromosome 3p)
• Papillary type, *met* gene (oncogene)

STAGING

• See TMN staging in Section VII.

SIGNS AND SYMPTOMS

• Localized

—Classic triad of flank pain, hematuria, and mass in 10% of patients
—Varicocele

• Metastatic

—Hemoptysis
—Bone pain
—Liver dysfunction
—40% have gross hematuria.
—Paraneoplastic syndromes in 10% of patients
—Anemia
—Hypercalcemia: PTH-LP or bone metastases
　—Rare form of prostaglandin-mediated hypercalcemia; responsive to Indocin
—Erythrocytosis: erythropoietin mediated
—Stauffer syndrome, reversible after nephrectomy for localized disease
　—Altered liver function; elevated alkaline phosphatase; prolonged partial thromboplastin time

• Fever

PATHOPHYSIOLOGY

• Histologic types described by the AJCC

—Malignant: clear cell, papillary, chromophobe, collecting-duct carcinoma
—Benign: oncocytoma, papillary adenoma, metanephric adenoma

CAUSES/RISK FACTORS

• Environmental/substance: smoking, petrochemicals, phenacetin, diuretics, cadmium exposure
• Chronic hemodialysis, obesity
• Hereditary forms

—VHL; germline mutation in VHL gene; characterized by
　—Multiple bilateral renal cancers and cysts
　—CNS hemangioblastoma, retinal angioma, endolymphatic sac tumor
　—Pancreatic neuroendocrine tumor; pheochromocytoma, epididymal cystadenoma
　—Risk of each tumor type is dependent on the type of germline mutation. Missense mutations are associated with pheochromocytoma, and deletions are associated with CNS disease.
—Hereditary papillary renal cancer; germline mutation in *met* gene
—Hereditary renal oncocytoma

COMPLICATIONS

• Fatigue, weight loss
• Tumor rupture, metastases
• Hematuria, paraneoplastic syndromes
• Surgical: anesthetic complications; incisional hernia, hemorrhage, pneumonia, pulmonary embolus

DIFFERENTIAL DIAGNOSIS

• See also Section I, "Renal Masses—Benign and Malignant."
• Metastasis, lymphoma, transitional cell carcinoma of renal pelvis
• Sarcoma, Wilms' tumor, angiomyolipoma
• Abscess, xanthogranulomatous pyelonephritis
• Renal tuberculosis, infected renal cyst
• Pseudotumor (hypertrophied column of Bertin)

 Database

HISTORY

• Smoking, petrochemical exposure
• Symptoms of metastatic disease

—Headache, altered mental status, bone pain, pathologic fracture, back pain, hemoptysis

• Fatigue, ECOG performance status, fever, nightsweats, weight loss
• Family history of renal cancers: VHL, HPRC, HRO
• Medical history: dialysis, drug use, smoking, petrochemical exposure

PHYSICAL EXAMINATION

• Fever, jaundice
• Hypertension: ? renin mediated
• Palpable masses or lymphadenopathy
• Painful sites of metastatic disease
• Varicocele

—Associated with vena caval or renal vein thrombus, obstructing venous drainage
—Dose not decompress in supine position
—Lung auscultation: pleural effusion or metastases

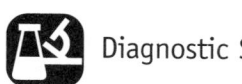 ## Diagnostic Studies

LABORATORY TESTING

- CBC: anemia, polycythemia
- Liver function tests, PT, PTT; alkaline phosphatase with bony metastasis, Stauffer syndrome, or liver metastasis
- Calcium: hypercalcemia, mediated by PTH-LP, bony metastases; rarely vitamin D or prostaglandin mediated
- BUN, creatinine

—Assess renal function to estimate residual function after renal surgery.
—Creatinine clearance if better estimate of renal function needed
—Urinalysis: About 40% of patients have gross hematuria; a higher percentage have microscopic hematuria.

IMAGING

- CT the abdomen, with and without contrast.
- Ultrasound: Differentiate a cystic from a solid renal mass.

—Transesophageal ultrasound is useful to evaluate the proximal extent of a supradiaphragmatic tumor thrombus.

- Chest x-ray
- MRI: can evaluate mass; very useful in evaluation of caval or renal vein thrombus; MRI brain if CNS metastasis suspected
- Arteriogram: prior to partial nephrectomy
- Bone scan: if alkaline phosphatase elevated or symptoms present

SPECIAL STUDIES: N/A

 ## Treatment

GENERAL MEASURES

- The mainstay of clinically localized RCC is radical or partial nephrectomy.
- General medical examination to assess overall health before surgery

MEDICAL

- Adjuvant therapies have thus far not been beneficial.
- IL-2 is currently under investigation in the setting of local disease spread.

SURGICAL

- Stages T1, T2, and T3a, T4

—Radical nephrectomy is the gold standard.
—A partial nephrectomy or enucleation can be considered in small lesions (<4 cm).
—Cryotherapy or radiofrequency ablation for small lesions is investigational.

- Stages T3b, T3c

—Radical nephrectomy with removal of renal vein or vena caval thrombus
—Control of all veins draining into the vena cava prior to cavotomy
—Hypothermia and cardiac arrest may be needed to remove a thrombus extending to the right atrium.

- Regional lymphadenectomy: No studies have shown a survival benefit in prophylactic lymph node dissection.
- Solitary kidney, bilateral disease, hereditary syndromes

—Radical nephrectomy may necessitate dialysis.
  —Most transplant centers will wait 1 to 2 years before considering transplantation.
  —Low-risk population (nondiabetic, Caucasian, ages 20–44 years); 5-year survival after transplantation is 86%.
  —Partial nephrectomy or enucleation of tumors will spare normal renal parenchyma and preserve quality of life.
  —Some centers follow patients with hereditary RCC until the largest tumor is 3 cm in diameter before recommending surgery; metastases have not yet been reported with this novel approach.

ALTERNATIVE THERAPIES: N/A

PATIENT EDUCATION

- Discussions of screening asymptomatic family members in hereditary forms

 ## Follow-Up

MONITORING

- Five-year disease-specific survival for N0-M0 disease from the SEER database

—T1: 92%; T2: 88%; T3: 65%; T4: 26%

- CT abdomen and chest x-ray at 3 to 6 months post-op and at 1 year post-op; also liver function test, CBC, creatinine/BUN
- Evaluation of bone pain, CNS symptoms, or other signs of recurrence or metastases

PREVENTION

- Cigarette smoking
- Environmental exposure

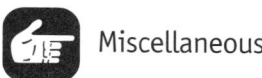 ## Miscellaneous

SYNONYMS

- Hypernephroma, Grawitz tumor

ASSOCIATED CONDITIONS

- Hematuria, paraneoplastic syndromes, metastases, hereditary renal cancer syndromes

NOTES

- See also Section I, "Renal Masses—Benign and Malignant," and Section II, "Renal Cell Carcinoma—General."

ABBREVIATIONS

- VHL, von Hippel-Lindau disease; HPRC, hereditary papillary renal cancer; HRO, hereditary renal oncocytoma; AJCC, American Joint Committee on Cancer; PTH-LP, parathyroid hormone-like protein

REFERENCES

Bassil B, Dosoretz DE, Prout GR. Validation of the tumor, nodes, and metastasis classification of renal cell carcinoma. *J Urol* 1985;134:450.

Belldegrun A, deKernion JB. Renal tumors. In: Walsh PC, Retik AB, Vaughan ED, Wein AJ, eds. *Campbell's Urology*, 7th ed. Philadelphia: WB Saunders, 1998.

Guinan PD, et al. Renal cell carcinoma: Tumor size, stage, and survival. *J Urol* 1995;153:901.

Hafez KS, Novick AC, Campbell SC. Patterns of recurrence and guidelines for follow-up after nephron sparing surgery for sporadic renal cell carcinoma. *J Urol* 1997;157:2067.

Lerner SE, et al. Disease outcome in patients with low stage renal cell carcinoma treated with nephron sparing or radical surgery. *J Urol* 1996;155:1868.

Author: McClellan M. Walther

Renal Cell Carcinoma—Metastatic (N+, M+)

 Basics

DESCRIPTION

• Malignant neoplasm arising from proximal renal tubular epithelium

EPIDEMIOLOGY

• 26,000 estimated new cases in 1998
• 10,000 estimated deaths in 1998
• Ratio of men to women: 2:1
• Peak incidence during fifth to seventh decade of life
• Blacks and Whites have similar incidence; Hispanics have one-third higher rates.

GENETICS

• Sporadic form associated with mutations on chromosome 3p12-p26 region
• Familial form associated with mutations on chromosome 3p21.1-p12 region
• Associated with genetic mutations such as von Hippel-Lindau disease
• Majority of tumors overexpress c-myc and EGFR and underexpress HER-2

STAGING

• See TNM classification in Section VII.

SIGNS AND SYMPTOMS

• Up to 66% detected as incidental renal mass

—60% of patients have gross or microscopic hematuria.
—40% of patients have pain, abdominal mass, or both.
—10% to 15% of patients have the classic triad of gross hematuria, flank pain, and palpable mass.

• Classic presentation frequently a sign of advanced disease

—20% have hypertension.
—Can present with bone pain, dyspnea, cough, or weight loss from metastatic lesions
—Paraneoplastic syndromes common, including erythrocytosis, hypercalcemia, hypertension, neuromyopathy, amyloidosis, and nonmetastatic hepatic dysfunction (Stauffer syndrome)

PATHOPHYSIOLOGY

• Adenocarcinoma arising from proximal convoluted renal tubular epithelium
• Usually unilateral, but 2% bilateral
• Originates in the cortex and grows into the perinephric tissue
• Grossly yellow to orange due to high lipid content
• Five histologic cell types: clear, granular, chromophobe, tubulopapillary, and sarcomatoid
• Sarcomatoid variant associated with more aggressive tumor and worse prognosis
• No true capsule; pseudocapsule composed of compressed parenchyma and fibrous tissue
• No side or site preference
• The mode of spread is via direct extension, propagation into the renal vein, or hematogenous spread.
• The most common sites of metastasis are the lung, liver, subcutaneous tissue, and central nervous system.

CAUSES/RISK FACTORS

• Smoking: twofold increase in risk
• Von Hippel-Lindau disease, with incidence of 28% to 45%
• Acquired renal cystic disease, with incidence of 4% to 9%
• Adult polycystic kidney disease
• Abuse by phenacetin-containing analgesics
• Radiographic agent: colloidal thorium dioxide
• Higher incidence in shoe workers, leather tanners, and workers exposed to cadmium, various petroleum products, and asbestos

COMPLICATIONS

• Metastatic spread to the lungs, liver, brain, or elsewhere
• Tumor necrosis, resulting in severe pain
• Invasion into the renal vein and the inferior vena cava, with obstruction of blood flow
• Complications related to treatment

DIFFERENTIAL DIAGNOSIS

• Benign renal cyst, oncocytoma, cortical adenoma, hamartoma (angiomyolipoma), fibroma, lipoma, other benign tumor
• Malignant metastatic, sarcoma, lymphoblastoma, adrenal carcinoma, large transitional cell carcinoma of the kidney, nephroblastoma (Wilms' tumor)

 Database

HISTORY

• Smoking: increases risk by twofold
• Other associated tumors, such as cerebellar hemangioblastoma and retinal angiomata (von Hippel-Lindau disease)
• History of horseshoe kidney or polycystic kidney disease: Both can increase risk.
• Family history of RCC: rare cases of familial RCC
• Flank pain, hematuria, weight loss, fever, cough, dyspnea, bone pain

PHYSICAL EXAMINATION

• Flank or abdominal mass
• The sudden development of a varicocele in men is not uncommon.

Diagnostic Studies

LABORATORY TESTING

- Urinalysis: hematuria seen in 60% of patients
- Complete blood count: Anemia occurs in 30% of patients due to the anemia of chronic disease.
- May also see erythrocytosis
- Sedimentation rate: elevated in 55% to 75% of patients
- Serum calcium: Hypercalcemia occurs in 3% to 13% due to paraneoplastic effects.
- Liver function tests: abnormal in up to 14% due to nonmetastatic hepatic dysfunction (Stauffer syndrome)

IMAGING

- CT scan is the most sensitive and cost-effective single imaging modality.
- Ultrasound is useful to evaluate cystic masses.
- Any non-simple cyst by ultrasound requires a CT scan.
- CT findings: heterogeneous low-density mass in the cortex of the kidney that enhances with IV contrast

—85% of solid renal masses that enhance with IV contrast are RCCs.
—CT is the method of choice to define renal vein involvement, perinephric spread, and lymph node involvement.

- CNS imaging is essential in patients with symptoms of advanced disease.
- Helical (spiral) chest CT scan to detect pulmonary metastases
- Bone scan to rule out bony metastases
- MRI is useful for documenting inferior vena cava involvement.
- Angiography is reserved for solitary kidneys where partial nephrectomy is being considered.

SPECIAL STUDIES

- The cavogram useful to determine the precise involvement of the renal vein and inferior vena cava, but is rarely necessary now, due to MRI.
- FNA is of limited benefit: It is useful to differentiate primary RCC from metastatic tumors.

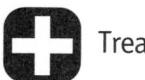 ## Treatment

GENERAL MEASURES

- Local disease is best managed by radical nephrectomy with total tumor excision.
- Partial nephrectomy is limited to patients with bilateral disease or a solitary kidney.
- Metastatic spread is treated using IL-2– or interferon-alpha–based immunotherapy, with limited success
- Many experimental protocols exist that combine surgical and immunotherapy.

MEDICAL

- RCCs express MDR-1, making chemotherapy largely unsuccessful; response rates are 10%, and duration is <6 months.
- Hormone therapy (antiestrogens, progesterones, androgens): first thought to have 0% to 33% response rate; now has little-to-no benefit
- Immunotherapy treatment of choice
- Response to treatment defined as complete (CR) (no residual tumor) or partial (PR) (regression of metastatic tumor sites by 50% or greater)
- Interferon-alpha with CR of 1%, PR of 15% to 20%
- IL-2 approved by the FDA with CR of 5%, PR of 10% to 15%

—Can be given in high-dose, low-dose, bolus, or continuous infusion
—Associated with significant toxicity, including capillary leak, acute renal failure, hypotension, respiratory distress
—Should only be administered in centers with experience with IL-2, due to toxicity
—Treatment-related mortality between 1% and 2%
—Newer protocols looking at combinations of IL-2 and interferon-alpha, and 5-FU, look promising.

SURGICAL

- Radical nephrectomy is the gold standard for localized disease.

—May be needed for palliation (i.e., bleeding, pain) in patients with advanced disease

- Isolated solitary metastasis (i.e., lung) can be resected and provide improved survival rates.

ALTERNATIVE THERAPIES

- Radiation can palliate painful bony or CNS metastasis.
- Experimental protocols

—Combination of IL-2, interferon-alpha, and 5-FU promising
—Dendritic cell therapy, gene therapy, and tumor vaccines

PATIENT EDUCATION

- 5-year survival

—Stage I (T1, N0, M0): 60% to 82%
—Stage II (T2, N0, M0): 47% to 80%
—Stage III (N+, M0): 35% to 51%
—Stage IV (N+ or M+): 0% to 20%

- National Kidney Cancer: (800)850-9132; http://www.nkca.org

 ## Follow-Up

MONITORING

- No universal, agreed-upon follow-up schedule

—After surgery, every 3 months for the first year suggested, with serum chemistries and chest x-ray

PREVENTION

- Little is known. Stop smoking, as smoking increases risk by twofold.

 ## Miscellaneous

SYNONYMS

- Clear cell carcinoma, hypernephroma, alveolar carcinoma, internist's tumor

ASSOCIATED CONDITIONS

- Hypertension in up to 40% of patients
- Numerous paraneoplastic syndromes: hypercalcemia, erythrocytosis, elevated sedimentation rate, hypertension
- Sudden onset of varicocele not uncommon
- Cerebellar hemangioblastoma and retinal angiomata in patients with von Hippel-Lindau disease

NOTES: N/A

ABBREVIATIONS

- FNA, fine-needle aspiration; IL-2, interleukin-2; MDR, multidrug resistance; RCC, renal cell carcinoma

REFERENCES

Belldegrun A. Advanced renal cell carcinoma. *Semin Urol Oncol* 1996;14:195.

deKernion JB, Belldegrun A. Renal tumors. In: Walsh PC, Retik AB, Vaughan ED, Wein AJ, eds. *Campbell's Urology*, 7th ed. Philadelphia: WB Saunders, 1998:2283–2326.

Dreicer R, Williams RD. Renal parenchymal neoplasms. In: Tanagho EA, McAninch JW, eds. *Smith's General Urology*, 14th ed. Norwalk, CT: Appleton & Lange, 1995:372–391.

Authors: Stephen J. Freedland and Arie S. Belldegrun

Renal Cell Carcinoma—Pediatric

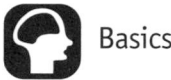 Basics

DESCRIPTION

- Malignant tumor (nephroblastoma or Wilms' tumor) arising from metanephric blastema

EPIDEMIOLOGY

- Most common urologic malignancy in children
- Seven new cases per million children per year
- 350 new cases reported annually; 8% of solid childhood cancers
- Ratio of boys to girls: 0.97:1.0
- Peak incidence in third year of life: 90% of patients less than 7 years
- No racial predisposition

GENETICS

- 1% of patients with familial form
- Autosomal dominant with varying penetrance
- Two tumor suppressor genes identified

—WT1 maps to *11p13* and WT2 maps to *11p15*

STAGING

- Based on clinical and pathologic features
- Most common staging method is NWTS (National Wilms' Tumor Study)

—Stage I: tumor limited to the kidney and completely excised with renal capsule intact
—Stage II: tumor beyond kidney and completely excised
—Stage III: Residual nonhematogenous spread of tumor after surgical resection can be in regional lymph nodes, peritoneal contamination, or positive margins.
—Stage IV: hematogenous metastases
—Stage V: bilateral renal involvement at time of diagnosis

SIGNS AND SYMPTOMS

- Most commonly present as asymptomatic renal mass: seen in 75% of patients

—25% to 63% have hypertension due to elevated renin.
—33% have abdominal pain.
—25% have microscopic hematuria.

- Common findings include distension, anorexia, nausea, vomiting, and fever.

PATHOPHYSIOLOGY

- Blastoma arising from proximal metanephric blastema
- Usually unilateral, but 10% bilateral
- Grossly large multiloculated, gray or tan, with areas of hemorrhage and necrosis
- Malignant cells are pluripotent.
- Most commonly see blastemal, epithelial, and/or stromal elements
- Most common diagnostic feature is nephrogenic cells with tubuloglomerular pattern with background of stromatogenic cells
- Three cell types have a worse prognosis (anaplastic, clear cell carcinoma, and malignant rhabdoid tumors) and are treated more aggressively; these account for 10% cases and 60% of deaths.
- Unfavorable histology (UH) includes anaplastic, clear cell carcinoma, and malignant rhabdoid tumors.
- All other histologic types are considered favorable (FH).
- No true capsule; fibrous pseudocapsule occasionally seen
- No side or site preference
- 10% to 15% of patients have metastatic disease at presentation.
- The most common site is the lung (85%–95%) or liver (10%–15%)
- Regional lymphatics involved in 25% of patients

CAUSES/RISK FACTORS

- 1% have familial; typically younger with bilateral and multicentric disease
- Autosomal dominant with varying penetration
- Children of machinists with higher risk

COMPLICATIONS

- Metastatic spread to the lungs, liver, or elsewhere
- Hemorrhage into the tumor with or without necrosis, causing pain
- Subcapsular hemorrhage, causing pain, fever
- Intraperitoneal rupture, causing an acute abdomen
- Tumor necrosis, resulting in severe pain
- Complications related to therapy

DIFFERENTIAL DIAGNOSIS

- Benign renal mass: hydronephrosis, polycystic kidney, congenital mesoblastic nephroma, multicystic dysplastic kidney, renal abscess, mesenteric cyst, choledochal cyst, intestinal duplication cyst, splenomegaly
- Malignant renal mass: renal cell carcinoma, neuroblastoma, rhabdomyosarcoma, lymphoma, lymphosarcoma, hepatoblastoma

 Database

HISTORY

- Parents' occupation: children of machinists higher risk
- Family history of nephroblastoma: 1% of cases are familial.
- Pseudohermaphroditism: associated with increased risk
- Flank pain, hematuria, fever, increasing abdominal girth

PHYSICAL EXAMINATION

- Abdominal mass
- 15% of patients with associated anomalies

—Sporadic aniridia: 33% risk of nephroblastoma
—Hemihypertrophy in 3% of patients
—Musculoskeletal anomalies in 3% of patients
—Hamartomas in 8% of patients
—Genitourinary anomalies in 4% of patients

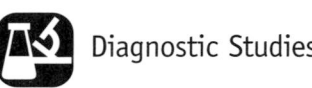 Diagnostic Studies

LABORATORY TESTING

- Urinalysis: hematuria seen in 25% of patients
- Complete blood count: may rarely see erythrocytosis due to erythropoietin production
- Liver and renal function tests: baseline pretreatment
- Urinary catecholamines to rule out neuroblastoma

IMAGING

- Classically, IVP is the test of choice.
- IVP shows deformation and distortion of the calyceal morphology by an intrarenal mass.
- 10% have nonvisualization of the affected kidney due to complete urinary outflow blockage. Today, ultrasound, CT scan, MRI, and IVP are all useful.
- KUB may demonstrate an egg-shell pattern around the tumor: represents old hemorrhage.
- If a stippled pattern is present, neuroblastoma is likely.
- Ultrasound is useful to rule out hydronephrosis, renal agenesis, or multicystic kidney disease.
- The tumor has a heterogeneous echo pattern due to necrosis and hemorrhage.
- MRI is not useful to establish diagnosis, but is useful in following patients postoperatively.
- Chest x-ray to rule out metastatic spread to the lungs
- Any questionable chest x-ray findings require a chest CT scan.

SPECIAL STUDIES

- Rarely necessary

Treatment

GENERAL MEASURES

- Primary treatment is surgical excision.
- Patients are staged based on pathologic and surgical findings.
- Treatment is tailored to each stage.
- Treatment consists of chemotherapy with or without RT.
- As survival improves, the goal is to minimize toxicity of treatment.

MEDICAL

- Primary surgical excision is used for staging.
- Treatment is based on stage, and stratified based on histology.
- RT is begun 1 to 3 days after surgery.
- Chemotherapy is started postoperatively once bowel function has returned.
- Actinomycin-D 15 g/kg/d for 5 consecutive days; repeat at 6 weeks, 3 months, and thereafter, at 12- to 13-week intervals.
- Vincristine 1.5 mg/m^2 weekly for 8 to 10 weeks initially; thereafter, at the beginning and end of each course of actinomycin-D
- Doxorubicin 20 mg/m^2/d for 3 days every 12 weeks, beginning 6 weeks after the first course of actinomycin-D
- Treatment recommendations are based on NWTS-III.
- Stage I FH/UH

—No RT; actinomycin-D and vincristine for 6 months

- Stage II FH, no RT

—Actinomycin-D and vincristine for 15 months

- Stage III FH

—RT 1000 cGy to flank
—Actinomycin-D, vincristine, and doxorubicin for 15 months

- Stage IV FH

—RT 1000 cGy to flank and 1200 cGy to the lungs
—Actinomycin-D, vincristine, and doxorubicin for 15 months

- Stage II–IV UH

—RT with 1000 cGy to flank
—Actinomycin-D, vincristine, doxorubicin, and ± cyclophosphamide for 15 months

- Stage V: Treatment is individualized.

SURGICAL

- Primary treatment is complete resection of tumor.
- Radical nephrectomy via transabdominal approach with observation of intraabdominal organs
- Exploration of contralateral kidney prior to nephrectomy
- It is not essential to obtain negative surgical margins, as preoperative chemotherapy and radiation therapy can shrink the tumor.
- Avoid intraperitoneal tumor spillage.
- Lymphadenectomy is of limited benefit; biopsy grossly enlarged nodes.

ALTERNATIVE THERAPIES

- NWTS-IV looking at minimizing toxicity while retaining efficacy

PATIENT EDUCATION

- 4-year survival from NWTS-III

—Stage I FH: 97%; stage II FH: 92%; stage III FH: 84%; stage IV FH: 83%
—Stage I–III UH: 68%; stage IV UH: 55%

- Clear cell carcinoma: 75%
- Rhabdoid sarcoma: 25%

Follow-Up

MONITORING

- No established guidelines for follow-up
- Most patients are followed by the NWTS.

PREVENTION

- None known

Miscellaneous

SYNONYMS

- Wilms' tumor

ASSOCIATED CONDITIONS

- See Physical Examination in "Database" section.
- Associated with Beckwith-Wiedemann syndrome (visceromegaly, omphalocele, hemihypertrophy, microcephaly, mental retardation, and macroglossia)
- Thirty-fold increase in incidence of neurofibromatosis
- 15% of patients successfully treated develop a second malignancy.

NOTES: N/A

ABBREVIATIONS

- cGY, centigray; FH, favorable histology; NWTS, National Wilms' Tumor Study; UH, unfavorable histology; WT, Wilms' tumor

REFERENCES

Dreicer R, Williams RD. Renal parenchymal neoplasms. In: Tanagho EA, McAninch JW, eds. *Smith's General Urology*, 14th ed. Norwalk, CT: Appleton & Lange, 1995:372–391.

Snyder HM, D'Angio GJ, Evans AE, Raney RB. Pediatric oncology. In: Walsh PC, Retik AB, Vaughan ED, Wein AJ, eds. *Campbell's Urology*, 7th ed. Philadelphia: WB Saunders, 1998:2210–2256.

Authors: Stephen J. Freedland and Arie S. Belldegrun

Renal Cysts

 Basics

DESCRIPTION

• Fluid-filled, epithelial-lined masses involving the renal parenchyma, which may or may not communicate with the collecting system. These can be congenital or acquired. Distinct from peripelvic and parapelvic cysts that do not involve the renal parenchyma

EPIDEMIOLOGY

• Congenital: autosomal dominant polycystic kidney disease (ADPKD) (adult population): 10% of renal failure patients in the United States
• Autosomal recessive polycystic kidney disease (ARPKD) (pediatric population): 1 in 40,000 live births
• Acquired simple cystic disease: Approximately one-half of the population over the age of 50 has one or more cysts.
• Acquired cystic disease of dialysis: Incidence increases with time on dialysis (both hemodialysis and intraperitoneal).

GENETICS

• Applicable to congenital cystic disease only
• Autosomal dominant usually manifested in adulthood: responsible gene localized to chromosome 16

—Autosomal recessive usually manifested in childhood: gene not identified

STAGING

• See Bosniak classification, below.

SIGNS AND SYMPTOMS

• ADPKD

—Hypertension, hematuria, UTI, urolithiasis, renal insufficiency, Berry aneurysms, enlarged kidneys

• ARPKD

—Renal failure, failure to thrive: if manifested at birth, usually die within 2 months; if manifested later, will develop liver failure secondary to hepatic fibrosis

• Simple cystic disease

—Usually asymptomatic; incidental finding on imaging
—Acquired cystic disease of dialysis
—Usually asymptomatic; incidental finding on imaging

PATHOPHYSIOLOGY

• ADPKD

—Multiple cysts of varying size communicating with nephron, massively enlarged kidneys
—Cysts of other organs, including liver, pancreas, spleen, lung
—Aneurysms of circle of Willis, colonic diverticula, mitral valve prolapse
—ARPKD
—Multiple, small, subcapsular cysts representing dilated collecting tubules, hepatic fibrosis

• Simple cystic disease

—Varying size, fibrous wall with single layer of cuboidal epithelium
—Distinct from peripelvic cysts (See Section II, "Renal Cysts—Peripelvic and Parapelvic.")

• Acquired cystic disease of dialysis

—Mainly cortical and multiple, usually less than 1 cm in size, often contain calcium oxalate crystals, increased risk of developing renal cell carcinoma

CAUSES/RISK FACTORS

• ADPKD

—A genetic defect may result in an abnormality of the basement membrane or extracellular matrix.

• ARPKD

—Mechanism of genetic defect unknown

• Simple cystic disease

—Aging

• Acquired cystic disease of dialysis
• Duration of dialysis and possible uremia toxin may contribute to cyst formation.

COMPLICATIONS

• ADPKD

—Renal failure, UTI, urolithiasis hypertension, cerebrovascular accident

• ARPKD

—Renal failure, hepatic failure, and death

• Simple cystic disease

—None

• Acquired cystic disease of dialysis

—Malignant transformation in 25%

DIFFERENTIAL DIAGNOSIS

• See also Section I, "Renal Masses—Benign and Malignant."
• Simple vs. complex cyst
• Peripelvic/parapelvic cyst
• Cystic renal cell carcinoma
• Solid renal mass: renal cell carcinoma, oncocytoma, angiomyolipoma
• Renal abscess

 Database

HISTORY

• Pain, hematuria, colic: might relate to stone disease, malignancy, ADPKD
• GI complaints: might relate to malignancy or enlarged kidneys of ADPKD
• Weight loss or constitutional symptoms if malignancy suspected

—If in renal failure, duration of dialysis
—Family history of hypertension or renal failure, ADPKD

PHYSICAL EXAMINATION

• Blood pressure is elevated in ADPKD.
• Palpable abdominal or flank mass in ADPKD or malignancy
• Adenopathy in malignancy
• Palpable liver or spleen in ADPKD
• Murmurs in ADPKD

Diagnostic Studies

LABORATORY TESTING

• Urinalysis: hematuria in ADPKD or malignancy, proteinuria in renal failure, pyuria in infection
• Creatinine: commonly elevated if ADPKD or ARPKD

IMAGING

• Renal ultrasound criteria for simple cyst; if these criteria are not met, then go to thin-section CT.

—Absence of internal echoes
—Sharply defined thin, smooth wall, and distinct margin
—Through transmission with acoustic enhancement behind cyst
—Spherical or slightly ovoid shape

• Thin-section CT scan before and after IV contrast if indeterminate by ultrasound

—Sharply defined thin, smooth wall, and distinct margin
—Spherical or slightly ovoid shape
—Homogeneous content
—Hounsfield unit density ranging from −10 to +20 without enhancement after IV contrast

• Bosniak classification of renal cysts

—Type I: Fulfill ultrasound or CT criteria for simple cyst: benign
—Type II: minimal complexity, such as internal, thin-walled septa or small calcifications: benign
—Type III: more extensive calcifications or thickened septa: suspicious for malignancy, warrants surgery
—Type IV: mural nodules with enhancement consistent with cystic neoplasm: surgery warranted

SPECIAL STUDIES

• Arteriography rarely utilized today

 Treatment

GENERAL MEASURES

• ADPKD

—Screen family members by ultrasound; 50% of children will be affected.

• ARPKD

—Supportive care for pulmonary, renal, hepatic, and cardiac failure

• Simple cystic disease

—None

• Acquired cystic disease of dialysis

—If hematuria associated with heparinization of dialysis, conversion to peritoneal dialysis

MEDICAL

• ADPKD

—Blood pressure control critical to avoid worsening renal failure
—Treat UTI aggressively to avoid worsening renal failure.

• ARPKD

—If patient survives, needs treatment for renal, hepatic, and cardiac failure

• Simple cystic disease: N/A
• Acquired cystic disease of dialysis

—Treatment for chronic renal failure

SURGICAL

• ADPKD

—Unroofing of cysts if severe pain
—Nephrectomy if severe hematuria

• ARPKD

—Splenic vein to left renal vein shunt if severe portal hypertension

• Simple cystic disease

—Partial nephrectomy warranted if Bosniak type III or IV

• Acquired cystic disease of dialysis

—Nephrectomy warranted if malignancy suspected
—Embolization or nephrectomy if refractory hematuria

ALTERNATIVE THERAPIES: N/A

PATIENT EDUCATION

• ADPKD

—Genetic counseling and screening of family members

• ARPKD

—Poor prognosis, early death

• Acquired cystic disease of dialysis

—Onset of hematuria warrants attention and the need to exclude malignancy.

 Follow-Up

MONITORING

• ADPKD

—Aggressive blood pressure control

• ARPKD

—Rare long-term survival

• Simple cystic disease

—None unless symptoms change

• Acquired cystic disease of dialysis

—Annual ultrasound to assess for malignancy

PREVENTION: N/A

 Miscellaneous

SYNONYMS: N/A

ASSOCIATED CONDITIONS

• Renal failure: ADPKD, ARPKD

NOTES

• See also Section II, "Renal Cysts—Peripelvic and Parapelvic," "Polycystic Kidney Disease—Autosomal Dominant," and "Polycystic Kidney Disease—Autosomal Recessive."

ABBREVIATIONS

• ADPKD, autosomal dominant polycystic kidney disease; ARPKD, autosomal recessive polycystic kidney disease

REFERENCES

Bosniak MA. The current radiological approach to renal cysts. *Radiology* 1986;158:1.

Glassberg K. Renal dysplasia and cystic disease of the kidney. In: Walsh PC, Retik AB, Stamey TA, Vaughan ED Jr, eds. *Campbell's Urology*, 6th ed. Philadelphia: WB Saunders, 1992:1443–1495.

Author: Joseph C. Presti, Jr.

Renal Cysts—Peripelvic and Parapelvic

 Basics

DESCRIPTION

• A peripelvic and/or parapelvic renal cyst really describes the location of a simple parenchymal cyst. A renal sinus cyst is not a cyst derived from the renal parenchyma and probably develops from the lymphatic system.

EPIDEMIOLOGY

• Most common renal mass, generally of no clinical significance
• Simple renal cysts

—Incidence increases with age; most commonly seen in individuals over 50 years of age
—Very rare in children

GENETICS: N/A

STAGING

• Bosniak: categorization of cystic renal masses

—Category I: simple benign cyst meeting all CT or sonographic criteria
—Category II: benign simple cystic lesions minimally complicated (septated cysts), minimally calcified cysts, infected cysts, high-density cysts
—Category III: complicated cystic lesions that demonstrate findings seen in malignancy, that require surgical intervention (resection for benign disease or nephrectomy for malignant disease)
—Category IV: obvious malignant lesion with cystic details necessitating nephrectomy

SIGNS AND SYMPTOMS

• Generally asymptomatic
• Does not cause hematuria
• Incidental finding on some radiographic test

PATHOPHYSIOLOGY

• The predominant type of renal sinus cyst appears to be one derived from the lymphatics.
• Most often, these cysts are multiple, and often they are bilateral. The majority appear after the fifth decade, and they may be associated with inflammation, obstruction, or a calculus.
• Considered as an anomaly that is acquired
• Generally not palpable in an adult
• Only the very large ones may produce some sort of flank pain.
• May obstruct the intrarenal collecting system
• Round, tense, and thin-walled; fluid-filled; hollow
• The diameter of the cavity can range from millimeters to centimeters.

CAUSES/RISK FACTORS: N/A

COMPLICATIONS: N/A

DIFFERENTIAL DIAGNOSIS

• Complicated renal cysts, multilocular
• Renal sinus cysts, derived from the lymphatics
• Abscesses
• Hematomas
• Infarcts
• Localized inflammatory pseudotumors
• Angiomyolipomas
• Lymphoma
• Cystic Wilms' tumor
• Calyceal diverticulum, smooth intrarenal sac that connects with the pelvicalyceal system by a narrow channel (neck)
• Pyeloureteric duplication
• Chronic dialysis patients have a high likelihood of developing cysts in their native kidneys (35%–80%). 100-fold increased risk of developing renal cell cancer in these cysts when compared with the general population

 Database

HISTORY

• No typical findings

PHYSICAL EXAMINATION

• Generally not palpable in an adult

Diagnostic Studies

LABORATORY TESTING

- If cyst fluid aspirated

—Normal: Cystic fluid should appear as clear, straw-colored.
- Low level of fat, low level of protein, no blood, negative cytology

—Malignant cysts
- Murky aspirate, often bloody, high concentration of fat and protein, positive cytology

—Inflammatory cyst
- Purulent aspirate, generally no blood present, moderately elevated fat and protein, high levels of lactate dehydrogenase and amylase; cytology shows many inflammatory cells; bacterial culture will more than likely be positive.

IMAGING

- Real-time ultrasound (US)

—Very good but sometimes unable to identify a cyst clearly (20%–40% risk of error), demonstrates a smooth, thin-walled structure with no internal echoes and posterior acoustic enhancement

- Intravenous urogram (IVU)

—Tomographic pictures depict renal mass often with calyceal stretching; need further diagnostic testing

- Computerized tomography (CT scan)

—Can elucidate and clarify most ultrasound indeterminate masses

- Magnetic resonance imaging (MRI)

—Can be used in place of CT scan, especially with a patient with severe contrast allergy or compromised renal function, using intravenous gadolinium evaluating fat-suppressed T1-weighted images

SPECIAL STUDIES

- Renal arteriography: avascular, sharply defined radiolucent mass with a thin wall

 ## Treatment

GENERAL MEASURES

- Observation is the rule. The vast majority of simple renal cysts do not require treatment.
- Cyst aspiration should generally be limited to ruling out infection, obstruction by the cyst, or cysts that are suspicious for malignancy.
- Percutaneous drainage will provide symptomatic relief for a large cyst causing flank pain; however, recurrence is common.

—Ultrasonic guided cyst puncture with fluid aspiration and sclerosis
—Cyst fluid should then be microscopically evaluated for sediment.
—Cyst fluid should be sent for cytology.

MEDICAL: N/A

SURGICAL

- Partial excision with marsupialization is considered the treatment of choice.

—For those cysts that are recurrent after a failed attempt at percutaneous drainage
—For those cysts that are not manage by percutaneous drainage
—If cyst fluid is bloody or blood stained or if sediment is questionable, further testing and possible surgical exploration may be necessary.

- Three methods for percutaneous endoscopic treatment of a renal cyst:

—Direct transcystic
—Direct transparenchymal
—Indirect

- Laparoscopic procedure with a four-port transperitoneal or a retroperitoneal technique

ALTERNATIVE THERAPIES: N/A

PATIENT EDUCATION: N/A

 ## Follow-Up

MONITORING

- Ultrasound

—Most commonly used modality

PREVENTION: N/A

 ## Miscellaneous

SYNONYMS

- Terms used in the literature to describe cysts adjacent to the renal pelvis or within the hilum: peripelvic cyst, parapelvic cyst, renal sinus cyst, parapelvic lymphatic cysts, hilus cysts, cysts of the renal hilum, and peripelvic lymphangiectasis

ASSOCIATED CONDITIONS: N/A

NOTES

- See also Section I, "Renal Masses—Benign and Malignant," and Section II, "Renal Cysts."

ABBREVIATIONS: N/A

REFERENCES

Amis ES Jr, Cronan JJ, Pfister RC. Needle puncture of cystic renal masses: A survey of the Society of Uroradiology. *AJR* 1987;148:297.

Bosniak NA. The current radiological approach to renal cysts. *Radiology* 1986;158:1.

Dalton D, Neiman J, Grayhack JT. The natural history of simple renal cysts: A preliminary study. *J Urol* 1986;135:905.

Author: E. James Seidmond

Renal Dysplasia, Hypodysplasia, and Hypoplasia

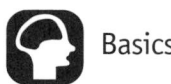

Basics

DESCRIPTION

- Dysplasia is abnormal or primitive tissue development, and is a histologic diagnosis only, not a disease.

—Multicystic dysplastic kidney (MCDK)

- Hypoplasia represents small kidneys that have subnormal calyces and nephrons without dysplasia.

—True hypoplasia
—Oligomeganephronia
—Ask-Upmark kidney (segmental hypoplasia)

- Hypodysplasia represents small kidneys that have subnormal calyces and nephrons with dysplasia.

—With normal ureteral orifice
 —With ureteropelvic or ureterovesical junction obstruction or primary obstructive megaureter
 —Without obstruction
—With abnormal ureteral orifice
 —With lateral ectopia, usually associated with reflux
 —With medial or caudal ectopia and ureteroceles
—Urethral obstruction
—Prune-belly syndrome
—Aplastic dysplasia (renal aplasia)

EPIDEMIOLOGY

- MCDK

—1 in 4300 live births
—Males more than females; left side more common than right

- Oligomeganephronia

—The majority are sporadic, without associated anomalies.
—Male-to-female ratio: 3:1
—Present before 2 years of age

- Ask-Upmark kidney

—Present generally after 10 years of age
—Female-to-male ratio: 2:1

- Hypodysplasia

—Incidence related to underlying condition (i.e., ureterocele)

GENETICS

- A majority of dysplastic and hypoplastic kidneys are sporadic and nongenetic.
- Familial adysplasia: occurrence of renal agenesis, dysplasia, MCDK, or aplasia in family

—Autosomal dominant

STAGING: N/A

SIGNS AND SYMPTOMS

- MCDK; unilateral

—Abdominal mass
 —Less often vomiting, failure to thrive, flank pain, infection, hematuria, proteinuria, hypertension in adulthood

- Ask-Upmark kidney (segmental hypoplasia) usually first presents with signs of hypertension.

—Headaches, encephalopathy, and/or retinopathy

- All bilateral disorders generally present with signs of renal insufficiency.

—Dehydration, failure to thrive, hypertension, growth retardation, polyuria, polydipsia

PATHOPHYSIOLOGY

- Normal metanephric differentiation requires induction by the ureteric bud.
- The branching of the collecting system, as well as nephron formation, are determined by the ureteric bud.
- Epithelial–mesenchymal interactions and peptide growth factors play a central role in nephrogenesis.
- Obstruction at specific stages may produce hypodysplasia.
- Mackie and Stephens "Bud Theory"

—An abnormal ureteric bud can lead to renal dysplasia, as well as an ectopic orifice.
—In duplex systems, the degree of ureteral ectopia correlates with dysplasia.

- All dysplastic conditions

—Varying degrees of corticomedullary differentiation
—Varying degrees of atrophic, cystic, undifferentiated, and abnormally differentiated nephronic elements
—May be areas of cartilaginous metaplasia

- Multicystic dysplastic kidney

—Kidney size is variable: small to enormous.
—Grossly multiple cysts of varying size, no lobar organization
—Occasionally, small islands of renal tissue
—Primitive ductules and cartilage
—Atretic ureter (possible cause or associated maldevelopment)

- Obstructive renal dysplasia

—Secondary to neurogenic bladder, PUV, or ureteral obstruction
—The peripheral cortex is most severely involved.
—Cystic with distension of collecting tubules

- Aplastic dysplasia: a nubbin of nonfunctioning tissue

—Possibly an involuted MCDK

- Hypoplasia

—Small kidneys that have subnormal calyces and nephrons without dysplasia

- True hypoplasia
- Oligomeganephronia

—Decreased number of nephrons with hypertrophy of each nephron
—Fewer than six calyces
—Small renal artery
—No dysplasia
—Enormous glomeruli and elongated tubules

- Ask-Upmark kidney (segmental hypoplasia)

—Most likely an acquired lesion secondary to reflux
—Deep groove(s) on cortical surface of kidney
—Under the groove are tubules resembling thyroid tubules.
—Inflammatory cells and fibrotic glomeruli
—Arteriosclerosis
—Juxtaglomerular hyperplasia

CAUSES/RISK FACTORS

- Ureteral abnormalities
- Ureteral anomalies
- Prune belly syndrome

COMPLICATIONS

- Renal failure
- MCDK

—Contralateral kidney abnormalities: 20% to 75%
—Contralateral reflux: 10% to 20%
—Associated gastroenterologic and cardiac abnormalities common

DIFFERENTIAL DIAGNOSIS

- MCDK

—Autosomal recessive polycystic kidney disease
 —US: bilateral, enlarged kidneys; cysts less than 2 cm; dilated intrahepatic biliary ducts
—Autosomal dominant (adult) polycystic kidney disease
 —US: bilateral enlarged kidneys; extrarenal cysts

- Hypodysplasia

—Reflux nephropathy
 —US: polar scarring over calyces
 —VCUG: reflux

Renal Dysplasia, Hypodysplasia, and Hypoplasia

 Database

HISTORY

- Renal disease

—Polyuria, polydipsia, flank pain, headaches, fatigue

- Bladder disease

—Dysuria, hematuria, nocturia, incontinence

PHYSICAL EXAMINATION

- Weight and height (growth chart)
- Blood pressure
- Eyes: papillary edema, retinopathy
- Oral: dehydration
- Abdomen: palpable kidneys, distended bladder
- Extremities: edema

 Diagnostic Studies

LABORATORY TESTING

- Urinalysis

—Hematuria, proteinuria, low specific gravity

- Serum creatinine, BUN and electrolytes

—Uremia, hyperkalemia

IMAGING

- Multicystic dysplastic kidney

—US shows no normal parenchyma, noncommunicating cysts.

- Hypoplasia

—US: small kidneys
—Retrograde pyelogram shows a reduced number of calyces.

- Dysplasia

—US: diffusely hyperechoic, cortical cysts

SPECIAL STUDIES

- Biopsy
- Cystoscopy

 Treatment

GENERAL MEASURES

- MCDK

—VCUG to rule out contralateral reflux
—Nuclear renal scan if hydronephrosis cannot be ruled out

MEDICAL

- If reflux, antibiotic prophylaxis
- If impending or existent renal insufficiency, nephrology consultation

SURGICAL

- Nonfunctional kidney: nephrectomy for hypertension, abdominal pain, chronic infections
- Ureteral reimplantation for reflux
- MCDK

—Indications for nephrectomy: hypertension, abdominal pain, chronic infections, increasing size
—3% to 7% incidence of nodular blastema
  —Development of Wilms' tumor is anecdotal.
  —The literature does not support routine removal of MCDKs.

ALTERNATIVE THERAPIES

- Renal transplantation

PATIENT EDUCATION

- Depends on underlying etiology

 Follow-Up

MONITORING

- Blood pressure and growth chart at least annually
- Serum creatinine, BUN, and electrolytes at least annually
- Urinalysis and culture at least annually
- Bilateral disease: US at least annually
- MCDK

—US every 2 years to ensure involution

PREVENTION: N/A

 Miscellaneous

SYNONYMS: N/A

ASSOCIATED CONDITIONS

- MCDK: Meckel-Gruber syndrome, Jeune asphyxiating thoracic dystrophy, and Aellweger cerebro-hepatorenal syndrome
- Oligonephronia: limb deformities and branchio-oto-renal syndrome

NOTES

- See also Section II, "Multicystic Dysplastic Kidney."

ABBREVIATIONS

- MCDK, multicystic dysplastic kidney; PUV, posterior urethral valves

REFERENCES

Glassberg KI. Renal dysplasia and cystic disease of the kidney. In: Walsh PC, Retik AB, Vaughan ED, Wein AJ, eds. *Campbell's Urology,* 7th ed. Philadelphia: WB Saunders, 1998:1757.

Watkins SL, Avner ED. Renal dysplasia and cystic disease. In: Barnah TM, Avner ED, Harmon WE, eds. *Pediatric Nephrology,* 4th ed. Baltimore: Williams & Wilkins, 1994:467.

Authors: Eric A. Kurzrock and Laurence S. Baskin

Renal Ectopia

 Basics

DESCRIPTION

• A kidney that lies outside the renal fossa

EPIDEMIOLOGY

• Incidence: 1 in 500 to 1000 autopsies
• Left side slightly more than right
• No sex preference
• Bilateral in 10%

GENETICS

• None known

STAGING

• Can be pelvic, lumbar, crossed, or thoracic

SIGNS AND SYMPTOMS

• Often asymptomatic, incidental finding
• Pelvic kidneys have poor drainage of urine that predisposes to infection and stones.
• Occasionally

PATHOPHYSIOLOGY

• Distinct entity from renal ptosis

—A ptotic kidney is in the normal position, but can move to a lower position in the pelvis with positional change.
—The renal artery of the ptotic kidney is in the normal position.

• The renal artery of an ectopic kidney is in an aberrant location.

—An ectopic artery can arise from the lower aorta or iliac vessels.

• Thoracic ectopia can be acquired or congenital.

—Acquired: kidney herniates through congenital defect in diaphragm (foramen of Bochdalek)

• Often associated with a fusion abnormality (crossed renal ectopia, horseshoe kidney) and mal-rotation of the renal pelvis
• Genital abnormalities can be associated.

CAUSES/RISK FACTORS

• Abnormal fetal ascent of the kidney

COMPLICATIONS

• Contralateral renal agenesis in 10%
• Vesicoureteral reflux in 70%
• Hydronephrosis in 56% of ectopic kidney and in 26% of contralateral non-ectopic kidney

—37% due to ureteropelvic junction obstruction
—15% due to ureterovesical junction obstruction
—26% vesicoureteral reflux in ectopic kidney, 60% in contralateral kidney

• Pelvic kidneys may interfere with vaginal delivery in up to one-third of patients.
• Misdiagnosis of a "tumor mass"

DIFFERENTIAL DIAGNOSIS

• Pelvic: opposite sacrum
• Abdominal: above iliac crest
• Cephaloid: subdiaphragmatic
• Thoracic: above diaphragm
• Crossed: contralateral

—With fusion (90%)
—Without fusion (10%)
—Solitary crossed (rare)

• Bilateral crossed (rarest)

 Database

HISTORY

• Usually asymptomatic, unless presents because of infection or stones

PHYSICAL EXAMINATION

• Usually normal
• Occasionally palpable mass

Diagnostic Studies

LABORATORY TESTING

- Usually unremarkable

IMAGING

- Excretory urography

—The pelvic kidney is often difficult to visualize over the bony pelvis.
—The contralateral renal unit may be hypertrophied.

- Ultrasound or CT can usually identify the location of the kidney.
- Any imaging study that demonstrates a unilateral kidney should prompt a search for an ectopic contralateral unit.
- VCUG to rule out reflux (preset in up to 70%)
- A retrograde pyelogram may be necessary to define anatomy.

SPECIAL STUDIES: N/A

 ## Treatment

GENERAL MEASURES

- Normally no treatment necessary unless symptomatic

MEDICAL: N/A

SURGICAL

- In pregnancy, cesarean section may be necessary if the pelvic kidney interferes with delivery.
- Pyeloplasty may be necessary.
- ESWL or endourologic procedure for calculi

ALTERNATIVE THERAPIES: N/A

PATIENT EDUCATION

- Discuss the condition with the patient and family.

 ## Follow-Up

MONITORING

- Periodic ultrasound or KUB to monitor for hydronephrosis or stones

PREVENTION: N/A

 ## Miscellaneous

SYNONYMS: N/A

ASSOCIATED CONDITIONS

- Crossed renal ectopia, horseshoe kidney

NOTES

- See also Section II, "Renal Fusion Abnormalities."

ABBREVIATIONS: N/A

REFERENCES

Gleason PE, et al. Hydronephrosis in renal ectopia: Incidence, etiology and significance. *J Urol* 1994;151:1660–1661.

Kelalis P, King L, Belman B, eds. *Clinical Pediatric Urology,* 3rd ed., vol 1. Philadelphia: WB Saunders. 1992:507–514.

Author: Hyman H. Rabinovitch

Renal Fusion Abnormalities

 Basics

DESCRIPTION

- Congenital joining of the kidneys
- Renal fusion with crossed renal ectopia; the kidney crosses the midline to lie on the side opposite of its UVJ.
- *Horseshoe kidney:* where an isthmus of renal parenchyma or fibrous tissue joins the lower poles (90%) of the two kidneys. It is the most common fusion anomaly.

EPIDEMIOLOGY

- About 1 per 1000 have some type of renal fusion anomaly.
- Crossed renal ectopia about 1 in 7000

—Slight male predominance
—Crossing left to right is more frequent than right to left.

- Horseshoe kidney: 1 to 4 in 1000

—2 to 3× more common in males

GENETICS

- None known

STAGING: N/A

SIGNS AND SYMPTOMS

- Crossed renal ectopia

—Most asymptomatic, occasional abdominal mass
—Many have extraurologic abnormalities, and 65% may exhibit other genitourinary anomalies.

- Horseshoe kidney

—One-third have no symptoms.
—Abdominal pain due to ureteropelvic junction obstruction or calculi

- May have associated gastrointestinal complaints

PATHOPHYSIOLOGY

- Fusion of the two metanephroi occurs early in embryologic development; therefore, the fused kidney rarely ascends out of the pelvis.
- Aberrant blood supply form iliac and lower aorta
- The fused renal mass almost always has two complete collecting systems and ureters.
- Ureters are usually orthotopic, and the pelvis is anteriorly located.

—Ureters must pass over the fused isthmus or fibrous tissue and may become obstructed.
—Ureters can also be obstructed by aberrant vessels.

- Most crossed ectopic kidneys fuse with the contralateral kidney (95%).

—Typically, the ectopic kidney upper pole is fused with the lower pole of the contralateral kidney ("lump" or "pancake kidney").
—Four types of crossed ectopia commonly described:
  —Crossed ectopia with fusion: 85% to 90%
  —Crossed ectopia without fusion: 10%
  —Solitary kidney, crossed ectopia very rare
  —Bilateral (criss-) crossed ectopia (very rare)

CAUSES/RISK FACTORS

- Increased incidence of fusion in

—Trisomy: 18% to 20%
—Turner syndrome: 7% horseshoe kidney
—Neural tube defects

COMPLICATIONS

- Pain
- Obstruction
- Calculi
- Infection

DIFFERENTIAL DIAGNOSIS

- Malrotated kidneys may give the radiographic appearance of horseshoe kidney.

 Database

HISTORY

- Usually no symptoms
- Can have complaints relating to stone or infection
- Symptoms mimicking peptic ulcer or cholelithiasis

PHYSICAL EXAMINATION

- Usually unremarkable
- Occasionally, palpable mass in lower abdomen

Diagnostic Studies

LABORATORY TESTING

- Urinalysis normal unless stone, obstruction, or infection
- Renal function is usually normal.

IMAGING

- Excretory urography: horseshoe kidney

—Horsehoe kidney demonstrates incomplete rotation of the collecting system.
—Reversal of normal calyceal axis (lower pole calyx more medial than upper pole calyx)
—Mild dilation of the pelvis and or ureters can be seen.

- Excretory urography: crossed fused ectopia

—One ureter will cross the midline to empty orthotopically.

- VCUG to evaluate for reflux
- Ultrasound/CT is usually needed to define anatomy and evaluate for mass, if clinically indicated.
- Renal scan to assess function

SPECIAL STUDIES

- Arteriography essential if surgery planned

 ## Treatment

GENERAL MEASURES

- Usually no therapy needed in the absence of symptoms

MEDICAL: N/A

SURGICAL

- Pyeloplasty for UPJ obstruction
- ESWL for urolithiasis

ALTERNATIVE THERAPIES

- Routine division of the isthmus is no longer performed for horseshoe kidney.

PATIENT EDUCATION

- Discuss the condition with the patient and family.

 ## Follow-Up

MONITORING

- KUB and ultrasound

PREVENTION: N/A

 ## Miscellaneous

SYNONYMS

- Crossed fused renal ectopia: "pancake kidney," "lump kidney," "horseshoe kidney"

ASSOCIATED CONDITIONS

- May see increased incidence of skeletal and cardiovascular anomalies

NOTES

- See also Section II, "Renal Ectopia."

ABBREVIATIONS: N/A

Reference

Kelalis P, King L, Belman B, eds. *Clinical Pediatric Urology,* 3rd ed., vol 1. Philadelphia: WB Saunders. 1992:520–527.

Author: Hyman H. Rabinovitch

Renal Infarction

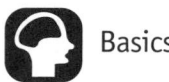 Basics

DESCRIPTION

• Obstruction of blood flow to the kidney or portion of the kidney that results in tissue necrosis

EPIDEMIOLOGY

• Difficult to classify because up to 75% of patients have the incorrect diagnosis made at presentation
• Predominant age: elderly

GENETICS: N/A

STAGING: N/A

SIGNS AND SYMPTOMS

• Nonradiating flank pain
• Abdominal pain
• Nausea and vomiting
• Fever
• Decreased urine output
• Anuria
• Hypertension
• Leukocytosis
• Albuminuria
• Increased serum LDH, AST, ALT

PATHOPHYSIOLOGY

• Acute

—Traumatic: subintimal bleeding due to stretching of the renal artery
—Embolic: complete or partial blockage of renal blood flow, leading to ischemia

• Chronic

—Slow growth of blockage due mostly to atherosclerotic disease associated with increased collateral formation

CAUSES/RISK FACTORS

• Emboli
• Atherosclerosis
• Trauma
• Renal artery thrombosis
• Renal vein thrombosis
• Collagen vascular disease
• Intimal dissection
• Renal artery aneurysm
• Sickle cell disease
• Endocarditis
• Iatrogenic: angiography/angioplasty

COMPLICATIONS

• Azotemia
• Hypertension
• Postinfarction syndrome (leukocytosis, pain, nausea, and vomiting)

DIFFERENTIAL DIAGNOSIS

• Renal calculi
• Pyelonephritis
• Acute abdomen
• Cholecystitis
• Lumbar radiculopathy
• Myocardial infarction

 Database

HISTORY

• Cardiac disease: 90% of patients with renal infarction have underlying cardiac disease.

—Atrial fibrillation
—Prosthetic valves
—Bacterial endocarditis
—Recent myocardial infarction

• Recent trauma?
• Gross hematuria?
• Fever?
• Decreased urine output or anuria?
• Flank pain or renal calculi

PHYSICAL EXAMINATION

• Abdominal pain: rebound or guarding, to distinguish from acute abdomen
• Flank ecchymosis: may suggest trauma
• Abdominal bruit: possible abdominal aortic aneurism or renal artery stenosis

Diagnostic Studies

LABORATORY TESTING

- WBC elevation seen in >70%
- Hematocrit may decrease from trauma.
- Urinalysis

—Hematuria: microscopic seen in 80%
—Albuminuria: 1 to 4+ in >90%

- Creatinine: usually normal in the acute setting
- LDH, ALT, AST: elevated in 100%, 83%, and 66%, respectively

IMAGING

- Computerized tomography: first line for screening

—Can demonstrate obstruction and can distinguish infection from infarction
—Shows the demarcation in a partial infarction
—Can visualize hematoma and collecting system injury. Demonstrates the "cortical rim" sign

- Intravenous pyelography: nonvisualization of the affected side on delayed films. Poor choice in the acute setting if renal infarction is considered
- Ultrasound: can aid in defining obstruction. At present, no role in the acute evaluation

SPECIAL STUDIES

- Angiography: superior to computerized tomography for imaging vascular injury and is the "gold standard" to prove the diagnosis. Can be combined with therapeutic maneuvers (see below).

 Treatment

GENERAL MEASURES

- Recusation and stabilization of the patient
- Timing is of the essence because the warm ischemic time of the human kidney is 1 hour.

MEDICAL

- General supportive measures, including hemodialysis, if needed
- Anticoagulation: if no contraindication. Use heparin 80-U/kg bolus, followed by continuous infusion to maintain the serum partial thromboplastin time at twice normal.

SURGICAL

- Revascularization: if performed rapidly in the appropriate patient
- Prognostic indicators for successful revascularization

—Arteriogram showing well-developed collaterals
—Renin-mediated hypertension
—Normal renal size
—Preexisting atherosclerosis
—Radioisotope uptake by the affected kidney
—Presence of nephrogram on intravenous pyelography

- Young patients who can undergo operation within 6 hours of the time of the injury have potential for a successful outcome, and many authorities believe this group should be treated operatively.
- Patients with bilateral thrombosis or thrombosis of a solitary kidney should have aggressive therapy, including surgery, due to the poor outcome with conservative treatment.

ALTERNATIVE THERAPIES

- Thrombolytic therapy: Administer within a rapid time frame. The most commonly used agents are urokinase, streptokinase, or tissue plasminogen activator. Usually delivered by selective renal infusion to minimize the systemic effects
- Balloon catheter angioplasty

PATIENT EDUCATION: N/A

 Follow-Up

MONITORING

- Monitor anticoagulation.
- Establish diuresis.
- Treat the underlying conditions (i.e., atrial fibrillation).
- Follow long term for hypertension and for stabilization of renal function

PREVENTION

- Chronic anticoagulation for cardiac or thrombotic conditions
- Decrease risk factors for atherosclerosis (i.e., stop smoking).

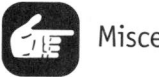 Miscellaneous

SYNONYMS: N/A

ASSOCIATED CONDITIONS: N/A

NOTES

- Infarction secondary to embolism or trauma tends to do poorly with operative intervention, due to poorly formed collaterals, while infarction from thrombosis does better, due to preformed collaterals.

ABBREVIATIONS

- AST, aspartate aminotransferase; ALT, alanine aminotransferase

REFERENCES

Hall SK. Acute renal vascular occlusion, an uncommon mimic. *J Emerg Med* 1993;11:691.

Lang EK, Sullivan J, Frentz G. Renal trauma: Radiologic studies: Comparison of urographic, computerized tomography, angiography and radionuclide studies. *Radiology* 1985;154:1.

Lessman RK, Johnson SF, Coburn JW, et al. Renal artery embolism, clinical features and long term follow-up in 17 cases. *Ann Intern Med* 1978;89:477.

Lumerman JH, Smith AD. Complete and partial renal infarction. *Am Urol Assoc Update* 1997;16:186.

Ouriel K, Andrus CH, et al. Acute renal artery occlusion: When is revascularization justified? *J Vasc Surg* 1987;5:348.

Authors: Jeffrey H. Lumerman and Arthur D. Smith

Renal Oncocytoma

 Basics

DESCRIPTION

• Oncocytoma is a generally benign tumor of the kidney, but it may also occur in the salivary, parathyroid, adrenal, and thyroid (Hurthle-cell) glands.

EPIDEMIOLOGY

• 3% to 7% of renal cortical tumors
• Male:female ratio: 2:1
• Median age is 62; range is 15 to 94 years.
• Bilaterality: 6% of cases
• Multifocality: either unilateral or bilateral; has been coined *oncocytomatosis*

GENETICS

• Most frequent genetic abnormalities

—Loss of chromosome 1p
—Loss of Y chromosome in males

STAGING: N/A

SIGNS AND SYMPTOMS

• Typically asymptomatic and are incidentally found
• Gross or microscopic hematuria, abdominal pain, and flank mass are reported with very low incidence.

PATHOPHYSIOLOGY

• Gross pathology

—Tumors have a well-formed capsule.
—Cross-section demonstrated tan-to-brown without central necrosis or hemorrhage.
—Medium and large tumors may have pathognomonic central stellate scars, which sometimes can be diagnosed on CT, MRI, and occasionally, US.

• Microscopic pathology

—May originate from the distal convoluted renal tubule in contrast to renal cell carcinomas, which arise from proximal convoluted renal tubules
—Characterized by an abundance of mitochondria
—Large polygonal cells with bright granular, eosinophilic cells called "oncocytes"
—Nuclei are uniform.
—Mitoses rare
—Grade I: well-differentiated cells with regular nuclei and abundant cytoplasm
—Grade II: more variation in the nuclei and cytoplasm
—Grade III: degeneration to significant nuclear pleomorphism and possible mitotic activity

• Rare reports of malignant/metastatic oncocytoma

—Unclear if many of these are actually low-grade oncocytic renal cell carcinomas

CAUSES/RISK FACTORS

• Unknown

COMPLICATIONS: N/A

DIFFERENTIAL DIAGNOSIS

• There are no completely reliable clinical or radiographic criteria that distinguish oncocytoma from carcinomas (see also Section I, "Renal Masses—Benign and Malignant").
• Renal cell carcinoma

—Many contain granular cells alone or in combination with spindle cells or clear cells.

• Adenoma
• Angiomyolipoma
• Rhabdoid tumor of the kidney
• Metastatic cancer (e.g., breast, lung, GI tract, lymphoma)

 Database

HISTORY

• None particularly pertinent

PHYSICAL EXAMINATION

• Generally well-appearing individual
• A palpable or ballotable flank mass is rare.

Diagnostic Studies

LABORATORY TESTING

- General laboratory values (CBC, chemistry panel, LFTs) are usually normal.

IMAGING

- Renal ultrasound

—Appear as solid renal mass of variable size and shape

- CT scan and MRI

—May reveal a central stellate scar

- Nuclear renal scan

—Not useful in diagnosis

- Angiography

—Often reveals a lucent rim sign
—Homogenous capillary nephrogram phase
—Absence of wildly aberrant neoplastic vessels
—"Spoke-wheel" pattern of feeding arteries

SPECIAL STUDIES

- Needle aspirations/biopsies

—May be useful when contemplating nephron-sparing surgery
—Reserved for the elderly or poor surgical candidates, to confirm diagnosis

- Antibody studies

—Tumor cells react to cytokeratin antibodies, but not to vimentin antibodies.

- Nuclear morphology (electron microscopy)

—Demonstrates abundant mitochondria with endoplasmic reticulum or Golgi apparatus
—Used to differentiate between a typical renal oncocytoma and low-grade oncocytic renal cell carcinoma

- Flow cytometry

—Has demonstrated aneuploidy and tetraploidy in some cell populations
—Conflicting data make this study an unreliable prognostic indicator.

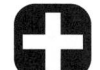 ## Treatment

GENERAL MEASURES

- When diagnosis is unclear, obtain a metastatic work-up.

MEDICAL

- No current medical management exists.

SURGICAL

- Mainstay of treatment: radical nephrectomy

ALTERNATIVE THERAPIES

- Renal-sparing surgery when the preoperative diagnosis is clearly oncocytoma

—Enucleation
—Partial nephrectomy

PATIENT EDUCATION

- Patients should be well informed about the surgical risks, which increase with the size of the tumor.

 ## Follow-Up

MONITORING

- Generally, due to the benign nature of oncocytoma, follow-up is minimized after nephrectomy.
- Exceptions

—Large tumors may have metastatic potential.
—Multifocality
　—Mandates annual surveillance of the contralateral kidney, preferably with renal ultrasound
—Renal-sparing surgery
　—Should have periodic follow-up

- Imaging modalities for follow-up

—Renal ultrasound is the preferred modality, due to less radiation exposure and excellent sensitivity.
—MRI and CT scan are alternate modalities.

PREVENTION

- None known

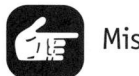 ## Miscellaneous

SYNONYMS: N/A

ASSOCIATED CONDITIONS: N/A

NOTES

- See also Section I, "Renal Masses—Benign and Malignant."

ABBREVIATIONS: N/A

REFERENCES

Lieber M. Renal oncocytoma. *Urol Clin North Am* 1993;20(2):355–359.

Weirich G, Glenn G, Junker K, et al. Familial renal oncocytoma: Clinicopathological study of five families. *J Urol* 1998;160(2).

Authors: J. Bryan Ellsworth, Byron D. Joyner, and J. Brantley Thrasher

Renal Papillary Necrosis

 Basics

DESCRIPTION

- Ischemic necrosis of the renal papillae

EPIDEMIOLOGY

- Female-to-male ratio: 1.1:1.0
- Mean age: 57
- Most are radiographic asymptomatic diagnoses.

GENETICS

- None known

STAGING: N/A

SIGNS AND SYMPTOMS

- Episode of gross hematuria
- Renal colic and flank pain
- Sepsis with ureteral obstruction and infection

PATHOPHYSIOLOGY

- Renal medulla and papilla are vulnerable to ischemic necrosis.

—Relative hypoxia due to slow rate of blood flow in the vasa recta
—Hypertonic environment

CAUSES/RISK FACTORS

- Diabetes mellitus

—Associated vascular disease

- Pyelonephritis
- Sickle cell trait or disease

—Sickling is intensified in a hypoxic hypertonic environment.

- Analgesic abuse, particularly phenacetin

—Concentrated in the kidney, especially the papilla

- Urinary tract obstruction

—Reduces blood flow

- Lupus nephritis
- Wegener's granulomatosis
- Renal artery stenosis
- Idiopathic

COMPLICATIONS

- Ureteral obstruction

—Severe sepsis if infection present

- <5% risk of renal failure

—Comorbidities contribute to risk.

DIFFERENTIAL DIAGNOSIS

- Nephrolithiasis
- Urothelial neoplasms
- See also Section I, "Filling Defect—Upper Urinary Tract."

 Database

HISTORY

- Gross hematuria
- Colicky flank pain

PHYSICAL EXAMINATION

- Costovertebral angle tenderness
- Fevers/chills if infected and obstructed

 Diagnostic Studies

LABORATORY TESTING

- Urinalysis

—Many red blood cells per high power field
—Epithelial cells and casts may be seen.

IMAGING

- Intravenous pyelogram

—Gold standard radiologic examination
—Medullary form of papillary necrosis
—Detachment of necrotic central portion of pyramid tips
—Appears as round or oval cavity
—Papillary form of papillary necrosis
—A larger portion of the entire papilla is necrotic.
—Detachment begins in the region of calyceal fornices.
—Triangle-shaped defect

- Ultrasound is usually not the study of choice.
- CT scan

—Ring shadows in medullae
—Contrast-filled clefts in renal parenchyma
—Renal pelvic filling defects

- Retrograde pyelogram

—Use when renal function is poor.

SPECIAL STUDIES: N/A

Treatment

GENERAL MEASURES

- Adequate oral or intravenous hydration

MEDICAL

- Antibiotics for associated urinary tract infection/pyelonephritis
- Long-term management of diabetes

SURGICAL

- Ureteral catheterization to relieve obstruction
- Percutaneous nephrostomy for immediate decompression in presence of infection
- Ureteroscopic extraction of sloughed papilla

ALTERNATIVE THERAPIES

- Nephrectomy or partial nephrectomy

—Long-term remission is possible because recurrences are usually unilateral.

PATIENT EDUCATION

- Avoid frequent use of nonsteroidal/analgesic medication.
- Strict control of diabetes
- Adequate oral fluid intake

 Follow-Up

MONITORING

- Follow symptoms for relief of flank pain.
—Imaging, if indicated
- Monitor urinalysis.

PREVENTION

- Hydration
- Control diabetes.
- Avoid excessive nonsteroidal medications.

 Miscellaneous

SYNONYMS

- Medullary necrosis, sloughed renal papilla

ASSOCIATED CONDITIONS

- Diabetes, urinary tract infection, pyelonephritis, analgesic abuse, flank pain, hematuria

NOTES

- Essentially a pathologic and radiographic diagnosis

ABBREVIATIONS: N/A

REFERENCES

Griffin MD, Bergstralhn EJ, Larson TS. Renal papillary necrosis: A sixteen-year experience. *J Am Soc Nephrol* 1995;6(2):248–256.

Schaeffer AJ, Del Greco F. Other renal diseases of urologic significance. In: Walsh PC, Retik AB, Stamey TA, Vaughn ED Jr, eds. *Campbell's Urology*, 6th ed. Philadelphia: WB Saunders, 1992:2079–2080.

Segasothy M, Abdul Samad S, Zulfiqar A, Shaariah W, Morad Z, Prasad Menon S. Computed tomography and ultrasonography: A comparative study in the diagnosis of analgesic nephropathy. *Nephron* 1994;66(1):62–66.

Authors: Gregory L. Chen and Demetrius H. Bagley

Renal Sarcomas

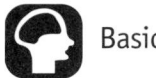 Basics

DESCRIPTION

- Sarcomas of the kidney are rare solid tumors representing less than 1% of all renal malignancies.

—Occur predominantly in children, but may be seen in adults
—Category includes Wilms' tumor, leiomyosarcoma, rhabdomyosarcoma, liposarcoma, fibrosarcoma, renal myxoma, and angiosarcoma, but not sarcomatoid renal cell carcinoma

EPIDEMIOLOGY

- Renal sarcomas: 1% of renal cancers in adults; leiomyosarcoma the most common

—Leiomyosarcomas are more common in women.

- Wilms' tumor: primarily in children, with median age of 3.5 years; 5% to 6% of all neoplasms in children

—Associated with aniridia, hemihypertrophy, and Beckwith-Wiedemann syndrome
—Inherited genetic predisposition in 2% of cases

- No identifiable environmental risk factors in either children or adults

GENETICS

- The inheritance pattern of Wilms' tumor in children follows a two-hit mutational model.
- 30% of Wilms' exhibit loss on 11p; candidate tumor suppressor gene, WT1
- WT1: located at 11p13 close to the region altered in the Beckwith-Wiedemann syndrome
- ? Another Wilms' tumor gene localized to chromosome 1
- Unknown for adult renal sarcomas

STAGING

- Staging system (stages I–IV) established by the National Wilms' Tumor Study Group (NWTSG) and defines role of radiation therapy and chemotherapy for Wilms' tumor patients (see Section II, "Wilms' Tumor")
- Adult renal sarcomas: no staging system

SIGNS AND SYMPTOMS

- Asymptomatic abdominal mass: the most common presentation
- Microhematuria: 25% of children, but gross hematuria is rare in children and adults.
- Signs of vena caval obstruction: varicoceles, hepatomegaly, ascites

PATHOPHYSIOLOGY

- The order of frequency for adult sarcomas is leiomyosarcoma, liposarcoma, and fibrosarcoma, followed by very rare lesions, such as rhabdomyosarcoma and angiosarcoma.
- Often highly cellular and demonstrate many mitoses

- Differentiate adult sarcomas from sarcomatoid renal cell carcinoma by staining for low-molecular-weight cytokeratins.
- Adult mesenchymal tumors: benign cystic nephroma, fibroepithelial polyps, and angiomyolipomas
- Wilms' tumor: categorized into favorable or unfavorable histology, with distinct implications for treatment

—Unfavorable histology: extreme nuclear atypia or anaplasia in more than one region of the tumor or in any extrarenal site

CAUSES/RISK FACTORS

- Specific etiology: unknown
- Risk factors: family history of Wilms' tumor or history of a contralateral renal sarcoma

COMPLICATIONS

- Disseminated disease: lymphatic and pulmonary disease
- Hypertension, erythrocytosis, hypercalcemia, and Cushing syndrome
- Significant bleeding may develop from angiosarcomas.

DIFFERENTIAL DIAGNOSIS

- Child: A renal mass in a child is a Wilms' tumor until proven otherwise (>90% of renal cancer in children).
- Adult: A solid mass may represent a renal cell carcinoma, transitional cell carcinoma, or metastatic lesion.
- A benign angiomyolipoma must be distinguished from a liposarcoma.
- For diagnosis of a primary renal sarcoma in an adult, a metastatic sarcoma must be ruled out, the lesion must arise from the renal parenchyma, and a sarcomatoid variant of renal cell carcinoma must be excluded.

 Database

HISTORY

- Age and sex of the patient

—Wilms' tumor presents earlier in males than in females.
—Mean age of diagnosis of Wilms' tumor: 34.9 months

- Family history
- History of mental retardation or the presence of genitourinary anomalies

—Benign renal hamartomas are associated with tuberous sclerosis in adults.
—Wilms' tumor is associated with hypospadias, cryptorchidism, and pseudohermaphroditism.

- Complaints of abdominal pain, weight loss, pulmonary symptoms

—Acute pain may indicate tumor rupture.
—Shortness of breath may indicate lung metastases or congestive heart failure from IVC obstruction.

PHYSICAL EXAMINATION

- Abdominal palpation for renal mass and contralateral renal unit or hepatomegaly
- Head and neck examination

—Lymphadenopathy or associated macroglossia

- Genitourinary examination

—Identify hypospadias or undescended testes.

 Diagnostic Studies

LABORATORY TESTING

- Serum chemistry: BUN, creatinine, calcium, and liver function studies

—Document function of contralateral renal unit; rule out hypercalcemia.

- Hemoglobin, coagulation studies
- Urinalysis: may demonstrate microhematuria or pyuria

IMAGING

- Abdominal CT or MRI

—Size and local extent of the renal mass, the status of the contralateral renal unit, retroperitoneal adenopathy
—IV contrast with either the CT or MRI is important for imaging the liver for metastatic spread or IVC extension.

- Renal ultrasound: initial diagnosis/differential diagnosis of a cystic renal mass
- A plain chest radiograph is adequate to rule out pulmonary metastases in both adult sarcomas and pediatric Wilms' tumor.
- Metastases to the bone are rare; therefore, a bone scan is not required unless the patient complains of specific bone pain.

SPECIAL STUDIES: N/A

Treatment

GENERAL MEASURES

• The initial therapeutic approach for adult renal sarcomas involves surgical resection after adequate radiologic staging.
• Disease eradication depends on complete extirpation.
• Chemotherapy has failed to alter the natural history of these lesions.
• Combination therapy with radiation and chemotherapy is important only in Wilms' tumor.

MEDICAL

• Vincristine and dactinomycin for 6 months, given as pulse-intensive regimens, are successful for stages II–IV Wilms' tumor in children with a favorable histology.

—Cyclophosphamide is added to the regimen for an unfavorable histology.

• The role of chemotherapy in adult Wilms' tumor is uncertain.
• No effective agents exist for other adult renal sarcomas.

SURGICAL

• Radical nephrectomy with limited regional lymphadenectomy is the standard approach.
• Wide local excision may include a bowel resection or hepatic resection.
• The surgical approach is dictated by the location and size of the lesion in both children and adults.
• A thoracoabdominal incision may be best for adult sarcomas, while a midline incision is appropriate for pediatric Wilms' tumors.
• Avoid tumor spillage in Wilms' tumor, with adequate inspection of the contralateral kidney.

ALTERNATIVE THERAPIES

• No studies of combination chemoradiation followed by surgical excision in adult renal sarcomas
• Current clinical trials for pediatric Wilms' tumor are focused on reduction of treatment intensity for patients with a favorable stage and histology.

PATIENT EDUCATION

• Adult patients should be educated about the guarded prognosis of renal sarcomas, unless discovered at an early stage.

—A majority of patients manifest metastatic disease within 2 years, but late recurrences are known with adult Wilms' tumor.
—The contralateral recurrence rate is unknown, and as such, the other kidney should be followed closely.

• Pediatric patients should expect a greater than 90% cure rate with favorable Wilms' tumors.
• Late tumor recurrence has been documented; therefore, patients should be followed for 5 to 10 years.
• Secondary malignancies may develop in the radiation field after approximately 20 years.
• Contralateral renal function may be altered by chemotherapy, but it is most often only proteinuria.
• The risk of Wilms' tumor in the offspring of survivors is estimated at 2%, and may be greater in patients with bilateral or familial disease.

Follow-Up

MONITORING

• Adults: close follow-up for 2 to 5 years

—Chest radiographs every 3 to 6 months
—Abdominal MRI: best for the remaining renal unit and hepatic recurrence every 3 to 6 months
—No specific tumor markers for renal sarcomas
—Length of follow-up is uncertain, but the contralateral kidney should be examined intermittently for life.

• Pediatric Wilms' tumor: radiologic follow-up as adults

—Children should also be examined for renal dysfunction, endocrinologic abnormalities such as ovarian or testicular failure following radiation therapy, and cardiac dysfunction for 10 to 15 years.

PREVENTION: N/A

Miscellaneous

SYNONYMS

• Kidney cancer, nephroblastoma

ASSOCIATED CONDITIONS

• Wilms' tumor is associated with Beckwith-Wiedemann syndrome, Denys-Drash syndrome, AGR syndrome (aniridia, genitourinary malformations, and mental retardation), hemihypertrophy, and hypospadias.

NOTES

• See also Section II, "Wilms' Tumor."

ABBREVIATIONS: N/A

REFERENCES

Grignon DJ, McIsaac GP, Armstrong RF, Wyatt JK. Primary rhabdomyosarcoma of the kidney. A light microscopic, immunohistochemical, and electron microscopic study. *Cancer* 1998;62:2027–2032.

Hentrich MU, Meister P, Brack NG, Lutz LL, Hartenstein RC. Adult Wilms tumor. *Cancer* 1995;75:545–551.

Tsuda N, Chowdhury PR, Hayashi T, et al. Primary renal angiosarcoma: A case report and review of the literature. *Pathol Int* 1997;47(11):778–783.

Wiener JS, Coppes MJ, Ritchey ML. Current concepts in the biology and management of Wilms Tumor. *J Urol* 1998;159:1316–1325.

Author: Daniel B. Rukstalis

Renal Tubular Acidosis

 Basics

DESCRIPTION

• Renal tubular acidosis (RTA) is a clinical syndrome characterized by a defect in urinary acidification (H+ ion secretion), hypokalemic hyperchloremic nonanion gap metabolic acidosis, increased pH of the urine, and increased predisposition for urinary stone disease. The basic defect lies in the renal tubules, which results in abnormal H+ secretion and urinary acidification. Four major types of RTA:
• Type I, distal
• Type II, proximal
• Type III (mixed)
• Type IV (secondary to diabetic nephropathy and interstitial renal disease)

EPIDEMIOLOGY

• RTA I: more common in adults (two-thirds adults, one-third children) and women; endemic in certain regions of Thailand
• RTA II: usually associated with Fanconi syndrome; urinary loss of glucose, amino acids, uric acid, phosphate, and bicarbonates

GENETICS

• RTA I: usually sporadic or secondary to other systemic/renal disorders; autosomal dominant variant rare
• Familial RTA usually occurs in childhood; sporadic and secondary RTA I occurs at any age.

STAGING: N/A

SIGNS AND SYMPTOMS

• Hypokalemic hyperchloremic metabolic acidosis, urinary pH of 5.5 or more, and nephrocalcinosis and/or nephrolithiasis
• Some patients may present with hypokalemic paralysis, vomiting, diarrhea, failure to thrive (in children), and associated Fanconi syndrome (type II).

PATHOPHYSIOLOGY

• Type I (distal) tubular acidosis: Distal nephrons are unable to maintain a proton gradient due to the permeability defect, the proton pump secretory defect, the voltage dependent defect, and carbonic anhydrase deficiency. There is a normal capacity to reabsorb filtered bicarbonate, but urinary pH is consistently above 6.0.
• Type II (proximal) tubular defect: Proximal tubules are unable to reabsorb bicarbonate.
• Type III tubular acidosis: mixed defect
• Type IV: usually secondary to diabetic nephropathy and interstitial renal disease

CAUSES/RISK FACTORS

• Genetic
• Secondary to obstructive uropathy, pyelonephritis, acute tubular necrosis, analgesic nephropathy, renal transplantation, sarcoidosis, idiopathic hypercalcemia and primary hyperparathyroidism, diabetic nephropathy, and sometimes in association with Fanconi syndrome (Type II)

COMPLICATIONS

• Nephrocalcinosis, nephrolithiasis, metabolic acidosis, and failure to thrive (in children)

DIFFERENTIAL DIAGNOSIS

• Other causes of metabolic acidosis
• Calcium phosphate stones
• Recurrent stones: >2 per year
• Bilateral stones
• Medullary nephrocalcinosis
• Medullary sponge kidney
• Hypocitraturia <0.5 mmol/24 h
• Hypokalemia
• Chronic pyelonephritis
• Azotemia

 Database

HISTORY

• History of hematuria, urinary tract infections, passage of stones in urine
• History of recurrent, familial, or childhood renal stone disease
• Ask about diabetes mellitus, sarcoidosis, obstructive uropathy, renal transplantation, and analgesic abuse.

PHYSICAL EXAMINATION

• Urologic examination of genitalia, suprapubic area for swelling and tenderness
• Examination for osteomalacia, hypokalemic muscle weakness, and growth retardation
• Examination for other renal and systemic diseases, such as renal failure, diabetes, sarcoidosis, primary parathyroidism, etc.

Diagnostic Studies

LABORATORY TESTING

• Blood: renal function test, electrolytes, blood gases: for hypokalemic, hyperchloremic, nonanion gap metabolic acidosis
• Urine pH (fasting, under oil, pH meter)

—pH of more than 5.5: complete type I RTA
—pH more than 5.5, but systemic acidosis mild or absent: ammonium chloride loading test and measure urinary bicarbonates; pH does not decrease to less than 5.5: incomplete type I RTA
—If bicarbonaturia present: bicarbonate loading test; if fractional excretion of bicarbonate 15% at normal serum bicarbonate: type II RTA
—Hyperkalemia: type IV RTA

IMAGING

• Plain x-ray: for nephrocalcinosis and nephrolithiasis
• Intravenous pyelogram: for stone, medullary sponge kidney, papillary necrosis, nephrocalcinosis, obstructive uropathy

SPECIAL STUDIES

• Ammonium chloride loading test for incomplete type I RTA
• Bicarbonate loading test for type II RTA
• Stone analysis

 ## Treatment

GENERAL MEASURES

• Identifiable causes, such as obstructive uropathy or drug-induced RTA, should be corrected or eliminated.
• If there is no identifiable etiology, then direct treatment to correction of acidosis.

MEDICAL

• Alkali therapy decreases stone formation and growth, prevents nephrocalcinosis, normalizes growth retardation in children, and corrects hypokalemia in most cases.
• Oral alkali therapy in the form of potassium bicarbonate or citrate in both type I and type II RTA with the goal of treatment to restore urinary citrate to high-normal levels, and not simply correct the metabolic acidosis
• Type I (distal) RTA treatment is generally lifelong.

—1 to 2 mmol/kg/d of oral bicarbonate or citrate in 2 to 3 divided doses in adults
—2 to 3 mmol/kg/d in children

• Type II (proximal) RTA

—The dosage of alkali required may be as high as 15 mmol/kg/d due to the severe bicarbonate wasting.
—Adults with bicarbonate levels >10 mEq/mL and no evidence of bone disease may not require treatment.
—Supplemental potassium, vitamin D, and phosphate may become necessary.

• Type IV RTA treatment is directed toward correction of hyperkalemia rather than acidosis.

—Dietary potassium restriction
—Thiazide or loop diuretics
—Mineralocorticoid replacement in cases of adrenal disease or hyporeninemia (fludrocortisone 0.1 mg/d)

SURGICAL

• Management of stone by lithotripsy, percutaneous nephrolithotomy, and, rarely, open surgery

ALTERNATIVE THERAPIES: N/A

PATIENT EDUCATION: N/A

 ## Follow-Up

MONITORING

• Spot urine testing for NAG (N-acetyl-β-D-glucosaminidase) has eliminated the need for 24-hour urine collection.

—Levels increased secondary to renal tubular cell damage and hypercalciuria

• Urinary calcium excretion

—Should be kept below 0.05 mmol/kg/d in infants and children

• Potassium levels should be monitored during alkali therapy and replaced appropriately.

PREVENTION

• See above.

 ## Miscellaneous

SYNONYMS: N/A

ASSOCIATED CONDITIONS

• See above.

NOTES: N/A

ABBREVIATIONS

• RTA, renal tubular acidosis; NAG, N-acetyl-β-D-glucosaminidase

REFERENCES

Kinkead TM, Menon M. Renal tubular acidosis. AUA Update Series, Vol. XIV, Lesson 7, 1995.

Menon M, Parulkar BG, Drach GW. Urinary lithiasis: Etiology, diagnosis, and medical treatment. In: Walsh PC, Retik AB, Vaughan ED, Wein AJ, eds. *Campbell's Urology,* 7th ed. Philadelphia: WB Saunders, 1998.

Pohlman T, Hruska KA, Menon M. Renal tubular acidosis. *J Urol* 1984;132:431.

Authors: Javid Javidan, Ashutosh Tewari, and Mani Menon

Renal Vein Thrombosis

 Basics

DESCRIPTION

• Renal vein thrombosis (RVT) is acute or chronic blood clot in one or both renal veins. May extend into the vena cava

EPIDEMIOLOGY

• Newborns and infants: commonly associated with asphyxia, dehydration, shock and sepsis; usually acute and unilateral; 30% bilateral

—Male-to-female ratio: 2:1 in the neonate, with no sex predisposition beyond age 1

• Adults: associated with nephrotic syndrome, renal carcinoma, oral contraceptives, steroids, or renal transplantation; usually chronic and unilateral

GENETICS: N/A

STAGING: N/A

SIGNS AND SYMPTOMS

• Infant: severe illness typical, occasional colicky pain

—60% enlarged kidneys on physical examination; gross hematuria and microangiopathic hemolytic anemia and thrombocytopenia

• Adult: depends on onset of RVT

—Acute RVT: sudden flank pain, costovertebral angle tenderness, and gross hematuria
—Chronic RVT: generally asymptomatic; proteinuria and microscopic or gross hematuria

PATHOPHYSIOLOGY

• Newborn: diminished intrarenal blood flow due to hypovolemia (sepsis, dehydration, diarrhea)

—Initiates thrombosis of the intrarenal venous radicles. Both antegrade and retrograde spread results in RVT.
—May become bilateral, produce vena caval occlusion and renal artery thrombosis
—65% in neonates, 30% beyond 1 year of age

• Adults: most often unilateral; acute and chronic forms

—Acute: severe hydration, sudden hypercoagulability, renal vein obstruction from tumor or transplant rejection
—Chronic: nephrotic syndrome (most often membranous glomerulonephritis)
  —Slow onset allows the development of collateral venous kidney drainage; therefore, symptoms are rare.
—Nephrotic syndrome: alterations in coagulation system that favors thrombosis
  —RVT in the nephrotic syndrome: 5% to 62%
  —RVT highest in nephrotic syndrome due to membranous nephropathy; however, membranoproliferative glomerulonephritis, lipoid nephrosis, and amyloidosis have also been associated with high rates of RVT.

CAUSES/RISK FACTORS

• Infants

—Dehydration: diarrhea, vomiting, and shock
—Maternal diabetes, polyhydramnios, and toxemia
—Cyanotic congenital heart disease with resultant polycythemia
—Performance of angiocardiography
—Acute hypoxia, birth trauma
—Sickle cell disease
—Cytomegalovirus

• Adults

—Nephrotic syndrome
—Trauma shock, sepsis, dehydration
—Oral contraceptives, steroids
—Renal transplantation, particularly in patients receiving treatment with OKT-3 and cyclosporine
—Abdominal tumors, especially renal cell carcinoma
—Use of angiographic contrast agents

COMPLICATIONS

• The kidney may recover completely, atrophy to a small scarred kidney, or recover partially, resulting in renovascular hypertension or chronic tubular dysfunction.
• Nephrectomy may be required if renovascular hypertension or chronic infection develops.
• Consumptive coagulopathy, pulmonary embolism

DIFFERENTIAL DIAGNOSIS

• Hemolytic–uremic syndrome
• Hydronephrosis, urolithiasis
• Renal cystic disease
• Wilms' tumor
• Abscess
• Hematoma

 Database

HISTORY

• Infant

—Risk factors: mother's history, birth, and early postnatal course
—Gross hematuria

• Adult

—Risk factors should be explored.
—Sudden onset of hematuria and flank pain should raise the question of renal vein thrombosis, as should a history of nephrotic syndrome in the presence of hematuria.

PHYSICAL EXAMINATION

• Infant

—Unilateral, or often bilateral, flank masses. Evidence of dehydration and cyanotic heart disease

• Adult

—Evidence of blunt trauma, abdominal mass
—Edema suggestive of nephrosis

Diagnostic Studies

LABORATORY TESTING

- Infants

—Thrombocytopenia, leukocytosis, hemolytic anemia
—Consumptive coagulopathy (prolonged clotting time, elevated fibrinogen and fibrin split products)
—Proteinuria
—Elevated BUN and creatinine

- Adult

—Proteinuria and microscopic hematuria
—Hemolytic anemia, consumptive coagulopathy, and thrombocytopenia may be present.
—Elevated BUN and creatinine; hypoalbuminemia

IMAGING

- Infant

—Ultrasonography: diffuse renal enlargement, nonspecific renal echo patterns, and thrombosis within the renal vein
—IVP (if performed): delayed opacification and renomegaly
—A renal scan may be obtained to assess the function of the involved kidney.
—The extent of thrombus may be assessed by duplex ultrasonography, and only rarely will CT, MRI, or renal venography be required for confirmation of the diagnosis or determination of the extent of thrombus.

- Adult

—IVP: faint or absent excretion of contrast and congested, enlarged kidney due to congestion
  —Collateral circulation causes the collecting system opacification to varying degrees.
  —The renal pelvis is usually stretched, distorted, and blurred, occasionally leading to confusion with polycystic disease.
  —Notching of the ureter: collateral circulation
—Complete nonfunction may require retrograde pyelography that demonstrates a compressed, stretched, and distorted collecting system.
—Inferior vena cavography with selective catheterization of the renal vein is the gold standard for the diagnosis.
—Duplex ultrasonography is helpful, especially in the transplanted kidney.
—MRI: excellent imaging; avoids contrast MRI; CT findings are similar in noninvasive evaluation of acute RVT.
  —Object of low attenuation within the renal vein and/or inferior vena cava and proximal venous enlargement
  —Capsular venous collaterals, thickened Gerota's fascia and pericapsular stranding

SPECIAL STUDIES: N/A

 ## Treatment

GENERAL MEASURES

- Evaluate and treat all underlying causes.
- Aggressive rehydration and treatment of sepsis, diarrhea, and electrolyte abnormalities

MEDICAL

- Infants

—Thrombolytic agents (urokinase/streptokinase) reported but controversial
—Acute renal failure: peritoneal dialysis as necessary
—Systemic heparinization: prevents thrombus propagation into inferior vena cava (risk of propagation low with fluid and electrolyte repletion)

- Adults

—Unilateral RVT: heparin anticoagulation and long-term anticoagulation with warfarin
  —The optimum duration of anticoagulation therapy is unknown; many believe that anticoagulation should be continued until the chronic state of dehydration is reversed, as evidenced by maintenance of serum albumin levels above 2.5 g/L.
—Acute clot dissolution (streptokinase/urokinase), systemically or with selective renal vein infusion, may be useful, especially in RVT of a renal transplant.

SURGICAL

- Infants: no role for surgical thrombectomy in infants

- Adults

—Rarely used, because neither renal preservation nor improved survival documented
—Surgical thrombectomy may be theoretically useful in patients with acute bilateral RVT who are not expected to survive, especially if pulmonary emboli occur despite anticoagulation therapy.

ALTERNATIVE THERAPIES: N/A

PATIENT EDUCATION: N/A

 ## Follow-Up

MONITORING

- Infants

—Renal function may be followed, using nuclear scanning.
—Monitor blood pressure, because renovascular hypertension may occur after RVT, even with normal renal function.

- Adults

—Treat nephrotic syndrome.
—Because RVT may be asymptomatic, all patients with nephrotic syndrome should be monitored for the development of RVT-related hypertension and hematuria.

PREVENTION

- Adults

—Long-term anticoagulation seems appropriate, as RVT has recurred when patients discontinued anticoagulation.

 ## Miscellaneous

SYNONYMS: N/A

ASSOCIATED CONDITIONS: N/A

NOTES

- See Section II, "Nephrotic Syndrome."

ABBREVIATIONS: N/A

REFERENCE

Llach F, Nikakhtar B. Renal thromboembolism, atheroembolism, and renal vein thrombosis. In: Schrier RW, Gottschalk CW, eds. *Diseases of the Kidney,* 6th ed. 1997:1903–1913.

Author: James L. Mohler

Renovascular Hypertension

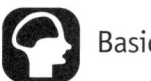 Basics

DESCRIPTION

- *Hypertension* (in adults) is defined by the World Health Organization as systolic BP >160 and/or diastolic BP >95.
- Repeated BP readings prior to evaluation
- Practical definition for renovascular RVH

—Correction of renal artery lesion, which relieves HTN
—The presence of renal arterial lesion alone does not define RVH.

EPIDEMIOLOGY

- 95% of HTN is essential.
- 3% to 5% of HTN is surgically correctable.
- RVH most common surgically correctable lesion
- Present in 2% of hypertensive population

GENETICS: N/A

STAGING: N/A

SIGNS AND SYMPTOMS

- HTN coexisting with

—Vascular insufficiency to other organs (e.g., carotid or coronary artery disease)
—Headaches, dizziness, palpitations, easy fatigability

- Symptoms of hypokalemia (muscle weakness, tetany, polyuria) and metabolic alkalosis
- Retinopathy (hemorrhages, exudates, or papilledema)
- Abdominal, flank, or carotid bruits

PATHOPHYSIOLOGY

- Two major pathologic entities: atherosclerosis and fibromuscular disease
- Atherosclerosis

—In 60% to 70%; intimal plaques; usually in proximal 2 cm
—Begins as smooth muscle proliferation
—Forms rounded mound in lumen with lipid deposition, necrosis, inflammation, and plaque formation
—Predominantly in males, older age groups progressive in 40%
—Attention to concurrent carotid and coronary atherosclerosis

- Fibromuscular disease

—In 30% to 40%; occurs in distal two-thirds, may be in segmental renal artery
—Intimal fibroplasia
  —Progressive intimal collagenous disease in children and young adults
—True fibromuscular hyperplasia
  —Progressive hyperplasia of smooth muscle and fibrous tissue
  —In children and young adults
  —Angiographically indistinguishable from intimal fibroplasia

—Medial fibroplasia
  —Most common fibrous lesion (75%–80%)
  —Typically in women, 20 to 50 years old
  —Fibrous rings with aneurysmal dilatation interspersed
  —Characteristic "string of beads" angiographic appearance
  —Rarely progresses after age 40
—Perimedial (subadventitial) fibroplasia
  —In young women
  —Dense collagen collar beneath vascular adventitia
  —Progressive, renal artery only; right more common than left
—Miscellaneous
  —Renal artery aneurysm, dissection, and embolism
  —Seen in diverse clinical settings

- Normal physiology

—Renin–angiotensin–aldosterone system is major hormonal system
—Regulates systemic BP and sodium/potassium balance
—Renin released by juxtaglomerular apparatus in response to
  —Baroreceptor mechanism at afferent arteriole: Increased pressure decreases renin.
  —Macula densa mechanism at distal tubule: Decreased salt intake increases plasma renin.
  —Beta-adrenergic receptor mechanism: Increased renin release from nerve stimulation is blocked by the beta-adrenergic blocker.
  —Cytosolic calcium and cAMP act as second messengers.
—Renin acts on angiotensinogen to produce angiotensin I (AI).
—AI converted to angiotensin II (AII) by angiotensin converting enzyme (ACE) in lung, plasma, and vascular endothelium
—AII acts as a direct vasoconstrictor.
  —Affects sodium and volume balance
  —Causes adrenal aldosterone release
—Aldosterone promotes tubular sodium reabsorption and potassium excretion.

- Pathophysiology

—Goldblatt HTN model (two types)
—The two-kidney, one-clip model reflects human renovascular HTN.
  —The pressure gradient across the affected renal artery causes increased renin secretion from and decreased renal blood flow to the damaged kidney.
  —Absent renin from opposite kidney
  —Elevated BP from AII vasoconstriction
—One-kidney, one-clip: volume expansion, normal or low renin
  —HTN unresponsive to ACE-inhibitors and AII antagonists, unless sodium depleted
  —20% of patients with RAS cured by angioplasty have normal plasma renin.
  —BP normalization from increased GFR and "pressure natriuresis"

CAUSES/RISK FACTORS

- Cigarette smoking

—Present in 74% of fibromuscular dysplasia and 88% of atherosclerosis
—Risk factor for atherosclerosis

- Genetic factors for fibromuscular dysplasia

COMPLICATIONS

- Cardiac disease: angina, myocardial infarct
- Retinal effects: blurred vision, scotomata, blindness
- Central nervous system dysfunction: dizziness, vertigo, tinnitus, syncope, cerebrovascular accident, encephalopathy
- Renal disease: mild azotemia to renal failure

DIFFERENTIAL DIAGNOSIS

- Essential HTN
- Renal parenchymal HTN
- Endocrine HTN (primary aldosteronism, Cushing syndrome, pheochromocytoma, oral contraceptive induced)

Database

HISTORY

- No pathognomonic clinical features
- HTN often in absence of family history of HTN
- Age of onset >45 years or <25 years
- Abrupt onset of moderate/severe HTN

—Absence of "labile phase" of essential HTN

- Development of severe or malignant HTN

—Usually BP >200/140; defined by papilledema, with retinal hemorrhages and/or exudates

- Headaches

—Typically occipital; more common than in essential HTN

- Cigarette smoking commonly associated with atherosclerosis and fibromuscular dysplasia
- Uncommon in Black race
- Good BP control with ACE inhibitors, and resistance or escaped control with diuretics or anti-adrenergics
- Flash pulmonary edema with bilateral renovascular disease
- Azotemia with bilateral disease
- Associated cardiac or carotid vascular disease

PHYSICAL EXAMINATION

- Retinopathy: papilledema, hemorrhages, exudates (secondary to focal spasm and narrowing of retinal vessels)
- Abdominal/flank bruits

—However, also present in normal elderly and some younger adults with no renovascular disease

 Diagnostic Studies

LABORATORY TESTING

- Serum electrolytes, blood urea nitrogen, and creatinine

—Hypokalemia (due to secondary hyperaldosteronism) is present in only 20%.
—Azotemia, especially with bilateral disease

- Peripheral plasma renin activity (PRA)

—Collect at noon after 4 hours of ambulation and off medications.
—Index against urinary sodium excretion
—20% false-negative result
—16% of essential HTN patients with elevated PRA
—May be impossible for patient to stop medications, i.e., invalidating test

- Differential split renal function studies

—Historical test
—Performed with infusion of inulin or para-aminohippuric acid and antidiuretic hormone during a diuresis
—Performed if unilateral parenchymal disease with isotopic renal scan

- Single-dose captopril test

—ACE inhibitor induces fall in BP and rise in PRA
—RVH patients treated with a beta-blocker still respond as above.
—Patients stop all medications except beta-blockers for 2 weeks.
—Remain on normal sodium diet
—Given 25 mg captopril (crushed and dissolved) after baseline PRA and BP
—In supine or semirecumbent position
—BP monitored for 1 hour, then final PRA measured
—Positive result
  —Post-captopril PRA >12 ng/mL/h
  —Absolute renin increase >10 ng/mL/h
  —400% or 150% renin increase if baseline PRA <3 ng/mL/h or >3 ng/mL/h, respectively

IMAGING

- Intravenous urogram

—Delayed calyceal uptake most reliable abnormality in RVH
—False-positive 13%, false negative 22%: unreliable and abandoned for diagnosis of RVH

- Radionuclide renogram

—Variability in results; unreliable for RVH

- Digital subtraction angiography

—Computer-assisted angiography
—5% to 20% not interpretable
—Requires good patient compliance
—Requires central venous access and large volume of contrast
—Sensitivity and specificity inferior to conventional angiography
—Can be performed in conjunction with renal vein renin sampling

- Captopril renogram

—ACE-I administration reduces RBF and GFR in the kidney with RAS.
—Isotope renogram performed before and after ACE-I given
—Acceptable sensitivity (67%–96%) and specificity (41%–100%) for RVH
—Prolonged time to maximal activity most common positive test criteria
—Less accurate if azotemia or bilateral RAS
—Differential renal vein renin levels still gold standard
—If high clinical risk and positive captopril renogram
  —May proceed to arteriography (without selective renal vein renin levels)

- Doppler ultrasound angiography

—Duplex scanning with B-mode ultrasound and Doppler
—Measures blood flow velocity
—Used to detect RAS; follow for progression and monitor after treatment.
—High-grade RAS correlates with
  —Peak systolic velocity 180 to 210 cm/s
  —Ratio to peak aortic velocity (>3.5)
  —Remains technically demanding and operator dependent
  —May be unsuccessful with obese patient or secondary to overlying bowel gas

- Spiral computed tomographic angiography

—Data obtained in single breath-hold
—Role undetermined
—Need for potentially nephrotoxic contrast agent
  —RVH patients with coexisting renal compromise

- Magnetic resonance angiography

—Measures absolute flow, GFR, tissue diffusion and perfusion
—Images vessels 1 to 2 mm in diameter
—Nephrotoxic contrast agent not necessary

SPECIAL STUDIES: N/A

(continued)

Renovascular Hypertension (continued)

 Treatment

GENERAL MEASURES

- Renovascular disease is progressive.
- Both HTN and progressive renal loss must be managed.

—Management, therefore, differs from that for essential HTN.

MEDICAL

- Indicated for patients awaiting definitive treatment, failing treatment, refusing treatment, or too ill for intervention.
- ACE-inhibitors, beta-adrenergic blockers, calcium channel blockers, or angiotensin receptor blockers may be used.
- ACE-inhibitors may cause irreversible progressive renal failure.
- Especially in bilateral disease or in patients with a solitary kidney; indicated for RVH secondary to atherosclerosis

—Study coronary and carotid arteries preoperatively

- Calcium channel blockers induce afferent arteriolar dilation.

—Preserve GFR when used with ACE-inhibitors.

SURGICAL

- Indications for surgery

—Poor HTN control after aggressive medical therapy
—Poor medical compliance
—Total renal artery occlusion/dissection
—Progressive loss of renal function
—Failure of PTRA
—Considerations in atherosclerosis
  —Study coronary and carotid arteries preoperatively.

- Bypass procedures

—Aortorenal, hepatorenal, splenorenal
  —Avoid the aorta for bypass if significant aortic disease exists.
  —Artificial graft (Dacron), autogenous artery (splenic, hypogastric), and autogenous saphenous vein as graft material

- Endarterectomy

—Especially for RAS secondary to occlusive atherosclerosis
  —Transaortic or renal approach

- Partial nephrectomy/nephrectomy

—When revascularization not technically feasible

- Cure and improvement of HTN and renal function in approximately 70% to 90%

ALTERNATIVE THERAPIES

- Percutaneous transluminal renal angioplasty (PTRA)

—Treatment of choice for mural dysplasia
—Approximately 90% success rate
—Variable response for atherosclerotic lesions
  —Best in short, nonostial lesions
  —Restenosis in 25% to 60% (nonostial) and 40% to 70% (ostial)

- Renal artery stenting

—Limited long-term follow-up
—Indicated for ostial lesions, not entirely open after angioplasty, intimal tear
  —84% cure of primary occlusion at 5 years in one study
  —BP improved in 60% and renal function improved or stabilized in 60% in another small series
  —Restenosis occurs by neointimal hyperplasia.
  —Randomized trials needed, with measurement of early and late restenosis rates

- Angioinfarction

—Patient resistant to medical therapy (minimal renal function, too ill for intervention)

PATIENT EDUCATION: N/A

Follow-Up

MONITORING

- BP and renal function
—Serum creatinine and GFR
- Follow-up angiography
—Early and late restenosis occurs between 6 and 48 months.

PREVENTION

- Cessation of cigarette smoking

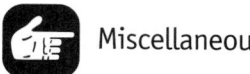 Miscellaneous

SYNONYMS: N/A

ASSOCIATED CONDITIONS

- Coexistent carotid, coronary, or aortic disease in atherosclerosis; progressive renal loss with HTN

NOTES

- RAS is not tantamount to renovascular HTN.
- See also Section I, "Hypertension—Urologic Considerations."

ABBREVIATIONS

- ACE, angiotensin converting enzyme; AI, angiotensin I; AII, angiotensin II; HTN, hypertension; PRA, plasma renin activity; PTRA, percutaneous transluminal renal angioplasty; RAS, renal artery stenosis; RBF, renal blood flow; RVH, renovascular hypertension

REFERENCES

Calligaro KD, Dougherty MJ, Dean RH. *Modern Management of Renovascular Hypertension and Renal Salvage.* Baltimore: Williams & Wilkins, 1996.

Libertino JA. Renovascular surgery. In: Walsh PC, Retik AB, Vaughan ED, Wein AJ, eds. *Campbell's Urology,* 7th ed. Philadelphia: WB Saunders, 1997.

Vaughan ED Jr, Sosa RE. Renovascular hypertension. In: Walsh PC, Retik AB, Vaughan ED, Wein AJ, eds. *Campbell's Urology,* 7th ed. Philadelphia: WB Saunders, 1997.

Authors: Michael R. Bernstein and S. Bruce Malkowicz

Retroperitoneal Abscess

 Basics

DESCRIPTION

• An abscess in the retroperitoneal space, with the following boundaries: superiorly, the diaphragm; inferiorly, the pelvic diaphragm; anteriorly, the parietal peritoneum; and posteriorly, the investing fascia of posterior body wall muscles (iliacus, psoas, quadratus lumborum, and transversalis muscles)

EPIDEMIOLOGY

• 0.9 to 4.0 cases per 10,000 hospital admissions

GENETICS: N/A

STAGING: N/A

SIGNS AND SYMPTOMS

• Fever, chills
• Generalized malaise, anorexia, weight loss
• Diffuse abdominal pain
• Tachycardia, tachypnea

PATHOPHYSIOLOGY

• Produced by pyogenic bacteria generally and fungi occasionally

—Common: *E. coli*, *Proteus*, and *Staphylococcus aureus*

• Starts as a focal accumulation of neutrophils in a space created by liquefactive necrosis of the native cells in the tissue
• May expand due to progressive necrosis of surrounding cells; may become walled off by connective tissue (barrier to further spread)

CAUSES/RISK FACTORS

• Causes

—GU: renal/perirenal infection
—GI: appendicitis, enteritis/colitis, pancreatic abscess, diverticulitis, GI malignancies
—TB, osteomyelitis, epidural abscess with extension

• Risk factors that contribute to abscess formation

—GU: urolithiasis, UTI, urinary tract obstruction, polycystic kidney disease, renal/ureteral surgery
—Diabetes mellitus
—GI surgery
—Retroperitoneal hematoma

COMPLICATIONS

• Fistula to skin, bowel, or chest (empyema)
• Sepsis/septic shock
• Death

DIFFERENTIAL DIAGNOSIS

• Retroperitoneal hematoma
• Retroperitoneal urinoma
• Retroperitoneal tumor, primary or secondary
• Retroperitoneal fibrosis

 Database

HISTORY

• Previous urologic disease?

—UTI, nephrolithiasis, urinary tract obstruction, polycystic kidney disease, renal or ureteral surgery, trauma (especially penetrating trauma) to urinary tract

• Gastrointestinal conditions?

—Inflammatory diseases such as appendicitis, enteritis, pancreatitis, diverticulitis
—Malignancies, GI surgery, GI trauma?

• Other associated conditions?

—Diabetes mellitus immunosuppression, TB, osteomyelitis, retroperitoneal bleeding

PHYSICAL EXAMINATION

• Flank and/or costovertebral angle tenderness
• Lower abdominal, groin, and/or upper thigh tenderness (due to irritation to retroperitoneal nerves)
• Pleuritic chest pain (due to irritation of diaphragm)
• Positive psoas sign (increased abdominal pain on patient raising the thigh against the examiner's hand), suggesting irritation of the psoas muscle

 Diagnostic Studies

LABORATORY TESTING

• CBC: leukocytosis (absolute neutrophil count >10,000/(L), anemia (hemoglobin <14 g/dL in adult males or <12 in adult females)
• Sedimentation rate: elevation (>15 mm/h in males or >20 mm/h in females if age <50 years; >20 mm/h in men or >30 mm/h in women if age >50 years)
• Urine: urinalysis (pyuria or hematuria)
• Urine culture and sensitivity

IMAGING

• Abdominal plain film: obliteration of psoas muscle border on affected side, displacement of bowel gas and/or kidney, ileus, perinephric gas
• Ultrasonography: gas and fluid collection(s)
• IVP: poor or nonfunctioning renal unit, ureteral dilation and/or deviation
• CT (most sensitive radiographic study): air–fluid levels within retroperitoneum

SPECIAL STUDIES

• Ultrasound or CT-guided needle aspiration

Treatment

GENERAL MEASURES

• Promptness in diagnosis is necessary to prevent significant morbidity and mortality.
• Definitive therapy: antibiotics in combination with drainage

MEDICAL

• Antibiotic therapy: broad-spectrum coverage prior to percutaneous or open surgical drainage

—Choice based on culture and sensitivity of abscess specimen (most common organisms: *E. coli, Proteus,* and *S. aureus*)
—Continue until there is resolution of all systemic signs of sepsis; therapy usually fails without drainage.

SURGICAL

• Indications

—Large abscess(es)
—Percutaneous drainage option with high risk and/or low chance of success (e.g., in cases with large multiloculated abscess or in those with thick, purulent material)
—Recurrence after percutaneous drainage
—Presence of nonfunctioning kidney with nephrectomy planned
—Presence of pancreatic or carcinomatous abscess or associated bowel fistula

• Approaches include flank, anterior (subcostal or midline), and posterior (dorsal lumbotomy); the extraperitoneal route is preferable.
• Obtain abscess specimens for Gram stain and aerobic and anaerobic culture and sensitivity studies.
• Thoroughly explore, debride, and irrigate the abscess cavity, and use drain(s) such as the Penrose drain, communicating the abscess cavity to the exterior.

ALTERNATIVE THERAPIES

• Percutaneous drainage (ultrasound or CT-guided) with placement of indwelling catheter communicating with abscess collection: more effective for small, nonloculated abscess

PATIENT EDUCATION: N/A

 Follow-Up

MONITORING

• Repeat imaging (ultrasound or CT) to assess the retroperitoneum after initial percutaneous or open surgical drainage is necessary within a few days (time interval dependent on clinical status).
• Drains are left in place until both of the following occur: external drainage stops/becomes clear and collapse of abscess cavity is documented on imaging.

PREVENTION

• Early intervention/management and/or close monitoring of predisposing conditions such as renal/perirenal infections, obstructive uropathy, nephrolithiasis, GI inflammatory diseases, etc.

 Miscellaneous

SYNONYMS: N/A

ASSOCIATED CONDITIONS

• See Causes/Risk Factors in "Basics" section.

NOTES

• Once multiple organ system failure occurs, overall mortality of retroperitoneal abscess remains >50% despite aggressive therapy. See also Section I, "Retroperitoneal Mass."

ABBREVIATIONS: N/A

REFERENCES

Craig MC, et al. Diseases of the retroperitoneum. In: Gillenwater JY, Grayhack JT, Howards SS, Duckett JW, eds. *Adult and Pediatric Urology,* 3rd ed. St. Louis: Mosby, 1996.

Knol JA, et al. Inguinal anatomy and abdominal wall hernias. In: Greenfield LJ, et al., eds. *Surgery: Scientific Principles and Practice.* Philadelphia: Lippincott-Raven, 1997.

Shaff MI, et al. Computed tomography and magnetic resonance imaging of the acute abdomen. *Surg Clin North Am* 1988;68:233.

Wittmann DH, et al. Peritonitis and intraabdominal infection. In: Schwartz SI, et al., eds. *Principles of Surgery.* New York: McGraw-Hill, 1994.

Authors: Thomas H.S. Hsu and Inderbir S. Gill

Retroperitoneal Fibrosis

 Basics

DESCRIPTION

• Retroperitoneal fibrosis (RPF) is characterized by encasement of the retroperitoneal structures, with extensive woody fibrous tissue and subacute inflammation. It usually exhibits a perivascular distribution, involving the aorta and inferior vena cava as well ureters and psoas muscle. Severe cases of RPF may involve the intestinal mesentery, portal/hepatic system, diaphragm, or iliac vessels.

EPIDEMIOLOGY

• 2:1 male-to-female predominance
• RPF most common in fifth to sixth decades; can be seen at any age

GENETICS

• Unknown

STAGING: N/A

SIGNS AND SYMPTOMS

• Pain

—Generally vague and nonspecific
—Dull, insidious pain in the lumbosacral region, flank, lower abdomen, periumbilical area, groin, or testes is not affected by movement or straining.
—Not generally relieved with narcotics, but may respond to NSAIDs

• Anuria

—Patients with advanced disease may present with signs of renal failure, such as anuria, hiccups, and other muscle twitches.
—Lower extremity symptoms: Lower extremity edema, varicosities, thrombophlebitis, or ischemic pain may occasionally be present.
—Other symptoms: malaise, anorexia, weight loss, low-grade fever, nausea, or vomiting

PATHOPHYSIOLOGY

• Gross appearance

—RPF appears as a thick, woody-hard plaque engulfing the retroperitoneal structures.

• Microscopic appearance

—Early process, the "cellular phase": collagen, fibroblasts, and cellular infiltrate suggesting a subacute nonspecific inflammatory reaction (polys, lymphocytes, eosinophils, or plasma cells). More advanced RPF, the "fibrotic phase": exhibits avascular, acellular, hyalinized fibrosis

• Pathogenesis

—Fibrosis is first seen around the aorta; the ureters are the first structures to be functionally compromised.
—The fibrotic process causes progressive medial deviation of the ureter and subsequent ureteral obstruction. Compression of the great vessels may also occur.

CAUSES/RISK FACTORS

• Most cases: no etiologic factor identified; therefore, the disease is termed *idiopathic retroperitoneal fibrosis*.
• The most common, identifiable risk factors are medications.

—Prolonged methysergide (Sansert) therapy for migraine headaches
—Others reported: LSD, methyldopa (Aldomet), phenacetin, metoprolol, amphetamines

• Other causes: malignancy (solid tumors, lymphomas), aortitis, sclerosing cholangitis, perianeurysmal inflammation, Crohn disease or other inflammatory bowel disease, thrombophlebitis, Riedel's thyroiditis, retroperitoneal hemorrhage, urinary extravasation, trauma, radiation therapy, surgery, collagen vascular disease, asbestos exposure, and fat necrosis

COMPLICATIONS

• Ureteral obstruction

—Half to two-thirds of patients: The process of fibrosis pulls the middle third of the ureter toward the midline and can eventually lead to hydronephrosis and renal failure. One-third of patients have a nonfunctioning kidney at the time of presentation.

• Vascular obstruction

—Obstruction of the inferior vena cava or iliac vessels may cause venous congestion of the lower extremities.
—Less commonly, compression of the aorta or iliac vessels may cause lower extremity ischemia.

DIFFERENTIAL DIAGNOSIS

• Medial deviation of the ureters

—Malignancies, aneurysms, bladder diverticulum, and prior surgery
—20% of normal individuals have medial deviation of the ureters, especially on the right.
—CT or MRI is needed to differentiate between these causes of medial deviation and RPF.

• Retroperitoneal mass

—Malignant processes: lymphoma, multiple myeloma, retroperitoneal sarcoma, or extensive metastatic retroperitoneal adenopathy
—Usually, malignancies are associated with more rapid development of symptoms and more significant discomfort.
—Masses of vascular origin: aneurysm, pseudoaneurysm of a prior graft, and hematoma
—Urinoma: history of trauma, stones, recent instrumentation, or recent surgery
—Retroperitoneal abscess: Suspect in patients who are acutely ill with a clinical presentation consistent with sepsis.

 Database

HISTORY

• Pain duration and location?
• Urinary symptoms or diminished frequency?
• Gastrointestinal symptoms such as weight loss, nausea, anorexia, vomiting
• Lower extremity symptoms of swelling or pain
• Significant medical history?

—Malignancies, collagen vascular disease, fibrotic processes, inflammatory bowel diseases, asbestos exposure, radiation therapy

• History of trauma with hematoma or urinary extravasation?
• Significant surgical history?

—Any abdominal, particularly vascular or endoscopic, procedures should be noted.

• Medications, especially ergot compounds (methysergide, LSD) (see list above)

PHYSICAL EXAMINATION

• There are no distinct features; appear weak and chronically ill if azotemia and gastrointestinal disturbances

—Pallor: Anemia is associated with renal insufficiency.
—Edema: fluid overload from renal failure

• Vital signs: Temperature may be elevated; hypertension is present in 47% of patients.
• Abdominal examination: mas tenderness, CVA tenderness, or bruit
• Lower extremities: edema, varicosities, coolness, pulses

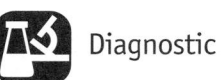 Diagnostic Studies

LABORATORY TESTING

• No tests are diagnostic.

—Azotemia, hyperkalemia, and other electrolyte abnormalities if bilateral obstruction
—ESR is usually elevated.
—CBC: leukocytosis, eosinophilia, and/or normocytic normochromic anemia

• Elevated serum antibodies to ceroid, procollagen III, and anticardiolipin (investigational)

IMAGING

• Excretory urography

—Medial deviation and tapering of the middle third of the ureter beginning at the third or fourth lumbar vertebra
—Varying degrees of hydronephrosis; may see nonfunctioning kidney

• Ultrasound

—Smooth-bordered, irregular, echo-free mass centered on the sacral promontory
—More useful for following the response of hydronephrosis to therapy

- CT

—Symmetric, geometrically shaped mass encasing the retroperitoneal structures, with attenuation numbers similar to muscle
—Allows CT-directed biopsy of the mass

- MRI: Similar to CT; may give better definition of the extension, shape, and contour of the fibrosis
- Nuclear medicine

—Diuretic scintigraphy: kidney function and obstruction
—Gallium scintigraphy: assesses the intensity and activity of the disease and response to treatment

- Angiography

—Venography may be useful in evaluating the level of extrinsic compression or presence of thrombosis.
—Arteriography may occasionally be useful in patients with evidence of arterial compromise.

SPECIAL STUDIES

- Retrograde pyelography: Confirm medial deviation of the ureters and stent placement.

 ## Treatment

GENERAL MEASURES

- Stop any potential mediations (methysergide).
- Low-protein, sodium-restricted diet for patients with renal insufficiency
- Treatment generally involves a combination of medical and surgical therapies.
- Biopsy may be necessary to rule out malignancy (needle, open or laparoscopic).

MEDICAL

- Steroids

—Even if surgery planned; sometimes resolution of obstruction
—Best in patients with multiple system involvement, particularly gastrointestinal complaints
—If active inflammation or intense uptake on gallium scintigraphy, more likely to respond

- Other immunosuppressive medications

—Steroids most common; drugs such as azathioprine reportedly effective

- Tamoxifen: reported for radiation-induced RPF or idiopathic RPF
- Other cytoreductive medications: methotrexate, cyclophosphamide, penicillamine

SURGICAL

- Temporary diversion

—If acutely ill; in combination with medical therapy, usually steroids
—Ureteral stents
  —Retrograde placement usually easy
  —Helpful to localize ureter within the hardened mass of RPF during procedures
—Percutaneous nephrostomy: rarely necessary

- Ureterolysis

—Transabdominal midline approach through the posterior peritoneum between the duodenum and inferior mesenteric vein
—Exposure of the proximal dilated ureter facilitates identification of the encased portion.
—Laparoscopic ureterolysis has been described as a less morbid alternative.

- Transposition: done at time of ureterolysis to avoid recurrence

—Performed bilaterally, even with unilateral disease, due to inevitable contralateral ureteral obstruction with progressive RPF
—Methods
  —Intraperitoneal placement of ureters
  —Lateral placement with retroperitoneal fat interposed between the ureters and the fibrosis
  —Ureters wrapped with omentum

- Other genitourinary procedures from severe RPF and ureteral obliteration

—Ileal ureteral interposition graft, autotransplantation, urinary diversion

- Arterial compression may require surgical mobilization of the aorta or common iliac arteries.

ALTERNATIVE THERAPIES

- Observation: may be a role in patients on methysergide after discontinuation if renal function is not diminished. These patients should be monitored for resolution of hydronephrosis. If the hydronephrosis does not resolve, standard combined medical and surgical interventions should be employed.

PATIENT EDUCATION

- Patients with RPF should avoid medications implicated in RPF.
- Instruct in the signs and symptoms of renal insufficiency.

 ## Follow-Up

MONITORING

- Renal function: ultrasound for hydronephrosis; creatinine

PREVENTION

- Most cases are idiopathic; preventive measures are difficult.
- Avoid methysergide; sumatriptan is now available for migraine sufferers.

 ## Miscellaneous

SYNONYMS

- Ormond disease, periureteritis fibrosa, periureteritis plastica, chronic periureteritis, sclerosing retroperitoneal granuloma, fibrous retroperitonitis

ASSOCIATED CONDITIONS: N/A

NOTES

- Example images are available via the Internet.

—www.med.univ-rennes1.fr/cerf/iconocerf/idx/u/retroperitoneal_space_fibrosis.html

ABBREVIATIONS

- RPF, retroperitoneal fibrosis; LSD, lysergic acid diethylamide; ESR, erythrocyte sedimentation rate

REFERENCES

Kottra JJ, Dunnick NR. Retroperitoneal fibrosis. *Radiol Clin North Am* 1996;34:1259–1275.

Oosterlink W, Derie A. New data on diagnosis and medical treatment of retroperitoneal fibrosis. *Acta Urol Belg* 1997;65:3–6.

Resnick, MI, Kursh ED. Extrinsic obstruction of the ureter. In: Walsh PC, Retik AB, Vaughan ED, Wein AJ, eds. *Campbell's Urology*, 7th ed. Philadelphia: WB Saunders, 1998.

Authors: Martha K. Terris and Howard N. Winfield

Retroperitoneal Sarcomas

 Basics

DESCRIPTION

- Primary malignant tumors arising from mesodermal tissues

EPIDEMIOLOGY

- Rare: <1% of adult tumors
- Occur in fourth and fifth decades
- Equal sex distribution
- No racial predilection

GENETICS: N/A

STAGING

- Histologic grade and margin of resection are the most important prognostic considerations.
- For high-grade tumors, a second factor for metastatic disease is size (>5 cm).

—Liver more common site of metastasis than is lung

SIGNS AND SYMPTOMS

- Abdominal mass and pain (frequently back pain) most common
- Other symptoms: weight gain or loss, increased abdominal girth, gastrointestinal and genitourinary symptoms, fever, and anorexia
- Presentation and physical findings vary widely, depending on location of the tumor and displacement, or more rarely, invasion of normal structures, thereby interfering with normal physiologic processes.

PATHOPHYSIOLOGY

- Most common: liposarcoma
- Other histologic types in order of incidence: leiomyosarcoma, fibrosarcoma, rhabdomyosarcoma, lymphangiosarcoma, myxosarcoma
- Malignant mesenchymoma

—Very rare high-grade tumor with poor prognosis and that contains two or more distinct subtypes of sarcoma

- Sarcomas classified as low-, moderate-, and high-grade based on demonstration of mitoses within the resected tumors

—Rhabdomyosarcomas are always designated as high grade, regardless of mitotic rate.
—Fine-needle biopsy is seldom adequate to define tumor grade.
—The surgical biopsy site must be completely excised in continuity at the time of the definitive resection.

- Growth is centrifugal and associated with creation of a pseudocapsule comprised of compressed adjacent normal tissue that also contains viable tumor cells.

—Rarely invade the adjacent neurovascular structures

- Nodal metastases occur <2%; lymphadenectomy only indicated if regional lymph nodes are clinical involved

CAUSES/RISK FACTORS

- Generally unknown

—Rare cases of fibrosarcoma reported several decades following retroperitoneal radiation therapy for seminoma

- Recent studies indicate different pathogenic mechanisms in liposarcoma subgroups based on differential *p53* expression.

COMPLICATIONS

- Gastrointestinal and genitourinary obstruction and associated symptoms

DIFFERENTIAL DIAGNOSIS

- Other malignant primary retroperitoneal tumors

—Lymphoma, teratoma, hemangiopericytoma, angiosarcoma, fibrohistiocytoma, schwannoma, pheochromocytoma

- Metastatic tumors to the retroperitoneum

—Bladder, prostate, cervix, colon, testis, ovary

- Retroperitoneal infections
- Benign retroperitoneal tumors of mesodermal, neural, vascular, and embryonal remnant origin
- Benign retroperitoneal processes

—Retroperitoneal fibrosis, lymphocele, and pelvic lipomatosis

 Database

HISTORY

- Insidious onset of symptoms

—May be identified incidentally associated with evaluation for concomitant pathology
—Symptoms related to size and location of tumor

PHYSICAL EXAMINATION

- Palpable mass noted on examination

—Usually firm and nontender; borders may be indistinct, if demonstrable
—Malignant retroperitoneal tumors are usually hard and have irregular borders on palpation.

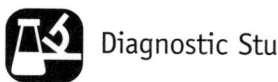 ## Diagnostic Studies

LABORATORY TESTING

- No definitive markers

—Check renal and liver function studies.

IMAGING

- CT scan or MRI to evaluate to local extent of the tumor

—MRI may give addition information over CT scan with regard to vascular structures.

- Preoperative evaluation should include a functional renal study (nephrectomy may be necessary).
- Gastrointestinal imaging, depending on consideration for operative approach, may be necessary.
- Extent of disease evaluation to exclude the presence of metastatic sites indicated prior to exenterative surgery

SPECIAL STUDIES

- Angiography and/or venography is still sometimes required if the operative plan anticipates a major vascular resection with graft reconstruction.

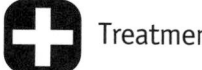 ## Treatment

GENERAL MEASURES

- Complete surgical excision remains the primary mode of therapy, with survival documented only in those patients with complete tumor extirpation.

—5% local recurrence per year following "complete" surgical excision
—40% local recurrence seen in patients with no evidence of disease at 5 years, at 10-year follow-up
—Incomplete resection of high-grade sarcomas leads to poor survival beyond 2 years.
—Reexcision and radiation therapy for local recurrences have been successfully employed in patients treated initially with primary local excision, for low- to moderate-grade sarcomas.

- Radiation therapy

—Neoadjuvant (tumor downstaging for organ preservation), intraoperative, and adjuvant techniques using external beam and brachytherapy approaches: occasional efficacy (reduction in local recurrence rate) in the management of large, high-grade retroperitoneal sarcomas

MEDICAL

- Tumors have demonstrated little chemosensitivity to date, although some new combination regimens have reported limited success.

—Used primarily for metastatic or incompletely resected local disease
—Agents with activity include Adriamycin, cisplatin, ifosfamide, paclitaxel, and docetaxel.

SURGICAL

- Surgery frequently requires sacrifice of major portions of the gastrointestinal and/or genitourinary systems, as well as portions of major vascular channels.

—Localized metastatic disease is also approached surgically, if it is felt possible to totally remove all demonstrable tumor.

ALTERNATIVE THERAPIES: N/A

PATIENT EDUCATION: N/A

 ## Follow-Up

MONITORING

- Because of the high incidence of local recurrence, even at 10-year follow-up, patients must be closely monitored with appropriate radiologic studies long term (i.e., CT abdomen).

PREVENTION: N/A

 ## Miscellaneous

SYNONYMS: N/A

ASSOCIATED CONDITIONS

- Increased sarcoma risk in Gardner syndrome, neurofibromatosis, tuberous sclerosis, Li-Fraumeni syndrome, patients treated for retinoblastoma in childhood, or previous exposure to ionizing radiation.

NOTES

- See also Section I, "Retroperitoneal Mass."

ABBREVIATIONS: N/A

REFERENCES

Eilber FR, Eckardt J. Surgical management of soft tissue sarcomas. *Semin Oncol* 1997;24:526–533.

Heslin MJ, Lewis JJ, Nadler E, et al. Prognostic factors associated with long-term survival for retroperitoneal sarcoma: Implications for management. *J Clin Oncol* 1997;15:2832–2839.

Resnick MI, Kursh ED. Diseases of the retroperitoneum. In: Walsh PC, Retik AB, Vaughan ED, Wein AJ, eds. *Campbell's Urology*, 7th ed. Philadelphia: WB Saunders, 1998:403–422.

Author: Richard E. Greenberg

Rhabdomyosarcoma—Pediatric (Sarcoma Botryoides)

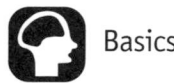 Basics

DESCRIPTION

• Malignancy arising from any part of the body containing embryonal mesenchyme. Sarcoma botryoides are polypoid tumors ("cluster of grapes") arising in hollow organs.

EPIDEMIOLOGY

• Rhabdomyosarcomas account for 4% to 8% of all malignant disease in children under 15 years of age.
• The genitourinary region makes up 20%.
• Common sites include the prostate, bladder (arising from the area of the trigone), and vagina.

GENETICS

• Familial aggregations with other sarcomas, breast cancers, and brain tumors
• Increased incidence with neurofibromatosis
• Congenital anomalies not common

STAGING

• IRS clinical classification (see Section III)

SIGNS AND SYMPTOMS

• Dependent on the site of origin

—Large, palpable abdominal mass single most common presentation for rhabdomyosarcoma

• Bladder or prostate

—Strangury
—Urinary retention
—Incontinence
—Infection
—Hematuria
—Tumor prolapsing through the urethra

• Vagina

—Bloody, foul-smelling discharge
—Tumor prolapsing through the vagina

PATHOPHYSIOLOGY

• Three common histologic types

—Embryonal
  —Polypoid form: sarcoma botryoides
  —Resembles skeletal muscle in the 7- to 10-week-old fetus
  —Accounts for two-thirds of all GU rhabdomyosarcomas
—Alveolar
  —Resembles skeletal muscle in the 10- to 21-week-old fetus
  —More commonly seen in tumors of the trunk and extremities
—Pleomorphic
  —Comprises only 1% of all childhood cases
  —Usually found in adults

CAUSES/RISK FACTORS

• None known

COMPLICATIONS: N/A

DIFFERENTIAL DIAGNOSIS

• Prolapsing ectopic ureterocele
• Urethral prolapse
• Transitional carcinoma of the bladder
• Neurofibroma of the urethra
• Fibromas and fibromatous polyps of the urethra
• Leiomyomas of the urethra
• Hamartomatous polyps
• Hydrocolpos
• Paraurethral cyst
• Imperforate hymen
• Uterovaginal prolapse
• Bladder prolapse

 Database

HISTORY

• Symptoms of lower urinary tract obstruction?

—Urinary retention
—Strangury
—Gross hematuria

• Is there a bloody or foul-smelling vaginal discharge?
• Is there a prolapsing urethral or vaginal mass?

PHYSICAL EXAMINATION

• Abdominal and bimanual examination

—Palpable mass

• Examination of the introitus

—Presence of prolapsing mass or "cluster of grapes"

Rhabdomyosarcoma—Pediatric (Sarcoma Botryoides)

 Diagnostic Studies

LABORATORY TESTING

- Urinalysis and urine culture
—Presence of hematuria or infection
- Complete blood count (CBC)
—Presence of anemia
- BUN/creatinine
—Presence of renal failure secondary to obstruction

IMAGING

- Magnetic resonance imaging
- CT scan of chest, abdomen, and pelvis: Evaluate for metastasis.
- Intravenous urography: bladder filling defect; evaluate for obstruction.
- Ultrasonography
- Bone scan: metastatic evaluation

SPECIAL STUDIES

- Cystoscopy and biopsy
—Recommended for visible intravesical mucosal tumors
- Perineal or extraperitoneal suprapubic biopsy
—Percutaneous approach for large abdominal masses
- Laparotomy or laparoscopy
—Rarely indicated
- Bone marrow biopsy or aspirate
—Useful in clinical staging

 Treatment

GENERAL MEASURES

- Based on findings from IRS trials (I-II)
—IRS-IV now underway
- Multimodal approach using chemotherapy, radiation therapy, and surgery

MEDICAL

- Multiagent chemotherapy for all patients
—IRS-IV trial: randomized to one of three regimens
  —VAC (vincristine, actinomycin D, cyclophosphamide)
  —VAI (vincristine, actinomycin D, ifosfamide)
  —VIE (vincristine, actinomycin D, etoposide)
- Radiotherapy
—Based on IRS clinical classification (See Appendix)
  —Group I: no radiation therapy
  —Group II: standard-dose therapy of 5040 cGy (180 cGy for 28 days)
  —Group III: randomized between standard dose of 5040 cGy vs. hyperfractionated therapy of 5940 cGy (110 cGy twice a day for 54 fractions)

SURGICAL

- Primary surgical treatment is restricted to tumor biopsy or limited local resection.
- Limited, conservative (bladder salvage) surgery if possible after intense multiagent chemotherapy
- Long-term results suggest that approximately 50% of patients retain their bladders.

ALTERNATIVE THERAPIES: N/A

PATIENT EDUCATION: N/A

 Follow-Up

MONITORING

- Long-term follow-up is essential.
—Recurrence of tumor usually within 2 years
—Secondary malignancy related to cyclophosphamide and radiotherapy

PREVENTION: N/A

 Miscellaneous

SYNONYMS

- Malignant rhabdomyoma, myelosarcoma, rhabdomyoblastoma, botryoid tumor

ASSOCIATED CONDITIONS

- Reduced functional capacity of bladder secondary to radiotherapy, surgery, and chemotherapy. Psychosocial issues related to extensive pelvic surgery resulting in impotence and change in body image. Chemotherapy may induce sterility.

NOTES

- See also Section II: "Bladder Tumors—Benign and Malignant, General."

ABBREVIATIONS

- IRS, Intergroup Rhabdomyosarcoma Study

REFERENCES

Andrassy RJ, et al. Conservative surgical management of vaginal and vulvar pediatric rhabdomyosarcoma: A report from the Intergroup Rhabdomyosarcoma Study III. *J Pediatr Surg* 1995;30;1034.

Atra A, et al. Conservative surgery in multimodal therapy for pelvic rhabdomyosarcoma in children. *Br J Cancer* 1994;70;1004.

Snyder HM III, et al. Pediatric oncology. In: Walsh PC, Retik AB, Vaughan ED, Wein AJ, eds. *Campbell's Urology,* 7th ed. Philadelphia: WB Saunders, 1998.

Snow B. Tumors of the lower urinary tract. In: Kelalis PP, et al., eds. *Clinical Pediatric Urology.* Philadelphia: WB Saunders, 1992.

Authors: John W. Colberg and Robert M. Weiss

Scrotum—Squamous Cell Carcinoma

 Basics

DESCRIPTION

• Squamous cell carcinoma of the scrotum is an environmentally induced cancer with a high metastatic potential.

EPIDEMIOLOGY

• Typically presents in sixth decade
• Incidence: 0.2 to 0.3 per 100,000 men over 35 years
• 20 times more common in the United Kingdom than in the United States
• Lower social class related to higher incidence
• Urban population higher incidence than rural
• Lower incidence among Blacks

GENETICS

• Possible HPV subtype 6 and 11 relationship

STAGING

• A1: localized to scrotal wall
• A2: locally extensive tumor invading adjacent structures (testis, spermatic cord, penis, pubis, perineum)
• B: metastatic disease involving inguinal lymph nodes only
• C: metastatic disease involving pelvic lymph nodes without evidence of distant spread
• D: metastatic disease beyond the pelvic lymph nodes, involving distant organs

SIGNS AND SYMPTOMS

• Usually a solitary, slow-growing pimple, wart, or nodule on anterolateral aspect of scrotum
• Ulceration of lesion at 6 months with raised, rolled edges; seropurulent discharge; and an indurated base
• Patients typically present late to physician, at around 8 to 10 months after self-treatment with ointments
• 50% to 60% have palpable inguinal adenopathy at presentation.
• 25% have inguinal metastasis at presentation.
• No predilection for a side, when occupational exposure is excluded

PATHOPHYSIOLOGY

• Squamous cell carcinoma: Most are well or moderately well differentiated and contain focal areas of keratosis.
• Surrounding epidermis frequently shows hyperkeratosis, acanthosis, and dyskeratosis.
• A diffuse lymphocytic infiltrate may be present.

CAUSES/RISK FACTORS

• Chemical/mechanical irritation

—Soot: chimney sweepers
—Oil/petroleum: machine workers (mule-spinners, lathe workers, pressmen)

• Poor hygiene
• Repeated trauma
• Psoralens and ultraviolet A radiation (PUVA)
• Human papillomavirus virus (HPV) subtypes 6 and 11

COMPLICATIONS

• Lymphedema, lymphoceles, wound infections, and femoral hernias after ilioinguinal lymph node dissections

DIFFERENTIAL DIAGNOSIS

• Benign lesions

—Sebaceous cysts, eczema, nevus, psoriasis, folliculitis, syphilis, tuberculous epididymitis with a draining sinus, and periurethral abscess

• Malignant lesions

—Basal cell carcinoma, malignant melanoma, Paget disease, and various sarcomas

 Database

HISTORY

• History of sexually transmitted diseases: warts (HPV), trauma, occupational exposure to chemical/mechanical irritants
• Change in size of lesion, ulceration? Fever?

PHYSICAL EXAMINATION

• Examination of external genitalia, inguinal lymph nodes, and distant lymph nodes

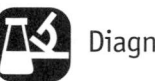 Diagnostic Studies

LABORATORY TESTING

• WBC to rule out infectious process
• Urinalysis and urine culture, if indicated

IMAGING

• CT scan can help assess size of nodes and extent, but cannot differentiate inflammation vs. metastasis.
• Lymphangiography is accurate in delineating metastatic vs. inflammatory nodes, but cannot detect micrometastasis.

SPECIAL STUDIES

• HPV testing

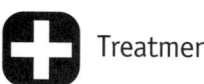 Treatment

GENERAL MEASURES: N/A

MEDICAL

- Broad-spectrum antibiotics for 6 weeks in patients with lymphadenopathy

SURGICAL

- Primary lesion

—Wide local excision of lesion with a 2-cm margin of skin and dartos to negative margin
—Small lesions may be primarily closed.
—Large lesions may require split-thickness skin grafts, local flaps, or testicular implantation into the subcutaneous thighs.
—Excision of scrotal contents is rarely indicated, except when directly involved.
—Local recurrence rates reported at 21% to 40%

- Regional lymph nodes

—If palpable lymphadenopathy resolves after an antibiotic course, or was never present, then a superficial inguinal lymph node biopsy should be performed.
    —Ipsilaterally if initial lesion lateral
    —Bilaterally if initial lesion at median raphe
—If palpable lymphadenopathy persists after a course of antibiotics, then a bilateral superficial inguinal lymph node biopsy should be performed.
—Subsequent ilioinguinal lymphadenectomy should only be carried out on the side of the positive biopsy.
    —A contralateral superficial inguinal lymph node biopsy should be performed at the time of unilateral ilioinguinal lymphadenectomy.
    —If there is a positive frozen section, then a bilateral ilioinguinal lymphadenectomy should be performed
—Surgical ilioinguinal lymphadenectomy: two different incision approaches
    —An oblique incision parallel to the inguinal ligament for the inguinal nodes
    —A low midline incision for the pelvic lymph nodes
    —All obturator and external iliac nodes from the common iliac artery bifurcation to the node of Cloquet: the femoral canal should be removed, with free communication between the inguinal area and the pelvis.

- Survival at 5 years

—Stage A: 70% to 80%
—Stage B: 40% to 50%
—Stage C: rare survival
—Stage D: rare survival

ALTERNATIVE THERAPIES

- Radiation therapy has not been effective and is reserved for recurrences and poor surgical candidates.
- Combination chemotherapy (cyclophosphamide, vincristine, methotrexate, and 5FU) has had minimal success in advanced disease.
- Bleomycin as single agent has been reported successful in two cases.

PATIENT EDUCATION

- Self-examinations for local recurrence of lesion and lymphadenopathy

 Follow-Up

MONITORING

- Periodic follow-up for monitoring of local recurrence of lesion and lymphadenopathy

PREVENTION

- Decrease exposure to risk factors and improve hygiene.

 Miscellaneous

SYNONYMS

- Potts disease, chimney sweeps disease, mule-spinners disease

ASSOCIATED CONDITIONS: N/A

NOTES

- See also Section I, "Scrotum—Mass and/or Pain (Acute Scrotum)."
- First occupationally related cancer; described in chimney sweeps

ABBREVIATIONS: N/A

REFERENCES

Lowe FC, Klein LT. Squamous cell carcinoma of the scrotum. In: Crawford D, Das S, eds. *Urological Diseases,* 2nd ed. Baltimore: Williams & Wilkins, 1997, 545–549.

Lowe FC. Squamous cell carcinoma of the scrotum. *Urol Clin North Am* 1992;19(2):397–405.

Lowe FC. Squamous cell carcinoma of the scrotum. *Urology* 1995;25(1).

Oesterling JE, Lowe FC. Squamous cell carcinoma of the scrotum. AUA Update Series Volume IX, Lesson 23, 1990, 178–183.

Authors: Michael C. Kearney and Franklin C. Lowe

Seminal Vesiculitis (Pyospermia)

 Basics

DESCRIPTION

- Pyospermia is the presence of white cells in a semen sample (usually >10 per HPF) and is associated with infection/inflammation of the seminal vesicals.

EPIDEMIOLOGY

- Found on infertility evaluation
- 10% to 20% of men presenting for infertility evaluation

GENETICS

- Unknown

STAGING: N/A

SIGNS AND SYMPTOMS

- Patients are generally asymptomatic.
- Symptomatic patients: see specific infection

PATHOPHYSIOLOGY

- The source of leukocytes is not established.
- Leukocytes are easily confused with immature sperm cells on microscopy. Special stains are required to confirm.
- Pyospermia is more common in infertility patients than in fertile men.
- Pyospermia is associated with decreased sperm counts and decreased motility.
- Pyospermia is an adverse prognostic factor for IVF.

CAUSES/RISK FACTORS

- Unknown

COMPLICATIONS

- Chronic pain (controversial)
- Infertility (controversial)

DIFFERENTIAL DIAGNOSIS

- Prostatitis
- Epididymitis
- Immature germ cells in semen

 Database

HISTORY

- Voiding symptoms (urgency, frequency, dysuria)
- Genital tract pain
- Urethral discharge
- Medical or surgical history

—UTI, STD, hernia surgery, vasectomy, varicocelectomy, etc.

PHYSICAL EXAMINATION

- Genital examination

—Vas, epididymis, testis: looking for tenderness, swelling

- Rectal examination

—Prostate size, texture (boggy?), tenderness

 Diagnostic Studies

LABORATORY TESTING

- UA, culture
- Semen analysis

—Excess white cells noted
—Antileukocyte monoclonal antibodies: One-third of patients with round cells on semen analysis have true pyospermia.

- Semen culture: rarely grows other than normal genital flora

IMAGING

- Not specifically indicated

—Transrectal ultrasound may rarely be used.

SPECIAL STUDIES: N/A

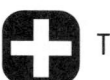 Treatment

GENERAL MEASURES

- Supportive care

MEDICAL

- Controversial
- There is no evidence that antibiotics are helpful in this situation, but they are commonly given.

—Antibiotic choice and course as for prostatitis (quinolone, sulfa-trimethoxasole, etc).

SURGICAL: N/A

ALTERNATIVE THERAPIES: N/A

PATIENT EDUCATION: N/A

 Follow-Up

MONITORING

- Follow-up UA and SA to evaluate for persistent pyospermia or signs of infection

PREVENTION

- Unknown

 Miscellaneous

SYNONYMS

- Pyospermia

ASSOCIATED CONDITIONS

- Infertility

NOTES

- See also Section I, "Infertility."

ABBREVIATIONS

- SA, semen analysis; IVF, in vitro fertilization

REFERENCES

Bar-Charma N, et al. Infection and pyospermia in male infertility: Is it really a problem? *Urol Clin North Am* 1994;21(3):469.

Sigman L, Lopes L. The correlation between round cells and white blood cells in the semen. *J Urol* 1993;149(5 Part 2):1338.

Wolff H. The biologic significance of white blood cells in semen. *Fertil Steril* 1995;63(6):1143.

Author: David E. McGinnis

Sexual Abuse—Pediatric

 Basics

DESCRIPTION

• Exploitation of a child for gratification or profit. The abuse comprises a spectrum that includes exhibitionism, pornography, fondling, or intercourse

EPIDEMIOLOGY

• An estimated 25% of girls and 10% of boys are sexually abused at least once prior to the age of 16 years.
• Abuse may occur at any age, and girls appear to be more frequently affected than boys.

GENETICS: N/A

STAGING: N/A

SIGNS AND SYMPTOMS

• Gynecologic/urologic

—Recurrent urinary tract infections
—Hematuria
—Dysuria
—Chronic pelvic pain
—Urinary retention
—Enuresis
—Dysfunctional voiding
—Vaginal discharge or bleeding

• Gastrointestinal

—Constipation/encopresis
—Anal/rectal pain
—Anal/rectal bleeding

• Psychological

—Headaches
—Eating disorders
—Behavioral disturbances
—Alteration in school performance

PATHOPHYSIOLOGY: N/A

CAUSES/RISK FACTORS

• Socioeconomic factors

—Affects all socioeconomic strata
—Increased risk occurs in families with
  —Social isolation
  —Adolescent parents
  —Parents with a history of being abused
  —Parental violence
  —Parental mental illness
  —Overcrowding
  —Alcohol and drug abuse
  —Child with prematurity or congenital malformations

COMPLICATIONS

• Psychological impact
• Enuresis, voiding dysfunction
• Encopresis, constipation

DIFFERENTIAL DIAGNOSIS

• Congenital hemangiomas
• Streptococcal infection of genitalia
• Straddle injury
• Urethral caruncle or prolapse
• Lichen sclerosis
• Congenital vaginal, anal, and urethral abnormalities

—Periurethral bands
—Intravaginal ridges
—Anterior midline perineal folds

• Medical conditions

—Crohn disease
—Hemolytic–uremic syndrome
—Chronic constipation
—Neurogenic patulous anus

 Database

HISTORY

• Child reporting abuse

—Statements made by the child may be admissible in civil court and should be recorded in a verbatim manner.

• Caregiver presents with direct allegations of sexual abuse
• Complaints directly related to sexual abuse, such as vaginal discharge, rectal bleeding
• Complaints not related to abuse, such as UTI, enuresis, encopresis, abdominal pain, hematuria, urinary retention (this is the most common presentation to the urologist)
• No complaints, but physical examination is suspicious

PHYSICAL EXAMINATION

• The examination may be normal, as healing occurs quickly.
• Definitive findings

—Presence of sperm or semen
—Positive culture for *Neisseria gonorrhoeae*, syphilis, or *Chlamydia*

• Suggestive findings

—Bites, chafing, bruising, abrasions of inner thigh and genitalia
—Abnormal hymen (scarred, distorted, or torn)
—Injury or scar of posterior fourchette
—Enlarged hymenal opening for age (normal after age 5: equals age in millimeters)
—Anal gapping, skin tags, rectal tears, perianal scars, bites
—Perineal condylomata
—Vaginal or rectal discharge or bleeding

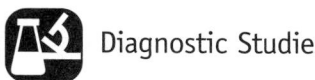 Diagnostic Studies

LABORATORY TESTING

- Girls

—Culture the endocervix, vagina, rectum, and pharynx for *Neisseria gonorrhoeae* and *Chlamydia trachomatis*.
—Evaluate vaginal secretions for *Trichomonas* and *Gardnerella vaginalis*.
—Pregnancy test in pubertal girls
—Culture herpetic lesions if present
—Urine culture

- Boys

—Culture the urethra, rectum, and pharynx for *Neisseria gonorrhoeae* and *Chlamydia trachomatis*.
—Urine culture
—Culture herpetic lesions if present

Imaging

- No routine imaging necessary unless physical abuse is also present

SPECIAL STUDIES

- Internal pelvic examination under anesthesia if vaginal bleeding, suspicious foreign body, or chronic vaginal discharge is present

 Treatment

GENERAL MEASURES

- If the physician is comfortable with the diagnosis of sexual abuse, then a referral to a local/state protective services agency should be made.
- If the physician is suspicious that sexual abuse has occurred, then referral to a child abuse specialist is indicated.

MEDICAL

- As needed to treat pain if trauma is present

SURGICAL

- Vaginal and anal lacerations may require endoscopic evaluation and closure under general anesthesia.

ALTERNATIVE THERAPIES

- All cases of suspected child abuse must be reported to the local/state authorities. When making a referral, the physician should stress to the family that no allegations are being made; rather, the issue needs to be further evaluated and that the physician must comply with state laws.
- Statements made by the child during the clinic visit may be admissible in civil court and should be recorded in a verbatim manner.
- Vaginal and anal lacerations often heal quickly; thus, when present, they should be photographed.

PATIENT EDUCATION

- Information is available from the Attorney General's Task Force on Child Abuse and Neglect.

 Follow-Up

MONITORING

- Antibiotic therapy and follow-up cultures in those with sexually transmitted diseases
- Follow up to ensure healing of traumatized tissues.
- Behavioral therapy for voiding dysfunction

PREVENTION

- Prevention is difficult, but an awareness of the magnitude of the problem will keep physicians clued to subtle signs and symptoms. Inclusion of the anal and genital examination in the yearly physical will help identify cases early.

 Miscellaneous

SYNONYMS

- Sexual abuse, child pornography, fondling

ASSOCIATED CONDITIONS: N/A

NOTES: N/A

ABBREVIATIONS: N/A

REFERENCES

Bays J, Chadwick D. Medical diagnosis of the sexually abused child. *Child Abuse Negl* 1993;17:91–110.

Ellsworth PI, Merguerian PA. Recognition and management of suspected child sexual abuse. AUA Update Series, Volume XIV, Lesson 3, 1995:273–280.

Finkelhor D. *Sexually Victimized Children*. New York: Free Press, 1976.

Herman-Giddens ME, Frothingham JE. Prepubertal female genitalia: Examination for evidence of sexual abuse. *Pediatrics* 1987;80(2):203–208.

Muram D. Child sexual abuse—Genital tract findings in prepubertal girls. The unaided medical examination. *Am J Obst Gynecol* 1989;60:328–333.

Authors: Paul A. Merguerian and Pamela I. Ellsworth

Sickle Cell Disease—Urologic Considerations

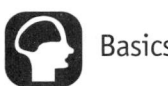 Basics

DESCRIPTION

• Sickle cell (SC) disease is a chronic hemoglobinopathy transmitted genetically and marked by severe chronic hemolytic anemia and periodic acute painful episodes. The heterozygote is termed *sickle cell trait* and usually has no symptoms.

EPIDEMIOLOGY

• Prevalence estimated at approximately 8% of African Americans

—8% to 10% of African Americans have the SC trait.
—25% to 30% of Western Africans have the SC trait

• Approximately 4000 to 5000 pregnancies are at risk of SC disease.
• Worldwide distribution parallels that of malaria.
• Life expectancy: men, 42 years; women, 48 years

GENETICS

• Autosomal co-dominant inheritance pattern
• The allele is on chromosome 11.

—Several haplotypes; allelic with beta-thalassemia

• SC disease: inheritance of 2 alleles, all RBCs contain HbS
• SC trait: from 1 allele, 40% of Hb is HbS

STAGING: N/A

SIGNS AND SYMPTOMS

• Varies by organ system (see below for urologic organs involved)

PATHOPHYSIOLOGY

• Sickling of RBCs caused by HbS

—Substitution of valine for glutamate at sixth amino acid position
—HbS tetramer: The deoxygenated state polymerizes into double-stranded filaments and bundles.

• Vaso-occlusion occurs at the postcapillary sphincter.
• Chronic anemia is the hallmark of the disease; RBC mean lifespan: 17 days
• SC trait (heterozygote) usually asymptomatic

CAUSES/RISK FACTORS

• Family history of disease

COMPLICATIONS

• Nephropathy

—Renal insufficiency
  —Vaso-occlusion in renal medulla secondary to hypertonicity, inducing HbS sickling
  —Progressive cortical infarction leads to CRF; average age of onset: 23 years

—Hyposthenuria, inability to maximally concentrate urine in the face of dehydration or vasopressin
  —Usually associated with renal insufficiency; able to dilute urine
—Associated impairment of K excretion
  —Risk of hyperkalemia with alpha-blockers, captopril, or K-sparing diuretics
—Renal biopsy: focal and segmental glomerulosclerosis, membranous glomerulopathy, or MPGN
—Proteinuria can progress to full-blown nephrotic syndrome.

• Hematuria

—Microscopic or gross hematuria; mechanism unknown
—Source rarely identified; ? due to papillary necrosis
—Usually unilateral, left-sided in origin in 80% of cases
—More common in men than in women
—Usually remits with conservative measures (e.g., bedrest, hydration) but recurrence noted in approximately 50% of cases

• Papillary necrosis

—Due to medullary ischemia from sickling in vasa recta
—Radiologic diagnosis with contrast can be difficult, due to poor concentrating ability of the kidneys from renal insufficiency.
—Can be a cause of hematuria; it is of prime importance to rule out this entity in settings of hematuria in sickle patients.
—Can obstruct if sloughed papillae block the UPJ

• Priapism

—Affects approximately 66% of SC disease patients
—Two age peaks; onset usually after puberty
  —5 to 13 years and 21 to 29 years
—Initiating factors: nocturnal penile tumescence and sexual arousal
—Typically, bicorporal involvement
  —Less common tricorporal (greater risk of impotence)
—Pathophysiology: engorgement and sludging of the corpora, with no outflow and low-flow state
—The major risk is fibrosis and subsequent impotence; children have a greater chance of recovery and subsequent erectile function.

• Impotence

—Fibrosis as a result of recurrent episodes of priapism

• Retarded sexual maturation

—Primary hypogonadism, due to testicular ischemia or infarction, hypopituitarism, or hypothalamic insufficiency
—Correlates with the degree and severity of the sickle disease

• Infertility

—Complication of hypogonadism and direct testicular insult by ischemia and infarction

• Urinary tract infection

—Usually caused by *E. coli,* other gram-negatives
—Can lead to more serious infections or bacteremia

• Renal tubular acidosis

—Incomplete distal RTA (type IV) from progressive medullary infarction
—Inability to lower urine pH to <5
—Can develop hyperchloremic metabolic acidosis in SC disease and renal insufficiency
—*Not* associated with nephrolithiasis

• Acute urinary retention

—Related to acute, painful SC; transient, resolves with resolution of the acute episode

• Renal medullary carcinoma: rare;? association with SC trait

DIFFERENTIAL DIAGNOSIS

• SC trait

—8% to 10% of African Americans; few associated complications

• HbSC disease: milder course than SC disease
• SC beta-thalassemia: severity related to presence or absence of HbA
• SC anemia with coexistent beta-thalassemia
• SC hereditary persistence of fetal Hb: rare complications
• SC-Hb Lepore disease: vaso-occlusive complications known to occur
• SC-Hb D disease: similar to SC disease
• SC-Hb O Arab disease: moderately severe form of hemolytic anemia
• SC-Hb E disease

 Database

HISTORY

• African-American descent (even among Caucasians)?
• Prior episodes of sickle complications and outcomes?
• Timing of sexual maturation?
• Determine time length of any priapism episodes.

PHYSICAL EXAMINATION

• Look for staging of sexual maturation.
• Palpate testes in men to check for atrophy
• In cases of priapism, examine the glans to determine bicorporal or tricorporal involvement.

 Diagnostic Studies

LABORATORY TESTING

• Complete blood count: degree of anemia
• Peripheral blood smear: presence of sickled or deformed RBCs
• Hb electrophoresis: types and percentages of Hb present

- Sickle cell prep: rapid determination of SC disease vs. trait vs. normal
- UA: hematuria, proteinuria, or infection

—Urine culture: infection if indicated by UA or symptoms

- Creatinine levels of blood and urine

—Monitor for renal insufficiency, and calculate GFR as needed.

- ABG on corporal blood aspirates in priapism setting to check for high- vs. low-flow state

—pH remaining at <7.10 (acidotic) suggests a low-flow state.

IMAGING

- IVP as indicated for hematuria; may not be useful in progressive renal insufficiency (poor concentrating ability limits visualization)
- US: noninvasive; look for renal source of hematuria if renal insufficiency precludes contrast use.

SPECIAL STUDIES

- Cystoscopy: as needed for hematuria
- Retrograde pyelograms: upper tract sources of bleeding if IVP limited or suspect papillary necrosis
- Ureteroscopy: for hematuria as indicated
- Renal biopsy: as needed for specific glomerulopathies
- Impotence evaluation by nocturnal penile tumescence testing or MRI is rarely useful as an additive beyond the information gained by history and physical examination.

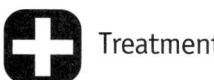 Treatment

GENERAL MEASURES

- Bed rest: limits hematuria and exacerbations of pain episodes
- Aggressive hydration: counters dehydration, increases perfusion, and improves blood rheology
- Metabolic alkalinization limits further sickling
- Pain control

—Narcotics for pain: Risk of addiction is negligible in the acute setting; PCA for inpatients

MEDICAL

- Simple transfusion

—Improves blood rheology; increases proportion of RBCs with normal Hb to decrease SC sludging
—Indications: acutely (priapism, life-threatening hemorrhage), and preoperatively if indicated by procedure

- Exchange transfusion

—Indications as for simple transfusion
—Used when needed for improved rheology if simple transfusion fails
—Risk of cerebrovascular accidents with increased hematocrit, causing a relative hyperviscosity (ASPEN syndrome)

- Antibiotics

—As needed for infections
—Perioperative and periprocedural use: recommended for invasive urologic procedures

- Special considerations

—Hematuria
  —Diuresis with IV hydration is standard.
  —Alkalization decreases sickling and hematuria.
  —Aminocaproic acid is used to induce thrombosis and control persistent and threatening hematuria, but it can cause clot formation in the urinary tract.
  —Persistent or life-threatening hematuria may necessitate nephrectomy.
—Priapism (see Section I)
  —Prompt corporal irrigation is important to induce detumescence and remove old clotted blood.
  —Use α-adrenergic agents for corporal injection to decrease inflow to the corpora, aiding in detumescence.
  —Impotence due to fibrosis as a complication can be managed by implantation of a penile prosthesis after the process stabilizes for 6 months.
—Delayed sexual maturation
  —Gonadotropic supplementation by testosterone is used, as needed, to induce sexual characteristics, and it may improve fertility in select patients.

SURGICAL

- May be needed for priapism or obstruction due to sloughed papilla

ALTERNATIVE THERAPIES: N/A

PATIENT EDUCATION

- Maintain hydration and prevent dehydration.
- Risks: renal insufficiency; impotence with priapism episodes
- Report significant events/complications promptly for treatment (i.e., priapism or hematuria)
- Genetic counseling for patients who want to have children
- Need for yearly health maintenance evaluations, including laboratory evaluation

 Follow-Up

MONITORING

- Hematology consultation is essential for management.
- Yearly labs: CBC, creatinine
- Urologic follow-up, as needed

—Priapism: episodes and degree and progression of fibrosis; erectile dysfunction and therapy
—Hematuria evaluation: in older patients after the acute setting to rule out other important pathology

- Psychological counseling: as needed to cope with chronic condition

PREVENTION

- Avoid situations that precipitate sickling episodes (dehydration, hypoxia, cold, infections, fever, acidosis)

 Miscellaneous

SYNONYMS: N/A

ASSOCIATED CONDITIONS

- Erectile dysfunction

NOTES

- See also Section I, "Priapism."

ABBREVIATIONS

- CRF, chronic renal failure; MPGN, membranoproliferative glomerulonephritis; PCA, patient-controlled analgesia; RTA, renal tubular acidosis; SC, sickle cell

REFERENCES

Allon M. Renal abnormalities in sickle cell disease. *Arch Intern Med* 1990;150:501–504.

Burnett AL, et al. Evaluation of erectile function in men with sickle cell disease. In: Walsh PC, Retik AB, Vaughan ED, Wein AJ, eds. *Campbell's Urology,* 7th ed. Philadelphia: WB Saunders, 1998.

Embury SH. Sickle cell disease. In: Hoffman R, ed. *Hematology: Basic Principles and Practices,* 2nd ed. New York: Churchill Livingstone, 1995.

Fowler JE, et al. Priapism associated with the sickle hemoglobinopathies; prevalence, natural history and sequelae. *J Urol* 1991;145:65–68.

Siegel JF, et al. Association of sickle cell disease, priapism, exchange transfusion and neurological events: ASPEN syndrome. *J Urol* 1993;150(Pt 1): 1480–1482.

Authors: Jonathan D. Block and Ronald P. Kaufman, Jr.

Spermatic Cord Tumors

 Basics

DESCRIPTION

- Firm, often painless groin or extratesticular scrotal mass, usually a sarcoma

EPIDEMIOLOGY

- Can occur at any age
- Peaks at ages 16 to 19 and greater than 50

GENETICS

- Unknown

STAGING

- AJCC/TNM available, but not frequently used

SIGNS AND SYMPTOMS

- Firm mass either paratesticular or in inguinal canal

PATHOPHYSIOLOGY

- Sarcomas

—Rhabdomyosarcoma, 29%; leiomyosarcoma, 24%; liposarcoma, 19%; fibrosarcoma, 10%; malignant fibrous histiocytoma, 7%

- Desmoid tumors at this location should be distinguished from reactive processes, such as pseudosarcomatous myofibroblastic proliferation (so-called proliferative funiculitis) and inflammatory fibrous pseudotumor, all of which exhibit fibroblastic/myofibroblastic differentiation.

CAUSES/RISK FACTORS

- Unknown

COMPLICATIONS

- Very rare

DIFFERENTIAL DIAGNOSIS

- Incarcerated inguinal hernia
- Epididymitis
- Spermatocele, hydrocele
- Lipoma of spermatic cord
- Adenomatoid tumor of epididymis
- Desmoid tumors
- Proliferative funiculitis
- Inflammatory fibrous pseudotumor
- See also Section I, "Spermatic Cord Mass."

 Database

HISTORY

- How long has the mass been present?

—Sudden onset suggests an incarcerated hernia.

- Any change in mass size?

—Long-term presence without change in size suggests, but does not guarantee, a benign pathology

- Any weight loss or bone pain?

—Evaluate for metastatic disease.

PHYSICAL EXAMINATION

- Palpate the testes bilaterally.

—Clearly delineate the mass as extratesticular.

- Palpate the supraclavicular, axillary, and inguinal lymph nodes.

—Evaluate for metastatic disease

 Diagnostic Studies

LABORATORY TESTING

- If the mass is not clearly extratesticular, obtain testis tumor markers (alpha-fetoprotein, beta-hCG, and LDH) prior to exploration.

IMAGING

- Scrotal ultrasound

—All noncystic, extratesticular masses should be explored.

- Chest x-ray to evaluate for pulmonary metastases
- CT abdomen/pelvis with oral and intravenous contrast

—Evaluate for metastatic disease in retroperitoneal lymph nodes.

SPECIAL STUDIES: N/A

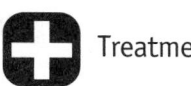 Treatment

GENERAL MEASURES

• Wide local excision for primary tumors

—Combined radiation, chemotherapy, and surgery for metastatic disease

MEDICAL

• Aggressive ifosfamide- or Adriamycin-based chemotherapy for metastatic disease

SURGICAL

• Inguinal exploration with possible biopsy and high spermatic cord ligation for treatment of local disease
• A frozen-section analysis, particularly of liposarcomas, can give falsely benign reports.
• Retroperitoneal lymph node dissection

—Recommended for
—Rhabdomyosarcoma and other high-grade sarcomas in absence of obviously positive retroperitoneal lymph nodes on CT scan
—Leiomyosarcomas in face of positive CT in absence of other metastatic disease

ALTERNATIVE THERAPIES: N/A

PATIENT EDUCATION

• Low-grade tumors at high risk for local recurrence
• High-grade tumors at high risk for recurrent local and metastatic disease

 Follow-Up

MONITORING

• History and physical examination, chest x-ray every 3 months; CT abdomen and pelvis every 6 months

PREVENTION

• Unknown

 Miscellaneous

SYNONYMS: N/A

ASSOCIATED CONDITIONS: N/A

NOTES

• See also Section I, "Spermatic Cord Mass" and "Groin Mass."

ABBREVIATIONS: N/A

REFERENCES

Grey LF, Sorial RF, Shaw WH. Spermatic cord sarcoma: Leiomyosarcoma and retroperitoneal lymph node dissection. *Urology* 1986;27:28.

Russo P, Brady MS, Conlon K, et al. Adult urological sarcoma. *J Urol* 1992;147:1032.

Schwartz SL, Swierzewski, SJ, Sondak VK, Grossman HB. Liposarcoma of the spermatic cord: Report of 6 cases and review of the literature. *J Urol* 1995;153:154.

Takahashi S, Tsukamoto T, Lieber MM. Genitourinary sarcomas in adults. In: Vogelzang NJ, Shipley WU, Scardino PT, Coffey DS, eds. *Comprehensive Textbook of Genitourinary Oncology*. Baltimore: Williams & Wilkins, 1996:1124–1139.

Author: Michel S. McGuire

Spermatocele

Basics

DESCRIPTION

• A painless mass in the caput or head of the epididymis that contains fluid and spermatozoa

EPIDEMIOLOGY

• Since spermatozoa appear after puberty, these lesions are never seen in children.
• Maximum incidence occurs in the fourth and fifth decades.
• No racial predilection

GENETICS

• Unknown

STAGING: N/A

SIGNS AND SYMPTOMS

• Usually not painful
• Palpable above the testis, in the region of the caput epididymis
• Will transilluminate with flashlight in dark room
• Can achieve a size that is uncomfortable in tight underwear or while sitting with crossed legs
• Usually can palpate the testis separately from spermatocele
• Feels like "a third ball" to the patient

PATHOPHYSIOLOGY

• Efferent duct of the epididymis becomes obstructed
• Cysts may be uni- or multilocated
• Covered with pseudostratified epithelium supported by a fibrous layer
• Liquid content has numerous spermatozoa, spermiophages, and sloughed cells
• May be the source of antisperm antibodies in the blood
• Rarely obstructing to other efferent ducts

CAUSES/RISK FACTORS

• Prior trauma of infection of scrotal contents is suggested as a cause, but most spermatoceles are idiopathic.
• Not related to prior vasectomy
• Suspected in some cases of DES exposure in utero

COMPLICATIONS

• Heavy feeling, only occasional pain
• Concern of being a testicular cancer
• Rarely cause of azoospermia in cases of solitary testis

DIFFERENTIAL DIAGNOSIS

• Hydrocele
• Hernia
• Testicular tumor
• Varicocele
• Young syndrome (bronchiectasis, absent cilia, epididymal distension, azoospermia)
• Bilateral congenital absence of vas with distension of epididymal caput

Database

HISTORY

• Patient discovers a painless scrotal mass on self-examination (usual presentation).

—Denies infection or trauma
—No urinary symptoms
—May be uncomfortable while sitting with crossed legs or in tight underwear

• Is there any change is size?

—No change in size by position (supine or erect)
—Progressive increase in size of mass over time, but may remain unchanged in size

• Birth history

—Was mother exposed to DES?

• Medical or surgical history

—Not related to prior hernia surgery or vasectomy
—Not specifically related to prior epididymitis

PHYSICAL EXAMINATION

• Transilluminate the mass.

—If it transilluminates and feels distinct from the testis, favor a spermatocele.

• Palpate the testis bilaterally.

—A spermatocele is distinctly palpable and separate from the testis.
—A spermatocele is soft, not hard (like a tumor) or nodular (like epididymitis).

• Examine the groin for an inguinal hernia.
• Examine for a varicocele while the patient stands upright and performs the Valsalva maneuver.

—A varicocele demonstrates a thrill from retrograde blood flow.

Diagnostic Studies

LABORATORY TESTING

- Urinalysis to rule out infection
- Tumor markers (beta-hCG, alpha-fetoprotein) if tumor suspected

IMAGING

- Scrotal ultrasound demonstrates a spermatocele in the head of the epididymis.

—May be the only imaging test needed
—Lesions as small as 2 mm are displayed.
—The echo texture of the underlying testis is normal.
—Spermatoceles and epididymal cysts have been reported in as many as 70% of men having high-resolution ultrasound.

- Magnetic resonance imaging

—Indicated if ultrasound results are equivocal
—Spermatoceles appear dark on T1-weighted images (similar to water).
—T2-weighted images show spermatoceles with a signal intensity similar to that of the testis.

SPECIAL STUDIES: N/A

 ## Treatment

GENERAL MEASURES

- No treatment necessary, unless the patient has discomfort
- Differentiate a spermatocele from testicular cancer.
- Surgery should be deferred if the patient is in his reproductive years, because surgery may lead to complete obstruction of all ductuli efferentia of the epididymis.
- Aspiration of a spermatocele may be a natural source of sperm for IUI, IVF, or ICSI.

MEDICAL: N/A

SURGICAL

- Spermatocelectomy is best accomplished with microsurgical dissection to remove all cystic structures and preserve the blood supply to the epididymis and testis.

—Multiple cysts may be seen with optical aids.
—Removal of even small spermatoceles can avoid recurrences.

ALTERNATIVE THERAPIES

- Aspiration or injection of a sclerosing agent should be discouraged, because it may provoke epididymitis.
- Planned aspirations may provide sperm in azoospermic men.
- In rare cases, the spermatocele may cause obstruction of the other efferent ducts of the epididymis. Surgery should proceed with caution.

PATIENT EDUCATION

- Patients should be told that these lesions are benign and that surgery is elective.
- Surgery may have negative reproductive consequences.

 ## Follow-Up

MONITORING

- Self-examinations are encouraged after demonstrating the anatomy of the scrotum and testis to patient.

—Comparative ultrasounds are suggested if there is a change in size or consistency.

PREVENTION: N/A

 ## Miscellaneous

SYNONYMS: N/A

ASSOCIATED CONDITIONS

- Epididymitis
- Young syndrome (bronchiectasis, absent cilia, obstructed epididymis)
- Congenital absence of the vas and distension of epididymal caput

NOTES

- Hydrocele fluid does not contain sperm; see also Section I, "Scrotum—Mass and/or Pain (Acute Scrotum)."

ABBREVIATIONS

- DES, diethylstilbestrol; hCG, human chorionic gonadotropin; IUI, intrauterine insemination; IVF, in vitro fertilization; ICSI, intracytoplasmic sperm injection

REFERENCES

Hricak H, Hamm B, Kim Bohyan. *Images of the Scrotum.* New York: Raven Press, 1995:146–147.

Jacobs SC, Casale AJ. Operations for hydroceles, spermatoceles and epididymal disorders. In: Fowler JE Jr, ed. *Urologic Surgery.* Boston: Little, Brown, 1992:570.

Nistal M, Paniagua R. *Testicular and Epididymal Pathology.* New York: Thieme-Stratton, 1994:282.

Werthman P, Hamilton, Yes L, Meldrum D, Rajfer J. Percutaneous sperm aspiration of a spermatocele for intracytoplasmic sperm injection. *J Urol* 1997;158:1524.

Author: Joel L. Marmar

Spinal Cord Injury—Urologic Considerations

 Basics

DESCRIPTION

• Spinal cord injury (SCI) alters lower urinary tract function based on level and completeness of injury.

—Lower (sacral) level injury: lower motor neuron lesion, bladder paralysis (detrusor areflexia [DA]), and retention
—Suprasacral injury: upper motor neuron lesion, reflexive and poorly controlled involuntary detrusor contraction (detrusor hyperreflexia [DH]), and incontinence
—Uncoordinated involuntary contraction of the sphincter mechanism, occurring simultaneously with uninhibited involuntary contraction of the bladder detrusor muscle (detrusor–sphincter dyssynergia [DSD]), prevalent in high thoracic and cervical-level SCI.
—Elevation of intravesical pressure causes significant morbidity in SCI.

EPIDEMIOLOGY

• Incidence: 32 new injuries per 1,000,000 population
• Prevalence: 906 per 1,000,000 population
• 85% of injuries: at/above T12
• 55% in quadriplegia, 45% in paraplegia
• 54% of injuries neurologically incomplete, 46% complete

GENETICS: N/A

STAGING

• ASIA Impairment Scale of SCI

—A: complete. No sensory or motor function is preserved in the sacral segments S4-S5.
—B: incomplete. Sensory but not motor function is preserved below the neurologic level and extends through the sacral segments S4-S5.
—C: incomplete. Motor function is preserved below the neurologic level, and the majority of key muscles below the neurologic level have a muscle grade less than 3.
—D: incomplete. Motor function is preserved below the neurologic level, and the majority of key muscles below the neurologic level have a muscle grade greater than or equal to 3.
—E: normal. Sensory and motor function is normal.

SIGNS AND SYMPTOMS

• Three phases of neurologic/urologic dysfunction after SCI

—Spinal shock phase: immediately after injury
—Flaccid paralysis, no reflex activity below the neurologic level of the lesion
—Duration variable: 6 weeks to 6 months
—Bladder areflexic with urinary retention
—Recovery phase: Reflex activity returns below the level of the lesion.
—Bladder/sphincter function variable, unpredictable
—Stable phase: no further recovery; bladder and sphincter function stabilize.
—Neither neurologic level of lesion nor the patient's symptoms accurately predict urinary function.
—Cervical/high thoracic-level injury: DH common, with associated DSD
—Lower thoracic and lumbar-level injury: variable urinary function
—Sacral-level injury: DA predominates
—Note: Low-level lesions may have DH, while upper level lesions may have DA.

• Urinary urgency, frequency, nocturia: difficulty inhibiting reflex detrusor contraction (DH)
• Incontinence

—DH: urge incontinence
—Intrinsic sphincteric deficiency (ISD): stress incontinence

• Urinary tract infection (UTI): urosepsis possible, especially with DSD
• Incomplete bladder emptying, elevated residual, retention: DSD or DA
• Renal insufficiency: late complication

—Renal scarring: recurrent pyelonephritis
—Renal pressure atrophy: sustained elevated intravesical pressure

• Urolithiasis: urinary stasis with or without chronic infection
• Hematuria: UTI, urolithiasis, urinary retention, bladder cancer (chronic inflammation, indwelling catheterization)

PATHOPHYSIOLOGY

• DH: uncontrolled reflex bladder contraction

—Collateral sprouting of new neural pathways
—Loss of inhibitory impulses from cortical centers; primitive reflex pathways

• DSD: abnormal reflexive sphincter contraction during involuntary detrusor contraction

—Functional bladder outflow obstruction, elevated intravesical pressure
—Secondary damage: pressure, infection, urolithiasis
—DH must be present for DSD. DH may occur without DSD.
—10% to 20% of patients have internal (bladder neck) sphincter dyssynergia with external sphincter dyssynergia
—Elevated intravesical pressure >40 cm H_2O responsible for sequelae of DH-DSD

• DA

—Interruption of sacral reflex arc; no detrusor contraction
—Low-pressure storage (volumes up to 500 mL)
—Adrenergic overgrowth: decreased bladder compliance, elevated storage pressure

• Autonomic dysreflexia: potentially life threatening

—Lesions at T6 and higher
—Exaggerated sympathetic outflow produced by noxious stimulus below the lesion (i.e., bladder distention)
—Reflex vasoconstriction below the level of the lesion: paroxysmal hypertension
—Parasympathetic outflow cannot bypass the neurologic lesion; modulating parasympathetic discharge effects are limited to above the level of the lesion: diaphoresis, vasodilatation, piloerection.
—Reflex bradycardia from marked hypertension
—Requires immediate attention
—If during urologic procedure
—Stop procedure, drain bladder; usually effective
—Nifedipine (10 mg SL), nitrates (NTG 0.4 mg SL), or intravenous agents (nitroprusside) may be required.

• ISD damage to sacral cord

CAUSES/RISK FACTORS

• Multiple etiologies for SCI

—Arachnoiditis, arteriovenous malformation, congenital malformation (myelodysplasia)
—Guillain-Barré, herniated intervertebral disc, cord infarct
—Plaques of multiple sclerosis, spinal stenosis
—Transverse myelitis, trauma, tumor

COMPLICATIONS

- Bladder wall thickening, detrusor hypertrophy, diverticula

—Bladder wall fibrosis, decreased compliance, vesicoureteral reflux: all associated with chronic catheter

- Recurrent UTI

—Males febrile with parenchymal involvement; abscess formation possible
  - —Prostatitis, epididymo-orchitis, pyelonephritis
    - —Female febrile UTI: pyelonephritis

- Urolithiasis: urinary stasis, chronic infection (urea-splitting organisms)

—Bladder, renal, ureteral: may complicate UTI with obstruction

- Urinary retention
- Hydroureteronephrosis

—Intravesical pressure >40 cm H_2O impairs ureteral urine flow.
—Ureteral dilatation impairs the ureterovesical junction to prevent reflux.
—Vesicoureteral reflux predisposes to chronic pyelonephritis, renal staghorn calculus.
—Renal insufficiency, pressure atrophy, chronic infection

- Neoplastic transformation: associated with chronic catheter

—Chronic inflammation: squamous metaplasia in 80%, squamous cell carcinoma in 5%

- Tissue erosion: chronic catheters cause hypospadias, complete disruption of the urethra from the meatus to the bladder neck, and intractable incontinence.

DIFFERENTIAL DIAGNOSIS

- A comprehensive urologic evaluation is required in SCI to rule out other conditions.
- Incomplete bladder emptying

—BPH, prostate cancer
—Urethral stricture
—Bladder/urethral tumor: benign or malignant

- Urinary incontinence

—Pelvic floor prolapse, urethral hypermobility, cystocele
—Intrinsic sphincteric deficiency: trauma, previous surgery
—Fistula formation: especially in females (vesicovaginal, etc.)

 Database

HISTORY

- Neurologic disease: onset, duration
- Voiding symptoms

—Irritative: frequency, urgency, nocturia
—Incontinence: urge, stress
—Obstructive: hesitancy, intermittency, slow stream, straining

- Method of urinary management

—Condom catheter urinary collection
—Intermittent self-catheterization
—Indwelling urethral or suprapubic catheter
—Credé, Valsalva voiding

- Urinary tract infection

—Severity of infection: febrile, hospitalization, IV antibiotics required?
—Frequency of recurrence

- Urolithiasis

—Episodes, surgical intervention, calculus composition

- Autonomic dysreflexia (AD): associated with urination

PHYSICAL EXAMINATION

- Fever: parenchymal urinary tract infection

—Men: prostate, testes/epididymis, renal
—Women: renal

- Hypertension: AD with manipulation of the GI/GU systems
- Generalized edema: severe renal insufficiency
- Palpable flank mass: hydronephrosis
- Flank tenderness: ureteral obstruction, pyelonephritis
- Abdominal mass: distended bladder, urinary retention
- Incontinence of urine

—Spontaneously
—Stress maneuvers: Marshall test
—Abdominal/pelvic palpation/compression

- Testicular mass

—Epididymo-orchitis/epididymitis; secondary abscess, etc.

- Prostate mass/nodule: focal prostatitis

—Neurologic: sacral root
  —Perianal sensation
  —Anal tone, sphincter control
  —Bulbocavernosus reflex: contraction of anal sphincter with stimulation of glans penis/clitoris

 Diagnostic Studies

LABORATORY TESTING

- Blood studies

—Serum chemistry: renal function, creatinine, electrolyte levels
—Complete blood count: elevated WBC, secondary anemia due to decreased renal function or chronic infection

- Urine studies

—Urine analysis
  —Proteinuria: renal dysfunction
  —Pyuria, nitrite, leukocyte esterase: acute or chronic infection
  —Hematuria: infection or lithiasis

IMAGING

- Renal ultrasound: to screen calculus, hydronephrosis, mass
- Excretory urography

—Contraindicated with serum creatinine >2.0
—Delayed excretion of contrast with high urinary-storage pressures
—Hydroureteronephrosis
  —Marked elevation of intravesical pressure (i.e., DH/DESD) or calculi
—Bladder thickening, trabeculation, diverticulum, incomplete emptying

- Voiding cystourethrogram

—Bladder thickening, trabeculation, diverticulum, incomplete emptying
—Ureter: vesicoureteral reflux, hydroureter, hydroureteronephrosis
—Urethra: usually normal; rule out stricture.
  —DH + DESD: prostatic urethra dilated; membranous urethra persistently narrow, stenotic, nonrelaxing
—Nuclear medicine renal scan
  —Quantification of glomerular filtration rate (GFR)
  —Sequential studies detect deterioration of renal function.
  —Furosemide wash-out analysis (1 mg/kg IV) determines obstruction: half-life >20 minutes.

(continued)

Spinal Cord Injury—Urologic Considerations (continued)

SPECIAL STUDIES

- Videourodynamics: essential to determine effective urologic management for all patients with neurogenic lower urinary tract dysfunction. Periodic reevaluation to confirm acceptable intravesical pressure and prevent upper urinary tract damage
  - Medium-fill cystometry at 50 cc/min
    - DH: uninhibited involuntary detrusor contraction; voiding pressure >60 cm H_2O in men, 40 cm H_2O in women
    - DH + DSD: uninhibited involuntary detrusor contraction; intravesical pressure >40 cm H_2O during storage, >60 cm H_2O during voiding
    - DA: no detrusor contraction with filling, usually up to maximum of 600 mL. Storage pressure <30 cm H_2O
    - DA with decreased compliance: gradually increasing intravesical pressure during filling despite absent detrusor contraction. Storage pressure >40 cm H_2O is associated with upper tract deterioration.
  - Fluoroscopy
    - Intravesical pressure normal (DH, DA): bladder walls smooth, spherical; bladder neck closed at rest; reflux absent
    - DH: bladder neck funneling with detrusor contraction; voiding complete without reflux
    - DA: bladder neck closed throughout filling
    - ISD: bladder neck slightly open at rest; opens further with Valsalva efforts, incontinence
    - DH + DSD: storage: bladder walls trabeculated; "Christmas tree" configuration, diverticula; voiding: dilated prostatic urethra, narrow membranous urethra, normal bulbous and pendulous urethra; ureter: vesicoureteral reflux with or without hydronephrosis
  - Urethral pressure profile
    - DA: stable throughout study
    - DH: stable with filling, isobaric with intravesical pressure during voiding
    - DH + DESD: sustained or accentuated pressure during involuntary, uninhibited detrusor contraction
  - Sphincter electromyography
    - Polyphasic potentials, fibrillation, positive sharp waves
    - DH + DESD: accentuated with involuntary uninhibited detrusor contraction
- Cystoscopy for coexisting pathology
- DH + DESD
  - Normal penile urethra; spastic, nonrelaxing, stenotic membranous urethra
  - Dilated prostatic urethra with bladder trabeculation/diverticuli

 Treatment

GENERAL MEASURES

- Urodynamics are essential to determine lower urinary tract function/dysfunction and to plan urologic management.
- Control intravesical pressure: protects upper tracts
- Spontaneous voiding with continence is possible with DH controlled medically.
- Urinary drainage: intermittent catheterization or external collection appliance
- Indwelling catheterization: Avoid due to complications (UTI, erosion, calculi, etc.).
- Intermittent self-catheterization: most effective treatment; requires low storage pressure

- Urinary tract colonized; treat only symptomatic UTI.
- If unable to self-catheterize urethra: Consider continent catheterizable stoma.
- Males unable to self-catheterize
  - Condom catheter if storage/detrusor leak point pressure <40 cm H_2O, voiding pressure <60 cm H_2O
  - Outlet obstruction (BPH, DSD, etc.) requires medical or surgical treatment.
  - Ileal conduit "bladder chimney" if cannot maintain appliance
- Females unable to catheterize urethra or stoma: incontinent ileal "bladder chimney" urostomy
- Incontinence or elevated intravesical pressure due to poor compliance or hyperreflexia
  - Reduce storage pressure: Continence between catheterizations preserves upper urinary tracts.
  - Augmentation cystoplasty if anticholinergic therapy ineffective

- Lower urinary tracts that cannot be reconstructed require cystectomy and urinary diversion.

- Incontinent urostomy: continuous leakage into appliance
- Continent urinary reservoir

MEDICAL

- Anticholinergics to improve urinary storage pressure/decrease involuntary contraction

- Oxybutynin 5 mg po tid-qid
- Propantheline bromide 15 mg po bid-tid
- Hyoscyamine 0.375 mg po bid-tid
- Tolterodine 2 to 4 mg po bid

- Alpha-adrenergic blockers: decrease internal sphincter function, lower voiding pressure; ineffective for DESD

- Doxazosin 2 to 8 mg po qd
- Terazosin 2 to 5 mg po qd-bid
- Prazosin 1 mg po tid
- Tamsulosin 0.4 mg po od
- Phenoxybenzamine 10 mg po bid (nonselective)

- Botulinum toxin injection into external sphincter for DSD: short-lived; requires repeated injection

SURGICAL

• Endoscopic sphincter ablation: only males with DSD; requires condom catheter

—Electrosurgical or Nd:YAG laser sphincterotomy: Incise the external sphincter from the bulbous urethra to the mid-prostatic urethra; incise the prostate and bladder neck if internal sphincter dyssynergia is present.
—Sphincter stent prosthesis: bridges mid-prostatic to bulbous urethra
   —Suprapubic tube cystostomy may be required in the perioperative period.
—Augmentation cystoplasty: The bladder is incised in a clamshell fashion to disrupt detrusor contraction; an intestinal segment is used to patch the bladder, increasing urinary storage with decreased pressure.
   —Intermittent catheterization for urinary drainage
   —Limited dexterity mandates construction of a continent catheterizable stoma for the urinary reservoir, especially in females.
—Ileal conduit cutaneous vesicostomy: "bladder chimney"
   —Conduit of ileum connecting dome of bladder to anterior abdominal wall; urostomy requires stomal appliance
   —Useful for those unable to perform self-catheterization (i.e., quadriplegia)
—Cystectomy with continent urinary reservoir
   —Ileal or colon pouch; continent catheterizable stoma (appendix or tapered ileum) on abdomen
—Cystectomy with ileal urostomy

ALTERNATIVE THERAPIES

• Vanilloid agents: suppress uninhibited involuntary detrusor contraction in patients refractory to anticholinergic therapy

—Capsaicin, resiniferotoxin: applied intravesically, requires repeated instillation

• Sacral deafferentation with sacral nerve root stimulation

—Deafferentation with dorsal rhizotomy abolishes spontaneous detrusor contraction, improving urinary storage.
—Nerve root stimulation allows control over detrusor contraction
—Obstruction by the sphincter may require sphincteric ablation.

PATIENT EDUCATION

• Explain the potential dangers of untreated neurogenic lower urinary tract dysfunction, especially renal failure, infection, and urinary lithiasis.

 Follow-Up

MONITORING

• Annual evaluation

—Videourodynamic testing: Assure low intravesical pressure.
—Upper tract imaging (US, ExU) to rule out upper tract changes (calculi, hydronephrosis)
—Serum chemistry to confirm normal renal function and electrolyte balance

PREVENTION: N/A

 Miscellaneous

SYNONYMS

• Neurogenic bladder (general)
• DH: overactive bladder, spastic bladder, hyperactive bladder, hypertonicity of bladder, uninhibited neurogenic bladder
• DA: motor neurogenic bladder, flaccid bladder, paralysis of bladder, sensory neurogenic bladder, autonomic neurogenic bladder
• DSD: reflex neurogenic bladder

ASSOCIATED CONDITIONS

• Neurogenic impotence

NOTES

• See also Section I: "Neurogenic Bladder."

ABBREVIATIONS

• ASIA, American Spinal Injury Association; DA, detrusor areflexia; DH, detrusor hyperreflexia; DSD, detrusor–sphincter dyssynergia; DESD, detrusor–external sphincter dyssynergia; ISD, intrinsic sphincter deficiency

REFERENCES

Blaivas JG. Spinal cord injury. In: Blaivas JG, Chancellor MB, eds. *Atlas of Urodynamics*. Baltimore: Williams & Wilkins, 1996:160–173.

Bors E, Comarr AE. *Neurological Urology*. Baltimore: University Park Press, 1971.

Chancellor MB, Blaivas JG. Spinal cord injury. In: Chancellor MB, Blaivas JG, eds. *Practical Neurourology: Genitourinary Complications in Neurologic Disease*. Boston: Butterworth-Heinemann, 1995: 99–118.

McGuire EJ, Savastano JA. Urodynamics and management of the neuropathic bladder in spinal cord injury patients. *J Am Paraplegia Soc* 1985;8:28.

Watanabe T, Rivas DA, Chancellor MB. Urodynamics of spinal cord injury. *Urol Clin North Am* 1996;23:459.

Yalla SV, Fam BA. Spinal cord injury. In: Krane RJ, Siroky MB, eds. *Clinical Neuro-Urology*. Boston: Little, Brown, 1991:319–332.

Authors: David A. Rivas and Patrick J. Shenot

Stroke—Urologic Considerations

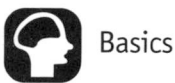 Basics

DESCRIPTION

- Cerebrovascular accidents (CVAs), typically caused by thrombotic or hemorrhagic brain injury, can cause transient or permanent urinary tract dysfunction.

EPIDEMIOLOGY

- Prevalence: over age 65, 60/10,000; over age 70, 95/10,000
- United States: 550,000 per year, resulting in 150,000 deaths and 300,000 disabled victims
- 10% return to normal; 40% have mild residual impairment; 40% require special care; 10% need institutionalization lifelong.
- Urinary incontinence (UI) and urinary retention (UR) typically develop in the recovery period.

GENETICS

- More common in African Americans

STAGING: N/A

SIGNS AND SYMPTOMS

- Acute UR after CVA: due to cerebral shock

—Factors contributing to UR: impaired consciousness, restricted mobility, inability to communicate, acute overdistention of bladder

- UI occurs in 38% to 60% in recovery period

—UI: poor prognostic indicator of recovery and survival
—Frequency, urgency, and urge incontinence most common
—Factors contributing to UI: severe motor deficits, altered mental status, dysphagia, preexisting lower urinary tract pathology

PATHOPHYSIOLOGY

- Acute UR: detrusor areflexia, presumably from "cerebral shock"

—UR usually resolves in days to weeks.

- UI is multifactorial, and depends on the location of the CVA.

—The pontine micturition center (PMC) coordinates the micturition reflex.
—The cerebral cortex and midbrain send a tonic inhibiting signal to the PMC.
—The hypothalamus and pons are facilitatory.
—Basal ganglia: both facilitatory and inhibitory functions
—Cerebellum: inhibitory during bladder filling and facilitatory during voiding
—Difficult to predict effect of CVA on LUT function (complex neurointegration)
—Cortical and capsular CVAs: disinhibition of the micturition reflex: detrusor hyperreflexia and uninhibited relaxation of the external sphincter

- Common urodynamic findings with CVAs

—Normal bladder and normal sphincter
—Detrusor hyperreflexia/normal sphincter
—Detrusor areflexia/normal sphincter
—Detrusor–sphincter dyssynergia is rare after a CVA.
—Diminished bladder contractility (often due to preexisting conditions)

CAUSES/RISK FACTORS

- UI after CVA

—Detrusor hyperreflexia: disinhibition of PMC and facilitation of micturition reflex
—Uninhibited sphincter relaxation
—Detrusor areflexia or diminished contractility: generally resolve

- Cognitive deficits: altered mental status, neglect, proprioceptive loss, aphasia
- Motor deficits: impaired mobility
- Altered sensation: proprioceptive loss; loss of sensation
- Preexisting LUT pathology: 15% have UI prior to CVAs.

—Benign prostatic hyperplasia/bladder outlet obstruction (BOO)
—Preexisting detrusor instability
—Intrinsic sphincter deficiency
—Diabetic cystopathy
—Detrusor hypocontractility

COMPLICATIONS

- Early: if bladder drainage not provided

—Acute overdistention injury, UTI, acute renal failure, incontinence

- Late: if LUT dysfunction not addressed

—Urinary incontinence, skin breakdown, renal insufficiency, UTI, diminished quality of life, institutionalization

DIFFERENTIAL DIAGNOSIS

- Rule out other causes of UI or LUT dysfunction.

—Transient or reversible causes of UI: common in elderly ("DIAPERS")
   —**D**elirium
   —**I**nfection
   —**A**trophic urethritis/vaginitis
   —**P**harmaceuticals
   —**P**sychological problems, severe depression
   —**E**xcess urine output (e.g., congestive cardiac failure, hyperglycemia)
   —**R**estricted mobility
   —**S**tool impaction
—Fixed causes of UI
   —BOO, intrinsic sphincter deficiency, urethral hypermobility/pelvic prolapse, GU malignancy
   —Stones, diabetic cystopathy, spinal cord lesions (spinal stenosis, disc herniation, and multiple sclerosis)
   —Concomitant neurologic disease (Parkinson disease, HIV, and peripheral neuropathy)

 Database

HISTORY

- Do symptoms suggest a reversible cause of UI?

—Acute change in mental status
—Dysuria, fevers, and chills
—Depression, poor mobility, constipation/obstipation

- Previous urologic complaints, symptoms, or UI?

—Suggest underlying/preexisting condition

- Assess list of new and old prescribed and over-the-counter medications

—Common cause of UI in the elderly

- Medical and surgical history

PHYSICAL EXAMINATION

- Assess the abdomen for bladder distention.
- Neurologic examination

—Attention to the lower extremities, perineum, and sphincter tone and reflexes.

- Assess the prostate for size and consistency.
- Pelvic examination in women
- Assess the chest for signs of congestive failure,
- Assess the lower extremities for edema.

—Fluid retention may result in postural diuresis and UI at night.

- Check post-void residual (PVR) urine if suspect incomplete emptying

 Diagnostic Studies

LABORATORY TESTING

- Urinalysis

—Make sure to check for proteinuria, glycosuria, and specific gravity

- Urine culture (if suspect UTI)
- BUN, creatinine, prostatic-specific antigen (if appropriate)

IMAGING

- IVP, CT scan, or ultrasound scan of abdomen and pelvis

—Rule out stones or cancer (if suspected)
—KUB to rule out impaction (if suspected)

- CT scan or MRI to rule out spinal pathology (if suspected)

SPECIAL STUDIES

- Urodynamics for more accurate assessment of LUT function

—Indications: confirm presence/etiology of LUT dysfunction; failure of conservative measures; surgical planning

- Voiding diary: Assess day-to-day function.

—Functional bladder capacity; fluid intake; time and frequency of incontinence; situation in which UI occurs; diurnal variation in urine output

Treatment

GENERAL MEASURES

- Initial goals

—Adequate bladder drainage by CIC or Foley catheter until patient resumes voiding
—Prevent acute complications: see above.

- Long-term goals

—Attain adequate bladder drainage
—Maintain urinary continence
—Prevent complications, minimize risk of infection, maintain renal function
—Improve quality of life

MEDICAL

- UR or PVRs are elevated (>150–200 cc): CIC is the best treatment.

—Indwelling Foley or suprapubic tubes are discouraged.
  —Last resort due complications (e.g., stones, UTI, etc.)

- If frequency, urgency, urge UI due to hyperreflexia

—Time voiding, prompted voiding, bladder training, and behavior modifications are the first line of management.
—Anticholinergics may be added as needed: Use them judiciously, because UR may be induced.
  —Oxybutynin 2.5 mg po bid to 10 mg po tid
  —Hycosamine 0.125 mg po bid to 0.375 mg po tid
  —Detrol (Tolterodine) 2 mg po bid
—Fluid restriction as needed (based on the voiding diary)
—Restricted mobility: Improve access to a bathroom; provide a commode, urinal, or assistance
—Condom catheter: undesirable; risk UTI and penile skin breakdown

- Hyperreflexia and detrusor–sphincter dyssynergia (usually with concomitant spinal cord lesion)

—CIC, anticholinergics

- Stress UI and hyperreflexia

—Behavior modification, as above, may be sufficient.
—Imipramine 10 mg po bid to 25 mg po tid; anticholinergic effect, may also increase outlet resistance

SURGICAL

- Indicated only for the treatment of other concomitant LUT dysfunction

—BOO in men unresponsive to medical management: BPH and stricture
—Stress UI in women unresponsive to medical management

- UDS before considering surgery
- Counsel the patient that surgery is indicated to correct certain LUT dysfunction; some symptoms may persist postoperatively.

ALTERNATIVE THERAPIES

- Continence pads should be used as an aid, not as a substitute for other measures.
- Biofeedback and electrical stimulation: unproved efficacy in this setting

PATIENT EDUCATION

- Patients should be counseled that, in the majority, UR will resolve and UI can be controlled.

 ## Follow-Up

MONITORING

- Patients performing CIC or with indwelling catheters should be followed at least biannually.

—Yearly: BUN, creatinine, renal ultrasound, UDS

- Hyperreflexia and adequate emptying can be followed yearly.

PREVENTION: N/A

 ## Miscellaneous

SYNONYMS: N/A

ASSOCIATED CONDITIONS

- Neurosurgical procedures and head trauma may imitate a CVA.

NOTES: N/A

ABBREVIATIONS

- BOO, bladder outlet obstruction; UI, urinary incontinence; UR, urinary retention; LUT, lower urinary tract; PVR, post-void residual; CIC, clean intermittent catheterization; UDS, urodynamic studies

REFERENCES

Burney TL, et al. Effects of cerebrovascular accidents on micturition. *Urol Clin North Am* 1996; 23:3.

Gelber DA, et al. Causes of urinary incontinence after acute hemispheric stroke. *Stroke* 1993; 3:378–382.

Khan Z, et al. Analysis of voiding disorders in patients with cerebrovascular accidents. *Urology* 1990;35:3.

Authors: Marko Gudziak and Valal K. George

Syphilis

 Basics

DESCRIPTION

• A sexually transmitted disease caused by Treponema pallidum, a spirochete
• Characterized by primary, secondary, latent, and tertiary stages
• Manifestations range from simple genital ulcer disease to systemic disease with life-threatening sequelae.

EPIDEMIOLOGY

• U.S. incidence peaked in the 1940s at 70 in 100,000; and was stable in 1993 at 12 in 100,000.
• Higher incidence in African Americans and youths.
• Incidence highest in southern states, higher in STD/HIV-positive patients.

GENETICS: N/A

STAGING

• Primary, secondary, and tertiary stages (see below)

SIGNS AND SYMPTOMS

• Primary: painless, usually solitary (60%) chancre with indurated edge on oral mucosa or genitalia (usually associated with nontender inguinal adenopathy)
• Secondary: constitutional symptoms, characteristic truncal and palmar/plantar erythematous rash, condyloma lata (sessile perianal warts: may be confused with condyloma acuminata)
• Latent (asymptomatic): "early" if <1 year, "late" if >1 year
• Tertiary: benign tertiary characterized by parenchymatous gummas
• Neurosyphilis: myriad neurologic symptoms secondary to meningovascular or parenchymatous brain disease; or tabes dorsalis: damage to dorsal columns
• Cardiovascular: luetic aneurism (aortic root), myocarditis

PATHOPHYSIOLOGY

• The chancre has a high concentration of spirochetes and appears 9 to 90 days (mean: 21) following exposure.
• Untreated, progresses to secondary in 6 to 24 weeks, and then becomes latent
• Latent progresses to tertiary in one-third of patients (up to 20 years after exposure), regresses in one-third (with negative serology), and remains latent in one-third (asymptomatic with positive serology). One-half of tertiary is benign (parenchymal gummas), one-fourth is neurologic, and one-fourth cardiovascular.

CAUSES/RISK FACTORS

• Unprotected sex, prostitution

COMPLICATIONS

• Increased risk of contracting other STDs, including HIV
• Neurologic debilitation, death from complications of tertiary syphilis
• Jarisch-Herxheimer reaction: acute febrile illness with headache, myalgia; thought to be caused by lysis of treponemes
• May cause early labor in pregnant women

DIFFERENTIAL DIAGNOSIS

• Other STDs: herpes (usually tender, preceded by vesicles, shorter time from exposure, prominent constitutional symptoms, and tender lymphadenopathy), chancroid (painful ulcer and tender lymphadenopathy), lymphogranuloma venereum (associated with chlamydia infection with draining inguinal sinuses). Also consider trauma, fixed drug eruption, and fungal infection.

 Database

HISTORY

• History of other STDs
• Medications (fixed drug eruption?), history of trauma
• Review of systems: constitutional symptoms (herpes)
• History of recent sexual contacts, high-risk behaviors: Was there contact with someone with known infection? What was the timing of contacts and development of the chancre?
• Characteristics of the chancre: Is the chancre tender (chancroid, herpes)? Were there vesicles (herpes)?
• Symptoms of other STDs: Dysuria and urethral discharge may point to urethritis.

PHYSICAL EXAMINATION

• Careful examination of genitalia: solitary vs. multiple chancres and their location. Is the chancre tender? Does it have a clean base? Is the edge indurated? Is there associated inguinal lymphadenopathy, tender vs. non-tender?

Diagnostic Studies

LABORATORY TESTING

- Serologic tests
—Nontreponemal tests (RPR, VDRL)
  —Sensitive and used for screening
  —Treponemal tests (e.g., FTA-ABS, MHA-TP) are highly specific and confirm positive nontreponemal tests.
  —Nontreponemal tests correlate with disease activity and should revert to negative following treatment, but treponemal tests will stay positive in over 85%.
  —All STD patients should receive nontreponemal tests and HIV counseling.
- Microscopy
—Treponemes cannot be viewed with conventional means, but only with dark-field microscopy of a scraping of the chancre, the gold standard of diagnosis.

IMAGING: N/A

SPECIAL STUDIES

- CSF sampling for neurosyphilis: (+)VDRL of CSF is diagnostic, (−)FTA-Abs rules out neurosyphilis.

 Treatment

GENERAL MEASURES

- Treat all patients and known contacts. Retreat if a fourfold decrease in nontreponemal titer not achieved.

MEDICAL

- Penicillin (PCN) is the only proven treatment. Different stages require different doses.
- Primary, secondary, and early (<1 year) latent: benzathine PCN 2.4 million units IM × 1
- Late (>1 year) or indeterminate latent, tertiary (except neurologic): benzathine PCN 2.4 million units IM every week × 3
- Neurosyphilis: aqueous crystalline PCN-G 2.4 million units IV q4h × 10 days

SURGICAL: N/A

ALTERNATIVE THERAPIES

- Patients who report PCN allergy must be skin tested and desensitized. If they are truly allergic, give an alternate treatment.

—Doxycycline 100 mg bid × 14 days, or tetracycline 500 mg qid × 14 days

PATIENT EDUCATION: N/A

 Follow-Up

MONITORING

- Repeat the nontreponemal test at 1, 3, 6, and 12 months after treatment.
- Document a 4× decrease in titer. Retreat and evaluate for neurosyphilis if no decrease is seen.

PREVENTION

- Barrier protection during sex, avoidance of high-risk partners, abstinence. Treat all known contacts.

 Miscellaneous

SYNONYMS

- Vernacular: bad blood, big pox, birds in the blood

ASSOCIATED CONDITIONS: N/A

NOTES

- See also Section I, "Penis—Lesion."

ABBREVIATIONS: N/A

REFERENCES

Zenilman JM. Update on bacterial sexually transmitted diseases. *Urol Clin North Am* 1992;19: 25–34.

Parish LC, Seghal VN, Buntin DM. *Color Atlas of STDs*. Tokyo: Igaku–Shoin Medical Publishers, 1991.

Mandel GL, ed. *Atlas of Infectious Diseases,* vol 5, Sexually Transmitted Diseases, Rein MF, ed. 1996. Current Medicine, Philadelphia.

Authors: Jonathan F. Masoudi and S. Bruce Malkowicz

Testis—Cancer, General

 Basics

DESCRIPTION

- Malignant neoplasm of the testicle that is usually of germ cell origin

EPIDEMIOLOGY

- 1999 statistics: 7,400 new cases with 300 deaths
- Relatively uncommon (1% of all cancers in males)
- Most common neoplasm in young adult men
- Overall prevalence is 2 to 3 per 100,000
- In the age group of 15- to 34-year-old men, the incidence is approximately 62 per 100,000.

GENETICS

- Some suggestion of familial tendency, but controversial
- Abnormality of short-arm chromosome 12

STAGING

- See the appendix for TNM system.

PATHOPHYSIOLOGY

- Around 95% arise from germ cells and are malignant.
- Seminoma: most common (40%). The overall survival rate is 90%.
- Nonseminomatous germ cell tumor (NSGCT)

—Embryonal cell carcinoma (15%–20%)
—Teratoma (5%–10%)
—Choriocarcinoma (<1%)
—Yolk sac carcinoma (usually in children)

- 40% are of more than one histologic pattern. Most frequent: embryonal carcinoma and teratoma

—Secondary tumors may be seen occasionally in patients with leukemia, and to a lesser degree in other neoplasms (prostate, gastrointestinal tract, lung, kidney, neuroblastoma, and melanoma).

- 5% of testicular neoplasms arise from the gonadal stroma tumors; the majority are benign.

—Most are Leydig cell and Sertoli cell tumors.

CAUSES/RISK FACTORS

- Cryptorchidism

—10% of testicular cancer occurs in men with a history of an undescended testicle.

- 15% to 20% of testicular carcinoma may occur in the contralateral descended testicle.

—Probably associated with an endocrine imbalance or defect

- Exposure to DES in utero

COMPLICATIONS

- Metastasis, death, subfertility/infertility

DIFFERENTIAL DIAGNOSIS

- See also Section I, "Testicular Mass—Adult and Pediatric."
- Painless enlargement of the testicle

—May be noticed by patient, sexual partner, or occasionally by the health care provider
—Although most testicular neoplasms are painless, about one-fourth have some discomfort, and the diagnosis of epididymitis is often given, not infrequently delaying the diagnosis.

- Symptomatic hydrocele, hernia, benign testicular/epididymal lesion
- Epididymitis, torsion testicle or appendage (usually painful)

 Database

HISTORY

- Testicular cancer should be suspected in all men with a painless mass in the testicle.
- Weight loss and back or abdominal pain suggests metastasis.
- Epididymitis is also common in young men, but this condition is usually very painful.

PHYSICAL EXAMINATION

- Diagnosis of a testis tumor can usually be made on physical examination.
- An examination of both testes, using both hands, is essential.

—Testicular size, consistency, size and location of mass, tenderness

- Adenopathy, abdominal mass, lower extremity edema

Diagnostic Studies

LABORATORY TESTING

• Urinalysis may aid in cases of epididymitis.
• Markers for testis tumors can be divided into three groups:

—Serum protein markers: elevated in 50% to 70%; persistent elevation of one or more of these markers after orchiectomy indicates metastases.
  —Beta subunit of human chorionic gonadotropin (beta-hCG): half-life of 24 to 36 hours
  —Alpha-fetoprotein (AFP): half-life of 5 to 7 days
  —Lactic acid dehydrogenase (LDH): nonspecific; usually a marker of tumor bulk
  —Placental alkaline phosphatase: limited use at this time
—Cytogenetic markers: chromosomal marker on chromosome 12 (investigational)
—Molecular markers: investigational

IMAGING

• Ultrasound is the principal radiologic diagnostic test that can be used if there is a doubt.

—The lesion is usually hypoechoic, but not 100% accurate.

• A testicular MRI may be used at times, but is usually not necessary.
• Nuclear flow scan if torsion suspected
• The metastatic work-up usually includes chest x-ray, CT of the abdomen and pelvis, and sometimes CT of the chest.
• Lymphangiography has been replaced by CT scans in most centers. It may be used to guide postoperative abdominal radiation therapy.

SPECIAL STUDIES

• A needle biopsy, or other transscrotal procedure, of a suspected testicular malignancy is contraindicated.

 Treatment

GENERAL MEASURES

• Radical orchiectomy is the initial treatment, even in the presence of metastasis.

—Additional therapy is based on the type of tumor and the stage. Usually combination of medical, surgical, and radiation management
  —Clinical stage I disease limited to the testicle: no evidence of lymphatic spread
  —Clinical stage II: clinical or radiographic evidence of lymphatic spread below the diaphragm
—Clinical stage III: evidence of supradiaphragmatic or extranodal metastases

• Commonly, testicular cancer is divided into seminoma and nonseminomatous germ cell tumors.

• Seminoma
—Most clinical stage I patients
  —Radiation therapy to the retroperitoneal subdiaphragmatic lymphatics; standard of care since the 1920s
  —Dose is approximately 2500 cGy.
  —Surveillance is an option, but morbidity of radiation is so low that most physicians recommend radiation.
  —Studies to further reduce the radiation therapy dose are underway in some centers.
  —Two cycles of chemotherapy; but there is no long-term follow-up in these nonrandomized trials.
—Stage II and III seminomas: usually treated with cisplatin-based combination chemotherapy

• Nonseminomatous germ cell tumors (NSGCTs)

—Risk factors to be considered in deciding treatment:
  —Vascular invasion, primary tumor stage (pT 2 or greater), percentage of embryonal cancer, preoperative and postoperative tumor markers, and presence of choriocarcinoma are all considered a high risk for observation.
—Stage I: 70% of clinical stage I is cured by orchiectomy.
  —Surveillance after orchiectomy is an option; the patient must agree to close follow-up.
  —Wide support for this in Europe
  —Retroperitoneal node dissection or laparoscopic retroperitoneal lymph node dissection.
  —Chemotherapy is an option, but is not the treatment of choice for stage I disease.
—Stage II: Divide into low-volume (IIA) and high-volume (IIB: nodes 2–5 cm in diameter; and IIC: >5cm) disease.
  —IIA: node dissection or chemotherapy
  —IIB, IIC: Three to four cycles of chemotherapy (cisplatin, bleomycin, etoposide [PEB]), particularly if the tumor markers do not return to normal levels following orchiectomy
  —If residual nodal therapy is seen on CT scan, and tumor markers return to normal levels, resection of the mass is generally advocated.
—Stage III: as for IIC

MEDICAL
• See above

SURGICAL
• See above

ALTERNATIVE THERAPIES: N/A

PATIENT EDUCATION: N/A

 Follow-Up

• Optimal timing for follow-up is not well defined; most relapses occur in the first 6 months.
• Nevertheless, recurrent disease has been seen at 3 and 4 years after orchiectomy.
• Patients who have had definitive treatment should be followed closely with a PE, chest x-ray, and tumor markers every month for 1 year, then at 3-month intervals for 3 years, and then yearly.
• Surveillance protocols in lieu of definitive treatment will require the above plus CT scans every 2 to 3 months for the first year and then every 4 to 6 months from the second to the fourth year.

 Miscellaneous

SYNONYMS

• Testicular tumor, cancer, neoplasm, seminoma, nonseminomatous germ cell tumor, germ cell tumors

ASSOCIATED CONDITIONS: N/A

NOTES

• See other specific tumor types in Section II.

ABBREVIATIONS

• NSGCT, nonseminomatous germ cell tumor

REFERENCE

Carroll PC, Presti JC, and Guest Editors. Entire issue. *Urol Clin North Am* 1998;25:365–544.

Author: David C. McLeod

Testis—Carcinoma In Situ

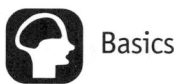 Basics

DESCRIPTION

• A precursor of all histologic variants of testicular germ cell tumors, except spermatocytic seminoma

EPIDEMIOLOGY

• General population: 0.8% of adult males, roughly paralleling the incidence of invasive germ cell tumors
• Typical age of diagnosis: 18 to 50 years; peak incidence: 30 to 35 years
• Associated with

—Cryptorchidism: 2% to 3%
—Contralateral testis tumor: 5% to 6%
—Infertility: 1%
—Gonadal dysgenesis: approximately 100%
—Testicular feminization: approximately 25%
—Extragonadal germ cell tumor: approximately 50%

• Postpubertal diagnosis: The disease course for prepubertal CIS has not been adequately delineated.
• No known cases of spontaneous regression

GENETICS

• Unknown

STAGING: N/A

SIGNS AND SYMPTOMS

• None, unless related to associated testicular tumor or feminization

PATHOPHYSIOLOGY

• Congenital

—Malignant gonocytes, which arise early in fetal life

• Acquired

—*p53* mutations: 66% of CIS specimens showed mutation of the *p53* gene.
—Numerical aberration in the number of copies in chromosome 1 associated with CIS

• Histopathology

—Typically malignant germ cells in a single row along the tubular membrane, with Sertoli cells the only other cell type
—Large nucleus, with multiple nucleoli
—High intracellular glycogen levels
—Occasionally found in tubules with spermatogenesis, or several rows of CIS germ cells

• Also called intratubular germ cell neoplasia

CAUSES/RISK FACTORS

• Congenital

—Cryptorchidism
—Gonadal dysgenesis
—Testicular feminization syndrome
—Gonadal dysgenesis

• Acquired

—Germ cell tumor
—Testicular atrophy

COMPLICATIONS

• Progression to invasive germ cell tumor

—100% progression to invasive disease if not treated

DIFFERENTIAL DIAGNOSIS

• Invasive germ cell tumor

 Database

HISTORY

• Infertility, germ cell tumor, cryptorchidism

—Poor semen analysis associated with CIS

• Surgical history

—Orchidopexy, orchiectomy

PHYSICAL EXAMINATION

• Testicular examination

—Atrophy, irregularity, or mass

Diagnostic Studies

LABORATORY TESTING

• None are specific for CIS.

—AFP, bhCG not elevated unless associated with testicular malignancy

IMAGING

• Ultrasound

—Testes have a more irregular pattern.
—Microcalcification (microlithiasis) may be associated with CIS.

• Magnetic resonance imaging

—Significant differences are noted between T1 relaxation times of normal testicles and ones with CIS.

SPECIAL STUDIES

• Semen analysis

—DNA flow cytometry to evaluate for hyperdiploid aneuploidy
—Bilateral CIS associated with azoospermia

• Testicular biopsy is the confirmatory study.

—Should not be fixed in formalin (obscures detail)
  —Can use either Bouin's, Stiena, Cleland, or Lillie
—Diagnosis by light microscopy
—Immunohistochemical markers include
  —Placental alkaline phosphatase, monoclonal antibody M2A, monoclonal antibody 43-9F, monoclonal antibody TRA-1-60
—Due to the diffuse nature of CIS, it is usually seen on random biopsy, even if present in only 5% of tubules.
—Needs to be at least 3 mm × 3 mm × 3 mm
  —No seeding has been noted with transscrotal biopsy for CIS.

 ## Treatment

GENERAL MEASURES

• Bilateral biopsy if US shows no mass
• Presence and status of contralateral testicle

—Normal contralateral testicle: orchiectomy
—No contralateral testicle: radiation therapy
—Contralateral tumor: contralateral orchiectomy, with ipsilateral radiation
—Contralateral CIS: bilateral radiation therapy

MEDICAL

• Radiation therapy

—20 Gy (2 Gy × 10 days) is curative, while preserving endocrine function to prevent lifelong testosterone replacement.
  —No contralateral germ cell tumors were noted with bilateral testicular radiation of 30 Gy (expected 5%–6% contralateral tumors) in PTS followed for 30 years.

SURGICAL

• Orchectomy: inguinal incision between internal and external ring, early vascular control, removal of testis with tunica intact

—Only if contralateral testis is normal

ALTERNATIVE THERAPIES

• Chemotherapy

—Not advised; multiple documented cases with persistence of CIS after curative chemotherapy for nodal disease secondary to contralateral germ cell tumor

PATIENT EDUCATION

• Instruct in testicular self examination.
• Some have advocated offering bilateral testicular biopsy to patients with a history of cryptorchidism when they are 18 to 20 years old.

 ## Follow-Up

MONITORING

• Negative biopsy for CIS

—If biopsy after the age of 18 is negative, risk of development of CIS and testicular germ cell tumor exceedingly rare, follow-up not needed

• Positive biopsy for CIS

—No reported cases of failure with either orchiectomy or radiation therapy; routine follow-up

PREVENTION: N/A

 ## Miscellaneous

SYNONYMS

• Intratubular germ cell neoplasia

ASSOCIATED CONDITIONS

• Testis germ cell tumor, cryptorchidism, infertility

NOTES

• See also Section I, "Testicular Mass—Adult and Pediatric," and Section II, "Testis Tumor—Adult, General" and "Testis Tumors—Pediatric, General."

ABBREVIATIONS

• CIS, carcinoma in situ

REFERENCE

Van Echten J. Cytogenetic evidence that carcinoma in situ is the precursor lesion for invasive testicular germ cell tumors. *Cancer Genet Cytogenet* 1995;85(2):133–137.

Authors: Jonathan Walker and John Lynch

Testis—Choriocarcinoma

 Basics

DESCRIPTION

- Choriocarcinoma is one of the histologic types of nonseminomatous germ cell tumor (NSGCT). Pure testicular choriocarcinomas are quite rare, but choriocarcinoma may be a component of mixed germ cell testicular tumors.

EPIDEMIOLOGY

- Incidence: Pure choriocarcinoma accounts for <1% of all nonseminomatous tumors; it may co-exist with other histologic types in up to 30% to 40% of NSGCTs.
- Age range (as for NSGCT): 18 to 25; predominantly Caucasian patients, rare in Blacks and Asians

GENETICS

- Isochromosome of the short arm of chromosome 12p, I(12p), identified as a specific genetic marker of germ cell tumors. In tumors not demonstrating this, there is excess 12p genetic material.
- Nonrandom genetic loss from chromosome 12q (a possible tumor-suppressor gene site) has also been reported.
- A few cases of familial incidence have been reported.

STAGING

- See TNM classification in Section VII.

SIGNS AND SYMPTOMS

- May present as a small, intratesticular mass. Frequently, the primary tumor cannot be palpated and does not distort the testis.
- Evidence of metastatic disease (weight loss, abdominal mass)

—Evidence of a "burned-out" primary may sometimes be found on orchiectomy, with no viable tumor present.
—Occasionally, no primary can be located, in spite of metastasis.

- Patients may present with advanced distant metastatic disease seemingly out of proportion to the small primary.
- Gynecomastia may be a feature (high levels of beta-hCG elaborated).

PATHOPHYSIOLOGY

- Must demonstrate two distinct cell types: syncytiotrophoblasts and cytotrophoblasts. Concomitant hemorrhage is common and often readily apparent on gross examination.
- Choriocarcinoma is the embryonic analogue of placental components.
- Pure choriocarcinoma always spreads unaltered as choriocarcinoma.

—Spread by lymphatic channels, but also by hematogenous routes, which accounts for its rapid and diffuse metastatic potential

CAUSES/RISK FACTORS

- As for other NSGCTs: Cryptorchidism may increase risk 4 to 80 times. Up to 10% of patients with testis tumor have a history of cryptorchid testis.
- A history of maternal exposure to DES, previously suspected to predispose to tumor development, does not increase risk of tumor development.
- Cryptorchidism
- Family history
- Testicular microlithiasis: One study has shown a 40% incidence of concomitant testis tumor.

COMPLICATIONS

- Complications are as for standard treatment (surgical and chemotherapeutic) for NSGCT.

DIFFERENTIAL DIAGNOSIS

- See also Section I, "Testicular Mass—Adult and Pediatric."

—Other NSGCT and seminoma
—Testicular lymphoma
—Adenomatoid tumor of testis

 Database

HISTORY

- A testis mass may be subtle or impalpable in choriocarcinoma.
- Patients may present with pulmonary metastases or other evidence of metastatic disease.
- A work-up for gynecomastia may lead to the diagnosis.
- Loss of libido or sexual dysfunction in an otherwise healthy-appearing young man

PHYSICAL EXAMINATION

- Neck: Evaluate for cervical/supraclavicular adenopathy.
- Breasts: gynecomastia
- Abdomen: retroperitoneal or liver masses
- Testis: intratesticular mass

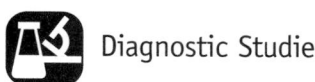 ## Diagnostic Studies

LABORATORY TESTING

- CBC, multichannel chemistry (for liver function tests, LDH, alkaline phosphatase)
- Testicular tumor markers

—Beta-subunit human chorionic gonadotropin levels (beta-hCG) may be extremely high (>10,000; normal ≤5.0). Alpha-fetoprotein (AFP) should be normal (<20 IU) in pure choriocarcinoma.

—Both seminomas and NSGCTs express placental alkaline phosphatase (PLAP). Seminomas do not express keratins, but embryonal carcinomas, yolk-sac tumors, and choriocarcinomas express low-molecular-weight keratins. These may be helpful in identifying poorly differentiated extragonadal tumors of germ cell origin.

IMAGING

- Diagnostic

—Testicular ultrasound: may show single or multiple masses, usually hypoechoic. Cystic changes may be common. When the primary tumor is impalpable, ultrasound may direct orchiectomy of the appropriate testis.

—Chest x-ray: may reveal multiple metastatic nodular lesions with indistinct borders

- Staging

—CT scan of chest: to evaluate mediastinal and pulmonary involvement

—CT scan of abdomen: to evaluate retroperitoneal nodes and other organs

—CT scan of head: to rule out brain metastases

SPECIAL STUDIES: N/A

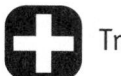 ## Treatment

GENERAL MEASURES

- Orchiectomy of the involved testis, if a primary tumor can be identified, followed by diagnostic staging evaluation and, usually, chemotherapy

MEDICAL

- Chemotherapy: Platinum-based combination chemotherapy, such as BEP (bleomycin–etoposide–cisplatinum) is primary therapy, especially in tumors presenting with advanced disease.
- Regimens using combinations with ifosfamide and carboplatin, combined with either etoposide or vinblastine, are employed in "poor-risk" patients. Patients presenting with pure choriocarcinoma and diffuse metastatic disease would be considered to fall into this category.
- Second-line regimens: high-dose platinum-based compounds combined with etoposide, ifosfamide, Cytoxan, and paclitaxel, coupled with bone marrow transplant stem cell rescue. 10% to 25% cure rates

—Pure choriocarcinoma is so rare, no series to evaluate treatment have been possible.

SURGICAL

- If all lesions identifiable on staging evaluations regress, and if tumor markers (beta-hCG) have normalized, close monitoring is generally accepted. If residual masses in the mediastinum or retroperitoneum persist, surgical excision is recommended.

ALTERNATIVE THERAPIES

- Historically, choriocarcinomas have not responded to radiation therapy, usually because the disease is too diffuse at the time of diagnosis. There may be selected instances in which palliative radiotherapy may be indicated, such as in brain metastases.

PATIENT EDUCATION

- As with all testis tumors, testicular self-examination should be taught to groups of young men at risk.

 ## Follow-Up

MONITORING

- Conventional testis tumor follow-up is recommended: every 3 months for 2 years, then every 6 months for 2 years, then annually for life.
- Follow-up should include tumor markers, chest x-ray, and interval CT scans of the chest, abdomen, and brain.

PREVENTION

- Note: Orchiopexy of the maldescended testis does not prevent the development of testis tumor, but it does provide access to the testis for examination and early detection of masses that might develop.

 ## Miscellaneous

SYNONYMS

- Malignant teratoma, trophoblastic (MTT)

ASSOCIATED CONDITIONS

- Cryptorchidism, gynecomastia, sexual dysfunction

NOTES

- See also Section I, "Testicular Mass—Adult and Pediatric," and Section II, "Testis Tumor—Adult, General" and "Testis Tumors—Pediatric, General."

ABBREVIATIONS

- NSGCT, nonseminomatous germ cell tumor

REFERENCES

Bosl GJ, Motzer RJ. Testicular germ-cell cancer. *N Engl J Med* 1997;337:242.

Richie JP. Neoplasms of the testis. In: Walsh PC, Retik AB, Vaughan ED, Wein AJ, eds. *Campbell's Urology*, 7th ed. Philadelphia: WB Saunders, 1998.

Steinfield AD. Testicular germ cell tumors: Review of contemporary evaluation and management. *Radiology* 1990;175:603.

Author: Donald F. Lynch, Jr.

Testis—Embryonal Carcinoma

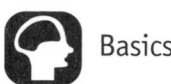 Basics

DESCRIPTION

• Most common histologic subtype of nonseminomatous germ cell tumor (NSGCT)

EPIDEMIOLOGY

• Annual age-adjusted incidence of all testicular cancers: 3.7 in 100,000
• Approximately 5500 cases per year
• Testes tumors: approximately 1% to 2% of all neoplasms in males. Germ cell: approximately 97%
• Mostly in the 20- to 40-year age group
• Second most common germ cell tumor (26%) following seminoma (42% cases)
• African Americans have one-third the incidence of American Whites.
• Bilateral: approximately 2% to 3% of cases. More common in right testicle

GENETICS

• No evidence of familial disease; 5% of patients with testicular cancer develop cancer in the contralateral testis.
• Short-arm chromosome 12 (p12): presence of isochromosome 12
• Rearrangements of short- and long-arm chromosome 1

STAGING

• See TNM classification in Section VII.

—Stage A: testis only; stage B: retroperitoneal disease; stage C: metastatic disease (i.e., above diaphragm)

SIGNS AND SYMPTOMS

• Painless testicular enlargement
• Testicular ache, pain in approximately 10% of cases
• Symptomatic metastases in 10% to 20% of cases (cough, dyspnea, abdominal mass, nodal enlargement, lumbar pain, lower extremity swelling)
• Gynecomastia (5%); infertility

PATHOPHYSIOLOGY

• Pure embryonal carcinomas: 3% of all germ cell tumors
• Including mixed tumors, embryonal cells are present in 45% of tumors.
• Gross: small gray-white lesion that does not replace the entire testis. Irregular margins with extensive hemorrhage and necrosis are common.
• Microscopic: pleomorphic cells with indistinct cellular borders. May present in cords, glands, sheets, or papillary structures. Mitotic figures and giant cells abound.
• The histology of metastases may be different from that of primary tumor.
• More aggressive and radioresistant than seminomas. 50% to 60% have metastases at presentation.
• Lymphatic spread is most common.

—The first site of metastasis is the retroperitoneum.
   —Left-sided tumors: spread to preaortic, para-aortic lymph nodes
   —Right-sided tumors: interaortocaval nodes; once in the retroperitoneum, may spread from right-sided lymph nodes to the left paraaortic and preaortic nodes
—Second most common site of metastasis: lungs

• Relapse risk high with embryonal; overall 35% to 40% relapse rate with vascular, lymphatic, tunical, or epididymal invasion

CAUSES/RISK FACTORS

• Cryptorchydism: 10 to 40× increased incidence
• Testicular atrophy (nonspecific or mumps-related)
• Estrogen exposure (conflicting data)
• Contralateral testicular tumor: bilateral in 3.5% of cases

COMPLICATIONS

• 50% of men are subfertile at the time of diagnosis.
• Retroperitoneal lymph node dissection: <10% loss of ejaculation with nerve-sparing procedure due to sympathetic injury. Risk of small bowel obstruction, ileus, lymphocele, vascular injury, neurologic injury (lumbar vessels).
• Chemotherapy: bleomycin (pulmonary fibrosis), etoposide (myelosuppression, alopecia, secondary leukemia), cisplatinum (renal insufficiency, nausea, vomiting, neuropathy), ifosfamide (hemorrhagic cystitis), vinblastine (neuromuscular toxicity)

DIFFERENTIAL DIAGNOSIS

• See also Section I, "Testicular Mass—Adult and Pediatric."

—Hydrocele, testicular torsion, epididymitis, hernia, spermatocele
—Carcinoma in situ: 50% progress to invasive disease.
—Embryonal carcinoma: 20% to 25% of tumors
—Seminoma: 40% of tumors (pure: 85%; anaplastic: 5%–10%; spermatocytic: 5%–10%); teratocarcinoma (25%–30%), teratoma (5%–10%), choriocarcinoma (1%), Leydig cell tumor, Sertoli cell tumor
—Polyembryoma

 Database

HISTORY

• History of undescended testis found in 10% of patients
• Previous testicular malignancy: Approximately 5% will develop another tumor.
• DES exposure in utero

PHYSICAL EXAMINATION

• Full physical examination with emphasis on chest, abdomen, urologic (careful testicular examination with transillumination), and nodal examination

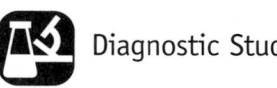 Diagnostic Studies

LABORATORY TESTING

• Serum markers

—Alpha-fetoprotein (AFP)
   —Produced by fetal gut, liver, and yolk sac. Half-life of approximately 5 days. Elevated in 80% of embryonal carcinoma, also yolk sac and teratoma. Absent in pure seminoma, pure choriocarcinoma
—Beta-human chorionic gonadotropin (beta-hCG)
   —Normally secreted by placental syncytiotrophoblast. Consists of alpha and beta chains. Alpha chain analogous to luteinizing hormone and thyroid-stimulating hormone. Half-life of approximately 24 to 36 hours. Elevated in 60% of all NSGCT, 30% of pure seminomas, all choriocarcinomas. May be positive in other visceral malignancies
—Lactic dehydrogenase (LDH)
   —Most useful when other markers are negative. Isoenzymes elevated in 60% of NSGCT. Relates to tumor bulk
—Placental-like alkaline phosphatase (PLAP). Most useful to diagnose seminomas when markers are negative (positive in 60%–80% of seminomas). False-positive in smokers

IMAGING

• Initial studies

—Scrotal US: first-line imaging tool. Sensitivity: 98%; specificity: 57%. Therefore, difficult to differentiate between benign and malignant masses. Typically of mixed echogenicity (seminomas are hypoechoic)
—Chest radiography: Lung metastases are found in 10% patients at presentation.
—Abdominal and pelvic CT scans: routine to evaluate retroperitoneum. Very sensitive but not specific (30% false-negatives). After chemotherapy, cannot distinguish teratoma, necrosis, and fibrosis
—Chest computerized tomography: very sensitive. Routine in large centers

SPECIAL STUDIES

• Lymphangiography: not routine. Replaced by CT scanning
• MRI: in selected cases

 Treatment

GENERAL MEASURES

• Stages A, B1, B2

—Traditional: radical orchiectomy and nerve-sparing retroperitoneal lymph node dissection (RPLND). RPLND may be transabdominal or thoracoabdominal. Bilateral dissection above inferior

520

mesenteric artery (IMA), unilateral below IMA. Stage I relapse rate: 8% to 10%
—Watchful waiting after radical orchiectomy. 20% to 40% relapse rate, more than 90% within first year. No good studies to date
    —If confined to the testis, only <6 positive nodes, or no nodes >2 cm (stages I, IA), may be observed.
    —If >6 positive nodes or any node >2 cm (stage IIB), recommend chemotherapy with bleomycin, etoposide (VP-16), cisplatinum (BEP) in two cycles. Each cycle consists of bleomycin (30 U on days 2, 9, 16), etoposide (100 mg/m² on days 1–5), and cisplatinum (20 mg/m² on days 1–5).

- Stages B3, C

—Traditional: inguinal orchiectomy and BEP in two cycles
    —Complete response: surveillance
    —Partial response: RPLND. If residual cancer is present, repeat chemotherapy with vinblastine, ifosfamide, and cisplatinum (VIP). Must add Mesna to reduce incidence of hemorrhagic cystitis. No therapy indicated if specimen shows teratoma, retroperitoneal fibrosis
    —Treatment failure: VIP chemotherapy, autologous bone marrow transplant

- Poor response to chemotherapy: >35 years old, high tumor volume, interval >3 weeks between orchiectomy and chemotherapy, extrapulmonary metastases

MEDICAL

- See above

SURGICAL

- See above

ALTERNATIVE THERAPIES

- External beam radiation

—Prophylactic irradiation usually reserved to treat relapse after RPLND and chemotherapy. 4000 to 5000 cGy
—Complications: early: nausea, skin erythema, reduction in spermatogenesis; late (uncommon): impaired spermatogenesis, secondary malignancies, gastrointestinal effects (peptic ulcer disease, hemorrhagic gastritis)

PATIENT EDUCATION

- University of Pennsylvania Cancer Center: www.oncolink.com
- American Cancer Society: (800)ACS-2345; www.cancer.org
- National Cancer Institute: (800)4-CANCER; www.nci.nih.gov

 Follow-Up

MONITORING

- In patients managed with surveillance

—First 2 years
    —Monthly visits, with serum tumor markers, chest radiography, and abdominal radiography
    —Abdominal and pelvic CT scans every 3 months
—Third year
    —Visits every 3 months, with serum markers and chest radiography
    —Abdominal and pelvic CT scans at 6-month intervals
—Fourth year
    —Visits every 4 months, with serum markers and chest radiography
    —Abdominal and pelvic CT scans at 6-month intervals
—Fifth year and beyond, if no relapse
    —Visits every 6 months, with serum markers and chest radiography
    —Abdominal and pelvic CT scans at 6-month intervals

- After RPLND

—40% relapse post-RPLND with surveillance only (stages B1, B2). Monitoring controversial
—Chest x-ray and serum markers every other month for first 2 years, then less intense. Cross-sectional imaging every 6 months
—Reliable patients who will follow up for at least 2 years: chemotherapy for documented relapse (four courses of BEP). Otherwise, if follow-up is not guaranteed, suggest two courses of adjuvant BEP post-RPLND.

PREVENTION

- Self-examination of contralateral testis

 Miscellaneous

SYNONYMS: N/A

ASSOCIATED CONDITIONS: N/A

NOTES

- See Section II for other testis tumor types.

ABBREVIATIONS

- BEP, bleomycin, etoposide, cisplatinum; NSGCT, nonseminomatous germ cell tumor; RPLND, retroperitoneal lymph node dissection

REFERENCES

Donohue JP, et al. Retroperitoneal lymphadenectomy in clinical stage A testis cancer (1965–1989): Modifications of technique and impact on ejaculation. *J Urol* 1993;149:237–243.

Donohue JP, et al. Stage I nonseminomatous germ cell testicular cancer—Management options and risk benefit considerations. *World J Urol* 1994;12:170–177.

Mostofi FK. Testicular tumors. Epidemiologic, etiologic and pathologic features. *Cancer* 1973;32:1186.

Williams SD, et al. Treatment of disseminated germ cell tumors with cis-platinum, bleomycin, and either vinblastine or etoposide. *N Engl J Med* 1987;316:1435.

Authors: Ricardo F. Sánchez-Ortiz and S. Bruce Malkowicz

Testis—Endodermal Sinus Tumor (Yolk Sac Tumor)

 Basics

DESCRIPTION

- A type of nonseminomatous germ cell tumor (NSGCT) of the testicle
- 80% of testicular endodermal sinus tumors (ESTs) are stage I at diagnosis (unlike extratesticular ESTs, which often present at a more advanced stage).
- Chemotherapy has greatly improved the prognosis in children with ESTs. Age is an important prognostic variable. Overall relapse-free survival for patients under age 1 is 78% but decreases to 25% for patients older than 2 years.

EPIDEMIOLOGY

- Although rare, it is the most common pediatric testis tumor.
- Incidence is approximately 40% to 60% of pediatric testicular neoplasms (incidence of testicular neoplasms in general is 1.1 per million U.S. Whites under the age of 15 years).
- Median age at diagnosis: 24 months
- Right- and left-sided tumors occur with equal frequency.
- <1% of cases have bilateral testicular involvement at presentation.

GENETICS

- A deletion event on the short arm of chromosome 1—at 1p36.3—has been implicated in pediatric gonadal pure yolk sac tumors (YSTs).
- No report of familial clusters

STAGING

- See TNM classification in Section VII.
- Stage I: tumor limited to one (or both) testis, which is removed by high inguinal orchiectomy; no clinical, radiographic, or histologic evidence of residual disease beyond the testis; serum alpha-fetoprotein (AFP)-negative postoperatively
- Stage II: transscrotal tumor aspiration, biopsy of tumor within the scrotal sac or scrotal orchiectomy; microscopic residual disease within the scrotum or high in the spermatic cord (less than 5 cm from the proximal end); microscopic retroperitoneal lymph node involvement (lymph nodes <2 cm in diameter, but histologically positive for tumor) or serum AFP-positive more than 4 weeks after orchiectomy
- Stage IIA: gross retroperitoneal lymph node involvement (lymph nodes >2 cm in diameter and histologically positive for tumor)
- Stage III

—A: extraabdominal lymph node metastases
—B: Extranodal metastases are present (liver, lung, peritoneum, bones, bone marrow, or brain).

SIGNS AND SYMPTOMS

- Testicular enlargement, usually painless
- Abdominal swelling: secondary to lymphadenopathy or malignant ascites
- Lymphadenopathy
- Acute abdominal pain, weight loss, fatigue
- Transillumination negative (hydrocele, if present, does not exclude tumor)

PATHOPHYSIOLOGY

- Histology

—Hallmark is presence of eosinophilic, PAS-positive inclusions in the cytoplasm of clear cells
—Intracellular and intercellular hyaline droplets present
—Cytoplasmic inclusions resist diastase digestion.
—Cytoplasmic inclusions shown to contain AFP
—AFP is usually made by yolk sac cells in the embryo and usually disappears from serum by 3 months of age.
—Polyvesicular vitelline tumor: Variant of YST that is predominantly cystic (may have more favorable prognosis with this histologic subtype)

- Pathophysiology

—Current opinion supports Teilum's theory (1959): ESTs derived from yolk sac elements that were present in early embryonic life

CAUSES/RISK FACTORS

- Unknown

COMPLICATIONS: N/A

DIFFERENTIAL DIAGNOSIS

- NSGCTs, seminomatous germ cell tumors, benign tumors of testis, paratesticular lesion/tumors, infection, epididymitis–orchitis, torsion, hydrocele, spermatocele, hematoma

 Database

HISTORY

- Often, a history of minor trauma calls attention to a painless testicular mass.
- Fatigue, weight loss

PHYSICAL EXAMINATION

- General examination for lymphadenopathy
- Abdominal mass
- Scrotal examination

—Palpate the testicle, epididymis, and cord to localize the mass.
—Note any tenderness.
—Transillumination
—Examine the contralateral testicle.

Testis—Endodermal Sinus Tumor (Yolk Sac Tumor)

 ## Diagnostic Studies

LABORATORY TESTING

- Urinalysis may contain white cells and bacteria in inflammatory lesions such as epididymitis; usually normal with tumor
- AFP

—The only useful marker for yolk sac carcinoma

- Beta-hCG

—To rule out mixed tumor
—Although not synthesized by yolk sac, rarely may be elevated if tumors contain syncytiotrophoblast cells

- LDH may be a nonspecific marker for tumor burden
- Alkaline phosphatase and other liver function abnormalities if liver involved

IMAGING

- US scrotal: often suggestive of diagnosis

—Essential examination if a hydrocele precludes examination of the testicle

- CT of pelvis and abdomen to evaluate retroperitoneal lymph nodes and liver
- Chest x-ray or CT of chest to evaluate for pulmonary metastasis

SPECIAL STUDIES: N/A

 ## Treatment

GENERAL MEASURES

- Counseling: surgery; potential chemotherapy; need for strict surveillance and follow-up; further surgery after radical orchiectomy, when needed; fertility; sperm banking, where appropriate

MEDICAL

- Chemotherapy

—All patients with stage II or III disease should be treated with combination chemotherapy using vincristine, dactinomycin, and cyclophosphamide (VAC) *or* cisplatin, vinblastine, and bleomycin (PVB) for 1 year. There is a 58% salvage rate with these chemotherapeutic regimens.

- Radiation

—Very limited role
—Reserved for bulky disease and localized tumor in the retroperitoneum that is refractory to chemotherapy

SURGICAL

- Radical orchiectomy

—Alone for stage I disease

- Retroperitoneal lymphadenectomy

—No routine role, as has a high complication rate and is of little proven benefit in stage I disease

- Second-look laparotomy

—If rising AFP, suspicious CT findings, no obvious metastatic disease

ALTERNATIVE THERAPIES: N/A

PATIENT EDUCATION

- Patients and their families should understand and agree to the need for strict surveillance and follow-up.
- Testicular self-examination of remaining testicle monthly

 ## Follow-Up

MONITORING

- Strict follow-up is essential. This is especially true for stage I patients treated with radical orchiectomy alone. A formal protocol should be followed to track and monitor patients.

—One month postorchiectomy: chest and abdominal CTs and serum AFP determination
—Surveillance (nonsurgical) as per NSGCT
  —Year 1: monthly chest x-ray and AFP; 3-monthly CT scans of chest and abdomen
  —Year 2: every 2-month chest x-ray and serum AFP, and every 6-month abdominal and chest CT
  —Year 3 and beyond: Recurrence is unlikely, and studies are arranged every 6 months.

PREVENTION: N/A

 ## Miscellaneous

SYNONYMS

- Yolk sac tumor; childhood endodermal sinus tumor (CEST); orchidoblastoma; infantile adenocarcinoma of the testis; testicular adenocarcinoma with clear cells

ASSOCIATED CONDITIONS

- Increased incidence of genitourinary anomalies reported, including inguinal hernia, duplex collecting systems, renal ectopia, hypospadias, renal agenesis

NOTES

- See also Section I, "Testicular Mass—Adult and Pediatric," and Section II, "Testis Tumor—Adult, General" and "Testis Tumor—Pediatric, General."

ABBREVIATIONS

- EST, endodermal sinus tumor; YST, yolk sac tumor; CEST, childhood endodermal sinus tumor

REFERENCES

Connolly JA, Gearhart JP. Management of yolk sac tumors in children. *Urol Clin North Am* 1993; 20(1):7–14.

Snyder HM III, et al. Pediatric oncology. In: Walsh PC, Retik AB, Vaughan ED, Wein AJ, eds. *Campbell's Urology,* 7th ed. Philadelphia: WB Saunders, 1997.

Authors: Owen Prowse and Laurence Klotz

Testis—Leydig Cell Tumors

 Basics

DESCRIPTION

- The majority of testicular neoplasms are derived from germ cells. 4% to 10% of testicular tumors are from non–germ cells. Non–germ cell tumors tend to develop over a long period of time. Leydig cell (interstitial cell) tumors make up approximately 90% of non–germ cell tumors. These tumors are usually benign, however 7% to 10% of Leydig cell tumors metastasize in adults only.

EPIDEMIOLOGY

- 1% to 3% of testicular neoplasms
- Ages range from 2 to 90 years.
- Most common between ages 20 and 50
- Single most common tumor in the sex cord stromal category
- 20% are pediatric and present commonly between the ages of 5 and 10.

GENETICS

- Questionable association with Klinefelter syndrome
- Reported almost exclusively in White males
- Associated with unilateral renal agenesis

STAGING

- TNM classification for testicular tumors, Section VII

SIGNS AND SYMPTOMS

- Adults

—Painless testicular enlargement, firm and nontender
—Gynecomastia
  —Most common symptom
  —15% to 20% of patients
  —Result from elevated human chorionic gonadotropin (hCG) and/or elevated estrogen levels
—Infertility: 10% of cases
—Loss of libido
—10% of patents present with symptoms related to metastatic disease at the time of diagnosis.
  —Back pain
  —Cough
  —Dyspnea and hemoptysis in advanced pulmonary disease
  —Anorexia/nausea/vomiting
  —Lower extremity swelling

- Children

—Often small and difficult to detect
—Isosexual pseudoprecocity
  —Elevated testosterone production/elevated 17-ketosteroid production
  —Secondary to androgen hormone production by neoplasm
  —Prominent external genitalia
  —Libido evident
  —Mature masculine voice
  —Pubic hair (precocious puberty)

PATHOPHYSIOLOGY

- Solid, well-circumscribed tumor
- Yellow-to-gray nodular appearance
- 0.5 to 10.0 cm in size; 3% bilateral
- Hemorrhage and necrosis unusual but may be present
- Crystals of Reinke

—Pathognomonic for Leydig cell tumor
—Intracytoplasmic, eosinophilic, rod-shaped structure
—30% to 40% of specimens

- Von Hanseman cells

—Cells with abundant granular eosinophilic cytoplasm

- 60% secrete testosterone and/or corticosteroids.
- 50% secrete estrogen.

CAUSES/RISK FACTORS

- No definitive cause
- Viral-like particles in Leydig cell tumors have been noted.
- Elevated levels of beta-hCG and estrogen in maternal and fetal blood are associated with Leydig cell hyperplasia.
- No association with cryptorchidism

COMPLICATIONS

- Persistent gynecomastia following tumor resection

DIFFERENTIAL DIAGNOSIS

- Epididymitis or epididymo-orchitis is the most common misdiagnosis in patients with testis tumors.
- Hydrocele is the second most common misdiagnosis in patients with testis tumors.
- Leydig cell hyperplasia

—Secondary to elevated gonadotropins
—Common in patients with Klinefelter syndrome

- Adrenogenital syndrome

—Hyperplastic nodules
—Bilateral, multifocal
—Absent Reinke crystals

- Malignant lymphoma

—Epididymis, spermatic cord, and tubule invasion noted with 4% of lymphomas
—Usually bilateral

- Metastatic tumor to testis
- Paraneoplastic syndromes may mimic gynecomastia secondary to Leydig cell tumors.
- Other primary testicular neoplasms (i.e., germ cell, other sex cord, mixed-cell types)
- Plasmacytomas

 Database

HISTORY

- An incorrect diagnosis is made in up to 25% of patients with testicular neoplasms.
- Symptoms of orchitis or epididymitis
- History of undescended testis: 5% to 10% of cases
- Past trauma
- Pain, weight loss, malaise

PHYSICAL EXAMINATION

- Palpable, painless testicular mass: 80% to 90% of cases
- Supraclavicular nodes palpable
- Gynecomastia
- Groin, flank, or abdominal mass
- Virilizing effects in children

Diagnostic Studies

LABORATORY TESTING

- B-hCG, AFP, LDH, cell count, UA, chemistries, and CBC are minimal recommended laboratories for any suspected testicular neoplasm.
- Follicle-stimulating hormone (FSH), luteinizing hormone (LH), and serum testosterone are useful to differentiate the primary from the secondary testis effect.
- Urinary 17-ketosteroids
- Serum and urinary estradiol

IMAGING

- Testicular ultrasound
—Solid hypoechoic mass
- CT scan of abdomen and chest to evaluate lymphatic spread

SPECIAL STUDIES

- Selective venous sampling of gonadal vein
—Detect excess endocrine production
- MRI: not frequently used; however, may detect some tumors undetected by ultrasound

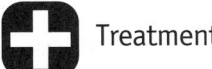 ## Treatment

GENERAL MEASURES

- Metastatic disease
—10% of cases
—Persistent estrogen levels in serum of micrometastatic disease
—Responds poorly to radiation and chemotherapy, yet preferred if RPLND positive
—Median survival: 4 years
- Benign/local disease in majority of patients; good prognosis

MEDICAL

- Ortho-Para DDD: some evidence of benefit

SURGICAL

- Radical inguinal orchiectomy
—Definitive method of diagnosis and treatment for stages I, II neoplasm
- RPLND if suspicion of malignancy by CT criteria
—Postoperative decline in estrogen levels
—May have residual gynecomastia after removal of tumor

ALTERNATIVE THERAPIES: N/A

PATIENT EDUCATION

- Important to perform routine examination of testicles

 ## Follow-Up

MONITORING

- Follow-up visits should include careful examination of the remaining testis, the abdomen, and regional lymph nodes.
- RPLND patients should be followed every 3 months for 2 years, then every 6 months for 3 years, and then yearly.
- Tumor markers, serum testosterone, and 17β-estradiol at routine visits
- CT imaging of lung and abdomen
- CBC, electrolytes, and endocrine levels should be performed at routine visits.

PREVENTION: N/A

 ## Miscellaneous

SYNONYMS

- Interstitial cell tumor

ASSOCIATED CONDITIONS: N/A

NOTES

- See also Section II, "Testis Tumor—Pediatric, General."

ABBREVIATIONS

- RPLND, retroperitoneal lymph node dissection

REFERENCES

Bertram KA. Treatment of malignant Leydig cell tumor. *Cancer* 1991;68(10):2324–2329.

Ernstoff MS. *Urologic Cancer.* Boston: Blackwell Science, 1997:525–527.

Richie JP. Neoplasms of the testis. In: Walsh PC, Retik AB, Vaughan ED, Wein AJ, eds. *Campbell's Urology,* 7th ed. Philadelphia: WB Saunders, 1998:2411–2452.

Robertson CA. Gynecomastia. *J Urol* 1989;142:1325–1327.

Young RH. *Testicular Tumors.* Chicago: ASCP Press, 1990:101–104.

Authors: Chris B. Threatt and Cary N. Robertson

Testis—Seminoma

 Basics

DESCRIPTION

• Seminoma is a germ cell tumor of the testicle which is composed of cells that are considered the malignant counterpart of gonocytes.

EPIDEMIOLOGY

• Seminoma is the most common testicular cancer.
• Peak incidence among men aged 20 to 40
• Four to five times more common among White men in comparison to African-American men.
• Increasing incidence in the United States, United Kingdom, and Denmark
• Patients who have had one seminoma are at an increased risk of developing a contralateral seminoma.

GENETICS

• Unknown

STAGING

• See the appendix for TNM classification.

SIGNS AND SYMPTOMS

• Usually presents as a painless swelling in the scrotum

—Pain, "heaviness," and "tenderness" are less common complaints.

• A history of antecedent testicular trauma is probably coincidental, not causative.

PATHOPHYSIOLOGY

• Divided by latest AFIP fascicle into two subtypes: classical and spermatocytic
• The spermatocytic subtype is rare, usually appears in the elderly, and has a better prognosis.
• Of note, the newest Armed Forces Institute of Pathology fascicle does not include a category of "anaplastic seminoma" because the mitotic rate criterion of Mostofi bears no prognostic significance.

Leeds Consensus Conference (1989)

I	No evidence of metastases
II	Metastases confined to nodes
IIA	Maximum diameter ≤2 cm
IIB	Maximum diameter >2 to 5 cm
IIC	Maximum diameter >5 to 10 cm
IID	Maximum diameter >10 cm
III	Supradiaphragmatic and infradiaphragmatic nodes; abdominal status: A, B, C, D
IV	Extralymphatic metastases

CAUSES/RISK FACTORS

• Origin probably related to gonadal dysgenesis
• Increased incidence of seminoma in patients with maldescended testes
• Males with cryptorchidism may have an increased risk of developing seminoma that is 35 times higher than in the normal population.
• A correlation exists between carcinoma in situ of the testis and the development of invasive testicular neoplasia.

COMPLICATIONS

• Involvement of retroperitoneal lymph nodes may produce backache.
• Widely disseminated parenchymal disease in lungs, liver, bone, or even brain is very rare but, if present, may produce systemic symptoms.
• Prophylactic mediastinal irradiation (PMI) is no longer incorporated into therapeutic protocols because of risks of late cardiac toxicity.

DIFFERENTIAL DIAGNOSIS

• See Section I, "Testicular Mass—Adult and Pediatric."

 Database

HISTORY

• Symptoms of acute pain, backache, systemic symptoms?
• Is there a change in the size of the scrotum caused by swelling?
• Birth history: maldescended testis, cryptorchidism, etc.?
• History of inguinal surgery (which might have disrupted the lymphatics)?

PHYSICAL EXAMINATION

• Palpate the testes bilaterally.
• Transilluminate the mass.
• Examine the groin for evidence of surgical scar.
• Inspect for lymphedema of the groin and lower extremities.

Diagnostic Studies

LABORATORY TESTING

- Complete blood count and chemistry screen
- Pulmonary/renal function tests for patients who may receive chemotherapy
- Beta-hCG and AFP to rule out nonseminomatous germ cell tumor

—Note: Seminoma can rarely have elevated beta-hCG but never elevated AFP.

- Placental alkaline phosphatase (now considered useful only for monitoring response to therapy if elevated at the outset)

IMAGING

- Transscrotal ultrasound: often diagnostic of a neoplasm
- Chest radiograph: to rule out metastasis
- CT scans of abdomen, pelvis, thorax

SPECIAL STUDIES

- Pedal lymphangiogram

—Useful historically for identification of retroperitoneal metastasis

—Primary use today for radiation therapy planning

 ## Treatment

GENERAL MEASURES

- Seminoma is an exquisitely radiosensitive tumor.
- Standard treatment of patients with stage I (no obvious metastasis) seminoma is postoperative (orchiectomy) radiotherapy to paraaortic and ipsilateral pelvic nodes. With appropriate radiation techniques, survival rates at 5 years approach 100%.

MEDICAL

- Standard treatment for stage II (retroperitoneal adenopathy) and above (pulmonary or visceral metastasis) is platinum-based chemotherapy (e.g., BEP).

SURGICAL

- Radical inguinal orchiectomy with high ligation of the spermatic cord (although transscrotal biopsy no longer thought to be associated with increased risk of local recurrence)

ALTERNATIVE THERAPIES

- Three large series (from Toronto, Royal Marsden Hospital, and Danish Cooperative Group) now suggest that selected stage I patients can be managed with surveillance as opposed to radiotherapy.

—Although failure rates following surveillance approach 15%, most patients can be salvaged by chemotherapy.

- Some radiotherapy centers are also willing to treat stage I disease by directing beams only to the paraaortic nodes.

PATIENT EDUCATION: N/A

 ## Follow-Up

MONITORING

- Annual surveillance for early-stage patients treated by irradiation. More frequent follow-up (including interval CT scans for those managed expectantly)

PREVENTION: N/A

 ## Miscellaneous

SYNONYMS: N/A

ASSOCIATED CONDITIONS: N/A

NOTES: N/A

ABBREVIATIONS

- BEP, bleomycin, etoposide, cisplatin; AFP, alpha-fetoprotein; hCG, human chorionic gonadotropin

REFERENCES

Coia LR, Hanks GE. Complications from large field intermediate dose infradiaphragmatic irradiation: An analysis of patterns of care outcome studies of Hodgkin's disease and seminoma. *Int J Radiat Oncol Biol Phys* 1988;15:29.

Thomas GM. Consensus statement on the investigation and management of testicular seminoma: EORTC genito-urinary group monograph 7. In: Newling DW, Jones WG, eds. *Prostate Cancer and Testicular Cancer*. New York: Wiley-Liss, 1990.

Authors: Benjamin W. Corn and Richard K. Valicenti

Testis—Sertoli Cell Tumor

 Basics

DESCRIPTION

• Rare non–germ cell tumor. Sertoli cells are supporting cells of the testes. They play a major role in the microenvironment of the seminiferous epithelium.

EPIDEMIOLOGY

• Comprise 0.4% to 1.5% of all primary testicular neoplasms
• Age range: newborn to the 90s
• 10% are malignant.
• Only 100 cases reported

GENETICS

• Unknown

STAGING

• TNM classification: See Section VII.

SIGNS AND SYMPTOMS

• Painless, slow-growing scrotal mass

—Bilateral in 40% to 50% of large-cell calcifying Sertoli cell tumors

• Feminization (gynecomastia) secondary to estrogen production in up to 25% of general Sertoli cell tumors
• Precocious puberty

—More commonly in large-cell calcifying Sertoli cell tumor variant

PATHOPHYSIOLOGY

• Subtypes

—General Sertoli cell tumors (40% occur in prepubertal patients)
—Large-cell calcifying Sertoli tumors (primarily in patients younger than 20 years of age)
—Sclerosing Sertoli cell tumors (confined exclusively to men 18–80 years of age)

• Grossly, tumors are well demarcated, hard, and yellow/white to tan. Size is variable. General and large-cell calcifying variants may achieve massive proportions (up to 20 cm); sclerosing tumors are small (0.4–1.5 cm).
• Histologically, all tumors contain epithelial components resembling Sertoli cells and stroma.

—Enormous potential for variation in both epithelial and stromal differentiation
—Call-Exner–like bodies occasionally seen within tubules

• Malignancy determined by presence of metastases (lymph nodes, bone, and lung)

—Occurs almost exclusively in adults with general Sertoli cell tumors (up to 30%)
—Large size, poor tumor demarcation, invasion of adjacent structures, blood vessel and lymphatic invasion, and increased mitotic activity are suggestive of malignancy.
—Sclerosing and large-cell calcifying variants have a low malignant potential.

CAUSES/RISK FACTORS

• A majority arise in normal intrascrotal testes; occurrence has been reported in cryptorchid or maldescended testes.
• Large-cell calcifying Sertoli cell tumors can be associated with Carney syndrome, tuberous sclerosis, and the Peutz-Jeghers syndrome.

—Tumors are usually bilateral and multifocal, and show familial occurrence.
—36% are associated with extragonadal manifestations.

COMPLICATIONS

• Subferitlity

DIFFERENTIAL DIAGNOSIS

• See also Section I, "Testicular Mass—Adult and Pediatric."
• Epididymo-orchitis
• Testicular torsion
• Inguinal hernia
• Hydrocele
• Spermatocele
• Paratesticular tumor
• Trauma

 Database

HISTORY

• Age of patient?

—Important in assessing malignant potential

• Presence of gynecomastia, precocious puberty, or feminizing signs?
• Symptoms of urinary tract infection, epididymitis, or pain?
• History of trauma?
• Family history or history of dysplastic complex syndromes?

PHYSICAL EXAMINATION

• General appearance

—Evidence of dysplastic syndromes (tuberous sclerosis, Carney syndrome)
    —Cutaneous myxomas and pigmented lesions of the face and mucosa
—Signs of feminization

• Palpation of testes and cord structures

—Solid, painless testicular mass
—Size of tumor(s)
—Presence of bilateral masses

• Breast examination

—Presence of gynecomastia (palpable breast tissue)

Diagnostic Studies

LABORATORY TESTING

- Standard germ cell tumor markers (alpha-fetoprotein, beta-human chorionic gonadotropin, and placental alkaline phosphatase) are typically negative.
- Sex hormones (estrogen and testosterone)
—In absence of clinical features, not helpful preoperatively
—May be used postoperatively to follow tumors with malignant potential

IMAGING

- Scrotal ultrasonography
—General and sclerosing Sertoli cell tumors demonstrate mixed echogenicity.
—Large-cell calcifying Sertoli cell tumors exhibit increased vascularity and hyperechoic areas with curvilinear shadowing secondary to calcifications.
- Chest radiography: metastatic potential
Bone scan: metastatic evaluation
- CT scan of abdomen and pelvis: evidence of nodal involvement

SPECIAL STUDIES: N/A

 ## Treatment

GENERAL MEASURES

- Surgery is the initial treatment of choice.
- The treatment and prognosis of metastatic disease are uniformly poor.

MEDICAL

- Chemotherapy for metastatic disease
—Cisplatin based
—No dramatic response has been reported.
- Radiotherapy
—Limited experience

SURGICAL

- Radical orchiectomy
—Initial procedure of choice through inguinal incision
- Retroperitoneal lymph node dissection in presence of retroperitoneal lymph node involvement
—Limited experience but may be beneficial

ALTERNATIVE THERAPIES: N/A

PATIENT EDUCATION

- Testicular self-examination monthly, starting in high school

 ## Follow-Up

MONITORING

- Long-term clinical surveillance required
—Recurrence 15 years after initial presentation has been reported.

PREVENTION: N/A

 ## Miscellaneous

SYNONYMS

- Androblastoma, gonadal stromal tumor (prepubertal patients), Sertoli cell–mesenchyme tumor

ASSOCIATED CONDITIONS

- Tuberous sclerosis, Carney syndrome

NOTES : N/A

ABBREVIATIONS: N/A

REFERENCES

Nogales FF, et al. Malignant large cell calcifying Sertoli cell tumor of the testis. *J Urol* 1995;153; 1935–1937.

Ritchie JP. Neoplasms of the testes. In: Walsh PC, Retik AB, Vaughan ED, Wein AJ, eds. *Campbell's Urology,* 7th ed. Philadelphia: WB Saunders, 1998.

Authors: John W. Colberg and Robert M. Weiss

Testis—Teratoma, Mature and Immature

 Basics

DESCRIPTION

- A teratoma is a tumor composed of all three germ layers: ectoderm, mesoderm, and endoderm. A teratoma of the testis can occur in both children and adults. In prepubertal children, it is a benign tumor; in adults, it behaves as a malignant neoplasm.

EPIDEMIOLOGY

- Peak incidence in young adult males: age 15 to 35
- Lower incidence among Black men than among white men
- Pure teratoma: 5% to 10% of all germ cell tumors (GCTs)
- Teratoma: present in 48% of mixed GCTs
- 1% to 2% of patients with a testicular teratoma will develop a contralateral tumor.

GENETICS

- Chromosome (12p) alteration in 80% of GCTs, including teratomas

STAGING

- Several staging systems are in use; TNM is the most widely used.
- Clinical staging systems

—TNM: See Section VII.
—Boden-Gibb: stage I: confined to the testis; stage II: spread to regional nodes; stage III: spread beyond retroperitoneal nodes/metastatic dx

- Pathologic staging system

—TNM: See Section VII.
—Walter Reed: See Section III.

SIGNS AND SYMPTOMS

- Painless testicular swelling most common
- Lump or nodule; painful swelling (10%); gynecomastia (5%)
- Symptoms of advanced (10%–15%)

—Backache (bulky retroperitoneal disease); neck mass (supraclavicular adenopathy)
—Lower extremity swelling (venous obstruction); cough or dyspnea (pulmonary metastasis)
—Bone pain (skeletal metastasis)

PATHOPHYSIOLOGY

- Gross

—Heterogeneous mass; larger than other GCTs (5–10 cm)
—Firm, solid areas with intervening cysts; hemorrhage and necrosis, common

- Micro

—Mature teratoma: cystic epithelial areas lined by respiratory or gutlike or squamous epithelium with well-formed adjacent fibroelastic or smooth muscle stroma with cartilage or other tissue elements
—Immature teratoma: more primitive epithelial structures

CAUSES/RISK FACTORS

- Cryptorchidism: 3 to 14 increased incidence relative to general population
- Nonspecific or mumps-associated atrophy: potential risk
- Possibly maternal exposure to estrogens during pregnancy
- Trauma: prompts evaluation; not a causative factor

COMPLICATIONS

- Local complications due to growth of extratesticular teratoma

DIFFERENTIAL DIAGNOSIS

- See Section I, "Testicular Mass—Adult and Pediatric."

 Database

HISTORY

- Undescended testes?
- Previous testicular tumor?
- Maternal DES exposure?

PHYSICAL EXAMINATION

- Bimanual palpation of testes and scrotal contents

—Examine the normal testis first, noting consistency and size.

- Any firm, hard, or fixed area should be considered suspicious.
- Determine involvement of the cord, scrotal investments, or skin.
- Abdomen: masses; supraclavicular nodes: adenopathy
- Gynecomastia; extremities for edema

Diagnostic Studies

LABORATORY TESTING

- Testicular markers: AFP and hCG (oncofetal substances), LDH (cellular enzyme)

IMAGING

- Testicular ultrasound: occult testicular neoplasm
- Chest x-ray: minimal assessment of lung parenchyma and mediastinal structures
- CT of thorax

—More sensitive than chest x-ray, increased detection of pulmonary metastasis

- CT scan of abdomen

—Identifies retroperitoneal adenopathy (nodes 1 cm or larger)
—Replaced IVP and pedal lymphangiography as procedure of choice for evaluation of retroperitoneum

SPECIAL STUDIES

- Testicular biopsies of the affected testis should not be performed, as they may open up routes for secondary tumor spread.
- Consider a biopsy of the contralateral testis to detect ITGCN.

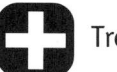 ## Treatment

GENERAL MEASURES

- Radical orchiectomy

—Transinguinal approach; provides histologic diagnosis and local staging

- Further treatment dependent on stage

—Stage I: surveillance vs. RPLND
  —16% to 19% occult retroperitoneal disease
  —Relapse 20% when managed by surveillance
—Stage II a (low-volume <2 cm): RPLND
—Stage II b (>2 cm, bulky nodes): RPLND and BEP × 2 cycles
—Stages II c/III: BEP × 4 cycles
  —CR→observe
  —PR→RPLND→cancer→VIP
  —PR→RPLND→teratoma or fibrosis→observe

MEDICAL

- Adjuvant chemotherapy

—BEP: bleomycin (B) 30 U; etoposide (E) 100 mg/m²; cisplatin (P) 20 mg/m²

- Salvage VIP (per cycle): VP-16 (etoposide) 75 mg/m²; ifosfamide 1.2 g/m²; cisplatin 20 mg/m²

SURGICAL

- RPLND

—Transabdominal or thoracoabdominal approach
—Morality rate: 1%
—Morbidity ranges 5% to 25%; atelectasis, pneumonitis, ileus, lymphocele, or pancreatitis

ALTERNATIVE THERAPIES

- Radiation of retroperitoneal nodes

—Outside of North America, management included routine postorchiectomy radiotherapy for clinical stage I.

PATIENT EDUCATION

- Testicular self-examination

 ## Follow-Up

MONITORING

- First year: monthly chest x-ray, tumor markers
- Year 2: bi-monthly chest x-ray, tumor markers
- CT scan of abdomen every 2 to 3 months first 2 years, and at least every 6 months thereafter

PREVENTION: N/A

 ## Miscellaneous

SYNONYMS

- Teratoma differentiated

ASSOCIATED CONDITIONS

- Impaired fertility

NOTES

- There is a risk, after chemotherapy, of malignant transformation of a teratoma to sarcoma or carcinoma.
- A teratoma may grow rapidly (growing teratoma syndrome) and become less amenable to complete surgical excision.

ABBREVIATIONS

- AFB, alpha-fetoprotein; BEP, bleomycin, etoposide, cisplatin; CR, complete response; DES, diethylstilbestrol; dx, disease; GCTs, germ cell tumors; ITGCN, intratubular germ cell neoplasm; PR, partial response; RPLND, retroperitoneal lymph node dissection; VIP, VP-16, ifosfamide, cisplatin

REFERENCES

Brodsky GL. Pathology of testicular germ cell tumors. *Hematol Oncol Clin North Am* 1991;5(6): 1095.

Heidenreich A, et al. The role of retroperitoneal lymphadenectomy in mature teratoma and the testis. *J Urol* 1997;157:160.

Ilson DH, et al. Genetic analysis of germ cell tumors: Current progress and future prospects. *Hematol Oncol Clin North Am* 1991;5(6):1271.

Leibovitch I, et al. Adult primary pure teratoma of the testis: The Indiana experience. *Cancer* 1995;75:2244.

Walsh PC, Retik AB, Vaughan ED, Wein AJ, eds. *Campbell's Urology*, 7th ed. Philadelphia: WB Saunders, 1998:2411–2452.

Authors: Corlis L. Archer and Gabriel P. Haas

Testis Tumor—Adult, General

 Basics

DESCRIPTION

• Testicular cancer is the most common malignancy in males 15 to 35 years old.
• Improved early detection, accurate staging, and multidisciplinary treatment has resulted in a significant decrease in mortality.

EPIDEMIOLOGY

• 7400 cases of malignant tumors per year in the United States with 300 deaths

—Incidence: Whites, 3.7 in 100,000; Blacks, 0.9 in 100,000

• Highest incidence: Europe, 8.6 in 100,000
• Lowest incidence: Africa and Asia
• More common on right (53%), 2% to 3% bilateral

GENETICS

• Possible increased incidence in siblings and sons (British reports)

STAGING

• TNM classification of AJCC: See the appendix.
• Boden-Gibb classification older system

—Stage I: testis only
—Stage II: retroperitoneal micrometastasis A; nodes 2 to 5 cm B; nodes >5 cm C
—Stage III: metastasis above diaphragm/visceral involvement

• Metastatic spread to regional (retroperitoneal) lymph nodes

—Right testicle drains into interaortocaval nodes, then to precaval, preaortic, and paracaval nodes
—Left testicle drains into left paraaortic and then to preaortic nodes

• Inguinal metastasis (uncommon) if

—Tunica albuginea invasion
—Previous orchiopexy or inguinal herniorrhaphy (altered lymphatic drainage)

• Distant metastasis

—Lung is most common, followed by liver, bone, brain, kidney, adrenal, GI tract, and spleen

• Choriocarcinoma is an exception, with early hematogenous spread.

SIGNS AND SYMPTOMS

• Local symptoms

—Painless nodule, mass, or firmness is most common (50%–55%)
—Dull ache or heaviness (30%–35%)
—Acute pain (10%)
—Huge scrotal or groin mass (rare)

• Symptoms due to metastasis (10%) to lungs (cough, dyspnea, hemoptysis), supraclavicular nodes (neck mass), or massive retroperitoneal involvement (anorexia, nausea, vomiting, back pain)
• Gynecomastia or painful breasts in 5% (systemic endocrine manifestation)
• Signs

—Mass, nodule, or swelling (65%–70%)
—Tenderness (15%–20%)
—Tender or enlarged breasts (3%–5%)
—Abdominal or neck mass
—Pleural effusion or other pulmonary findings

PATHOPHYSIOLOGY

• Germ cell tumors (seminoma, embryonal carcinoma, teratoma, choriocarcinoma, yolk sac): 90% to 95% of tumors
• "Mixed" germ cell tumors common (60%)
• Non–germ cell tumors (Leydig cell, Sertoli cell, gonadoblastoma) 5% to 7%
• Paratesticular and secondary tumors (lymphoma, metastasis) are rare.
• Seminoma

—Most common type (35%–65%); three subtypes:
    —Typical (85%); 10% produce human chorionic gonadotropin (hCG) (syncytiotrophoblasts).
    —Anaplastic (5%–10%); increased metastasis; 30% of seminoma deaths
    —Spermatocytic (2%–10%); most common germ cell tumor after age 65; low metastatic potential (? benign)

• Embryonal carcinoma; present in 40% of germ cell tumors
• Yolk sac tumor

—Most common in children; often in mixed tumors
—92% stain for alpha-fetoprotein (AFP)

• Choriocarcinoma

—Pure form is rare; usually fatal (pulmonary/brain metastasis)

• Teratoma

—Component of 10% to 25% of adult tumors (pure form: 3% in adults, 38% in children)
—The adult teratoma has malignant potential (benign in children).

• Leydig (interstitial) cell tumors (2%–3%)

—No association with cryptorchidism
—10% are malignant, but no reliable criteria are available. (Before puberty, 100% benign)

• Sertoli cell tumors (1%); 90% are benign.

CAUSES/RISK FACTORS

• Cryptorchidism

—Present in 7% to 10% of cases
—Risk is 4 to 14 times higher than normal.
—Seminoma most common
—Orchiopexy does not prevent tumor formation, but allows for easier examination.

• Trauma

—No relationship (may bring attention to an enlarged or painful testis)

• Hormonal factors

—Exogenous estrogen causes maldescent and dysgenesis of the testis.
—Children of women treated with DES (3%–5%) Atrophy, idiopathic, or due to infectious agents (mumps): may increase risk

COMPLICATIONS: N/A

DIFFERENTIAL DIAGNOSIS

• Epididymitis, epididymo-orchitis, torsion, hydrocele, hernia, spermatocele, hematoma
• Any firm intratesticular mass is cancer until proven otherwise.

Database

HISTORY

- Change in testicular size or texture; duration of symptoms (delay in diagnosis is very common)
- Pain in scrotum; heaviness or dull ache in testis or lower abdomen
- Previous inguinal/scrotal surgery
- History of infertility (3% of patients)
- History of cryptorchidism
- Testicular tumor in father or siblings

PHYSICAL EXAMINATION

- Begin with the normal contralateral testis.
- The testis is examined between the thumb and the first two fingers of both hands.
- Any firm or hard area in the testis is considered cancer.
- Examine the testis for

—Size, consistency, texture, mobility, mass or nodule
—Hydrocele
—Separation from the epididymis or spermatic cord
—Scrotal skin involvement
—Scrotal ultrasound is considered by many to be an extension of the physical examination.

- A complete nodal examination is required.

—Abdominal, inguinal, or supraclavicular mass

- Gynecomastia
- Pleural effusion, wheezing

 Diagnostic Studies

LABORATORY TESTING

- hCG and AFP levels prior to orchiectomy

—Monitored during follow-up for recurrence

- hCG

—Half-life: 24 to 36 hours
—Elevated in 40% to 60% of patients with testis cancer, and in 100% of choriocarcinomas
—Elevated in 10% to 15% of "pure" seminomas

- AFP

—Half-life: 5 to 7 days
—Elevated in 50% to 70% of patients with testis cancer
—Produced by yolk sac tumors, embryonal carcinoma, teratocarcinoma
—Not elevated in pure seminoma or pure choriocarcinoma

- One or both markers will be elevated in 85% to 90% (depends on stage)
- 10% to 15% of nonseminomas will have normal markers, even at the advanced stage.
- Leydig cell tumors may exhibit elevated serum and urinary estrogen.
- LDH, placental alkaline phosphatase (PLAP), neuron-specific enolase, and GGT: limited clinical use as markers

IMAGING

- Scrotal ultrasonography

—80% of testis tumors are hypoechoic, 20% are hypo- and hyperechoic.
—80% to 90% accurate in detecting neoplasm
—Echo patterns are not specific for histologic type.

- Abdominal CT scan

—For staging of retroperitoneal lymph nodes and abdominal viscera
—Accuracy is about 70% to 90% (depends on stage)
—Cannot detect micrometastasis in normal-sized lymph nodes

- Plain chest radiograph

—Lungs are the most common site of recurrence after retroperitoneal lymph node dissection (RPLND).
—For staging of intrathoracic metastasis and follow-up after orchiectomy
—A chest CT scan may be needed for patients with a high risk of recurrence or with advanced initial disease.

SPECIAL STUDIES: N/A

 Treatment

GENERAL MEASURES

- The patient is counseled regarding

—Loss of a testis
—Impact on fertility (50% may have subfertile semen parameters at presentation)
—Possible loss of ejaculation (RPLND)
—Risk of recurrence and options for initial or subsequent treatment

- Treatment options depend on clinical stage and tumor type.
- Nonseminomas

—Stage I (testis only)
 —30% of clinical stage I patients are understaged.
 —High risk of metastasis if primary tumor has vascular/lymphatic invasion, high proportion of embryonal carcinoma
 —Absence of yolk sac tumor
 —Risk of recurrence helps in selecting therapy.
 —Surveillance with a rigorous follow-up protocol after orchiectomy for low-risk, highly reliable patients
 —Nerve-sparing RPLND should preserve ejaculation in 90% to 100% and eliminate the need for rigorous follow-up.
 —Recurrence after either of the above options can be salvaged with chemotherapy.
 —Primary chemotherapy can also be offered to high-risk patients.
—Stage II (retroperitoneal micrometastasis A; nodes 2–5 cm B; nodes >5 cm C)
 —For IIA (nonbulky): RPLND with or without adjuvant chemotherapy, or primary chemotherapy and RPLND for residual mass
 —For bulky disease: primary chemotherapy followed by RPLND for residual mass
—Stage III
 —Primary chemotherapy followed by RPLND for residual mass

- Seminomas

—Stages I and IIA (nonbulky)
 —External beam radiation to retroperitoneal and ipsilateral ilioinguinal nodes
 —Contralateral inguinal region is included if a history of inguinal or scrotal procedures
—Stages IIB (bulky) and III
 —Primary chemotherapy
 —A residual mass rarely requires RPLND or radiation.

(continued)

MEDICAL

• Seminomas are highly sensitive to radiation and platinum-based chemotherapy.
• Nonseminomas are less sensitive to radiation, but are highly responsive to platinum-based chemotherapy.

SURGICAL

• Radical inguinal orchiectomy

—A 5- to 7-cm incision is made over the inguinal canal.
—The external oblique is fascia incised, and ilioinguinal nerve is preserved.
—A rubber tourniquet is applied around the spermatic cord at the internal inguinal ring to prevent tumor dissemination during manipulation.
—Deliver the testis into the operative field. Ligate and divide the spermatic cord at the internal ring.
—Leave a long tail of silk suture at the stump of the spermatic cord to facilitate removal of the entire cord during RPLND (if needed).
—Complications, such as inguinoscrotal or retroperitoneal hematoma due to inadequate hemostasis, are uncommon.

• RPLND

—A midline incision is made from the xiphoid to the pubis.
—A posterior peritoneal incision is made around the right colon and cecum to the ligament of Treitz.
—The root of the mesentery is lifted away from the posterior abdominal wall.
—Bowel, based on superior mesenteric pedicle, is lifted up and placed on the chest.
—Lymphatic tissue is removed from around the vena cava and aorta with the "split and roll" maneuver.
—The upper limit is just above the renal vessels.
—The lateral limit is the lateral border of each ureter.
—The inferior limit is the bifurcation of the common iliac artery.
—The ipsilateral spermatic cord is removed.
—For low-stage retroperitoneal disease, a modified nerve-sparing dissection is performed:
　—Full dissection is carried down to the origin of the inferior mesenteric artery.
　—Below this level, dissection is limited to the ipsilateral half of the aorta and common iliac artery.
　—The sympathetic plexus, present on the anterior surface of aorta, is spared to preserve ejaculation (85%–95%).
—Prospective nerve-sparing RPLND
　—Individual sympathetic nerve fibers are identified and tagged.
　—Lymphatic tissue is removed from around these nerves.
　—In addition to stage I, this is also suitable for selected stage II disease.
　—Ejaculation is preserved in over 95%.
—Complications (5%–20%) include ileus, atelectasis, pneumonitis, lymphocele, pancreatitis, and vascular or bowel injury.

• Laparoscopic node dissection is under study.

ALTERNATIVE THERAPIES: N/A

PATIENT EDUCATION

• Delay in diagnosis has been the rule rather than the exception.
• Public education campaign to emphasize testicular self-examination and early physician consultation
• Patients should perform monthly self-examination of the remaining testis.

Follow-Up

MONITORING

• Tumor marker levels, a chest radiograph, and an abdominal CT scan are used to monitor response to therapy.

—At least 5-year follow-up is recommended for most patients.
—Frequent chest x-rays and tumor markers for first 2 years
—Failure to normalize AFP and hCG levels indicates residual viable tumor.
—A rise in tumor markers often precedes clinically detectable disease.
—10% to 20% of postchemotherapy RPLND patients will have viable tumor despite normal markers.

PREVENTION: N/A

 Miscellaneous

SYNONYMS: N/A

ASSOCIATED CONDITIONS

• Cryptorchidism, subfertility

NOTES

• See Section II for specific tumor types.

ABBREVIATIONS

• RPLND, retroperitoneal lymph node dissection

REFERENCES

Baniel J, Roth BJ, Foster RS. Cost and risk benefit in the management of clinical stage II non-seminomatous testicular tumors. *Cancer* 1995;75:2897.

Donohue JP, Zachary JM, Maynard BR. Distribution of nodal metastases in non-seminomatous testis cancer. *J Urol* 1982;128:315.

Jewett MAS, Torbey C. Nerve-sparing techniques in retroperitoneal lymphadenectomy in patients with low-stage testicular cancer. *Semin Urol* 1988;6:233.

Mostofi FK, Sesterhenn IA. Anatomy and pathology of testis cancer. In: Vogelzang NJ, Scardino PT, Shipley WU, Coffey DS, eds. *Comprehensive Textbook of Genitourinary Oncology.* Baltimore: Williams & Wilkins, 1996:953–967.

Richie JP. Neoplasms of the testis. In: Walsh PC, Retik AB, Vaughn ED, Wein AJ, eds. *Campbell's Urology,* 7th ed. Philadelphia: WB Saunders, 1998:2411–2452.

Authors: Badar M. Mian and William R. Morgan

Testis Tumor—Pediatric, General

 Basics

DESCRIPTION

- Painless scrotal mass within the testis

EPIDEMIOLOGY

- 1% to 2% of all pediatric solid tumors
- 2% of all testicular tumors
- 77% of all pediatric testicular masses are malignant.
- Annual incidence: 0.5 to 2.0 per 100,000 children
- Peak age of incidence: 2 years
- Incidence of germ cell tumors not as great as in adults
- A greater percentage of benign intratesticular lesions in children compared with adults
- Rare in Black and Asian children

GENETICS

- Gonadoblastomas are associated with the 45XO/46XY karyotype in intersex patients with gonadal dysgenesis.
- Yolk sac tumors of the testis have structural abnormalities of loci on chromosomes 1p, 6q, and 3p.

STAGING

- Intergroup staging system

—Stage 1: limited to testis (testes), completely resected by high inguinal orchiectomy; no clinical, radiologic, or histologic evidence of disease beyond the testis; tumor markers normal after appropriate half-life decline (alpha-fetoprotein [AFP], 5 days; beta-human chorionic gonadotropin [bhCG], 16 hours). Patients with normal or unknown tumor markers at diagnosis must have a negative ipsilateral retroperitoneal node sampling to confirm stage 1 disease.
—Stage 2: transscrotal orchiectomy; microscopic disease in scrotum or high in spermatic cord (≤5 cm from proximal end); retroperitoneal lymph node involvement (≤2 cm) and/or persistently elevated or increased tumor markers
—Stage 3: retroperitoneal lymph node involvement (≤2 cm) but no visceral or extraabdominal involvement
—Stage 4: distant metastasis, including liver

SIGNS AND SYMPTOMS

- 87% with painless scrotal mass
- 7% to 25% have a secondary hydrocele; most common misdiagnosis
- If painful, may be associated with torsion or hemorrhage into tumor
- If hormonally functional, may see signs of precocious puberty and gynecomastia (gonadal stromal tumors)
- Secondary tumors of the testis (lymphomas/leukemias) may present with a testicular mass.
- Males with congenital adrenal hyperplasia may present with precocious puberty and testicular masses.

PATHOPHYSIOLOGY

- Classification based on germ cell and non–germ cell origin of tumor (American Academy of Pediatrics Prepubertal Testis Tumor Registry)

—Germ cell tumor (yolk sac tumor): 77%
—Gonadal stromal tumor: 8%
—Gonadoblastoma: 1%
—All others (lymphoma, leukemia, etc.): 14%

- 29% of prepubertal tumors are of non–germ cell origin; many can be enucleated with testicular salvage.
- Gonadal stromal tumors may be hormonally active with precocious puberty and gynecomastia (increased penile size, pubic hair, deepened voice).
- Leydig cell tumors: Reinke crystalloids, seen in 35% of adults, are rarely seen in children.
- Testis tumor of the adrenogenital syndrome (TTAGS) is benign and usually suppressible with glucocorticoids.
- Sertoli cell tumor: benign if <5 years of age; when hormonally active, causes gynecomastia
- Yolk sac tumor: 82% of germ cell tumors; associated with elevated AFP in 80% of patients

—AFP is normally elevated in the neonate; its half-life is 5 days; persistent elevation beyond five half-lives implies metastatic disease.
—bhCG secreted by the syncytiotrophoblast (half-life: 16 hours); rarely elevated in prepubertal children with yolk sac tumors
—Metastasis by hematogenous and lymphatic spread
—Yolk sac elements will stain positive for AFP on immunohistochemical staining.

- Teratoma: second most common testis tumor in children

—Not associated with elevated AFP and does not stain positively for AFP
—Metastasis from a teratoma in prepubertal children has not been reported.
—Testis-sparing enucleation via an inguinal incision is possible.

CAUSES/RISK FACTORS

- Cryptorchidism: Data apply to *all* patients (pediatric and adult).

—7% to 10% of patients with testicular tumor have a history of cryptorchidism.
—The relative risk of testis cancer in patients with cryptorchidism is 3 to 14 times the expected incidence.
—Earlier orchiopexy may have a favorable influence on reducing the risk of developing a tumor in adulthood.

- Maternal diethylstilbestrol treatment
- Nonspecific or mumps-associated atrophy of the testis

COMPLICATIONS

- Precocious puberty with gonadal stromal tumors
- Gynecomastia with gonadal stromal tumor
- Mortality rate with yolk sac tumors: 1% to 15%, dependent on stage

DIFFERENTIAL DIAGNOSIS

- Hernia/hydrocele: may be seen conjointly with a testicular tumor
- Epididymitis diagnosed prepubertally is usually associated with a urinary tract infection.
- Torsion of spermatic cord: more common at puberty; acute onset of pain
- Paratesticular rhabdomyosarcoma: The testis is normal by ultrasound examination, which depicts the extratesticular origin of the tumor.
- Varicocele: typically seen in older boys; changes with Valsalva and supine position

 Database

HISTORY

- History of undescended testicle?
- Asymptomatic scrotal mass in majority of patients
- Acute pain associated with hemorrhage into tumor
- Breast tenderness with gynecomastia

PHYSICAL EXAMINATION

- Hard mass confined to the testis (intratesticular)
- Negative transillumination
- The testis may feel normal with small, hormonally active tumors.
- Palpate the abdomen/nodes to rule out lymphatic metastases.
- Palpate the supraclavicular nodes to rule out lymphatic metastasis.
- Evaluate for signs of precocious puberty and gynecomastia.

Diagnostic Studies

LABORATORY TESTING

- Serum tumor markers AFP, bhCG

—Extreme elevations of AFP are normal in the perinatal period up to 8 months of age.
—AFP is not elevated in 20% of patients with yolk sac tumor.
—Obtain prior to orchiectomy in all patients with a testicular mass

- Serum testosterone, LH, FSH levels if gonadal stromal tumor suspected

—Testosterone is elevated and gonadotrophin suppressed with Leydig cell tumor

- Serum estrogen and progesterone are elevated in patients with gynecomastia

IMAGING

- Testicular ultrasound: distinguishes intratesticular from extratesticular location of the mass

—Most extratesticular lesions (hernia, varicocele) are benign.
—Near 100% sensitivity for detecting testicular neoplasia
—No sonographic feature discriminates between benign and malignant intratesticular tumors.
—If the testis is not palpable due to a hydrocele, sonography is recommended.

- Chest x-ray

—Evaluate for pulmonary metastases in patients with yolk sac tumors.

- CT scan of pelvis and abdomen with contrast

—Evaluate the retroperitoneum for evidence of lymph node metastasis.
—Evaluate the liver and other solid organs for metastasis.

- Depending on signs and symptoms, specific tests, such as a bone scan, may be needed to stage the disease.

SPECIAL STUDIES: N/A

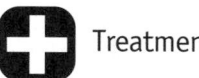 ## Treatment

GENERAL MEASURES

- All intratesticular masses are assumed to be malignant until proven otherwise.
- Specific treatment of malignant tumors (Yolk sac tumor) is stage-specific and multimodal (surgery, chemotherapy, and radiation).

MEDICAL

- Chemotherapy is based on tumor histology and stage.

—Yolk sac tumor stage 2: 1 year of vincristine, actinomycin D, and cyclophosphamide (VAC); or cisplatin, vinblastine, and bleomycin (PVB)
—Yolk sac tumor stage 3: combination therapy VAC or PVB, with or without radiation therapy with or without cytoreductive surgery

SURGICAL

- All intratesticular masses are explored through an inguinal incision, with early control of spermatic vessels.

—Testis-sparing surgery is possible in children with teratomas, Leydig cell tumors, TTAGS, and epidermoid cysts.
—Frozen sections to confirm benign nature of mass. All other lesions removed by radical orchiectomy

- Retroperitoneal lymph node dissection (yolk sac tumor)

—Reserved for patients with postchemotherapy residual retroperitoneal disease and postchemotherapy elevated AFP
—Not necessary in the majority of children, as 80% present with stage 1 disease

ALTERNATIVE THERAPIES: N/A

PATIENT EDUCATION

- All patients with an undescended testis need to be instructed at an appropriate age in self-examination for testicular masses.

 ## Follow-Up

MONITORING

- Dependent on stage of disease and pathologic diagnosis
- Stage 1 yolk sac tumor testis

—Monthly AFP and chest x-rays for 1 year
—CT abdomen every 3 months for 1 year, then every 6 months for 2 years

PREVENTION

- Early correction of an undescended testicle may decrease the malignant potential; more importantly, it allows easy palpation of the testicle.

 ## Miscellaneous

SYNONYMS

- Endodermal sinus tumor, infantile embryonal carcinoma

ASSOCIATED CONDITIONS

- Secondary malignancy of the testis due to acute lymphoblastic leukemia

NOTES

- See also Section I, "Testicular Mass—Adult and Pediatric" and specific tumor types in Section II.

ABBREVIATIONS

- TTAGS, testis tumor of the adrenogenital syndrome; LH, luteinizing hormone; FSH, follicle-stimulating hormone; VAC, vincristine, actinomycin D, cyclophosphamide; PVB, cisplatin, vinblastine, bleomycin

REFERENCES

Connolly JA, Gearhart JP. Management of yolk sac tumors in children. *Urol Clin North Am* 1993;20:7.

Grady RW, Ross JH, Kay R. Patterns of metastatic spread in prepubertal yolk sac tumor of the testis. *J Urol* 1995;153:1259.

Kay R. Prepubertal testicular tumor registry. *Urol Clin North Am* 1993;20:1.

Skoog SJ. Benign and malignant pediatric scrotal masses. *Pediatr Clin North Am* 1997;44:1229.

Author: Steven J. Skoog

Torsion—Testicular

 Basics

DESCRIPTION

• Testicular torsion is a vascular event that involves cessation of blood flow to the testis, ultimately leading to testicular loss, unless timely intervention occurs. Two distinct types occur: extravaginal torsion (prenatal and neonatal) and intravaginal torsion (all age groups).

EPIDEMIOLOGY

• Most common age: early puberty
• Second most common: newborn
• Occurrence: 1 in 4000 males

GENETICS

• Unknown

STAGING: N/A

SIGNS AND SYMPTOMS

• Acute onset of testicular pain

—Nausea, vomiting
—Inguinal, abdominal pain

• Scrotal swelling/asymmetric

—Erythema of scrotal skin
—High-riding/elevated testis

PATHOPHYSIOLOGY

• Extravaginal torsion

—Lack of testicular fixation in the scrotum allows the testis, spermatic cord, and tunica vaginalis to twist, often to the level of the internal ring.

• Intravaginal torsion

—The spermatic cord twists inside the tunica vaginalis due to its high insertion on the cord, allowing the testis to turn freely within the scrotum. The testis has a more transverse lie ("bell clapper deformity") and is more prone to twist.
—Often occurs around puberty due to increase in testicular size

• Vascular compromise results in rapid onset of swelling, and subsequent tissue necrosis after 6 to 8 hours.

CAUSES/RISK FACTORS

• Extravaginal: antenatal/neonatal: incomplete testicular descent
• Intravaginal: horizontal lie to testis

COMPLICATIONS

• Hemorrhage
• Reactive hydrocele
• Loss of testis/necrosis
• Contralateral torsion
• A retained necrotic testis may be at risk for tumor formation; a postpubertal necrotic testis may lead to antisperm antibodies.

DIFFERENTIAL DIAGNOSIS

• Torsed appendage to testis, epididymitis
• Hydrocele
• Epididymitis, orchitis, epididymo-orchitis
• Inguinal hernia
• Varicocele, spermatocele
• Testicular trauma
• Testis tumor
• Idiopathic scrotal edema
• Henoch-Schönlein purpura

 Database

HISTORY

• Acute onset of testicular pain, associated with nausea and vomiting, may awaken the patient from sleep.

—Suggests testicular torsion

• Mild onset over a few days: suggests torsion of testicular appendage
• Urinary tract symptoms: suggests epididymitis and/or orchitis, but cannot rule out torsion
• History of trauma: suggests testicular injury; cannot rule out torsion
• Prior inguinal/scrotal surgery: cannot rule out torsion
• Prior episodes of scrotal pain/swelling: suggest intermittent testicular torsion

PHYSICAL EXAMINATION

• Observation

—The patient that ambulates easily usually does not have testicular torsion.
—Observe scrotal asymmetry, position of testes (i.e., dependent vs. high-riding/elevated in scrotum), and scrotal erythema.
—The "blue dot sign" suggests a torsed appendix testis.

• Palpate the normal testis first; look for horizontal position.
• Palpate the involved testis carefully, the lower pole first: If tender, suspect testicular torsion; if the upper aspect is tender, consider a torsed appendage.
• Palpate the spermatic cord: If tender, consider testicular torsion.
• Prehn's sign: See Section III.
• Palpate the scrotal wall: If thickened and the testis is not tender, consider idiopathic scrotal edema.
• Hard, nontender testis: Consider a testicular tumor and/or antenatal/neonatal torsion (young infant).
• A large hydrocele is nonspecific.

Diagnostic Studies

LABORATORY TESTING

• Urinalysis, urine culture if infection suspected; positive results do not rule out testicular torsion.

IMAGING

• Technetium-99m pertechnetate radionuclide scanning to determine presence or absence of perfusion
• Color flow Doppler ultrasonography; may be technically difficult in small patients
• MRI: provides detailed anatomic information; availability, interpretation, or cost may be problematic.

SPECIAL STUDIES: N/A

 ## Treatment

GENERAL MEASURES

• Prompt referral to urology or pediatric urology
• If the index of suspicion is high for testicular torsion, surgical intervention should proceed promptly.

MEDICAL: N/A

SURGICAL

• Extravaginal

—Prompt surgical intervention to reduce torsion is indicated if the event is felt to be acute ($<$8 hours) and salvage is possible. Otherwise, removal of the necrotic testis and contralateral orchidopexy are indicated.

• Intravaginal

—Prompt surgical exploration to detorse testis, if salvageable, or remove necrotic testis, orchidopexy for contralateral testis

• Orchidopexy: creation of subdartos scrotal pouch, with or without three-point suture fixation of testis

ALTERNATIVE THERAPIES: N/A

PATIENT EDUCATION

• Parents and older children should seek medical attention immediately for scrotal pain and/or swelling.

 ## Follow-Up

MONITORING

• Periodic follow-up to assess testis and/or testes for atrophy and/or pubertal development

PREVENTION

• Perform orchidopexy of contralateral side at time of surgery

 ## Miscellaneous

SYNONYMS: N/A

ASSOCIATED CONDITIONS

• Cryptorchidism, vanishing testis (antenatal torsion), testicular trauma, Henoch-Schönlein purpura

NOTES

• See also Section I, "Testis and Genital Pain—Chronic," and Section III, "Torsion—Testicular Appendages."

ABBREVIATIONS: N/A

REFERENCES

Caldamone AA, Valvo JR, Altebarmakian VK, Rabinowitz R. Acute scrotal swelling in children. *J Pediatr Surg* 1984;19(5):581–584.

Ehrlich RM, ed. Neonatal testicular torsion. *Dialogues Pediatr Urol* 1991;14(5):1–8.

Kass EJ, Lundak B. The acute scrotum. *Pediatr Clin North Am* 1997;44(5):1251–1266.

Rabinowitz R, Hulbert WC. Acute scrotal swelling. *Urol Clin North Am* 1995;22(1):101–105.

Schimmel MS, Prat O. Perinatal acute scrotum: Controversies in the management of torsion of the testis. *AJDC* 1993;147:933–934.

Authors: Michael G. Packer and Mark R. Zaontz

Transplant Rejection—Renal

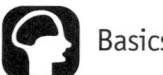

Basics

DESCRIPTION

• A transplanted kidney's functional and structural demise due to immune responses by the recipient. There are three types:

—Hyperacute (minutes to weeks following transplantation)
—Acute (weeks to months following transplantation)
—Chronic (months to years following transplantation)

EPIDEMIOLOGY

• 14% rejection rate in first year for those rejection-free at discharge

GENETICS

• Likelihood of rejection: cadaver transplant greater than living, nonrelated transplant, which is greater than living, related transplant
• Increased level of graft survival with increased degree of HLA cross-matching

STAGING: N/A

SIGNS AND SYMPTOMS

• Fever, symptoms of influenza, pain/swelling over graft site, oliguria, fluid retention/weight gain, increased blood pressure

PATHOPHYSIOLOGY

• Hyperacute: mediated by preformed cytotoxic antibodies against graft (develop after prior transfusion, transplantation, child birth)
• Acute: mediated by mononuclear cell infiltration and vasculitis (T-cell recognition and activation by foreign antigen presented by MHC proteins of presenting cells)
• Chronic: interstitial fibrosis, vascular changes, minimal mononuclear cell infiltration

CAUSES/RISK FACTORS

• Failure of immune suppression, resulting in T-cell stimulation against donor antigens
• Prior rejection episodes: development of HLA antibodies

COMPLICATIONS

• Graft failure, development of new anti-HLA antibodies, hypertension (HTN)

DIFFERENTIAL DIAGNOSIS

• Pyelonephrosis
• Acute tubular necrosis (ATN)
• Cyclosporin A (CsA) toxicity
• Obstructive uropathy
• Technical complications

—Arterial or venous thrombus, arterial stenosis, urinary obstruction (early posttransplant)
—Glomerulonephritis
—Recurrence of original disease

Database

HISTORY

• Suspect diagnosis of rejection if

—Classic signs/symptoms, or
—Fever, creatinine rise >25% over 1 to 2 days, and CsA levels normal

PHYSICAL EXAMINATION

• Tenderness/erythema at site of graft

Diagnostic Studies

LABORATORY TESTING

- Rising BUN/creatinine

—Note: baseline may be elevated; a creatinine rise greater than 25% over 1 to 2 days suggests rejection.

- Urinalysis with culture

—Rule out pyelonephritis.

- CsA levels

—Suspect CsA toxicity if abnormal levels
—Trough 12 to 18 hours after oral dose, 12 hours after IV dose
—Reference range: 150 to 400 ng/mL

IMAGING

- Renal scan: decreased renal blood flow/glomerular filtration rate

—Progressively worsens on serial examinations (stabilizes in ATN)

- Renal ultrasound

—Rule out obstructive uropathy.
—Assess for diminished vascular flow.
—Detect graft swelling (graft may be small/atrophic in chronic rejection).

SPECIAL STUDIES

- Needle biopsy of transplant kidney (confirmation of rejection)

—Repeat biopsies may be required.
—Subendothelial vascular mononuclear cell infiltrates are characteristic.

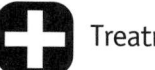 Treatment

GENERAL MEASURES

- Attempt to reverse rejection through medical therapy; graft removal may be necessary.

MEDICAL

- Hyperacute rejection: refractory to immunosuppression and requires immediate removal of transplanted kidney

—Can result in DIC if not removed promptly

- Acute rejection: pulse-dose steroids (protocols may vary between institutions)

—Solu-Medrol 500 mg IV qd × 3 days; then prednisone taper

- Chronic rejection: no effective therapy. Avoid excessive immunosuppression.
- If incomplete or no response to steroid therapy, then antilymphocyte antibody therapy with ATG or OKT3 (protocols may vary between institutions)

—ATG (polyclonal antithymocyte antibodies) at 15 to 30 mg/kg qd for 10 days
  —Must institute CMV prophylaxis with ganciclovir; follow WBC with differential and platelets
  —Continue immunosuppression with CsA and steroids
—OKT3 (monoclonal anti-CD3 antibodies) at 5 mg qd for 10 to 14 days
  —Must institute CMV prophylaxis with ganciclovir and follow biweekly CD3 levels
  —Continue immunosuppression with CsA.
    —Significant first-dose reactions are possible. Pulmonary edema: must have a clear chest x-ray less than 24 hours prior to dosing OKT3; fever, chills: steroid, Benadryl, acetaminophen prophylaxis

SURGICAL

- Allograft nephrectomy

—Remove a symptomatic, irreversibly rejected kidney transplant.
—Remove an asymptomatic, chronically rejected kidney to withdraw immunosuppression and prevent further development of anti-HLA antibodies.

ALTERNATIVE THERAPIES: N/A

PATIENT EDUCATION

- Transplant team-teaching about immunosuppressive regimens

 Follow-Up

MONITORING

- Determination of adequate immunosuppression and CsA levels

PREVENTION

- As above

 Miscellaneous

SYNONYMS

- Graft rejection

ASSOCIATED CONDITIONS: N/A

NOTES

- See prescribing information in Section V.

ABBREVIATIONS

- CsA, cyclosporin A

REFERENCES

Sunthanthiran M. Acute rejection of renal allografts: Mechanistic insights and therapeutic options. *Kidney Int* 1997;51:1289–1304.

Sunthanthiran M, Strom T. Mechanisms and management of acute renal allograft rejection. *Surg Clin North Am* 1998;78(1):77–94.

Authors: John Oh and Leonard G. Gomella

Transurethral Resection Syndrome

 Basics

DESCRIPTION

• Syndrome characterized by mental confusion, nausea, vomiting, and hypertension during TURP when irrigation fluid enters the intravascular space

EPIDEMIOLOGY

• 2% to 10% of patients undergoing TURP

GENETICS: N/A

STAGING: N/A

SIGNS AND SYMPTOMS

• Lacks a stereotypical presentation
• Occurs as quickly as 15 minutes up to 24 hours postoperatively
• Nausea, vomiting, and confusion most common neurologic symptoms
• Blurred vision, chest pain, and fatigue also seen

PATHOPHYSIOLOGY

• Syndrome secondary to acute changes in intravascular volume and plasma solute concentrations from irrigant fluid absorption

—Irrigants used during procedure, including water (hemolytic), glycine, sorbitol, and mannitol, are electrically nonconducting but osmotically active fluids.
—Fluid either gains direct intravascular access to the prostatic venous plexus or is slowly absorbed from the retroperitoneal and perivesical space.

• Intravascular volume shifts

—Intravascular volume expansion
    —Hypertension or hypotension can occur.
    —Rapid volume expansion from the absorbed irrigant can explain hypertension and reflex bradycardia.
    —The patient with poor left ventricular function may develop pulmonary edema from volume overload.
    —Rapid volume overload and electrolyte changes result in frequent arrhythmias.
—Factors contributing to volume gain
    —Intravesicular pressure: governed by the height of the irrigation bag
    —Number of prostatic sinuses opened
    —ADH produced from stress of surgery

• Plasma solute effect

—Solute changes alter neurologic function are independent of volume-related effects.
—CNS symptoms may be caused by derangements of sodium, osmolality, ammonia, and glycine.
—Hyponatremia
    —Caused by irrigant absorption (dilutional hyponatremia)
    —Most likely cause of transurethral (TUR) syndrome
    —15% of patients have serum sodium concentrations <125 mmol/L.

—Causes visual aberrations, encephalopathy, pulmonary edema, cardiovascular collapse, seizure, and death
—Hypo-osmolality
    —Derangement of CNS function is not hyponatremia per se, but hypo-osmolality.
    —The blood–brain barrier is essentially impermeable to sodium, but not water.
    —The brain reacts to sustained hypo-osmotic stress by decreasing intracellular Na/K/Cl concentration to decrease intracellular osmolality and prevent intracerebral swelling.
    —With *acute* osmotic change, this mechanism is not fast enough, and CNS edema occurs.
    —Cerebral edema can increase intracerebral pressure, with resulting hypertension and bradycardia (Cushing reflex).
    —Hyponatremia is a reflection of the degree of hypoosmolality and volume overload.
—Hyperammonemia
    —Glycine in the irrigant gains intravascular access and is metabolized by the liver to two toxic metabolites: glyoxylic acid and ammonia.
    —Hyperammonemia may contribute to alterations of CNS function.
—Hyperglycinemia
    —Glycine is a major inhibitory neurotransmitter.
    —Has a role in seizures and encephalopathy
    —Inhibitory transmitter in the retina; may cause visual aberrations
    —Metabolized to oxalate, which may precipitate in the kidney and cause renal damage

CAUSES/RISK FACTORS

• Elevated pressure of irrigant solution (height of bag >40 cm above level of prostate)
• Lengthy resection (>90 minutes)
• Type of resecting equipment (best to use continuous-flow resectoscope)
• Quality of the resection (number of opened prostatic sinuses)
• Volume of tissue resected (>45 g)

COMPLICATIONS

• Cerebral edema and associated complications
• Cardiopulmonary collapse
• Renal failure
• Death

DIFFERENTIAL DIAGNOSIS

• Myocardial infarction
• CVA
• Acute hemorrhage
• Narcotic overdose
• Seizure disorder

 Database

HISTORY

• Symptoms during surgery

—Prickling sensation in the skin
—Uneasiness, chest pain, confusion

• Symptoms after surgery

—Nausea, confusion, vomiting

PHYSICAL EXAMINATION

• Nonspecific, often clammy
• A neurologic examination may reveal loss of orientation but usually no focal signs.

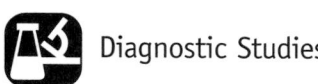 Diagnostic Studies

LABORATORY TESTING

- Serum sodium concentration <125 mEq

IMAGING: N/A

SPECIAL STUDIES: N/A

 Treatment

GENERAL MEASURES

- Supportive care to maintain pulmonary and hemodynamic stability

MEDICAL

- Correction of volume overload

—Furosemide 20 mg IV to promote diuresis; repeat as needed
—Furosemide is usually successful for mild degrees of hyponatremia, without a need for hypertonic saline.

- Correction of sodium deficit

—Calculate Na deficit: (pre-op Na − post-op Na) × ECF
—Extracellular fluid (ECF) compartment calculated by multiplying body weight by 20%
—Replace Na deficit with 3% saline that contains 513 mEq/L of Na.
—Replace Na deficit over 3 to 6 hours, with frequent monitoring of serum sodium.

SURGICAL: N/A

ALTERNATIVE THERAPIES

- Treatment of hyperammonemia when glycine used in irrigant

—Neurologic signs/symptoms may be secondary to hyperammonemia.
—L-arginine acts in the liver by preventing hepatic release of ammonia and accelerates ammonia conversion to urea.
—Give (postoperatively) L-arginine 4 g (20 mmol) IV over 3 minutes and repeat, or give 38-g (180-mmol) infusion over 120 minutes.

PATIENT EDUCATION

- Patients undergoing TUR should be made aware of the risk of TUR syndrome.

 Follow-Up

MONITORING

- Serial serum sodiums intraoperatively and postoperatively
- Hemodynamic monitoring, if necessary

PREVENTION

- Recognition of the syndrome
- Experience with transurethral resection
- Limit the resection time to <90 minutes.
- Monitor serum electrolytes for longer resections.

 Miscellaneous

SYNONYMS

- TUR syndrome

ASSOCIATED CONDITIONS

- Benign prostatic hypertrophy

NOTES: N/A

ABBREVIATIONS: N/A

REFERENCES

Gravenstein D. Transurethral resection of the prostate syndrome: A review of the pathophysiology and management. *Anesth Analg* 1997;84(2):438.

Olsson J, Nilsson A, et al. Symptoms of the transurethral resection syndrome using glycine and the irrigant. *J Urol* 1995;154(1):123.

Sacks SA. The transurethral resection syndrome. AUA Update Series, Volume 4, Lesson 40, 1985.

Authors: Stephen D.W. Beck and Michael O. Koch

Tuberculosis—Genitourinary

 Basics

DESCRIPTION

- Urinary tract infection with *Mycobacterium tuberculosis;* common in the prostate, bladder, and epididymis. Over the last 30 years, major changes have occurred in the approach to genitourinary tuberculosis (GU TB). As a result, the morbidity and mortality associated with the disease has been greatly reduced.

EPIDEMIOLOGY

- Predominate age group: 20 to 40 years
- 2:1 ratio of male-to-female incidence
- During the past 10 to 15 years, there has been an increase in cases secondary to the spread of diseases from other parts of the world and the AIDS epidemic.

GENETICS: N/A

STAGING: N/A

SIGNS AND SYMPTOMS

- No classical clinical picture, and most symptoms are of bladder origin.
- Vague, nonspecific complaints such as malaise, lethargy, weight loss, and low-grade fevers are common.
- Initial symptoms may be minimal, even in the presence of extensive disease.
- Common to see recurrent urinary tract infections with *E. coli*
- Usually no clinical symptoms until TB involves the calyces or the pelvis of the kidney
- Dysuria from seeding of the bladder with TB
- Chronic cystitis unresponsive to therapy
- Painful swollen testis
- Suprapubic pain when disease is extensive
- Chronic draining scrotal sinuses should be considered tuberculosis in origin until proven otherwise.
- Nocturia, hematuria

PATHOPHYSIOLOGY

- Invasion of GU organs is by ascent (prostate to bladder) or descent (kidney to bladder, prostate to epididymis).
- The kidney and prostate are the primary sites of TB infection in the GU tract.
- Tuberculomas develop in glomerular capillaries as a result of hematogenous seeding from the lungs.
- Renal TB may take years to develop in a patients with a normal immune system.
- Normal renal parenchyma is slowly replaced by caseous material, and calcium is laid down as part of the reparative process.
- Large calcifications in the prostate should suggest TB.
- Perinephric abscess is rare but may develop.
- Ureters undergo fibrosis, resulting in shortening and straightening.
- Involvement of the testis is unusual.

- Involvement of prostatic ducts and seminal vesicles may occur.

—The prostate may feel hard and nodular.

- Bacille Calmette-Guérin (BCG) therapy for bladder cancer can cause disseminated disease mimicking TB.

CAUSES/RISK FACTORS

- Immunocompromised states
- Poor living conditions/poverty
- Malnutrition
- Chronic TB infection

COMPLICATIONS

- Ureteral TB

—Stricture formation
—Hydronephrosis
—Complete nonfunctioning of an affected kidney (autonephrectomy) described

- Renal TB

—Obliteration of the renal and psoas shadow on plain radiographs
—A perinephric abscess may cause an enlarging mass in the flank.

- Genital TB

—Sterility a consequence
—An abscess of the epididymis may erode through the scrotal wall or testis, creating a sinus tract and drainage.

- Bladder TB

—Stenosis of ureterovesical junction
—Fibrosis and contraction of bladder

DIFFERENTIAL DIAGNOSIS

- Chronic nonspecific cystitis or pyelonephritis
- Nonspecific epididymitis
- Urinary bilharziasis (schistosomiasis)
- Amicrobic cystitis
- Necrotizing papillitis
- Medullary sponge kidney
- Renal stones or nephrocalcinosis
- Disseminated coccidioidomycosis

 Database

HISTORY

- Men commonly present with epididymitis.
- Bacterial cystitis may be superimposed on bladder TB.
- History of or exposure to TB
- Determine last PPD testing results

PHYSICAL EXAMINATION

- Painful swollen testis
- Nontender, enlarged epididymis with a beaded or thickened vas deferens
- A nodular and indurated prostate and thickened seminal vesicles on DRE mimic neoplasm.
- An upper abdominal bruit may be an indication of advanced renal disease.
- Thickening or coarseness of the epididymis or prostate nodularity

Diagnostic Studies

LABORATORY TESTING

- Routine urinalysis, standard culture

—Urine is usually sterile on routine cultures; however, 20% of patients will have a superimposed bacterial cystitis or urinary tract infection with *E. coli*.

- Specific staining of urine for acid-fast bacteria and mycobacterial culture
- First morning specimen offers highest yield of TB
- A minimum of three early-morning urine specimens are recommended.

—Acid-fast stains from a 24-hour urine specimen are positive in 60% of cases.
—High index of suspicion for persistent pyuria without bacteria on repeated cultures (stain with methylene blue)

- CBC, electrolytes, erythrocyte sedimentation rate (measure monthly as indicator of response to therapy)

IMAGING

- Chest plain film
- KUB

—Enlargement of one kidney
—Punctuate calcifications in the renal parenchyma
—Large calcified structures in the prostatic
—Renal stones in 10%
—Obliteration of the psoas shadow due to perinephric abscess

- Excretory urogram

—Mandatory study; "moth-eaten appearance in ulcerated calyces"
—Dilation of upper tract secondary to ureteral stricture
—Obliteration of calyces
—Loss of kidney function due to complete occlusion or renal destruction

- Retrograde pyelography

—Selective culture for TB
—Assessment of ureteral

- CT scan

—Option if IVP contraindicated
—Useful in delineating disease in seminal vesicles
—Limited value in early management

SPECIAL STUDIES

- Tuberculin skin test

—Induration >10 mm in diameter is considered a positive reaction.
—A positive reaction indicates exposure, not necessarily active disease.
—May be negative in a patient with miliary TB, AIDS, or advanced age
—A negative tuberculin skin test makes the diagnosis of TB unlikely.

—Must not have had BCG vaccine or therapy in the past

- Cystoscopy

—TB appears as a patchy erythematous ulceration with exudate.
—Demonstrates extent of disease
—Biopsy for tissue confirmation
—TB may mimic transitional cell cancer or carcinoma in situ

 Treatment

GENERAL MEASURES

- Treat active disease promptly in an outpatient setting. Supervision of a urologist (optional) to ensure compliance and to monitor for complications from chemotherapy
- It is no longer necessary to manage in an inpatient setting unless compliance is an issue.

MEDICAL

- Notes: Current antituberculous drugs are isoniazid, rifampin, streptomycin, pyrazinamide, and ethambutol

—Patient with uncomplicated TB infection
  —Isoniazid, rifampin, and pyrazinamide once a day in the morning, 3 times a week, for 2 months. Followed by isoniazid and rifampin once a day, 3 times a week, for 4 months. 1 g of vitamin C, 3 times a week, for 4 months with above regimen
—Patient with complicated TB infection
  —Add streptomycin to the above for very intense infection or severe bladder symptoms.

- Steroids

—No place in initial therapy
—For acute TB cystitis or stricture at distal ureter
—Prednisone 20 mg po tid

SURGICAL

- Nephrectomy

—Symptomatic (hypertension or obstruction) nonfunctioning kidney with extensive disease
—Coexistent renal cell carcinoma
—Perform 4 to 6 weeks after start of antituberculous drugs

- Epididymectomy

—Indicated for caseating abscess unresponsive to chemotherapy

ALTERNATIVE THERAPIES: N/A

PATIENT EDUCATION

- Completion of TB regimens long term is essential.

 Follow-Up

MONITORING

- All patients should be seen 3, 6, and 12 months after completion of therapy.
- IVP should be performed for rising creatinine or for renal involvement.
- Three consecutive early-morning urine cultures should be examined.
- An initially elevated ESR should be repeated.

PREVENTION: N/A

 Miscellaneous

SYNONYMS: N/A

ASSOCIATED CONDITIONS

- AIDS, immunocompromised states

NOTES: N/A

ABBREVIATIONS

- TB, tuberculosis

REFERENCES

Gow JG. AUA Update Series, Volume XI, Lesson 26, 1992, 201–208.

Gow JG. Genitourinary tuberculosis. In: Walsh PC, Retik AB, Vaughan ED, Wein AJ, eds. *Campbell's Urology,* 7th ed. Philadelphia: WB Saunders, 1998:807–834.

Mehta JB, et al. Epidemiology of extrapulmonary tuberculosis: A comparative analysis with pre-AIDS era. *Chest* 1991;99:1134.

Tanagho EA, McAninch JW. *Smith's General Urology.* Norwalk, CT: Appleton & Lange, 1995.

Authors: C.B. Threatt and C.N. Robertson

Urachal Abnormalities

 Basics

DESCRIPTION

• Congenital urachal abnormalities can be divided into four types:

—Urachal sinus is the most common urachal abnormality and consists of the channel resulting from spontaneous drainage of a urachal cyst to the umbilicus.
—Urachal cyst: persistence of part of this channel between the bladder and umbilicus lacking communication to either structure. The second most common urachal anomaly
—Patent urachus: persistence of the urachal channel between the bladder and umbilicus. The most uncommon type of urachal abnormality
—Urachal diverticulum of the bladder. May result from drainage of a urachal cyst to the bladder but is more commonly seen patients with neurogenic bladders, where it is of little clinical consequence

EPIDEMIOLOGY

• Asymptomatic abnormalities are quite common (particularly urachal diverticulae of the bladder).
• Symptomatic problems of the urachus: occur in 1 in 5000 newborns and account for 3 of every 200,000 general hospital admissions
• A patent urachus and urachal sinus both present in early infancy.
• Urachal cysts most commonly cause symptoms in older children. A patent urachus is slightly more common in boys, but a urachal sinus occurs slightly more often in girls.

GENETICS

• Not generally associated with any single syndrome, many patients with urachal problems are found to have coexisting congenital abnormalities of other systems.

STAGING: N/A

SIGNS AND SYMPTOMS

• Patent urachus: clear fluid draining from the umbilicus in the newborn period
• Urachal sinus: may present in infancy or later with umbilical drainage or nonspecific periumbilical erythema
• Symptomatic urachal diverticula of the bladder: UTI is the most common presentation.
• Urachal cyst: most commonly presents in an older child with signs of suppuration (calor, rubor, dolor) in the lower abdominal wall. Occasionally, a urachal cyst will present as an asymptomatic midline lower abdominal mass.

PATHOPHYSIOLOGY

• The urachus is a tubular connection between the allantoic stalk and the dome of the bladder.
• One-third of adults have microscopic patency of this channel.
• Faulty resolution of this connection results in urachal abnormalities.
• The urachus lies in the space of Retzius between the peritoneum and transversalis fascia (median umbilical ligament).
• The umbilicovesical fascia surrounds the urachus; this fascia extends laterally to the obliterated umbilical arteries.
• This self-contained space limits the spread of suppuration when the urachal remnants become infected.
• Infected urachal cyst: *Staphylococcus* sp. most common, followed by *Streptococcus fecalis* and *Escherichia coli*

CAUSES/RISK FACTORS

• Bladder outlet obstruction causes anatomic persistence of the urachus.

—15% of patients with urachal problems have bladder outlet obstruction; most prune-belly or triad syndrome
—Babies with significant urethral obstruction (i.e., posterior urethral valves) generally have no urachal problems.

COMPLICATIONS

• Except for the drainage of urine and urine infections, patients with a patent urachus have few short-term complications.

—Urachal cysts do present with infection in an infraumbilical mass. These may rupture into the peritoneal cavity and cause peritonitis. Deaths have been reported.
—Persistent urachal tissue at the dome of the bladder can degenerate in adults to mucin-producing adenocarcinoma.

DIFFERENTIAL DIAGNOSIS

• Umbilical granulomas can cause weeping and serous drainage of the umbilical stump.
• Omphalitis (cellulitic infection of all cord structures) can also occur in newborns.
• Persistence of the omphalomesenteric duct can result in soiling of the umbilicus with enteric contents.
• Vitelline duct cyst (Rosen's cyst) can present with signs of suppuration in the lower abdomen.
• Acute appendicitis is quite similar in presentation to an infected urachal cyst, though most often the patient with acute appendicitis will not demonstrate a midline lower abdominal mass. Ovarian cysts can sometimes present with a lower abdominal mass that can be confused with a urachal cyst.

 Database

HISTORY

• Older children with urachal cysts uniformly give a history of lower abdominal pain, typically of a few days duration, but occasionally more chronic in nature. Patients with an infected urachal cyst can complain of voiding symptoms secondary to a UTI.
• Babies with a patent urachus generally have always drained clear fluid from the umbilicus.
• Patients with a urachal sinus can develop umbilical drainage (often purulent) and often give a history of periumbilical pain and tenderness.
• Urachal diverticulae in the bladder most commonly present with symptoms of UTI.

PHYSICAL EXAMINATION

• Urachal cysts typically are diagnosed when they become infected. They demonstrate the combination of a midline lower abdominal mass associated with signs of anterior peritoneal irritation (tenderness, guarding). Rarely, the cyst can rupture into the abdominal cavity, with resultant signs of generalized peritonitis with sepsis.
• Babies with a patent urachus will demonstrate clear fluid at the umbilicus. Passage of a small sound through the urachus to the bladder should be possible.
• Patients with a urachal sinus will often demonstrate granulation tissue and inflammation at the umbilicus. Drainage of the umbilicus is common, but not as marked as in the patients with a patent urachus. Fever may be present.

 Diagnostic Studies

LABORATORY TESTING

• Leukocytosis is often present with infected urachal cysts.
• The urinalysis and culture will often be positive with symptomatic urachal remnants.

IMAGING

• Urachal cysts are best imaged with ultrasound, though, in the patient with signs of acute abdomen, the CT scan will also demonstrate well the pathologic anatomy.
• Clearly, a sinogram is diagnostic in demonstrating the communication between the umbilicus to the bladder found in patients with a patent urachus. A sinogram also shows the pathologic anatomy of the urachal sinus; in this case, the patency of the tract ends before connecting with the bladder. The sinogram will also differentiate the presence of an omphalomesenteric duct as the cause of umbilical drainage.

—Voiding cystography is necessary to show the urachal diverticulum; the cystogram will also demonstrate a patent urachus. Typically, the cystogram is negative in patients with either a urachal cyst or a urachal sinus.

SPECIAL STUDIES: N/A

 Treatment

GENERAL MEASURES

• Broad-spectrum antibiotics is the first step in management of most urachal problems.

MEDICAL

• Generally, medical management of urachal abnormalities has no merit, except in the case of urachal diverticulae of the bladder that are causing no symptoms.

SURGICAL

• Except for the asymptomatic urachal diverticulum, the treatment of all urachal abnormalities is surgical, i.e., complete excision of the abnormal structure, including a cuff of bladder. Historically, patients with infected urachal cysts were treated first with incision and drainage, followed by delayed resection of all cyst remnants. However, complete one-stage excision of all infected urachal remnants following administration of broad-spectrum antibiotics is preferable when possible.

ALTERNATIVE THERAPIES

• Laparoscopic excision of urachal remnants is possible and may be preferred when there is no active suppuration.

PATIENT EDUCATION

• Umbilical inflammation and drainage should be evaluated promptly.

 Follow-Up

MONITORING

• Adequate surgical resection should obviate long-term medical follow-up.

PREVENTION: N/A

 Miscellaneous

SYNONYMS

• Urachal anomalies, umbilical cysts

ASSOCIATED CONDITIONS

• Umbilical granulomas, omphalitis, prune-belly syndrome, patent omphaloenteric ducts

NOTES

• See also Section II, "Urachal Carcinoma."

ABBREVIATIONS: N/A

REFERENCES

Cilento BG, Bauer SB, Retik AB, Peters CA, Atala A. Urachal anomalies: Defining the best diagnostic modality. *Urology* 1998;52:120.

Mesrobian H, Zacharias A, Balcom A, Cohen R. Ten years of experience with isolated urachal anomalies in children. *J Urol* 1997;158:1316.

Scharli AF. Vitello-intestinal disorders. In: Freeman N, Burge D, Griffiths M, Malone P, eds. *Surgery of the Newborn*. Edinburgh: Churchill Livingstone, 1994:243–253.

Author: George F. Steinhardt

Urachal Carcinoma

 Basics

DESCRIPTION

• Urachal carcinoma is a rare tumor, predominantly adenocarcinoma. Frequently, the prognosis is poor, due to delayed diagnosis. Occurs at any site in the urachus between the umbilicus and the bladder attachment

EPIDEMIOLOGY

• Annual incidence: 1 in 5 million, or 0.01% of adult cancers; 0.17% to 0.34% of bladder cancers and 20% to 39% of bladder adenocarcinomas
• Most common in fifth to seventh decades
• Males predominate

GENETICS: N/A

STAGING

• TNM stage as in bladder cancer (see Section VII)

SIGNS AND SYMPTOMS

• Hematuria: either gross or microscopic

—Gross or microscopic mucus

• Irritative voiding symptoms
• Abdominal and/or suprapubic pain
• Suprapubic mass (especially with sarcoma in child)
• Umbilical discharge of blood or pus
• Incidental finding on imaging study

—Bladder or suprapubic mass possibly with stippled calcification

PATHOPHYSIOLOGY

• Mucin-producing adenocarcinomas predominate (70%).

—Acini lined with malignant columnar epithelium without basement membrane
—Colloid carcinoma or signet ring pattern

• Other cell types: non–mucin-producing adenocarcinomas (15%), sarcomas, TCCs, and squamous cell carcinomas
• Any section of urachus involved: frequently in dome of bladder

—A supravesical tumor has an irregular capsule.
—Intravesical tumor not encapsulated, lying beneath a layer of normal urothelium

• Invades muscularis propria and perivesical fat, often with demarcation from surface epithelium
• Local invasion to space of Retzius, anterior abdominal wall, peritoneum, and umbilicus
• Metastases to iliac and inguinal lymph nodes, lung, omentum, liver, and bone delayed

CAUSES/RISK FACTORS

• A urachus derived from cloaca has glandular epithelium.
• Adenomatous hyperplasia, cysts, or calculi may predispose.
• Carcinogenic pathways and genetic defects unknown
• Cancer in an exstrophic bladder may be urachal in origin.

COMPLICATIONS

• Hemorrhage
• Infection
• Locoregional organ involvement: of bladder, pelvis, abdominal wall
• Metastatic disease

DIFFERENTIAL DIAGNOSIS

• Primary bladder adenocarcinoma
• Adenocarcinoma local invasion or metastatic involvement

—Colorectal
—Ovarian, endometrial, or cervical
—Prostate

• Primary TCC with adenomatous metaplasia

 Database

HISTORY

• Age of the patient?

—Sarcoma common in young

• Is hematuria present?

—Indicates invasion of the bladder

• Presence of pneumaturia?

—Suggests enterovesical fistula with invasion of bowel, or conversely, that arises in bowel and is not urachal

• Irritative voiding symptoms?

—Possible urinary infection, perhaps secondary to fistula

• Does mass change in size?

—A urachal cyst may shrink intermittently as contents discharge.

• History of bowel or ovarian cancer?

—Indicates potential for secondary involvement of bladder by local recurrence or metastases or nonurachal tumor

• Multisystem symptom inventory

PHYSICAL EXAMINATION

• Multisystem examination

—Evaluate for signs of catabolism, anemia, and metastatic disease.
—Evaluate for comorbidity and anesthetic risk.

• Palpate the suprapubic mass.

—Involving abdominal wall? Define margins.

• Bimanual vaginal and/or rectal examination

—If the mass is palpable, is it mobile or adherent to the pelvic wall?

• Exclude GYN or rectal tumor mass

Diagnostic Studies

LABORATORY TESTING

- Urinalysis
- Urine culture to exclude infection
- Urine cytology

—Differentiate from TCC.

- Routine hematology
- Renal function tests (creatinine and blood urea nitrogen)

—Possible renal impairment from ureteral obstruction

- Hepatic function tests (transaminases, alkaline phosphatase, albumin and bilirubin)

—Possible hepatic impairment from metastases

- Other laboratory tests
- Serum CA-125 elevated in some urachal carcinomas
- Endoscopy

—Cystoscopy
  —Tumor on anterior wall or dome may be submucosal, papillary, polypoid, or fungating.
  —Biopsy tumor and adjacent "normal" bladder epithelium

IMAGING

- Abdominal ultrasonography

—Useful to screen for hydronephrosis and evaluate nature of suprapubic mass

- Excretory urography

—Upper urinary tract integrity
—As initial evaluation of hematuria, may reveal bladder mass or ureteral obstruction

- Abdominal CT or MRI

—Excellent assessment of local tumor extent and metastases

- Isotope bone scan, chest radiograph, or CT as metastatic evaluation

SPECIAL STUDIES

- Histopathology to identify tumor cell type

—Confirm consistent with urachal origin
—If adenocarcinoma, differentiate between mucin-producing, signet ring cell, and mucin-nonproducing

- Immunohistochemistry when urachal origin of adenocarcinoma in doubt

—Staining by antibodies for CEA, PSA, OC125, and vimentin: indicates origin from urachus or bowel, prostate, ovary, and uterus, respectively

 ## Treatment

GENERAL MEASURES

- A localized tumor requires prompt resection. Transurethral surgery alone is inadequate.
- A metastatic tumor requires chemotherapy and perhaps focal radiation.
- Systemic evaluation or supportive management as needed

—Cardiorespiratory assessment
—Treat the infection.
—Nutritional support
—Enterostomal consultation

MEDICAL

- Chemotherapy indicated in locally extensive or metastatic disease

—Multidrug regimens, including "FAM" (5-fluorouracil, doxorubicin, and mitomycin-C)
—Novel agents (e.g., paclitaxel, gemcitabine)

SURGICAL

- En bloc excision of the tumor is imperative: includes web of posterior rectus sheath and peritoneum bounded laterally by the obliterated umbilical arteries (median umbilical ligaments) and entire urachus with umbilicus and bladder dome segment
- Partial cystectomy adequate for small and well-differentiated tumor, especially mucinous adenocarcinoma
- Radical cystectomy with urinary diversion for larger and poorly differentiated tumors, especially non–mucin-producing or signet ring cell

ALTERNATIVE THERAPIES

- External beam radiation therapy

—As adjuvant for locally aggressive tumors
—Symptomatic metastatic lesions

PATIENT EDUCATION

- Patients are advised regarding patterns of recurrence and follow-up requirements.

 ## Follow-Up

MONITORING

- Periodic evaluation on biannual to annual schedule

—Constitutional and general physical assessment
—Metastatic survey
—Pelvic imaging with CT or MRI to assess local recurrence
—If the bladder is retained, screen for recurrence.
  —Urinalysis and cytology
  —Cystoscopy

PREVENTION: N/A

 ## Miscellaneous

SYNONYMS: N/A

ASSOCIATED CONDITIONS

- Urachal cyst, bladder exstrophy

NOTES

- Early diagnosis makes cure likely. See also Section II, "Urachal Abnormalities."

ABBREVIATIONS

- CEA, carcinoembryonic antigen; TCC, transitional cell carcinoma

REFERENCE

Sheldon CA, Clayman RV, Gonzalez R, Williams RD, Fraley EE. Malignant urachal lesions. *J Urol* 1984;131:1.

Authors: John A. Heaney and Mark S. Ernstoff

Ureter and Renal Pelvic Tumors—General

Basics

DESCRIPTION

- 5% of all urothelial tumors; most commonly transitional cell carcinoma (TCC)

EPIDEMIOLOGY

- Male-to-female ratio: 2:1; White-to-Black ratio: 2:1
- Rare before 40 years, with peak incidence in sixth to seventh decade
- Balkan nephropathy: endemic to Bulgaria, Greece, Romania, and Yugoslavia

—Associated with upper tract urothelial tumors. Tumors are often multiple, bilateral, and indolent. Renal-sparing surgery is indicated where possible.

- 5-year survival rate: stage I, 80%; stage II, 50%; stages III and IV, <10%

GENETICS

- Most have no family history of disease.
- Certain familial cancer syndromes show an increased incidence of TCC (Lynch type II).
- Familial clustering exists, but it is difficult to determine if it is related to environmental factors.
- Data are inconclusive on a direct genetic relationship.
- Low-grade superficial TCC: loss of *p15* and *p16* (chromosome 9p)
- High-grade TCC: loss of *p53* (chromosome 17p)
- Amplification and overexpression of normal genes that code for growth factors or their receptors

—EGF-R (on chromosome 7): trisomy 7 associated with TCC
—Erb-2 mutations associated with TCC

STAGING

- See TNM classification in the appendix.

SIGNS AND SYMPTOMS

- Hematuria: most common presenting complaint (75% of patients)
- Dull flank pain due to the gradual distention of collecting system (30% of patients)
- Asymptomatic: incidental diagnosis in 10% to 15%
- Rarely, patients present with signs of advanced disease (abdominal or flank mass, anorexia, etc.).

PATHOPHYSIOLOGY

- >90% of upper tract urothelial tumors are TCC.
- Squamous cell carcinoma (SCC): 7%; associated with long-term infection, inflammation, and calculi
- Rarer tumors include adenocarcinoma, inverted papilloma, sarcoma, and carcinosarcoma.
- Up to 50% of ureteral TCCs are multicentric.
- Tumors of the ureter tend to be less invasive and smaller than those of the renal pelvis.

CAUSES/RISK FACTORS

- Smoking: Risk ranges from 2.6 to 8.0; risk increases with higher dose and duration of tobacco use.
- Occupational exposure: similar to that for bladder cancer; approximately 20% of TCCs, with disease latency of 30 to 50 years. Most chemicals are aromatic amines (aniline dyes [color fabrics]), 2-naphthylamine, 4-aminobiphenyl, 4-nitrobiphenyl, 4,4-diaminobiphenyl, 2-amino-1-naphthol, soot from coal, combustion gas, and aliphatic hydrocarbons.
- High-risk occupations: autoworkers, leather workers, painters, truck drivers, metal workers, machinists, dry cleaners, dental technicians, beauticians, and physicians
- Relative risk of disease following exposure: 4.0 to 5.5
- Coffee: minor contribution, with relative risk of 1.3
- Analgesic abuse: all components implicated; highest risk with phenacetin abuse; latency of 25 years (dose of 10–15 g over 10 years); tend to be women who present with high-stage tumors. Relative risk: 2.4 for men and 4.2 for women
- Infectious agents: chronic bacterial infection with calculi and obstruction; increased risk of SCC
- Cyclophosphamide: hemorrhagic cystitis and carcinoma; 9 times increased risk of carcinoma after exposure; latency of 6 to 13 years

COMPLICATIONS

- Local invasion of renal parenchyma or surrounding structures (including renal veins, vena cava)
- Visceral metastases, most commonly to liver, lung, and bone
- Lymphatic spread to paraaortic, paracaval, and pelvic nodes
- 30% to 50% risk for bladder TCC and 1% risk of contralateral upper tract TCC. Conversely, those with bladder TCC are at very low risk of upper tract tumors.
- Following treatment: perforation with extraluminal spillage of tumor, and ureteral stricture

DIFFERENTIAL DIAGNOSIS

- Extrinsic masses: parapelvic cyst, vascular impressions
- Intrinsic lesions

—Benign ureteropelvic junction obstruction, renal cell carcinoma, suburothelial hemorrhage, radiolucent calculus, blood clot, malacoplakia, fungal ball, sloughed renal papilla
—Less commonly: fibroepithelial polyp, air bubble, granuloma, leukoplakia, hemangioma, cholesteatoma, and leiomyoma

Database

HISTORY

- Age and sex of patient? Uncommon before the age of 40, peak incidence in mid-60s
- Hematuria: most common presenting symptom
- Flank or abdominal pain: presenting symptom in one-third of patients
- Tobacco use: occupational exposure (up to 20% of TCCs)
- History of analgesia abuse in past: dose-related effect; phenacetin is most common
- History of recurrent infections and staghorn calculi: SCC

PHYSICAL EXAMINATION

- Usually normal; flank or abdominal mass with advanced disease
- Weight loss

Diagnostic Studies

LABORATORY TESTING

- Urinalysis: hematuria (gross or microscopic)
- Cytopathology

—Voided specimen: low sensitivity for upper tract TCC; ureteral catheterization specimens are more sensitive.
—Accuracy increases with increasing grade of tumor.

IMAGING

- Intravenous pyelogram (IVP)

—50% to 75%: radiolucent filling defect; is irregular and continuous with the wall. 10% to 30% show obstruction or nonvisualization of the collecting system, which indicates more invasive disease.
—Examine the contralateral kidney for function.

- Retrograde urography: better visualization than IVP (>75% accuracy)
- Antegrade pyelography

—Used only if not possible to visualize collecting system via retrograde approach. Risk of seeding of tumor cells along the tract is small but real. CT may eliminate the need for antegrade pyelography.

- CT: useful for both diagnosis and staging of tumors
- Ultrasound or MRI: of little use in upper tract tumors

SPECIAL STUDIES

- Ureteroscopy and nephroscopy

—Diagnostic accuracy of 58% to 83%. Not accurate for staging TCCs due to difficulty in determining the depth of invasion, particularly renal pelvic TCC

- Brush biopsy

—High positive predictive value, overall accuracy of 78%; significant risk of bleeding and ureteral perforation

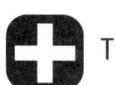 Treatment

GENERAL MEASURES

- The standard treatment is nephroureterectomy.
- Indications for conservative, renal-sparing surgery include a single kidney, bilateral disease, reduced or nonfunction of the contralateral kidney, and a tumor of low grade and stage.
- Survival is more closely related to stage and grade of tumor than to the treatment modality.
- Recurrence rate is reduced with more aggressive resection of tumor: 48% recurrence with nephrectomy, 32% with nephrectomy plus partial ureterectomy, 24% with nephrectomy plus subtotal ureterectomy, and 12% with nephroureterectomy.

- If positive cytology is the only sign of upper tract TCC, only close follow-up is required (IVP, retrograde, flexible ureteroscopy where indicated).

MEDICAL

- Chemotherapy: comparable to that for TCC of the bladder; useful adjuvantly in high-risk patients and may be of benefit for palliation with metastatic disease

SURGICAL

- Total nephroureterectomy and excision of cuff of bladder; either with two incisions or TUR of orifice plus flank incision (for proximal tumors only)

—80% to 90% 5-year survival (low grade and stage)
—30% to 75% recurrence rate in ureteral stump
—Radical lymphadenectomy not shown to improve survival

- A partial nephrectomy may be indicated with a single kidney.
- Segmental ureteral resection: option for solitary low-grade upper and mid-ureteral lesions

—Recurrence rate of 6%; higher if multifocal

- Distal ureterectomy and ureteroneocystostomy: distal, solitary ureteral lesions

ALTERNATIVE THERAPIES

- Endoscopic resections: for low-grade, superficial, or solitary kidney

—Risk of perforation higher than that in bladder (overall complication rate: 7%)
—Requires close follow-up due to high recurrence rate

- Radiation therapy: can be used for advanced tumors not amenable to surgery
- Angioinfarction: for incurable disease in those deemed unfit for surgery
- Instillation therapy with bacillus Calmette-Guérin (BCG) or mitomycin

—Appears to be safe, but indications and outcome not clearly defined
—May be useful in multiple superficial tumors or bilateral disease

PATIENT EDUCATION

- Avoid or limit tobacco and chronic analgesia use.
- Avoid occupational exposure to implicated toxins.

 Follow-Up

MONITORING

- Cystoscopy with cytology every 3 to 6 months for 2 to 3 years, then yearly
- Ureteroscopy is more sensitive than radiologic techniques for follow-up of upper tract TCC

PREVENTION

- Complete avoidance of tobacco products
- Occupational protection from chemicals implicated in urothelial tumors
- Early evaluation of hematuria

 Miscellaneous

SYNONYMS: N/A

ASSOCIATED CONDITIONS

- Ballcan nephropathy

NOTES

- See also Section I, "Filling Defect—Upper Urinary Tract," and Section II, "Ureter and Renal Pelvis—Transitional Cell Carcinoma" and "Ureter and Renal Pelvis—Squamous Cell Carcinoma."

ABBREVIATIONS

- TCC, transitional cell carcinoma; SCC, squamous cell carcinoma; MVAC, methotrexate, vinblastine, doxorubicin, cisplatin; BCG, bacillus Calmette-Guérin

REFERENCES

Messing EM, Catalona WJ. Urothelial tumors of the urinary tract. In: Walsh PC, Retik AB, Vaughan ED, Wein AJ, eds. *Campbell's Urology*, 7th ed. Philadelphia: WB Saunders, 1997.

Simons JW, Marshall FF. Transitional cell carcinoma of the renal pelvis and ureter. *Clin Oncol* 1997;65:1412–1417.

Tawfiek ER, Bagley DH. Upper-tract transitional cell carcinoma. *Urology* 1997;50(3):321–329.

Authors: Owen Prowse and Laurence Klotz

Ureter and Renal Pelvis—Squamous Cell Carcinoma

 Basics

DESCRIPTION

• Squamous cell cancer (SCC) arising in the collecting system (calyces, infundibuli, renal pelvis, ureters)

EPIDEMIOLOGY

• <1% of all GU malignancies
• 6% to 15% of all primary neoplasms of the upper urinary tract
• The small number of cases at any one institution makes characterization difficult.
• Associated with chronically infected/irritated states; e.g., renal tuberculosis, stones, staghorn calculi, strictures
• Most often occurs in the fifth decade of life

GENETICS

• No genetic basis
• No conclusive gender difference

STAGING

• Analogous to bladder cancer
• See TNM classification for renal pelvis and ureter in the appendix.

SIGNS AND SYMPTOMS

• Ureteral obstruction is the main presentation.

—Most commonly abdominal or flank pain (82%)
—Pain may be sharp, dull, constant, or intermittent.

• Others present with gross or microscopic hematuria.
• Others present with an abdominal/flank mass.

—Mass secondary to ureteral obstruction and high-grade hydronephrosis

• Urinary tract infections

—Due to stasis and obstruction of the urinary tract

• Constitutional symptoms are nonspecific and associated with advanced disease.

—Anorexia, lethargy, weight loss

PATHOPHYSIOLOGY

• SCC of the urinary tract is commonly associated with chronically infected states.

—Renal calculi, staghorn calculi, tuberculosis, schistosomiasis

• This chronic exposure is hypothesized to lead to malignant degeneration, although never definitively demonstrated.

—Irritation causes de-differentiation of normal transitional epithelium.
—These de-differentiated cells then undergo dysplastic changes with continued irritation.
—Dysplastic changes eventually result in transformation into SCC.

CAUSES/RISK FACTORS

• Strong association with SCC of the pelvis and renal calculi (40%–80%)

—Calculi are the source of irritation to the normal epithelium.

• Any chronically infected state

—Recurrent pyelonephritis
—Struvite stone
—Renal tuberculosis
—Parasitic infections (e.g., schistosomiasis)
—Renal tuberculosis

• Chemical carcinogens may be risk factors, although never definitively demonstrated.

—Cigarette smoking, benzene chemical exposure, petroleum products

COMPLICATIONS

• Renal insufficiency, metastatic disease

DIFFERENTIAL DIAGNOSIS

• Upper urinary tract filling defect or renal pelvic mass on imaging

—Inflammatory lesion
—Malakoplakia
—Fungal lesion
—Other malignancies
  —Transitional cell carcinoma (most commonly)
  —Adenocarcinoma of the upper urinary tract

 Database

HISTORY

• Age of the patient

—Most presenting in the fifth generation

• History of recurrent infections
• Systemic/renal tuberculosis or recent exposure
• Hematuria

—May be secondary to irritation (e.g., stones) or secondary to bleeding tumor
—May not be reported by the patient, as it may be microscopic only

• Flank or abdominal pain

—Usually secondary to renal obstruction
—May be typical renal colic or may be dull nonspecific pain

• With advanced disease, constitutional symptoms may prevail.

PHYSICAL EXAMINATION

• Most commonly present with a completely normal physical examination
• Findings related to advanced disease states

—Abdominal pain or costovertebral angle tenderness (CVA tenderness)
—Flank mass secondary to renal obstruction and hydronephrosis

Diagnostic Studies

LABORATORY TESTING

• Almost all have irregular urinalysis.

—Hematuria in 87%
—Pyuria (>8 WBCs/HPF) in 83%

• Serum chemistries are usually within normal limits.

—May have tumor-associated hypercalcemia, which resolves after tumor excision

• Blood urea nitrogen and creatinine may be elevated.

—Chronic infection and scarring
—Renal obstruction

IMAGING

• Cannot make diagnosis from radiographic studies

• IVP, angiography, and ultrasound are not diagnostic.

—Common findings: hydronephrosis, nonexcretion of contrast material, renal stones, filling defects

• MRI/MRA or CT scan should be performed if surgery is planned.

—Provides the surgeon with useful data
　—Size and extent of the tumor
　—Vascular pattern of the tumor
　—Presence of metastases
　—State of the native renal unit

SPECIAL STUDIES

• Diagnosis is made by histologic examination of the lesion.

—An endoscopic biopsy is extremely useful with rigid and flexible ureteroscopy.

• Diagnosis is commonly made following definitive surgery (e.g., nephrectomy).
• Cytology should be performed in all suspected patients; difficult to interpret unless experienced cytologist

 ## Treatment

GENERAL MEASURES

• Treatment of choice is surgical excision (radical nephroureterectomy).
• Infected patients all require broad-spectrum antibiotics pre- and postoperatively.

MEDICAL

• Adjuvant chemotherapy and radiotherapy: marginal results

—Average survival is short, with high-grade and high-stage disease.

• Survival is most dependent on the stage at the time of diagnosis.

—Distant metastases are commonly noted at the time of tissue diagnosis.
　—Lymph nodes (regional), lung, bone, liver, ipsilateral adrenal gland

• If survival rates are to be improved, adjuvant chemotherapy should be considered for most patients following resection.

SURGICAL

• Surgical treatment is performed if surgical candidate (co-morbid medical conditions)

—Similar to transitional cell carcinoma for same location and stage
—Cystoscopy as part of staging/treatment

• Nephroureterectomy is the treatment of choice.

—A bladder cuff is typically excised with the specimen.

• A curative resection is often difficult due to high-stage disease, frequently noted at the time of diagnosis.
• Surgery is frequently required for palliation of symptoms.

—Patients with severe hematuria
—Septic patients have a small chance of survival without excision of the infected tissue and associated stone (if present).

ALTERNATIVE THERAPIES: N/A

PATIENT EDUCATION: N/A

 ## Follow-Up

MONITORING

• Follow with cystoscopy and urine cytology: every 3 months for the first 2 years.
• A metastatic work-up should by performed semi-annually.
• Local urothelial recurrence is as high as 20%.

—Imaging and cytology to detect recurrence/metastatic disease

PREVENTION

• Thorough endoscopic examination with biopsy (as necessary) for all patients undergoing treatment of staghorn calculi to rule out neoplasm

 ## Miscellaneous

SYNONYMS: N/A

ASSOCIATED CONDITIONS

• Staghorn and renal calculi

NOTES

• See also Section I, "Filling Defect—Upper Urinary Tract," and Section II, "Ureter and Renal Pelvic Tumors—General" and "Bladder Cancer—Squamous Cell Carcinoma."

ABBREVIATIONS: N/A

REFERENCES

Li MK, Cheung WL. Squamous cell carcinoma of the renal pelvis. *J Urol* 1987;138:269–271.

Nativ O, Reiman HM, Lieber MM, Zincke H. Treatment of primary squamous cell carcinoma of the upper urinary tract. *Cancer* 1991;68:2575–2578.

Papadopoulos I, Wirth B, Weichert-Jacobson K, Loch T, Wacker H. Primary squamous cell carcinoma of the ureter and squamous adenocarcinoma of the renal pelvis: 2 case reports. *J Urol* 1996;155(1):288–289.

Authors: Mitchell C. Fraiman and Michael Grasso III

Ureter and Renal Pelvis—Transitional Cell Carcinoma

 Basics

DESCRIPTION

• Transitional cell carcinoma (TCC), a urothelial neoplasm of the ureter and intrarenal collecting system, accounts for more than 90% of upper tract urothelial tumors.

EPIDEMIOLOGY

• 10% of renal tumors are renal pelvic tumors.
• 5% of urothelial tumors are found in the upper urinary tract.
• 3:1 ratio of men to women
• 2:1 ratio of Whites to Blacks
• Peak incidence of 10 per 100,000 per year in 75- to 79-year-old white men
• Mean age of 65
• Incidence is increasing.

GENETICS

• Lynch syndrome II: The familial cancer syndrome with colonic tumors and extracolonic (commonly endometrial) cancers may increase the risk for upper tract TCC.

STAGING

• See TNM Staging for renal pelvis and ureter in the appendix.

SIGNS AND SYMPTOMS

• 75% of patients present with gross or microscopic hematuria.

—Dull flank pain in 30% secondary to gradual obstruction

• Acute colic can occur secondary to passage of clots.

—Abdominal or flank mass, weight loss, anorexia, bone pain in advanced disease

• 10% to 15% are asymptomatic and found on imaging studies.

PATHOPHYSIOLOGY

• Grading based on the degree of tumor cell anaplasia
• Carcinoma in situ (CIS): poorly differentiated TCC confined to the urothelium

—Grade 0: papilloma or papillary lesion with a fibrovascular core covered by normal bladder mucosa
—Grade I: well differentiated with a thin fibrovascular stalk and thickened urothelium containing more than seven cell layers, cells with slight anaplasia and pleomorphism
—Grade II: moderately differentiated, loss of cell polarity, higher nuclear–cytoplasmic ratio, more frequent mitotic figures, nuclear pleomorphism and prominent nucleoli
—Grade III: poorly differentiated, no differentiation from basement membrane to urothelial surface, marked nuclear pleomorphism, high nuclear–cytoplasmic ratio, frequent mitosis

—The ABO blood group antigen may be of prognostic significance.

• DNA flow cytometry: aneuploid cells correlated with grade, stage, and worse survival

—An S-phase (DNA synthesizing fraction) >10% indicates a more aggressive tumor with potential for invasion.
—p53 mutations may have prognostic value.

CAUSES/RISK FACTORS

• Cigarette smoking: largest risk factor; risk increases 3× over nonsmokers.

—Ureteral tumors > renal pelvic > bladder
—Cessation for more than 10 years reduces risk by 50% to 60%.

• Coffee drinking: 1.3 relative risk in persons drinking >7 cups per day
• Analgesic abuse: relative risk of 2.4 for men, 4.2 for women
• Papillary necrosis and phenacetin abuse are independent, synergistic risk factors.

—Balkan nephropathy: In families, incidence is 100 to 200 times greater, although bladder cancer incidence is unchanged.
—Tumors are low grade, commonly multiple and bilateral; consider nephron-sparing approaches.

• Occupational exposures are similar to those for bladder cancer: chemicals, petrochemicals, plastics, coal, coke, asphalt, and tar; relative risk 4.0 to 5.5
• Cyclophosphamide: metabolite acrolein associated with high-grade, aggressive urothelial tumors

COMPLICATIONS

• Gross hematuria with clots
• Urinary obstruction with compromise of renal function
• Caudal recurrence in distal ureter or bladder
• Lymphatic extension, most commonly to paraaortic, paracaval, and ipsilateral common iliac and pelvic lymph nodes

DIFFERENTIAL DIAGNOSIS

• Based on imaging studies

—TCC
—CIS
—Squamous cell carcinoma
—Adenocarcinoma
—Nonurothelial tumors
  —Malignant: renal cell carcinoma, sarcoma, carcinosarcoma, angiosarcoma
  —Benign leiomyoma, neurofibroma, plasmacytoma, inverted papilloma, fibroepithelial polyp, ureteritis cystica
—Radiolucent stone (uric acid, cysteine)
—Blood clot
—Fungus ball/aspergillosis
—Sloughed papilla
—Crossing lower pole vessel
—Air bubble
—Granuloma, hemangioma, renal tuberculosis, cholesteatoma

 Database

HISTORY

• Age and history of cigarette smoking, coffee drinking
• Occupation (industry, chemicals, paints)
• Medications: analgesics (i.e., phenacetin, aspirin), cyclophosphamide
• Gross hematuria, flank pain
• Family history: Balkan family, colonic malignancy

PHYSICAL EXAMINATION

• Costovertebral tenderness with obstruction
• Weight loss
• Flank or abdominal mass

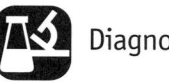 Diagnostic Studies

LABORATORY TESTING

• Urinalysis: gross or microscopic hematuria
• Voided urine cytology: insensitive test for upper tract TCC
• Catheterized ureteral or renal pelvis washing with saline, 65% to 73% sensitive
• Brush biopsies 91% sensitive, 88% specific, 89% accurate, risks perforation and bleeding
• Ureteroscopic cup biopsies: most sensitive
• Electrolytes, liver function tests usually normal unless metastasis and/or obstructed

IMAGING

• Chest x-ray
• Excretory urography

—Filling defect in 50% to 75% of patients: irregular and attached to collecting system wall
—10% to 30% of patients will have obstruction or nonvisualization of the collecting system.
—Study the contralateral side, as contralateral tumors will change management.

• Retrograde urography

—Use dilute contrast (one-half to one-third).
—Inject through the bulb tip or open-ended catheter to fill the entire collecting system (10–15 cc).
—Avoid extravasation of contrast, perforation, or overfilling.

• Computer tomography

—Can be done as alternative to excretory urography, but less sensitive
—Small tumors may be missed because of volume averaging.
—A noncontrast study done first will differentiate uric acid stones from tumors.
—TCC is relatively hypovascular (average Hounsfield units: 46; range: 10–70).
—Helpful for metastatic staging in advanced disease

- Ultrasound

—Can help distinguish stone from tumor in renal pelvis and intrarenal collecting system, not ureter
—Endoluminal ultrasound: may be used as an adjunct to ureteroscopy to define tumor size and invasion at the time of ureteroscopy

SPECIAL STUDIES

- Cystoscopy

—Necessary to rule out coexisting bladder tumors

- Ureteroscopy

—Valuable for direct visual diagnosis, saline washing, cup biopsy, and treatment of certain patients
—Diagnostic accuracy >90%

- Experimental laboratory studies: ABO blood group antigens, DNA flow cytometry, DNA synthesizing (S-phase) fraction, *p53* abnormalities

 ## Treatment

GENERAL MEASURES

- Although nephroureterectomy with a bladder cuff is the standard treatment of upper tract TCC, indications for conservative surgery may include

—Solitary kidney, renal insufficiency, poor candidate for open surgery, bilateral upper tract TCC, low-grade, low-stage disease (controversial)

- In general

—Patients with low-grade, low-stage tumors do well with conservative or radical surgery.
—Patients with intermediate-grade tumors do better with radical surgery.
—Patients with high-grade, high-stage tumors do poorly with either type of surgery.

MEDICAL

- Instillation of bacille Calmette-Guérin (BCG), mitomycin, or thiotepa as an adjunct may be helpful for multiple recurrences. BCG may be useful with CIS.
- Radiation as a postoperative adjuvant treatment may reduce local recurrence rates and improve survival.
- MVAC chemotherapy may have limited benefit as an adjuvant therapy in advanced disease.

SURGICAL

- Endoscopic tumor resection and ablation

—Percutaneously or ureteroscopically
—Best for low-grade, low-stage tumors in select patient groups
—Techniques include electrosurgical resection, biopsy and fulguration, and laser coagulation and ablation with Nd:YAG or holmium:YAG.
—Local recurrence is 40% after treatment of renal pelvic tumors and 25% after treatment of ureteral tumors.
—Asynchronous bladder tumors occur in 39% after upper tract endoscopic treatment.
—Requires vigilant postoperative surveillance with cystoscopy, ureteroscopy, cytology, and pyelograms
—Segmental resection or distal ureterectomy with bladder cuff
  —Successful for low-grade, low-stage lesions
—Open resection of renal pelvis tumors: high recurrence rate, less desirable option
—Partial nephrectomy: 38% recurrence, less desirable option
—Nephroureterectomy with bladder cuff
  —Standard treatment for upper tract TCC
  —Avoid transection of the ureter.
  —Anterior cystotomy is preferred to remove epithelium adjacent to the ureteral orifice.
  —Lymphadenectomy may be of benefit in high-stage tumors.

ALTERNATIVE THERAPIES: N/A

PATIENT EDUCATION

- Smoking cessation; avoid excessive analgesic use.
- Emphasize the importance of surveillance.

 ## Follow-Up

MONITORING

- Cystoscopy and cytology every 3 months for 2 years or until tumor-free, then every 6 months for 2 years, then yearly thereafter
- If conservative treatment performed, ureteroscopy every 3 months until upper tract is clear, then every 6 months

PREVENTION

- Avoid cigarette smoking, analgesic abuse, and occupational chemical exposure.

 ## Miscellaneous

SYNONYMS

- Upper tract tumor, filling defect

ASSOCIATED CONDITIONS

- Transitional cell carcinoma of the bladder, tobacco abuse, analgesic abuse, Balkan nephropathy

NOTES

- See also Section I, "Filling Defect—Upper Urinary Tract," and Section II, "Ureter and Renal Pelvic Tumors—General."

ABBREVIATIONS

- TCC, transitional cell carcinoma; CIS, carcinoma in situ

REFERENCES

Bagley DH. Treatment of upper urinary tract neoplasms. In: Smith AD, et al., eds. *Smith's Textbook of Endourology.* St. Louis: QMP, 1996:474–487.

Blute ML. Treatment of upper urinary tract transitional cell carcinoma. In: Smith AD, et al., eds. *Smith's Textbook of Endourology.* St. Louis: QMP, 1996:352–365.

Keeley FX, Kulp DA, Bibbo M, McCue PA, Bagley DH. Diagnostic accuracy of ureteroscopic biopsy in upper tract transitional cell carcinoma. *J Urol* 1997;157:33–37.

Messing EM, Catalona W. Urothelial tumors of the renal pelvis and ureter. In: Walsh PC, Retik AB, Vaughan ED, Wein AJ, eds. *Campbell's Urology,* 7th ed. Philadelphia: WB Saunders, 1998:2383–2394.

Authors: Gregory L. Chen and Demetrius H. Bagley

Ureter—Ectopic

 Basics

DESCRIPTION

- Any ureter whose orifice terminates anywhere other than the normal trigonal position is considered ectopic. However, clinically, an ectopic ureter implies a ureter that terminates at the bladder neck or distally into one of the mesonephric duct structures.

EPIDEMIOLOGY

- Incidence: 1 in 2000 births (0.05%)
- 10% bilateral
- 80% with a duplicated renal system

GENETICS

- Unknown

STAGING: N/A

SIGNS AND SYMPTOMS

- Continuous incontinence only in girls, if ureter drains distal to sphincter
- Persistent vaginal discharge if ureter drains in vagina
- Acute or recurrent urinary tract infection (UTI)
- Urgency and/or frequency
- Epididymitis or discomfort during ejaculation in males

PATHOPHYSIOLOGY

- Congenital: The ureter terminates in an abnormal location.
- In duplex kidneys, the ureter drains the upper pole.
- Ureteral orifice termination differs in males and females
—Males
  —Urethra (proximal to external sphincter)
  —Prostatic utricle
  —Seminal vesicle
  —Ejaculatory duct
  —Vas deferens
—Females
  —Urethra (proximal or distal to sphincter)
  —Vestibule
  —Vagina
  —Cervix or uterus
  —Gartner's duct

CAUSES/RISK FACTORS: N/A

COMPLICATIONS

- The ureter may reflux or be obstructed.
- Possible hydronephrosis and/or hydroureter
- May present with renal hypoplasia or dysplasia
- The more caudal the ureteral opening, the greater the degree of renal maldevelopment.

DIFFERENTIAL DIAGNOSIS

- Ureterocele
- Megaureter
- Ureteral diverticula

 Database

HISTORY

- Prenatal hydronephrosis?
—Serves to initiate postnatal evaluation
- Continuous urinary incontinence in a female?
—Ectopic ureter ends below external sphincter
- Continuous vaginal discharge?
—Ectopic ureter ends in mesonephric structures
- Epididymitis in a prepubertal boy?
—Ureter ends in a wolffian duct remnant
- Recurrent urinary urgency, frequency?
—Ureter may end in bladder neck region

PHYSICAL EXAMINATION

- Examine perineal and genital skin in girls
—If maceration is present, suggests irritating effect of ectopic ureter draining urine continuously
- Direct visualization of the vulva
—May reveal urinary dribbling

 Diagnostic Studies

LABORATORY TESTING

- Urinalysis and urine culture if UTI suspected

IMAGING

- Abdominal ultrasound
—Dilated pelvis and collecting system (upper pole if a duplex system)
—Dilated ureter behind a normal bladder
—A large ectopic ureter may press against the bladder and create an indentation.
- Excretory urography of a duplex system
—Poorly or nonvisualizing upper pole
—The upper pole displaces the lower pole downward and outward (drooping lilly appearance).
—The lower pole pelvis and upper portion of its ureter may be farther from the spine than on the contralateral side.
—The lower pole ureter may be tortuous due to its wrapping around a markedly dilated upper pole ureter.
—May see ureter entering ectopic location
- Excretory urography of a single system
—Poorly or nonvisualizing renal system, may see ureter entering ectopic location
- Voiding cystogram
—May show reflux into the ectopic ureter
—May show reflux into the lower pole ureter of duplex systems in 50% of cases
- DMSA renal scan
—Performed if renal parenchyma is difficult to localize
—Estimates degree of function of renal moiety drained by ectopic ureter
- MRI, CT
—Performed if renal parenchyma and/or ectopic ureter is difficult to localize

SPECIAL STUDIES

- Vaginoscopy
—Careful inspection may reveal an ectopic ureter.
- Cystourethroscopy
—Indigo carmine may be helpful in detecting an ectopic ureter.

Treatment

GENERAL MEASURES

• Treatment modality depends on various parameters.

—Gender, and location of ectopic ureter
—Associated pathology, e.g., reflux
—Degree of function in renal moiety

MEDICAL

• Treat UTIs, if any.
• Place on prophylactic antibiotics such as amoxicillin, trimethoprim sulfmethoxazole, nitrofurantoin

SURGICAL

• If minimal function present (<10%) in renal moiety drained by ectopic ureter, partial (duplex system) or total (single system)

—Heminephrectomy
  —Flank approach to expose upper pole vessels
  —The kidney is retracted gently and the upper pole vessels ligated.
  —The capsule is separated from the upper pole parenchyma.
  —The upper pole parenchyma and ureter are transected.
  —The stripped off capsule is used for closure.
  —Important to preserve lower pole parenchymal and ureteral vasculature
—Nephrectomy
  —Performed using surgeon's preferred approach
  —The ectopic obstructed ureter is resected if it refluxes.
  —A second incision may be needed, e.g., Gibson.
  —Care is needed to avoid injury to lower pole ureteral vessels and vas in males.
  —Resection is performed to the level of the bladder.

• Function is adequate for renal preservation: A ureteropyelostomy or ureteral reimplantation is performed.

—Ureteropyelostomy
  —A dorsal lumbotomy or flank approach is used.
  —The upper ureter is isolated, and the kidney is gently retracted.
  —The upper ureter is anastomosed widely to the lower pole renal pelvis in a tension-free manner.
—Common sheath ureteral reimplantation
  —For a duplicated system
  —Preferred approach if the lower pole ureter refluxes
—Solitary ureteral reimplantation
  —Performed for single systems only

• Bilateral ectopic ureters

—A poorly developed bladder neck leads to incontinence and a small bladder capacity.
—Ureteral reimplantation and bladder neck reconstruction are performed.
—May need bladder augmentation

ALTERNATIVE THERAPIES: N/A

PATIENT EDUCATION

• Parents should be instructed in the natural history and treatment options for children with this condition.

 Follow-Up

MONITORING

• Intravenous pyelogram or ultrasound and cystogram postoperatively
• Discontinue antibiotic prophylaxis if there is no reflux or obstruction.
• Ultrasound 1 year after surgery

PREVENTION: N/A

 Miscellaneous

SYNONYMS

• Orthotopic ureter

ASSOCIATED CONDITIONS

• Dysplastic kidney, contralateral reflux, urethral duplication, imperforate anus, tracheoesophageal fistula

NOTES

• A high index of suspicion is essential for diagnosing this condition.

ABBREVIATIONS: N/A

REFERENCES

Ahmed S, Barker A. Single-system ectopic ureters: A review of 12 cases. *J Pediatr Surg* 1992;27:491.

el Ghoneimi A, Miranda J, Truong T, Monfort T. Ectopic ureter with complete ureteric duplication: Conservative surgical management. *J Pediatr Surg* 1996;31:467.

Gharagozloo AM, Lebowitz RL. Detection of a poorly functioning malpositioned kidney with single ectopic ureter in girls with urinary dribbling: Imaging evaluation in five patients. *AJR* 1995; 164:957.

Plaire JC. Management of ectopic ureters: Experience with the upper tract approach. *J Urol* 1997;158:1245.

Author: Anthony Atala

Ureter—Malignant Obstruction

 Basics

DESCRIPTION

- Impairment of urinary drainage through the ureter(s) due to cancer. This can be intrinsic obstruction (a mass inside the ureter) or extrinsic obstruction (compression from tumor outside the ureter, usually metastatic or directly extending from another primary cancer).

EPIDEMIOLOGY

- Intrinsic ureteral tumors

—Incidence less than 0.5 per 100,000 in males
—Average age of occurrence: 65 years
—Male:female ratio: 2:1
—White:Black ratio: 2:1
—Occurs in 2% to 4% of individuals with history of bladder cancer
—Incidence of bilateral ureteral tumors: 1%

- Extrinsic tumors

—5% to 10% of retroperitoneal fibrosis is malignant.
—60% to 70% occur within 2 years of diagnosis of primary cancer.
—Can occur 20 years or more after diagnosis of primary cancer

GENETICS

- Intrinsic tumors

—Endemic nephropathy in Balkan countries with high incidence of primary ureteral cancer
—Incidence of bilaterality: 10% in Balkans vs. 1% elsewhere
—Loss of genetic material in chromosome 9 is thought to initiate superficial papillary transitional cell tumors.
—Inactivation of *p53* tumor suppressor gene important in invasive tumors

- Extrinsic: N/A

STAGING

- Intrinsic tumors: See TNM system in Section VII (similar to primary bladder cancer staging)
- Extrinsic tumors obstructing one or both ureters are staged according to the status of the primary tumor.

SIGNS AND SYMPTOMS

- Intrinsic obstruction

—75% of patients experience gross hematuria.
—30% of patients experience flank pain.
—10% to 15% present with fever due to infection associated with the obstruction.
—Some are asymptomatic.
—The few (<1%) with bilateral obstruction may experience uremic symptoms from renal insufficiency.

- Extrinsic obstruction

—Similar symptoms to intrinsic obstruction
—Symptoms may be masked by symptoms from the primary tumor or other metastases to bone or other sites.

PATHOPHYSIOLOGY

- Intrinsic malignant ureteral obstruction

—90% due to transitional cell carcinoma (TCC) originating from the urothelium
—5% to 8% due to squamous cell carcinoma (SCC) originating from the urothelium
—2% to 5% due to other cell types arising from urothelium or smooth muscle/adventitia of ureteral wall
—Obstruction results when sufficient compromise of the ureteral lumen has occurred to interfere with urine drainage from the kidney to the bladder.

- Extrinsic malignant ureteral obstruction

—Metastatic cancer to lymph nodes near the ureter impinges on the ureteral wall, sometimes circumferentially.
—Direct extension from another primary tumor compresses the ureter or invades its wall and compromises the ureteral lumen.
　　—The most common sites of cancers causing extrinsic ureteral obstruction are (in decreasing order of incidence) cervix, prostate, bladder, colon, ovary, uterus, stomach, breast, lymph nodes, pancreas, lung, gallbladder, testis, and small bowel.

CAUSES/RISK FACTORS

• Intrinsic obstruction (primary ureteral tumors)

—Cigarette smoking is the single most important risk for developing primary ureteral cancer.
  —Risk shown proportional to amount of tobacco use
  —Duration of exposure to tobacco less well correlated with risk
—Occupational exposure to chemicals, plastics, coal, tar, and asphalt also increases risk.
—Analgesic abuse (phenacetin) correlated with risk of ureteral cancer
—Chronic infection and chronic urolithiasis increase the risk of ureteral cancer (SCC and adenocarcinoma).

• Extrinsic obstruction: N/A

COMPLICATIONS

• Chronic ureteral obstruction results in gradual loss of ipsilateral renal function.

—Total obstruction for more than 6 weeks may result in complete and irreversible loss of all function for that kidney.
—Bilateral obstruction may result in uremia requiring dialysis to sustain life.

• Partial obstruction of a ureter from a malignant process, extrinsic or intrinsic, may predispose to infection and life-threatening urosepsis with the need for immediate drainage to avoid death.

DIFFERENTIAL DIAGNOSIS

• See also Section I, "Hydronephrosis—Adult."
• Intrinsic ureteral obstruction

—Ureteral calculus
—Blood clot
—Papillary necrosis
—Stricture (usually malignant) or secondary to instrumentation

• Extrinsic malignant ureteral obstruction

—Benign, idiopathic retroperitoneal fibrosis
—Endometriosis
—Nearby infection (diverticulitis, abscess, etc.) with inflammatory reaction
—Scarring from other causes (radiation, prior surgery, or trauma)
—Iatrogenic (inadvertent ligation of ureter during surgery)
—Benign, adjacent processes with mass effect (lymphocele, aortic aneurysm)

 Database

HISTORY

• History of gross hematuria or flank pain?

—Episodic or chronic?
—Was the gross hematuria total (throughout the stream)?
  —Total favors bladder, ureteral, or renal origin
—Any colicky pain?
  —Colic favors bleeding from the kidney or ureter.

• Has the patient any history of malignancy, especially one of urinary tract or reproductive tract origin?

—Was there exposure to tobacco or analgesics, or any occupational exposure to chemicals, plastics, or petroleum derivatives?

• Prior urologic surgery, trauma, or history of nephrolithiasis?

PHYSICAL EXAMINATION

• Inspect the flanks.

—Asymmetry or ecchymosis might indicate a retroperitoneal mass or bleed.

• Palpate and percuss costovertebral angles (CVAs) and flanks bilaterally.

—CVA tenderness suggests a process affecting the ipsilateral kidney, such as obstruction.

• Palpate the abdomen for a mass.

—A mass in the abdomen can indicate cancer, an obstructed kidney, or both.

• Palpate for adenopathy that might provide evidence of advanced cancer.

(continued)

Ureter—Malignant Obstruction (continued)

 Diagnostic Studies

LABORATORY TESTING

• Urinalysis for microhematuria

—Crystals might suggest a stone rather than a tumor.

• Urine cytology

—A positive cytology suggests a urothelial cancer in the bladder, the ureter, or the renal collecting system.

IMAGING

• An intravenous urogram (IVU) will demonstrate a filling defect or a narrowing, suggesting a possible cancer.

—Complete obstruction may result in nonvisualization of that ureter and kidney on IVU.

• Retrograde pyelography (RP) can provide more detail than IVU but is more invasive.

—Shows details when diminished renal function precludes satisfactory contrast excretion through the ureter
—A filling defect or extrinsic compression typically has irregular edges typical of malignancy.
—There may be ureteral dilation distal to a ureteral tumor.

• Abdominal ultrasonography may show an obstructed (hydronephrotic) kidney, an abdominal mass, or an intraureteral filling defect (if larger than 0.5 cm).
• Computerized tomography (CT) can provide more detail than an abdominal ultrasound and can often a resolve a small calculus or other benign process and help differentiate it from a malignant one.

SPECIAL STUDIES

• Ureteral brushing and/or ureteroscopy with biopsy can help with the diagnosis of a malignant, intrinsic ureteral lesion.
• CT-guided needle aspiration and/or a needle core biopsy may be considered for extrinsic compression of the ureter to differentiate between a malignant retroperitoneal process and a benign one.

 Treatment

GENERAL MEASURES

• Immediate relief of obstruction: retrograde passage of a ureteral stent or by percutaneous nephrostomy; this is especially urgent with bilateral ureteral obstruction.

—Simple relief of obstruction with a tube does not cure the malignant process; it temporizes.
—A stent, if used only for palliation, must be changed every few months due to encrustation.
—An internal stent may be passed later, after percutaneous nephrostomy relieves obstruction, improves renal function, and/or permits associated ureteral edema to diminish.

MEDICAL

• Chemotherapy is appropriate for cancers that are not surgically resectable.

—Cancers such as lymphomas and metastatic testis cancer are examples where ureteral obstruction can resolve, in many cases, due to effective chemotherapy.

• Immunotherapy for uroepithelial ureteral cancers must be regarded as still investigational.

—Bacille Calmette-Guérin and interferon are effective for noninvasive urothelial cancers in the bladder and may hold promise in other parts of the urinary tract.

• With metastatic prostate cancer obstruction (and is still androgen-sensitive), hormonal therapy can relieve ureteral obstruction.

SURGICAL

- Intrinsic obstruction

—Normal kidney and ureter on the contralateral side: High-grade ureteral tumors require nephroureterectomy.
—Low-grade, small ureteral tumors: resected with reconstitution of ureteral continuity and preservation of the ipsilateral renal unit
—Local destruction of intraureteral tumors with cautery or laser is rarely feasible unless very small, and only in very select circumstances.

- If the malignancy is extrinsic and resectable, then primary surgical resection is best.

—Devascularization of the ureter or other ureteral injury may complicate the surgery.
—For tumors whose resection requires resection of part of the ureter, reconstruction must be balanced with the risks/benefits of en bloc nephroureterectomy to effect cure.

- For extrinsic compression from hormone-dependent, metastatic prostate cancer, "indirect" surgery can achieve relief of ureteral obstruction by means of bilateral orchiectomy to eliminate testosterone from the circulation.

ALTERNATIVE THERAPIES

- Primary radiation therapy can be effective for radiosensitive tumors causing malignant ureteral obstruction.

PATIENT EDUCATION

- Patients experiencing a primary ureteral cancer should be educated regarding the risk of recurrence due to continued smoking or exposure to other risk factors, where applicable.
- Patients with extrinsic cancer compressing the ureter who are palliated with a stent should be educated regarding the need for periodic changing of the stent.

 Follow-Up

MONITORING

- IVU or RP to look for recurrent obstruction or tumor

—Timing should be individualized to the disease process that produced the original obstruction.

- A renal ultrasound or renal scan to monitor for recurrent obstruction

—Less specific than IVU or RP but can pick up early recurrence of obstruction
—Ultrasound avoids radiation exposure and radiographic contrast.
—A renal scan shows differential function and requires no bowel preparation.

- Urinalysis to pick up new instance of microhematuria, which should raise suspicion of recurrence
- Urine cytology may pick up a recurrence of urothelial tumor.

PREVENTION

- Avoid risk factors, such as smoking, that predispose to urothelial cancer formation.

—A good diet and other habits may decrease the risk of other cancer, such as colon cancer, which can spread and obstruct the ureter.

 Miscellaneous

SYNONYMS: N/A

ASSOCIATED CONDITIONS

- Obstruction of colon or other abdominal organs due to malignancy
- Chronic anemia, if persistent, chronic bleeding
- Uremia, if bilateral ureteral obstruction

NOTES

- See also Section I, "Hydronephrosis—Adult."

ABBREVIATIONS

- TCCU, transitional cell cancer, ureter

REFERENCES

Huffman JL. Management of upper tract transitional cell carcinoma. In: Vogelzang NJ, et al., eds. *Comprehensive Textbook of Genitourinary Oncology.* Baltimore: Williams & Wilkins, 1996: 388–404.

Morrison AS. Advances in the etiology of urothelial cancer. *Urol Clin North Am* 1984;11:557–566.

Resnick MI, Kursh ED. Extrinsic obstruction of the ureter. In: Walsh PC, Retik AB, Vaughan ED, Wein AJ, eds. *Campbell's Urology,* 6th ed. Philadelphia: WB Saunders, 1992:560–564.

Author: Mark J. Noble

Ureterocele

Basics

DESCRIPTION

- Cystic dilatation of the distal segment of ureter
- Wide spectrum of anatomic variants and clinical presentations
- Multiple classification schema of ureteroceles exist. Ureteroceles may be classified: intravesical (entirely within the bladder) or ectopic (some portion of the ureterocele at the bladder neck or urethra); single system or duplex system (ureter to upper pole segment almost always involved); stenotic (small intravesical ureteral orifice), sphincteric (ureteral orifice within urethral sphincter), sphincterostenotic (small ureteral orifice within urethral sphincter), or cecoureterocele (intravesical ureteral orifice with a blind submucosal segment of ureterocele extending into the urethra)
- Complete ureteral duplication in 80%
- Hydroureteronephrosis of the upper pole moiety of a duplicated system is the classic finding. Reflux in the ipsilateral lower pole moiety is usually present.
- Simple single-system ureteroceles are usually associated with good renal function, while ectopic single system ureteroceles are usually associated with poor renal function and renal dysplasia.

EPIDEMIOLOGY

- Incidence: 1 in 500 to 4000 (autopsy reports)
- Caucasian predominance
- Female-to-male ratio: 6:1
- Left-to-right ratio: 1:1; bilateral 10%
- Most commonly presents in infancy
- Ectopic ureteroceles associated with the upper pole of a duplex system are most often present in infancy or childhood.
- Simple single-system ureteroceles most often present in adulthood and are usually asymptomatic.
- Ectopic single-system ureteroceles are more common in males and are associated with additional congenital anomalies.
- Larger ureteroceles present earlier.

GENETICS

- Multifactorial inheritance proposed
- Rare case reports of familial occurrence

STAGING: N/A

SIGNS AND SYMPTOMS

- Presentation is variable, depending on the anatomy of the ureterocele.

—Urosepsis in the first few months of life is the most common presentation.
—Palpable abdominal mass; abdominal, flank or pelvic pain
—Ureterocele prolapse through the urethra (in girls) and visible at introitus
—Urinary incontinence due to ectopia of ureteral orifice beyond urethral sphincter in females

- Pyelonephritis; hematuria

—Failure to thrive; elevated blood pressure
—Urinary retention due to infravesical obstruction by ureterocele
—Hemorrhagic infarction of prolapsed ureterocele (rare)

- Increasingly detected in fetuses on antenatal ultrasound by the presence of a cystic bladder mass associated with hydroureteronephrosis

PATHOPHYSIOLOGY

- Ureterocele histology: abnormal musculature, characterized by an incomplete muscular coat
- Trigone distortion and detrusor hypertrophy
- Upper pole ureters insert inferomedially and lower pole ureters insert superolaterally on the trigone (Weigert-Meyer rule).
- Reflux is present in 50% of ipsilateral lower pole moieties in the duplex system and in 10% to 25% of contralateral kidneys.
- Renal dysplasia is seen in 40% of upper pole moieties associated with duplex system ureteroceles.

CAUSES/RISK FACTORS

- Simple and ectopic ureteroceles are likely to represent different embryologic defects.
- Etiology is unknown, but there are several theories, including

—Congenital defect
  —Incomplete dissolution of Chwalla's membrane during development
  —Altered development of ureteral bud
  —Inadequate muscularization
  —Acquired defect (rare): *Schistosoma haematobium* infection; trauma

COMPLICATIONS

- Pyelonephritis, leading to renal scarring and renal failure or urosepsis
- Vesicoureteral reflux, ipsilateral lower pole (50%) and contralateral (25%)
- Hydronephrosis, ipsilateral and contralateral
- Bladder outlet obstruction, due to prolapsing ureterocele
- Infarction of prolapsed ureterocele (rare)
- Hemorrhage and bleeding of ureterocele (rare)

DIFFERENTIAL DIAGNOSIS

- Pseudoureterocele (ectopic ureter)
- Prolapsed urethra
- Bladder diverticulum
- Mesonephric duct cysts
- Urethral and bladder polyps
- Edema secondary to recent trauma/stone passage
- Transitional cell carcinoma

Database

HISTORY

- Recurrent urinary tract infections
- Periurethral mass
- Incontinence
- Abdominal mass
- Abdominal or flank pain
- Failure to thrive
- Hematuria

PHYSICAL EXAMINATION

- Genitourinary and abdominal examination
- Blood pressure

Diagnostic Studies

LABORATORY TESTING

- Serum creatinine: Follow total renal function.
- Urinalysis and urine culture

IMAGING

- Imaging studies must be performed with the bladder distended and empty, because ureteroceles can be compressed by a full bladder and, thus, may be missed.
- Antenatal ultrasound

—Dilated renal collecting system (single or duplex)
—Intravesical cystic dilatation
—Septations within bladder (representing ureterocele walls)
—Any abnormal antenatal ultrasound findings mandate a comprehensive postnatal evaluation.

- Renal/bladder ultrasound

—Usually first study performed
—If a ureterocele is suspected in a neonate, this study should be performed within 24 to 48 hours of birth.
—Well-defined cystic intravesical mass near bladder base
—Hydroureteronephrosis (especially upper pole moiety)
—Duplex renal moiety (distinct renal pelvices separated by parenchyma)
—Thinning of renal parenchyma of dilated moiety

- Voiding cystourethrogram (VCUG)

—Defines size and position of ureterocele
—Defines reflux in ipsilateral and contralateral systems
—Defines degree of detrusor backing for ureterocele. Eversion of a ureterocele may be seen with poor detrusor backing.

- Intravenous pyelogram (IVP)

—Not routinely performed in children
—A classic finding is a filling defect in the bladder base, seen as a round radiopacity surrounded by a radiolucent rim.
—If the affected renal moiety's function is poor:
  —Non-opacification of upper pole system
  —A reduced number of calyces suggests renal duplication with poor function of the upper pole.
  —Downward and laterally displaced lower pole moiety ("drooping lilly" sign)
  —The lower pole ureter may be laterally displaced and looped around the dilated upper pole ureter.
—If the affected renal moiety's function is good
  —The contrast-filled ureterocele is separated from medium in the bladder by a thin, lucent halo of the ureterocele wall ("spring-onion" or "cobra-head deformity" sign).

- Cystoscopy

—Findings are variable.
—Ureteroceles are best seen with an empty bladder and manual pressure on the flank.
—May be necessary to rule out pseudoureteroceles and bladder diverticulum
—Rarely is retrograde pyelography required to define the anatomy of a nonrefluxing ipsilateral lower pole moiety.

SPECIAL STUDIES

- Radionuclide renal scan

—DMSA scans evaluate the renal parenchyma in ipsilateral and contralateral moieties to define baseline renal function.
—DTPA or MAG-3 scans evaluate drainage from the collecting system to rule out obstruction and define the function of separate renal moieties.
—Often demonstrates minimal or no function in the upper pole moiety of the duplicated system
—A single intravesical system is usually associated with good renal function.

 Treatment

GENERAL MEASURES

- Individualize treatment. Each ureterocele is a unique embryologic anomaly with regard to anatomy, pathophysiology, and renal function.
- Management commonly involves surgery.
- Prior to surgical intervention, the anatomy of the urinary tract must be delineated as clearly as possible.
- If the renal parenchyma appears abnormal on ultrasound examination, then ipsilateral and contralateral renal function must be assessed.
- Always assume significant obstruction is present.
- Antibiotic prophylaxis until definitive treatment is performed
- Bladder outlet obstruction and vesicoureteral reflux should be minimized.
- Continence should be maintained.
- Total renal function must be protected and preserved.

MEDICAL

- Prophylactic therapy

—Low incidence of urinary tract infection while on prophylaxis
—May be used to delay surgical intervention until bladder enlarges

- Antibiotics

—Ampicillin
  —Infants <3 months of age; 10 to 15 mg/kg qd
—Trimethoprim-sulfamethoxazole (TMP-SMX)
  —Patients >3 months; 5 cc/10 kg qd

(continued)

Ureterocele (continued)

SURGICAL

- Endoscopic ureterocele incision

—Replaced transurethral resection (or unroofing) of entire ureterocele (procedure associated with an unacceptable rate of reflux)

—A small endoscopic incision or puncture made inferomedially on anterior wall of simple ureterocele above the bladder neck

—For ectopic ureteroceles, the incision must be sufficiently proximal to ensure patency and drainage above the bladder neck.

—Effective method of decompression in the face of sepsis

—Useful in neonates as part of staged reconstruction

—Highly successful for small, single-system intravesical ureteroceles, with low reported incidence of iatrogenic reflux and incontinence (<10%) and need for secondary procedures (10%–15%)

—In ectopic ureteroceles, higher incidence of failure to relieve obstruction (10%–25%), iatrogenic reflux (20%–50%), and secondary procedures (50%–90%). May still be the initial procedure of choice in these patients, to postpone a definitive procedure until bladder enlarges

—Never definitive if renal scarring or damage is severe

—In cecoureteroceles, this procedure can increase the degree of bladder outlet obstruction, as the distal segment can retain urine.

- Upper to lower ureteropyelostomy (ureteroureterostomy)

—Indicated for upper pole moieties with good renal function

—Not advised if upper pole function is questionable or poor

—Improves drainage for upper segment

—Single abdominal incision

—Good success in decompression (96%)

—High ureteroureterostomy preferable to avoid "yo-yo" reflux, which can complicate a low ureteroureterostomy

—The primary complication is development of strictures at the site of the anastomosis of a large upper pole ureter to a delicate lower pole ureter.

—Risk of reflux, UTI, and damage to other renal moiety

—Additional surgery may be required if the upper pole ureteral stump refluxes following a prior endoscopic incision.

- Nephroureterectomy (simplified approach)

—Heminephroureterectomy in a duplex system, or total nephroureterectomy in a single system

—Single abdominal incision

—A ureterocele may become a small bladder diverticulum.

—Procedure of choice for patients with small duplex-system ureterocele with dysplastic upper pole moiety and no vesicoureteral reflux

—70% of preexisting reflux in an ipsilateral or contralateral ureter is still present after surgery.

—10% to 50% require a second definitive procedure.

—Poor success rate in ureteroceles with high-grade reflux (grades III–V)

- Complete reconstruction

—Definitive procedure required in some cases

—Nephroureterectomy (partial in a duplex system, or total in a single system) through flank incision + ureterocele excision + ipsilateral/contralateral ureteral reimplant via lower abdominal incision

—Ureters can be tapered if dilated.

—May be required in patients with severe ipsilateral lower pole reflux (grades IV, V), large ureteroceles, and prolapsed ureteroceles

—May not be possible in neonates, secondary to small bladder size

—Formidable reconstructive surgery

—Reflux, incontinence in experienced hands <10%

—Risk of damage to bladder neck continence mechanisms

—Risk of damage to ipsilateral ureter

—Risk of vesicovaginal fistula, diverticula

- Percutaneous diversion

—Temporary procedure if renal function is in question

—May be used for acute urosepsis, unresponsive to antibiotics

—Rarely needed for an obstructed system, since endoscopic incision is simple

—High complication rate in infants

ALTERNATIVE THERAPIES

- Observation

—Consider in asymptomatic patients with mild or good renal function, in whom the ureterocele is small and associated with minimal reflux or obstruction (incidentally picked up as a filling defect on an IVP or ultrasound).
—If mild vesicoureteral reflux is present, then patients must be monitored for spontaneous resolution.
—Not an option in patients with significant hydronephrosis, reflux, or urinary tract infections

PATIENT EDUCATION

- Families need to understand that multiple procedures may be required in the treatment of ureteroceles.

 Follow-Up

MONITORING

- Periodic renal and bladder ultrasound
- VCUG
- Serum creatinine (if bilateral)
- Urine should be checked every 3 months, and urinary tract infections should be treated aggressively in children prior to definitive treatment.

PREVENTION

- Antibiotic prophylaxis can prevent UTI.

 Miscellaneous

SYNONYMS: N/A

ASSOCIATED CONDITIONS

- Duplex renal systems, vesicoureteral reflux, renal dysplasia

NOTES: N/A

ABBREVIATIONS

- DMSA, dimercaptosuccinic acid; DTPA, diethylenetriamine pentaacetic acid; MAG-3, mercaptoacetyltriglycine; VCUG, voiding cystourethrogram

REFERENCES

Coplen DE, Duckett JW. The modern approach to ureteroceles. *J Urol* 1995;153:166–171.

Gonzales ET. Ureteroceles. In: King LR, ed. *Urologic Surgery in Infants and Children*. Philadelphia: WB Saunders, 1998:78–95.

Pfister C, Ravasse P, Barret E, Petit T, Mitrofanoff P. The value of endoscopic treatment for ureteroceles during the neonatal period. *J Urol* 1998; 159:1006–1009.

Roy GT, Desai S, Cohen RC. Ureteroceles in children—An ongoing challenge. *Pediatr Surg Int* 1996;12:44–48.

Authors: Ganesh V. Raj and John S. Wiener

Urethra—Abscess (Periurethral Abscess)

 Basics

DESCRIPTION

• A life-threatening infection of the male urethra and periurethral tissues associated with urinary infection and urethral stricture disease

EPIDEMIOLOGY

• More likely in diabetics or in groups at high risk for sexually transmitted disease

GENETICS: N/A

STAGING: N/A

SIGNS AND SYMPTOMS

• Scrotal swelling (94%)
• Fever (70%)
• Acute urinary retention (19%)
• Spontaneously drained abscess (11%)
• Obstructed Foley or suprapubic tube (8%)
• Dysuria (6%)
• Urethral discharge (5%)

PATHOPHYSIOLOGY

• Occurs with periurethral extravasation of infected urine in men
• High-pressure voiding behind a stricture leads to extravasation of urine.
• Difficult dilation of urethral stricture causes urethral disruption, which leads to extravasation of infected urine into tissues during voiding.
• Can progress to Fournier disease, especially if immunocompromised
• Bladder instability associated with recurrent PUA
• Contributing factors include history of

—Gonorrhea (38%)
—Previous periurethral abscess (34%)
—Urethral stricture disease (28%)
—Diabetes mellitus (13%)

CAUSES/RISK FACTORS

• Urinary tract infection
• Urethral stricture disease
• Urethral dilation
• Neurogenic bladder
• Diabetes mellitus
• Previous PUA

COMPLICATIONS

• Sepsis, acute renal failure, death (1.6%), progression to necrotizing fasciitis
• Recurrent periurethral abscess, candidemia, bladder stone
• Necrosis of corpora spongiosa
• Urethrocutaneous fistula (watering-pot perineum); extensive skin loss
• Gastrointestinal bleeding

DIFFERENTIAL DIAGNOSIS

• Perirectal abscess
• Follicular abscess
• Fournier's gangrene
• Urethral carcinoma
• Carcinoma of perianal glands
• Pneumoscrotum
• Diffuse body edema secondary to congestive heart failure
• Drug allergy

 Database

HISTORY

• Symptoms of urinary tract infection

—Imitative voiding symptoms, hematuria, foul-smelling urine, fever, and chills
—Gonococcal or nongonococcal urethritis, other STDs

• Neurogenic bladder

—Symptoms of urgency or urge incontinence; an unstable bladder can leak urine into urethral tissue, causing recurrence.
—Catheter placement or use of intermittent catheterization
—Use of anticholinergic medications to relieve bladder urgency

• History of any type of surgery (especially GU) or known urethral stricture disease

—Previous surgery may be associated with urethral instrumentation, urethral dilation, or catheterization, all potential sources of urethral stricture or disruption.
—Pelvic radiation, cause of urethral stricture

• Diabetes

PHYSICAL EXAMINATION

• Fever, hypotension, tachycardia, or symptoms of possible sepsis
• Palpate the penile shaft and perineum for masses and tenderness.
• Scrotal/penile swelling: Urinary extravasation confined to Buck's fascia presents with localized penile swelling.
• Scrotal edema, foul-smelling phlegmon, or fluctuance indicates urinary extravasation into the periurethral tissues. Abscess formation may occur (77%).
• Necrotic tissue associated with gangrene or fasciitis (frank necrosis or discoloration) can extend around the rectum or up the abdominal wall (23%). Crepitation suggests gas gangrene.
• Palpable suprapubic mass with urinary retention
• Rectal examination, primarily to exclude perirectal abscess, evaluate for perianal carcinoma

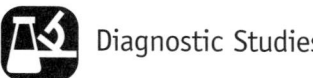 **Diagnostic Studies**

LABORATORY TESTING

- Urinalysis, urine culture and sensitivity for primary or secondary UTI due to PUA
- Wound culture: gangrene/fasciitis; gram-negative rods and anaerobes are most commonly found.
- Blood culture as part of sepsis work-up
- Coagulation profile/bleeding studies: sepsis-related coagulopathy
- BUN, creatinine

—Dehydration, renal failure
—The aminoglycoside dosage may need to be altered.

IMAGING

- Retrograde urethrogram (RUG)

—Urethral stricture and fistulas; urinary extravasation is diagnostic.
—Bladder stones
—Subcutaneous air associated with wet gangrene

SPECIAL STUDIES: N/A

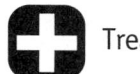 **Treatment**

GENERAL MEASURES

- General medical examination
- Supportive measures, as needed, for diabetes, hypotension, renal failure, or septic shock

MEDICAL

- Broad-spectrum antibiotic coverage

—Cephalosporin and aminoglycoside for treatment of sepsis
—Patient sent home on oral cephalosporin until wound clean and healing

SURGICAL

- Incision and drainage of abscess with radical debridement of necrotic tissue

—Pack the wound open with dilute Betadine- or hydrogen peroxide–soaked gauze.
—The testicles may be completely exposed and require delayed placement in the scrotum or staggered thigh pouches.
—Additional anesthetic debridement as the margin between necrotic and viable tissue becomes apparent
—May need skin graft to cover skin loss or secondary closure of scrotal defect
—Daily dressing changes and whirlpool baths to remove purulent and necrotic tissue

- Biopsy to exclude urethral or perianal cancer
- Urinary diversion

—Suprapubic tube initially; historically, urinary diversion was performed with a perineal urethrostomy; not associated with recurrent PUA
—Perineal urethrostomy as a secondary procedure, particularly in patients with an unstable bladder or where adequate urinary diversion has not occurred

- Cystoscopy

—Evaluation of urethral stricture disease after complete resolution of infection
—Long-term management of urethral stricture disease can range from conservative (intermittent catheterization) to surgery on a stricture at least 6 months after the infection and phlegmon are completely resolved.

ALTERNATIVE THERAPIES: N/A

PATIENT EDUCATION

- Explain the need for potential future surgical intervention.

 Follow-Up

MONITORING

- Stricture disease: retrograde urethrogram to evaluate stricture disease after infection resolved
- Uroflowmetry
- Urinary tract infection: Evaluate urine periodically to minimize the chance of recurrent PUA.

PREVENTION

- Adequate urinary diversion; divert urine from the healing urethral phlegmon.
- Recurrent PUAs occur in as many as 19% of patients.
- Sterilize the urine.
- Rehabilitation of urethral stricture

—Internal urethrotomy
—Staged urethral repair
—Intermittent catheterization; neurogenic bladder
—Perineal urethrostomy; unstable bladder, perineal induration that is slow to resolve

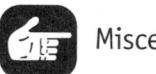 **Miscellaneous**

SYNONYMS

- Scrotal fasciitis

ASSOCIATED CONDITIONS

- Urethral stricture, urinary infection, diabetes, Fournier's gangrene, watering-pot perineum

NOTES

- See also Section I, "Urethral Mass," and Section II, "Fournier's Gangrene."

ABBREVIATIONS

- PUA, periurethral abscess

REFERENCES

Baker WJ, Wilkey JL, Barson LJ. An evaluation of the management of peri-urethral phlegmon in 272 consecutive cases at the Cook County Hospital. *J Urol* 1949;61:943–948.

Campbell MF. Periurethral phlegmon (urinary extravasation): A study of 135 cases. *Surg Gynecol Obstet* 1929;48:382–389.

Tashiro S, Hinman F. Periurethral and perirectal infections: Pathological and clinical differentiation. *J Urol* 1947;57:338–355.

Walther MM, Mann BB, Finnerty DP. Periurethral abscess. *J Urol* 1987;138:1167–1170.

Author: McClellan M. Walther

Urethra—Carcinoma, General

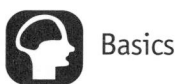 Basics

DESCRIPTION

• Urethral cancer is an uncommon malignant neoplasm originating within the surface cells of the urethral tract. Urethral cancer may occur anywhere from the neck of the bladder to the external meatus. The most common form, in both men and women, is squamous cell carcinoma (SCC).

EPIDEMIOLOGY

• Rare cancer: only 0.1% to 0.2% of all gynecologic malignancies
• Unique urologic malignancy because it is more common in women than in men (3:1)
• Women: higher prevalence among Whites; men: no racial predisposition

GENETICS: N/A

STAGING

• See TNM classification in the appendix.

SIGNS AND SYMPTOMS

• Often insidious at onset
• Symptoms usually first attributed to stricture disease
• Men: A majority present with a palpable urethral mass or obstruction.

—Urethral stricture, bleeding, perineal pain, or a new onset urethral fistula in an elderly man suggests the possibility of urethral cancer.

• Women: A majority present with urinary frequency, hesitancy, obstruction, and a palpable urethral mass or induration.

PATHOPHYSIOLOGY

• Urethral location

—Men: bulbomembranous (60%), penile (30%), prostatic (10%)
—Women: anterior urethra (distal one-third), 20% to 40%; posterior urethra (proximal two-thirds), 60% to 80%

• Spread/extension

—Men and women: spread by direct extension to adjacent structures
—Lymphatic metastases (both sexes)
  —Anterior urethra: to superficial and deep inguinal LN
  —Posterior urethra: to external iliac, obturator, and hypogastric LN
  —Palpable inguinal LN in approximately 20% of men, and approximately 30% of women— these almost always represent metastatic disease.
  —Metastasis outside the pelvis at initial presentation is uncommon.
—Hematogenous spread is uncommon, except in advanced cases of disease.

• Subtypes
—Men: 80% SCC, 15% transitional cell carcinoma (TCC), 5% adenocarcinoma (AC)
—Women: 60% SCC, 20% TCC, 10% AC, 8% undifferentiated tumors and sarcomas, 2% melanomas
  —In general, cancers of the anterior urethra are low grade and less extensive.
  —Cancers of the proximal or entire urethra are usually high grade and locally advanced.

• 5-Year survival rates

—Stages I and II (localized): 60% to 100%
—Stages III and IV (advanced): <40%

CAUSES/RISK FACTORS

• Urethral caruncle

—Benign uropathy frequently seen in postmenopausal women
—2.4% of all patients diagnosed with a urethral caruncle will have coincident in situ or invasive urethral cancer.
—Necessary to get tissue biopsy in women with urethral caruncle to rule out malignancy

• Condylomata acuminata

—Caused by human papilloma virus (HPV) infection
—HPV has been found within the urothelial cells of patients with TCC of the urethra.

• Diverticula

—Possible relationship between urethral diverticula and the harboring of clear-cell AC of the urethra

COMPLICATIONS

• Urethral stricture
• Fistula formation

DIFFERENTIAL DIAGNOSIS

• Caruncle
• Urethral prolapse
• Leukoplakia
• Stricture
• Fistula
• Erosion
• Periurethral abscess
• Inflammatory phlegmon
• Nephrogenic adenoma (rare)

 Database

HISTORY

• Age, sex, and race of the patient?

—Urethral cancer is most common in White women.
—No race predisposition in men
—Average age: >50 years (both sexes)

• Irritative symptoms or hematuria?

—Most present with frequency, hesitation, obstruction, and/or a palpable urethral mass or induration.
—Hematuria in a patient with a diverticula is suspicious for carcinoma.

• History of bladder cancer?

—Correlation of urethral cancer in both men and women with bladder cancer

• History of proliferative lesions of the urinary tract?

—Caruncles, papillomas, adenomas, and polyps have been associated with subsequent malignancy.
—Leukoplakia of the urethra is considered a premalignant lesion.

• History of STD, urethritis, stricture, or diverticula?

—The incidence of urethral stricture in men with urethral cancer ranges from 24% to 76%.
—Urethral stricture, bleeding, perineal pain, or fistula in an elderly man: Examine for urethral cancer.

PHYSICAL EXAMINATION

• Palpation

—Perineal mass, urethral mass
—Submucosal mass in the anterior vaginal wall with possible involvement of the vulva
  —May be difficult to differentiate urethral cancer from tumors originating in the vulva or vagina
—Inguinal lymph nodes palpable in 20% of men, 30% of women

• Pelvic/perineal examination best under anesthesia

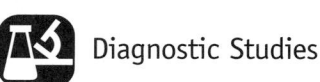 Diagnostic Studies

LABORATORY TESTING

• Urinalysis: dipstick and microanalysis for RBCs
• Urine cytology may be positive.

IMAGING

• Excretory urography

—Possibility of a coexisting genitourinary tract neoplasm or ureteral obstruction

• Voiding cystourethrogram

—Visualization of the posterior urethra in men, entire urethra in women
—Helpful in evaluating strictures, fistulas, diverticula, and neoplasms

• Retrograde urethrography

—Visualization of the anterior urethra in men
—Helpful in evaluating stricture, fistulas, diverticula, and neoplasms

• CT or MRI of abdomen/pelvis

—Useful in evaluating soft-tissue and lymph node involvement

• Bone scan and barium enema: only in symptomatic patients

SPECIAL STUDIES

- Cystourethroscopy with tissue biopsies (gold standard for diagnosis)
- Cystoscopy

—Papillary growth within the urethra; soft fungating mass that bleeds easily
—Ulcerative lesions may produce a foul-smelling discharge.

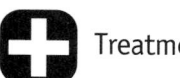 ## Treatment

GENERAL MEASURES

- The most important prognostic indicator for control and survival is the anatomic location and extent of tumor invasion.

MEDICAL

- Chemotherapy

—Role is undefined
—Significant antitumor activity has been demonstrated with mitomycin C, 5-fluorouracil, and several multidrug combinations; may enhance the effects of radiation therapy

SURGICAL

- Surgery is the treatment of choice for male urethral cancer, while radiation therapy is an option for primary female urethral neoplasms.
- Female urethral cancer may require radical cystectomy.
- Male urethral cancer by location

—Meatal/distal urethra (30%)
  —Transurethral resection, local excision with end-to-end anastamosis, partial amputation, or radical amputation with/without emasculation
  —Tumor infiltrating the corpus/locally to the distal half of the urethra requires partial penectomy with 2-cm margins to the visible/palpable tumor.
  —A proximal urethra or an entire urethra necessitates total penectomy/perineal urethrostomy
  —Ilioinguinal lymph node dissection only if inguinal nodes are palpable
—Bulbomembranous urethra (60%)
  —Radical cystoprostatectomy, pelvic lymphadenectomy, total penectomy, and possible scrotectomy offer the best long-term disease control and lowest incidence of recurrence
  —The excision may be extended to include subsymphyseal resection of the pubic arch and urogenital diaphragm.

—Prostatic urethra (10%)
  —Rare location; TUR of superficial lesion if the prostatic stroma is uninvolved
  —If prostatic involvement, cystoprostatectomy and total urethrectomy
—Subcutaneous penectomy
  —Intermediate alternative to patients that lies between limited local excision and total penectomy
  —Nonfunctional penis remains, but improved psychological outcome, reconstructive potential, and cosmetic appearance, without compromising tumor removal

ALTERNATIVE THERAPIES

- Radiation (women)

—Early lesions of the distal urethra (<4 cm) and of low tumor grade (T1, T2, T3, N0)
  —Interstitial radioactive implant (brachytherapy)
  —5-year survival rates: 70% to 80%
—Moderately advanced lesions involving the entire urethra (>4 cm) and of high tumor grade (T2, T3, N0-N1)
  —Combination of brachytherapy plus external beam radiation of primary tumor and regional lymph nodes
  —5-year survival rates: 40% to 50%
—Advanced local or regional disease involving adjacent organs, or massive nodal disease (advanced T3, T4, N2-N3)
  —Pelvic exenteration with external beam radiation
  —5-year survival rates: 7% to 19%
—Radiation in male urethral carcinoma: primarily palliative, occasionally as an adjunct to surgical resection
—Complications from radiation include bowel obstruction, fistula formation, urethral stricture, and incontinence.

PATIENT EDUCATION

- Urethral cancer is aggressive and is associated with significant morbidity and mortality.
- The earlier the diagnosis is made and the sooner treatment is begun, the better the survival rate.

 ## Follow-Up

MONITORING

- Most local recurrences occur within the first 1 to 2 years after treatment.
- Cystourethroscopy and urine cytology every 6 months; additional biopsies as necessary, based on these results

PREVENTION: N/A

 ## Miscellaneous

SYNONYMS: N/A

ASSOCIATED CONDITIONS

- Urethral stricture, urethral diverticula, leukoplakia

NOTES: N/A

ABBREVIATIONS

- SCC, squamous cell carcinoma; TCC, transitional cell carcinoma; AC, adenocarcinoma; HPV, human papilloma virus; CIS, carcinoma in situ

REFERENCES

Bird E, Coburn M. Phallus preservation for urethral cancer: Subcutaneous penectomy. *J Urol* 1997; 158:2146–2148.

Garden AS, Zagars GK, Delclos L. Primary carcinoma of the female urethra. *Cancer* 1993;71: 3102–3108.

Mostafi FK, et al. Carcinoma of the male and female urethra. *Urol Clin North Am* 1992;19: 347–358.

Rajan N, et al. Carcinoma in female urethra diverticulum: Case reports and review of management. *J Urol* 1993;150:1911–1914.

Tran LN, Krieg RM, Szabo RJ. Combination chemotherapy and radiotherapy for a locally advanced squamous cell carcinoma of the urethra. *J Urol* 1995;153:422–423.

Walsh PC, Retik AB, Vaughan ED, Wein AJ, eds. *Campbell's Urology*, 7th ed. Philadelphia: WB Saunders, 1998:3401–3409.

Authors: Greg Adey and Leonard G. Gomella

Urethra—Caruncle

Basics

DESCRIPTION

• Smooth, friable tissue located at distal posterior urethral in females

EPIDEMIOLOGY

• Postmenopausal woman: most common
• Child-bearing years: seldom seen
• Rare in childhood

GENETICS: N/A

STAGING: N/A

SIGNS AND SYMPTOMS

• Soft, smooth fleshy lesion at distal posterior urethral wall, usually bright red tissue

—May have sessile or pedunculated appearance
—<1 to 2 cm in size

• Symptoms: variable

—Most asymptomatic
—Irritative voiding symptoms (frequency, dysuria, urgency)
—Contact tenderness (sensitivity): i.e., clothing, touch
—May become secondarily infected: Ulceration and urethral bleeding (spotting) may develop.

PATHOPHYSIOLOGY

• Urethral caruncle felt to develop from an ectropion of posterior urethral wall secondary to retraction and postmenopausal vaginal atrophy
• Histology: usually vascular pyogenic granulation tissue covered by transitional or stratified squamous epithelial with loose connective tissue

—Papillomatous: most common; granulomatous and angiomatous subtypes also seen

CAUSES/RISK FACTORS

• Irritation/infection stimulates caruncle growth.

—Chronic cystitis, urethritis, cystocele associated with urethral caruncle

• Retraction of posterior urethral wall
• Postmenopausal vaginal atrophy (lack of estrogen)

COMPLICATIONS

• Can lead to bleeding and ulceration

DIFFERENTIAL DIAGNOSIS

• Urethral carcinoma

—Uncommon tumor; half arise in the distal third of the urethra.
—Peak incidence: fifth to seventh decade
—Tender, indurated mass
—Bleeding, frequency, and dysuria common
—Marshall et al. (1960) (1 out of 40 women diagnosed with urethral caruncle clinically had biopsy-proven malignant tumor)

• Urethral prolapse

—Primarily premenarcheal female (Black > White)
—Annular rosette appearance rather than posterior-only location of caruncle
—Usually paler appearance than caruncle
—Thrombosis of venous plexus (seen in elderly women): sudden pain and recent appearance of prolapse
—May appear edematous or ulcerated: necrosis sometimes seen

• Other: hemangioma, condylomatous polyps, papillomas, and cysts

Database

HISTORY

• Age of female

—Caruncle and urethral carcinoma seen most commonly in postmenopausal woman

• Irritative voiding symptoms (frequency, urgency, dysuria)
• Vaginal spotting
• The introital meatus may be sensitive to touch.

PHYSICAL EXAMINATION

• Vaginal introital inspection: urethra, labia, vagina, bimanual examination, inguinal node palpation

—Urethral caruncle usually visualized posteriorly (<2 cm)

• A small Q-tip in the urethra assists in location of the lesion.
• The urethral meatus may be sensitive to touch.

Diagnostic Studies

LABORATORY TESTING

- Usually not helpful

IMAGING: N/A

SPECIAL STUDIES

- Urethroscopy

—Caruncle and prolapse: distal urethra only; urethral carcinomas usually involve the more proximal urethra.

- Diagnostic biopsy (local/sedation)
- Excisional biopsy

 Treatment

GENERAL MEASURES

- Asymptomatic patients: reassure
- Symptomatic or large caruncle

—Topical estrogen or oral (sub-bleeding dosage)
—Surgical treatment
  —Surgical excision (leave Foley 1–3 days)
  —Fulguration (after biopsy)
  —Cryoablation

MEDICAL

- Topical estrogen or oral (sub-bleeding dosage)

SURGICAL

- Surgical excision (leave Foley 1–3 days)
- Fulguration (after biopsy)
- Cryoablation

ALTERNATIVE THERAPIES: N/A

PATIENT EDUCATION: N/A

 Follow-Up

MONITORING

- Periodic physical examination to assess for change in size or symptoms
- Reevaluate if spotting or irritative voiding symptoms reappear.
- Postexcision: Monitor for urethral stenosis.

—May need urethral dilation if voiding symptoms occur (decreased force of stream, hesitancy)

PREVENTION

- Avoid irritation from tight-fitting clothing

 Miscellaneous

SYNONYMS: N/A

ASSOCIATED CONDITIONS: N/A

NOTES

- See also Section I, "Urethral Mass."

ABBREVIATIONS: N/A

REFERENCES

Aagaar J, Bruskewitz R. Urethral caruncle. In: *Current Therapy in Genitourinary Surgery,* 2nd ed. 1992:164–165.

Marshall FC, Uson AC, Melicow MM. Neoplasms and caruncles of the female urethra. *Surg Gynecol Obstet* 1960;110:723.

Vela-Navarrete R. Caruncle and prolapse of the urethral mucosa. *Female Urol* Raz S, ed. 2nd Edition, 1983;10:560–563.

Author: Todd C. Igel

Urethra—Diverticula, Female

 Basics

DESCRIPTION

• A collection of urine and/or pus, adjacent to and connecting with the urethra

EPIDEMIOLOGY

• Reported incidence: 1.4% to 5%
• Mean age at diagnosis: 45 years
• May be more common in Black women

GENETICS

• Unknown

STAGING: N/A

SIGNS AND SYMPTOMS

• The 3Ds are classically described, but in clinical practice, symptoms are variable.

—Dysuria
—Dyspareunia
—Dribbling (especially post-void dribbling)

• Frequency, urgency, dysuria (about 50% of patients)
• Recurrent urinary tract infections (about 40% of patients)
• Vaginal wall pain and/or swelling
• Hematuria (rare presentation)
• May be asymptomatic incidental finding

PATHOPHYSIOLOGY

• Congenital (uncommon)
• Acquired

—Histology: "false diverticulum" of fibrous tissue; may lack epithelium
—Diverticulum contained within periurethral fascia

CAUSES/RISK FACTORS

• The usual explanation is abscess of the periurethral glands, which ruptures into the urethral lumen.

COMPLICATIONS

• Recurrent urinary tract infections
• Stone in diverticulum (1%–10% of cases)
• Bladder outlet obstruction
• Carcinoma in diverticulum (rare)

DIFFERENTIAL DIAGNOSIS

• Vaginal wall cyst or abscess that does not communicate with the urethra
• Skene's gland abscess
• Ectopic ureterocele
• Urethral or vaginal neoplasm

 Database

HISTORY

• Dysuria

—Most common description: pain during voiding; persists a few minutes after voiding

• Incontinence: possible causes

—Urine leaking from diverticulum
—Concomitant stress or urge incontinence

• Dyspareunia
• Recurrent urinary tract infections

PHYSICAL EXAMINATION

• Inspect the anterior vaginal wall.

—Many (but not all) diverticula are visible as a suburethral midline mass.

• Palpate the anterior vaginal wall.

—In some cases, the only sign of diverticulum is point tenderness on the urethra.
—The mass may be palpable.
  —Is it tender?
  —Does it compress? (If not, consider a vaginal wall cyst or an obstructed diverticulum.)
  —Classic finding: Palpating the mass expresses urine or pus from urethral meatus.
  —Induration suggests a stone or neoplasm.

• Assess bladder neck mobility.
• Observe for stress incontinence.
• Evaluate for other pelvic pathology (e.g., prolapse).

 Diagnostic Studies

LABORATORY TESTING

• Urinalysis, urine culture
• Preoperative tests appropriate to patient's age and medical condition

IMAGING

• A voiding cystourethrogram (VCUG) is the most helpful study.

—Sensitivity approximately 90%
—Evaluate size, position, configuration, and number of diverticula.

• Double-balloon urethrogram

—Painful; sensitivity not better than VCUG

• Vaginal ultrasound

—Sensitivity similar to VCUG
—Painful if diverticulum is tender

• Pelvic magnetic resonance imaging (MRI)

—Almost 100% accuracy but expensive
—Not painful unless vaginal coil is used

SPECIAL STUDIES

• Cystoscopy

—Less sensitive than VCUG in detecting diverticulum
—To see the entire urethra, use a scope with a flush end.
—Main value: to rule out concomitant pathology

• Urodynamic studies.

—Not needed for straightforward cases
—Helpful if incontinence is also present

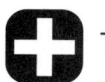 ## Treatment

GENERAL MEASURES

• Preoperative evaluation appropriate to age and medical condition

MEDICAL

• Treat the infection with appropriate antibiotics.

SURGICAL

• If very distal, may be marsupialized
• Usual procedure: key principles

—Excise the diverticulum completely.
—Close the urethral defect without tension.
—Cover with multiple layers (periurethral fascia, vaginal wall flap, consider Martius flap).
—Avoid overlapping suture lines.
—Small urethral catheter (12Fr to 14Fr) and suprapubic tube
—Aggressive anticholinergics (e.g., belladonna and opium suppositories) to prevent bladder spasms

• If stress incontinence is present, a bladder neck suspension or sling may be done at the same procedure.

ALTERNATIVE THERAPIES: N/A

PATIENT EDUCATION: N/A

 ## Follow-Up

MONITORING

• After surgery, do a VCUG before having the patient resume voiding.
• No coitus or tampons for at least 6 weeks

PREVENTION: N/A

 ## Miscellaneous

SYNONYMS: N/A

ASSOCIATED CONDITIONS: N/A

NOTES: N/A

ABBREVIATIONS

• VCUG, voiding cystourethrogram

REFERENCES

Ganabathi K, et al. Experience with the management of urethral diverticulum in 63 women. *J Urol* 1994;152:1445.

Leach GE, et al. LNSC$_3$; a proposed classification system for female urethral diverticula. *Neurourol Urodyn* 1993;12:523.

Leach GE, et al. Surgery for vesicovaginal and urethrovaginal fistula and urethral diverticulum. In: Walsh PC, Retik AB, Vaughan ED, Wein AJ, eds. *Campbell's Urology*, 7th ed. Philadelphia: WB Saunders, 1998.

Raz S. *Atlas of Transvaginal Surgery*. Philadelphia: WB Saunders, 1992.

Raz S, et al. Female urology. In: Walsh PC, Retik AB, Stamey TA, Vaughan ED, eds. *Campbell's Urology*, 6th ed. Philadelphia: WB Saunders, 1992.

Author: Deborah R. Erickson

Urethral Stricture

 Basics

DESCRIPTION

- Narrowing of the urethral lumen

EPIDEMIOLOGY

- Very prevalent in ancient times
- Progressively less common in the twentieth century with the advent of good management of urethritis

GENETICS

- No genetic issues have been identified.
- Congenital strictures are rare and may be linked with persistence of Chwalla's membrane.

STAGING

- No universal system
- Descriptive: Consider a location along the urethra.

—Meatus and fossa navicularis
—Pendulous (proximal, mid and distal)
—Bulbar and membranous

- Descriptive

—Length of stricture
—Nature of stricture (e.g., fibrous).

SIGNS AND SYMPTOMS

- Obstructive voiding

—Usually slow onset
—Delayed recognition, especially in young, in which symptoms occur very late due to capacity of bladder to compensate

- Other

—Urinary tract infection
—Urethral bleeding
—Epididymitis
—Urethrocutaneous fistula (extreme cases)

PATHOPHYSIOLOGY

- Etiology

—Impacts the type of stricture and the management
—Scar forms circumferentially in response to injury of epithelial lining of urethra
—Usually bonding, spongy tissue of urethral bed with epithelial layer
—Contracting down into smaller circumference; hence stricture
—The opening into spongy tissue gives rise to the possibility of extravasation.

- Types

—Congenital: rare, soft, often without spongiofibrosis
—Inflammatory
  —Used to be most common
  —Associated with STDs such as gonorrhea or nonspecific urethritis (chlamydial)
  —May involve long segments, often include bulbar urethra
—Ischemic: observed in cardiac bypass patients, ischemia was presumed cause; less common now
—Traumatic
  —Most common type in the United States
  —Blunt perineal: "straddle" injury where the urethra is trapped against the symphysis pubis; usually partial tear
  —Penetrating: gunshot wounds with varying degrees of tissue injury according to projectile and velocity
  —Iatrogenic: instrumentation: usually found at meatus or penoscrotal junction
  —Pelvic fracture: motor vehicle accidents and industrial injuries. Up to 10% of pelvic fractures will have urethral injury, which may vary from simple contusion through partial tear to complete transection with separation of the urethral ends.

CAUSES/RISK FACTORS

- Hazardous activity: unprotected sex, street fighting, motor vehicle accidents
- Urogenital instrumentation

—Catheterization
—Cystoscopy or other instrumentation (TURP, TURBT, etc.)

COMPLICATIONS

- Urinary obstruction

—Changes in voiding
  —Bladder hypertrophy/trabeculation
—Inability to instrument
  —Promotes formation of false passages on instrumentation
—Recurrent infections or stone formation

- Erectile dysfunction

—After traumatic urethral injury to the base of the penis
—Especially involving fractures of the pubic rami
—Occurs with surgical repair of urethral tear

DIFFERENTIAL DIAGNOSIS

- Benign prostatic hyperplasia
- Bladder infection
- Prostatic carcinoma
- Prostatitis
- Functional bladder disorder
- Urethral carcinoma

 Database

HISTORY

- Obstructive voiding: decrease in stream, frequency

—Bladder hyperactivity
—Frequent bladder infection; epididymitis

- Mechanism of injury

—Recent trauma
—Distant trauma or infection
—Instrumentation

- History of STD such as GC

PHYSICAL EXAMINATION

- Usually no specific findings, except with trauma
- Evidence of perineal trauma

—Hematoma of subcutaneous tissue: spreading without limit
—Hematoma of deep tissues: spread delimited by Buck's fascia, "butterfly hematoma"
—Urinoma: spread delimited by damage of the multiple layers of tissue in the penis

- Evidence of epididymitis

Diagnostic Studies

LABORATORY TESTING

- Nothing special, except as indicated by the associated circumstances (STDs, etc.)

IMAGING

- Retrograde urethrography

—Dilute (50%) intravenous contrast
—Introduced through the meatus with partially inflated Foley catheter or other nozzle
—Must fill entire urethra
—May observe some natural extravasation into bulbospongiosus with higher pressures and prostatic and bladder neck spasm

- Excretory urography and ultrasonography

—Not specific for urethra; may see some Doppler changes during voiding

- Magnetic resonance imaging: has reported utility

SPECIAL STUDIES

- Uroflowmetry: may indicate obstructive pattern
- Endoscopy

—Cystoscopy allows direct visualization of the stricture.
—With acute trauma: Identification of urethral discontinuity may permit direct cannulation of the proximal segment, thereby avoiding later intervention.

 ## Treatment

GENERAL MEASURES

- Urethral dilation

—Most conservative; may be repeated indefinitely; may be taught to patient; may cause false passages

- Urethrotomy

—The blind Otis urethrotomy is an historical curiosity.
—Optical or visual urethrotomy; cold knife or with vaporizing laser
   —With or without stenting (catheter)

- Urethral stent

—Most aggressive nonsurgical option; full utility not established; not favored for posttraumatic urethral disruption

MEDICAL

- Infection

—Include management of infection in all management strategies.

SURGICAL

- Meatal strictures: often after circumcision; meatotomy; balanitis xerotica obliterans

—Meatoplasty or pedicle island flap

- Pendulous urethral strictures: often after instrumentation and infection

—Onlay urethroplasty
—Staged repair in complex strictures
—Skin graft coverage may be required.

- Bulbar strictures: often due to urethral trauma

—Primary anastomosis for short strictures
—Onlay with pedicled island or free graft
—Two- and multistage repairs may be needed.

- Posterior urethral strictures: often due to pelvic fracture

—Most difficult to access
—Early realignment vs. drainage and late repair
   —"Cut-to-the-light" option: extended visual urethrotomy
   —Complex late repairs
   —High chance of erectile dysfunction at initial injury and repair

ALTERNATIVE THERAPIES: N/A

PATIENT EDUCATION: N/A

 ## Follow-Up

MONITORING

- High recurrence rate

—Flow rate changes are late; self-dilation is possible; endoscopic evaluation is definitive.

- Urethrography: no less traumatic than endoscopy

PREVENTION: N/A

 ## Miscellaneous

SYNONYMS: N/A

ASSOCIATED CONDITIONS

- STDs; see also Section II, "Balanitis Xerotica Obliterans."

NOTES

- Recurrence rates can be high after primary stricture repair. See also Section I, "Urethral Discharge."

ABBREVIATIONS: N/A

REFERENCES

Morehouse DD. Current indications and techniques of two-stage repair for membranous urethral strictures. *Urol Clin North Am* 1989;16:325.

Turner-Warwick R. Principles of urethral reconstruction. In: Webster GD, Kirby R, King LR, et al., eds. *Reconstructive Urology*. Oxford: Blackwell Scientific, 1993.

Author: Jeremy P.W. Heaton

Urethral Syndrome

 Basics

DESCRIPTION

- Entity in which patients suffer from frequency, urgency, and dysuria without objective urologic findings

EPIDEMIOLOGY

- More common in women during reproductive years
- Sometimes called prostatodynia in men
- Uncommon in children and the elderly

GENETICS: N/A

STAGING: N/A

SIGNS AND SYMPTOMS

- Frequency
- Urgency
- Dysuria/back or suprapubic pain
- Hesitancy

PATHOPHYSIOLOGY

- Unknown
- No consistent pathogen identified
- Some patients may be sensitive to dietary and or urinary pH changes.

CAUSES/RISK FACTORS

- History of prior urinary tract infection
- Women of child-bearing age
- Obstruction (urethral stenosis or glandular enlargement along the urethra)
- Psychogenic
- Neurogenic

COMPLICATIONS

- While there are no direct complications related, can cause significant quality-of-life problems

DIFFERENTIAL DIAGNOSIS

- Urinary tract infection
- Tumor
- Stone
- Interstitial cystitis
- STD
- Vaginitis
- Hormonal imbalance (estrogen deficiency)
- Cervicitis
- Chemical irritants (douches, spermicidal foams, contact allergies)

 Database

HISTORY

- Urinary complaints of dysuria, frequency, hesitancy: nonspecific
- May have history of UTIs
- Usually first seen by primary medical doctor or gynecologist
- There should be no history of lupus, neurologic disorders (MS), or trauma.
- Inquire about any foods that may exacerbate symptoms (i.e., cola, tea, coffee, fruits, etc.).

PHYSICAL EXAMINATION

- Specific physical findings are usually absent.
- Urologic/gynecologic examination
- Neurologic examination

 Diagnostic Studies

LABORATORY TESTING

- Urine analysis and culture should be negative.
- Swab cultures (*Trichomonas, Chlamydia,* etc.), if clinically indicated

IMAGING

- Intravenous urography with a post-void film

—If abnormal UA; not essential for diagnosis

SPECIAL STUDIES

- Uroflowmetry if incontinence is a major component; otherwise of no value
- Cystoscopy to rule out other disorders, such as tumor or interstitial cystitis
- These studies should be performed if symptoms persist more than 6 to 9 months.

Treatment

GENERAL MEASURES

- Conservative treatment always favored at first, since spontaneous resolution common
- Surgical correction of urethral stenosis (if present)
- Fulguration, resection, or cryoablation (not fully accepted due to side effects) of cystoscopically apparent trigonitis or urethritis if symptoms persist

MEDICAL

- Empiric antibiotics such as Bactrim at first. Erythromycin if no pyuria in UA
- Bladder washing with DMSO or antiinflammatory agents (not widely accepted)
- Anticholinergics, alpha-blockers, and skeletal muscle relaxants

SURGICAL

- Up to 65% of patients improved after surgery (in limited studies) if a treatable cause was found.
- Variable and controversial reports of urethral dilation relieving symptoms in women
- Urethral syndrome

ALTERNATIVE THERAPIES

- Observation: 85% to 100% improvement occurred in one study; this is the most important intervention.
- Biofeedback
- Dietary modification; avoidance of caffeine, certain fruits and vegetables
—Urinary alkalinization (i.e., water with baking soda) occasionally beneficial
—Specific dietary agents to identify and avoid
  —Beverages: alcoholic, caffeinated
  —Additives: spicy foods, vinegar, citric acid, aspartame, saccharine, artificial coloring in foods
  —Fruits: apples, bananas, citrus fruits, grapes, strawberries, and juices from these
  —Milk/dairy products: aged cheeses, eggs, sour cream, yogurt
  —Vegetables: lima beans, onions, rhubarb, most nuts
  —Meats/fish: aged, smoked, or canned products

PATIENT EDUCATION

- Reassure the patient after all other diagnoses are excluded.

Follow-Up

MONITORING

- Return visits if symptoms do not improve
- Consider a repeat cystoscopy in 1 year if symptoms do not improve and the first cystoscopy was unremarkable.
- Postoperative follow-up if surgical procedure is indicated

PREVENTION

- No prevention known at this time

Miscellaneous

SYNONYMS: N/A

ASSOCIATED CONDITIONS: N/A

NOTES

- This is a diagnosis of exclusion; see also Section I, "Dysuria," and Section II, "Interstitial Cystitis."
- If a correctable cause is found, then the diagnosis of urethral syndrome does not apply.

ABBREVIATIONS: N/A

REFERENCES

Brumfitt W, Hamilton-Miller JMT, Gillespie WA. The mysterious urethral syndrome. *BMJ* 1991b; 303:719–720.

Latham RH, Stamm WE. Urethral syndrome in women. *Urol Clin North Am* 1984;11:95–101.

Zufall R. Ineffectiveness of treatment of urethral syndrome in women. *Urology* 1978;12:337–339.

Authors: Pasquale Casale and Leonard G. Gomella

Urethritis—Gonococcal and Nongonococcal

 Basics

DESCRIPTION

• Gonococcal (GU) and nongonococcal (NGU) urethritis in men are sexually transmitted diseases usually characterized by dysuria and associated with urethral discharge. *Neisseria gonorrhoeae* (gram-negative diplococci) on Gram stain or cultured differentiates GU from NGU.

EPIDEMIOLOGY

• Gonorrhea is the most common reportable disease in the United States.
• Gonorrhea is most common in teenagers and in racial and ethnic minorities.
• Young men are prime candidates for contracting NGU.
• NGU more often affects men of higher economic status than does GU.

GENETICS: N/A

STAGING: N/A

SIGNS AND SYMPTOMS

• GU

—Urethral discharge: usually purulent, copious, and green, yellow, or white

• Infrequently may be scant, watery, or absent

—Dysuria usually as mild-to-severe burning. May present as urethral itching and occasionally no symptoms other than urethral staining on undershorts
—The pendulous urethra may be tender to palpation.
—Rarely presents with systemic symptoms

• NGU

—Urethral discharge: usually mild to moderate, clear or whitish. On rare occasion may be thick and purulent. May be absent or only noted as stain on undershorts
—Dysuria: may present as mild burning or not present at all
—Urethral itching may be the only complaint.
—Rarely presents with systemic symptoms

PATHOPHYSIOLOGY

• GU caused by *N. gonorrhoeae*
• NGU caused by several bacteria; most common:

—*Chlamydia trachomatis,* recovered in 25% to 60% of heterosexual men with NGU
—Other organisms that may be involved include *Ureaplasma urealyticum, Trichomonas vaginalis,* herpes simplex virus, and cytomegalovirus.

• Both GU and NGU are sexually transmitted diseases acquired during intercourse.
• The usual incubation period is 3 to 10 days for GU and 7 to 21 days for NGU.
• The urethra is the most common site of infection in all men.
• NGU occurs more than 50% of the time.
• *C. trachomatis* is cultured from the urethra in 4% to 35% of men with gonorrhea.

CAUSES/RISK FACTORS

• GU

—The risk of infection following a single episode of intercourse with an infected partner is approximately 17%.
—Risk increases as the number of sexual contacts increases.
—May also be transmitted through oral/anal sex with infected partner

• NGU

—Urethritis in homosexual males is more likely to be gonococcal than nongonococcal.

COMPLICATIONS

• GU

—Periurethritis, which may lead to abscess
—Urethral fibrosis, leading to stricture
—Epididymitis, which may lead to infertility or testicular atrophy
—Prostatitis, which may lead to abscess if untreated

• NGU

—Emotional problems are common. Fear of loss of sexual function or guilt may produce depression.
—May result in epididymitis and or nonbacterial prostatitis
—Usually does not cause severe physical complications in men

DIFFERENTIAL DIAGNOSIS

• Reiter syndrome: urethritis associated with conjunctivitis, arthritis, and reactive tenosynovitis

—No growth on culture, minimal number of leukocytes in urethral smear or urinalysis

 Database

HISTORY

• GU and NGU

—Relationship to sexual activity: when, type (vaginal, anal, oral)
—First episode or recurrent
—Number of sexual partners
—Severity of symptoms, i.e., burning, itching, frequency and urgency of urination
—Description of discharge: scant or copious, purulent or clear; when noted (morning, constant, any time)
—Symptoms relating to other body systems: GI, bronchopulmonary, musculoskeletal, cutaneous, neurologic

• GU symptoms are usually more severe; urethral discharge is purulent and more copious than with NGU, which is often more scant and watery.

PHYSICAL EXAMINATION

• GU and NGU

—Abdomen and flanks palpated for masses, tenderness, and bladder distention
—Scrotal contents examined for testicular and epididymal size, consistency, and tenderness
—Digital rectal examination for prostatic size, consistency, and tenderness; a prostatic smear should be obtained.

Diagnostic Studies

LABORATORY TESTING

- UA

—Fifteen or more polymorphonuclear leukocytes in high power fields of spun sediment in the first-void urine specimen correlate with urethritis.
—A positive leukocyte esterase dipstick test in the absence of urinary tract infection suggests urethritis.

- GU

—Gram-stained urethral smear and plated culture (Thayer-Martin) obtained 1 to 4 hours after voiding
  —Calcium alginate swab inserted 2 to 4 cm into urethra used to obtain specimen
—Leukocyte esterase urine dipstick test
—Midstream urinalysis to rule out urinary tract infection

- NGU

—Same as above to rule out GU
—Endourethral swab for *C. trachomatis* culture

IMAGING: N/A

SPECIAL STUDIES: N/A

 ## Treatment

GENERAL MEASURES

- GU

—Sexual intercourse should be avoided until cure.
—Sexual partners should be evaluated and treated.

- NGU

—Is the syndrome caused by different organisms that respond differently to treatment, and are and results inconsistent?
—Current recommendations from the Centers for Disease Control and Prevention are based on chlamydial infection.
—Sexual intercourse should be avoided or condoms used until cure: Sexual partners should be evaluated and treated.

MEDICAL

- GU

—Ceftriaxone 125 mg IM once

- NGU

—Azithromycin 1 g oral once, or doxycycline 100 mg oral qid × 7 days

SURGICAL: N/A

ALTERNATIVE THERAPIES

- GU

—Ciprofloxacin 500 mg once
—Ofloxacin 400 mg once
—Cefixime 400 mg oral once
—Spectinomycin 2 g IM once

- NGU

—Erythromycin 500 mg oral × 7 days
—Ofloxacin 300 mg oral bid × 7 days

PATIENT EDUCATION

- Patients should be instructed regarding the proper use of condoms.
- Having multiple sexual partners increases the risk: Patients should be instructed to inform sexual partners regarding evaluation and treatment.

 ## Follow-Up

MONITORING

- GU: Negative urethral smear and culture post-therapy
- NGU: Negative urethral smear and culture post-therapy

PREVENTION

- GU and NGU

—Proper use of condoms, if multiple sexual partners

 ## Miscellaneous

SYNONYMS: N/A

ASSOCIATED CONDITIONS

- Urethral stricture

NOTES

- See also Section I, "Urethral Discharge."

ABBREVIATIONS

- GU, gonococcal urethritis; NGU, nongonococcal urethritis

REFERENCES

Berger RE. Sexually transmitted diseases: The classic diseases. In: Walsh PC, Retik AB, Vaughan ED, Wein AJ, eds. *Campbell's Urology,* 7th ed. Philadelphia: WB Saunders, 1998:663–668.

Berger RE, Rothman I. Sexually transmitted diseases in males. In: Tanagho EA, McAninch JW, eds. *Smith's General Urology,* 14th ed. Norwalk, CT: Appleton & Lange, 1995:262–266.

Drugs for sexually transmitted diseases. *Med Lett* 1995;37:117–119.

Author: Leonard H. Finkelstein

Urolithiasis—Adult, General

 Basics

DESCRIPTION

• Urolithiasis may occur in any portion of the urinary tract and may be associated with mild-to-severe symptoms

EPIDEMIOLOGY

• More common in Caucasians than African Americans
• Peak incidence: fourth to sixth decades
• Within the United States, more common in the Northwest, Southeast, and Southwest

GENETICS

• In general, urolithiasis is associated with a polygenic defect and partial penetrance.
• Cystinuria, an unusual cause of urolithiasis, is a homozygous recessive disorder.
• Renal tubular acidosis is inherited and is associated with urolithiasis.

STAGING: N/A

SIGNS AND SYMPTOMS

• Upper urinary tract calculi

—Renal colic is classically associated with sudden-onset, severe flank pain over the affected side.
—Pain may radiate to the ipsilateral anterior lower abdominal quadrant, groin, or scrotum (labia in females).
—Patient unable to find comfortable position; pain not improved by lying still
—Associated nausea, vomiting common
—Microscopic or gross hematuria almost always present
—Fever or elevated white blood cell count if associated infection
—May be asymptomatic if stone not causing obstruction

• Lower urinary tract calculi

—May be asymptomatic
—Sudden interruption of urinary stream as stone acutely obstructs bladder neck; may lead to moderate-to-severe pain when voiding
—Microscopic or gross hematuria

PATHOPHYSIOLOGY

• Urolithiasis results from several factors:

—Supersaturation: Urine becomes oversaturated with certain types of crystal (i.e., uric acid, cystine), which then come out of solution; the saturation level is variably pH dependent, based on type of crystal

• Inhibitor deficiency: Inhibitors may limit crystal growth and aggregation (citrate and magnesium important inhibitors of urolithiasis).

CAUSES/RISK FACTORS

• Upper urinary tract calculi

—Calcium oxalate stones most common; also uric acid, cystine, struvite (magnesium ammonium phosphate), calcium phosphate
—Calcium stone formation may be due to dietary excess, hyperparathyroidism, sarcoidosis, multiple myeloma, leukemia, inappropriate loss of calcium in urine through renal tubules (renal leak), excessive intestinal absorption, inadequate levels of stone inhibitors in urine, or idiopathic.
—Uric acid stone formation may be due to dietary excess, gout, myeloproliferative disorders, chronic dehydration, Lesch-Nyhan syndrome, ingestion of uricosuric drugs (salicylates, thiazides), or idiopathic.
—Struvite stones are associated with urinary tract infection with urease-splitting organisms (*Proteus, Klebsiella,* and others), leading to alkaline urine and magnesium ammonium phosphate crystallization.
—Cystine stones are rare and associated with an inherited disorder of renal tubular reabsorption of cystine.

• Lower urinary tract calculi

—Bladder stones seen in patients with foreign material in bladder; inadequate bladder emptying as in neurogenic bladder or chronic bladder outlet obstruction (most often due to benign prostatic hyperplasia)

COMPLICATIONS

• Acute pain, necessitating hospitalization or intervention to remove stone

—Renal dysfunction (rare if two functioning kidneys present)

• Pyelonephritis, sepsis

—Dehydration secondary to nausea, vomiting
—Chronic urinary tract infection (associated with struvite stones)

DIFFERENTIAL DIAGNOSIS

• Flank/abdominal pain due to upper tract urolithiasis

—Bowel obstruction
—Appendicitis
—Mesenteric ischemia
—Abdominal aortic aneurysm
—Musculoskeletal causes of back pain
—Pyelonephritis

• Hematuria due to urolithiasis

—See Section I, "Hematuria—Adult (Gross and Microscopic)."

• Filling defect (see Section I, "Filling Defect—Upper Urinary Tract")

 Database

HISTORY

• Acute onset of severe pain; if stone partially obstructive, may have more chronic, mild-to-moderate pain

—Pain radiates to groin or lower abdomen

• Gross hematuria may be present.
• Any previous history of kidney stones or urinary tract infections?
• Family history of urolithiasis?
• Any change in urination?

—Frequency and urgency suggests stone in distal ureter or bladder calculi.

• Any history of neurogenic voiding dysfunction or obstructive urinary symptoms?

PHYSICAL EXAMINATION

• Fever present if associated infection

—Moderate, deep tenderness in flank common; greater tenderness suggests possible pyelonephritis.

• An abdominal mass suggests another cause for pain besides urolithiasis.

—Elevated heart rate and blood pressure secondary to pain

Diagnostic Studies

LABORATORY TESTING

- Urinalysis

—Microscopic hematuria unless stone has caused complete obstruction and no urine from affected side; pyuria may be present to mild degree, if significant pyuria suggests concomitant urinary tract infection

—Crystalluria may provide important information regarding the type of calculus present.

- Leukocytosis may be present if secondary infection

—Elevated creatinine may be present if bilateral obstruction or stone in solitary kidney

IMAGING

- Assessment of acute renal colic may be carried out using several different techniques:

—Computerized tomography (CT): noninfused helical CT scanning: rapid study, no need for contrast
  —First-line test of choice for most patients with acute renal colic; all stones are readily visible.
  —Pathology in other abdominal organs can also be assessed; the degree of hydronephrosis and size and location of stones can be reliably determined.
  —No information regarding renal function
—Intravenous pyelography
  —Requires IV contrast; delayed x-rays needed if high-grade obstruction present and contrast not immediately excreted; some stones radiolucent; can assess renal function
—Ultrasonography
  —Noninvasive; operator dependent; generally cannot visualize ureter in adult; its use in this setting largely superseded by availability and greater information provided by CT
—Retrograde pyelography
  —Invasive; allows for simultaneous removal of stone and/or placement of ureteral stent to relieve obstruction

SPECIAL STUDIES: N/A

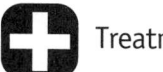 Treatment

GENERAL MEASURES

- Stones <4 to 5 mm likely to pass; stones >1 cm unlikely to pass spontaneously
- Indications for intervention

—Fever and/or infection
—Intractable pain
—Unable to tolerate oral fluid and at risk for dehydration
—Progressive renal deterioration; obstruction of solitary functioning kidney

MEDICAL

- Patients with evidence of active urinary tract infection should be treated with broad-spectrum antibiotics.
- Hydration and adequate pain control
- Drinking excessive amounts of fluids does not increase the likelihood of stone passage.
- Patients with a likelihood of spontaneously passing a stone (<4–5 mm in size) may be sent home with analgesics; should be instructed to return if pain worsens, or severe vomiting or fever
- Controversy exists regarding maximum period of observation of partially obstructing stone without development of significant irreversible renal dysfunction; generally should intervene if stone has not passed within 4 to 6 weeks

SURGICAL

- Patients with active UTI/sepsis: obstructed kidney drained by placement of ureteral stent or percutaneous nephrostomy tube

—Calculi in kidney: ESWL with or without stent placement
—Ureteral calculi: ESWL or ureteroscopic stone removal; the approach depends on size and location of stone, availability of ESWL, and patient and physician preference.
—Stent placement in anticipation of ureteral dilation and subsequent spontaneous stone passage is an option for patients with smaller ureteral calculi.

ALTERNATIVE THERAPIES: N/A

PATIENT EDUCATION

- The most important measure to avoid future stone episodes is increased fluid intake.

 Follow-Up

MONITORING

- If the stone is passed or extracted, it should be analyzed to determine stone type.

—Metabolic evaluation to assess etiology of stone formation and design preventive measures (dietary modifications, drugs) should be performed after the patient returns to baseline status; many are sometimes deferred with the first stone episode.

- Urinalysis and/or culture to assure resolution of infection and hematuria

PREVENTION

- Increased fluid intake is the single most important measure to avoid recurrent stone formation.

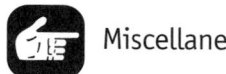 Miscellaneous

SYNONYMS: N/A

ASSOCIATED CONDITIONS

- Renal tubular acidosis, sarcoidosis, chronic diarrheal states, ileostomy, chronic UTI

NOTES

- See Sections II and III for details on specific types of stones; see Section II, "Urolithiasis—Pediatric."

ABBREVIATIONS

- ESWL, extracorporeal shock wave lithotripsy

REFERENCES

Preminger GM. Medical management of urinary calculus disease. Part 1: Pathogenesis and evaluation. AUA Update Series, Volume 14, Lesson 5, 1996.

Preminger GM. Medical management of urinary calculus disease. Part 2: Classification of metabolic disorders and selective medical management. AUA Update Series, Volume 14, Lesson 6, 1995.

Author: Glenn S. Gerber

Urolithiasis—Calcium Oxalate/Phosphate

 Basics

DESCRIPTION

• Formation of calcium salts in the urinary tract may result in a urinary stone.
• Calcium oxalate in its pure form or mixed with calcium phosphate (hydroxyapatite) is the most common type of renal calculus seen in industrialized countries.

EPIDEMIOLOGY

• Urinary tract stone disease affects 1% to 5% of the population in industrialized countries.
• U.S. annual stone incidence: 16.4 in 10,000
• One in 8 men and 1 in 20 women stone during lifetime
• The recurrence rate without treatment for calcium oxalate stones is 10% at 1 year, 35% at 5 years, and 50% at 10 years.
• Stone incidence by composition: calcium oxalate: 30% to 35%; mixed calcium oxalate and calcium phosphate: 30% to 35%

GENETICS

• Calcium oxalate: multifactorial; hypercalciuria an autosomal dominate trait
• Idiopathic hypercalciuria: 5% to 10% of normals and 50% with calcium nephrolithiasis
• Familial tendency to form stones

STAGING: N/A

SIGNS AND SYMPTOMS

• See Section II, "Urolithiasis—Adult."

PATHOPHYSIOLOGY

• Hypercalciuria may be heterogeneous in origin.
• Normocalcemic hypercalciuria (idiopathic hypercalciuria): 30% to 60% of all patients with calcium oxalate stones

—Absorptive hypercalciuria (AH)
  —Intestinal hyperabsorption of calcium; increased circulating calcium
  —Hypercalciuria is secondary to increased filtered load and reduced renal tubular reabsorption due to ↓ PTH.
  —Renal loss of calcium compensates for increased absorption and maintains normal serum calcium.
  —Hypercalciuria: >4 mg/kg body weight/24 h on a random diet (greater than 250 mg/24 h in women and 300 mg/24 h in men), or per Pak et al. (1975): >200 mg/24 h after a modified stone diet of 1 week's adherence to 400-mg calcium and 100-mEq sodium intake per day
  —AH type I: severe form; persistent hypercalciuria >200 mg/24 h on random diet or restricted diet with normocalcemia and normal or slightly ↓ PTH level; 2-hour fasting urinary calcium is normal.

  —AH type II: mild form; hypercalciuria on random diet but normocalciuria on calcium/sodium-restricted diet, normocalcemia and normal PTH level
  —AH type III: Vitamin D–dependent hypercalciuria, renal phosphate "leak"; low serum phosphate, elevated urinary phosphate, and calcium-enhanced vitamin D3 synthesis by the kidney lead to increased intestinal calcium absorption.
—Renal hypercalciuria (renal leak)
  —Impaired renal tubular reabsorption of calcium
  —Decreased in serum calcium; ↑ PTH; ↑ Vitamin D3, and increase in intestinal hyperabsorption
  —Serum calcium is normal, and the mild elevation in PTH is secondary.
  —Urinary calcium remains elevated on both random and restricted diets; 2-hour fasting urinary calcium is increased.
—Resorptive hypercalciuria
  —Primary hyperparathyroidism
  —Elevated serum and urinary calcium secondary to ↑ PTH secretion, causing excessive resorption of bone and an increased intestinal hyperabsorption of calcium due to action of ↑ PTH and increased renal synthesis of vitamin D3
  —2-hour fasting urinary calcium is increased.
—Unclassified hypercalciuria
  —Hypercalciuria with normal serum calcium, normal PTH, and increased 2-hour fasting urinary calcium
  —Use of sodium cellulose phosphate may help to distinguish AH by eliminating the problem of inadequate dietary preparation prior to fast and load calcium studies, renal hypercalciuria by reducing the suppressive effect of absorbed calcium on parathyroid stimulation.
—Other causes of calcium oxalate nephrolithiasis
  —Hyperuricosuria (urinary uric acid >600 mg/24 h
  —Only abnormality in 10% of calcium nephrolithiasis
  —Up to 40% of calcium stone-formers with other physiochemical abnormalities
  —May initiate calcium oxalate stone formation by direct induction of heterogeneous nucleation of calcium oxalate crystals, or by absorption of certain macromolecular inhibitors

—Hyperoxaluria
  —Urinary oxalate in excess of 45 mg/24 h
  —Mild hyperoxaluria (45–80 mg/24 h) is as important a risk factor for idiopathic calcium oxalate stones as hypercalciuria and is found in 37% of patients with calcium oxalate stones.
  —Activity of stone disease correlates better with level of urinary oxalate than calcium.
  —Most common cause is intestinal hyperabsorption of oxalate: ileal disease (enteric), inflammatory bowel disease; gastric or small bowel resection; jejunoileal bypass
  —Bile salts and fatty acids increase large-bowel oxalate absorption.
  —Fat malabsorption causes calcium to complex with bile acids and form calcium soap, which reduces the amount of free calcium in the intestinal lumen, which can complex with oxalate, and increases oxalate availability for absorption.
  —Stone formation is secondary to hyperoxaluria but is also contributed to by low-volume urinary output, low citrate secondary to hypokalemia, and chronic metabolic acidosis.
  —Low magnesium levels may also be secondary to intestinal malabsorption.
—Primary hyperoxaluria type I
  —Autosomal recessive, secondary defect of enzyme alanine–glyoxalate aminotransferase (AGT)
  —Increased urinary levels of oxalic, glycolic, and glyoxylic acids.
  —Clinically, nephrocalcinosis, tissue deposition of oxalate, and renal failure, with death by age 20 if untreated
  —Two-thirds have undetectable AGT on liver biopsy, and glyoxylate is oxidized to oxalate.
—Primary hyperoxaluria type II
  —Rare deficiency of D-glycerate dehydrogenase and glyoxalate reductase
  —Only 21 cases reported
  —Increased urinary oxalate and glycerate with nephrocalcinosis and renal failure
—Less common causes of hyperoxaluria
  —Excessive dietary intake of oxalate-rich foods (dark green vegetables, tea, cola, concentrated fruit juices, chocolate)
  —Substrate excess, vitamin C ingestion greater than 1000 mg/24 h
  —Pyridoxine (vitamin B6) deficiency ethylene glycol toxicity; converted in liver to glycoaldehyde and glycolic acid methoxyflurane anesthesia; converted in liver to oxalate

—Hypocitraturia
  —Less than 220 mg/24 h
  —Sole abnormality in 10% and identified with other causes of calcium nephrolithiasis in 15% to 60% of patients
  —Acidosis most important etiologic factor in hypocitraturia
  —Acidosis reduces urinary citrate secondary to the increase renal tubular reabsorption and decreased synthesis.
  —Causes of metabolic acidosis: inflammatory bowel disease, chronic diarrhea; thiazide-induced hypokalemia, and intracellular acidosis; purine-rich diet (high acid-ash); strenuous physical exercise (lactic acidosis); renal tubular acidosis (type I, distal); increased sodium intake. UTI with bacteria degrading citrate lowers urinary saturation of calcium salts by forming soluble complexes with calcium.
—Hypomagnesuria
  —Less than 50 mg/24 h
  —May coexist with hypocitraturia in two-thirds of patients
  —May coexist with low volume (less than 1 L/24 h) in 40% of patients
  —Exact pathogenesis is not known; may be of dietary origin
  —A common cause is inflammatory bowel disease and malabsorption.

CAUSES/RISK FACTORS

- Drach classification: intrinsic or extrinsic

—Intrinsic risk factors: hereditary/genetic
  —Polygenic defect with partial penetrance
  —Hypercalciuria inherited as autosomal dominant trait
  —Urinary calculi are rare in Native Americans, Blacks, and native-born Israelis.
  —Blacks have a higher prevalence of stones associated with infection.
  —Age of peak incidence: 20 to 40 years
  —Male-to-female ratio: 3:1; females have a higher incidence of infection stones or defects causing stones, such as cystinuria or hyperparathyroidism.
  —Studies suggest that higher levels of testosterone may increase endogenous liver production of oxalate to account for the higher incidence in males.
  —Coincident illness: inflammatory bowel disease, chronic pancreatitis, chronic diarrheal states, hyperparathyroidism medullary sponge kidney, recurrent UTI

—Extrinsic risk factors
  —Geography/climate
  —Stones are more prevalent in the United States in the mountainous Northwest, tropical Southeast, and arid Southwest.
  —Increased heat/humidity in the summer months has been associated with a higher incidence.
  —Higher temperature increases perspiration, leading to concentrated urine and increased crystallization.
  —Increased exposure to sunlight may lead to increased production of vitamin D3 and increased urinary calcium excretion.
  —Diet: Increased dietary protein, oxalates, refined sugars, and calcium, and decreased fiber intake are all risk factors.
  —A high-protein diet causes increased fixed-acid load and may cause mild resorption of bone and reduced renal tubular reabsorption of calcium, resulting in increased urinary calcium, decreased urinary pH and citrate excretion, and elevated urinary uric acid.
  —A high salt intake increases urinary calcium and decreases citrate.
  —Calcium restriction may be ineffective for patients who may be normocalciuric, and without oxalate restriction may lead to increased urinary oxalate, since less calcium is available in the intestinal lumen to bind oxalate and prevent its absorption.
  —An increase in urinary oxalate produces a greater stone risk with respect to urinary saturation of calcium oxalate than does an equimolar increase in urinary calcium.
—Water intake
  —Fluid consumption, especially of water, to produce greater than 2 L/24 h of urine output, reduces risk.
  —Urine dilution may increase ion activity and dilute urinary inhibitors, increasing risk of crystallization.
  —Dilution effects are probably offset by the reduced time that free crystals remain in the urinary tract.
  —Water hardness is caused by dissolved calcium and magnesium.
  —The harder the water, the worse it tastes.
  —Studies conflict on whether stones are more prevalent in areas with hard or soft water.
—Occupation
  —Stones are more likely in patients with sedentary occupations than in manual laborers.
  —Stones are more likely in white-collar than in blue-collar workers.
  —May be more related to diet than activity; upper socioeconomic individuals may have diets rich in animal protein.

COMPLICATIONS

- Pain, hematuria, infection, loss of renal function

DIFFERENTIAL DIAGNOSIS

- Hypercalcemia: primary hyperparathyroidism, RTA, vitamin D excess, immobilization, sarcoidosis, metastatic malignancies, milk–alkali syndrome, hyperthyroidism, myxedema, adrenal insufficiency, furosemide administration
- Filling defect: See Section I, "Filling Defect—Upper Urinary Tract."
- Flank pain: See Section I, "Flank Pain"

(continued)

Urolithiasis—Calcium Oxalate/Phosphate (continued)

 Database

HISTORY

• Review stone history, family history of stones, and the intrinsic and extrinsic risk factors noted above.

PHYSICAL EXAMINATION

• Look for coincident illness.

 Diagnostic Studies

• In deciding which kidney stone-formers need a metabolic evaluation, several points should be kept in mind:

—A predisposing urinary abnormality or underlying disease is identified in 80% to 90% of patients.
—A prescribed treatment program may need to be maintained for life.
—50% to 60% of patients pass only one stone in their lifetime.
—Involve your patient in the decision to do a work-up; explain risk and benefits of an extensive evaluation.

• Criteria for medical evaluation

—Recurrent stone formation
—Metabolically active (demonstrate x-ray evidence of new stone formation or stone growth within the past year or the documented passage of a new stone or gravel)
—Positive family history
—History of major stone complications
—Solitary kidney
—Age at onset less than 20 years
—Significant number of intrinsic or extrinsic risk factors
—History of metabolic stone (uric acid or cystine), infection stone (struvite), or pure calcium phosphate stone (rule out RTA or hyperparathyroidism)

LABORATORY TESTS

• Stone analysis
• SMA20
• Urinalysis, urine culture
• 24-hour urine (volume, calcium, oxalate, citrate, sodium, phosphate, magnesium, pH, uric acid, sulfate)
• Lab data are best obtained on a diet at least 1 month after acute stone passage or 1 week after IVP studies.
• Have the patient discontinue any medications that may affect the tests (vitamins, antacids, diuretics, acetazolamide, allopurinol, or other stone medications).
• When hypercalciuria is identified on a random diet, the patient should be placed on a 1-week modified diet: restrict calcium to 400 mg and sodium to 100 mEq per day.
• After 1 week on a modified diet, repeat 24-hour urine for volume, calcium, sodium, and oxalate, and obtain a serum calcium and PTH to help classify the type of hypercalciuria.
• A calcium fast and load test (as per Pak et al.) may further characterize hypercalciuria (see reference).

IMAGING

• IVP, ultrasound, and spiral CT are all useful imaging.

SPECIAL STUDIES: N/A

Treatment

GENERAL MEASURES

- Should be tailored to patient need
- First-time stone-formers at low risk for recurrence should follow a conservative approach.
- Conservative treatment (appropriate for all stone-forming patients, regardless of the etiology of their stone disease)

—High fluid intake, at least 8 to 10 (10-oz) glasses/day (water is best): "Drink to keep urine clear."
—Sodium restriction: Avoid salty foods and the salt shaker.
—Oxalate restriction: Avoid excessive oxalate sources.
—Protein restriction: 8 oz of meat, chicken, or fish per day; have a "vegetarian day" each week.
—Avoid extremes of calcium intake. One serving with each meal is generally acceptable; avoid late at night; avoid stone-provoking drugs, calcium supplements, vitamin D, p-binding antacids, furosemide, uricosuric agents, and triamterene.

MEDICAL

- Selective treatment (for recurrent or at high risk for recurrence)

—Absorptive hypercalciuria type I
—Dx: urinary calcium >300 mg/24 h on random diet and >200 mg/24 h on restricted diet; normal serum calcium and PTH
—Rx: sodium cellulose phosphate (2.5–5.0 g with each meal)
—Restrict dietary oxalate.
—Magnesium supplementation
—Long-term use can induce a negative calcium balance; need to monitor bone density
—Thiazide (does not correct cause of AH, possible rebound)
—Hydrochlorothiazide (HCTZ) 50 mg bid
—Trichlormethiazide (Naqua) 2 to 4 mg/d; reduce salt intake.
—Potassium citrate supplementation (20 mEq bid)
—Absorptive hypercalciuria type II
—Dx: urinary calcium >300 mg/24 h on random diet and <200 mg/24 h on restricted diet; normal serum calcium and PTH; and no evidence of bone disease
—Rx: moderate dietary calcium restriction (600 mg per day or 1 to 2 servings of dairy with meals); sodium restriction; thiazide as above if conservative approach not effective; potassium citrate supplementation
—Absorptive hypercalciuria type III
—Dx: urinary calcium >300 mg/24 h, increased urinary phosphate, normal serum calcium and PTH, decreased serum phosphate
—Rx: orthophosphate (Neutra-Phos-K) 250 to 500 mg tid/qid

—Renal hypercalciuria
—Dx: urinary calcium >300 mg/24 h on random diet and >200 mg/24 h on restricted diet; normal serum calcium and slightly increased PTH
—Rx: thiazide, increases tubular reabsorption; hydrochlorothiazide 50 mg bid; trichlormethiazide (Naqua) 4 mg/d potassium citrate supplementation (Polycitra K syrup 15–30 mL bid; Polycitra K crystals 1 packet bid; Urocit K 10–20 mEq bid); sodium restriction (2-g sodium diet; keep urinary sodium <100 mg/d)
—Hyperuricosuric calcium nephrolithiasis
—Dx: low-volume 24-hour urine, chronic urinary acidity pH <6.0, hx animal protein excess, urinary uric acid >600 mg/24 h
—Rx: increased fluid intake; reduced dietary purine, especially red meat; urinary alkalization (raise pH to 6.5–7.0), potassium citrate; reduce endogenous uric acid production (allopurinol 300 mg/d); if serum uric acid >8 mg/dL, if urinary uric acid >800 mg/24 h
—Hypocitraturic calcium nephrolithiasis
—Dx: urinary citrate <220 mg/24 h, evidence of RTA, chronic diarrhea, or thiazide treatment
—Rx: potassium citrate, increases intracellular pH, which increase citrate production
—Hyperoxaluria
—Dx: urinary oxalate >45 mg/24 h, hx dietary oxalate excess
—Rx: high fluid intake; low-oxalate diet; calcium supplementation (calcium citrate, Tums); therapy to control diarrhea pyridoxine (vitamin B6), 100 to 800 mg/d
—Type I RTA
—Dx: inability to acidify urine pH >5.5, (serum K, CO_2, low urinary citrate)
—Rx: potassium citrate

SURGICAL

- See Section II, "Urolithiasis—Adult, General."

ALTERNATIVE THERAPIES: N/A

PATIENT EDUCATION

- Stress need for adequate hydration

 Follow-Up

MONITORING

- Patients with recurrent stones on medical therapy require regular follow-up to monitor their progress.

PREVENTION

- Hydration is effective at minimizing stone risk.

 Miscellaneous

SYNONYMS: N/A

ASSOCIATED CONDITIONS: N/A

NOTES: N/A

ABBREVIATIONS

- AH, absorptive hypercalciuria; PTH, parathyroid hormone; RTA, renal tubular acidosis

REFERENCES

Menon M, Parulkar BG, Drach GW. Urinary lithiasis: Etiology, diagnosis and medical management. In: Walsh PC, Retik AB, Vaughan ED, Wein AJ, eds. *Campbell's Urology*, 7th ed. Philadelphia: WB Saunders, 1998.

Pak CYC, et al. A simple test for the diagnosis of absorptive, resorptive and renal hypercalciurias. *N Engl J Med* 1975;292:497.

Preminger GM. Medical management of urinary calculus disease. Part I: Pathogenesis and evaluation. AUA Update Series, Volume XIV, Lesson 5, 1995.

Preminger GM. Medical management of urinary calculus disease. Part II: Classification of metabolic disorders and selective medical management. AUA Update Series, Volume XIV, Lesson 6, 1995.

Author: John J. Pahira

Urolithiasis—Cysteine and Cystinuria

 Basics

DESCRIPTION

- Cysteine stones are only seen in patients who have cystinuria
- Cysteine stone formation is a common problem in homozygotes

EPIDEMIOLOGY

- 1% to 2% of urinary calculi in the overall stone-patient population
- Worldwide prevalence of homozygous cystinuria varies from 1 in 7000 to 1 in 100,000.
- Heterozygous cystinuria 1 in 20 to 1 in 200

GENETICS

- The homozygous recessive state excretes >400 mg cystine per day. Carries a substantial risk for stone formation
- Heterozygotes generally excrete 100 to 300 mg cystine per day. Only rarely form cystine stones

STAGING: N/A

SIGNS AND SYMPTOMS

- Same as any stone-former; although, because of the genetic basis, cystinurics may present in the pediatric age group. However, stone formation usually begins in the second or third decade.

PATHOPHYSIOLOGY

- Inherited genetic mutation that codes for a defect of small intestinal mucosal absorption and renal tubular absorption of the four dibasic amino acids (COLA):

—Cystine, ornithine, lysine, and arginine

- Only cystine is relatively insoluble across the normal urinary pH range.

—This results in supersaturation and crystallization of cystine stones.

- Increased urine pH increases solubility and decreases stones

CAUSES/RISK FACTORS

- The only known risk factor for cystine stones is inheritance of the genetic mutation.

COMPLICATIONS

- Recurrent stone disease

—Potential for obstruction or infection
—Irreversible loss of renal function is rare with contemporary diagnosis and treatment.

DIFFERENTIAL DIAGNOSIS

- Cystine stones may be confused with calcium oxalate/phosphate stones, magnesium-ammonium-calcium phosphate stones, or uric acid stones, though clinical distinction should be apparent.

 Database

HISTORY

- Age of onset of stones

—May be pediatric or geriatric; usually second or third decade

- Family history of stones

—Particularly siblings

- May be asymptomatic or, with an acute episode, usual symptoms of stones, including hematuria, flank pain, etc.

PHYSICAL EXAMINATION

- Often no particular findings
- May be consistent with acute stone episode (CVA tenderness, etc.)

 Diagnostic Studies

LABORATORY TESTING

- Urinalysis

—Hexagonal crystals are diagnostic.
—24-hour urine for quantitative cystine determination
  —Normal: 40 to 60 mg/g creatinine
  —Increased: heterozygotes 100 to 300 mg/g creatinine/d; homozygotes >400 mg/g creatinine

- Stone analysis

—Cystine alone
—Cystine combined with calcium oxalate/phosphate or struvite

IMAGING

- Plain radiographs

—Homogeneous, lightly opaque stone
—May take on a "staghorn" appearance with rounded edges and "daughter" stones proximal to an obstructing pelvic or infundibular stone

- Ultrasound appearance

—Highly echogenic with acoustic shadowing

- CT appearance (without intravenous contrast)

—High Hounsfield units, essentially indistinguishable from other types of stones

SPECIAL STUDIES: N/A

Treatment

GENERAL MEASURES

- Hydration
—Urinary output to exceed 2 L per day
- Salt restriction
—Dietary sodium increases cystine excretion.

MEDICAL

- Urinary alkalization to a pH range of 7.5 to 8.0 to increase urinary solubility

—Start with potassium citrate, 10-mEq tablets, 2 tablets qid, and adjust as necessary.
—Alternatives are balanced citrates and sodium bicarbonate, though the sodium load should be considered.

- Thiol derivatives will decrease urinary cystine excretion by binding to cystine to form cysteine. This is then relatively soluble.

—Alpha-mercapto-proprionylglycine (Thiola)
  —The best agent
  —800 to 1200 mg daily in 4 divided doses is generally adequate.
  —Titrate to keep urinary cystine excretion <400 mg daily.
  —Side effects include gastrointestinal intolerance, rash, arthralgia, leukopenia, proteinuria, and nephrotic syndrome.
  —Pyridoxine supplementation should be given to prevent vitamin B6 deficiency.
—D-penicillamine (Cuprimine) 1 to 2 g daily in divided doses may be used as an alternative, but the incidence and severity of these same side effects are higher than with Thiola.

- Captopril is also a thiol derivative, which can decrease urinary cystine.

—25 to 50 mg tid can be given for those patients who fail fluids, alkalization, and standard thiols, or when any cystinuric requires antihypertensive medication.

SURGICAL

- Shock wave lithotripsy

—Cystine stones do not reliably fragment with extracorporeal shock wave lithotripsy.
—This treatment is generally limited to cystine stones <1.0 to 1.5 cm.
- Percutaneous management

—Percutaneous management is the mainstay of treatment for most large cystine stones in the kidney.
—With percutaneous access, cystine stones may be fragmented readily with ultrasound, holmium laser, electrohydraulic lithotripsy, or Lithoclast.
- Ureteroscopy

—Approach of choice for most ureteral cystine stones that fail to pass spontaneously
—A ureteroscopic approach may also be used to access some pyelocalyceal cystine stones.
—The holmium laser is the intracorporeal lithotriptor of choice with ureteroscopic access.

ALTERNATIVE THERAPIES

- Dietary methionine restriction

—Generally unpalatable and rarely adhered to. Urinary cystine levels will fall only negligibly.

PATIENT EDUCATION

- Explain that this is a congenital problem.

—Advise regarding the importance of lifelong monitoring and treatment.

 Follow-Up

MONITORING

- See the patient every 6 to 12 months.

—KUB or ultrasound at those intervals, depending on metabolic activity
- Serum studies and urinalysis at regular intervals to follow patients on thiol derivatives

PREVENTION

- Same as treatment

—Hydration and alkalization
—Thiols for patients who fail hydration and alkalization

 Miscellaneous

SYNONYMS: N/A

ASSOCIATED CONDITIONS: N/A

NOTES

- See also Section II, "Urolithiasis—Adult, General" and "Urolithiasis—Pediatric."

ABBREVIATIONS: N/A

REFERENCES

Chow GK, Streem SB. Medical management of cystinuria: Results of contemporary clinical practice. *J Urol* 1996;156:1576.

Streem SB. Medical and surgical management of cystine stones. *Probl Urol* 1993;7(4):523.

Author: Stevan B. Streem

Urolithiasis—Infectious (Struvite)

 Basics

DESCRIPTION

- *Infectious calculi* usually refers to those that are composed of magnesium ammonium phosphate (struvite) or magnesium ammonium phosphate and calcium phosphate (triple phosphate) and that result from chronic infections with urease-producing bacteria.

EPIDEMIOLOGY

- 15% to 20% of upper urinary tract calculi
- More common in women

GENETICS: N/A

STAGING: N/A

SIGNS AND SYMPTOMS

- Infection symptoms

—Frequency, urgency, dysuria
—Fever
—Flank pain: dull ache or colic

- Hematuria

PATHOPHYSIOLOGY

- Urease-producing bacteria

—Hydrolyze urea into NH_3 and CO_2
—Common organisms include *Proteus, Klebsiella, Serratia, Pseudomonas,* and *Staphylococcus.*
—*E. coli* may rarely produce urease.

- Struvite crystallization occurs with an alkaline pH and supersaturation with OH^-, NH_4^+, and CO_3^-.

CAUSES/RISK FACTORS

- Neurogenic voiding dysfunction
- Indwelling catheters
- Urinary diversions

—All are at high risk for urinary tract infections.
—May have urease-producing bacterial infections without any anatomic or functional abnormality

COMPLICATIONS

- Obstruction
- Pyonephrosis
- Parenchymal or perinephric abscess
- Urosepsis

DIFFERENTIAL DIAGNOSIS

- Staghorn calculi of other compositions

—Uric acid
—Cystine

- Urolithiasis of any etiology with secondary infection with any type bacteria
- A stone acts as foreign body, making eradication difficult.

 Database

HISTORY

- Infection

—Acute or chronic symptoms
—Frequency, urgency, dysuria
—Persistent, difficult to eradicate

- Flank pain

—Colic or dull ache

- May be entirely asymptomatic

—Stones may grow to a massive size without symptoms.

PHYSICAL EXAMINATION

- Flank mass/tenderness

—Perinephric abscess

 Diagnostic Studies

LABORATORY TESTING

- Urinalysis

—Pyuria
—Hematuria

- Urine culture and sensitivity

—Often persistence of same organism despite appropriate antibiotics

IMAGING

- Intravenous urography or plain abdominal radiograph

—Staghorn calculus
  —Hallmark of struvite stone formation
  —Density depends on carbonate apatite content
  —May be laminated
—Needed to define intrarenal anatomy
—To assess renal function

- Radionuclide renography

—To define renal function if poor on IVU

- Computerized tomography/spiral CT

—To define extent of stone
—To evaluate parenchymal and perinephric involvement
—To evaluate adjacent organs and structures

SPECIAL STUDIES: N/A

Treatment

GENERAL MEASURES

- Goals of therapy

—Eliminate the infection.
—Remove all stones.
—Preserve renal function and parenchyma.

- Maintain high urine output.
- Acidify the urine.

MEDICAL

- Antibiotics

—May slow stone growth and ameliorate symptoms
—Cannot sterilize urine in presence of stone
—Penicillin and derivatives useful for *Proteus*
—Always check sensitivities.

- Acetohydroxamic acid

—Inhibition of bacterial urease
—Neurologic, hematologic, and dermatologic side effects are common.

SURGICAL

- Shock wave lithotripsy

—May be used as primary therapy for delicate or partial staghorn calculi
   —If little stone burden
   —Often requires adjunctive use of retrograde catheter or stent

- Percutaneous nephrostolithotomy

—Particularly useful for debulking of large staghorn calculi
—Frequently in combination with or as sandwich therapy around shock wave lithotripsy
—Combination less morbid than either modality alone

- Ureteroscopy: useful for ureteral fragments
- Anatrophic nephrolithotomy

—Rarely indicated today; mostly of historical interest
—Bivalve kidney to remove all stones

- Nephrectomy

—For poorly functioning or nonfunctioning kidney
—For management of refractory pyonephrosis, perinephric abscess

ALTERNATIVE THERAPIES

- Renal irrigation

—Hemiacidrin or Suby G solution; useful as adjunct to surgery

PATIENT EDUCATION

- Management usually requires referral to a tertiary care setting due to specialized techniques and instrumentation.

 Follow-Up

MONITORING

- Surveillance urine cultures

—At least monthly after treatment, especially after discontinuing antibiotics, until proven sterile for several months

PREVENTION

- Suppressive antibiotics for 3 to 6 months after stone removal
- High urine output
- Urinary acidification
- Evaluate for other underlying metabolic disorders.

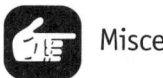 Miscellaneous

SYNONYMS

- Staghorn calculus; struvite stones

ASSOCIATED CONDITIONS

- Neurogenic bladder, urinary diversion

NOTES

- See also Section II, "Urolithiasis—Adult, General" and "Urolithiasis—Pediatric."

ABBREVIATIONS: N/A

REFERENCES

Lingeman JE, Newmark JR, Wong MYC. Classification and management of staghorn calculi. In: Smith AD, ed. *Controversies in Endourology*. Philadelphia: WB Saunders, 1995:136–145.

Menon M, Parulkar BG, Drach GW. Urinary lithiasis: Etiology, diagnosis and medical management. In: Walsh PC, Retik AB, Vaughan ED, Wein AJ, eds. *Campbell's Urology*, 7th ed. Philadelphia: WB Saunders, 1998:2661–2733.

Sequra JW, Preminger GM, Assimos DG, et al. Nephrolithiasis clinical guidelines panel summary report on the management of staghorn calculi. *J Urol* 1994;151:1648–1651.

VanArsdalen KN, Banner MP, Pollack HM. Radiographic imaging and urologic decision making in the management of renal and ureteral calculi. *Urol Clin North Am* 1990;17:171–190.

Author: Keith VanArsdalen

Urolithiasis—Pediatric

 Basics

DESCRIPTION

• Urinary stone formation in children is the clinical manifestation of a number of different disorders. Metabolic disorders and anatomic anomalies are common, so complete metabolic and anatomic evaluations are necessary in pediatric stone-formers.
• Classification: infection, anatomic, metabolic, or idiopathic

EPIDEMIOLOGY

• Rare in industrialized countries
• Geographic differences

—Middle/Far East: bladder stones; male predominance; ammonium acid urate and oxalate; lower socioeconomic strata
—Europe: more than in United States; male predominance, usually <5 years; mostly upper tract (infectious: *Proteus*); magnesium ammonium phosphate
—United States (rare): 1/50 of adult urolithiasis population; rare secondary to infection; higher percentage of metabolic stone-formers; calcium oxalate

GENETICS

• Cystinuria: autosomal recessive
• Xanthinuria: autosomal recessive
• Renal tubular acidosis (RTA): autosomal dominant in small subset of patients
• Primary hyperoxaluria: autosomal recessive

STAGING: N/A

SIGNS AND SYMPTOMS

• Varies from silent occurrence with microscopic hematuria to acute renal colic. Staghorn calculi present insidiously.

PATHOPHYSIOLOGY

• Stone formation: same as adults

—Urinary crystals bind to form a nidus, which grows to form a stone.
—Solute concentration (state of hydration), urinary pH, concentration of crystallization inhibitors, presence of infection, and urinary obstruction contribute to stone formation.
—Crystallization of uric acid and cystine are enhanced in acidic urine.
—Infection stones (magnesium ammonium phosphate) are formed in alkaline urine.
—Calcium oxalate urolithiasis is not affected by urinary pH.

• Infection

—Magnesium ammonium phosphate (struvite) and calcium phosphate stones
—Urea-splitting organisms
—Younger patients
—Vesicoureteral reflux in ±15% of patients; recurrence rate: 14%

• Anatomic

—Congenital anomalies of the urinary tract: UPJ obstruction, neurogenic bladders, and following bladder neck surgery
—High recurrence rate (27%)

• Metabolic stone formation
—Cystinuria
    —Autosomal recessive disorder of amino acid transport
    —Excessive excretion of dibasic amino acids: cystine, ornithine, lysine, and arginine (COLA)
    —The homozygote is the stone-former; the heterozygote is the carrier of the gene.
    —The homozygote excretes large amounts of dibasic amino acids; the heterozygote excretes levels greater than normal individuals.
—RTA
    —Type I RTA: disorder of hydrogen ion excretion; hyperchloremic acidosis; urinary calcium loss leads to growth retardation/osteomalacia; hypercalciuria with diminished citrate excretion leads to stone formation (nephrocalcinosis); calcium phosphate stones; acquired: dysproteinemias, lupoid hepatitis, Sjögren syndrome, Wilson disease, primary biliary cirrhosis, jejunoileal bypass
—Hypercalcemia/hypercalciuria
    —Hypercalcemia: common: immobilization ("latent" stone-former); rare: primary hyperparathyroidism; sarcoidosis; hypervitaminosis D; milk-alkali syndrome
    —Hypercalciuria: absorptive hypercalciuria vs. renal hypercalciuria; postfurosemide stone formation (in premature infants); inhibition of chloride absorption by furosemide causes hypercalciuria; diminished urinary output (<1.5 cc/kg/h), alkaline urine, and prolonged furosemide use are risk factors.
—Uric acid lithiasis
    —Uncommon
    —Secondary to myeloproliferative (purine turnover) or intestinal tract (fluid and bicarbonate losses) disease
—Primary hyperoxaluria: two types of enzymatic disorders:
    —Type 1, glycolic aciduria: deficiency of alanine—glyoxylate aminotransferase of liver cells (increased urinary oxalic and glycolic acids)
    —Type 2, L-glyceric aciduria; deficiency of D-glyceric dehydrogenase; increased endogenous production of oxalate with hyperoxaluria, urolithiasis, nephrocalcinosis, and renal injury; oxalosis: deposition of calcium oxalate in extrarenal sites when renal insufficiency is present

- Idiopathic stones

—Similar to adult stone-formers
—Calcium oxalate stones
—Diagnosis of exclusion
—Categories: hypercalciuria, hyperoxaluria, hyper-uricosuria, hypocitruria

CAUSES/RISK FACTORS

- Endemic stones: dietary factors
- Urinary tract infection, urinary obstruction
- Family history, genetic predisposition

COMPLICATIONS

- Acute ureteral obstruction and colic, hematuria, loss of renal function, perpetuation of urinary tract infection, loss of school/work time

DIFFERENTIAL DIAGNOSIS

- Causes of hematuria (see Section I, "Hematuria—Pediatric")
- Causes of acute abdominal pain (see Section I, "Flank Pain")

 Database

HISTORY

- Family history: cystinuria, uric acid lithiasis, primary hyperoxaluria, RTA
- History: prematurity, use of diuretics, history of immobilization, low fluid intake
- Dietary habits, age of onset
- Previous intestinal or urinary disorders or surgery

PHYSICAL EXAMINATION

- Nonspecific, costovertebral angle tenderness, or abdominal signs
- Fever, suggesting urinary tract infection

 Diagnostic Studies

LABORATORY TESTING

- Urinalysis: Look for crystals.

—Cystine: hexagonal crystals, best seen with infrared spectrography

- RTA: second morning voided specimen; pH >5.5
- Serum electrolytes and creatinine

IMAGING

- Ultrasound, intravenous pyelogram, nonenhanced helical computerized tomography
- Voiding cystourethrography essential in all children with stones

SPECIAL STUDIES

- Cyanide nitroprusside test to detect cystine (positive with values greater than 75 mg/g creatinine)

—Note: false positives in Fanconi syndrome or Wilson disease
—Confirm a positive test with 24-hour collection.

- 24-hour urine collection for calcium, creatinine, citrate, cystine, oxalate, phosphate, uric acid

—Cystine: >400 mg cystine/d (normal: 50 mg/d)

- RTA: inability to form acid urine pH (<5.5) in the presence of systemic acidosis

—Ammonium chloride loading test (100 mg/kg/24 h) to confirm RTA (solution: 500 mg/5 cc)

- Renal leak hypercalciuria: elevated urine calcium after fasting ("fasting hypercalciuria")
- Calcium/creatinine ratio (normal: <0.2)
- Fasting-calcium loading test (Pak test)

—Calcium- and sodium-restricted diet for 7 days prior to test
—Hydration, calcium load of 14.3 mg/kg
—4-hour urine collection
    —Absorptive hypercalciuria: normal fasting urine calcium excretion, hypercalciuria with calcium load
    —Renal hypercalciuria: Fasting urine calcium is elevated.

(continued)

Urolithiasis—Pediatric (continued)

 Treatment

GENERAL MEASURES

- Hydration: essential in the management of all stone-formers

—Fluid intake should be 50 cc/kg/24 h, drinking every hour while awake, and awakened halfway through the sleep cycle to drink two glasses of water; maintain a urine output of 35 mL/kg/d.

- Dietary restrictions

—Cystinuria: Restrict dietary methionine and sodium; this is a difficult diet, particularly in children.
—Uricosuria: Restrict dietary protein (meats, peanuts, etc.).

- Early ambulation after orthopedic procedures or fractures
- Infection stones: complete stone clearance and prevention of further infection

MEDICAL

- Infection stones

—Broad-spectrum antibiotics, with specificity to *Proteus* urinary tract infection
—Long-term antibiotic prophylaxis after stone clearance

- Metabolic stone disease
- —Cystinuria
    —Alkalinization to maintain pH above 7.8: sodium bicarbonate 12.6 g/24 h (not ideal because of sodium load); potassium citrate 1.2 to 1.7 mEq of base/kg/24 h divided into 4 doses (Polycitra K: 2 mEq base and 2 mEq potassium/mL). Confirm pH with Nitrazine paper; watch for calcium phosphate stones.
    —Chelating agents: D-penicillamine 20 to 50 mg/kg/d divided into 3 to 4 doses (see Section V for dosing information); alpha-mercapto-propionylglycine (Thiola) 15 mg/kg/d into 3 to 4 divided doses (see Section V for dosing information)
- —RTA: potassium citrate 0.5 to 3.0 mEq/kg/24 h divided into 4 doses (corrects systemic acidosis)
- —Absorptive hypercalciuria: low-calcium diet (400–600 mg/d)
    —Neutral phosphate (orthophosphate) 25 to 35 mg/kg/24 h divided into 4 doses
- —Renal leak hypercalciuria
    —Thiazide diuretics (increase calcium uptake in distal tubule)
    —Hydrochlorothiazide 2 mg/kg/d
    —Potassium citrate 1.0 mEq/kg/d
- —Postfurosemide calcium stones: hydrochlorothiazide 2 mg/kg/d
- —Uric acid stones
    —Alkalinization of urine to pH 6.5 (higher pH may lead to formation of calcium phosphate stones)
    —Potassium citrate 0.5 to 0.9 mEq/kg/d
    —IV alkalinization: 1/6 molar lactate at 0.5 to 1.0 cc/kg/h for hospitalized patients in acute renal colic
    —Allopurinol 200 mg/d
- —Primary hyperoxaluria
    —Pyridoxine 1.5 to 3.0 mg/kg
    —Magnesium oxide 6.5 mg/kg/d
    —Orthophosphate 25 to 35 mg/kg/d (adjust to renal function and GFR)

- Idiopathic stones
- —Hypercalciuria
    —Thiazide diuretics (hydrochlorothiazide 0.7 mg/kg/24 h)
    —Low-sodium diet
    —Potassium citrate 0.5 to 0.9 mEq/kg/d divided into 4 doses
    —Orthophosphate 25 to 35 mg/kg/d (if thiazide therapy fails)
- —Hyperoxaluria
    —Orthophosphate 25 to 35 mg/kg/d
    —Potassium citrate 0.5 to 0.9 mEq/kg/d
- —Hyperuricosuria
    —Diet adjustment
    —Alkalinization: potassium citrate 0.5 to 0.9 mEq/kg/d
- —Hypocitruria: potassium citrate 0.5 to 0.9 mEq/kg/d

SURGICAL

- Correct the obstruction, if present.
- Endourologic management is now possible with new smaller instrumentation.

—Percutaneous nephrostolithotomy: small peel-away sheaths and pediatric offset lenses (9Fr–16Fr); ultrasonic probes or electrohydraulic lithotripsy; particularly effective for infection stones. Preoperative nephrostomy tube (2–3 days) recommended

—Retrograde ureteroscopy (flexible and rigid): used in children as young as 3 years; rigid (6.9Fr) and flexible (7Fr) scopes allow treatment of ureteral stones. Preoperative stent placement is advocated in lieu of in situ ureteral orifice dilation. Vaporize the stone with a holmium laser.

—ESWL: safe for children. post-ESWL renal growth and function demonstrated; protect posterior basilar lung regions with foam pads. Ineffective for large cystine stones (>1 cm)

    —Not applicable in primary hyperoxaluria, nephrocalcinosis, and renal insufficiency (may worsen renal failure)

—Open surgery: an option; may complicate management in recurrent stone-formers

ALTERNATIVE THERAPIES: N/A

PATIENT EDUCATION

- Chronic conditions require patient/parent education, encouragement of increased fluid (water) intake, and special diets.

 Follow-Up

MONITORING

- All of these patients are presumed to be recurrent stone-formers. They need serial renal imaging with ultrasound or nonenhanced helical CT scanning.

PREVENTION

- See General Measures in the "Treatment" section.

 Miscellaneous

SYNONYMS: N/A

ASSOCIATED CONDITIONS: N/A

NOTES

- See also Section II, "Urolithiasis—Adult, General."

ABBREVIATIONS

- UPJ, ureteropelvic junction

REFERENCES

Cohen TD, et al. Pediatric urolithiasis: Medical and surgical management. *Urology* 1996;47:292.

Diamond DA, Menon M. Pediatric urolithiasis. AUA Update Series, Volume X, Lesson 40, p 314, 1991.

Resnik MI. Cystine stones. In: Siedmon J, Hanno P, eds. *Current Urologic Therapy*. Philadelphia: WB Saunders, 1994:167–169.

Smith LH, Segura JW. Urolithiasis. In: Kelalis P, et al., eds. *Clinical Pediatric Urology*. Philadelphia: WB Saunders, 1992:1327–1352.

Author: T. Ernesto Figueroa

Urolithiasis—Staghorn

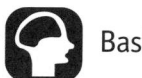 **Basics**

DESCRIPTION

- Branching calculi that fill the majority of the intrarenal collecting system

EPIDEMIOLOGY

- Occurs with chronic UTI
- More common in women

GENETICS

- No genetic basis

STAGING

- Complete staghorns involve the renal pelvis and branch into minor/major infundibulum and calyces.
- Partial staghorn: incomplete filling of the intrarenal collecting system
- Measured most commonly by their longest diameter

—Computer-assisted volumes have also been used to better estimate stone burden.

- Broad branches vs. tight narrow branches

—Tight branches and associated infundibular stenosis: more difficult to treat

SIGNS AND SYMPTOMS

- The majority are symptomatic.

—Recurrent urinary tract infection (UTI) (99%)
—Recurrent fever of unknown cause
  —Evaluation demonstrates the unsuspected staghorn calculus.
—Hematuria
—A palpable mass
  —A mass is secondary to renal obstruction and hydronephrosis.
—Flank pain: often not present
—Constitutional symptoms are associated with infected states.
  —Malaise, fever/chills, diaphoresis

PATHOPHYSIOLOGY

- Most staghorn calculi are composed of struvite-infected material.

—Magnesium–ammonium–phosphate

- UTI important in pathogenesis

—Bacteria reside inside of the stones.
—Bacteria produce urease.
  —Proteolytic enzyme: hydrolyzes urea into ammonia, bicarbonate, and carbonate
  —Urease production: mostly *Proteus* species; some *Pseudomonas, Klebsiella, Staphylococci, E. coli,* etc.

—Bicarbonate causes alkaline urine, and this induces supersaturation of the urine.

- Crystallization is enhanced by stasis caused by obstruction or pyelocalyceal paralysis (from bacterial endotoxins).
- Chronic infections lead to stone formation.

—This cycle involves infundibular obstruction with or without stricture, possibly hydronephrosis, further stone formation and obstruction, and loss of renal parenchyma.

- Metabolic calculi (calcium) can also form a staghorn.
- Staghorn stones may be mixed (e.g., struvite and calcium oxalate or calcium phosphate)

CAUSES/RISK FACTORS

- Recurrent UTIs

—Propagated by states of stasis and/or obstruction
  —Reflux of urine; neurogenic bladder; preexisting stone disease; stricture disease
—Most in women: UTIs more common in women
—Metabolic disorders such as hyperoxaluria, cystinuria, or hypercalciuria

COMPLICATIONS

- Perinephric abscess, loss of renal function, and XGP (no renal function or blood flow on nuclear medicine scan)

- Factors that predispose to renal deterioration include solitary kidney, recurrent stones, complete staghorns, neurogenic bladder, and refusal of treatment.

- Urothelial malignancies (squamous cell carcinoma most common)

DIFFERENTIAL DIAGNOSIS

- Filling defect in the upper urinary tract collecting system

—See Section I, "Filling Defect—Upper Urinary Tract."
—Urothelial lesions (e.g., inflammatory, malignant)

- Stones
- Blood clots

 Database

HISTORY

- Usually discovered during a diagnostic work-up for recurrent urinary tract infections

—History of prior calculi?
—Constitutional signs, including fever, malaise?
—Hematuria?
—Flank pain or abdominal mass?
—Neurogenic bladder?

- Undiagnosed severe metabolic disorders

—Cystinuria
—Primary hyperoxalosis
—Primary hyperparathyroid

PHYSICAL EXAMINATION

- May have costovertebral angle tenderness
- Palpable mass: high-grade hydronephrosis

Diagnostic Studies

LABORATORY TESTING

- Assess existing renal function

—BUN and creatinine

- CBC, urinalysis, and urine culture are all essential.

IMAGING

- Must have functional renal study; nonfunction with XGP

—Excretory urogram
—Nuclear medicine scan
—CAT scan with and without intravenous contrast

- Plain films of the abdomen may demonstrate the presence of a large calculus.

—Stones in the presence of *Proteus* or *Klebsiella* UTIs are likely struvite stones.
    —Lightly calcified and relatively less dense on plain film
—Stones in the presence of *Pseudomonas,* some *Streptococcus* and *Staphylococcus*
    —Relatively dense: increased calcium content

- If surgical intervention is planned, additional imaging is helpful.

—CT/spiral CT scan with and without intravenous contrast
    —Provides three-dimensional location of the stone
    —Evaluation of the cortical thickness
    —Rule out the possibility of a coexisting perirenal abscess.

SPECIAL STUDIES

- A retrograde ureteropyelogram may be necessary prior to planning surgical treatment.

—Delineation of the collecting system
—Rule out infundibular stenosis.
—Rule out ureteral stricture disease.

 ## Treatment

GENERAL MEASURES

- Removal of all stone and infectious material is required.

—The stone may regrow over weeks if not completely cleared.
—Infection will persist because the stone itself is infected.

- Broad-spectrum antibiotics are needed prior to stone manipulation and treatment.

MEDICAL

- Observation with supportive care (e.g., hydration and antibiotics)

—Reserved for those patients who would not tolerate any of the above surgical therapies
—28% of patients with staghorn calculi died while on one long-term watchful waiting.

SURGICAL

- First-line therapy: endoscopic clearance via percutaneous nephrostolithotomy

—Complementary endoscopes and lithotrites are applied.
—Combine with ESWL for tightly branched stones.
—Ureteroscopy: helpful in complex cases (e.g., bleeding diathesis, co-morbid conditions, obesity)

- ESWL as monotherapy is *not* the treatment of choice for an infected staghorn.
- Open surgery is reserved for special cases.

—Nephrectomy: option for kidney with very poor function, if contralateral kidney normal
—Stones that would require multiple percutaneous nephrostomies (3–4) to gain access
—Tight infundibular stenosis: severe stenosis requiring infundibuloplasty

ALTERNATIVE THERAPIES: N/A

PATIENT EDUCATION

- Patients with chronic UTIs should have routine upper tract imaging.

 ## Follow-Up

MONITORING

- Patients are monitored postoperatively with routine renal ultrasound and plain films (imaging).
- Serial urine cultures are obtained to ensure a noninfected state.

PREVENTION

- Once the stone burden is cleared, prevent further infections.

—Low-dose sulfa-based or nitrofurantoin antibiotics: useful during the first 6 months of follow-up.

Miscellaneous

SYNONYMS: N/A

ASSOCIATED CONDITIONS

- Recurrent UTI

NOTES

- See also Section II, "Urolithiasis—Adult, General" and "Urolithiasis—Pediatric."

ABBREVIATIONS

- XGP, xanthogranulomatous pyelonephritis

REFERENCES

Blandy JP, Singh M. The case for a more aggressive approach to staghorn stones. *J Urol* 1976;115(5):505–506.

Segura JW, et al. Nephrolithiasis Clinical Guidelines Panel summary report on the management of staghorn calculi. The American Urological Association Nephrolithiasis Clinical Guidelines Panel. *J Urol* 1994;151:1648–1651.

Segura JW. Staghorn calculi. *Urol Clin North Am* 1997;24(1):71–80.

Teichman JMH, Long RD, Hulbert JC. Long-term renal fate and prognosis after staghorn calculus management. *J Urol* 1995;153(5):1403–1407.

Authors: Mitchell C. Fraiman and Michael Grasso III

Urolithiasis—Uric Acid

 Basics

DESCRIPTION

• Urinary stones composed of uric acid

EPIDEMIOLOGY

• 1 in 1000 adults
• 5% to 10% of renal stones
• Incidence equal among men and women
• More common in Jews and Italians

GENETICS

• The familial variety is autosomal dominant.

STAGING: N/A

SIGNS AND SYMPTOMS

• Flank pain with obstruction, passage, or presence of renal stones
• Fever, chills, and sepsis with infection and obstructing stone

PATHOPHYSIOLOGY

• Uric acid crystallization caused by the supersaturation of urine with respect to undissociated uric acid
• Uric acid is a weak acid with limited solubility and two dissociable protons.
• pKa 1 is 5.5; pKa 2 is 10.3 (nonphysiologic)
• At a pH of 5.35, half of the uric acid is urate salt and half is free uric acid.
• At a pH of 6.5, 90% of the uric acid is soluble.
• Uric acid may serve as a nidus for calcium oxalate stone formation.

CAUSES/RISK FACTORS

• Excretion of excessively acidic urine
• Strenuous exercise, dehydration
• Crohn disease, regional ileitis
• Ulcerative colitis, ileostomy, short-bowel syndrome
• Hyperuricosuria, gout
• Purine gluttony
• Inborn errors of metabolism

—Lesch-Nyhan syndrome: hypoxanthine—guanine phosphoribosyl transferase deficiency (HGPRT)
—Phosphoribosylpyrophosphate synthetase overactivity
—Glucose-6-phosphate deficiency

• Myeloproliferative states: neoplasia, leukemia, hemolytic anemia, chemotherapy
• Decreased urinary volume

COMPLICATIONS

• Renal and ureteral stones with pain, obstruction, or infection
• Staghorn calculus formation
• Bladder stones: outlet obstruction, infection

DIFFERENTIAL DIAGNOSIS

• Renal stones

—Uric acid
—Calcium oxalate monohydrate
—Calcium oxalate dihydrate
—Cysteine
—Struvite (magnesium ammonium phosphate)

• Filling defect on intravenous urogram (see also Section I, "Filling Defect—Upper Urinary Tract")

—Can be differentiated on noncontrast CT scan
    —Uric acid stone; urothelial neoplasm (e.g., transitional cell carcinoma)
    —Blood clot, fungus ball, sloughed renal papilla, crossing renal vessel

 Database

HISTORY

• Acute: pain, fever, chills, nausea, vomiting secondary to renal colic
• Purine gluttony

—Diet high in red meats, fish, and poultry

• Increased physical activity with dehydration; poor urine output; poor urine volume
• Gout, family history of uric acid stones
• Short-bowel syndrome, inflammatory bowel disease, ileostomy
• Myeloproliferative disorders

PHYSICAL EXAMINATION

• Costovertebral angle tenderness

Diagnostic Studies

LABORATORY TESTING

• Serum uric acid level may be normal or elevated >380 μmol/L or 6.4 mg/100 mL

—Latent hyperuricemia (borderline uric acid elevation) may require a purine loading test.

• Urinalysis

—pH: generally <5.8
—Presence of white blood cells, red blood cells
—Crystals: uric acid appearance of coffin-lid crystals

• 24-hour urine collection for uric acid, volume suggestive of uric acid

—Volume <2L/d; pH <6.0; uric acid >4.0 mmol/d

IMAGING

• KUB with tomograms: Uric acid stones may not be visible (noncalcified).
• Intravenous urogram
• Noncontrast abdominal CT scan/spiral CT: best test
• Renal ultrasound helps differentiate a non-calcified stone from other nonurolithiasis causes of the filling defect.

SPECIAL STUDIES

• Purine loading test: ingestion of 2-g purine bases

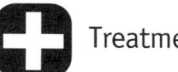 ## Treatment

GENERAL MEASURES

• Increase oral fluid intake to keep urine output greater than 2 L a day.
• Limit red meat, fish, and poultry in the diet.

MEDICAL

• Oral alkalinization therapy to maintain a urine pH of 6.5 to 7.0. May require 3 to 4 months to dissolve stone. Do not exceed pH 7, as stones of other composition can precipitate, such as calcium phosphate.
• Requires patient to self-monitor urine pH daily, with pH paper or Nitrazine paper
• Potassium citrate 30 to 60 mEq/d (Polycitra-K or Urocit-K)

—Alternative: sodium bicarbonate 650 mg every 6 to 8 hours

• For hyperuricemia or urinary uric acid secretion >1200 mg/d, treat with allopurinol 100 to 600 mg/d in additional to oral alkalinization.

—Allopurinol inhibits conversion of hypoxanthine and xanthine to uric acid. Side effects: skin rash, fever, or acute attack of gout

SURGICAL

• Extracorporeal shock wave lithotripsy, percutaneous ultrasonic lithotripsy, and ureteroscopic lithotripsy and extraction are all effective in stone removal, depending on stone burden.

ALTERNATIVE THERAPIES

• Alkalinization via a nephrostomy tube or ureteral stent is also an option.

PATIENT EDUCATION

• Importance of low-purine diet, adequate fluid intake, and proper monitoring of urine pH to keep it consistently at 6.5 to 7.0.

 ## Follow-Up

MONITORING

• Follow-up includes urinalysis for pH, crystals, red and white blood cells.
• Follow stone size with ultrasound or CT scans every 2 to 3 months on therapy.

PREVENTION

• Low-purine diet, adequate fluid intake, urinary alkalinization

 ## Miscellaneous

SYNONYMS

• Uric acid nephrolithiasis

ASSOCIATED CONDITIONS

• Gout, hyperuricemia, hyperuricosuria

NOTES

• See Section I, "Filling Defect—Upper Urinary Tract."

ABBREVIATIONS: N/A

REFERENCES

Low RK, Stoller ML. Uric acid-related nephrolithiasis. *Urol Clin North Am* 1997;24(1):135.

Menon M, Parulkar BG, Drach GW. Urinary lithiasis: Etiology, diagnosis and medical management. In: Walsh PC, Retik AB, Vaughn ED Jr, Wein AJ, eds. *Campbell's Urology,* 7th ed. Philadelphia: WB Saunders, 1998.

Authors: Gregory L. Chen and Demetrius H. Bagley

Vaginitis/Vulvovaginitis

 Basics

DESCRIPTION

• Inflammation or infection affecting the vagina, with a wide variety of etiologies and characterized by a vaginal discharge, pain, pruritis, and burning

EPIDEMIOLOGY

• Age dependent on etiology
• Incidence/prevalence

—Trichomonas: 2% to 5% of patients in a general gynecologic practice
—Yeast: 75% of women with at least one infection and 50% with at least two during their lifetime
—Atrophic: affects all women to some degree during their lifetime

GENETICS: N/A

STAGING: N/A

SIGNS AND SYMPTOMS

• Vaginal discharge: increased in amount, and change in odor or consistency
• Irritation of the vulvar skin
• Vaginal pain
• Pruritis
• Dyspareunia

PATHOPHYSIOLOGY: N/A

CAUSES/RISK FACTORS

• Foreign body: mostly in preadolescent female (cotton, toilet paper, etc.). Can occur in others, such as with retained tampon
• Atrophic vaginitis: mostly postmenopausal due to lack of estrogen production, allowing an increased vaginal pH and bacterial overgrowth coupled with mucosal thinning. Increased susceptibility to trauma and infection
• Bacterial infection: usually a polymicrobial disease not sexually transmitted. *Gardnerella vaginalis* most common. Also caused by *Mycoplasma hominis*, *Mobiluncus* species, *Peptostreptococcus*, and other anaerobes
• Fungal infections: including *Candida*. Increased in pregnancy, diabetes, steroid use, and after antibiotic therapy
• *Trichomonas vaginalis:* protozoan affecting the vagina and lower urinary tract. Sexually transmitted
• Including herpes, genital warts caused by human papilloma virus, gonorrhea, and *Chlamydia*

COMPLICATIONS

• Retained foreign bodies can lead to vaginal erosion or toxic shock syndrome.
• *T. vaginalis* can cause alterations in the epithelium of the cervix and vagina, leading to a false-positive cytology.
• STD: can lead to pelvic inflammatory disease

DIFFERENTIAL DIAGNOSIS

• Malignancy
• *Chlamydia*
• *Neisseria gonorrhoeae*
• Allergic reaction
• *Gardnerella vaginalis*
• *Trichomonas vaginalis*
• Vulvar dystrophy
• Bacterial infection
• *Candida*

 Database

HISTORY

• Prior vaginal infection
• Pregnancy
• Diabetes
• Steroid use
• Antibiotic use
• Sexually transmitted diseases or suspect sexual contacts
• Vaginal discharge: color, consistency, and odor
• "Lost tampon"

PHYSICAL EXAMINATION

• Examine the vulva, vagina, and cervix thoroughly.

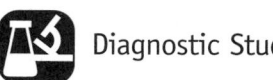 Diagnostic Studies

LABORATORY TESTING

• Cervical specimen for gonorrhea and chlamydia evaluation
• Potassium hydroxide prep

—"Whiff" test: characteristic fishlike smell with *Gardnerella*
—Observe on microscope for pseudohyphae and spores of *Candida*

• Saline wet prep

—Observe for motile trichomonads
—Clue cells: bacteria-covered epithelial cells characteristic of *Gardnerella*
—Note the number of leukocytes.
—Note the presence or absence of normal Lactobacillus.

• Urinalysis

—Culture: if dysuria is present

IMAGING: N/A

SPECIAL STUDIES: N/A

Treatment

GENERAL MEASURES

- Remove the foreign object, if present.
- Avoid intercourse.
- Sitz bath
- White vinegar douche: 60 mL/L water
- Keep the area clean and dry.
- Treat the partner, if indicated.

MEDICAL

- Bacterial

—*G. vaginalis*
  —Metronidazole 500 mg po bid for 7 days. May cause alcohol intolerance. Contraindicated in early pregnancy
  —Metronidazole 2g one time dose. Contraindicated in pregnancy
  —Metronidazole gel (0.75%, 5g) vaginally bid for 5 days
  —Clindamycin 300 mg bid for 7 days
  —Clindamycin gel (2%, 5g) vaginally once daily for 7 days. Good for use in early pregnancy

- Atrophic vaginitis

—Intravaginal estrogen cream 2 to 4 g/d vaginally. Contraindicated in patient with history of breast cancer
—Oral therapy
  —Conjugated estrogen (Premarin) 0.625 mg daily
  —Estradiol (Estrace) 1 mg daily

- *Candida*

—Miconazole nitrate (Monistat) vaginal suppository 200 mg at bedtime for 3 days, or cream (2%, 5g) intravaginally at bedtime for 7 days
—Clotrimazole (Gyne-Lotrimin) vaginal suppository 200 mg at bedtime for 3 days, or 500-mg tab one dose, or cream (1%, 5g) intravaginally at bedtime for 7 days
—Butoconazole nitrate (Femstat) (2% cream, 5g) intravaginally at bedtime for 3 days
—Terconazole (Terazol) 80-mg suppository, or 0.8% cream intravaginally at bedtime for 3 days
—Fluconazole (Diflucan) 150-mg tab po once
—Boric acid powder 600 mg in a gelatin capsule vaginally at bedtime for 2 weeks

- *T. vaginalis*

—Metronidazole 2 g orally once for patient and partner. May cause alcohol intolerance. Contraindicated in early pregnancy
—Metronidazole 500 mg po bid for 7 days
—Clotrimazole vaginal suppository once daily for 7 days. For use in pregnancy

- STDs: See specific chapters referring to these entities.

SURGICAL: *N/A*

ALTERNATIVE THERAPIES: *N/A*

PATIENT EDUCATION

- Keep the genital area clean and dry.
- Control medical problems (i.e., diabetes).
- Wear cotton underwear.
- Avoid broad-spectrum antibiotics.
- Patient information: American College of Obstetricians and Gynecologists (ACOG), 409 12th St. SW, Washington, DC 20024; (800)762-ACOG

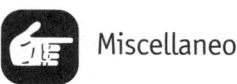 Follow-Up

MONITORING

- Follow the patient for symptom resolution.

PREVENTION

- See Patient Education in the "Treatment" section.

Miscellaneous

SYNONYMS: *N/A*

ASSOCIATED CONDITIONS: *N/A*

NOTES

- See Section I, "Dyspareunia."

ABBREVIATIONS: *N/A*

REFERENCES

Curry SL, Barclay DL. Benign disorders of the vulva and vagina. In: DeCherny AH, Pernoll ML, eds. *Current Obstetrics and Gynecologic Diagnosis and Treatment*. Norwalk, CT: Appleton & Lange, 1994:689–700.

MacKay HT. Gynecology. In: Tierney LM, McPhee SJ, Papadakis MA, eds. *Current Medical Diagnosis and Treatment*. Norwalk, CT: Appleton & Lange, 1998:694–696.

Roy S. Vulvovaginitis. In: Mishell DR Jr, Brenner PF, eds. *Management of Common Problems in Obstetrics and Gynecology*. Oxford: Blackwell Scientific, 1994:367–374.

Soper DE. Genitourinary infections and sexually transmitted diseases. In: Berek JS, Adashi EY, Hillard PA, eds. *Novak's Gynecology*. Baltimore: Williams & Wilkins, 1996:429–435.

Authors: Jeffrey H. Lumerman and Robert M. Moldwin

Varicocele—Adult

 Basics

DESCRIPTION

- A varicocele is the palpable or sometimes visible dilation of the pampiniform plexus of veins situated within the spermatic cord.

EPIDEMIOLOGY

- Varicoceles found in adolescents; rare prior to puberty. In these children, the presence of a varicocele should prompt a search for intraabdominal/retroperitoneal pathology. (See Section II, "Varicocele—Pediatric.")
- Found in 15% of all males; most common on left side
- Found in up to 40% of men with primary infertility; 80% with secondary infertility

GENETICS: N/A

STAGING: N/A

SIGNS AND SYMPTOMS

- Most asymptomatic
- If symptomatic: dull ache or pulling sensation
- Pain may be bilateral; does not radiate
- Recumbency relieves symptoms; pain is never present on awakening.
- Discomfort increases with standing, sitting, or exertion, especially when the activity is over a long period of time.

PATHOPHYSIOLOGY

- Varices

—Dilation of the pampiniform plexus of veins in the scrotum due to absent competent venous valves in the spermatic vein
—Lack of valves may be congenital (e.g., complete absence of valves) or acquired.
—When the spermatic vein is exposed to high venous pressures, especially in the left spermatic vein, which drains into the left renal vein, gradual dilation of the spermatic vein may cause valves to separate, with retrograde flow of blood.
—Rarely, a tumor or renal vein thrombus from the renal tumor may occlude the renal vein and cause a varix.

- Infertility due to varicoceles (several theories)

—Retrograde flow of renal and/or adrenal hormones with altered metabolism (i.e., corticosteroids) or altered blood flow (i.e., epinephrine, renin, PGE1) within the testes (current evidence weak)
—Hormonal dysfunction. Changes in the pituitary–testicular axis. Role unclear
—Testicular hypoxia. Unclear mechanism
—Increase testicular temperature.
  —Loss of countercurrent testicular cooling mechanism
  —The varix increases intratesticular temperature compared with controls (0.6°C–0.8°C).
  —Widely accepted explanation for varicocele subfertility

CAUSES/RISK FACTORS

- Congenital: absence of valves in the spermatic vein
- Acquired: loss of valvular competence or extrinsic compression by intraabdominal tumor, renal vein tumor thrombus

COMPLICATIONS

- Pain and infertility

DIFFERENTIAL DIAGNOSIS

- See Section I, "Scrotum—Mass and/or Pain (Acute Scrotum)."

 Database

HISTORY

- Patients present for evaluation of varices for one of four reasons: infertility, pain, adolescent growth retardation, or a varix diagnosed on routine physical examination.

—Infertility
  —Primary: failure to conceive despite >12 months of unprotected intercourse (varix found in 37%)
  —Secondary: those who have previously conceived (varix found in 80%)
—Pain: dull ache or heavy sensation, nonradiating, increasing during the course of the day with activity and standing, exaggerated with Valsalva or activity associated with straining (including sexual intercourse)
—Acute onset suggests obstruction of the renal vein or spermatic vein (i.e., tumor thrombus).

PHYSICAL EXAMINATION

- Examine in a warm room after the patient has been standing for 10 minutes (reduces the effect of cremasteric response and allows veins to fill).
- Inspection may identify large varices. Varices may be palpable with or without Valsalva.
- Elevation of the testes (shortens the cord)
- Perform a Valsalva maneuver (cremasteric muscle contracts with the internal oblique muscle during straining and shortens cord). Increased intraabdominal pressure distends the pampiniform plexus.

—Varix grading
  —Grade 1: varix palpable but only with Valsalva
  —Grade 2: varix palpable without the need of Valsalva
  —Grade 3: varix visible on inspection

- Examine for an abdominal mass.

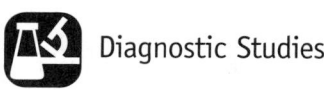 Diagnostic Studies

LABORATORY TESTING

- Urinalysis may suggest hematuria and a renal mass (rare cause).
- Only useful if associated with infertility
- Seminal fluid analysis

—Necessary prior to varix ligation to confirm male-factor subfertility
—Typical findings for male-factor infertility due to varicocele
  —Sperm density <20 million/mL; motility <60%; motile sperm/ejaculate <40 million

- Endocrine screen, as needed, to evaluate for infertility (FSH, LH, free and total testosterone, LH, estradiol)

IMAGING

- Doppler/ultrasound may be useful to exclude other intrascrotal pathologies: testicular tumor, epididymitis.
- Ultrasound with color Doppler: used to identify "subclinical" varices

—Defined as dilated pampiniform plexus veins, which were undetectable during physical examination but exhibited dilation with Valsalva to a caliber >2 mm during US examination and/or reverse flow with Valsalva during color Doppler examination

—The utility of repairing "subclinical" varices is controversial in male subfertility and of no value in men with orchalgia.

- Internal spermatic venography

—Internal spermatic venography is potentially both diagnostic and therapeutic.

- Abdominal imaging, if mass suspected

SPECIAL STUDIES

- Testes biopsy, if azoospermia present

 ## Treatment

GENERAL MEASURES

- Treat varix only if either male subfertility, pain, or, in the case of adolescents, testicular growth retardation
- No benefit in treating patients without signs or symptoms
- The efficacy of varix ligation in men with normal semen analysis is unproved, and repair should be recommended only after other factors (especially female subfertility) have been excluded.

MEDICAL

- Infertility: no medical therapy, except for approaches to improve sperm parameters

—In vitro fertilization as a means of overcoming male infertility has been successful, but is not cost effective and should be reserved for use in those cases in which female infertility demands advanced reproductive intervention (i.e., tubal obstruction).

- Pain: Analgesics are not durable and ultimately delay definitive therapy.

SURGICAL

- Operative therapy of varices may be categorized by anatomic site of varix ligation or by surgical technique.

—Anatomic site of ligation
  —Inguinal (Ivanissevitch): inguinal incision with ligation of the spermatic veins within the inguinal canal. Allows repair of coincident hernia
  —Retroperitoneal (Palermo or high ligation): muscle-splitting incision, exposure of the spermatic vessels with or without preservation of the spermatic artery. Mass ligation permitted at this level due to the presence of collateral arterial circulation (vasal artery, cremasteric artery) to cord structures distally. Preserve the spermatic artery whenever possible.
  —Subinguinal: the standard in recent years; incision over the cord below the external ring; here, the number of veins requiring ligation is greater than more cephalad; magnification is recommended to salvage the spermatic artery and lymphatics.
—Surgical techniques
  —Open with or without magnification: preservation of artery and lymphatics enhanced with magnification (loupes and operating microscope); small venous tributaries identified, reducing the probability of recurrence
  —Laparoscopic varix ligation: high ligation with minimally invasive technique; laparoscopic magnification, allows sparing of artery and lymphatics; recovery is rapid (regular activity in 4–6 days); no major advantage over subinguinal microscopic technique

ALTERNATIVE THERAPIES

- Interventional radiology

—Venography of the spermatic vein with occlusion (injection of boiling-hot contrast, coils, Gelfoam, balloon). Venous access through the femoral vein; the internal jugular offers some advantage in a right-sided varix.
—Recovery is 3 to 4 days, a slight advantage over surgery therapy; recurrence is reported in up to 20%, and above that reported for operative procedures using magnification (0.5%–1.5%).

- Scrotal hypothermia device (Zorgniotti): cools the scrotum by means of alcohol evaporation from an athletic support made damp via a reservoir worn on the waist band; fertility success equivocal

PATIENT EDUCATION: N/A

 ## Follow-Up

MONITORING

- Varicocele recurrence

—Monitor at 3-month intervals. Recurrence (due to increase in caliber of collateral veins/missed veins) is evident within 6 to 12 months.

- Infertility

—Semen analysis: 3-month intervals. In general, the response to varix ligation is demonstrable within 6 months, but an increase in sperm density and motility may require up to 1 year.

- Pain relief of pain will typically respond immediately after surgery. Follow-up may be curtailed in these patients.
- Rarely, testicular atrophy or a hydrocele can occur; spermatic artery and lymphatic preservation limits these complications.

PREVENTION: N/A

 ## Miscellaneous

SYNONYMS

- Varix, varicocele, varices (plural)

ASSOCIATED CONDITIONS

- Infertility

NOTES

- See Section II, "Varicocele—Pediatric."

ABBREVIATIONS: N/A

REFERENCES

Goldstein M, Gilbert BR, Dicker AP, Dwosh J, Gnecco C. Microsurgical inguinal varicocelectomy with delivery of the testis: An artery and lymphatic sparing technique. *J Urol* 1992;148:1808–1811.

Nagler HM, Zippe CD. Varicocele: Current concepts and treatment. In: Lipshultz LI, Howards SS, eds. *Infertility in the Male*, 2nd ed. St Louis: Mosby–Year Book, 1991.

Schlegel PN. Is assisted reproduction the optimal treatment for varicocele-associated male infertility? A cost-effectiveness analysis. *Urology* 1997;49:83–90.

Author: James F. Donovan

Varicocele—Pediatric

 Basics

DESCRIPTION

- A varicocele is an abnormal tortuosity and dilation of the veins of the pampiniform plexus of the spermatic cord.

EPIDEMIOLOGY

- Present in approximately 15% of adolescent boys but rare prior to puberty
- Left sided 78% to 93%, right 1% to 7%, bilateral 2% to 0%
- No racial, cultural, or geographic predilection

GENETICS

- Unknown

STAGING

- See Physical Examination in the "Database" section.

SIGNS AND SYMPTOMS

- Usually asymptomatic
- Discovered on routine physical examination
- May present as a scrotal mass
- Infrequent testicular discomfort

PATHOPHYSIOLOGY

- Hyperthermia: A varicocele causes an increase in scrotal temperature.

—Increased testicular arterial blood flow interferes with countercurrent heat exchange of the pampiniform plexus.
—Increased testicular temperature affects such temperature-dependent enzymes as DNA polymerase.
—Proliferation of germ cells may be affected by elevated temperature >33°C to 34°C.
—Increased testicular temperature induces apoptosis in germ cells.

- Venous stasis

—Venous hypertension alters composition of the interstitial space.
—Potential effects on Leydig, peritubular myoid, and Sertoli cell function
—Possible oxygen depletion in the testis

- Adrenal/renal reflux of toxic metabolites

—Reflux of blood from adrenal, renal veins demonstrated by venography
—Potential for exposure to adrenal/renal metabolites harmful to the testis
—This theory not supported by experimental animal studies

- Endocrine imbalances

—Decrease in intratesticular testosterone concentration
—Abnormal response to gonadotropin-releasing hormone (GnRH stimulation test)
—Impaired Leydig cell function will not support normal spermatogenesis.

—Diminished Sertoli cell response to follicle-stimulating hormone (FSH)

- Testicular paracrine imbalance

—Spermatogenesis requires intimate communication between different cell types within the testis.
—Paracrine substances (inhibin, activin) are required for cell-to-cell communication in the testis.
—The testicular environment produced by the varicocele adversely affects the synthesis and secretion of paracrine factors.

- Histology of the testis

—All cell types involved; changes increase with time
—Germ cell sloughing; maturation arrest
—Thickened basement membrane of seminiferous tubule
—Ultrastructural changes to Leydig and Sertoli cells

- Testicular hypotrophy/atrophy

—Significant testicular volume loss in 30% to 70% of adolescents with a varicocele
—The most rapid growth of the testis occurs between ages 11 and 16 years.
—Testicular hypotrophy is reversible in 80% of patients with a varicocele correction.

CAUSES/RISK FACTORS

- Unique anatomy of left testicular vein: elevated venous pressure

—8 to 10 cm longer than right
—Right-angle entry into left renal vein
—Lack of venous valves in proximal testicular vein
—Compression of left renal vein by superior mesenteric artery (nutcracker effect)

- Erect posture of humans (no varicoceles in four-legged animals)
- Increased testicular blood flow at puberty exceeds venous outflow capacity.
- Secondary causes: renal tumors with venous extension, retroperitoneal fibrosis, renal vein thrombosis

COMPLICATIONS

- Posttraumatic scrotal hematoma
- Thrombosis
- Testicular hypotrophy, atrophy
- Male-factor infertility

DIFFERENTIAL DIAGNOSIS

- Inguinal hernia
- Hydrocele
- Lipoma of cord (benign soft-tissue tumor)
- Epididymal cyst
- Spermatocele
- Paratesticular rhabdomyosarcoma

 Database

HISTORY

- Usually asymptomatic
- May change in size with position/Valsalva
- Heaviness or dull ache in scrotum
- Medical history

—A previous scrotal, inguinal surgery may affect surgical decisions.

PHYSICAL EXAMINATION

- Examine in warm room; upright and supine positions
- Paratesticular mass superior to testis: feels like "bag of worms"
- Negative transillumination; positive transillumination implies a hydrocele or hernia.
- Increases in size with Valsalva maneuver
- Varicocele grade by physical examination

—Grade 1: varicocele detected only by Valsalva maneuver
—Grade 2: nonvisible but palpable varicocele
—Grade 3: visible prior to palpation

- Estimate testicular size and consistency.

—Prader orchidometer, disk orchidometer
—The contralateral (right) testis serves as the normal control.
—A 2-cc or 20% size discrepancy is significant.

- Examine for a bilateral varicocele and lymphedema.

—If present, rule out a secondary varicocele.

- Solitary right varicocele: Rule out a renal, retroperitoneal tumor.

Diagnostic Studies

LABORATORY TESTING

• Semen analysis: not generally available in this age group

—No normal data due to variations in pubertal development

• GnRH stimulation test

—Exaggerated response with elevated LH, FSH
—Abnormal in 43% of adolescents with varicocele
—Not correlated with testicular atrophy
—Not correlated with future infertility in adolescents

IMAGING

• Testicular ultrasound

—Most accurate measure of testicular volume
—A 2-cm³ volume difference (L < R) is significant.
—Accurate assessment of catch-up growth following varicocelectomy

SPECIAL STUDIES: N/A

 ## Treatment

GENERAL MEASURES

• If asymptomatic and no testicular size discrepancy: Observe.

MEDICAL: N/A

SURGICAL

• Surgical indications

—Greater than 2-cm³ size difference in testicular volume
—Scrotal pain
—Bilateral varicoceles
—Abnormal spermiogram (rarely available; must be >17 years of age)

• The suprainguinal retroperitoneal approach (Palomo) with artery and vein ligation is the most common method of surveyed pediatric urologists.
• The microscopic inguinal/subinguinal technique has a similar varicocele persistence rate and hydrocele rate as the Palomo technique and preserves the testicular artery.
• The varicocele persists after surgery in 0.6% to 16% of adolescents, depending on the surgical approach.
• Postvaricocele hydrocele noted in 0.8% to 8.6%
• Postoperative catch-up growth of the left testis is seen in 80% of patients with a successful varicocelectomy.

ALTERNATIVE THERAPIES

• Radiographic embolization: rarely used, except for persistent varicocele in the pediatric population
• Laparoscopic varicocelectomy: rarely used due to potential for serious operative injury.

PATIENT EDUCATION

• Must carefully counsel patient and parents about the varicocele
• Get parents' advice separately on what to communicate to their son.

 ## Follow-Up

MONITORING

• Surgical patients (3 and 6 months postoperatively)

—Assess the catch-up growth of the left testis.
—Assess the possible complication of a hydrocele and a persistent varicocele.

• Observed patients (no testicular size discrepancy)

—Assess testicular size and development at 6- to 12-month intervals.
—Consider semen analysis at an appropriate age.

PREVENTION: N/A

 ## Miscellaneous

SYNONYMS

• Varix

ASSOCIATED CONDITIONS

• Secondary varicoceles due to renal tumors, retroperitoneal tumors, and venous thrombosis

NOTES

• At present, surgical correction of a varicocele is correlated only with catch-up growth of the left testis. Future fertility and paternity are not proven.

ABBREVIATIONS

• GnRH, gonadotropin-releasing hormone

REFERENCES

Kass EJ, Reitelman C. Adolescent varicocele. *Urol Clin North Am* 1995;22:151.

Skoog SJ, Roberts KP, Goldstein M, Pryor JL. The adolescent varicocele: What's new with an old problem in young patients? *Pediatrics* 1997;100:112.

Steno OP. Varicocele in the adolescent. *Adv Exp Med Biol* 1991;286:295.

Author: Steven J. Skoog

Vas Deferens—Congenital Absence/Obstruction

 Basics

DESCRIPTION

• The vas deferens is a thick, muscular tube that carries sperm from the cauda epididymis to the ejaculatory ducts in the prostate. Vasal obstruction may be congenital or acquired and, if bilateral, may result in infertility. The mesonephric duct is the common embryologic origin of the vas, the epididymis, and seminal vesicle, thus absence of the vas may indicate absence of epididymis and seminal vesicle. Congenital absence of the vas is rare and may be bilateral (CBAV) or unilateral.

EPIDEMIOLOGY

• CBAV occurs in 1.4% of the infertile male population and in 0.5% of male autopsies (25% of all patients with obstructive azoospermia).

GENETICS

• 60% to 80% with CBAV have the cystic fibrosis (CF) gene mutation; 15%, compound heterozygous; 65%, simple heterozygous; and 20%, no detectable mutation.
• 20% with no detectable CF mutations may harbor undefined CF gene alterations or another etiology of the vas aplasia.

STAGING: N/A

SIGNS AND SYMPTOMS

• If bilateral absence or obstruction

—Diminished semen volume (aspermia)
—Azoospermia
—Infertility (typical presentation)

PATHOPHYSIOLOGY

• If acquired obstruction

—Inflammatory obstruction: viral and bacterial infections (especially TB) (Note: STDs typically cause epididymal obstruction, not vasal.)
—Surgical obstruction: vasectomy, iatrogenic during another surgical procedure

• If congenital absence

—CF transmembrane conductase regulator (CFTR) dysfunction
  —The CF gene encodes for the CFTR, which is responsible for the regulation of chloride ion influx/efflux across the epithelial cell membrane.
  —The hypothesis is that a proper fluid milieu is essential for the optimal vasal morphogenesis; vasal maldevelopment may be the most sensitive urologic expression of CFTR dysfunction.
—Improper mesonephric duct development
  —Improper mesonephric duct development prior to week 7 of gestation might manifest with CBAV and renal agenesis.

CAUSES/RISK FACTORS

• If acquired

—History of operative procedures: hernial repair, renal transplant, other retroperitoneal or deep pelvic surgeries
—History of trauma to lower abdomen or pelvis

• If congenital absence

—CF

COMPLICATIONS

• Infertility, anxiety, and/or depression

DIFFERENTIAL DIAGNOSIS

• Vasal obstruction and CBAV should be differentiated from all other causes of azoospermia and/or aspermia.

—Anatomic (congenital/acquired): seminal vesical aplasia, ejaculatory duct obstruction (EDO), exstrophy/epispadias, BNO, vasectomy (includes inadvertent injury during other groin/scrotal procedures)
—Neuropathic: diabetic neuropathy of the sympathetic innervation, spinal cord injury, intraoperative injury to sympathetic chain, multiple sclerosis, myelodysplasia, idiopathic retrograde ejaculation, psychogenic
—Pharmacologic ejaculatory dysfunction: antipsychotics (major tranquilizers), antidepressants (tricyclic and monoamine oxidase inhibitors), antihypertensives, alcohol, baclofen, ε-aminocaproic acid, methadone, naproxen, DHT-inhibitors
—Hypogonadism
—Inflammatory: TB

 Database

HISTORY

• History of infertility: duration, prior pregnancies (present partner, another partner), previous treatments, evaluation and treatment of partner
• Sexual history: potency, lubricants, timing of intercourse, frequency of intercourse, frequency of masturbation
• Childhood and development: cryptorchidism, orchidopexy, herniorrhaphy, Y-V plasty of bladder neck, testicular torsion, onset of puberty
• Medical history: systemic illness (i.e., diabetes mellitus, multiple sclerosis), previous/current therapy
• Surgical history: orchiectomy (testicular cancer, torsion); retroperitoneal surgery; pelvic injury; pelvic, inguinal, or scrotal surgery; herniorrhaphy; Y-V plasty; transurethral prostate resection
• Infections: viral febrile, mumps orchitis, venereal, tuberculosis, small pox
• Gonadotoxins: chemicals (pesticides), drugs (chemotherapeutics, cimetidine, sulfasalazine, nitrofurantoin, alcohol, marijuana, androgenic steroids, cocaine), thermal exposure, radiation, smoking
• Family history: CF, androgen receptor deficiency
• Review of systems: respiratory infections, anosmia, galactorrhea, impaired visual fields, headaches

PHYSICAL EXAMINATION

• General examination

—Exclude hypogonadism signs (e.g., eunuchoidal skeletal proportion, loss of normal male hair distribution, and excessive wrinkling).
—Exclude other endocrine abnormalities: Skin pigmentation may be related to adrenal disease. Headache, visual field defects, or galactorrhea may point to a hypothalamic–pituitary abnormality.
—Gynecomastia may be a clue to testicular dysfunction, whether primary or secondary.

• Genital examination

—If obstruction: palpable vasa, normal-size testes, some degree of fullness to the epididymis
—If congenital absence: nonpalpable vasa or palpation of atretic vas streak, distended and firm epididymal remnant
—NB: Normal seminal vesicles are not palpable on a digital rectal examination.

Diagnostic Studies

LABORATORY TESTING

• Hormonal: FSH, LH, prolactin, and testosterone serum concentration measurements should be normal.
• Semen analysis: volume <1 cc; pH: acidic; fructose usually absent

IMAGING

• TRUS to demonstrate atrophic or aberrant seminal vesicles or EDO
• Vasography: preferably at the time of corrective surgery and only if testicular biopsy showed active spermatogenesis
• Renal ultrasound: In patients with detectable CF mutations, renal anomalies are unusual; however, 40% of patients with no CF mutations demonstrate unilateral renal agenesis.

SPECIAL STUDIES

• CF mutation analysis
• Testicular biopsy: active spermatogenesis

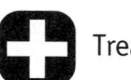 Treatment

GENERAL MEASURES

• Many patients will require assisted reproductive techniques (ARTs); however, patients whose obstruction was acquired after infection may not need them.
• Anatomic obstruction may respond to surgical repair.

MEDICAL

• Prompt antibiotic therapy in men with genital tuberculosis or other bacterial infections can maintain fertility and may preclude the need for later surgical intervention.

SURGICAL

• CAVD

—Microsurgical sperm aspiration from the caput epididymis or efferent ductules for use in ICSI
—Testicular aspiration of sperm for ICSI

• Vasal occlusion: epididmovasostomy, vasovasostomy, or IVF with ICSI

ALTERNATIVE THERAPIES

• Artificial insemination by sperm donor (AID).
• Adoption might be considered.

PATIENT EDUCATION

• Educate the patient on the implications for fertility; encourage genetic counseling for CF.

 Follow-Up

MONITORING

• Follow-up semen analysis 3 to 4 months after vasectomy reversal/vasoepidymostomy

PREVENTION

• Genetic counseling

—CF mutation analysis of both partners should be attempted before ART. If both are positive, then amniocentesis or chorionic villous sampling might be recommended to define the genetic status of the fetus. Additionally, the couple may consider alternate means of conception (e.g., AID).
—Alternatively, preimplantation genetic diagnosis of each embryo can be performed with uterine transfer of only embryos that are not at risk for CF/CBAVD development.

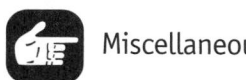 Miscellaneous

SYNONYMS: N/A

ASSOCIATED CONDITIONS

• If congenital

—Seminal vesicles are hypoplastic or absent in up to 90% of cases.
—Upper urinary tract abnormalities in 20% of CAVD

NOTES

• See also Section I, "Infertility."

ABBREVIATIONS

• CBAV, congenital bilateral absence of the vas deferens; BNO, bladder neck obstruction; LND, lymph node dissection; DHT, dihydrotestosterone; ICSI, intracytoplasmic sperm injection; EDO, ejaculatory duct obstruction; ART, assisted reproductive technique; IVF, in vitro fertilization; AID, artificial insemination donor

REFERENCES

Honig S, et al. Ultrasonographic renal and seminal vesicle anomalies in patients with congenital absence of the vas deferens. *J Urol* 1991;145:453A.

Silber S, et al. Absence of the vas deferens: The fertilizing capacity of human epididymal sperm. *N Engl J Med* 1990;323:1785.

Authors: Ehab A. El-Gabry and Irvin H. Hirsch

Vesicoureteral Reflux—Adult

 Basics

DESCRIPTION

• Vesicoureteral reflux (VUR) is the retrograde passage of urine from the bladder into the ureter. Refluxed urine often reaches the renal pelvis and calyces.

EPIDEMIOLOGY

• 5% of adults have VUR (may be high due to the increased likelihood of work-up given a typical history).
• 85% of childhood reflux occurs in girls; probably similar in adults
• Reflux is more common in Whites than in Blacks.

GENETICS

• Having a parent or sibling with VUR increases the risk.
• Important in pediatrics, where asymptomatic renal scanning may occur; less important in adults

STAGING

• VUR is graded I–V, based on a contrast voiding cystourethrogram (VCUG).

—I: contrast seen in nondilated ureter
—II: ureter and nondilated renal pelvis and calyces
—III: mild-to-moderate ureteral and renal pelvic/calyceal dilation
—IV: moderate ureteral tortuosity and renal pelvic/calyceal dilation
—V: gross dilation of ureter, pelvis, and calyces, with loss of papillary impressions

SIGNS AND SYMPTOMS

• Adult VUR usually asymptomatic
• May complain of cystitis, often progressing to febrile UTI

PATHOPHYSIOLOGY

• Failure of development or breakdown of the distal ureteral antireflux mechanism

—Normally, the distal 4 to 5 cm of the ureter courses through the muscular wall of the bladder before reaching the bladder trigone. This tunnel prevents reflux of urine.
—A congenital lack of the intravesical tunnel is the most common etiology
—Other causes: disorders that cause elevated intravesical pressure (BPH, spinal cord injury, MS, and other neurologic diseases). Patients who have undergone urinary diversion (ileal conduit) or bladder replacement (orthotopic neobladder, catheterizable diversions) are, in many cases, expected to have VUR.

CAUSES/RISK FACTORS

• Environmental factors, medications, or chemicals do not cause VUR. Reflux may develop, however, in patients with neurogenic bladder disease who do not catheterize frequently enough to keep bladder storage pressure low.

COMPLICATIONS

• Pyelonephritis is most common. In the setting of chronic infections, patients can form renal stones and lose kidney function.

DIFFERENTIAL DIAGNOSIS

• Simple pyelonephritis
• Uncommonly, an adult will present with chronic renal failure due to previously undiagnosed VUR.

 Database

HISTORY

• Have infections been recurrent?
• Does simple cystitis lead to fever and flank pain?
• Lower urinary tract voiding symptoms to suggest outlet obstruction or neuropathic bladder

PHYSICAL EXAMINATION

• Costovertebral angle tenderness with pyelonephritis
• Digital rectal examination for BPH
• Neurologic impairment?

Diagnostic Studies

LABORATORY TESTING

• Blood testing not necessary, except for severe cases in which renal function should be evaluated
• Urinalysis and culture should demonstrate the presence of infection if the patient is symptomatic.
• Between infections, the urine will often be normal.

IMAGING

• VCUG: definitive test for identifying and grading the severity of reflux

—The occasional patient will not reflux during storage, but begin refluxing during voiding.

• A nuclear medicine cystogram is often performed as a follow-up test in children, but it provides less anatomic information than the VCUG.

SPECIAL STUDIES

• Patients with overt neurologic disease and VUR should undergo urodynamic testing (cystometrogram) to evaluate bladder storage pressure.

 ## Treatment

GENERAL MEASURES

• With the exception of pregnant women and those with neurologic disease, adult VUR typically does not require treatment.

MEDICAL

• Pregnant women with known VUR should be given antibiotic prophylaxis until delivery (e.g., amoxicillin 250 qd). Adult VUR does not otherwise require ongoing medical therapy.

SURGICAL

• Open ureteral reimplantation is 90% to 95% effective in eliminating reflux in adults. All techniques create a new ureteral tunnel through the muscular bladder wall.

ALTERNATIVE THERAPIES

• Bulking agents, such as injectable collagen, Teflon paste, and fat, may be injected through the cystoscope under the ureter near the orifice. Initial results are good; however, long-term follow-up is scant.

PATIENT EDUCATION

• Patients with known VUR should be instructed to seek immediate treatment for the symptoms of cystitis. Early treatment can often prevent pyelonephritis.

 ## Follow-Up

MONITORING

• Medical follow-up is unnecessary in patients without hypertension or proteinuria, unless the patient develops recurring infections, at which point repeat work-up is needed. Patients with intrinsic renal disease due to prior reflux (in childhood) require follow-up of blood pressure, creatinine, and urine protein.

PREVENTION

• With recurrent UTIs, trial of suppressive antibiotics

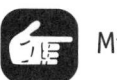 ## Miscellaneous

SYNONYMS

• Reflux

ASSOCIATED CONDITIONS

• See causes of high bladder storage pressure mentioned above.

NOTES

• See also Section II, "Vesicoureteral Reflux—Pediatric."

ABBREVIATIONS

• VUR, vesicoureteral reflux; VCUG, voiding cystourethrogram

REFERENCES

Bailey RR, Lynn KL, Robson RA. End-stage reflux nephropathy. *Ren Fail* 1994;16(1):27–35.

El-Khatib M, Packham DK, Becker GJ, Kincaid-Smith P. Pregnancy-related complications in women with reflux nephropathy. *Clin Nephrol* 1994;41(1):50–55.

Hall MK, Hackler RH, Zampieri TA, Zampieri JB. Renal calculi in spinal cord–injured patient: Association with reflux, bladder stones, and Foley catheter drainage. *Urology* 1989;34(3):126–128.

Zhang Y, Bailey RR. A long term follow up of adults with reflux nephropathy. *N Z Med J* 1995;108(998):142–144.

Author: Douglas F. Milam

Vesicoureteral Reflux—Pediatric

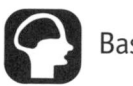 Basics

DESCRIPTION

• Vesicoureteral reflux (VUR) is an abnormal condition due to incompetence of the ureterovesical junction (UVJ), where urine flow occurs in a retrograde manner, and might lead to an upper tract pathology. It may be unilateral or bilateral, congenital or acquired.

EPIDEMIOLOGY

• 0.4% of normal population
• 50% of children with UTI
• 8% of adults with bacteriuria
• After age 6 months, the female-to-male ratio of infection with reflux is 10:1.

GENETICS

• Congenital VUR tends to be familial

—40% of asymptomatic siblings of children with VUR have reflux with some evidence of clinically silent scarring.
—Two-thirds of children with parents with known VUR have evidence of reflux.
—Analysis of 88 affected families indicated that the best model is that of a single dominant gene acting together with a random environmental effect.
—Computer modeling indicated that the gene frequency was 1 in 600 and that gene mutation is uncommon.

STAGING

• The grading system adopted by the International Reflux Study Committee is as follows:

—Grade I: reflux partly up to the ureter
—Grade II: reflux up to the pelvis and calyces without dilatation; normal calyceal fornices
—Grade III: same as grade II, but with mild or moderate dilatation and tortuosity of the ureter and no blunting of the fornices
—Grade IV: moderate dilatation and tortuosity of the ureter, pelvis, and calyces; complete blunting of fornices
—Grade V: gross dilatation and tortuosity of the ureter, pelvis, and calyces; absent papillary impressions in the calyces

SIGNS AND SYMPTOMS

• Symptomatic pyelonephritis: Adults usually present with chills, high fever, renal pain, nausea and vomiting, and symptoms of cystitis. Children usually present with fever only; however, abdominal pains and sometimes diarrhea may occur.
• Asymptomatic pyelonephritis: The incidental findings of pyuria and bacteriuria may be the only clues.
• Symptoms of cystitis only: Irritative voiding symptoms prevail: frequency, urgency, nocturia, burning micturition, and dysuria. Low back pain, suprapubic pain, urge incontinence and hematuria are common. Fever is unusual. These patients may have reflux with asymptomatic chronic pyelonephritis and bacteriuria that is resistant to anti-

microbial therapy or rapid recurrence of infection following treatment.
• Renal pain on voiding is rare.
• Uremia: This is the last stage of bilateral reflux.
• Hypertension: in the later stages of atrophic pyelonephritis
• Symptoms related to underlying disease

—Urinary tract obstruction: Girls may present with symptoms of hesitancy and intermittency secondary to spasm of periurethral striated muscle. In males, a slow stream may be due to posterior urethral valves (infants) or BPH (men over age 50).
—Spinal cord disease: Symptoms of neurogenic bladder may prevail: incontinence, urgency, retention, or large residual volume.

PATHOPHYSIOLOGY

• Reflux can damage the kidney through one of the following mechanisms:

—Infection: When reflux is present, bacteria reach the kidney, and since the urinary tract cannot empty itself completely, infection is perpetuated.
—Hydroureteronephrosis: Dilatation of the upper tract is usually associated with reflux for the following reasons:
    —Increased work load: In the presence of reflux, the ureter has to transport an increased volume of urine. This result in an eventual loss of its contractile power (decompensation), leading to stasis and dilatation.
    —High hydrostatic pressure: The transmission of the high intravesical pressure to the ureteral and pelvic walls results in marked stretching and dilation.
    —Weak ureteral musculature: In reflux, the ureteral wall is invariably deficient in musculature to some degree. This limits its ability to compensate for overwork and increased hydrostatic pressure, thus making it more ready to dilate if subjected to overload.

• Reflux nephropathy: Pyelointerstitial backflow or pyelotubular backflow under the high pressure of reflux would lead to extravasation of urine in the kidney interstitium, thus even sterile urine, if severe enough, may result in a marked inflammatory response, with eventual scarring and fibrosis.

CAUSES/RISK FACTORS

• Congenital causes: trigonal weakness (primary reflux), ureteral abnormalities (complete ureteral duplication, ectopic ureteral orifice, and ureterocele), Eagle-Barrett (prune belly) syndrome
• Vesical trabeculation: A heavily trabeculated bladder may be associated with reflux; causes include spastic neurogenic bladder and severe obstruction distal to the bladder.
• Inflammatory: edema of vesical wall secondary to cystitis
• Iatrogenic: prostatectomy, wedge resection of the posterior vesical neck, ureteral meatotomy, ureterocele resection
• Contracted bladder secondary to interstitial cystitis, TB, radiotherapy, carcinoma, or schistosomiasis

• Pregnancy: due to obstructive and hormonal factors
• Spinal cord disorders
• Urinary tract obstruction distal to bladder neck

COMPLICATIONS

• Pyelonephritis
• Hydroureteronephrosis
• Hypertension
• Uremia

DIFFERENTIAL DIAGNOSIS

• VUR should be differentiated from other causes of hydroureter nephrosis without reflux.

—Nonocclusive: functional vesicoureteral obstruction, low ureteral tone
—Occlusive: occlusion of the ureteral lumen from outside or inside (tumor, stone, foreign body) or secondary to scarring (TB, schistosomiasis)

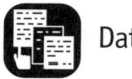 Database

HISTORY

• A history compatible with acute pyelonephritis or persistent recurrent cystitis suggests the presence of VUR (most commonly in females, particularly younger girls).
• Medical history: TB, schistosomiasis
• Surgical history: prostatectomy, wedge resection of the posterior vesical neck, ureteral meatotomy, ureterocele resection, or pervious radiation
• Family history: VUR
• Review of systems: spinal cord disease, urinary tract obstruction, and pregnancy

PHYSICAL EXAMINATION

• General examination: A neurogenic deficit compatible with a paretic bladder may be revealed.
• Abdominal and pelvic examination

—Inspection: A mass visible in the upper abdominal area may indicate hydronephrosis. Fullness in the costovertebral angle may be consistent with perinephric infection.
—Palpation: The finding of a soft or firm renal mass may suggest hydronephrosis. During an attack of acute pyelonephritis, renal tenderness may be elicited; however, chronic renal infection is usually painless. Palpation of the suprapubic area may reveal a distended bladder secondary to obstruction or neurogenic disease. A markedly thickened bladder caused by the posterior urethral valve in a male infant may be felt as a hard midline mass deep in the pelvis.
—Percussion: Percussion of the renal area may outline a hydronephrotic mass, both anteriorly and posteriorly. Pelvic percussion of this area may reveal a distended bladder.

Diagnostic Studies

LABORATORY TESTING

- UA: bacteruria and/or pyuria, particularly in females. Males may have sterile urine due to relatively sterile penile urethra.
- Kidney function tests: Creatinine levels may be elevated in the advanced stage of renal damage.

IMAGING

- X-ray: In case of a neurologic deficit, a plain film may reveal absence of the sacrum, spina bifida, or meningomyelocele.
- Excretory urograms: may show persistent dilation in areas of the ureter, hydronephrotic changes, or healed pyelonephritis (calyceal clubbing with narrowed infundibula or cortical thinning). However, a normal IVU does not rule out reflux. An IVU may also show a ureterocele or ureteral duplication (suggesting reflux in the lower pole of the kidney).
- Renal ultrasound: may show hydronephrotic changes of the kidney, or high residual bladder volume in cases of obstruction distal to bladder neck
- Cystography: simple, delayed, or voiding cystography may demonstrate reflux, as well as voiding cinefluoroscopy. The voiding phase of the cystogram may also reveal changes compatible with distal urethral stenosis in girls or changes diagnostic of posterior urethral valves in young boys.

SPECIAL STUDIES

- Urethral calibration: to rule out distal urethral stenosis (commonly in young girls suffering from UTI)
- Cystoscopy: to examine

—Morphology of the ureteral orifice: Normally, the orifice has the appearance of a volcanic cone; with progressive weakness, it first looks like a football stadium, and then like a horseshoe. The complete incompetent junction has the appearance of a golf hole.
—Position: The degree of the ureteral orifice lateralization correlates with the degree of ureterotrigonal weakness. (Weak ureteral orifices lie farther from vesical neck.)

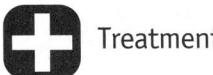 ## Treatment

GENERAL MEASURES

- Hot sitz baths, anticholinergics, and urinary analgesics are occasionally warranted for relief of cystitis in females.
- Antibiotic suppression is currently the most common form of therapy in the pediatric population.

MEDICAL

- Antimicrobial for UTI, followed by chronic suppressive therapy for at least 6 months

SURGICAL

- Surgical treatment is warranted if medical treatment fails, or if there is evidence of progressive renal damage.

—Temporary urinary diversion: In case of marked impairment of renal function or massive dilation of the ureters, a preliminary urinary diversion (e.g., cystostomy or nephrostomy) may be used until definitive relief of obstruction and ureterovesicoplasty can be done at the optimum time.

- Permanent urinary diversion: If successful ureterovesicoplasty cannot be accomplished, a Bricker type of diversion is indicated. In massively dilated and atonic ureters with poor renal function, ureterocutaneous diversion may be the procedure of choice.

—Other surgical procedures
  —Nephrectomy: is indicated in unilateral reflux with a severely damaged kidney and a contralateral normal one
  —Heminephrectomy: In a duplicate system with a functionless one pole, heminephrectomy with removal of its entire ureter may be attempted.
  —Transureteroureterostomy: may be tried in unilateral reflux
  —Ureterovesicoplasty: Any of the following approaches may be tried, with a high success rate: suprahiatal repair, infrahiatal repair, combined supra- and infrahiatal repair, or transtrigonal repair.

ALTERNATIVE THERAPIES

- Triple voiding or void by the clock methods may be tried in young children; however, they are generally less effective.
- An indwelling urethral catheter may be tried in infant girls.

PATIENT EDUCATION: N/A

 ## Follow-Up

MONITORING

- Follow-up after medical treatment should include a monthly UA, cystograms every 6 months, and an IVU or renal scan every 6 months until the patient is stable.

PREVENTION

- Maintenance of sterile urine may help reduce risks.

 ## Miscellaneous

SYNONYMS: N/A

ASSOCIATED CONDITIONS

- Spinal cord disease, duplicate ureters, ectopic ureteral orifice, ureterocele, prune-belly syndrome, obstructive urinary tract pathology

NOTES

- See also Section I, "Urinary Tract Infection—Pediatric," and Section II, "Vesicoureteral Reflux—Adult."

ABBREVIATIONS

- UVJ, ureterovesical junction; UTI, urinary tract infection; VUR, vesicoureteral reflux; TB, tuberculosis

REFERENCES

Bailey RR. The relationship of VUR to UTI and chronic pyelonephritis—reflux nephropathy. *Clin Nephrol* 1973;1:132.

Tanagho EA, Pugh RCB. The anatomy and function of the ureterovesical junction. *Br J Urol* 1963;35:151.

Authors: Ehab A. El-Gabry and Leonard G. Gomella

Von Hippel-Lindau Disease/Syndrome

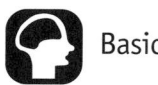 Basics

DESCRIPTION

- Von Hippel-Lindau disease/syndrome (VHL) is a hereditary neoplastic disorder characterized by clear-cell renal cell carcinoma (RCC), pheochromocytoma, pancreatic cysts and neuroendocrine tumors, brain and spinal cord hemangioblastomas, retinal angiomas, endolymphatic sac tumor, and papillary cystadenomas of the epididymis in males and the broad ligament in females.

EPIDEMIOLOGY

- Age at diagnosis varies from early childhood through about the seventh decade.
- Males and females are affected about equally.
- No apparent racial predilection
- 1 in 35,000 to 40,000 live births
- Estimate of between 6000 and 7000 individuals with VHL in United States

GENETICS

- VHL tumor suppressor gene identified at 3p25-26.
- Autosomal dominant inheritance
- 100% (126/126) of families' mutations identifiable
- New mutations and mosaics observed in some individuals

STAGING

- See TNM for renal cell carcinoma in the appendix.

SIGNS AND SYMPTOMS

- Dependent on affected sites
- RCC, clear-cell type (bilateral, multiple solid masses and cysts), occurs in 28% to 45% of all affected with VHL.

—Asymptomatic during much of growth. Large tumors may result in hematuria, flank pain, and a palpable mass. Metastatic RCC is found in some asymptomatic individuals.
—Mean age: 37. Also, teenage onset occurs; reported as young as age 15

- Pheochromocytoma of adrenal gland (may be bilateral and multifocal) in about 18%, extra-adrenal, and can become malignant

—Hypertension, headaches, palpitations, episodic sweating, anxiety attacks, personality changes; life-threatening conditions are hypertensive crises, myocardial infarction, cardiac failure, stroke, and metastatic disease.
—Earliest age of symptomatic onset reported as 8 years old; mean age, 20 years old

- Pancreatic neuroendocrine (also called islet cell) carcinoma in about 12%, microcystic adenoma, cysts in up to 93%

—Most are asymptomatic; may be location-related biliary obstruction or pancreatitis; diarrhea, steatorrhea, and diabetes due to cystic replacement of pancreas; early satiety or pain due to extrinsic compression; neuroendocrine carcinoma metastasis to liver and bone

- Retinal angiomas, also called hemangioblastomas, occur in 58% to 60%.

—Blurred or decreased vision, retinal detachment, eye pain, glaucoma, or blindness may result.
—About 5% under age 10, with rare diagnoses reported in 1- to 2-year-old infants

- Central nervous system hemangioblastomas occur in 60% to 65%.

—Brain hemangioblastomas (cerebellum > brain stem > cerebrum); may be associated cyst
—Headaches, vertigo, ataxia, vomiting, wide-based gait, slurred speech, nystagmus, and dysmetria; rarely occurring are papilledema, temporal lobe hemangioblastoma with seizures, and hemangioblastoma-associated erythrocytosis.
—Spinal cord hemangioblastoma; may be associated syringomyelia, cyst, and edema
　　—Localized pain, sensory loss, proprioception loss, paraparesis, hypertonia, muscle wasting

- Papillary cystadenoma of the epididymis (most often bilateral)

—Most are asymptomatic; rare report of infertility due to obstructive azospermia; atrophy of seminiferous tubules of the testicle may be seen.

- Endolymphatic sac tumor (ELST) in 10% to 12%

—Hearing decrease or loss, tinnitus, vertigo; less often, facial paresis
—Case reviewed with hearing loss at age 11, and ELST detected on MRI 3 years later

PATHOPHYSIOLOGY

- Hemangioblastomas

—Pathologically benign neoplasms occurring in brain, spinal cord, and retina almost exclusively
—Vascular lesion containing channels lined by cuboidal epithelium and interspersed with nests of foamy stromal cells and pericytes; mast cells may produce erythropoietin; commonly cystic areas
—CNS tumor cells resemble RCC histopathology.

- Renal cell carcinoma and cysts

—RCC, clear-cell type; complex cysts lined by clear cells; metastatic potential increases with size, especially when >3 cm.

- Pheochromocytoma

—Neural crest tumors arising in adrenal medulla chromaffin cells; occur extraadrenal as paragangliomas; generally encapsulated and highly vascular; microscopically, cells in round clusters are separated by endothelium-lined spaces; vessels containing norepinephrine and epinephrine seen on electron microscopy; metastasis reported

- Pancreatic neuroendocrine carcinoma (also called islet cell carcinoma)

—Well-demarcated, unencapsulated nodules made of nests of polygonal cells with vesicular nuclei; metastatic potential, especially to liver and bone

- Pancreatic cystic disease
- Benign cysts and cystadenomas: Cysts from 3 mm to >10 cm are epithelium-lined collections of serous fluid; serous cystadenoma or microcystic adenoma, a cluster of cysts separated by thickened walls of stroma arranged in stellate pattern with central nidus that may be calcified or scarlike

- ELST

—Inner ear tumor: sac at end of endolymphatic duct within the dura of posterior fossa
—Locally aggressive, usually slow growing, low-grade papillary adenocarcinoma; histologically resembling papillary cystadenoma of the epididymis

- Papillary cystadenoma of the epididymis and broad ligament

—Benign neoplasms: Epididymal cystadenoma are well circumscribed but unencapsulated; histologically, the tumor architecture is papillary and tubular, with a fibrous stroma. Rarely found in the broad ligament is a histologically identical lesion thought to be the female counterpart to the male epididymal cystadenoma.

Von Hippel-Lindau Disease/Syndrome

CAUSES/RISK FACTORS

- Inheritance of mutation in the VHL tumor suppressor gene predisposes to development of characteristic tumors of VHL.
- New heritable mutations may occur in the VHL gene of germ cells or in early embryonic cells.
- Sporadic clear-cell RCC and sporadic hemangioblastomas have been shown to have somatic mutations in both alleles of the VHL tumor suppressor gene.
- Preliminary unpublished studies appear to support the widely accepted view of cigarette smoking as a risk for the kidney cancer.
- A study of VHL gene somatic mutations in RCC occurring in industrial solvent workers implicates trichloroethene (TRI) as the possible mutagenic agent.

COMPLICATIONS

- Avoided in most with regular screening, early detection, and treatment
- *Caution:* Rule out pheochromocytoma before any surgical procedure or delivery of a child.
- Hypertensive crisis, myocardial infarction, and stroke due to pheochromocytoma
- Blindness, deafness, paralysis
- Obstructive hydrocephalus, cerebral hemorrhage
- Seizures are rare but occur with the less common cerebral tumors, especially temporal lobe.
- Cardiac failure due to chronic effect of pheochromocytoma
- Pancreatic insufficiency: exocrine and endocrine
- Biliary obstruction, jaundice, pancreatitis
- Hematuria
- Obstructive azospermia (quite rare)
- Metastasis from RCC, neuroendocrine carcinoma of pancreas, and, rarely, pheochromocytoma, and all associated morbidity and mortality of metastatic disease

DIFFERENTIAL DIAGNOSIS

- Multiple endocrine neoplasia when pheochromocytoma is manifestation in patient and/or family
- Non-VHL familial clear-cell RCC
- Polycystic kidney disease
- Sporadic neoplasms of same histopathology as characteristic tumors of VHL
- CNS hemangioblastoma vs. metastasis

 Database

HISTORY

- Family history of VHL or any of the characteristic VHL tumor types
- Medical history of the patient
- Surgical history: pathology reports to confirm histopathology of neoplasm(s)
- Review of systems: Inquire about the symptoms listed under Signs and Symptoms in the "Basics" section.

—For example, headaches, ataxia, blurred vision, hearing loss, anxiety attacks, flank pain, hypertension, hematuria

PHYSICAL EXAMINATION

- Retinal focused eye examination, indirect ophthalmoscopy (as needed, fluorescein angiography)
- Must include neurologic examination (including Romberg, tandem walk, coordination, sensory)
- Costovertebral angle palpation to assess for renal mass or tenderness
- Blood pressure and heart rate may be suggestive of pheochromocytoma.
- Scrotal examination to assess epididymis for tumors
- Cardiac and lung auscultation as first cardiopulmonary assessment, if surgery is needed

 Diagnostic Studies

LABORATORY TESTING

- 24-hour urinary test for catecholamines, VMA, and metanephrines

—Testing for functional pheochromocytoma
—May substitute blood catecholamines and/or metabolites
—May add glucagon stimulation or clonidine suppression test
—CBC (If elevated RBCs, measure erythropoietin.)

- Blood chemistries: attention to creatinine, BUN, and glucose
- Urinalysis: often normal, even when there are multiple renal tumors

IMAGING

- Magnetic resonance imaging with gadolinium: brain and spinal cord

—Hemangioblastomas, associated cysts; mainly cerebellum, also brain stem and cerebrum
—Spinal cord hemangioblastomas, syringomyelia, and edema
—Attention to region of internal auditory canal

- Computerized tomography of abdomen, with and without contrast

—Assessment of kidneys, pancreas, and adrenals for tumors and cysts

- Ultrasound of retroperitoneum

—Complements CT scan of abdomen to distinguish cysts vs. solid tumors
—Preliminary screen of children's kidney, pancreas, and adrenals

- Ultrasound of scrotal sacs to assess epididymis for cystadenomas

SPECIAL STUDIES

- Ophthalmoscopy of retina for every patient, and if needed, add fluorescein angioscopy
- MRI of abdomen (may substitute for or complement CT of abdomen)
- ^{131}I-MIBG (metaiodobenzylguanidine) scintigraphy for pheochromocytomas, adrenal and extraadrenal
- ENT examination and audiology: if hearing loss, vertigo, tinnitus
- MRI of internal auditory canal (IAC) to rule out ELST

(continued)

Von Hippel-Lindau Disease/Syndrome (continued)

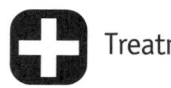 Treatment

GENERAL MEASURES

• Surgery is the mainstay of treatment, as described in the Surgical section below.

MEDICAL

• Current medical treatment is to replace or correct function after organ ablation or dysfunction due to disease, or following surgical removal as treatment.
• Antihypertensives until cause of hypertension is determined and eliminated
• Phenoxybenzamine preoperatively before pheochromocytoma resection
• If surgically addisonian, hydrocortisone and fludrocortisone replacement therapy
• Rarely, the patient becomes surgically anephric and requires dialysis.
• Pancreatic exocrine or endocrine insufficiency

—Pancreatic enzymes; insulin

• A clinical trial is planned for anti-VEGF (vasoendothelial growth factor)

SURGICAL

• Surgery is the mainstay of VHL treatment.
• Nephron-sparing surgeries (permit long-term use of native kidneys)

—When at least one tumor is greater than 3 cm
—Multiple bilateral primary renal tumors
—Some long-term renal transplants are known.

• Pheochromocytoma resection: increasingly partial adrenalectomies performed laparoscopically
• Neuroendocrine carcinoma (islet cell carcinoma) resection (type of surgical procedure dictated by tumor location and size)
• Neurosurgery when benign hemangioblastoma or associated cyst threatens function
• Neuro-otologic and neurosurgical resection of endolymphatic sac tumor selectively for hearing preservation and ablation of locally aggressive tumor.
• Laser or cryotherapy for retinal angiomas; rarely enucleation and prosthesis replacement

ALTERNATIVE THERAPIES

• Renal transplantation when there have been bilateral nephrectomies
• Hemodialysis in anephric patient while awaiting renal transplant
• Gamma knife therapy of carefully selected brain tumors

—Only after careful selection based on location, size, and without associated cyst

PATIENT EDUCATION

• Key to preventing morbidity and mortality
• Rule out pheochromocytoma prior to any surgery and in pregnancy.
• Inform of organs to be screened and frequency.
• Supply the patient with screening guidelines by patient age.

—Eye examinations beginning in infancy
—Pheochromocytomas have occurred as early as age 6.

• Advise against smoking cigarettes.
• Genetic counseling is essential.

—Inform the patient of the risk to relatives.
—Inform the patient of the economic and psychosocial impact of a genetic diagnosis.

• Physician and patient queries

—Locate clinical centers for families with VHL, with the assistance of
    —Genetic counselors, the Internet (see below), VHL Family Alliance (see below)
    —Call: NIH Patient Recruitment and Referral Center: (800)411-1222; in Washington, DC: (301)496-4891; e-mail: prrc@cc.nih.gov; www.cc.nih.gov

• Patient support group

—VHL Family Alliance: (800)767-4VHL or (617)232-5946; e-mail: info@vhl.org or www.vhl.org

• Genetic diagnostic laboratory

—University of Pennsylvania School of Medicine: (800)669-2172 or (215)573-9161

Von Hippel-Lindau Disease/Syndrome

 Follow-Up

MONITORING

- At least yearly, of all characteristic sites of VHL lesions
- More frequent monitoring of actively growing lesions

PREVENTION

- A study is planned to identify factors that stimulate development and growth of VHL tumors.
- Preliminary data suggest that cigarette smoking correlates with an increased incidence of renal tumors.

 Miscellaneous

SYNONYMS: N/A

ASSOCIATED CONDITIONS

- See Pathophysiology in the "Basics" section.

NOTES

- See also Section I, "Renal Masses—Benign and Malignant," and Section II, "Renal Cell Carcinoma—General."

ABBREVIATIONS

- VHL, von Hippel-Lindau disease/syndrome; ELST, endolymphatic sac tumor; VMA, vanillylmandelic acid

REFERENCES

Brauch H, et al. Exposure to trichloroethene is associated with mutations in the VHL gene of patients with renal cell cancer. AACR, New Orleans, March 28, 1998.

Choyke PL, et al. Von Hippel-Lindau disease: Genetic, clinical and imaging features. *Radiology* 1995;194:629–642.

Glenn GM, et al. Von Hippel-Lindau disease: Clinical review and molecular genetics. *Probl Urol* 1990;4(2):312–330.

Latif, et al. Identification of the von Hippel-Lindau disease tumor suppressor gene. *Science* 1993;260:1317–1320.

Linehan WM, Klausner RD. Renal carcinoma. In: Vogelstein B, Kinzler K, eds. *The Genetic Basis of Human Cancer*. New York: McGraw-Hill, 1998: 455–473.

Walther MM, et al. Parenchymal sparing surgery in patients with hereditary renal cell carcinoma. *J Urol* 1995;153:913–916.

Authors: Gladys M. Glenn and W. Marston Linehan

Wilms' Tumor

 Basics

DESCRIPTION

- A malignant tumor of the kidney, found most commonly in children

EPIDEMIOLOGY

- Cause of 90% of renal tumors in children
- Fourth most common pediatric tumor
- Median age: 3.5 years; 90% of cases before age 7
- Males and females equally affected
- Seen with increased frequency in children with

—Beckwith-Wiedemann syndrome: 1 in 10 children develop a tumor of the liver, adrenal cortex, or kidney.
—Hemihypertrophy (2%)
—Denys-Drash syndrome: pseudohermaphroditism, nephropathy, and Wilms' tumor
—WAGR syndrome: Wilms' tumor, sporadic aniridia (about one-third develop Wilms'), genitourinary malformations, mental retardation

- Younger patients (15 months) have a higher incidence of associated congenital anomalies (45%)

GENETICS

- WT1 gene: Denys-Drash and WAGR syndromes, chromosome 11p13
- WT2 gene: Beckwith-Wiedemann syndrome, chromosome 11p15

STAGING

- See the TNM system in Section VII.

SIGNS AND SYMPTOMS

- Most children are well-appearing and present with an abdominal mass.
- Vague abdominal pain, fever, pallor, anemia, malaise, anorexia
- Hypertension; may be renin mediated in 25% to 63% of patients
- Hematuria, constipation

PATHOPHYSIOLOGY

- An abnormal proliferation of metanephric blastema composed of three cell types: blastema, stroma, and epithelial cell types
- This triphasic tumor consists of a tubuloglomerular swirl of "nephrogenic" cells in a background of undifferentiated "stromagenic" cells. The nonepithelial component can further differentiate into striated muscle, adipose tissue, cartilage, or bone.
- About 5% of tumors are bilateral.
- Histologic types are divided into favorable and unfavorable, each requiring different treatment.

—Favorable: In NWTS-3, only 9% presented with metastatic disease.
—Unfavorable: anaplasia or sarcomatous
——Constituted about 12% of patients in NWTS-2, but half of deaths
—Rhabdoid tumor and clear cell sarcoma
——Renal tumors of poor prognosis are no longer considered to be Wilms'.

- Cystic nephroma is a rare cystic form of Wilms' tumor.

CAUSES/RISK FACTORS

- Associated with hemihypertrophy, Beckwith-Wiedemann syndrome, aniridia

COMPLICATIONS

- Treatment related
- Acute bone marrow suppression and hepatic toxicity are seen with radiation and chemotherapy.

—Doxorubicin: At least one episode of congestive heart failure in 32% after 15 years
—Etoposide, ifosfamide: nephrotoxicity

- Patients with bilateral renal tumors are at increased risk for end-stage renal disease.
- Radiation can affect organ growth and function.

—Spine: scoliosis
—Chest: interstitial pneumonitis in 12%; high mortality
—Abdomen: ovarian failure, enteritis

- Secondary malignancy (6%) in field of treatment: leukemia, sarcoma (especially osteogenic sarcoma), adenocarcinoma, brain tumor
- Late surgical toxicity: sepsis related to absence of spleen in patients undergoing splenectomy to remove the renal tumor; bowel obstruction

DIFFERENTIAL DIAGNOSIS

- Neuroblastoma, mesoblastic nephroma, rhabdomyosarcoma, hepatoblastoma, renal cell carcinoma, lymphoma, multicystic dysplastic kidney, polycystic kidney, ureteropelvic junction obstruction

 Database

HISTORY

- Enlarging abdominal girth localized to one side of abdomen in 75% of patients
- Abdominal pain, acute pain with fever, mass, anemia, and hypertension suggest a bleeding tumor.
- Gross hematuria is uncommon.
- Cough, pleural pain

PHYSICAL EXAMINATION

- Abdominal mass

—Firm, nontender, smooth mass on one side of abdomen. Most tumors are unilateral and do not cross the midline. (Note: Neuroblastomas are nodular and extend across the midline.)

- Varicocele associated with vena caval or renal vein thrombus
- Associated findings (congenital anomalies in 15%; GU anomalies in 4%)

—Hypospadias, cryptorchidism, renal fusion
—Aniridia (1 in 70 children with Wilms' tumor)
—Hemihypertrophy: associated with embryonal cancers: Wilms', adrenocortical neoplasms, hepatoblastoma

—Beckwith-Wiedemann syndrome
——Visceromegaly involving adrenal cortex, kidney, liver, pancreas, and gonads
——May also include omphalocele, microcephaly, macroglossia, and hemihypertrophy

 Diagnostic Studies

LABORATORY TESTING

- CBC: anemia, polycythemia (paraneoplastic syndrome)
- Liver function tests
- BUN, creatinine
- Serum calcium
- Coagulation screen
- Urinalysis: microscopic hematuria in a quarter of patients
- 24-hour urine for catecholamines

—Elevated excretion associated with neuroblastoma

IMAGING

- Ultrasound

—Performed initially to confirm solid renal mass; some Wilms' tumors are cystic.
—Doppler sonography to exclude tumor venous thrombus
——Evaluate the renal vein and vena cava for thrombus.

- Abdominal CT, with and without contrast: better abdominal staging
- IVP is used less frequently.

—Wilms' tumor sometimes associated with peripheral "eggshell" calcification on KUB
—Neuroblastoma associated with "salt and pepper" calcification pattern of tumor

- Abdominal MRI: to exclude tumor venous thrombus if other studies are not helpful
- Head MRI: Rhabdoid tumor is associated with brain metastases.
- Chest x-ray: most common site of metastases; chest CT is under evaluation.
- Metastatic bone survey/bone scan: Clear cell sarcoma is associated with bone metastases.
- Arteriography: except when other modalities do not image the tumor well or when partial nephrectomy is considered

SPECIAL STUDIES

- Bone marrow aspiration

—To exclude neuroblastoma cells if diagnosis in doubt

- Chromosome studies in patients with congenital anomalies suggestive of hereditary syndrome

Treatment

GENERAL MEASURES

• Treatment course is guided by stage of disease and histology (imaging and surgical resection/staging)
• Therapy based on series of NWTSG studies
• Bilateral renal disease, unresectable renal tumors, metastatic disease, or tumor thrombus above the hepatic veins are treated initially with chemotherapy.

MEDICAL

• Chemotherapy

—Pulse-intensive dactinomycin plus vincristine (18 weeks) for
  —Stage I favorable histology, age greater than 2 years, or tumor less than 550 g
  —Stage I anaplasia
  —Stage II favorable histology
—Pulse-intensive dactinomycin, vincristine, and doxorubicin (24 weeks) for
  —Stages III–IV favorable histology
  —Stages II–IV focal anaplasia
  —Stage V: Following chemotherapy, a second-look operation is performed to remove the tumor and attempt renal parenchyma–sparing surgery; aggressive therapy and/or radiation in patients not responding
—Dactinomycin, vincristine, doxorubicin, cyclophosphamide, mesna, and etoposide (24 weeks) for
  —Stages II–IV diffuse anaplasia
  —Stages II–IV clear cell sarcoma of the kidney
—Carboplatin, etoposide, and cyclophosphamide
  —Stages I–IV rhabdoid tumor

• Radiation

—Stage III favorable histology and stages II–III focal anaplasia
  —Abdominal radiation
—Stage IV favorable histology or focal anaplasia
  —Abdominal radiation based on local tumor stage
  —Whole lung radiation for patients with chest x-ray evidence of pulmonary metastases
—Stages II–IV diffuse anaplasia and all stages of clear cell sarcomatoid
  —Abdominal radiation
  —Whole-lung radiation for patients with chest x-ray evidence of pulmonary metastases
—All stages of rhabdoid tumor
  —Abdominal irradiation

SURGICAL

• Only surgical therapy for stage I favorable histology, age less than 2 years, tumor weight less than 550 g
• Abdominal exploration to exclude metastatic disease
• Gerota's fascia entered to examine both kidneys and tumors. Unlike in renal cell carcinoma, a radical nephrectomy has not been found necessary in Wilms' tumor.

• Unilateral tumor
—Nephrectomy after careful examination of contralateral kidney to exclude disease
• Bilateral tumors or tumor in solitary kidney
—Exploration of both kidneys is mandatory to diagnose bilateral disease.
  —Bilateral disease: chemotherapy followed by renal-sparing surgery
  —Partial nephrectomy initially, if very limited disease present
—Reexploration after chemotherapy for excision of residual disease
• Avoid tumor spill (sixfold increase in abdominal recurrence)
• Biopsy suspicious for lymphadenopathy
—Mark nodes with clips to guide radiation.
—Radical/routine lymph node dissection is not recommended.

ALTERNATIVE THERAPIES: N/A

PATIENT EDUCATION

• 4-year postnephrectomy survival in NWTS-3
—Favorable histology
  —Stage I: 96%; stage II: 92%
  —Stage III: 91%; stage IV: 81%
—Unfavorable histology
  —Stages I–III: 68%; stage IV: 55%

 ## Follow-Up

• Patients with hemihypertrophy/Beckwith-Wiedemann syndrome, WAGR syndrome, Denys-Drash syndrome, or sporadic aniridia need periodic screening for Wilms' tumor.

—Renal ultrasound every 3 months until age 7 years
—After age 7, physical examination every 6 months until adult

• Majority of Wilms' tumor recurrences within 2 years of nephrectomy

MONITORING

• Stage I

—Favorable histology, <24 months and tumor weight <550 g
  —Chest x-ray and abdominal ultrasound every 3 months first 2 years after diagnosis, then every 6 months for 1 year, then yearly for 2 years

• All others

—Chest x-ray 6 weeks and 3 months after surgery; then every 3 months for 15 months, every 6 months for 18 months, and yearly for 2 years
—Abdominal ultrasound every 3 months for 2 years, then every 6 months for 3 years

• Clear cell sarcoma

—Skeletal survey, bone scan, and brain MRI at diagnosis and every 6 months for 5 years
—Chest x-ray 6 weeks and 3 months after surgery; then every 3 months for 15 months, every 6 months for 18 months, and yearly for 2 years
—Abdominal ultrasound every 3 months for 2 years, then every 6 months for 3 years

• Rhabdoid tumor

—Brain MRI every 6 months for 5 years
—Chest x-ray 6 weeks and 3 months after surgery; then every 3 months for 15 months, every 6 months for 18 months, and yearly for 2 years
—Abdominal ultrasound every 3 months for 2 years, then every 6 months for 3 years

• Irradiated patients

—Skeletal x-ray of irradiated sites yearly to full growth, then every 5 years to detect secondary neoplasms

PREVENTION: N/A

 ## Miscellaneous

SYNONYMS

• Nephroblastoma, embryoma of the kidney, mixed tumor of the kidney

ASSOCIATED CONDITIONS

• Hemihypertrophy, Beckwith-Wiedemann syndrome, aniridia

NOTES

• See also Section II, "Renal Cell Carcinoma—Pediatric."
• The web site for the NWTSG is http://mule.fhcrc.org/nwtsg

ABBREVIATIONS

• NWTSG, National Wilms Tumor Study Group

REFERENCES

Paulino AC. Current issues in the diagnosis and management of Wilms tumor. *Oncology* 1996;10:1553–1571.

Petruzzi MJ, Green DM. Wilms tumor. *Pediatr Clin North Am* 1997;44:939–952.

Snyder HM, D'Angio GJ, Evans AE, Raney RB. Pediatric oncology. In: Walsh PC, Retik AB, Vaughan ED, Wein AJ, eds. *Campbell's Urology*, 7th ed. Philadelphia: WB Saunders, 1998.

Wiener JS, Coppes MJ, Ritchey ML. Current concepts in the biology and management of Wilms tumor. *J Urol* 1998;159:1316–1325.

Author: McClellan M. Walther

Short Topics
A to Z

11-Beta-hydroxylase Deficiency

 11-Beta-hydroxylase Deficiency

DESCRIPTION   Comprises 5% to 8% of congenital adrenal hyperplasia cases. Autosomal recessive disorder that manifests as childhood hypertension, hypokalemia, and muscle weakness. Low plasma renin activity is a hallmark. Afflicted females are virilized and may have male-appearing genitalia. Males may be hyperdeveloped. Diagnosed by high levels of deoxycorticosterone and/or 11-deoxycortisol in serum or their tetrahydrometabolites in a 24-hour urine

CAUSES

- Enzyme deficiency, leading to low cortisol levels and high ACTH level, causing adrenal hyperplasia

TREATMENT

- Oral hydrocortisone (10–20 mg/m^2/d)
- Refractory hypertension treated with spironolactone, amiloride, and/or calcium channel blockers
- Surgical correction of ambiguous genitalia in females
- Prenatally treated with steroid administration to mother

REFERENCE

Mantero F, Opocher G, Armanini D, Filipponi S. 11 beta-hydroxylase deficiency. *J Endocrinol Invest* 1995;18(7):545–549.

 21-Hydroxylase Deficiency

DESCRIPTION   Responsible for greater than 90% of congenital adrenal hyperplasia cases. The most common cause of female pseudohermaphrodism. Most have aldosterone deficiency, which can lead to a fatal salt wasting. Untreated are tall as children but short as adults. Females untreated may have secondary amenorrhea or polycystic ovarian syndrome. Males may have small testes with precocious secondary sexual characteristics. Diagnosed by elevated 17-alpha-hydroxyprogesterone levels in serum with ACTH stimulation test

CAUSES

- Enzyme deficiency, leading to low cortisol levels and high ACTH level, leading to adrenal hyperplasia

TREATMENT

- Oral hydrocortisone (10–20 mg/m^2/d)
- 9-Alpha-fluorohydrocortisone for salt wasters
- Surgical correction of ambiguous genitalia in females
- Prenatally treated with steroid administration to mother

REFERENCE

New MI. Steroid 21-hydroxylase deficiency (congenital adrenal hyperplasia). *Am J Med* 1995; 98(1A):2S–8S.

 5-Alpha-reductase Deficiency

DESCRIPTION   An autosomal recessive disorder characterized by a 46,XY male with an external female phenotype at birth, normally developed Wolffian structures, and bilateral testes residing outside the abdominal cavity. Hypoplasia or absence of the prostate and a blind ending vagina are common. Virilization occurs at puberty. Diagnosed by normal-to-high male plasma testosterone levels or abnormal ratios of serum testosterone to DHT (dihydrotestosterone) or abnormal ratios of urinary 5-alpha- to 5-beta-steroid metabolites

CAUSES

- Loss of DHT during fetal development

TREATMENT

- Male gender assignment: genital reconstruction and supplemental androgen
- Female gender assignment: orchiectomy, estrogen/progesterone therapy, and vaginoplasty

REFERENCE

Imperato-McGinley J. 5 alpha-reductase-2 deficiency. *Curr Ther Endocrinol Metab* 1997;6: 384–387.

 Aarskog Syndrome

DESCRIPTION   A malformation syndrome carried by both an X-linked and an autosomal dominant form. Primary diagnostic criteria include short stature, hypertelorism, short nose with anteverted nares, maxillary hypoplasia, a crease below the lower lip, mild interdigital webbing, clinodactyly, and shawl scrotum. Cardiac abnormalities are also reported.

SYNONYMS

- Faciodigitogenital syndrome

CAUSES

- Genetic with unknown pathogenesis

TREATMENT

- No specific treatment

REFERENCE

Teebi AS, Rucquoi JK, Meyn MS. Aarskog syndrome: Report of a family with review and discussion of nosology. *Am J Med Genet* 1993;46(5): 501–509.

 Abdominoperineal Resection— Urologic Considerations

DESCRIPTION   Commonly performed for rectal cancers in which the rectum, anus, and a portion of the sigmoid colon are removed. The extensive pelvic dissection can lead to a number of urologic problems. Impotence and urinary retention can occur in males, secondary to neural disruption. Urinary incontinence and altered sexual function may occur in females, secondary to removal of the anterior vaginal wall. Damage to the ureters is not uncommon during the procedure.

SYNONYMS

- Miles' resection
- Abdominal perineal proctosigmoidectomy

TREATMENT

- Stent placement preoperatively may help in identifying the ureters.
- TURP may be considered preoperatively in men with BPH.
- A penile prosthesis is often necessary for impotence.

REFERENCE

Kodner IJ, Fry RD, Fleshman JW, Birnbaum EH. Colon, rectum and anus. In: Schwartz SI, et al. *Principles of Surgery,* 6th ed. New York: McGraw-Hill, 1994.

 Accu-Dx (AuraTeck FDP)

DESCRIPTION   The AuraTeck FDP (PerImmune, Inc., Rockville, MD; marketed as Accu-Dx, Mentor Urology, Santa Barbara, CA) is a rapid immunoassay. It detects the urinary fibrin/fibrinogen degradation products associated with bladder cancer. This test has the advantage of being simple and rapid (7 minutes). A multicenter study reported a higher sensitivity of AuraTeck FDP than conventional urine cytology and hemoglobin dipstick in detecting bladder cancer. A higher sensitivity of the test to detect low-stage, low-grade disease was also noted.

REFERENCE

Schmetter BS, Habicht KK, Lamm DL, et al. A multicenter trial evaluation of the fibrin/fibrinogen degradation products test for detection and monitoring of bladder cancer. *J Urol* 1997;158: 801–805.

Acquired Renal Cystic Disease

DESCRIPTION The development of renal cysts in patients with long standing ESRD or severe chronic renal insufficiency. Usually asymptomatic, but can present with abdominal pain or hematuria. More common in males. Three to 6 times greater incidence of renal cell carcinoma over general population. Tumors tend to be very aggressive, with a high incidence of metastasis. (See also Section II, "Renal Cysts.")

CAUSES

• Unknown, but accumulation of toxins that are not filtered by dialysis is theorized.

TREATMENT

• Close follow-up for early detection of malignancy
• Renal transplantation can reverse growth of cysts, but malignancy can still occur.

REFERENCE

Glassberg KI, Filmer RB. Renal dysplasia, renal hypoplasia, and cystic disease of the kidney. In: Kelalis PP, et al. *Clinical Pediatric Urology*, 3rd ed. Philadelphia: WB Saunders, 1992.

 ## Actinomycosis—Renal

DESCRIPTION A chronic granulomatous infection by a member of the *Actinomyces* genus. No pathognomonic findings. Fibrosis and fistulas are common. Can present as sepsis with negative urine culture. Imaging can reveal renal abscesses and hydronephrosis. Diagnosed by gram-positive organisms on stain and prolonged incubation of bacteria. Microscopic examination of the organism can appear as yellow bodies called sulfur granules.

CAUSES

• Can reach kidney by hematogenous spread or instrumentation

TREATMENT

• Usually nephrectomy of involved unit
• Aggressive antibiotic therapy with penicillin or cephalosporin

REFERENCE

Ieven M, Verhoeven J, Gentens P, Goossens H. Severe infection due to *Actinomyces bernardiae:* Case report. *Clin Infect Dis* 1996;22(1):157–158.

 ## Adenomatous Polyps of the Urethra

DESCRIPTION Congenital, benign lesions that occur most frequently in the prostatic urethra. Have been reported in the anterior urethra. Present in the first decade of life, usually as obstruction. Hematuria and enuresis are also common. Diagnosis depends on VCUG, which will reveal a filling defect on cystourethroscopy.

TREATMENT

• Transurethral or suprapubic resection is curative.

REFERENCE

Ritchey ML, Andrassy RJ, Kelalis PP. Pediatric urologic oncology. In: Gillenwater JY, Grayhack JT, Howards SS, Duckett JW, eds. *Adult and Pediatric Urology*, 3rd ed. St Louis: Mosby, 1996.

 ## Adrenal Cysts

DESCRIPTION Rare (0.064%–0.18% on autopsy studies), more often detected on imaging. Most are asymptomatic. Can cause GI discomfort, pain if large, and even an acute abdomen with rupture or infection. Four major types: endothelial, pseudocyst, epithelial, and parasitic, in order of decreasing incidence

CAUSES

• Parasitic, primarily from *Equinococcus granulosus* infection
• Pseudocysts are thought to result from infarction or hemorrhage.

TREATMENT

• Larger than 3.5 cm: aspiration for fluid analysis and cytology to rule out malignancy
• Smaller than 3.5 cm: Observe with serial ultrasound or CT scan.

REFERENCE

Ulusoy E, Adsan O, Guner E, Cetinkaya M, Ataman T, Seckin S. Giant adrenal cyst: Preoperative diagnosis and management. *Urol Int* 1997;58(3): 186–188.

 ## Adrenal Cytomegaly

DESCRIPTION First described by Kampmeier in 1927. Found infrequently in children and adults. Microscopically, seen as foci of cells with large and often hyperchromatic nuclei involving mainly the cortex. Seen often in Beckwith-Wiedemann syndrome. Other possible associations include hemolytic disease of the newborn, erythroblastosis fetalis, and congenital rubella. Considered a benign lesion.

CAUSES

• Theorized origin by pathophysiologic condition that demands increased functional capacity and proliferation of adrenocytes

REFERENCE

Favar BE, Steele A, Grant JH, Steele P. Adrenal cytomegaly: Quantitative assessment by image analysis. *Pediatr Pathol* 1991;11(4):521–536.

 ## Adrenal Hypoplasia

DESCRIPTION Occurs as either primary or secondary defect. Adrenal hypoplasia congenita is an inherited disorder, which has been traced to the gene *DAX-1*. This gene is in close proximity to other genes encoding for glycerol kinase and Duchenne muscular dystrophy. Both of these diseases are seen in association with adrenal hypoplasia. Hypogonadotrophic hypogonadism is also a common finding. Can also occur as a result of lack of pituitary trophic signaling, as in pituitary agenesis. Can be detected by biochemical testing. Antenatal maternal estriol screening can also detect.

CAUSES

• X-linked inheritance of defective *DAX-1* gene

TREATMENT

• Replacement of adrenal hormones
• Must be detected early, or it can be fatal secondary to salt wasting.

REFERENCE

Marfin G, Sheaves R, Muscatelli F, et al. Gene deletion causing adrenal hypoplasia and hypogonadotrophic hypogonadism. *Clin Endocrinol* 1994;40(6): 807–808.

Adrenal Metastasis

DESCRIPTION The fourth most common site of metastatic spread of tumors. Common metastasis include lung and breast (most common), kidney, stomach, pancreas, and melanoma. See also Section I, "Adrenal Mass."

REFERENCE

Bostwick DG. Adrenal glands. In: Bostwick DG, Eble JN, eds. *Urological Surgical Pathology*. St Louis: Mosby, 1997:763.

 ## Adrenal Myelolipoma

DESCRIPTION Rare, nonfunctioning lesions composed of adipose and hematopoietic cells. Asymptomatic, except when very large or hemorrhage occurs. Can be diagnosed radiographically and is typically incidentally discovered. Ultrasound shows a highly echogenic mass. CT demonstrates density near that of fat. MRI T1-weighted images demonstrate high signal intensity, while T2-weighted images are moderately intense. See also Section I, "Adrenal Mass."

CAUSES

• Unknown

TREATMENT

• Excision of tumor if symptomatic or if diagnosis cannot be confirmed radiographically

REFERENCE

Kobayashi T, Kubota Y, Sasagawa I, et al. Adrenal myelolipoma with abdominal pain. *Urol Int* 1997; 58(4):254–256.

 ## Adrenalitis—Herpetic and Nonspecific

DESCRIPTION Inflammation of the adrenal gland. Can lead to primary adrenal insufficiency (Addison disease), which accounts for 80% of cases. Tuberculosis is the second leading cause, with the balance made up by fungal infections; hemorrhage, metastatic neoplasms; sarcoidosis; amyloidosis; and adrenal leukodystrophy. Autoimmune adrenalitis can be associated with thyroiditis, diabetes mellitus, pernicious anemia, vitiligo, hypoparathyroidism, and mucocutaneous candidiasis. HIV with opportunistic CMV adrenalitis accounts for the greatly increasing number of cases.

TREATMENT

• Replacement of hormones, as necessary
• Treatment of underlying cause, as indicated

REFERENCE

Kendall J, Loriaux DJ. Disorders of the adrenal cortex. In: Stein et al., eds. *Internal Medicine,* 4th ed. Boston: Little, Brown, 1994.

 ## Adrenoleukodystrophy

DESCRIPTION Rare, X-linked recessive metabolic disorder occurring in boys. Characterized by adrenal atrophy and widespread, diffuse cerebral demyelination. It produces mental deterioration, corticospinal tract dysfunction, and cortical blindness. There is laboratory evidence of adrenal cortical dysfunction. Two phenotypes, onset in childhood or young adulthood, exhibit hypogonadism. Death inevitably occurs within months of onset.

SYNONYMS

• Formerly called Schilder disease

CAUSES

• Defect theorized in peroxisomes, which handle long-chain fatty acids

TREATMENT

• Lorenzo's oil (mixture of glyceryltrioleate and glyceryl trierucate oil) has been tried in this disease, with some delay in neurologic symptoms.

REFERENCE

Adrenoleukodystrophy: Phenotype, genetics, pathogenesis and therapy. *Brain* 1997;120(8):1485–1508.

 ## Al Ghorab Corporal Shunt

DESCRIPTION To treat priapism, a small transverse incision is made on the dorsum of the glans. A section of septum between the glans spongiosa and the corpora cavernosa is removed to create a shunt.

REFERENCE

Thomas AJ. Surgery for priapism. In: Novick AC, Streem SB, Pontes JE, eds. *Stewart's Operative Urology*. Baltimore: Williams & Wilkins, 1989: 826–832.

 ## Alagille Syndrome

DESCRIPTION Autosomal dominant disorder associated with abnormalities of the liver, heart, eye, skeleton, and kidneys. A characteristic facial appearance is also seen. Renal abnormalities are not specific but include dysplasia and renal failure.

SYNONYMS

• Alagille-Watson syndrome

CAUSES

• Autosomal dominant disorder mapped to chromosome 20

TREATMENT

• Renal replacement therapy as needed

REFERENCE

Krantz JD, Piccoli DA, Spinner NB. Alagille syndrome. *J Med Genet* 1997;34(2):152–157.

 ## Alkaline Phosphatase— Urologic Considerations

DESCRIPTION Enzyme produced in many tissues, such as bone, liver, placenta, and intestine. Can monitor progression of metastatic cancer to bone (such as prostate cancer). Bone source can be distinguished from other sources by its heat lability compared with other forms. Also has been recommended by some authors as a useful tool for monitoring seminoma

REFERENCE

Koshida K, Uchibayashi T, Yamamoto H, Hirano K. Significance of placental alkaline phosphatase in the monitoring of patients with seminoma. *Br J Urol* 1996;77(1):138–142.

Alkaptonuria

DESCRIPTION An inborn error of metabolism wherein homogenistic acid (HGA) accumulates in the body and is excreted in a large amount in the urine. If allowed to stand, the urine gradually turns dark. Alkali can accelerate this process. Ochronosis (deposition of a bluish-black pigment noted in the connective tissue) may lead to arthropathy. Of urologic interest, renal failure occurs, rarely, with long-standing disease. Even more rarely, stones from HGA can occur.

CAUSES

• Single gene defect causing absence of homogentisic acid oxidase

TREATMENT

• Symptomatic treatment

REFERENCE

Venkataseshan VS, Chandra B, Graziano V, et al. Alkaptonuria and renal failure: A case report and review of the literature. *Mod Pathol* 1992;5(4): 464–471.

 Alpha-fetoprotein (AFP)

DESCRIPTION Single-chain glycoprotein (MW 70,000) that aids in the management of testicular cancer. Normally produced by the liver, yolk sac, and GI tract of the fetus. Half-life is 5 days. Normal level is 11 ng/mL. Can be elevated in 38% of cases of embryonal cell carcinoma, 64% of teratocarcinoma, and yolk sac tumors. Other reasons for elevation include hepatoma, neural tube defects, fetal death, ataxia–telangiectasia, some cases of benign hepatic disease.

REFERENCE

Ritchey ML, Andrassy RJ, Kelalis PP. Pediatric Urologic Oncology. In: Gillenwater JY, Grayhack JT, Howards SS, Duckett JW, eds. *Adult and Pediatric Urology*, 3rd ed. St Louis: Mosby, 1996.

 Alport Disease

DESCRIPTION Consists of hereditary nephritis, high-frequency neural hearing loss, and ocular abnormalities. Can present as hematuria, proteinuria, or uremia. Family history is crucial in diagnosis. The nephritis is progressive, usually resulting in renal failure by the third decade. Males are more severely affected.

CAUSES

• Genetic mutation on a single locus on the X chromosome

TREATMENT

• Renal replacement therapy, as needed

REFERENCE

Roy S, Noe HN. Renal disease in childhood. In: Walsh PC, Retik AB, Vaughan ED, Wein AJ, eds. *Campbell's Urology*, 7th ed. Philadelphia: WB Saunders, 1998.

 Alstrom-Edwards Syndrome

DESCRIPTION Characterized by retinitis pigmentosa, nerve deafness, obesity, diabetes, renal failure, and hypergonadotropic hypogonadism. The associated nephropathy may be a form of juvenile nephronophthisis. No chromosome abnormalities are seen.

SYNONYMS

• Alstroms syndrome

TREATMENT

• No treatment is available for infertility.

REFERENCE

Nistal B, Paniagua R. Non-neoplastic diseases of the testes. In: Bostwick, et al. *Urologic Surgical Pathology*, 1st ed. St Louis: Mosby, 1997.

 Aminoaciduria

DESCRIPTION Excretion of an overabundance of amino acids in the urine. Found in association with renal tubular acidosis, Fanconi syndrome, and other primary renal tubular disturbances. May also occur secondary to other diseases that affect the kidney, such as diabetes mellitus and diabetes insipidus

REFERENCE

Neithercut WD, Spooner RJ, Hendry A, Dagg JH. Persistent nephrogenic diabetes insipidus, tubular proteinuria, aminoaciduria, and parathyroid hormone resistance following long term lithium administration. *Postgrad Med J* 1990;66(776): 479–482.

 Ammonium Chloride Loading Test

DESCRIPTION Acid loading test to rule out distal renal tubular acidosis. Performed by giving 0.1 g/kg ammonium chloride oral solution over 45 minutes after a 6-hour fast. 100 mL of water are given every hour during the test. Urine pH is measured hourly for 4 hours. Serum bicarbonate values are taken at hours 2 and 4 to ensure adequate acidification (<16 mmol/L). The normal result is urine pH <5.4. Distal RTA exists if pH >5.4. (See also Section II, "Renal Tubular Acidosis.")

REFERENCE

Osther PJ, Hansen AB, Rohl HF. Screening renal stone formers for distal renal tubular acidosis. *Br J Urol* 1989;63(6):581–583.

Ammonium Urate Urolithiasis

 Ammonium Urate Urolithiasis

DESCRIPTION Extremely rare form of stone disease (<0.5%), endemic in countries with poor nutrition. In contrast to uric acid stones, these grow only in urine with pH <6.5. Caused mostly by infection, usually mixed with struvite stones.

TREATMENT

- Treat infection, increase urine output to >2.5 L/d. Chemolitholysis not possible and intervention may be necessary. Encourage a balanced diet.

 Anderson-Hynes Pyeloplasty

DESCRIPTION Used to treat UPJ obstruction. The ureteropelvic junction is excised, and excess renal pelvis is removed. The widely spatulated ureter is reanastomosed to the renal pelvis with interrupted chromic suture, and the excess renal pelvis is closed with simple or running suture. After nephrostomy, a ureteral stent is placed.

REFERENCE

Kay R. Procedures for ureteropelvic junction obstruction. In: Novick AC, Streem SB, Pontes JE, eds. *Stewart's Operative Urology*. Baltimore: Williams & Wilkins, 1989:220–233.

 Angiokeratoma of Fordyce

DESCRIPTION Vascular malformation of subepidermal blood vessels with an overlying epidermal proliferative reaction. Capillary ectasia is present in the papillary dermis. Typically, numerous dark red to blue dome-shaped papules are linearly arranged on the scrotum and, less commonly, on the penis. In women, one larger vulvar papule is typical. Usually asymptomatic, but can cause annoying bleeding. Typically seen in older patients, these are distinct form congenital scrotal hemangiomas (see Section III, "Scrotum—Hemangioma")

SYNONYMS

- Fordyce's angiokeratoma

CAUSES

- Possibly from high regional venous pressure (i.e., varicocele)

TREATMENT

- Electrosurgery and lasers are effective, but rarely necessary.

REFERENCE

Schiller PI, Itin PH. Angiokeratomas: An update. *Dermatology* 1996;193(4):275–282.

 Angiolymphoid Hyperplasia—Penile

DESCRIPTION A subtype of a broad class of histiocytoid hemangiomas in which four features are found: (1) vacuolated histiocytoid cells, (2) tumor vessels that are thick-walled or capillaries consisting only of histiocytoid endothelial cells, (3) interstitial eosinophils, and (4) lymphoid infiltrates. Usually confined to the skin of one area of the body

SYNONYMS

- Pseudopyogenic (or atypical pyogenic) granuloma
- Inflammatory angiomatous nodule
- Subcutaneous angioblastic hyperplasia with eosinophilia
- Epithelioid hemangioma
- Intravenous atypical vascular proliferation

CAUSES

- Unknown etiology

TREATMENT

- Local surgical excision
- Laser (CO_2) has been successfully used.

REFERENCE

Allen PW, Ramakrishna B, MacCormac LB. The histiocytoid hemangiomas and other controversies. *Pathol Ann* 1992;27[Pt 2]:51–87.

 Angiomyxoma—Perineal

DESCRIPTION Benign lesion, which rarely metastasizes. Rarely occurs in the pelvic soft tissues. Characterized by slow, infiltrative growth. May present as mass in the pelvis. Histologically, demonstrates wavy collagen fibrils related to the myxoid change. Multiple prominent blood vessels are also seen. Occurs mainly in females. Can be quite locally aggressive with frequent local recurrence

CAUSES

- Unknown

TREATMENT

- Wide local excision with close postoperative monitoring

REFERENCE

Hong RD, Outwater E, Gomella LG. Aggressive angiomyxoma of the perineum in a man. *J Urol* 1997;157(3):959–960.

 Angiosarcoma—Genitourinary

DESCRIPTION Very rare malignancy. Grossly, appears as well-circumscribed mass or diffusely fungating tumor. Microscopically, shows numerous vascular channels. Stains positively for factor VIII immunohistochemically. Can be widely metastatic and have persistent local recurrence

CAUSES

- Uncertain
- Bladder angiosarcoma has been reported postradiation for treatment of other malignancy.

TREATMENT

- Radical resection of affected area (penectomy, cystectomy with diversion)
- Lymph node dissection for presence of lymphadenopathy
- Adjuvant radiation and/or chemotherapy for metastatic disease

REFERENCE

Webber RJS, Alsaffar N, Bisset D, Langlois NEI. Angiosarcoma of the penis. *Urology* 1998;51: 130–131.

 Anterior Urethral Valves

DESCRIPTION Much less common than posterior urethral valves. Obstruction of the anterior urethra usually associated with a urethral diverticulum. Usually presents with voiding symptoms or bulging diverticulum on ventral shaft with voiding. Diagnosed by VCUG and renal US. Retrograde urethrogram may miss valve. May be associated with reflux, but less so than with PUV. Renal deterioration is less common than with PUV.

CAUSES

- Diverticulum acting as valve, although cusps without diverticulum have been reported

TREATMENT

- Foley catheter if azotemia occurs
- Endoscopic valve fulguration or single-stage urethroplasty if urethra adequate
- Staged urethroplasty for large diverticulum
- Vesicostomy for reflux or persistent azotemia

REFERENCE

Van Savage JG, Khoury AE, McLorie GA, Bagli DJ. An algorithm for the management of anterior urethral valves. *J Urol* 1997;158[3 Pt 2]: 1030–1032.

Antiandrogen Withdrawal Syndrome

DESCRIPTION   Decrease of PSA levels occurs in 15% to 40% of patients on withdrawal of nonsteroidal antiandrogen in patients treated for advanced prostate cancer with total androgen blockade. Possibly caused by a mutation in the androgen receptor, which then acts to stimulate growth of tumor when bound by the agent. Initially reported for flutamide, bicalutamide and nilutamide have also shown this effect. This effect should be sought before adding other more cytotoxic agents to patients with hormone refractory prostate cancer, and could partially explain the activity of some salvage therapies.

REFERENCE

Smith DC. Secondary hormonal therapy. *Semin Urol Oncol* 1997;15(1):3–12.

 ### Antisperm Antibodies

DESCRIPTION   Develop when there is disruption in the blood testis barrier and may be a cause of infertility. Serum antisperm antibody levels are not as useful as the antibodies in the semen. Can be measured by immunobead testing. The higher the percentage of sperm binding to the bead, the lower the probability of pregnancy. Scoring varies by lab, but normal generally considered to be <10% of sample binding to the bead. (see also Section I, "Infertility," and Section III, "Semen Analysis—Abnormal" and "Semen Analysis—Technique and Normal Values")

CAUSES

- Ductal obstruction (i.e., vasectomy)
- Infection
- Cryptorchidism
- Varicocele
- Idiopathic

TREATMENT

- Condoms, antibiotics, steroids, and sperm washing have all been utilized with variable results. Most effective at the present time are assisted reproductive techniques such as in vitro insemination.

REFERENCE

Turek P. Immunopathology and infertility. In: Lipshultz, Howards SS, eds. *Infertility in the Male,* 3rd ed. St Louis: Mosby, 1997.

 ### Arteriovenous Malformation—Renal

DESCRIPTION   Presents commonly with hematuria. Associated signs and symptoms can include symptoms of CHF, cardiomegaly, diastolic hypertension, and abdominal or flank bruits. Gold standard for diagnosis remains angiography, demonstrating simultaneous visualization of major arteries and veins. CT scan and IVP may reveal a mass lesion, delayed nephrogram, or a filling defect.

SYNONYMS

- Arteriovenous fistula, renal
- Renal AVM

CAUSES

- Uncertain but can be congenital or acquired
- Acquired due to trauma, needle biopsy, percutaneous renal surgery, inflammation

TREATMENT

- Smaller lesions can be adequately treated with embolization.
- Larger lesions should be treated with either partial or total nephrectomy.

REFERENCE

Vasavada SP, Manion S, Flanigan RC, Novick AC. Renal arteriovenous malformations masquerading as renal cell carcinoma. *Urology* 1995; 46(5):716–721.

 ### Artificial Insemination

DESCRIPTION   The process by which semen is introduced into the female reproductive tract by artificial means, for the purpose of improving the chance for conception in fertile couples with patent tubes. Variations include controlled ovarian hyperstimulation, intrauterine insemination (IUI), direct intraperitoneal insemination (DIPI), a combination of IUI and DIPI, fallopian tube sperm perfusion (FSP), and peritoneal oocyte and sperm transfer. Other related means of improving fertility include in vitro fertilizations, such as zygote intrafallopian transfer (ZIFT) and tubal embryo stage transfer (TEST) techniques.

REFERENCE

Abyholm T, Tanbo T. GIFT, ZIFT, and related techniques. *Curr Opin Obstet Gynecol* 1993; 5:615–622.

 ### Ask-Upmark Kidney

DESCRIPTION   Small kidneys with areas of normal architecture separated by grooves overlying dilated calices without pyramids. The parenchyma of the grooved areas contain thyroid-like tubules and lack glomeruli. Usually unilateral and associated with vesicoureteral reflux. Commonly presents as malignant hypertension, but cases of nonmalignant hypertension and recurrent UTIs occur

SYNONYMS

- Segmental renal hypoplasia

CAUSES

- Unknown, but vesicoureteral reflux and ascending infection have been implicated

TREATMENT

- Nephrectomy of the affected side for refractory hypertension

REFERENCE

Zezulka AV, Arkell DG, Beevers DG. The association of hypertension, the Ask-Upmark kidney and other congenital abnormalities. *J Urol* 1986;135(5):1000–1001.

 ### Asopa Hypospadias Repair

DESCRIPTION   The dorsal preputial foreskin's inner rectangular graft is tubularized to form the neourethra, and the outer opposing skin, which shares the same blood supply, serves as the outer penile shaft skin cover.

REFERENCE

Wacksman J. Use of the Hodgson XX (modified Asopa) procedure to correct hypospadias with chordee: Surgical technique and results. *J Urol* 1986;136(6):1264–1265.

Aspergillosis—Genitourinary

 Aspergillosis—Genitourinary

DESCRIPTION Only *Candida* infections are more common opportunistic infections in the urologic population than aspergillosis. It affects patients with diabetes and malignancy and immunosuppressed patients (HIV, renal transplant). Can cause renal parenchymal disease or obstructive uropathy. The prostate has been a rare site of infection. Renal aspergilloma or pseudotumor has been reported in patients with AIDS. Urine cultures can be negative, but aspiration and cytology can demonstrate typical septated hyphae. Therapy is systemic amphotericin B and at least 3 months of itraconazole. Amphotericin B irrigations into the involved renal unit have been used to supplement the systemic therapy.

REFERENCE

Wise GJ, Freyle J. Changing patterns in genitourinary fungal infections. AUA Update Series, Volume XVI, Lesson 1, 1997.

 Aspermia

DESCRIPTION No ejaculate. (See also Section I, "Infertility" and "Retrograde Ejaculation," and Section III, "Semen Analysis—Technique and Normal Values," "Semen Analysis—Abnormal," and "Ejaculation—Decreased or Absent.")

CAUSES

• Retrograde ejaculation, failure of seminal emission

—Surgical (bladder neck dysfunction secondary to TURP, TUIP, retroperitoneal lymph node dissection)
—Medication (Thorazine, alpha-blockers, Aldomet, imipramine alpha-blockers)

• Radical prostatectomy
• Complete bilateral obstruction of ejaculatory duct
• Congenital anorchidism, imperforate anus, and other congenital anomalies

TREATMENT

• See Section III, "Ejaculation—Decreased or Absent."

REFERENCE

Dunetz GN, Krane RJ. Successful treatment of aspermia secondary to obstruction of ejaculatory duct. *Urology* 1986;27(6):529–530.

 Asthenospermia

DESCRIPTION A general term for defects in sperm movement. A decrease in sperm motility to <50% or 60% of normal. Can be detected on semen analysis and can be a cause of male factor infertility. (See also Section I, "Infertility," and Section III, "Semen Analysis—Abnormal" and "Semen Analysis—Abnormal.")

CAUSES

• Antisperm antibodies
• Infection
• Hypoandrogenic state
• Varicocele (most common surgically correctable abnormality)
• Partial ejaculatory duct obstruction
• Immotile cilia (Kartagener syndrome and immotile cilia syndrome)
• Idiopathic

TREATMENT

• Aimed at offending agent (i.e., antibiotics for infection, sperm washing for antibodies, varicocelectomy)
• Interest has been noted in vitamins C and E and other free radical scavengers

REFERENCE

Meacham RB, Lipschultz LI, Howards SS. Male infertility. In: Gillenwater JY, Grayhack JT, Howards SS, Duckett JW, eds. *Adult and Pediatric Urology*, 3rd ed. St Louis: Mosby, 1996.

 Athletic Hematuria

DESCRIPTION Hematuria, microscopic or gross, can be noted in athletes engaged in high-intensity or long-duration exercise. Usually benign in course. Repeated episodes of hematuria may cause anemia in some athletes. Theorized causes include foot-strike hemolysis, renal ischemia, release of a hemolyzing factor, direct trauma to bladder or kidney, dehydration, myoglobinuria, increased circulation, and NSAIDs. Important to diagnose, in order to prevent costly and invasive work-up

TREATMENT

• Adherence to sensible training guidelines
• Hydration

REFERENCE

Jones GR, Newhouse I. Sport-related hematuria: A review. *Clin J Sport Med* 1997;7(2):119–125.

 Atopic Dermatitis (Eczema)

DESCRIPTION Chronic pruritic eczematous condition that affects characteristic sites. In adults, the genitalia is a common site. Patients present with itching, excoriation, edema, erythema, and scaling. As the disease progresses, the skin undergoes lichenification (thickening). The cause is unknown, but there is a familial association with this and other atopic diseases (allergic rhinitis, asthma).

SYNONYMS

• Eczema
• Disseminated neurodermatitis
• Atopic eczema
• Besnier's purigo

TREATMENT

• Topical corticosteroids such as triamcinolone 0.1% bid; nighttime sedation with antihistamines or other agent. Treat stress and remove irritants (soaps, solvent, fabrics made of wool or nylon).

REFERENCE

Edwards L, Lynch PJ. In: *Principles and Practice of Dermatology*. 1998:960–961.

 Atypical Adenomatous Hyperplasia of the Prostate

DESCRIPTION Some lesions can be confused with low-grade prostate cancer on small needle biopsy samples. The differential of these confusing lesions includes atypical adenomatous hyperplasia of the prostate, sclerosing adenosis, postatrophic hyperplasia, basal cell hyperplasia, and others that must be differentiated from low-grade prostatic carcinoma. Histologically, AAH is a crowded focus of small glands. It has not yet been definitively associated with an increased risk of prostate cancer. However, there is evidence suggesting that AAH may be seen with low-grade adenocarcinoma arising in the transition zone. To maximize yield, it is recommended to stain for $34\beta E12$, which detects basal cell–specific cytokeratin. If basal cell staining is present, this helps to rule out carcinoma. Although the biologic significance of AAH is uncertain, its light microscopic appearance and immunophenotype allow it to be distinguished from carcinoma in most cases. The lesion appears to be distinct from atypical small acinar proliferation (ASAP), which appears to be associated with prostate cancer. (See also Section III, "Atypical Small Acinar Hyperplasia—Prostate (ASAP)" and "Postatrophic Hyperplasia of the Prostate Gland.")

SYNONYMS

- Small gland hyperplasia
- Atypical adenosis
- Atypical small acinar hyperplasia

REFERENCES

Bostwick DG. Neoplasms of the Prostate. In: Bostwick DG, ed. *Urologic Surgical Pathology*, 1st ed. St Louis: Mosby, 1997; Grignon DJ, et al. Atypical adenomatous hyperplasia of the prostate: A critical review. *Eur Urol* 1996;30(2): 206–211.

 ## Atypical Small Acinar Proliferation—Prostate (ASAP)

DESCRIPTION Prostate needle biopsies occasionally contain cells identified as atypical small acinar proliferation (ASAP) that is suspicious for but not diagnostic of malignancy. A controversial lesion, it appears that many patients with this diagnosis will ultimately have prostate cancer diagnosed (up to 45% in some series), prompting many to recommend that ASAP be treated like high-grade PIN. (See also Section III, "Atypical Adenomatous Hyperplasia" and "Postatrophic Hyperplasia of the Prostate.")

REFERENCE

Bostwick DG, MacLennan GT. Atypical small acinar proliferation of the prostate suspicious for malignancy in prostate biopsies: Histologic features and clinical significance. *Mod Pathol* 1997;10:70.

 ## AUA Symptom Index

DESCRIPTION Standardized instrument to assess the degree of prostatism (bladder outlet obstruction) in men. Originally sponsored and developed by the American Urologic Association, it is now used widely used. (See Section VII for a copy of the questionnaire.) The AUA Index consists of seven questions that assess emptying, frequency, intermittency, urgency, weak stream, and straining, with each graded on a score of 0 to 5. Score can range from 0 to 35. The index currently categorizes symptoms as

- Mild (score ≤7)
- Moderate (score 8–19)
- Severe (score 20–35)

The I-PSS is identical to the AUA index, except that it adds a single question to assess the quality of life based on the patient's perception of the problem. This is scored from 0 (or "delighted') to 6 (or "terrible').

SYNONYMS

- International Prostate Symptom Score (I-PSS), BPH Symptom Index

REFERENCE

Recommendations of the International Science Committee: The evaluation and treatment of lower urinary tract symptoms (LUTS) suggestive of benign prostatic obstruction. Proceedings of th 4th International Consultation on BPH, Paris, 1997.

 ## Azoospermia

DESCRIPTION The absence of viable sperm on semen analysis causes male factor infertility. When first noticed, the sample should be centrifuged and the pellet examined for the presence of sperm. If present, a work-up for oligospermia should be performed. A postejaculate urinalysis should be obtained to rule out retrograde ejaculation (i.e., the urine contains significant numbers of sperm, 10–15/HPF). If absent, a physical examination for the presence of vas deferens and hormone studies are indicated. (See Section I, "Infertility," and Section III, "Semen Analysis—Abnormal.")

CAUSES

- Congenital absence of vas deferens
- Ductal obstruction
- Germ cell failure
- Testicular failure
- Hypogonadotropic hypogonadism
- Gonadotoxins
- Idiopathic

TREATMENT

- Treatment is based on the underlying cause.

REFERENCE

Sigman M, Howards SS. Male infertility. In: Walsh PC, Retik AB, Vaughan ED, Wein AJ, eds. *Campbell's Urology*, 7th ed. Philadelphia: WB Saunders, 1998.

 ## Balanitis—Zoon's

DESCRIPTION Can be confused clinically with erythroplasia of Queyrat. Grossly, appears as a shiny, glazed-red macular erythematous lesion with multiple pinpoint, bright red "cayenne pepper" spots. Histologically, has subepidermal inflammatory infiltrate of plasma cells and dermal red cell extravasation. No malignant transformation reported.

SYNONYMS

- Balanoposthitis chronica circumscripta plasma cellularis
- Plasma cell balanitis

CAUSES

- Possibly *Mycobacterium smegmatis*
- Heat
- Poor hygiene
- Constant friction

TREATMENT

- Circumcision

REFERENCE

Jolly BB, Krishnamurty S, Vaidyanathan S. Zoon's balanitis. *Urol Int* 1993;50(3):182–184.

Balkan Nephropathy

DESCRIPTION An interstitial nephropathy that is endemic to the Balkan republics of Yugoslavia, Bulgaria, and Romania. Afflicts mainly the middle-aged rural populations. Slowly progressive. May eventually end in ESRD. Anemia, proteinuria, and hypertension can be severe. Renal biopsy has no specific markers for the disease. A strong association with increased incidence of upper tract transitional cell carcinoma (TCC) has been documented. Bladder TCC incidence is normal.

CAUSES

- No proven etiologic entity is known.
- Mycotoxin, long-acting virus, or hereditary causes are theorized.

TREATMENT

- Aggressive surveillance for TCC
- Renal replacement therapy, as necessary

REFERENCE

Plestina R. Some features of Balkan endemic nephropathy. *Food Chem Toxicol* 1992;30(3): 189–192.

Barcat-Redman Hypospadias Repair

 Barcat-Redman Hypospadias Repair

DESCRIPTION In a modification of the Mathieu procedure, this repair mobilizes the posterior urethral plate and splits the glans in addition to the parameatal flap. The full-thickness parameatal and urethral plate grafts are tubularized together and laid to rest in the new urethral groove.

REFERENCE

Duckett JW. Hypospadias. In: Walsh PC, Retik AB, Vaughan ED, Wein AJ, eds. *Campbell's Urology*, 7th ed. Philadelphia: WB Saunders, 1998:2093–2119.

 Bartter Syndrome

DESCRIPTION Congenital abnormality, which usually presents in childhood with metabolic acidosis, hyperreninemic hyperaldosteronism, and hypokalemia. Presenting symptoms are muscle weakness, polyuria, and sometimes growth retardation. Patients are normotensive. Renal biopsy reveals juxtaglomerular hyperplasia. Defective platelet aggregation and decreased vascular responsiveness to pressors are also noted.

CAUSES

- Decreased sodium transport in the thick ascending loop of Henle
- Decreased vascular responsiveness and increased prostaglandin secretion may also play a role.

TREATMENT

- Incurable
- Potassium supplementation, prostaglandin synthesis inhibitors, aldosterone antagonists, and ACE inhibitors can help greatly to ameliorate symptoms.

REFERENCE

Clive DM. Bartter's syndrome: The unsolved puzzle. *Am J Kidney Dis* 1995;25(6):813–823.

 Basal Cell Hyperplasia—Prostate

DESCRIPTION Multifocal lesion, which demonstrates small nests of uniform cells with dark, round nuclei and scant cytoplasm. The basement membrane is prominent. Occurs in context with benign prostatic hyperplasia. Must be differentiated from low-grade adenocarcinoma, transitional cell carcinoma, squamous metaplasia, and adenoid cystic carcinoma. Has no known malignant potential

CAUSES

- Unknown
- May be related to inflammation or ischemia

REFERENCE

Golomb J, Lewin KJ. Basal cell hyperplasia of prostate: An elusive lesion? *Urology* 1992; 40(3):245–248.

 bcl-2—Urologic Considerations

DESCRIPTION The protein product of the gene *bcl-2* acts as an apoptosis-blocking agent. Seems to be required for normal morphogenesis of the kidney, and seems unimportant as a prognostic factor in renal cell carcinoma. Seen in higher levels in prostatic intraepithelial hyperplasia but variable in prostate cancer. Levels increase during XRT. Expression is increased in high-grade bladder tumors.

REFERENCE

King ED, Matteson J, Jacobs SC, Kyprianou N. Incidence of apoptosis, cell proliferation and bcl-2 expression in transitional cell carcinoma of the bladder: Association with tumor progression. *J Urol* 1996;155(1):316–320.

 Beckwith-Wiedemann Syndrome

DESCRIPTION Characterized by macroglossia, abdominal wall defects, and neonatal hypoglycemia. Other characteristic features include gigantism, earlobe creases and pits, facial nevus flammeus, and prominent eyes with infraorbital creases. Most ominous is the increased risk of neoplasia, of which Wilms' tumor, adrenal cortical carcinoma, and hepatoblastoma are most common. Mental retardation is not associated.

SYNONYMS

- EMG (exomphalos, macroglossia, gigantism) syndrome

CAUSES

- Most cases are sporadic, but a genetic cause is widely suspected.

TREATMENT

- Close follow-up early in life for tumor surveillance

REFERENCE

Weng EY, Mortier GR, Grahan JM Jr. Beckwith-Wiedemann syndrome. An update and review for the primary pediatrician. *Clin Pediatr* 1995;34(6):317–326.

 Beer's Nephroureterectomy

DESCRIPTION Refers to a retroperitoneal two-incision approach to a nephroureterectomy through a flank and a separate Gibson or a midline Czerny incision

REFERENCE

Bergman H, Lockhart J. Surgery of the ureteral stump. In: Kaufman JJ, eds. *Current Urologic Therapy*. Philadelphia: WB Saunders, 1986: 212–214.

Behçet Disease

DESCRIPTION　A syndrome characterized by oral and genital ulcers, uveitis, and nonmucous membrane skin lesions of unknown etiology. Lesions on the genitalia are herpetiform and can be painful. Other genital ulcers, such as syphilis, herpes, and chancroid, must be ruled out first.

TREATMENT

• Lesions are treated with local moisture-retaining dressings, topical anesthetics, and local injection of steroids. Occasionally, systemic immunosuppressive agents may be used.

REFERENCE

Margolis DJ. Cutaneous diseases of the male external genitalia. In: *Campbell's Urology,* 7th ed. Walsh PC, Retik AB, Vaughan ED, Wein AJ, eds. Philadelphia: WB Saunders, 1998.

 Bellini Duct Carcinoma

DESCRIPTION　A variant of renal cell carcinoma in which the cell of origin is the collecting duct. Very few cases reported in literature. Immunohistochemically stains with high-molecular-weight keratin and lectin. Histologically, cells demonstrate intracytoplasmic mucicarminophilic material, which is not seen in RCC.

SYNONYMS

• Collecting duct carcinoma

CAUSES

• Uncertain

TREATMENT

• Radical nephrectomy for localized disease
• Chemotherapy (interferon-alpha based) for metastatic disease

REFERENCE

Kirkali Z, Celebi I, Akan G, Yorukoglu K. Bellini duct (collecting duct) carcinoma of the kidney. *Urology* 1996;47(6):921–923.

 Benchekroun Ileal Valve

DESCRIPTION　A hydraulic ileal valve is used as the continence mechanism in ileal or ileocecal reservoirs. As the reservoir fills, there is increased pressure in the valve. It is created by invaginating an ileal segment, which serves as the efferent continent limb.

REFERENCE

Benson MC, Olsson CA. Continent urinary diversion. In: Walsh PC, Retik AB, Vaughan ED, Wein AJ, eds. *Campbell's Urology,* 7th ed. Philadelphia: WB Saunders, 1998:3190–3245.

 Berger Disease (IgA Nephropathy)

DESCRIPTION　First described by Berger and Hinglas in 1968. The most common primary glomerulonephritis. Exhibits a wide variation in manifestation, ranging from a benign, indolent course to rapidly progressive renal failure. Commonly presents with hematuria, proteinuria, and abnormal urine sediment. Diagnosed by renal biopsy demonstrating IgA deposits in the mesangium on immunofluorescence staining.

SYNONYMS

• Idiopathic immunoglobulin A nephropathy

TREATMENT

• Recent promise seen in corticosteroids, fish oil, and ACE inhibitors
• Research in high-dose immunoglobulins
• Renal transplant for cases of renal failure

REFERENCE

Donadio JV Jr, Grande JP. Immunoglobulin A nephropathy: A clinical perspective. *J Am Soc Nephrol* 1997;8(8):1324–1334.

 Beta-hCG (Human Chorionic Gonadotropin)

DESCRIPTION　Glycoprotein with MW 38,000, half-life of 2 days. It is produced normally by the syncytiotrophoblast cells in pregnancy. Composed of two subunits, alpha and beta. The beta subunit is identical to a subunit of LH. Urologic uses include staging and follow-up of testicular cancer (100% of choriocarcinoma, 7% of seminoma, 60% of embryonal). Has been produced by urothelial tumors and secreting polyembryoma. Can be given exogenously to stimulate Leydig cells in secondary hypogonadism and facilitate descent of undescended testicles. The hCG test is used to determine the presence of undescended testicles.

REFERENCE

McAninch JW. Disorders of the testis, scrotum, and spermatic cord. In: Tanagho EA, McAninch JW, eds. *Smith's General Urology,* 14th ed. Norwalk, CT: Appleton & Lange, 1995.

 Bethanechol Supersensitivity Test

DESCRIPTION　A variation of urodynamic testing wherein bethanechol is administered subcutaneously 20 minutes before testing. Usually considered when normal bladder contraction is weak or absent. If positive, a rise in filling pressure of more than 20 cm of water and a shift in the filling curve to the left are noted. A positive test represents bladder denervation. No change during the test represents myogenic damage.

REFERENCE

Snyder JA, Lipsitz DU. Evaluation of female urinary incontinence. *Urol Clin North Am* 1991; 18(2):197–209.

Biothesiometry—Penile

DESCRIPTION Simple, inexpensive method of testing vibratory sensitivity threshold in evaluating neurogenic causes of impotence. Performed by measuring vibratory thresholds, usually in at least three different areas of the body, such as the medial malleolus, fingertips, and glans penis. Probably not as accurate and reproducible as other forms of neurologic testing, such as tibial evoked potentials, pudendal evoked potentials, and bulbocavernosus reflex latency

REFERENCE

Bemelmans BL, Hendrikx LB, Koldewijn EL, Lemmens WA, Debruyne FM, Meuleman EJ. Comparison of biothesiometry and neuro-urophysiological investigations for the clinical evaluation of patients with erectile dysfunction. *J Urol* 1995;153(5):1483–1486.

 ## Bladder Agenesis

DESCRIPTION Rare and usually lethal congenital abnormality that has been reported in fewer than 20 living patients. Associated abnormalities include renal agenesis, retroiliac ureters, crossed fused renal ectopia, malrotation of the gut, colonic duplication, anal atresia, intraperitoneal iliac arteries, and bicornuate uterus.

CAUSES

• Urogenital sinus abnormality during weeks 5 to 7 of development

TREATMENT

• Separation of urinary and fecal stream
• Other reconstructive surgeries as appropriate

REFERENCE

Kaefer M, Adams MC. Penis and bladder agenesis in a living male neonate. *J Urol* 1997;157(4):1439–1440.

 ## Bladder Ears

DESCRIPTION Transient bladder outpouching into the inguinal ring of male infants less than 6 months old. This close association of the bladder with the internal ring resolves spontaneously. Inguinal herniorrhaphy in male infants can result in significant bladder damage if bladder ears are present. Can differentiate from bladder diverticula by absence of definable neck

REFERENCE

Redman JF, Jacks DW, O'Donnell PD. Cystectomy: A catastrophic complication of herniorrhaphy. *J Urol* 1985;133(1):97–98.

 ## Bladder Hernia

DESCRIPTION Most are found in the inguinal or femoral region and are often associated with bladder outlet obstruction in men. Up to 10% of all inguinal hernias can contain some degree of bladder herniation. Rarely, massive herniation may be found with significant portions on the bladder and distal ureter descending into the scrotum. In women, herniation of the bladder into the anterior vaginal wall is technically a cystocele.

TREATMENT

• Repair of inguinal hernia with reduction of bladder herniation

REFERENCE

Amis ES, Newhouse JH, eds. *Essentials of Uroradiology,* 1st ed. Boston: Little-Brown, 1991:289.

 ## Bladder Hypoplasia

DESCRIPTION Lack of development of urinary bladder, leading to inadequate function and storage capacity. Results from either the failure of production or storage of urine or from complete bypass of the bladder. Causes include urogenital sinus abnormalities, severe epispadias, bilateral renal agenesis, severe renal dysplasia, and bilateral ureteral ectopia

TREATMENT

• Bladder reconstruction with bowel segments is employed.

REFERENCE

Canning DA, Koo HP, Duckett JW. Anomalies of the bladder and cloaca. In: Gillenwater JY, Grayhack JT, Howards SS, Duckett JW, eds. *Adult and Pediatric Urology,* 3rd ed. St Louis: Mosby, 1996.

 ## Bladder—Inflammatory Pseudotumor

DESCRIPTION A benign spindle cell lesion in patients who have not had surgery (as opposed to postoperative spindle cell nodule). Most patients are from 20 to 50 and present with gross hematuria. The lesion is nodular or pedunculated, but some may be sessile and invade the muscularis propria. This is a benign lesion, but it must be differentiated from myxoid sarcomatoid carcinoma and myxoid leiomyosarcoma.

TREATMENT

• Resection is the treatment.

REFERENCE

Young RH, Eble JN. Non-neoplastic disorders of the urinary bladder. In: Bostwick DG, Eble JN, eds. *Urologic Surgical Pathology,* 1st ed. St Louis: Mosby, 1997.

 ## Bladder Leiomyoma

DESCRIPTION Most common mesodermal tumor of the bladder. Very rare overall with fewer than 200 cases reported. Presents as mass or with voiding symptoms. Ultrasound reported to be useful for visualizing lesion. Differentiated from leiomyosarcoma on basis of nuclear abnormalities

CAUSES

• Unknown

TREATMENT

• Pedunculated lesions are amenable to transurethral resection.
• Sessile or large tumors may require partial cystectomy.

REFERENCE

Kabalin JN, Freiha FS, Niebel JD. Leiomyoma of bladder. Report of two cases and demonstration of ultrasonic appearance. *Urology* 1990;35(3):210–212.

Bladder Leiomyosarcoma

DESCRIPTION Rare malignancy that is more common in men than in women. Grossly, appears as subcutaneous nodule or ulcerative mass. Usually presents with hematuria and sometimes voiding symptoms. Histologically, appears with spindle shaped cells. Differentiated from leiomyoma by nuclear abnormalities

TREATMENT

• Partial cystectomy has been advocated for favorably placed lesions.
• Radical cystectomy for large or unfavorably located tumors

REFERENCE

Swartz DA, Johnson DE, Ayala AG, Watkin DL. Bladder leiomyosarcoma: A review of 10 cases with 5 year follow-up. *J Urol* 1985;133(2): 200–202.

 Bladder—Lymphoma

DESCRIPTION Involvement of the bladder is usually secondary to systemic disease. Primary lymphoma of the bladder is exceedingly rare. Most patients are female in the seventh to eighth decade. Patients typically present with gross hematuria. The tumors can be single or multiple, sessile or papillary. Most common types are large cell and small cell lymphocytic lymphoma.

TREATMENT

• Radiotherapy has been the treatment of choice for localized lymphoma; systemic therapy if the bladder is not the primary site

REFERENCE

Ohsawa M, et al. Malignant lymphoma of the bladder: Report of three cases and a review of the literature. *Cancer* 1993;72:1969–1974.

 Bladder—Metastasis

DESCRIPTION The bladder may become involved by metastatic cancer from nearly any site. The most common are thought to be the prostate, ovary, uterus, breast, kidney, lung, and stomach. Others include melanoma, leukemia, and lymphoma.

REFERENCE

Messing EM, Catalona W. Urothelial tumors of the urinary tract. In: Walsh PC, Retik AB, Vaughan ED, Wein AJ, eds. *Campbell's Urology*, 7th ed. Philadelphia: WB Saunders, 1998.

 Bladder—Neurofibroma

DESCRIPTION Benign tumor of the nerve sheath from overgrowth of Schwann cells. Originate in bladder from ganglia in the wall. Can present in childhood as obstruction or voiding symptoms. Malignant degeneration is rare.

CAUSES

• Neurofibromatosis
• Sporadic

TREATMENT

• Conservative resection, as needed
• Severe obstruction or intolerable symptoms may require cystectomy.

REFERENCE

Winfield HN, Catalona WJ. An isolated plexiform neurofibroma of the bladder. *J Urol* 1985;134(3):542–543.

 Bladder—Pheochromocytoma

DESCRIPTION Similar to pheochromocytomas in other areas of body. 10% are malignant. Thought to arise from paraganglionic cells in bladder, usually around trigone. Most are hormonally active and can present with hypertension during bladder emptying and filling. Can appear as a submucosal tumor on cystoscopy. Late metastasis can occur, so long-term follow-up is warranted.

TREATMENT

• Partial cystectomy is the treatment of choice.
• TUR may cause a hypertensive crisis.

REFERENCE

Piedrola G, Lopez E, Rueda MD, Lopez R, Serrano J, Sancho M. Malignant pheochromocytoma of the bladder: Current controversies. *Eur Urol* 1997;31(10):122–125.

 Bladder—Sarcoma

DESCRIPTION Types of sarcoma that have been described in the bladder include angiosarcoma, leiomyosarcoma, rhabdomyosarcoma, liposarcoma, chondrosarcoma, and osteosarcoma. These, combined, account for less than 1% of all malignant tumors of the bladder. Usually present as with hematuria or voiding symptoms

TREATMENT

• Usually resistant to radiotherapy and chemotherapy
• Chemotherapy usually consists of vincristine, dactinomycin, and cyclophosphamide.
• Radical or partial cystectomy if confined.

REFERENCE

Raney B Jr, Heyn R, Hays DM, et al. Sequelae of treatment in 109 patients followed for 5 to 15 years after diagnosis of sarcoma of the bladder and prostate. A report from the Intergroup Rhabdomyosarcoma Study Committee. *Cancer* 1993;71(7):2387–2394.

Bladder—Small Cell Carcinoma (Oat Cell Carcinoma)

 Bladder—Small Cell Carcinoma (Oat Cell Carcinoma)

DESCRIPTION Rare aggressive malignancy with poor survival. Histologically, similar to small cell carcinoma of lung. Immunohistochemically stains for neuron-specific enolase. Usually presents with gross hematuria secondary to fungating lesion. Usually muscle invasive at diagnosis. Transitional cell carcinoma, squamous cell carcinoma, or adenocarcinoma can coexist. Extensive staging is warranted before treatment.

TREATMENT

• Partial or radical cystectomy
• Platinum-based chemotherapy has shown partial regression.

REFERENCE

Holmang S, Borghede G, Johansson SL. Primary small cell carcinoma of the bladder: A report of 25 cases. *J Urol* 1995;153:1820–1822.

 Bladder—Teardrop

DESCRIPTION Diffuse pelvic pathology can compress the bladder into a teardrop configuration on various imaging studies, such as excretory urography or cystogram. Causes include pelvic lipomatosis, pelvic hematoma, pelvic adenopathy, and enlarged pelvic vasculature (usually caused by vena cava obstruction). Occasionally, a muscular patient with a hypertrophied iliopsoas can cause this finding.

REFERENCE

Amis ES, Newhouse JH, eds. *Essentials of Uroradiology,* 1st ed. Boston: Little, Brown, 1991:287–288.

 Bladder—Villous Adenoma

DESCRIPTION Tumor that has histologic appearance identical to villous adenoma of the colon. Can also be seen in the urachus. Cystoscopically appears exophytic and papillary. Histologically, a mucous-secreting epithelium with goblet cells is seen.

TREATMENT

• Transurethral resection with possible cystectomy, if invasion is suspected

REFERENCE

Grignon DJ. Neoplasms of the urinary bladder. In: Bostwick, et al. *Urologic Surgical Pathology,* 1st ed. St Louis: Mosby, 1997.

 Blastomycosis—Genitourinary

DESCRIPTION *Blastomyces dermatitidis* is endemic in the Ohio, Mississippi, and Missouri river basins. Opportunistic infection in immunocompromised patients, particularly associated with prolonged steroid use (>2 months), HIV, solid tumors treated with radiation or chemotherapy, and end-stage renal and hepatic disease. GU blastomycosis tends to involve the prostate and epididymis and produces voiding complaints. Prostatic abscess can be seen. Up to 30% can have epididymal involvement. GU blastomycosis is a manifestation of systemic disease; it has been reported to be transmitted by sexual relations to the GU system of the partner.

TREATMENT

• Standard therapy is long-term amphotericin B for a total dose of 1 to 3 g.

REFERENCE

Wise GJ, Freyle J. Changing patterns in genitourinary fungal infections. AUA Update, Volume XVI, Lesson 1, 1997.

 Bleomycin Toxicity

DESCRIPTION Used in combination chemotherapy for testicular cancer as well as cervical, ovarian, squamous cell cancer, and lymphoma. Pulmonary fibrosis is a potentially lethal toxicity. Skin changes, alopecia, and stomatitis are common. Vascular toxicity, anaphylaxis, and Raynaud's phenomenon have been reported.

TREATMENT

• Attention to minimizing oxygen concentration and hydration status during surgery is essential.

REFERENCE

de Wit R, Stoter G, Kaye SB, et al. Importance of bleomycin in combination chemotherapy for good-prognosis testicular non-seminoma: A randomized study of the European Organization for Research and Treatment of Cancer Genitourinary Tract Cancer Cooperative Group. *J Clin Oncol* 1997;15(5):1837–1843.

 Blue Diaper Syndrome

DESCRIPTION Defect in tryptophan absorption in which the urine contains indoles, giving it a blue color. Similar to Hartnup disease. Chronic course is usual. Hypoplasia of the optic disc and abnormal eye movements have also been reported.

SYNONYMS

• Familial hypercalcemia with nephrocalcinosis and indicanuria
• Tryptophan malabsorption

CAUSES

• Defective tryptophan absorption

TREATMENT

• Low-tryptophan diet
• No treatment known for underlying defect

REFERENCE

Chen Y, Wu L, Xiong Q. The ocular abnormalities of blue diaper syndrome. *Metab Pediatr Systemic Ophthalmol* 1991;14(3–4):73–75.

Blue Dot Sign

DESCRIPTION A blue discoloration seen through the scrotal wall when the testes are tented against the skin. Indicates the presence of torsion of appendix testes or appendix epididymis. Should be sought during the evaluation of scrotal pain or swelling. The torsed appendix may swell to the size of the testicle itself.

TREATMENT

• If torsion of the cord can be ruled out by palpation of the unequivocally normal testicle, appendiceal torsion can be observed.

REFERENCE

Dresner ML. Torsed appendage. Diagnosis and management: Blue dot sign. *Urology* 1973; 1(1):63–66.

 Blue Nevus (Melanosis)— Urologic Considerations

DESCRIPTION Benign melanotic lesion of the prostate. Must be differentiated from malignant melanoma. Usually incidental finding after TURP. In prostate, the term *blue nevus* has been used when melanin is confined to ovoid or elongated melanocytes in the stroma, while the term *melanosis* has been used for those prostatic lesions that have melanin in both the stromal melanocytes and glandular epithelium. Has occurred in lesions with adenocarcinoma

REFERENCE

Muzaffar S, Aijaz F, Pervez S, Hasan SH. Melanosis of the prostate: A rare benign morphological entity. *Br J Urol* 1995;76(2):265–266.

 Boari-Ockerblad Flap

DESCRIPTION After appropriate bladder mobilization, a tonguelike flap of bladder based on the ipsilateral superior vesicle artery is incised. The base of the flap should be at least 4 cm, while the tip should be at least 3 cm. The tubularized flap is then anchored to the psoas minor tendon, and either direct or tunneled anastomosis with the ureter is then performed. Useful to reimplant the ureter when there is loss of the distal ureter

REFERENCE

Kay R. Reimplantation of the ureter. In: Novick AC, Streem SB, Pontes JE. eds. *Stewarts Operative Urology.* Baltimore: Williams & Wilkins, 1989:526–538.

 Bonney Test

DESCRIPTION A clinical test used for over 50 years for the diagnosis of stress incontinence and for the selection of patients for incontinence surgery. As originally described, the test consists of two parts.

• The patient coughs with a symptomatically full bladder, and simultaneous urine loss from the urethra is visually confirmed.
• The examiner elevates the bladder neck with a finger on either side of the urethra while the patient coughs again.
• If then the patient is continent, the test is considered positive and the patient is thought to have an anatomic defect correctable by surgical elevation of the bladder neck. Bonney cautioned that the fingers must be carefully placed to avoid compressing the urethra in the midline. Currently, the clinical utility has been questioned by many clinicians as a meaningful test.

SYNONYMS

• Marshall Test

REFERENCE

Miyazaki FS. The Bonney test: A reassessment. *Am J Obstet Gynecol* 1997;177(6):1322–1328; discussion 1328–1329.

 Bors-Comarr Classification of Voiding Dysfunction

DESCRIPTION Based on observations noted on spinal cord–injured patients. The system takes into account three main factors:

• Anatomic location of the lesion (upper motor neuron, lower motor neuron)
• Completeness of the lesion (partial vs. complete spinal cord injury)
• Presence of residual urine, which would mean "unbalanced," according to the definition
• Best applied to patients with a complete neurologic lesion after spinal shock has resolved.

REFERENCE

Wein AJ. Neuromuscular dysfunction of the lower urinary tract. In: Walsh PC, Retik AB, Vaughan ED, Wein AJ, eds. *Campbell's Urology,* 7th ed. Philadelphia: WB Saunders, 1998.

 Bosniak Classification

DESCRIPTION Classification system to differentiate renal cystic masses visualized on CT as benign or malignant. Cysts graded on scale from I to IV, with grade I having typical appearance of benign simple cyst, and grade IV having appearance of renal cell carcinoma. Classification based on homogeneity and complexity of cystic fluid, presence or absence of septations, calcifications, or solid components; and the density of cystic fluid as determined by Hounsfield units. (See also Section II, "Renal Cysts.")

• Type I: fulfills ultrasound or CT criteria for simple cyst—benign
• Type II: minimal complexity, such as internal, thin-walled septa, or small calcifications—benign
• Type III: more extensive calcifications or thickened septa—suspicious for malignancy, warrants surgery
• Type IV: mural nodules with enhancement consistent with cystic neoplasms—surgery warranted

REFERENCE

Bosniak MA. The current radiological approach to renal cysts. *Radiology* 1986;158(1):1–10.

Bourne Test

DESCRIPTION: A diagnostic test for the detection of colovesical fistulas. The test consists of radiography of centrifuged urine samples obtained immediately after a barium enema. In one series of 10 patients in 7/10, the Bourne test was the only positive evidence of an otherwise occult colovesical fistula later proven at surgery.

REFERENCE

Amendola MA, Agha FP, Dent TL, Amendola BE, Shirazi KK. Detection of occult colovesical fistula by the Bourne test. AJR *Am J Roentgenol* 1984:Apr;142(4):715–718.

 Boyarsky Guidelines for BPH

DESCRIPTION To provide reproducible guidelines for severity of symptoms of prostatism/BPH/LUTS, scored questionnaire formats have been developed. Traditional assessment tools include the Madsen-Iversen Point System and the Boyarsky Guidelines. These have been generally replaced by the AUA or IPSS questionnaires, but are used in several ongoing follow-up studies of BPH therapies. (See specific topics, Section III.)

REFERENCE

Boyarsky S, Jones G, Paulson DF, Prout GR Jr. A new look at bladder neck obstruction by the Food and Drug Administration regulators: Guidelines for investigation of benign prostatic hypertrophy. *Trans Am Assoc Genitourin Surg* 1976;68:29.

 Boyce Nephrotomy (Anatrophic Nephrolithotomy)

DESCRIPTION The longitudinal anatrophic nephrotomy takes advantage of a nearly avascular plane in the kidney, which can be used to remove staghorn calculi (Boyce anatrophic nephrolithotomy). The incision site in the lateral posterior surface of the kidney can be accurately identified by injecting indigo carmine in the posterior renal artery branch. Once the capsule is incised, the parenchyma is divided with the blunt end of the knife in the proper plain. Traditionally used for staghorn calculi

REFERENCE

Straffon RA. Anatrophic nephrolithotomy. In: Novick AC, Streem SB, Pontes JE, eds. *Stewarts Operative Urology*. Baltimore: Williams & Wilkins, 1989:191–197.

 Brenner's Tumors

DESCRIPTION Tumors of variable malignant potential of the ovary. Extraovarian and testicular origins have been reported. Usually presents as ovarian mass. Light microscopy demonstrates distinctive nests of transitional cells indistinguishable from urothelium. Classified as typical, metaplastic, proliferating, or malignant. Usually stains for carcinoembryonic antigen

CAUSES

• Theorized origin from a metaplastic process of coelomic epithelium

TREATMENT

• Usually surgical removal to assess malignant potential

REFERENCE

Caccamo D, Socias M, Truchet C. Malignant Brenner tumor of the testes and epididymis. *Arch Pathol Lab Med* 1991;115(5):524–527.

 Bricker Ureteral Anastomosis

DESCRIPTION A direct ureteral to small bowel end-to-side refluxing anastomosis incorporating full-thickness ureteral and intestinal wall. Used in ileal conduit construction

REFERENCE

McDougal WS. Use of intestinal segments and urinary diversion. In: Walsh PC, Retik AB, Vaughan ED, Wein AJ, eds. *Campbell's Urology*, 7th ed. Philadelphia: WB Saunders, 1998:3137–3144.

 Brigham Sling (Urethropexy)

DESCRIPTION Used to treat stress incontinence in women. A combined endoscopic needle sling procedure that utilizes a rectus fascial strip placed at the bladder neck through a vaginal incision. The fascial sling is held in place with needles placed through the anterior abdominal wall similar to the Stamey and Raz suspension needles.

REFERENCE

Loughlin KR. The Brigham sling. *Contemp Urol* 1998;10:69–75.

 British Testicular Tumor Classification

DESCRIPTION Used mainly in Great Britain and based on the concept that all nonseminomatous tumors represent displaced, nonorganized embryonic blastomeres and are therefore teratomas. Classifies disparate lesions under a common category. The World Health Organization classification is used in most of the rest of the world.

REFERENCE

Ulbright TM. Neoplasms of the testes. In: Bostwick, D, ed. *Urologic Surgical Pathology*, 1st ed. St Louis: Mosby, 1997.

Brunn's Nests

DESCRIPTION Discrete clusters of transitional cells residing within the lamina propria that have become separated from the epithelial surface. Variant of bladder epithelium being noted in 80% to 90% of normal bladders. May become involved with transitional cell carcinoma

SYNONYMS

• Von Brunn's nests

TREATMENT

• Controversial whether radical or conservative therapy is indicated if involved by TCC

REFERENCE

Dinney CP, Ramirez EI, Swanson DA, Ro JY, Babaian RJ, Von Eschenbach AC. Management of transitional cell carcinoma involving von Brunn's nests. *J Urol* 2995;153:944–949.

 Brushite

DESCRIPTION Mineral name for calcium hydrogen phosphate dihydrate stones. (See Section II, "Urolithiasis—Calcium Oxalate/Phosphate.")

 BTA Testing (BTA and BTA Stat Urine Test)

DESCRIPTION The BTA test (Bard, Redmond, Washington) is a latex agglutination assay that has recently been approved by the Drug and Food Administration (FDA). It qualitatively detects high-molecular-weight basement membrane complexes, present when the tumor cells become invasive and undergo proteolytic degradation.

• A comparison of BTA with bladder wash cytology, and reported a higher sensitivity of BTA (54% vs. 23%). However, BTA was associated with a high false-positive rate (specificity 9%). A multicenter trial conducted demonstrated a sensitivity of 40% and 16% were reported for BTA and urine cytology, respectively.
• The initial BTA test had two limitations: It is a latex agglutination test and it yielded high false-positive rates. Consequently, a new BTA test (BTA stat) was developed. The BTA stat is a monoclonal antibody immunoassay that detects the presence of newly identified human complement factor H-related protein (hCFhrp). A study of BTA stat reported higher sensitivity compared with cytology. BTA stat has also had higher sensitivity compared with the BTA test, (58% vs. 44%). The specificity of BTA stat was reported as 72% for benign genitourinary disease and 95% in healthy volunteers. The main advantage of the BTA test is that it can simply be performed in an office setting, and provides rapid results.

REFERENCE

Leyh H, Hall R, Mazeman E, Blumenstein B. Comparison of the Bard BTA test with voided urine and bladder wash cytology in the diagnosis and management of cancer of the bladder. *Urology* 1997;50:49–53.

 Burch Colposuspension

DESCRIPTION Through a Pfannenstiel incision and a retropubic exposure, the paravaginal fascia is fixed to Cooper's ligament. Used in treatment of stress incontinence in women

REFERENCE

Raz S, Stothers L, Chopra A. Vaginal reconstructive surgery for incontinence and prolapse. In: Walsh PC, Retik AB, Vaughan ED, Wein AJ, eds. *Campbell's Urology,* 7th ed. Philadelphia: WB Saunders, 1998:1066–1094.

 Buried Penis

DESCRIPTION Congenital anomaly exhibiting a deficiency of penile shaft skin and abnormal attachments of the tunica dartos to Buck's fascia. The normal penis is then entrapped within the subcutaneous tissue. Phimosis is also present. Balanitis occurs secondary to accumulation of urine in between the prepuce and the glans.

TREATMENT

• Surgical correction is very effective.

REFERENCE

Boemers TM, De Jong TP. The surgical correction of buried penis: A new technique. *J Urol* 1995;154:550–552.

 Buschke-Lowenstein Tumor

DESCRIPTION Nonmalignant penile or perineal lesion, which may be large and exophytic. May cause urethral erosion and fistulas. Can be very locally invasive and mistaken grossly for squamous cell carcinoma. Microscopically, broad rete pegs, filled with benign squamous cells and surrounded by a layer of inflammatory cells, are noted.

SYNONYMS

• Verrucous carcinoma
• Giant condyloma acuminata

CAUSES

• Possible role of human papilloma virus 6 and 11

TREATMENT

• Local excision after proving diagnosis

REFERENCE

Chu QD, Vezeridis MP, Libbey NP, Wanebo HJ. Giant condyloma accuminata (Buschke-Lowenstein tumor) of the anorectal and perianal regions. Analysis of 42 cases. *Dis Colon Rectum* 1994;37(9):950–957.

Byar's Flaps

 Byar's Flaps

DESCRIPTION The penile prepuce is split dorsally and transferred ventrally, yielding redundant ventral skin to be used in a second-stage hypospadias repair.

REFERENCE

Duckett JW. Hypospadias. In: Walsh PC, Retik AB, Vaughan ED, Wein AJ, eds. *Campbell's Urology*, 7th ed. Philadelphia: WB Saunders, 1998:2093–2119.

 Calcinosis—Idiopathic Scrotal

DESCRIPTION Occurs in preexisting epidermal cysts or in the dermis without cysts. Usually affects young men. Multiple cysts (greater than 50) are not uncommon. Calcifications range in size from a few millimeters to 3 cm. May represent epidermal cysts that have, over time, lost their normal wall and calcified

TREATMENT

• Surgical excision if symptomatic

REFERENCE

Ro JY, Amin MB, Ayala AG. Penis and scrotum. In: Bostwick, D. ed. *Urologic Surgical Pathology*, 1st ed. St Louis: Mosby, 1997.

 Calcium Load and Fast Studies

DESCRIPTION Performed to diagnose cause of hypercalciuria in stone-formers. One method is to place patients on a low-calcium, low-sodium diet for 1 week. A fast is performed from 9 PM to 9 AM. At 7 AM, patients empty their bladders. This urine is discarded. 600 mL of distilled water is then consumed. Urine is collected from 7 AM to 9 AM. At 9 AM, 1 g of calcium is consumed and urine is collected from that point until 1 PM. Urine samples are analyzed for calcium, creatinine, and cAMP. Results can then differentiate between absorptive hypercalciuria, renal hypercalciuria, and hyperparathyroidism.

REFERENCE

Menon M, Parulkar BG, Drach GW. Urinary lithiasis: Etiology, diagnosis, and medical management. In: Walsh PC, Retik AB, Vaughan ED, Wein AJ, eds. *Campbell's Urology*, 7th ed. Philadelphia: WB Saunders, 1998.

 Camey I Orthotopic Urinary Diversion

DESCRIPTION A 40-cm segment of ileum is chosen for an orthotopic urinary diversion, and the midportion is chosen so that it can reach the urethra. A LeDuc antireflux ureteral ileal anastomosis is carried out on each end of the ileal segment.

REFERENCE

Benson MC, Olsson C.: Continent urinary diversion. In: Walsh PC, Retik AB, Vaughan ED, Wein AJ, eds. *Campbell's Urology*, 7th ed. Philadelphia: WB Saunders, 1998:3190–3245.

 Camey II Orthotopic Urinary Diversion

DESCRIPTION The initial Camey diversion is modified by using 65 cm of ileum, which is detubularized along its antimesenteric border. It is folded into a U-shape configuration, the adjoining sides of the U are sutured, and the resulting bowel is then folded again to create a pouch anastomosed to the urethra with a LeDuc ureteral anastomosis.

REFERENCE

Benson MC, Olsson CA. Continent urinary diversion. In: Walsh PC, Retik AB, Vaughan ED, Wein AJ, eds. *Campbell's Urology*, 7th ed. Philadelphia: WB Saunders, 1998:3190–3245.

 Carcinoid Tumors—Genitourinary

DESCRIPTION Very rare in the GU tract. Have been described in the kidneys, ovaries, uterine cervix, urethra, testes, and bladder. May have associated carcinoid syndrome. Usually 5-hydroxyindoleacetic acid and argentaffin positive on special staining. Electron microscopy demonstrates granules similar to Kulchitsky cells.

TREATMENT

• Surgical excision

REFERENCE

Yang CH, Krzyzaniak K, Brown WJ, Kurtz SM. Primary carcinoid tumor of urinary bladder. *Urology* 1985;26(6):594–597.

 Carcinosarcoma—Bladder

DESCRIPTION Rare tumor that has elements of epithelial and mesenchymal origin. Usually bulky, fast growing, invasive tumors. Epithelial elements are typically transitional cell carcinoma, but can be any of the other tumor types. Mesenchymal elements are usually spindle cells with evidence of chondroid, osteoid, smooth muscle, or rhabdomyoblastic differentiation. Usually presents with painless, gross hematuria

TREATMENT

• Transurethral resection or radical cystectomy, as appropriate
• Chemotherapy and radiotherapy have been used for metastatic disease, with poor results

REFERENCE

Orsatti G, Corgan FJ, Goldberg SA. Carcinosarcoma of urothelial organs: Sequential involvement of urinary bladder, ureter, and renal pelvis. *Urology* 1993;41(3):289–291.

Carcinosarcoma—Prostate

DESCRIPTION Very rare tumor, similar to the carcinosarcoma of the bladder, these tumor are mixtures of epithelial and sarcomatous elements. The epithelial element in the prostate, however, is adenocarcinoma. Most differentiate from collision tumors, which are separate coexisting tumors of differing cell types. True carcinosarcomas have an intermixture of cells in the same tumor.

TREATMENT

• Radical prostatectomy, if organ-confined

REFERENCE

Nazzeer T, Barada JH, Fisher HA, Ross JS. Prostatic carcinosarcoma: Case report and review of literature. *J Urol* 1991;146(5):1370–1373.

 ## Carney Syndrome

DESCRIPTION First described by Carney in 1977. Triad consisting of gastric leiomyosarcoma, extraadrenal paraganglioma, and pulmonary chondroma. The syndrome is complete when two features are present. GI hemorrhage is a common presentation. Primarily affects young women. Elevated urinary catecholamines are found. Prognosis depends on malignant spread of tumors. Large cell, calcifying Sertoli cell tumor associated in male patients

TREATMENT

• Surgical removal of sarcoma and paraganglioma
• Radiotherapy and chemotherapy for unresectable disease

REFERENCE

Lancha C, Diez L, Mitjavila M, Rueda M, Crespo A. A case of complete Carney's syndrome. *Clin Nucl Med* 1994;19(11):1008–1010.

 ## Cat-eye Syndrome

DESCRIPTION Rare, congenital syndrome with features of anal atresia, vertical iridochoroidal coloboma, congenital heart disease, urinary tract abnormalities, and mild-to-moderate mental retardation. The urologic abnormalities reported include renal hypoplasia, chronic pyelonephritis, horseshoe kidney, hydronephrosis, and vesicoureteral reflux.

CAUSES

• Associated with abnormality of chromosome 22

TREATMENT

• Close monitoring of possible pyelonephritis is warranted.

REFERENCE

Bellinghieri G, Triolo O, Stella MC, et al. Renal function in an adult female with cat-eye syndrome. *Am J Nephrol* 1994;14(1):76–79.

 ## Caudal Regression Syndrome

DESCRIPTION First described by Duhamel in 1961. Features a wide array of abnormalities centering on the anorectal, urogenital, and lower spine areas. Severe cases demonstrate fusion of the lower limbs, sacral agenesis, imperforate anus, and absent GU tract (except gonads). In less severe cases, imperforate anus and/or sacral agenesis is seen. These, in turn, are associated with voiding dysfunction. Vesicoureteral reflux is also quite common.

SYNONYMS

• Caudal dysplasia sequence
• VACTERL syndrome (vertebral, anal, cardiac, tracheoesophageal, renal, and limb)

CAUSES

• Disordered embryogenesis during the fourth to fifth week of gestation

TREATMENT

• Management of myriad of problems with multidisciplinary approach

REFERENCE

Boemers TM, Van Gool JD, De Jong T, Bax KM. Urodynamic evaluation of children with the caudal regression syndrome (caudal dysplasia sequence). *J Urol* 1994;151:1038–1040.

 ## Cavernosography

DESCRIPTION Test used to evaluate veno-occlusive leak in erectile dysfunction. Performed by the injection of contrast material into the corpora cavernosa after the injection of a pharmacologic agent, such as papaverine, to stimulate erection. Any visualized leakage of contrast material outside the corpora could be a defect in the veno-occlusive mechanism. Typical leak points include the glans, corpus spongiosum, superficial or deep dorsal veins, and cavernous and crural veins.

REFERENCE

Lue TF, Broderick G. Evaluation and nonsurgical management of erectile dysfunction and priapism. In: Walsh PC, Retik AB, Vaughan ED, Wein AJ, eds. *Campbell's Urology*, 7th ed. Philadelphia: WB Saunders, 1998.

 ## Cavernosometry

DESCRIPTION Test used to evaluate veno-occlusive leak in erectile dysfunction. Performed by first stimulating erection, either by saline infusion into the corpora or injection of a pharmacologic agent. Intracorporeal pressure measurements are then recorded. The inability to raise ICP to levels equal to systolic blood pressure or a rapid drop of pressure after cessation of infusion is indicative of veno-occlusive dysfunction.

REFERENCE

Lue TF, Broderick G. Evaluation and nonsurgical management of erectile dysfunction and priapism. In: Walsh PC, Retik AB, Vaughan ED, Wein AJ, eds. *Campbell's Urology*, 7th ed. Philadelphia: WB Saunders, 1998.

Cecil Urethral Stricture Repair

 Cecil Urethral Stricture Repair

DESCRIPTION The stricture is first excised, and the defect is closed with urethral skin. In the second stage, a neourethra is created by tubularizing the ventral penile skin, as described by Thiersch. The penis is then buried in a midline scrotal incision. In the third stage, the penis is freed from the scrotum, using scrotal skin to cover the ventrum of the penis, and the scrotum is primarily closed.

REFERENCE

Devine CJ, Devine PC. Operations for urethral stricture. In: Novick AC, Streem SB, Pontes JE, eds. *Stewarts Operative Urology*. Baltimore: Williams & Wilkins, 1989:650–680.

 Cervical Cancer—Urologic Considerations

DESCRIPTION Iatrogenic complications regarding cervical cancer treatment are well documented. If pelvic exenteration is performed, urinary diversion is obligatory. Radical hysterectomy has risks of ureteral and bladder damage, as well as fistula, if combined with radiation. Radiation therapy also can be morbid with radiation cystitis, ureteral stricture, and fistula possibly resulting. The increased risk of bladder cancer after XRT is controversial.

REFERENCE

Magerina JF. Complication of irradiation and radical surgery for gynecologic malignancies. *Obstet Gynecol Surv* 1993;48(8):571–575.

 Charcot-Boettcher Crystals and Filaments

DESCRIPTION Cytoplasmic crystal-like filaments, 10 to 25 μm in length, which are found normally in Sertoli cells. Pathognomonic for Sertoli cell differentiation. They have been identified in Sertoli cell tumors, but most reports have not mentioned their presence.

REFERENCE

Santienmma V, Rosati P, Guerzoni C, et al. Human Sertoli cells in vitro: Morphological features and androgen-binding protein secretion. *J Steroid Biochem Mol Biol* 1992;43(5): 423–429.

 CHARGE Association

DESCRIPTION Refers to the association of coloboma, congenital heart disease, choanal atresia, retarded growth and development, structural brain abnormalities, and ear anomalies. Of urologic interest is the association with genital hypoplasia secondary to low androgen levels.

CAUSES

- Mostly sporadic, but familial has been reported
- Theorized to originate during a developmental error of neural crest elements at about the sixth week

TREATMENT

- Generally, early management of sensory defects is very important.
- Androgen replacement may be attempted for genital hypoplasia.

REFERENCE

Harvey AS, Leaper PM, Bankier A. CHARGE association: Clinical manifestations and developmental outcome. *Am J Med Genet* 1991;39: 48–55.

 Christmas Tree Bladder

DESCRIPTION A radiologic change in bladder wall due to detrusor muscle hypotrophy and fibrosis as a result of detrusor–sphincter dyssynergia. Also called "pine cone appearance."

REFERENCE

Nordling J, Olesen KP. Basic urographic and cystourethrographic patterns. In: Pollack HM, ed. *Clinical Urography*. Philadelphia: WB Saunders, 1990:1935–1979.

 Chronic Pelvic Pain Syndrome (CPPS)

DESCRIPTION A term previously used exclusively in gynecology but is now being applied to men with chronic abacterial prostatitis. Nonbacterial prostatitis or chronic pelvic pain syndrome occurs in men with no history of urinary tract infection and negative bacterial cultures of urine and prostatic fluid. The inflammatory type presents with genitourinary or rectal pain or voiding symptoms; the prostatic fluid contains inflammatory cells. Men with the noninflammatory type, whose prostatic fluid has no leukocytes, have similar symptoms, but pelvic pain is usually the predominant complaint. See Section II for prostatitis syndromes and Section III, "Prostatitis—NIH Classification System."

SYNONYMS

- Chronic abacterial prostatitis
- CPPS

TREATMENT

- Empiric 8- to 12-week course of antibiotics
- Consider prostatic massage, if no response
- High-dose alpha-blockers (Flomax, Cardura, Hytrin)
- Antiinflammatory agents, lifestyle changes, stress reduction, holistic therapies
- Finasteride has shown promise in one study.
- Transurethral microwave thermotherapy (TUMT) as a last option

REFERENCE

Leskinen M, Lukkarinen O, Marttila T. Effects of finasteride in patients with inflammatory chronic pelvic pain syndrome: A double-blind, placebo-controlled, pilot study. *Urology* 1999;53(3):502–505.

Churg-Strauss Syndrome

DESCRIPTION Vasculitis characterized by extravascular microscopic granulomas in the lungs, heart, gastrointestinal tract, and skin. Histologically, necrosis and intense eosinophilic infiltration accompanied by histiocytes are seen. Both necrotizing and eosinophilic granulomatous vasculitis usually involve small arteries and veins. There is often a history of atopy. Presents with fever and weight loss. Eosinophilia, anemia, and an elevated erythrocyte sedimentation rate are found. The prostate may be involved by the granulomatous process.

SYNONYMS

• Allergic angiitis and granulomatosis

TREATMENT

• Corticosteroids
• Cytotoxic drugs are being investigated.

REFERENCE

Langford CA, Sneller MC. New developments in the treatment of Wegener's granulomatosis, polyarteritis nodosa, microscopic polyangiitis, and Churg-Strauss syndrome. *Curr Opin Rheumatol* 1997;9(1):26–39.

 ## Chylous Ascites

DESCRIPTION Accumulation of lymphatic fluid in the peritoneal cavity, which can be fatal. In the urologic setting, it can occur after RPLND. Presents as increasing abdominal girth. Paracentesis may be diagnostic and therapeutic.

CAUSES

• Leakage of lymphatics after RPLND
• Inferior vena cava resection is also cited as a risk factor.

TREATMENT

• Conservative measures include a fat-free diet, diuretics, and administration of medium-chain triglycerides.
• TPN, peritoneovenous shunt, or surgery may be required.

REFERENCE

Baniel J, Foster RS, Rowland RG, Bihrle R, Donohue JP. Management of chylous ascites after retroperitoneal lymph node dissection for testicular cancer. *J Urol* 1993;150(5):1422–1424.

 ## Circumcision—Pediatric Issues

DESCRIPTION Removal of the foreskin has its benefits and complications. Meatal stenosis is a problem seen much more commonly in circumcised boys. Removal of too much foreskin, postcircumcision phimosis, and skin bridges are also risks. Circumcision is contraindicated when hypospadias is noted. Circumcision is indicated for phimosis and recurrent balanitis. Benefits include a decrease in UTIs in the first 6 months of life. A decrease in risk of sexually transmitted diseases and penile cancer is theorized. The American Academy of Pediatrics policy currently recommends neonatal circumcision as optional.

REFERENCE

Brown MR, Cartwright PC, Snow BW. Common office problems in pediatric urology and gynecology. *Pediatr Clin North Am* 1997;44(5):1091–1115.

 ## Cisplatin Toxicity

DESCRIPTION Very commonly used antitumor agent with significant adverse effects. Used in urology for transitional cell carcinoma and testicular cancer. Nephrotoxicity is cumulative and dose-dependent, and limits use. Other significant effects include myelosuppression, ototoxicity, GI disturbances, and neurotoxicity.

TREATMENT

• Amifostine has been used to limit toxicity.
• Use of other platinum-based compounds may decrease toxicity while maintaining efficacy.

REFERENCE

Schellens JH, Pronk LC, Verweil J. Emerging drug treatments for solid tumors. *Drugs* 1996;51(1):45–72.

 ## Clitoromegaly

DESCRIPTION Enlargement of the clitoris. When noted, must consider possibility of intersex. May be so severe as to appear as a normal male penis. Chordee usually present. (See also Section II, "Intersex Disorders.")

CAUSES

• Virilization most commonly secondary to congenital adrenal hyperplasia

TREATMENT

• The underlying cause must be addressed.

REFERENCE

Snyder HM. Intersex. Practical Cases in Urology, Series XIX, Course 4, 1996.

 ## Clonidine Suppression Test

DESCRIPTION Used to rule out pheochromocytoma. Clonidine (0.3 mg) is administered and plasma norepinephrine levels are then measured. Those patients with essential hypertension with an elevation of norepinephrine levels will experience a 50% decrease in this catecholamine level. Patients with pheochromocytoma will not be suppressed.

REFERENCE

Vaughan ED Jr, Blumenfeld JD. The adrenals. In: Walsh PC, Retik AB, Vaughan ED, Wein AJ, eds. *Campbell's Urology,* 7th ed. Philadelphia: WB Saunders, 1998.

Clostridium difficile Colitis—Urologic Considerations

 Clostridium difficile Colitis—
Urologic Considerations

DESCRIPTION   Potentially life-threatening infection of the colon due to overgrowth of *C. difficile*. Can be precipitated by antibiotic therapy. Has been reported in association with bowel preps in anticipation of surgery. Presents with diarrhea and abdominal pain without fever and chills. Diagnosed by classic endoscopic findings, culture of organism, or detection of toxin in stool

SYNONYMS

- Pseudomembranous enterocolitis

CAUSES

- Suppression of normal bowel flora by antibiotics

TREATMENT

- Removal of antibiotic therapy
- Vancomycin

REFERENCE

McDougal WS. Use of intestinal segments in the urinary tract: Basic principles. In: Walsh PC, Retik AB, Vaughan ED, Wein AJ, eds. *Campbell's Urology*, 7th ed. Philadelphia: WB Saunders, 1998.

 Cobb's Collar

DESCRIPTION   Congenital narrowing of the bulbar urethra. Can present as hematuria, UTI, or poor stream. Endoscopy and retrograde urethrogram reveal a bulbar urethral narrowing. The obstructing membrane is located just distal to the external sphincter and is reinforced by a fold extending from the verumontanum.

SYNONYMS

- Moorman's rings
- Congenital obstructive posterior urethral membrane

TREATMENT

- Endoscopic resection

REFERENCE

Dewan PA, Keenen RJ, Morris LL, Le Quesne GW. Congenital urethral obstruction: Cobb's collar or prolapsed congenital obstructive posterior urethral membrane (COPUM). *Br J Urol* 1994;73(1):91–96.

 Cobra Head Sign

DESCRIPTION   The radiologic appearance on an intravenous urogram (IVU) of an intravesical ureterocele of a single ureter in an adult, also called spring onion sign. The dilated ureterocele filled with contrast material protrudes into the bladder, which is also filled with contrast material, but is separated from it by a thin radiolucent halo. The ureterocele might be congenital or acquired, as in cases of trauma or inflammation.

REFERENCE

Nussbaum AR, Dort JP, Jeffs RD, et al. Ectopic ureter and ureterocele: Their varied radiographic manifestations. *Radiology* 1986; 159:227.

 Coccidiomycosis—Genitourinary

DESCRIPTION   Outbreaks of *Coccidioides immitis* infection common when exposed to dust that contains the spore. An opportunistic infection more common in patients <5 and >50 years; associated conditions include AIDS, steroid use, and chemotherapy for malignancy. After pulmonary inoculation, the patient can develop erythema nodosum (valley bumps or valley fever). Chest radiograph demonstrates infiltrates with cavitation. Serologic tests are available to help establish the diagnosis. Disseminated disease involves the kidney in up to 65%, the adrenal in 16% to 32%, and the prostate in 6%. Renal coccidiomycosis may cause similar changes as seen in renal TB (moth-eaten calyces, infundibular stenosis, ureteral stricture, and calcifications). Prostatic infection with occasional abscess, and scrotal infections with fistulas, have been reported. Epididymal and prostatic involvement can demonstrate necrotizing and nonnecrotizing granulomas.

TREATMENT

- Therapy includes up to 2 g of amphotericin, with 1 year of ketoconazole (200 mg/d).

REFERENCE

Wise GJ, Freyle J. Changing patterns in genitourinary fungal infections. AUA Update, Volume XVI, Lesson 1, 1997.

 Cohen ("Cross-Trigonal") Ureteral Reimplantation

DESCRIPTION   Through a transvesical approach, the ureter is mobilized from its hiatus and it is delivered through a submucosal tunnel across the trigone. A cross-trigonal reimplantation is then carried out.

REFERENCE

Kay R. Reimplantation of the ureter. In: Novick AC, Streem SB, Pontes JE, eds. *Stewarts Operative Urology*. Baltimore: Williams & Wilkins, 1989:526–538.

 Column of Bertin—Hypertrophied

DESCRIPTION   Normal anatomic structure of kidney, which, if enlarged, can be mistaken for a renal mass. Normally appears as granular material in the renal sinus, which is simply cortex. Located between the pyramids. (See also Section III, "Renal Pseudotumors.")

REFERENCE

Redman JF. Anatomy of the genitourinary system. In: Gillenwater JY, Grayhack JT, Howards SS, Duckett JW, eds. *Adult and Pediatric Urology,* 3rd ed. St Louis: Mosby, 1996.

 Condylomata Lata

DESCRIPTION   Flat condyloma. Moist or mucous papule found in the skin folds of syphilis patients. Reflects secondary stage of syphilis. Secretes serous fluid. Can be covered by a layer of epidermal debris. Represents the hematogenous spread of spirochetes. (See also Section II, "Syphilis.")

TREATMENT

- Treatment of the underlying syphilis

REFERENCE

Rein MF. Infections caused by *Treponema* (syphilis, yaws, pinta, bejel). In: Stein, et al. *Internal Medicine,* 3rd ed. Boston: Little, Brown, 1990.

Congenital Nephrosis

DESCRIPTION   Renal cystic disease that has two main forms: (1) congenital nephrosis Finnish and (2) diffuse mesangial sclerosis. Associated with enlarged placenta at birth. Dilation of proximal convoluted tubule. Severe proteinuria may lead to starvation of affected children. Ultrasound reveals higher kidney echogenicity than liver or spleen.

SYNONYMS

- Microcystic disease
- Familial nephrotic syndrome

CAUSES

- CNF: autosomal recessive
- DMS: possibly familial

TREATMENT

- Supportive therapy
- Renal replacement therapy, as needed

REFERENCE

Lippert M. Renal cystic disease. In: Gillenwater JY, Grayhack JT, Howards SS, Duckett JW, eds. *Adult and Pediatric Urology*, 3rd ed. St Louis: Mosby, 1996.

 Constipation—Urologic Considerations

DESCRIPTION   Infrequent large bowel movements affect the urinary tract by increasing the risk of urinary tract infection, contributing to urinary incontinence, and impairing the resolution of reflux in children. The exact pathophysiology is unclear, but a rectum distended with hard stool obviously displaces and distorts the bladder within the pelvis. Since the rectum and bladder share sacral nerve roots, overdistension of the rectum may interfere with bladder function at the cord level. Urodynamic studies in children with functional constipation have revealed uninhibited contractions and small bladder capacity, both of which improve with improved bowel function. In addition, the same holding behavior, which leads to functional constipation often, alters bladder habits as well. Treatment of bowel dysfunction alone will resolve chronic recurrent urinary tract infection and urinary incontinence in some children. It is important to rule out neurologic and bowel disease as causes of constipation before making the diagnosis of functional constipation.

TREATMENT

- Diet changes
- Laxatives, stool softeners
- Toilet schedules

REFERENCE

Loening-Baucke V. Urinary incontinence and urinary tract infection and their resolution with treatment of chronic constipation of childhood. *Pediatrics* 1997;100:228.

 Contact Dermatitis

DESCRIPTION   Contact dermatitis is caused by an external irritant or allergen, and the patient complains of itching and burning or stinging. The findings are inflammation, scaling, and crust formation. Extreme reactions can result in blistering and necrosis. Allergic agents typically induce a dermatitis after repeated contact with the skin.

CAUSES

- Common irritant agents cause immediate symptoms and include industrial chemicals, soaps, cleansing products, spermicides and lubricants, perfumes, urogenital secretions, and feces.
- Sensitizing (allergic) agents for the genital skin include cleansing agents and disinfectants; lubricants and emollients; spermicides and other topical ointments; perfumes and fragrances; latex and other types of rubber; clothing; dyes; poison ivy (direct contact or indirect contact from the hand); and metals such as nickel.

TREATMENT

- Attempt to identify and remove the offending agent from contact with the skin.
- Topical corticosteroids, emollients, and antihistamines give symptomatic relief. Severe allergic contact dermatitis may require oral corticosteroids.
- Severe reactions may require debridement and grafting.
- Patch testing uninvolved skin to common antigens is often helpful.

REFERENCE

Margolis DJ. Cutaneous diseases of the male external genitalia. In: Walsh PC, Retik AB, Vaughan ED, Wein AJ, eds. *Campbell's Urology*, 7th ed. Philadelphia: WB Saunders, 1998.

 Cordonnier and Nesbit Ureteral Anastomosis

DESCRIPTION   A direct ureteral colonic refluxing anastomosis incorporating full-thickness ureteral and intestinal wall.

REFERENCE

McDougal WS. Use of intestinal segments and urinary diversion. In: Walsh PC, Retik AB, Vaughan ED, Wein AJ, eds. *Campbell's Urology*, 7th ed. Philadelphia: WB Saunders, 1998:3137–3144.

 Corpora Amylacea

DESCRIPTION   Small, round, ovoid bodies, lamellar in structure, located in the alveoli of the prostate. Composed of lecithin, albumin, and nitrogenous substances, which may precipitate around sloughed epithelial cells. Become more common with age. Act as the nidus for prostatic calculi formation

REFERENCE

Drach GW. Urinary lithiasis: Etiology, diagnosis, and medical management. In: Walsh PC, Retik AB, Vaughan ED, Wein AJ, eds. *Campbell's Urology*, 7th ed. Philadelphia: WB Saunders, 1998.

 Cortical Necrosis—Acute

DESCRIPTION   Acute cortical necrosis is a rare form of acute renal failure, characterized by necrosis of the cortex with sparing of the medulla. It is thought to be the result of selective arterial spasm of the cortical vasculature with continued perfusion of the renal medulla via the medullary arterioles. Pathologically, there is necrosis of the glomeruli, tubules, and arterioles. A cortical rim sign can be seen on contrast-enhanced CT scan, indicating spared perfusion of the renal capsule.

CAUSES

- Factors that can predispose a patient to acute cortical necrosis: shock, placental abruption, peritonitis, transfusion reaction, pancreatitis, and toxins.

REFERENCE

Wilck EJ, Gerard PS. Acute cortical necrosis. *Urology* 1997;49(3):116.

Cowper's Gland Carcinoma

 Cowper's Gland Carcinoma

DESCRIPTION Rare tumor that can present obstructive symptoms, pain with defecation, or constipation. Most have a palpable perineal mass. Microscopically, appears as adenocarcinoma. However, local necrosis and tissue destruction may prevent exact localization of the site of origin.

TREATMENT

• Combined surgical and radiation therapy has been employed.

REFERENCE

Mitsumori K, Elwell MR. Tumours of the male accessory sex glands. *IARC Scientific Pub* 1994; 111:431–449.

 Credé Maneuver

DESCRIPTION Used to facilitate voiding in those patients with decreased bladder tonicity and low outlet resistance. Involves placement of the thumb of each hand over the left and right anterior superior iliac spine, and the fingers over the suprapubic area and pressed into the abdomen. Both hands are then pressed downward into the pelvis. May not be effective in emptying, as the external sphincter may contract during maneuver

SYNONYMS

• Manual compression of bladder

REFERENCE

Barbalias GA, Klauber GT, Blaivas JG. Critical evaluation of the Crede maneuver: A urodynamic study of 207 patients. *J Urol* 1993; 130(4):720–723.

 Cribriform Clear Cell Hyperplasia of the Prostate

DESCRIPTION May be misdiagnosed as cribriform carcinoma. Anticytokeratin staining of basal cell layer can distinguish from carcinoma. Also, cells lack cytologic atypia, which is in contrast to carcinoma. Natural history unknown. Usually found in central area of gland

REFERENCE

Epstein JI. Non-neoplastic diseases of the prostate. In: Bostwick, D. et al. *Urologic Surgical Pathology*, 1st ed. St Louis: Mosby, 1997.

 Cryptococcus—Genitourinary

DESCRIPTION Fungal infection that is considered opportunistic. *Cryptococcus neoformans* thrives in areas inhabited by birds. Pulmonary site is most common primary infection site. Immunocompromised patients develop disseminated disease (AIDS, transplant). Adrenal insufficiency has been reported, but the most common sites of GU involvement are the prostate and the kidney. Prostate may be a reservoir in patients with AIDS. Epididymis and penis have also been reported as sites. GU involvement is considered a manifestation of systemic disease.

TREATMENT

• Systemic antifungal therapy with IV amphotericin B, flucytosine, fluconazole, or combination of drugs
• Surgical drainage of large abscesses may be considered.

REFERENCE

Wise GJ, Freyle J. Changing patterns in genitourinary fungal infections. AUA Update Series, Lesson 1, Volume XVI, 1997.

 Culp-DeWeerd Pyeloplasty

DESCRIPTION A spiral incision is carried out over the anterior and medial aspect of the pelvis and continued down across a point beyond the UPJ obstruction. The apex of the flap is brought down to the apex of the ureterotomy, where a 5-0 chromic stay suture is placed. The posterior and anterior anastomoses are completed with interrupt 5-0 chromic sutures. Used for UPJ obstruction

REFERENCE

Kay R. Procedures for ureteropelvic junction obstruction. In: Novick AC, Streem SB, Pontes JE, eds. *Stewarts Operative Urology*. Baltimore: Williams & Wilkins, 1989:220–233.

 Cystadenocarcinoma—Genitourinary

DESCRIPTION Commonly seen in other organ systems, such as the ovary, pancreas, appendix, and thyroid. In the GU system, reported in testes, paratesticular structures, and kidney. Grossly, multilocular cystic masses are noted. Microscopically, cuboidal to columnar epithelium is seen lining the cysts. These cells can secrete serous or mucinous substances. Malignant cells will demonstrate multilayering of epithelium, nuclear atypia, and invasion of surrounding stroma.

TREATMENT

• Surgical resection

REFERENCE

Yu CC, Huang JK, Chiang H, Chen MT, Chang LS. Papillary cystadenocarcinoma of the epididymis: A case report and review of the literature. *J Urol* 1992;147(1):162–1625.

 Cystadenoma—Genitourinary

DESCRIPTION Occurs commonly in the epididymis and represents benign epithelial hyperplasia. Usually causes very few symptoms. Can be bilateral. May be associated with von Hippel-Lindau syndrome. Grossly, appears cystic. Microscopically, demonstrates cells with clear, vacuolated cytoplasm arranged in glandular or papillary structures. Appears as a cystic to solid mass at the head of the epididymis on ultrasound

TREATMENT

• Observation
• Radical orchiectomy, if diagnosis is in doubt

REFERENCE

Choyke PL, Glenn GM, Wagner JP, et al. Epididymal cystadenomas in von Hippel-Lindau disease. *Urology* 1997;49(6):926–931.

Cystic Fibrosis—Urologic Considerations

DESCRIPTION Genetic disease affecting 1 in 2000 Caucasian births, in which defective chloride transport across epithelium occurs. This leads to complications involving the pancreas, liver, salivary glands, and lungs. Urogenital findings include bilateral absence of the vas deferens leading to infertility. Abnormal development of the mesonephric system, inguinal hernias, hydroceles, and undescended testes are also seen. Risk of testicular cancer may be increased. (See also Section II, "Vas Deferens—Congenital Absence/Obstruction.")

REFERENCE

Milunsky JM, Milunsky A. Case report: Cystic fibrosis and embryonal carcinoma of the testes. *Am J Med Sci* 1996;311(4):191–192.

Cystic Nephroma

DESCRIPTION Described by Boggs and Kimmelsteil in 1956. Rare cystic tumor of unknown origin. Affects children and adults equally. Can present as abdominal mass, hematuria, or flank pain. Has thick capsule and septae containing mature structures. Imaging cannot reliably predict malignant potential. Usually unilateral. Can grow quite large and compress intraabdominal organs. Usually benign, but sarcomas and adenocarcinoma can exist in the walls of the cyst

SYNONYMS

- Multilocular cystic kidney
- Focal polycystic kidney
- Multicystic or cystic adenoma

TREATMENT

- Partial or radical nephrectomy

REFERENCE

Lippert M. Renal cystic disease. In: Gillenwater JY, Grayhack JT, Howards SS, Duckett JW, eds. *Adult and Pediatric Urology*, 3rd ed. St Louis: Mosby, 1996.

Cystinosis

DESCRIPTION May be confused with cystinuria. Characterized by the intracellular accumulation of excessive quantities of cystine, with deposits in the cornea, conjunctiva, bone marrow, lymph nodes, leukocytes, and internal organs. Daily excretion of cystine is only 5% to 10% of that found in cystinuria. Stone formation is rare. Varied range of severity. Severe forms go on to ESRD. Usually detected by routine eye examination

CAUSES

- Autosomal recessive metabolic disorder demonstrating defective lysosomal transport of cystine

TREATMENT

- Salt and water replacement
- Renal transplantation

REFERENCE

Jenkins AD. Calculus formation. In: Gillenwater JY, Grayhack JT, Howards SS, Duckett JW, eds. *Adult and Pediatric Urology*, 3rd ed. St Louis: Mosby, 1996.

Cystitis Cystica

DESCRIPTION Similar to von Brunn's nests, which are areas of benign urothelium in the submucosa, except that the centers of the nests have undergone eosinophilic liquefaction to form small cystic cavities. Found in 60% of normal bladders at autopsy. Cystoscopically appear as small pearly white or yellowish lesions, usually <5 mm, but are occasionally larger. No clear relation to malignant transformation

TREATMENT

- No specific treatment

REFERENCE

Eble JN, Young RH. Carcinoma of the urinary bladder: A review of its diverse morphology. *Semin Diagn Pathol* 199714(2):98–108.

Cystitis—Eosinophilic

DESCRIPTION Rare and severe form of allergic cystitis. First described by Brown in 1960. Symptoms include hematuria, urgency, dysuria, and suprapubic discomfort. UA may show eosinophiluria. Cystoscopic findings may reveal raised plaques or ulcers that mimic CIS or invasive bladder cancer. Hydronephrosis may be seen on IVU or ultrasound. Bladder biopsy revealing eosinophilic infiltrate is pathognomonic. IVU or renal ultrasound may demonstrate hydronephrosis.

CAUSES

- Patients with allergies, including food, are at increased risk.
- Parasitic infections
- Drugs, including methicillin, anthranilic acid, intravesical mitomycin, and thiotepa

TREATMENT

- Conservative medical management with oral antibiotics, antihistamines, and steroids
- A full allergy evaluation is required.

REFERENCE

Choe JM, Kirkemo AK, Sirls LT. Intravesical thiotepa-induced eosinophilic cystitis. *Urology* 1995;46(5):729–731.

Cystitis Follicularis

DESCRIPTION Presence of submucosal lymphoid follicles in the submucosa of the urothelium. May appear grossly as punctate, yellow submucosal nodules. Not associated with malignancy

SYNONYMS

- Bacteriuric bumps

CAUSES

- Chronic bacterial infections

TREATMENT

- Treatment of underlying infection

REFERENCE

Catalona WJ. Urothelial tumors of the urinary tract. In: Walsh PC, Retik AB, Vaughan ED, Wein AJ, eds. *Campbell's Urology*, 7th ed. Philadelphia: WB Saunders, 1998.

Cystitis Glandularis

 Cystitis Glandularis

DESCRIPTION Similar to von Brunn's nests, which are areas of benign urothelium in the submucosa, except that the transitional cells have undergone glandular metaplasia. A common lesion in the urothelium, it is usually only detected microscopically, but occasionally can appear as a grossly visible lesion. Typical cystitis glandularis is the most common form. Diffuse cystitis glandularis of the intestinal type is seen in chronically irritated bladders, and this type is associated with an increased risk of bladder cancer (adenocarcinoma) and is associated with pelvic lipomatosis.

TREATMENT

- No specific treatment
- May consider close follow-up due to cancer risk

REFERENCE

Eble JN, Young RH. Carcinoma of the urinary bladder: A review of its diverse morphology. *Semin Diagn Pathol* 1997;14(2):98–108.

 Cystitis—Viral

DESCRIPTION Can produce clinically significant symptoms, such as dysuria, hematuria, and frequency. Standard urine culture is negative. UA may show WBCs and RBCs. Cytology may be suspicious for malignancy, with abnormally large cells having prominent nuclei. Viral serum and urine studies and serum antibody titers may be helpful in the diagnosis. Usually affects children or immunocompromised adults

CAUSES

- Viremic spread to bladder of adenovirus, papovavirus, or influenza A

TREATMENT

- Usually self-limited

REFERENCE

Mininberg DT, Watson C, Desquitado M. Viral cystitis with transient secondary vesicoureteral reflux. *J Urol* 1982;127(5):983–985.

 Cystometrogram

DESCRIPTION Evaluates the filling and/or storage phases of detrusor function. Catheters to measure the vesical pressure and abdominal pressure and to fill the bladder with saline, water, or CO_2 are utilized. The bladder filling rate is anywhere between 25 and 100 mL/min. Simultaneous measurements of pressure and volume are recorded and a curve is created. Variables observed are compliance, contractility, sensation, and capacity. During filling, the bladder volumes are recorded at (1) the first sensation of filling, (2) sensation of urgency to void, and (3) sensation of maximum capacity. Coughing and the Valsalva maneuver should be utilized to uncover involuntary contractions. Abnormalities that may be detected include altered sensation, changes in detrusor compliance, disorders of detrusor contractility, and/or presence of involuntary detrusor contraction or detrusor areflexia.

REFERENCE

Steers WD, Barrett DM, Wein AJ. Voiding function and dysfunction. In: Gillenwater JY, Grayhack JT, Howards SS, Duckett JW, eds. *Adult and Pediatric Urology,* 3rd ed. St Louis: Mosby, 1996.

 Cystosarcoma Phyllodes— Prostate

DESCRIPTION Tumor commonly seen in breast but rarely in prostate. Can present with voiding symptoms. Grossly, tumor is unusually soft, cystic, and spongy. Microscopically, elongated cells with spindle-shaped nuclei and scant pale cytoplasm are seen. Can range from benign to malignant

TREATMENT

- Surgical resection

REFERENCE

Cacic M, Petrovic D, Tentor D, Hutinec Z, Jelasic D. Cystosarcoma phyllodes of the prostate. *Scand J Urol Nephrol* 1996;30(6):501–502.

 Cytokeratin Staining

DESCRIPTION Commonly used in prostate cancer diagnosis (i.e., differentiate PIN from basal cell hyperplasia or distinguish various forms of acinar proliferations that are not cancer on needle biopsy) $34\beta E12$, which detects basal cell specific cytokeratin, is commonly used. If basal cell staining is present, this helps to rule out carcinoma. Also used to examine lymph nodes or periprostatic tissues for prostate cancer. May increase accuracy of lymph node staging. Has shown promise in breast cancer staging, where up to one-third of patients have unsuspected micrometastasis to lymph nodes. Its utility in prostate cancer metastasis is being investigated.

REFERENCE

Moul JW, Lewis DJ, Ross AA, Kahn DG, Ho CK, McLeod DG. Immunohistologic detection of prostate cancer pelvic lymph node micrometastases: Correlation to preoperative serum prostate-specific antigen. *Urology* 1994;43(1):68–73.

 Cytology—Prostate

DESCRIPTION Examination of cells, usually obtained by fine-needle aspiration, for the detection of malignancy. Characteristics that can be determined include DNA ploidy status, cell cycle distribution, and cytologic grade. Advantages over standard pathologic techniques include ease and rapidity of technique. Combination with flow cytometry seems to increase accuracy. Experienced cytopathologists are necessary for reliability.

REFERENCE

Paz-Bouza JI, Orfao A, Abad M, et al. Transrectal fine needle aspiration biopsy of the prostate combining cytomorphologic, DNA ploidy status and cell cycle distribution studies. *Pathol Res Pract* 1994;190(7):682–689.

Cytology—Urinary

DESCRIPTION Microscopic examination of the urine, usually performed for the detection of malignant cells during follow-up of TCC. Criteria for malignancy include increased cytoplasmic-to-nuclear ratio, eccentric nucleus, nuclear pleomorphism and irregularity, hyperchromasia, chromatin clumping, nuclear crowding and overlapping, prominent nucleoli, mitotic figures, lack of cytoplasmic vacuolization, and loss of cell cohesion. Highly accurate (95%) in high-grade carcinoma and CIS but less (10% to 50%) accurate in low-grade bladder cancer. Also useful in detecting unresected residual tumor, and may predict future tumor recurrence after transurethral resection

REFERENCE

Hudson MA, Catalona WJ. Urothelial tumors of the bladder, upper tracts and prostate. In: Gillenwater JY, Grayhack JT, Howards SS, Duckett JW, eds. *Adult and Pediatric Urology*, 3rd ed. St Louis: Mosby, 1996.

 Cytomegalovirus—Urologic Considerations

DESCRIPTION Cytomegalovirus (CMV) is the most important infectious threat to renal transplant recipients. Risk factors include the serologic status of donor and recipient, as well as the immunosuppressive regimen utilized. Other effects include voiding dysfunction by invading peripheral nerves. Cytomegalovirus cystitis has been reported to occur in AIDS. One of the TORCH infections (toxoplasmosis, rubella, cytomegalovirus, herpes simplex I and II, and syphilis), which can cause fetal malformations. CMV has been associated with perinatal renal vein thrombosis.

TREATMENT

• Gancyclovir for transplant patients has been effective.

REFERENCE

Miles BJ, Melser M, Farah R, Markowitz N, Fisher E. The urological manifestations of the acquired immunodeficiency syndrome. *J Urol* 1989;142(3):771–773.

 Davis Intubated Ureterotomy

DESCRIPTION An incision is carried out over the strictured UPJ, and a nephrostomy is placed through a lower pole calyx. A stenting catheter is passed through the cortex of the kidney down the ureter and into the bladder. The stent can be removed after a minimum of 6 weeks, after which time the ureterostomy catheter is removed. An antegrade nephrostogram is done to assure patency of the ureter, after which the nephrostomy catheter is removed.

REFERENCE

Kay R. Procedures for ureteropelvic junction obstruction. In: Novick AC, Streem SB, Pontes JE, eds. *Stewarts Operative Urology*. Baltimore: Williams & Wilkins, 1989:220–233.

 De Toni-Fanconi-Debre Syndrome

DESCRIPTION Syndrome of multiple defects of tubular function, which is characterized by aminoaciduria, phosphaturia, glycosuria, osteomalacia, and renal tubular acidosis. The proximal renal tubule is shortened and replaced by a thin tubular structure, constituting the swanneck deformity.

TREATMENT

• Replacement of cation deficits (especially potassium)
• Correction of acidosis with bicarbonate or citrate
• Replacement of phosphate loss with isoionic neutral phosphate solution
• Encouragement of liberal calcium intake with added vitamin D

REFERENCE

Ogier H, Lombes A, Scholte HR, et al. de Toni-Fanconi-Debre syndrome with Leigh syndrome revealing severe muscle cytochrome c oxidase deficiency. *J Pediatr* 1988;112(5):734–739.

 Delayed Nephrogram

DESCRIPTION The delay of contrast appearance, which is typically appreciated within a few minutes of contrast injection. The most common cause is intraluminal obstruction of the collecting system by calculus, tumor, or clot. Other causes are listed below.

SYNONYMS

• Increasingly dense nephrogram

CAUSES

• Extraluminal obstruction of the collecting system by extrinsic mass
• Intrarenal obstruction, usually by precipitated substances in the tubules, such as Tamm-Horsfall protein
• Azotemia
• Hypotension
• Renal vein thrombosis
• Rarely, acute renal failure

REFERENCE

Friedenberg RM. Excretory urography in the adult. In: Pollack HM, et al. *Clinical Urography*, 1st ed. Philadelphia: WB Saunders, 1990.

 Desmoplastic Small Round Cell Tumor

DESCRIPTION Rare tumor that typically presents in the abdominal cavity but sometimes involves the GU system. Those patients with GU involvement seem to be younger men. Usually very aggressive. Histologically, irregular nests of small round cells surrounded by fibrous connective tissue. Immunohistochemical studies reveal both epithelial and nonepithelial origins.

CAUSES

• Theorized reciprocal translocation between chromosomes 11 and 22

TREATMENT

• Surgical resection and multidrug chemotherapy have been employed with poor success.

REFERENCE

Furman J, Murphy WM, Wajsman Z, Berry AD. Urogenital involvement by desmoplastic small round-cell tumor. *J Urol* 1997;158:1506–1509.

Diabetes Insipidus—Urologic Considerations

 Diabetes Insipidus—Urologic Considerations

DESCRIPTION One cause of polyuria. Distinguished as neurogenic and nephrogenic. Of urologic interest, IVP can show marked hydronephrosis, dilated ureters, and megacystis secondary to the great increase in urine flow. Signs include hypernatremia and hyperosmolarity. Diagnosed by the inability to concentrate urine despite water deprivation and administration of ADH

CAUSES

- Neurogenic: loss of ADH secretion from trauma, tumor, or iatrogenic reasons
- Nephrogenic: idiopathic, medications, obstructive uropathy

TREATMENT

- Neurogenic: Replace ADH.
- Nephrogenic: Remove the underlying cause: chlorothiazide with low-sodium diet.

REFERENCE

Schaeffer AJ, Del Greco F. Other renal diseases of urologic significance. In: Walsh PC, Retik AB, Vaughan ED, Wein AJ, eds. *Campbell's Urology*, 7th ed. Philadelphia: WB Saunders, 1998.

 Dietl's Crisis

DESCRIPTION The most severe manifestation of nephroptosis, originally described by Jozef Dietl in 1864. Classically, colicky flank pain, nausea, chills, tachycardia, oliguria and transient hematuria, or proteinuria was described. Physical examination would reveal an enlarged, tender kidney. Nephroptosis was thought to be a relatively common condition in women in the early twentieth century.

CAUSES

- Hydronephrosis secondary to vascular obstruction of the ureter

TREATMENT

- Manual reduction of the ptotic kidney was initially used.
- Nephropexy has been used for nephroptosis and was one of the most commonly performed operations of the early twentieth century.

REFERENCE

Moss S. Floating kidneys: A century of nephroptosis and nephropexy. *J Urol* 1997;158:699–702.

 Doppler—Penile

DESCRIPTION The current most widely utilized method to measure arterial flow and prove arterial insufficiency as an etiology in impotence. Allows visualization of individual arteries and measurement of flow. Performed in the flaccid and erect states (after the intracavernosal injection of vasoactive agents). An increase in mean arterial diameter of more than 75% of the flaccid value and a mean peak flow velocity of greater than 25 cm/s after vasoactive agent injection is used to determine adequate arterial capacity. A wide variability in some patients has been shown, however.

REFERENCE

Bertolotto M. Penile sonography. *Eur Urol* 1999;540:7–12.

 Down Syndrome—Urologic Considerations

DESCRIPTION Also known as trisomy 21. Most common trisomy. Brachycephalic skull; congenital nasal hypoplasia; broad, short hands; and genitourinary anomalies in the form of undescended testicles and a small penis. Males affected are hypogonadal. Smaller than average phallus. Approximately one-fourth will have cryptorchidism. Microscopic renal cysts, usually of the glomerular space, can also occur.

REFERENCE

Rabinowitz R. General consideration of congenital anomalies. In: Gillenwater JY, Grayhack JT, Howards SS, Duckett JW, eds. *Adult and Pediatric Urology*, 3rd ed. St Louis: Mosby, 1996.

 Drash Syndrome (Denys-Drash Syndrome)

DESCRIPTION First described by Drash in 1970, this syndrome consists of nephrotic syndrome, Wilms' tumor with or without male pseudohermaphroditism. Presents as a newborn with ambiguous genitalia. Streak gonads are common, and gonadoblastomas have been reported. Renal insufficiency begins in the first years of life.

SYNONYMS

- Denys-Drash syndrome

CAUSES

- Genetic defect, usually sporadic, found on the WT1 gene of chromosome 11

TREATMENT

- Renal replacement therapy, as needed
- Some have advocated nephrectomy at the time of transplant because of Wilms' tumor risk.

REFERENCE

Mueller RF. The Denys-Drash syndrome. *J Med Genet* 1994;31(6):471–477.

 Dribbling—Post-Void

DESCRIPTION A complaint of loss of urine that occurs after completion of voiding. The cause is thought to be retained urine in the urethra distal to the sphincter in men and retained urine in the vagina or urethral diverticulum in women. In men, a common complaint associated clinically with BPH

REFERENCE

Blaivas JG, et al. Urinary Incontinence. In: Walsh PC, Retik AB, Vaughan ED, Wein AJ, eds. *Campbell's Urology*, 7th ed. Philadelphia: WB Saunders, 1998:1020–1021.

Drooping Lily Sign

DESCRIPTION Excretory urographic description for the lower pole moiety in a duplicated collecting system. The nonfunctioning upper pole produces a mass effect that pushes the lower pole downward. The lower pole ureter tends to be orthotopic, while the upper pole is typically ectopic.

REFERENCE

Amis ES, Newhouse JH. *Essentials of Uroradiology,* 1st ed. Boston: Little, Brown, 1991:263.

 Drug Eruption—Fixed

DESCRIPTION This is a sharply localized dermatitis that characteristically recurs at the same site each time the offending drug is administered (penis most common site), with an acute phase followed by desquamation and hyperpigmentation. Symptoms usually appear after 6 hours, although lesions can occur 24 to 48 hours later. A macrophage migration inhibition factor (MIF) assay is essential for diagnosis.

CAUSES

- Common

—Phenolphthalein
—Trimethoprim-sulfamethoxazole
—Antipyrine
—Quinine
—Tetracycline
—Salicylates/NSAIDs
—Hydroxyzine hydrochloride

TREATMENT

- Discontinuation of the drug causing the reaction results in complete resolution of the fixed drug eruption. Supportive topical therapy (steroids), as needed

REFERENCE

Cohen HA, Barzilai A, Matalon A, Hewel L, Gross S. Fixed drug eruption of the penis due to hydroxyzine hydrochloride. *Ann Pharmacother* 1997;31(3):327–329.

 Dysfunctional Voiding

DESCRIPTION Syndrome wherein external sphincter dyssynergia is noted in the absence of an identifiable neurologic cause. Occurs in children. Usually brought to attention through UTIs or secondary enuresis. Originally described by Hinman and Bauman in 1973 after review of similar reported cases. Upper tract damage can occur. Diagnosed by videourodynamics or EMG readings during urodynamics

SYNONYMS

- Hinman-Allen syndrome
- Hinmann syndrome
- Nonneurogenic neurogenic bladder

CAUSES

- Theorized to be psychogenic in origin

TREATMENT

- Combination of medications, behavioral therapy, and intermittent catheterization
- Surgery for diversion may be required to protect upper tracts.

REFERENCE

Yang CC, Mayo ME. Morbidity of dysfunctional voiding syndrome. *Urology* 1997;49(3):445–448.

 Dysgerminoma

DESCRIPTION Malignant tumor of the ovary, which is roughly the counterpart of seminoma of the testes. Occurs in children and young women. Occasionally seen in gonadal dysgenesis or testicular feminization syndrome. Can present as pelvic mass or abdominal pain. Pure dysgerminomas do not secrete tumor markers such as AFP or hCG.

TREATMENT

- Surgical resection for local disease
- Radiation therapy or chemotherapy for advanced disease

REFERENCE

Berek JS. Ovarian cancer. In: Hacker NF, et al. *Essentials of Obstetrics and Gynecology,* 2nd ed. Philadelphia: WB Saunders, 1992.

 Dysraphism—Spinal

DESCRIPTION Most common cause of neurogenic bladder dysfunction in childhood. Defined as failure of closure of the vertebral canal during embryonic development, leading to spinal cord dysfunction. The most common dysraphism, myelodysplasia, includes meningoceles, myelomeningoceles, and lipomeningoceles. Reflux, continence, sexuality, and bowel function are often important issues with these patients. Many rarer forms also exist, including tight filum terminale, dermoid cysts, and aberrant nerve roots with varying levels of resulting dysfunction. See also Section II, "Myelodysplasia (Myelomeningocele)—Urologic Considerations," and Section III, "Tethered Cord Syndrome."

REFERENCE

Bauer SB. Neurogenic dysfunction of the lower urinary tract in children. In: Walsh PC, Retik AB, Vaughan ED, Wein AJ, eds. *Campbell's Urology,* 7th ed. Philadelphia: WB Saunders, 1998.

 Echinococcus—Renal

DESCRIPTION Infection of the kidney by *Echinococcus* is rare, comprising 2% of cases. Typically presents with dull flank pain. Diagnosis can be made by radiography. The Casoni skin test with hydatid fluid antigen can be helpful. If cysts rupture into the collecting system, scolices can be seen in the urine sediment.

TREATMENT

- Surgical resection, with care to prevent rupture of cysts and spillage of contents, to prevent anaphylaxis

REFERENCE

Perimenis P, Athanasopoulos A, Barbalias G. Unusual echinococcal cyst. *J Urol* 1991;146:1359–1360.

Edward Syndrome

 Edward Syndrome

DESCRIPTION   Also known as trisomy 18. High incidence of urologic abnormalities is noted. Horseshoe kidney and hydronephrosis are seen in about 50%. Hypospadias and cryptorchidism are also common. 90% of patients die within the first year, usually secondary to cardiopulmonary problems. Uterine and vaginal abnormalities are common in females.

REFERENCE

Rabinowitz R. General consideration of congenital anomalies. In: Gillenwater JY, Grayhack JT, Howards SS, Duckett JW, eds. *Adult and Pediatric Urology*, 3rd ed. St Louis: Mosby, 1996.

 Ejaculation—Decreased or Absent

DESCRIPTION   Results from retrograde ejaculation or failure of seminal emission (no expulsion of semen through vas into posterior urethra). Extreme form is aspermia (no ejaculate, see Section III). A postejaculation urine should be examined for sperm as for aspermia. (See also Section I, "Infertility" and "Retrograde Ejaculation," and Section III, "Semen Analysis—Technique and Normal Values" and "Semen Analysis—Abnormal.")

CAUSES

- Bladder neck procedures (TURP, TUIP)
- Medications (antipsychotics, antidepressants, antihypertensives, alcohol, baclofen)
- Neuropathic (diabetic, spinal cord injury, myelodysplasia, retroperitoneal lymphadenectomy, abdominopelvic surgery)
- Ejaculatory duct obstruction/absence

TREATMENT

- Sperm recovery from bladder and insemination for retrograde ejaculation
- Medications to achieve seminal emission and or antegrade ejaculation (pseudoephedrine 60 mg qid, ephedrine 25–50 mg qid, phenylpropanolamine 75 mg bid, imipramine 25 mg bid)
- Electroejaculation (commonly used in spinal cord injury)

REFERENCE

Shaban SF, et al. Treatment of abnormalities of ejaculation. In: Lipshultz L, Howards S, eds. *Infertility in the Male*, 3rd ed. St Louis: Mosby, 1997.

 Ejaculation—Painful

DESCRIPTION   Pain associated with or immediately after ejaculation. Can be iatrogenic, physiologic, or psychogenic in nature. In many patients with postejaculatory pain, the source of the pain appears to involve the involuntary spasm of certain muscles of the male genitalia, which can be triggered by a variety of psychosexual conflicts. The syndrome of postejaculatory pain is considered within a continuum of psychogenic ejaculatory disorders (i.e., premature ejaculation).

CAUSES

- BPH (in up to 15%)
- Prostatitis
- Seminal vesical calculi
- Postoperative (prostatectomy)
- Medications (antidepressants, psychotropic agents, alpha-agonists)
- Psychogenic

REFERENCE

Corriere JN Jr. Painful ejaculation due to seminal vesicle calculi. *J Urol* 1997;157(2):626.

 Electroejaculation

DESCRIPTION   Procedure for obtaining sperm for assisted reproductive technologies in patients who cannot ejaculate on their own, such as spinal cord injury patients. Typically used after failure of vibratory penile stimulation. General anesthesia used, except in cases of complete spinal cord compromise. Electrical probe placed in rectum, facing anteriorly. Electrical stimulation causes erection and ejaculation, after which ejaculate is collected. Sigmoidoscopy is performed before and after the procedure to rule out rectal injury.

REFERENCE

Ohl NA, Sankson J, Menge AC, McCabe M, Keller LM. Electroejaculation versus vibratory stimulation in spinal cord injured men; sperm quality and patient preference. *J Urol* 1997;157(6):2147–2149.

 Electromyography—External Sphincter

DESCRIPTION   Generally EMG is the measurement of bioelectric potentials generated by depolarization of muscle. During urodynamics, surface electrodes may be used to monitor the activity of the external sphincter. During filling, there should be increases in activity, which will reach maximum near capacity. During voiding, there should be sudden and persistent cessation of sphincter activity. When empty, baseline sphincter activity recurs. To assess external sphincter activity, the patient may be asked to interrupt voiding in the middle of the stream, at which point there should be an abrupt increase in sphincter activity that should be sufficient to stop the flow. Abnormal EMG patterns may be detected in detrusor-sphincter dyssynergia, voluntary contraction of the pelvic floor with the Valsava maneuver, and dysfunctional voiding, among others. May also be used as biofeedback therapy for dysfunctional voiding

REFERENCE

Steers WD, Barrett DM, Wein AJ. Voiding function and dysfunction. In: Gillenwater JY, Grayhack JT, Howards SS, Duckett JW, eds. *Adult and Pediatric Urology*, 3rd ed. St. Louis: Mosby, 1996.

 Elephantiasis—Scrotum

DESCRIPTION   End result of long-standing lymphatic obstruction. Scrotum and penis can become massively enlarged and debilitating. Uncommon in the United States. (See also Section I, "Edema—External Genitalia.")

CAUSES

- Filiarisis and other infectious causes
- Malignancy obstructing lymphatics
- Surgical therapy that has altered lymphatic drainage
- Idiopathic, such as Milroy disease

TREATMENT

- Drug therapy for any infectious etiology
- Surgery for resection of redundant scrotum with flap coverage of testes

REFERENCE

Apesos J, Anigian G. Reconstruction of penile and scrotal lymphedema. *Ann Plast Surg* 1991;27(6):570–573.

Elijalde Syndrome

DESCRIPTION   Autosomal recessive syndrome characterized by gigantism and renal dysplasia. Renal cysts are also common.

SYNONYMS

• Acrocephalopolydactylous dysplasia

REFERENCE

Lippert M. Renal cystic disease. In: Gillenwater JY, Grayhack JT, Howards SS, Duckett JW, eds. *Adult and Pediatric Urology,* 3rd ed. St Louis: Mosby, 1996.

 Encopresis—Urologic Considerations

DESCRIPTION   Children who are incontinent of stool, even with minor fecal soiling, usually have significant constipation. Occult pathology of the bowel or nervous system must be ruled out as a possible cause. Encopresis usually is helpful in identifying bowel problems when the parents of a child are not aware of the child's stool habits. Children with encopresis and constipation have a higher risk of urinary tract infection and urinary incontinence. Successful treatment of functional constipation will usually resolve encopresis and associated urinary tract problems.

TREATMENT

• Diet changes
• Laxatives, stool softeners
• Toilet schedules

REFERENCE

O'Regan S, et al. Constipation, bladder instability, urinary tract infection syndrome. *Clin Nephrol* 1985;23:152.

 Endocarditis Prophylaxis— Urologic Considerations

DESCRIPTION   Some physicians believe that antimicrobial prophylaxis before procedures that may cause transient bacteremia can cause endocarditis in patients with valvular heart disease. Enterococci as a cause of endocarditis are most often reported associated with genitourinary procedures. These recommendations are identical for both gastrointestinal and genitourinary procedures and are supported by the American Heart Association. The goal before any urologic procedure should always be a sterile urine culture; these are recommendations in the absence of an active infection. Below are the recommendations for both children and adults.

DRUG	*REGIMEN*
Adult patients	
Amoxicillin	2 g po 1 h before procedure
Ampicillin ± gentamicin	Ampicillin 2 g IM/IV ± gentamicin 1.5 mg/kg (120 mg max) IM/IV 30 min before procedure
If ampicillin/amoxicillin/penicillin allergic:	
Vancomycin ± gentamicin	Vancomycin 1 g IV slowly over 1 h ± gentamicin IV/IM (1.5 mg/kg, 80 mg max) 1 h before and repeated 8 h later

Pediatric patients
Follow above guidelines using the following dosages (do not exceed adult dose levels).

Ampicillin 50 mg/kg
Amoxicillin 50 mg/kg
Gentamicin 2 mg/kg
Vancomycin 20 mg/kg

REFERENCE

Dajani AS, et al. Prevention of bacterial endocarditis: Recommendations by the American Heart Association. *JAMA* 1997;277:1794.

 Endocervicosis—Bladder

DESCRIPTION   Rare mucinous analogue of endometriosis. Histologically demonstrates glandular lesions involving the bladder, with prominent endocervical-like epithelium. Benign condition only reported in women. Patients are presumed to have an underlying malignancy and are usually treated surgically. Presents with irritative voiding symptoms and pelvic pain

TREATMENT

• Transurethral resection or partial cystectomy is curative.
• Close follow-up is recommended

REFERENCE

Rodriguez R, Alfert H. Endocervicosis of the bladder: A rare mucinous analogue of endometriosis. *J Urol* 1997;157(4):1355.

 Endometrioid Carcinoma— Prostate

DESCRIPTION   Resembles endometrial adenocarcinoma of the female uterus. Accounts for 0.5% of prostatic adenocarcinomas almost exclusively found in older men. Cystoscopically, friable polypoid white masses can be seen extending from the ducts at or near the verumontanum. Pathologically, involves the large prostatic ducts and verumontanum and stains for PAP and PSA. Serum PSA levels are usually normal at the time of diagnosis unless widespread metastasis are present.

SYNONYMS

• Ductal carcinoma
• Papillary carcinoma
• Adenocarcinoma with endometrioid features

TREATMENT

• Same as standard adenocarcinoma of prostate, with similar prognosis or slightly worse prognosis. Hormonal therapy can palliate but not extend survival in advanced disease.

REFERENCE

Bostwick DG. Neoplasms of the prostate. In: Bostwick, et al. *Urologic Surgical Pathology,* 1st ed. St Louis: Mosby, 1997.

Epidermoid Cyst—Testicle

 Epidermoid Cyst—Testicle

DESCRIPTION   Accounts for approximately 1% of testicular tumors. Keratinizing, stratified, squamous cell–lined cysts supported by fibrous tissue. Considered special cases of teratoma, but not truly teratoma since only a single germinal layer and not the required two layers is represented. Benign in behavior. Ultrasound is suggestive of diagnosis but not usually definitive.

TREATMENT

• Inguinal orchiectomy
• Some advocate organ-sparing surgery if the diagnosis is definitively proven by frozen section.

REFERENCE

Heidenreich A, Engelmann UH, Vietsch HV, Derschum W. Organ preserving surgery in testicular epidermoid cysts. *J Urol* 1995;153(4): 1147–1150.

 Epididymis—Metastasis

DESCRIPTION   Extremely rare. Sources that have been reported include colon, stomach, kidney, prostate, carcinoid, and pancreatic tumors. Prognosis is related to that of the primary disease. Can present as pain and swelling or as incidental finding on orchiectomy for prostate cancer. Four mechanisms for spread have been proposed, including direct extension, retrograde venous extension, retrograde lymphatic extension, and arterial embolism.

REFERENCE

Talbot RW, McCann BG. Secondary prostatic tumor of the spermatic cord and epididymis 5 years after prostatectomy and vasectomy. *Br J Urol* 1979;51(1):48.

 Erythrasma

DESCRIPTION   Superficial, asymptomatic skin infection by a diphtheroid. Physical examination reveals sharply delineated, round to oval patches with scales in the intertriginous regions. Wood's lamp examination reveals coral-red fluorescence. Histologically, only the stratum corneum is affected, with all other layers normal. More common in tropical climates

CAUSES

• *Corynebacterium minutissimum*

TREATMENT

• Antibiotic therapy (erythromycin or tetracycline for 14 days)

REFERENCE

Ro JY, Amin MB, Ayala AG. Penis and scrotum. In: Bostwick, et al. *Urologic Surgical Pathology*, 1st ed. St Louis: Mosby, 1997.

 Extragonadal Germ Cell Tumors

DESCRIPTION   Rare entity representing 3% to 5% of all germ cell tumors. Most common sites include the mediastinum, retroperitoneum, sacrococcygeal region, and pineal gland. All tumor types reported, with seminoma most common. Can present with wide local invasion and advanced metastasis with few symptoms

TREATMENT

• Wide local excision, if feasible, with chemotherapy and radiation

REFERENCE

Richie JP. Neoplasms of the testes. In: Walsh PC, Retik AB, Vaughan ED, Wein AJ, eds. *Campbell's Urology*, 7th ed. Philadelphia: WB Saunders, 1998.

 Fabry Disease/Syndrome

DESCRIPTION   Consists of multiple cutaneous angiokeratomas, corneal opacification, and progressive renal insufficiency. Symptoms of severe burning pain in the extremities usually begin in the first decade. Can cause febrile episodes. The skin lesion is known as angiokeratoma corporis diffusum. Cardiovascular effects include coronary artery disease and congestive failure. Renal failure leads to uremia and hypertension in the third to fifth decade.

SYNONYMS

• Ceramide trihexoside lipidosis

CAUSES

• X-linked disorder that affects the alpha-galactosidase gene

TREATMENT

• Renal replacement therapy

REFERENCE

Eng CM, Desnick RJ. Molecular basis of Fabry disease: Mutations and polymorphisms in the human alpha-galactosidase A gene. *Hum Mutat* 1994;3(2):103–111.

 Faciodigital Syndrome

DESCRIPTION   Nine different types of faciodigital syndromes have been described. Type I is an X-linked dominant condition. Facial milia, orofacial defects such as cleft palate, hand deformities, including shortening of the phalanges, and CNS defects are noted. Of urologic interest, cystic kidney disease is found that greatly resembles autosomal dominant polycystic kidney disease in appearance and course.

TREATMENT

• Renal replacement therapy, as needed

REFERENCE

Leao MJ, Ribeiro-Silva ML. Orofaciodigital syndrome type I in a patient with severe CNS defects. *Pediatr Neurol* 1995;13(3):247–251.

Familial Testotoxicosis

DESCRIPTION   Cause of isosexual precocity. Autosomal dominant pattern. Markedly elevated levels of testosterone with normal LH secretion noted. Sleep-associated LH pulses are absent, however. Typically presents with family history and testicular enlargement around ages 3 to 4. Lack of testosterone response to hCG administration, despite a measurable increase in LH. Hyperplasia of Leydig cells is noted on biopsy.

TREATMENT

- Testolactone, a competitive inhibitor of aromatase, has been used in combination with spironolactone with some success.

REFERENCE

Aziz AA, Jafri SM, Haque NU. Testotoxicosis: Gonadotrophin-independent male sexual precocity. *Postgrad Med J* 1992;68(797):225–228.

 ## Fanconi Syndrome

DESCRIPTION   An acquired or inherited disorder characterized by abnormalities of renal proximal tubular function, including glucosuria, phosphaturia, aminoaciduria, and bicarbonate wasting. The aminoaciduria is generalized, and defects in uric acid, water, potassium, and sodium absorption can also occur. The basic abnormality is unknown. The hereditary form presents in infancy with proximal tubular acidosis, hypophosphatemic rickets, hypokalemia, polyuria, and polydipsia. In the nephropathic form, failure to thrive and growth retardation are common, with progressive renal failure. Diagnosed by demonstrating the abnormalities of renal function

CAUSES

- Inherited (usually seen with other disorder)
- Acquired (6-mercaptopurine or outdated tetracycline, renal transplantation, multiple myeloma, amyloidosis, intoxication with heavy metals or other chemical agents, and vitamin D deficiency)

TREATMENT

- Sodium bicarbonate for acidosis
- Renal transplantation has been successful.

REFERENCE

Bickel H, Manz F. Hereditary tubular disorders of the Fanconi type and the idiopathic Fanconi syndrome. *Prog Clin Biol Res* 1989;305:111–335.

 ## Fertile Eunuch Disease/ Syndrome

DESCRIPTION   Isolated LH deficiencies patients have eunuchoid proportions with variable degrees of virilization and, often, gynecomastia. Large testes and ejaculate containing a few sperm are present. Plasma FSH levels are normal, but both serum LH and serum testosterone concentrations are low normal.

SYNONYMS

- Isolated LH deficiency

TREATMENT

- Testosterone replacement
- hCG therapy may be useful.

REFERENCE

McClure RD. Male infertility. In: Tanagho EA, McAninch JW, eds. *Smith's General Urology,* 14th ed. Norwalk, CT: Appleton & Lange, 1995.

 ## Feulgen Staining

DESCRIPTION   This is a chromogenic reaction for quantitative staining of DNA that has gained wide acceptance for DNA cytometry. Currently, it is considered the only staining technique that is stoichiometric for DNA, which means that DNA staining is both quantitative and specific.

REFERENCE

Hardonk MJ, Van Duijn P. Studies on the Feulgen reaction with histochemical model systems. *J Histochem Cytochem* 1964;12:758.

 ## Fibroepithelial Polyp

DESCRIPTION   The most common benign ureteral tumor. Arises from the upper third of the ureter. Resembles a smooth nodule or may be pedunculated. Histologically, a central fibrous core surrounded by normal or hyperplastic urothelium. Presents with flank pain and hematuria, usually in a young adult. Radiographically, seen as smooth filling defects. Hydroureteronephrosis can be seen, as well as ureteral intussusception. Can recur locally

TREATMENT

- Ureteroscopic resection, open ureterotomy with polypectomy, or partial ureterectomy, if the diagnosis can be confirmed preoperatively

REFERENCE

Brady JD, Korman HJ, Civantos F, Soloway MS. Fibroepithelial polyp of the renal pelvis: Nephron-sparing surgery after false-positive biopsy for transitional cell carcinoma. *Urology* 1997;49(3):460–464.

 ## Fibrous Hamartoma of Infancy

DESCRIPTION   Uncommon subcutaneous proliferative lesion, usually found in the shoulder and axillary regions during the first 2 years of life. Reported to occur in the genital region and should be in the differential diagnosis. Histologically demonstrates mature adipose tissue, scattered mesenchymal cells, and bundles of fibrous tissue

TREATMENT

- Local excision is curative.

REFERENCE

Stock JA, Niku SD, Packer MG, Krous H, Kaplan GW. Fibrous hamartoma of infancy: A report of two cases in the genital region. *Urology* 1995;45(1):130–131.

 ## Fibrous Pseudotumor of Testicular Tunic

DESCRIPTION   Reactive, benign process of the tunica vaginalis where multiple firm nodules occur in the tunica or within it. Presents as testicular masses. May be difficult to distinguish from malignant processes. Histologically, can demonstrate granulation tissue, fibroblastic proliferation, and nodules of hyalinized tissue

SYNONYMS

- Fibrous pseudotumors
- Multiple fibromas of the tunica vaginalis testes
- Reactive periorchitis

CAUSES

- Sometimes associated with trauma or hydrocele

TREATMENT

- Orchiectomy usually necessary to confirm diagnosis

REFERENCE

Sajjad SM, Azizi MR, Llamas L. Fibrous pseudotumor of testicular tunic. *Urology* 1982;19(1):86–88.

Filariasis—Urologic Considerations

 Filariasis—Urologic Considerations

DESCRIPTION   The disease is transmitted by mosquitoes. *Wuchereria bancrofti* is found in many areas of the Caribbean, Venezuela, Colombia, the Guianas, Brazil, Central America, sub-Saharan Africa, North Africa, Turkey, and Asia. Filariasis (bancroftian, Malayan, and Timorian) is often asymptomatic. The parasite causes symptoms due to inflammation and dysfunction of the lymphatics, where the adult worms develop (fever, headache, myalgia, and lymphadenitis). In lymphatic disease, manifestations usually occur 3 months to 1 year after acquisition. Occasionally, moderate lymphadenopathy, particularly involving the inguinal lymph nodes, occurs. Inflammation of the lymphatics of the extremities and genitalia leads to retrograde adenolymphangitis. Epididymitis, orchitis, and funiculitis also can occur, along with fever, chills, and other nonspecific systemic symptoms. Lymphatic dysfunction, with resulting chronically progressive edema of the limbs and genitalia, is relatively infrequent in children. Elephantiasis can result from fibrosis caused by chronic dysfunction of the lymphatic channels. Chyluria can occur as a manifestation of bancroftian filariasis. Lymphatic filariasis must be diagnosed clinically because serologic assays are not available, and in elephantiasis the microfilariae may no longer be present. Eosinophilia of 25% frequently occurs in early disease.

TREATMENT

• Diethylcarbamazine citrate is the drug of choice. The late obstructive phase of the disease is not affected by chemotherapy.
• Ivermectin, an investigational drug in the United States, is effective against the microfilariae of *W. bancrofti,* but is unlikely to become the drug of choice for lymphatic filariasis.
• Complex, decongestive physiotherapy may be effective in treating elephantiasis.
• Plastic surgical repair of the genitalia gives variable results.
• Chyluria originating in the bladder responds to fulguration; chyluria originating in the kidney is much more difficult to correct.

REFERENCE

AAP 1997 Red Book: Report of the Committee on Infectious Diseases, 24th ed. Elk Grove, IL: American Academy of Pediatrics.

 Foley Y-V Pyeloplasty

DESCRIPTION   The triangular portion of the Y is incised in the dependent portion of the pelvis, with the apex pointing to the stricture, and a single 2- to 3-cm longitudinal incision is continued from the apex anteriorly down across the stricture to complete the Y configuration. The apex of the triangle flap is then brought down to the lower apex of the ureterotomy and a 5-0 chromic stay suture is placed. Interrupted 5-0 chromic sutures are used to complete the anastomosis. Used for UPJ repair

REFERENCE

Kay R. Procedures for ureteropelvic junction obstruction. In: Novick AC, Streem SB, Pontes JE, eds. *Stewarts Operative Urology.* Baltimore: Williams & Wilkins, 1989:220–233.

 Fossa Navicularis Diverticulum

DESCRIPTION   First described by Guerin (1864), this diverticulum is partially separated from the urethra by a septum. On VCUG, it can often be seen as a small spherical collection of contrast at the tip of the penis. Common anatomic finding with rare symptoms, including dysuria, gross hematuria, spotting of blood, or hematospermia

SYNONYMS

• Valve of Guerin
• Dorsal urethral diverticulum
• Lacuna magna

CAUSES

• Thought to result embryologically from incomplete breakdown of the wall between the ectoderm and urethra being formed by the urethral folds

TREATMENT

• If symptomatic, the wall can be divided with tenotomy scissors or under direct vision with a resectoscope.

REFERENCE

Seskin FE, Glassberg KI. Lacuna magna in 6 boys with post-void bleeding and dysuria: Alternative approach to treatment. *J Urol* 1994; 152(3):980–982.

 Fowler-Stephens Orchiopexy

DESCRIPTION   This procedure is used for the intraabdominal testes. It entails ligating the spermatic vessels and allows the testes to survive from the vasal and cremasteric collaterals. The operation was originally described as a two-stage procedure in which the vessels are divided, and then 6 months later the testes are brought down to the scrotum, after collaterals have become more well developed.

REFERENCE

Rozanski T, Bloom DA, Colodny A. Surgery of the scrotum and testis in children. In Walsh PC, Retik AB, Vaughan ED, Wein AJ, eds. *Campbell's Urology,* 7th ed. Philadelphia: WB Saunders, 1998:2193–2198.

 Fragile X Syndrome

DESCRIPTION   The most common cause of inherited mental retardation. The affected gene encodes a protein known as FMR1, which is required for normal cognitive development. Facial dysmorphism and bilateral macro-orchidism are also seen. Measurement of testis size in mentally retarded males has been suggested as a simple screening test for this condition.

REFERENCE

Hagerman RJ. Fragile X syndrome. Molecular and clinical insights and treatment issues. *West J Med* 1997;166(2):129–137.

 Fraily Syndrome

DESCRIPTION   A condition in which vascular obstruction of the superior infundibulum might lead to hydrocalyx, bleeding, and intermittent nephralgia infection. Vessels causing obstruction may be arteries, veins, or both. Impaired drainage on delayed films or isotope renography must be confirmed before surgery. On ultrasound, diuretics will accentuate the caliectasis. Surgery provides relief.

REFERENCE

Fraley EE. Vascular obstruction of superior infundibulum causing nephralgia: A new syndrome. *N Engl J Med* 1966;275:1403.

Frequency-Dysuria Syndrome

DESCRIPTION Occurs in children and women. Presents as complaints of frequency and dysuria. Evaluation finds no infectious, anatomic, functional, or physiologic abnormalities. (See also Section II, "Urethral Syndrome.")

SYNONYMS

• Urethral syndrome

CAUSES

• In childhood, hypercalciuria has been theorized.
• In adults, fastidial organism infection has been theorized.

TREATMENT

• Usually self-limiting with few sequelae but can be recurrent

REFERENCES

Brock JW III. The frequency and frequency dysuria syndromes of childhood: Hypercalciuria as a possible etiology. *Urology* 1994;44(3): 411–412.

Gillespie WA, Henderson EP, Linton KB, Smith PJ. Microbiology of the urethral (frequency and dysuria) syndrome. A controlled study with 5-year review. *Br J Urol* 1989;64(3):270–274.

 Furhmann Classification

DESCRIPTION Classification used to grade renal cell carcinoma. Based on the concept that nuclear features correlate with survival. Consists of four grades based on size, contour, and conspicuousness of nucleoli. Large series have confirmed the correlation with survival. Grade 1 is round, uniform nuclei with minute or absent nucleoli. Grade 2 is slightly irregular nuclei about 15 μm, with nucleoli visible at 400X. Grade 3 is more irregular nuclei, 20 μm, with nucleoli visible at 100X. Grade 4 is similar to grade 3, with bizarre feature noted.

REFERENCE

Eble JN. Neoplasms of the kidney. In: Bostwick D, ed. *Urologic Surgical Pathology,* 1st ed. St Louis: Mosby, 1997.

 Funiculitis

DESCRIPTION Inflammation of the spermatic cord. The entire spermatic cord is subject to inflammatory diseases, usually the result of trauma or pyogenic bacteria (termed *funiculitis*), and is occasionally seen with scrotal inflammation or epididymitis. Parasitic infections (filariasis, schistosomiasis) can also induce inflammatory changes in the cord (see Section I, "Spermatic Cord Mass").

REFERENCE

Sabiston D. *Textbook of Surgery,* 15th ed. Philadelphia: WB Saunders, 1997.

 Ganglioneuroblastoma—Adrenal

DESCRIPTION Tumor originating from neural crest cells. In a spectrum of diseases between neuroblastoma and ganglioneuroma. Varied in appearance and malignant potential. Prognosis and behavior depend on histology.

CAUSES

• Unknown, but has been reported to have a genetic predisposition

TREATMENT

• Surgical resection

REFERENCE

Snyder HM III, D'Angio GJ, Evans AE, Raney RB. Pediatric oncology. In: Walsh PC, Retik AB, Vaughan ED, Wein AJ, eds. *Campbell's Urology,* 7th ed. Philadelphia: WB Saunders, 1998.

 Ganglioneuroma—Adrenal

DESCRIPTION Tumor originating from neural crest cells. The benign counterpart of neuroblastoma. Does not metastasize but can locally recur after resection. Can be locally aggressive. Most commonly presents as abdominal mass. Histologically, composed of ganglion cells with abundant cytoplasm and large nuclei

CAUSES

• Unknown, but has been reported to have a genetic predisposition

TREATMENT

• Surgical resection

REFERENCE

Snyder HM III, D'Angio GJ, Evans AE, Raney RB. Pediatric oncology. In: Walsh PC, Retik AB, Vaughan ED, Wein AJ, eds. *Campbell's Urology,* 7th ed. Philadelphia: WB Saunders, 1998.

 Germ Cell Aplasia

DESCRIPTION Total absence of germ cells within a normal interstitium. Patients present with infertility. Testes are small to normal. Sperm analysis reveals azoospermia. Normal secondary sexual characteristics are present. LH and testosterone are normal, with variable elevations of FSH. May represent endpoint of various etiologies, resulting in this histologic appearance

SYNONYMS

• Sertoli cell-only syndrome

TREATMENT

• Adoption or use of banked sperm

REFERENCE

Nistal M, Jimenez F, Paniagua R. Sertoli cell types in the Sertoli-cell-only syndrome: Relationships between Sertoli cell morphology and aetiology. *Histopathology* 1990;16(2):173–180.

 Gibbon Classification of Voiding Dysfunction

DESCRIPTION Classification based in large part on the system proposed by Bors-Comarr. Five categories are proposed to be important: (1) Full general and neurologic diagnosis. (2) State of the bulbocavernosus and anal reflexes in cord injuries. (3) Presence or absence of reflex detrusor contractions. (4) Urodynamic findings. (5) Failure of storage, emptying, or control when dealing with incontinence

REFERENCE

Gibbon NOK. Nomenclature of neurogenic bladder. *Urology* 1976;8:423.

 Gibson Incision

DESCRIPTION A curvilinear incision is made starting 2 to 3 cm medial to the anterior superior iliac spine, running parallel to the inguinal ligament down to 2 to 3 cm superior and just lateral to the pubic tubercle. The external and internal obliques and the transversalis muscle are bluntly opened along their fibers. After transecting the transversalis fascia, the peritoneum is swept medially to expose the ureter at its midsection. Useful for distal ureteral stones and renal transplant

REFERENCE

Montague DK. Surgical incisions. In: Novick AC, Streem SB, Pontes JE, eds. *Stewarts Operative Urology.* Baltimore: Williams & Wilkins, 1989:15–40.

Gil-Vernet Orthotopic Urinary Diversion

 Gil-Vernet Orthotopic Urinary Diversion

DESCRIPTION   A continuous segment of terminal ileum, cecum, and ascending colon are isolated. The unit is rotated 180 degrees to allow anastomosis of the reduced end of the ascending colon to the urethra and the ureters to the terminal ileum.

REFERENCE

Benson MC, Olsson CA. Continent urinary diversion. In: Walsh PC, Retik AB, Vaughan ED, Wein AJ, eds. *Campbell's Urology*, 7th ed. Philadelphia: WB Saunders, 1998:3190–3245.

 Gil-Vernet Ureteral Reimplantation

DESCRIPTION   Through a transvesical approach, the ureters are dissected free from their hiatus. The principle involves advancing the ureters across the trigone to the midline such that both ureteral orifices are juxtaposed. A single incision is made in the trigone mucosa, which will serve to join traction sutures from each ureter that are anchored in the midline.

REFERENCE

Atala A, Keating MA. Vesicoureteral reflux and megaureter. In: Walsh PC, Retik AB, Vaughan ED, Wein AJ, eds. *Campbell's Urology*, 7th ed. Philadelphia: WB Saunders, 1998:1882–1896.

 Gittes Needle Urethropexy

DESCRIPTION   A Stamey needle is delivered through a stab incision at the upper border of the pubis, and it is transferred under digital guidance through the anterior vaginal wall at the level of the bladder neck. A no. 2 proline suture is used to suspend the bladder neck on both sides, and the vaginal sutures eventually cut through the wall and become buried in scar. Used to treat stress incontinence

REFERENCE

Raz S, Stothers L, Chopra A. Vaginal reconstructive surgery for incontinence and prolapse. In: Walsh PC, Retik AB, Vaughan ED, Wein AJ, eds. *Campbell's Urology*, 7th ed. Philadelphia: WB Saunders, 1998:1066–1094.

 Glenn-Anderson Ureteroneocystostomy

DESCRIPTION   Through a transvesical approach, the ureter is mobilized from its hiatus and advanced towards the bladder neck through a submucosal tunnel, where it is reimplanted. Used to reimplant ureter in reflux or resection of ureter

REFERENCE

Kay R. Reimplantation of the ureter. In: Novick AC, Streem SB, Pontes JE, eds. *Stewarts Operative Urology*. Baltimore: Williams & Wilkins, 1989:526–538.

 Glomerulcystic Disease

DESCRIPTION   Rare, bilateral cystic kidney disease. Presents most commonly in childhood with bilateral flank masses, which are large kidneys with many cysts. Seen rarely in adults with HTN, hematuria, and ESRD. Cysts are confined to the cortex and arise from Bowman's space. Renal biopsy may be necessary to confirm diagnosis. Radiologically similar to ADPKD

SYNONYMS

• Cortical microcystic disease

CAUSES

• Heritable (autosomal dominant)
• Sporadic

TREATMENT

• Renal replacement therapy if renal failure occurs

REFERENCE

Glassberg KI, Filmer RB. Renal dysplasia, renal hypoplasia, and cystic disease of the kidney. In: Kelalis PP, et al. *Clinical Pediatric Urology*, 3rd ed. Philadelphia: WB Saunders, 1992.

 Glycolic Aciduria

DESCRIPTION   Form of primary hyperoxaluria. Often presents with stone disease in childhood. Extensive nephrocalcinosis and renal failure are common. Most patients die prior to age 30.

SYNONYMS

• Type 1 hyperoxaluria

CAUSES

• Enzymatic deficiency of glyoxylate carboligase

TREATMENT

• Oral phosphates are usually unsuccessful.

REFERENCE

Drach GW. Urinary lithiasis: Etiology, diagnosis, and medical management, In: Walsh PC, Retik AB, Vaughan ED, Wein AJ, eds. *Campbell's Urology*, 7th ed. Philadelphia: WB Saunders, 1998.

 Glycosuria— Renal

DESCRIPTION   Normal urine contains small amounts of glucose. Increased amounts represent either inefficient handling by the tubule or hyperglycemia. Diabetes is the most common cause of glycosuria. Causes of primary glucosuria are either intestinal glucose–galactose malabsorption or benign familial renal glycosuria. Some substances are known to cause false-positive glucose readings on dipstick, such as ascorbic acid and salicylates. Medications such as ACE inhibitors may also have a direct effect on the kidney to cause glycosuria. Pregnancy can be causative. May also be part of Fanconi syndrome or RTA.

REFERENCE

Brodehl J, Demar BS, Hoyer PF. Renal glucosuria. *Pediatr Nephrol* 1987;1(3):502–508.

Goldston Syndrome

DESCRIPTION Rare syndrome with principal features of kidney, liver, and brain abnormalities. The kidneys are cystic and large bilaterally. Histologic lesions of the liver are triads with a double band of fibrous tissue without bile ducts. The brain shows the Dandy-Walker malformation, which is the cystic dilation of the fourth ventricle secondary to obstruction of the foramina of Luschka and Magendie.

TREATMENT
- Renal replacement therapy, as indicated
- Hydrocephalus requires a shunt.

REFERENCE
Gloeb DJ, Valdes-Dapena M, Salman F, O'Sullivan MJ, Quetal TA. The Goldston syndrome: Report of a case. *Pediatr Pathol* 1989;9(3): 337–343.

 Gonadoblastoma

DESCRIPTION Rare tumor comprising 0.5% of all testes tumors. Occurs almost always in gonadal dysgenesis. Presents either with palpable mass or virilization secondary to androgen production. Germ cells appear similar to seminoma. Tubules microscopically contain PAS-positive staining Call-Exner bodies.

SYNONYMS
- Tumors of dysgenetic gonads
- Mixed germ cell tumor
- Gonadocytoma

CAUSES
- Gonadal dysgenesis

TREATMENT
- Radical orchiectomy with possible contralateral orchiectomy secondary to high incidence of bilaterality

REFERENCE
Richie JP. Neoplasms of the testes. In: Walsh PC, Retik AB, Vaughan ED, Wein AJ, eds. *Campbell's Urology,* 7th ed. Philadelphia: WB Saunders, 1998.

 Goodpasture Syndrome

DESCRIPTION Characterized by a triad of pulmonary hemorrhage, iron deficiency anemia, and glomerulonephritis. Less than 1% of all cases of GN. Antibody production appears to be self-limited. Histologically, shows focal proliferative and necrotizing glomerular lesions that progress rapidly to diffuse proliferation with crescents. Immunohistochemical studies show diffuse linear deposition of IgG along the GBM. Primarily a disease of young white males (male–female ratio, 6:1) with a mean age of 21. About one-third of patients die of pulmonary involvement. Renal involvement is usually severe and progressive, with rapid development of oliguria and renal failure.

CAUSES
- Anti-GBM antibody deposition in the lungs and kidneys

TREATMENT
- Steroid pulse therapy with prednisone
- Plasma exchange therapy to remove circulating anti-GBM antibody
- Cyclophosphamide to inhibit further antibody production
- Renal replacement therapy for ESRD

REFERENCE
Couser WG. Glomerular diseases. In: Stein, et al. *Internal Medicine,* 4th ed. Boston: Little, Brown, 1994.

 Goodwin Ureteral Anastomosis

DESCRIPTION Through a transcolonic approach, a nonrefluxing anastomosis is performed by raising a tunnel of mucosa with a mosquito hemostat for a 3- to 4-cm distance, then exiting the bowel wall. The ureter is grasped and pulled through the tunnel. The spatulated ureter is anastomosed to the colonic mucosa while incorporating some muscularis for security.

REFERENCE
McDougal WS. Use of intestinal segments and urinary diversion. In: Walsh PC, Retik AB, Vaughan ED, Wein AJ, eds. *Campbell's Urology,* 7th ed. Philadelphia: WB Saunders, 1998:3137–3144.

 Gout—Urologic Considerations

DESCRIPTION Inherited disorder of purine metabolism, which is characterized by elevated serum urate levels and severe recurrent arthritis. Leads to increased risk of urate urolithiasis. Most patients with uric acid stones, however, do not have gout. May also produce a type IV RTA, resulting in hyperkalemia and a mild metabolic acidosis

TREATMENT
- Alkalinization of urine and increasing urine output help prevent stones.
- Allopurinol or following a low-purine diet will decrease serum urate levels.

REFERENCE
Jenkins AD. Calculus formation In: Gillenwater JY, Grayhack JT, Howards SS, Duckett JW, eds. *Adult and Pediatric Urology,* 3rd ed. St Louis: Mosby, 1996.

 Granulosa Cell Tumors

DESCRIPTION The most common ovarian neoplasm. Usually small, cystic, unilateral, and secretes estrogens. Present in childhood as precocious puberty or as postmenopausal bleeding in older women. During the reproductive years, prolonged and irregular bleeding and a pelvic mass are most common. Can also present with urinary symptoms. Rarely can be present in the testes

TREATMENT
- Surgical excision is usually curative.
- Close follow-up of the contralateral ovary is necessary.

REFERENCE
Chan YF, Restall P, Kimble R. Juvenile granulosa cell tumor of the testis: Report of two cases in newborns. *J Pediatr Surg* 1997;32(5): 752–753.

Griess Test

 Griess Test

DESCRIPTION Detects the presence of nitrite in urine, which is formed when bacteria reduce the nitrate normally present. Lower sensitivity and specificity than microscopy and culture. This test in combination with leukocyte esterase has been used to screen asymptomatic patients. Microscopy is indicated for the higher risk population for UTI.

REFERENCE

Schaeffer AJ. Urinary tract infections. In: Gillenwater JY, Grayhack JT, Howards SS, Duckett JW, eds. *Adult and Pediatric Urology,* 3rd ed. St Louis: Mosby, 1996.

 Hald-Bradley Classification of Voiding Dysfunction

DESCRIPTION Based on the anatomic location of the neurologic lesion. Broken down into five classes: (1) suprasacral, (2) suprasacral spinal, (3) infrasacral, (4) peripheral autonomic neuropathy, and (5) muscular lesions. Examples include coordinated voiding with hyperreflexia in suprasacral lesions, while muscular lesions may be a decompensated bladder from longstanding bladder outlet obstruction.

REFERENCE

Wein AJ. Neuromuscular dysfunction of the lower urinary tract. In: Walsh PC, Retik AB, Vaughan ED, Wein AJ, eds. *Campbell's Urology,* 7th ed. Philadelphia: WB Saunders, 1998.

 Hautmann Pouch

DESCRIPTION This ileal neobladder is created from 70 cm of ileum, starting 15 cm from the ileocecal junction. The bowel is opened up along the antimesenteric border, and the bowel is arranged into an M or W shape. The limbs are sutured to each other with absorbable suture material to form a broad ileal plate. A preselected segment is anastomosed to the urethra and the ureters are implanted in a LeDuc fashion. The plate is then closed into a pouch and anastomosed to the urethra.

REFERENCE

Benson MC, Olsson CA. Continent urinary diversion. In: Walsh PC, Retik AB, Vaughan DE, Wein AJ, eds. Campbell's Urology, 7th ed. Philadelphia: WB Saunders, 1998:3190–3245.

 Heikel-Parkkulainen Reflux Classification System

DESCRIPTION Described by Heikel and Parkkulainen in 1966. System used to grade vesicoureteral reflux based on ureteral diameter and pelvicalyceal dilatation. Gained much popularity in Europe. Later, features of this system were used to create the International Classification System, which is now the standard.

REFERENCE

Heikel RE, Parkkulainen KV. Vesico-ureteric reflux in children: A classification and results of conservative treatment. *Ann Radiol* 1966;9:37.

 Hematocele

DESCRIPTION Collection of blood within the layers of the tunica vaginalis. Can present as scrotal swelling and may be asymptomatic. May be difficult to distinguish from tumor. Ultrasound may be helpful.

CAUSES

- Trauma
- Infection
- Bleeding disorders
- Tumor
- Uremia, rarely

TREATMENT

- Conservative management if patient asymptomatic and diagnosis confirmed. Often, diagnosis by surgical exploration

REFERENCE

Leibovitch I, Ramon J, Ben Chaim J, Nass D, Goldwasser B. Chronic hematocele complicating renal failure and hemodialysis. *J Urol* 1991; 146(1):162–164.

 Hematuria—Loin Pain Syndrome

DESCRIPTION A cause of recurrent gross hematuria that may be confused with IgA nephropathy is the loin pain–hematuria syndrome. This disorder, which generally affects young women, is characterized by recurrent episodes of gross hematuria associated with dull unilateral or bilateral loin pain and sometimes low-grade fever. Blood pressure and renal function are usually normal. The syndrome has been associated most often with the use of oral contraceptive agents and generally resolves when these agents are discontinued. Recent literature has suggested that this syndrome is not a distinct clinicopathologic entity.

TREATMENT

- A concerted medical and psychological approach is advocated.

REFERENCE

Hall R, Lailis A, Rapoport A. Hematuria-loin pain syndrome: Its existence as a discrete clinicopathological entity cannot be supported. *Clin J Pain* 1997;13(2):171–177.

 Hemi-Kock Neobladder

DESCRIPTION An orthotopic neobladder is constructed based on the theme of the Kock pouch. In this diversion, a single intussuscepted ileal nipple valve is used to create a nonrefluxing ureteroileal anastomosis. The remainder of the pouch is made from a detubularized ileum, which is configured into a pouch and anastomosed to the urethra.

REFERENCE

Benson MC, Olsson CA. Continent urinary diversion. In: Walsh PC, Retik AB, Vaughan ED, Wein AJ, eds. *Campbell's Urology,* 7th ed. Philadelphia: WB Saunders, 1998:3190–3245.

Hemizona Assay

DESCRIPTION   Assesses the ability of sperm to bind to the zona pellucida of the egg. Performed by dividing in half intact zona pellucida and incubating separately with donor sperm and the patient's sperm. A hemizona index is derived by dividing the number of bound donor sperm by the number of bound patient sperm. An index below 0.60 is seen in males who failed in vitro fertilization. Limited by the availability of human ova. Since this technique potentially bypasses the step of zona binding, men whose sperm cannot bind may be good candidates for these procedures.

REFERENCE

Yao YQ, Yeung WS, Ho PC. The factors affecting sperm binding to the zona pellucida in the hemizona binding assay. *Hum Reprod* 1996;11(7): 1516–1519.

 Henoch-Schönlein Purpura

DESCRIPTION   A form of purpura with an underlying pathologic feature of vasculitis, affecting mainly small blood vessels. The disease is predominately seen in children. Clinically, the purpuric skin lesions are typically located on the lower extremities. However, the hands, arms, and trunk might be affected. Joint pain, abdominal pain, and gastrointestinal bleeding may be present. Hematuria denotes a renal lesion, which is usually reversible. Similar to IgA nephropathy, but somewhat more severe, particularly in adults. Progressive renal failure occurs in at least 25%. Kidney biopsy reveals segmental glomerulonephritis with crescents and mesangial deposition of IgA and sometimes IgG. Lab test would reveal high ESR and normal-to-high platelet count. If renal involvement is not severe, the disease will subside without sequelae within 6 weeks.

CAUSES

• Unknown.

TREATMENT

• Currently no effective treatment is available.
• Immunosuppressive drugs have shown some success in nephropathies caused by that disorder.
• Short courses of steroids may be useful in systemic manifestations.
• Cytotoxic agents are being investigated.

REFERENCE

Goldstein AR, et al. Long-term follow-up of childhood Henoch-Schönlein nephritis. *Lancet* 1992;330:280.

 Hepatorenal Syndrome

DESCRIPTION   Known as progressive oliguric renal failure complicating the course of end-stage liver disease. Usually poor prognosis for recovery of renal function, and for survival overall. Urine is characteristically hyperosmolar, with a high creatine-to-plasma ratio and a very low sodium concentration.

CAUSES

• Thought to be functional, due perhaps to discharge of the sympathetic nervous system and/or metabolic imbalances, including endothelin and nitric oxide

TREATMENT

• A transjugular intrahepatic portosystemic shunt has been attempted.
• Orthotopic liver transplantation

REFERENCE

Epstein M. Hepatorenal syndrome: Emerging perspectives. *Semin Nephrol* 1997;17(6):563–575.

 Hernia Uterine Inguinale

DESCRIPTION   Cause of male pseudohermaphroditism. Rare syndrome of the persistence of Müllerian ducts. Affected males are not ambiguous at birth and generally present later, most commonly with an inguinal hernia on one side and an impalpable contralateral testes. Hernia sac may contain uterus. Karyotype is 46,XY. The gonadal tissue is exclusively testicular. Both Wolffian and Müllerian duct derivatives are present, with a vas and epididymis alongside an ipsilateral uterus, fallopian tube, and upper vagina. Testes have malignant potential. No uterine or vaginal malignancies have been reported.

CAUSES

• Isolated defect in the production of Müllerian inhibition substance or the response to MIF

TREATMENT

• Sex assignment as male
• Primary or staged orchidopexy
• Müllerian structures do not require removal, as the vas may be damaged.

REFERENCE

Snyder HM. Intersex. Practical Cases in Urology. Series XIX, Course 4, 1996.

 Hidradenitis Suppurativa— Urologic Considerations

DESCRIPTION   A chronic suppurative disease of the apocrine gland–bearing areas of the body, such as the axilla, buttocks, and groin. Lesions resemble boils and can resolve without scarring but more typically result in fibrosis, keloids, and sinus tract formation. Mild cases resemble simple boils (furunculosis). Diagnosed primarily by location and clinical course. Pain, fluctuation, discharge, and sinus tract formation are characteristic. In chronic cases, coalescence of inflamed nodules may cause palpable cordlike bands. The condition may become extensive and disabling; if the pubic and genital areas are severely involved, walking may be difficult.

CAUSES

• Not primarily infectious; caused by plugging of the follicles
• Secondary infection can occur after the follicle plugs, with resultant inflammatory response.

TREATMENT

• Avoid irritants such as antiperspirants.
• Conservative treatment with rest, moist heat, and prolonged antibiotics (tetracycline or erythromycin)
• Oral isotretinoin and intralesional corticosteroids may be effective.
• Surgical excision and plastic repair of the affected areas may be necessary.

REFERENCE

Goldberg JM, Buchler DA, Dibbell DG. Advanced hidradenitis suppurativa presenting with bilateral vulvar masses. *Gynecol Oncol* 1996; 160(3):494–497.

 Hinman-Allen Syndrome

• See Section III, "Pseudodyssynergia (Hinman Syndrome)."

Histoplasmosis—Genitourinary

DESCRIPTION *Histoplasma capsulatum* grows in soil enriched by bird guano, with outbreaks reported in caves, construction sites, and on bird farms. Disseminated virulent disease is seen in AIDS, children, and immunosuppressed individuals. GU involvement is a manifestation of systemic disease and can result in sloughed papilla, prostatic obstruction, or prostatic abscess. Epididymitis can resemble sperm granulomas. Up to 7% can experience adrenal insufficiency from adrenal destruction.

TREATMENT

• Two grams of Amphotericin B with maintenance therapy with itraconazole to prevent relapse

REFERENCE

Wise GJ, Freyle J. Changing patterns in genitourinary fungal infections. AUA Update, Volume XVI, Lesson 1, 1997.

 Hodgkin Disease—Urologic Considerations

DESCRIPTION Type of lymphoma differentiated from other lymphomas partially on basis of presence of Reed-Sternberg cells. Has become one of the most curable forms of malignancy. Has many urologic associations. An association with higher incidence in renal cell carcinoma patients has been proposed. Treatment with radiation for Hodgkin may predispose to bladder cancer. Kidney and bladder have been reported to be primary sites of Hodgkin. Extensive retroperitoneal lymphadenopathy may cause ureteral obstruction. (See also Section III, "Lymphoma—Urologic Considerations.")

REFERENCE

Jones MW. Primary Hodgkin's disease of the urinary bladder. *Br J Urol* 1989;63(4):438.

 Hodgson's Type I Hypospadias Repair

DESCRIPTION Chordee is repaired. A longitudinal tube along the urethral axis is formed on the inner surface of the prepuce, which is then transferred to the ventrum through a buttonhole incision at the base of the tube. The proximal neourethra is anastomosed to the proximal native urethra, and the distal neourethral tube is used to create the meatus.

REFERENCE

Devine CJ, Horton CE. Repair of hypospadias and epispadias. In: Novick AC, Streem SB, Pontes JE, eds. *Stewarts Operative Urology*. Baltimore: Williams & Wilkins, 1989:689–714.

 Hodgson's Type II Hypospadias Repair

DESCRIPTION Hodgson modified type I for the very distal hypospadias where no chordee exists, and the native urethral plate remains intact. The inner surface of the prepuce is again transferred to the ventrum via a buttonhole at the base. In this repair, the prepuce flap is sutured onto the urethral plate.

REFERENCE

Devine CJ, Horton CE. Repair of hypospadias and epispadias. In: Novick AC, Streem SB, Pontes JE, eds. *Stewarts Operative Urology*. Baltimore: Williams & Wilkins, 1989:689–714.

 Hodgson's Type III Hypospadias Repair

DESCRIPTION This is modified for the more proximal hypospadias repair. Here, Hodgson creates the buttonhole at the base of the penis, and he creates a longer tubular neourethral that is based on preputial and shaft skin.

REFERENCE

Devine CJ, Horton CE. Repair of hypospadias and epispadias. In: Novick AC, Streem SB, Pontes JE, eds. *Stewarts Operative Urology*. Baltimore: Williams & Wilkins, 1989:689–714.

 Horseshoe Kidney

DESCRIPTION Most common fusion anomaly. Presents in 1 in 400 births, with a male predominance. Usually, true fusion of the lower poles, which may be composed of thick functioning parenchyma or merely a fibrous band. Associated anomalies are seen in one-third of patients and include multisystem disturbances of the skeletal and cardiovascular systems and gastrointestinal tract, as well as genitourinary abnormalities, such as an increased frequency of ureteral duplication, reflux, and dysplasia. Usually asymptomatic. Radiographic diagnosis can be made with IVP, which reveals deviation of the axis of the kidneys. Renal scan may be helpful in surgical decision making, if necessary.

CAUSES

• Fusion of poles during ascent of the kidneys

TREATMENT

• Pyeloplasty and ureteral implantation may be required for proven UPJ obstruction or severe reflux, respectively.
• Can affect management of many other disease conditions, such as neoplasm, aortic aneurysm, and transplantation

REFERENCE

Artioukh DY, Wake PN, Edwards PR, Moody AP. Problems of abdominal aortic aneurysm associated with horseshoe kidney. *Eur J Vasc Endovasc Surg* 1997;14(1):75–78.

 Horton-Devine "Flip-Flap" Hypospadias Repair

DESCRIPTION The distal ventral skin over the urethra is mobilized, and the distal urethra is also mobilized. Parallel incisions are made in the glans to create a urethral plate, and the proximal flap is flipped over and sutured onto the urethral plate. The wings of the glans are then approximated over this distal repair.

REFERENCE

Devine CJ, Horton CE. Repair of hypospadias and epispadias. In: Novick AC, Streem SB, Pontes JE, eds. *Stewarts Operative Urology*. Baltimore: Williams & Wilkins, 1989:689–714.

 Hounsfield Units

DESCRIPTION Named after Hounsfield, the inventor of the CT scanner, an arbitrary scale created to compare density of different substances seen on CT scan. Water is represented by 0 HU. Air is −1000 HU. Bone is 1000 HU. Fat is in the range of −100 to 0 HU, while water with electrolytes is slightly above 0 HU. Soft tissue is in the range of 35 HU.

REFERENCE

Miraldi F. Imaging principles in computed tomography. In: Haaga JR, et al. *Computed Tomography of the Whole Body*, 1st edition. St Louis: Mosby, 1983.

 HPC-1 (Hereditary Prostate Cancer 1 Locus)

DESCRIPTION Locus found on chromosome 1q24-25, which has been potentially linked to inherited prostate cancer. Families in which this altered gene is found were determined to have a lower age at diagnosis, a higher grade of cancer, and more cases of advanced disease than normal.

REFERENCE

Gronberg H, Isaacs SD, Smith JR, et al. Characteristics of prostate cancer in families potentially linked to the hereditary prostate cancer 1 (HPC1) locus. *JAMA* 1997;278(15):1251–1255.

HPV (Human Papilloma Virus)—Urologic Considerations

DESCRIPTION Family of virus, with double-stranded DNA, which cause various warts, papillomas, and cervical cancer. Types 6, 11, 42, and 44 are associated with condyloma acuminatum. Types 16, 18, 31, 33, 35, and 39 have an association with cancer. Types 6 and 11 have been associated with Buschke-Lowenstein tumor. Subclinical condyloma can be detected with application of 5% acetic acid and inspection with a magnifying glass. Associated also with bowenoid papulosis and squamous cell carcinoma of the penis and urethra. Bladder cancer association is controversial.

TREATMENT

- Podophyllin or trichloroacetic acid for condyloma
- Laser therapy also effective

REFERENCE

Myula M, Iwasaka T, Iguchi A, Nakamura S, Masaki Z, Sugimori H. Do human papillomaviruses have a role in the pathogenesis of bladder carcinoma? *J Urol* 1996;155(2):471–474.

 ## Hunner's Ulcer

DESCRIPTION Cystoscopic finding of ulceration of the bladder mucosa found in patients with interstitial cystitis. Fulfills the one of the NIH criteria for IC. Found in a variable number of patients with IC. First described by Hunner in 1918, when he noted the ulcer in association with the constellation of clinical findings of IC.

REFERENCE

Koziol JA, Adams HP, Frutos A. Discrimination between the ulcerous and the non-ulcerous forms of interstitial cystitis by noninvasive findings. *J Urol* 1996;155(1):87–90.

 ## Hutch Diverticulum

DESCRIPTION Herniation of the bladder mucosa through the weakest point of the hiatus, in the detrusor above the intramural ureter, producing "Hutch diverticulum" and reflux. The condition is usually due to a chronic increase in intravesical pressure as a result of bladder outlet obstruction.

REFERENCE

Hutch JA, Ayers RD, Loquvam GS. The bladder musculature with special reference to the uretero vesical junction. *J Urol* 1961;85:531.

 ## Hydatid Cyst (Hydatid Disease)

DESCRIPTION The hydatid is the larval form of *Echinococcus granulosus,* and the cysts represent a thick parasitic membrane that is enveloped in fibrous tissue. The cysts are fluid filled and contain the parasites. The cysts grow slowly over many years and typically involve the kidney (2% incidence with echinococcus), with cases of seminal vesical involvement also reported. Renal cysts may cause pressure and chronic pain but do not affect renal function. They may rupture, causing new "metastatic" cysts. Treatment is by surgical excision. (See also Section III, "Echinococcus—Renal.")

REFERENCE

Perimenis P, Athanasopoulos A, Barbalias G. Unusual echinococcal cyst. *J Urol* 1991;146:1359–1360.

 ## Hydrocalycosis

DESCRIPTION A relatively rare cystic dilation of a major calyx. A calyceal diverticulum is distal to a minor calyx, whereas the hydrocalyx is a dilation of a major calyx. Caused by a congenital anomaly secondary to acquired intriscis obstruction from a parapelvic cyst or crossing vessel. Differential diagnosis included megacalycosis, ureteral obstruction and hydronephrosis, calyceal clubbing due to pyelonephritis or medullary necrosis, renal TB, or calyceal diverticulum. Patients may complain of flank pain, hematuria, or infection.

TREATMENT

- Dismembered pyeloplasty or percutaneous treatment of the narrowed infundibulum.

REFERENCE

Bauer SB. Anomalies of the kidney and ureteropelvic junction. In: Walsh PC, Retik AB, Vaughan ED, Wein AJ, eds. *Campbell's Urology,* 7th ed. Philadelphia: WB Saunders, 1998

 ## Hypercalcemia—Urologic Considerations

DESCRIPTION In urology, generally the result of metastatic lesions to bone, hydrochlorothiazide therapy, hyperparathyroidism, or chronic renal failure. Symptoms include anorexia, weakness, somnolence, polyuria, and coma. May also occur as a paraneoplastic syndrome from renal cell carcinoma. Can lead to hypercalciuria, which can increase chances of urolithiasis

TREATMENT

- Initial therapy involves diuresis by nonthiazide diuretics and IV saline.
- Inorganic phosphate and EDTA may be used for an emergency.
- Mithramycin, steroids, and etidronate disodium have also been used.

REFERENCE

McDougal WS. Perioperative care. In: Gillenwater JY, Grayhack JT, Howards SS, Duckett JW, eds. *Adult and Pediatric Urology,* 3rd ed. St Louis: Mosby, 1996.

 ## Hyperkalemia—Urologic Considerations

DESCRIPTION Hyperkalemia usually occurs in urologic patients as a result of renal insufficiency, addisonian crisis, trauma, shock, and diabetic acidosis. Also can be a consequence of small bowel substitution used in urinary diversion. ECG changes are characteristic, including peaked T waves, long PR interval, long QRS complex, and absent P wave.

TREATMENT

- Calcium gluconate protects against arrhythmias.
- Sodium bicarbonate and glucose/insulin therapy can be used urgently.
- Kayexalate po or pr can be used.
- Dialysis for renal failure

REFERENCE

McDougal WS. Perioperative care. In: Gillenwater JY, Grayhack JT, Howards SS, Duckett JW, eds. *Adult and Pediatric Urology,* 3rd ed. St Louis: Mosby, 1996.

Hypernatremia—Urologic Considerations

 ## Hypernatremia—Urologic Considerations

DESCRIPTION Hypernatremia in the urologic patient can result from dehydration, diabetes insipidus, and sometimes Cushing syndrome and hyperaldosteronism.

TREATMENT
- Hydration when appropriate
- Treatment of underlying cause

REFERENCE

McDougal WS. Perioperative care. In: Gillenwater JY, Grayhack JT, Howards SS, Duckett JW, eds. *Adult and Pediatric Urology,* 3rd ed. St Louis: Mosby, 1996.

 ## Hyperoxaluria—Urologic Considerations

DESCRIPTION Greatest significance is increased urolithiasis. Caused by dietary excess, bowel disorders such as extensive ileal resection, and primary hyperoxaluria. Primary hyperoxaluria can be associated with ESRD secondary to stones and interstitial deposits of calcium oxalate.

TREATMENT
- Dietary restriction of oxalate
- Hydration to increase urine output
- Enteric hyperoxaluria requires intensive dietary and medical intervention.

REFERENCE

Parks JH, Coe FL. Pathogenesis and treatment of calcium stones. *Semin Nephrol* 1996;16(5): 398–411.

 ## Hyperparathyroidism—Urologic Considerations

DESCRIPTION Associated in the MEN1 syndrome. Also increases risk of urolithiasis. Usually exhibits elevated serum and urine calcium with an inappropriately normal or elevated serum PTH level

TREATMENT
- Parathyroidectomy
- Work-up for MEN when appropriate

REFERENCE

Jabbour N, Corvilain J, Fuss M, Kinnaert P, Van Geertruyden J. The natural history of renal stone disease after parathyroidectomy for primary hyperparathyroidism. *Surg Gynecol Obstet* 1991;172(1):25–28.

 ## Hyperspermia

DESCRIPTION A poorly understood and clinically insignificant condition characterized by an excessive volume of ejaculate

REFERENCE

Pavona, N et al. Observation of excessive volume of ejaculate during routine semen analysis: A personal perspective. *J Ejac Technol Urol* 1981;10:24.

 ## Hypocitraturia

DESCRIPTION May develop from distal renal tubular acidosis, chronic diarrhea, thiazide-induced, and gastrocystoplasty. May be idiopathic. Common cause of calcium urolithiasis

TREATMENT
- Correction of acidosis in RTA
- Replacement therapy with potassium citrate

REFERENCE

Bek-Jenson H, Fornander AM, Nilsson MA, Tiselius HG. Is citrate an inhibitor of calcium oxalate crystal growth in high concentrations of urine? *Urol Res* 1996;24(2):67–71.

 ## Hypokalemia—Urologic Considerations

DESCRIPTION Can result from excessive upper gastrointestinal losses, diarrhea, diuretic therapy, steroid administration, and hyperaldosteronism. Metabolic alkalosis is often associated. Other high-renin states, such as renin-secreting tumors, have been reported as a cause.

TREATMENT
- Potassium supplementation either with oral or IV forms
- Correction of underlying defect

REFERENCE

Kuchel O, Horky K, Cantin M, Roy P. Unilateral juxtaglomerular hyperplasia, hyperreninism, and hypokalaemia relieved by nephrectomy. *J Hum Hypertens* 1993;7(1):71–78.

 ## Hyponatremia—Urologic Considerations

DESCRIPTION Many causes exist, but an acute cause in urology is a result of excessive nonelectrolyte irrigant absorption during endourologic procedures. As the fluid is absorbed, volume expansion and dilutional hyponatremia occur. Known as TUR syndrome, nausea, mental confusion, and sensory disturbances are seen, and if allowed to progress, blindness, convulsions, hypotension, coma, oliguria, and death can occur. Other causes include nephrotic syndrome, renal failure, SIADH, adrenal insufficiency, diuretics, RTA, GI losses, and mineralocorticoid insufficiency.

TREATMENT
- Treat the underlying cause.
- For TUR syndrome, diuretics and hypertonic saline with close monitoring

REFERENCE

Rao PN. Fluid absorption during urological endoscopy. *Br J Urol* 1987;60(2):93–99.

 ## Ice Water Test

DESCRIPTION Performed after standard cystometrogram, may aid in differentiation of upper and lower motor neuron lesions. Ice water is rapidly instilled into the bladder and left for 1 minute. If the water is ejected or the bladder pressure rapidly rises, the test is positive. Most patients with upper motor neuron/suprasacral lesions have a positive test (i.e., Parkinson's, MS, CVA). Patients with lower motor neuron lesions almost never have a positive test.

REFERENCE

Webster GD, Kreder KJ. Neurologic evaluation. In: Walsh PC, Retik AB, Vaughan ED, Wein AJ, eds. *Campbell's Urology,* 7th ed. Philadelphia: WB Saunders, 1998:936.

Indiana Pouch

DESCRIPTION A urinary reservoir is created from the right colon, and the ileal cecal apparatus is used a continent catheterizable limb. Originally described by Gilchrist et al. in 1950, the pouch was modified by Rowland and co-workers at the University of Indiana. Modifications included detubularizing the colon with subsequent closure in a Heinecke-Mikulicz configuration, strengthening of the ileocecal valve with imbricating sutures (which were performed on the ileal limb), and a tunneled ureterocolonic anastomosis.

REFERENCE

Benson MC, Olsson CA. Continent urinary diversion. In: Walsh PC, Retik AB, Vaughan ED, Wein AJ, eds. *Campbell's Urology*, 7th ed. Philadelphia: WB Saunders, 1998:3190–3245.

 International Continence Society Classification of Voiding Dysfunction

DESCRIPTION The International Continence Society has proposed a classification based on the functional state of the bladder and urethra. Operates with a "three-by-three" system. Detrusor function is classified as overactive, normal, or underactive. The urethra function is classified as overactive, normal, or incompetent. Sensation is also graded as normal, hypersensitive, and hyposensitive.

REFERENCE

Steers WD, Barrett DM, Wein AJ. Voiding dysfunction: Diagnosis, classification, and management. In: Gillenwater JY, Grayhack JT, Howards SS, Duckett JW, eds. *Adult and Pediatric Urology*, 3rd ed. St Louis: Mosby, 1996.

 International Prostate Symptom Score (IPSS)

DESCRIPTION One of the best known tools for measurement of lower urinary tract symptoms. Important tool, since symptoms are a large source of morbidity for those with voiding difficulties. Also important is the follow-up of treatment for BPH, such as medications and TUR. A tool for selecting patients who require treatment and those who would benefit from treatment. (See also Section III, "AUA Symptom Index.")

REFERENCE

Hakenberg OW, Pinnock CB, Marshall VR. Does evaluation with the International Prostate Symptom Score predict the outcome of transurethral resection of the prostate? *J Urol* 1997;158(1):94–99.

 Inverted Papilloma—Ureter and Renal Pelvis

DESCRIPTION Rare lesions with presentation similar to other upper tract tumors. Considered by most to be benign. Can coexist with malignant tumors, however. Typically small (less than 3 cm), pedunculated, and polypoid. Muscularis invasion is not seen microscopically. Inverting cords and nests of urothelial cells continuous with the urothelium is typical. Male predominance

TREATMENT

• Local excision with close follow-up

REFERENCE

Spevack L, Herschorn S, Srigley J. Inverted papilloma of the upper urinary tract. *J Urol* 1995; 153(4):1202–1204.

 IRS (Intergroup Rhabdomyosarcoma Study) Clinical Classification

DESCRIPTION Classification system used in the Intergroup Rhabdomyosarcoma studies. Generally accepted staging system. See Section II, "Rhabdomyosarcoma—Pediatric (Sarcoma Botryoides)."

• Group I: Localized disease, completely removed, regional nodes not involved

—A: Confined to muscle or organ of origin
—B: Contiguous involvement with infiltration outside the muscle or organ of origin, as this group includes both gross impression of complete removal and microscopic confirmation of complete removal

• Group II

—A: Grossly removed tumor with microscopic residual disease; no evidence of gross residual tumor; no evidence of regional node involvement
—B: Regional disease, completely removed (regional nodes involved and/or extension of tumor into an adjacent organ; no microscopic residual disease)
—C: Regional disease with involved nodes, grossly removed, but with evidence of microscopic residual disease

• Group III: Incomplete removal or biopsy with gross residual disease
• Group IV: Distant metastatic disease present at onset

REFERENCE

Andrassy RJ, et al. Conservative surgical management of vaginal and vulvar pediatric rhabdomyosarcoma: A report from the Intergroup Rhabdomyosarcoma Study III. *J Pediatr Surg* 1995;30;1034.

 Jack Stones

DESCRIPTION Term that refers to irregular, spiculated calcium oxalate stones (which resemble children's jacks) that are sometimes seen in the bladder

REFERENCE

Amis ES, Newhouse JH, eds. *Essentials of Uroradiology*, 1st ed. Boston: Little, Brown, 1991:224.

Jeune Syndrome

 Jeune Syndrome

DESCRIPTION Form of lethal short-limbed dwarfism. Features include constriction of upper thorax and polydactyly. Autosomal recessive inheritance. Of urologic interest, renal dysplasia, sometimes leading to end-stage renal disease, is associated.

SYNONYMS

- Asphyxiating thoracic dysplasia

TREATMENT

- Renal replacement therapy, as needed

REFERENCE

Ring E, Zobel G, Ratschek M, Trop M, Wendler H. Retrospective diagnosis of Jeune's syndrome in two patients with chronic renal failure. *Child Nephrol Urol* 1990;10(2):88–91.

 Juvenile Nephronophthisis

DESCRIPTION Group of four diseases, known as the juvenile nephronophthisis—renal medullary cystic disease complex, that result in ESRD. Characterized by small reniform kidneys with cysts found at the corticomedullary junction. JN is the most common (1 in 50,000 births). Results in ESRD by age 14. Presents as failure to thrive, azotemia, polyuria, and polydipsia. Hypertension is less common. Microscopically, appears to be an interstitial nephritis with cysts. Ultrasound reveals muddling of corticomedullary junction and cysts. Retinitis pigmentosa hepatic fibrosis and Bardet-Biedl syndrome are associated. (See also Section III, "Medullary Cystic Kidney.")

SYNONYMS

- Medullary cystic renal disease

CAUSES

- Autosomal recessive disease mapped to chromosome 2

TREATMENT

- Renal replacement therapy, as needed

REFERENCE

Lippert M. Renal cystic disease. In: Gillenwater JY, Grayhack JT, Howards SS, Duckett JW, eds. *Adult and Pediatric Urology*, 3rd ed. St Louis: Mosby, 1996.

 Juxtaglomerular Cell Tumor—Kidney

DESCRIPTION Rare but important benign renal mass because of secretion of renin. Cause of surgically curable hypertension. Presents with severe diastolic hypertension, hypokalemia, and elevated plasma renin levels. Young, female patient is typical. CT, renal angiography and renal vein sampling may be helpful in localization.

TREATMENT

- Partial nephrectomy or enucleation is treatment of choice

REFERENCE

Remynse LC, Begun FP, Jacobs SC, Lawson RK. Juxtaglomerular cell tumor with elevation of serum erythropoietin. *J Urol* 1989;142(6):1560–1562.

 Kallmann Syndrome

DESCRIPTION Failure of GnRH secretion by the hypothalamus, leading to testicular failure. Cause of male infertility. Cleft palate, renal anomalies, microphallus, cryptorchidism, blindness, and deafness are also associated. Testes are also small. Delayed puberty is often a presenting sign.

SYNONYMS

- Hypogonadotropic hypogonadism with anosmia

CAUSES

- Defect in short arm of X chromosome with variable inheritance and penetrance

TREATMENT

- Androgens can virilize but will not promote spermatogenesis.
- hCG with FSH and LH may help fertility.

REFERENCE

Sigman M, Howards SS. Male infertility. In: Walsh PC, Retik AB, Vaughan ED, Wein AJ, eds. *Campbell's Urology*, 7th ed. Philadelphia: WB Saunders, 1998.

 Kaposi's Sarcoma—Urologic Considerations

DESCRIPTION Tumor of reticuloendothelial system, which presents as a raised, painful papule or ulcer with a bluish hue. Seen in United States most commonly in association with AIDS. Most common site in GU system is the penis, with a much higher incidence in homosexual males. May cause urethral obstruction. (See also Section II, HIV Infection—Urologic Considerations.")

TREATMENT

- Radiation therapy or penectomy (partial or total) aimed at palliation
- Proximal urethrostomy for obstruction not responsive to other treatment

REFERENCE

Angulo JC, Lopez JI, Unda-Urzaiz M, Larrinaga JR, Zubiaur CL, Flores NC. Kaposi's sarcoma of the penis as an initial urological manifestation of AIDS. A report of two cases. *Urol Int* 1991;46(2):235–237.

 Kegel Exercise

DESCRIPTION First described by Arnold Kegel in 1948, can be used as treatment for urinary incontinence. Modern cure/improvement rates range from 50% to 80%. Usually, regimen is multiple contraction of pubococcygeus three or more times a day. Biofeedback, electrical stimulation, and cystometry are adjuncts to the Kegel exercise, which seem to increase efficacy.

REFERENCE

Bump RC, Hurt WG, Fantl JA, Wyman JF. Assessment of Kegel pelvic muscle exercise performance after brief verbal instruction. *Am J Obstet Gynecol* 1991;165(2):322–327.

 Kelly Cystocele Repair

DESCRIPTION The procedure was initially described in 1912 for the repair of a cystocele and not incontinence. Through a midline vaginal incision, the "lateral tissues" were reapproximated with silk or linen with bites of 1.5 cm of tissue.

REFERENCE

Raz S, Stothers L, Chopra A. Vaginal reconstructive surgery for incontinence and prolapse. In: Walsh PC, Retik AB, Vaughan ED, Wein AJ, eds. *Campbell's Urology*, 7th ed. Philadelphia: WB Saunders, 1998:1066–1094.

Kerr's Kinks

DESCRIPTION Kinking of the renal pelvis due to a deformity of the pyelocalyceal system, caused by traction of a strictured infundibulum and parenchymal fibrosis of a tuberculous kidney. Leads to obstruction and dilatation of areas not directly affected by tuberculous ulcerations and eventual pressure atrophy of renal tissue

REFERENCE

Barrie HJ, Kerr WK, Gale GL. The incidence and pathogenesis of tuberculous strictures of the renal pelvis. *J Urol* 1967;98:584.

 ## Kibrick test

DESCRIPTION Test designed to evaluate circulating immune factors, helping to diagnose a cause for infertility. Dilutions of serum from both partners are combined with semen samples in a medium with an agglutinating gelatin. Agglutination will occur if antibodies in the serum are reactive against the sperm. Controls are usually also run with the samples to prevent errors.

REFERENCE

Ainmelk Y, Nemirovsky M, Belisle S, Kandalaft N, McClure D, Elhilali M. Primary infertility: Correlation between sperm migration test and humoral immunity. *Int J Fertil* 1982;27(1):52–55.

 ## Kidney—Metastasis

DESCRIPTION May present as a renal mass and grossly appear as renal primary neoplasm. Discovered most often at autopsy; incidence of about 7% in autopsy series. Frequently asymptomatic, but flank pain, hematuria, or hemorrhage may occur. Common tumors found are lung (bronchogenic carcinoma most common), ovary, bowel, breast, and lymphoma. Virtually any origin is possible.

REFERENCE

Belldegrun A, deKernion JB. Renal tumors. In: Walsh PC, Retik AB, Vaughan ED, Wein AJ, eds. *Campbell's Urology*, 7th ed. Philadelphia: WB Saunders, 1998.

 ## Klinefelter Syndrome

DESCRIPTION Syndrome characterized by small, firm testes, gynecomastia, and elevated urinary gonadotropins; 1 out of 600 male births. Usually presents as incomplete virilization, infertility, or rarely as male pseudohermaphroditism. Mental retardation is associated. FSH is markedly elevated. Azoospermia is seen on sperm analysis. A testicular biopsy usually shows sclerosis of tubules.

CAUSES

• Nondysjunction of meiotic chromosome, resulting in XXY karyotype

TREATMENT

• No treatment can improve spermatogenesis.

REFERENCE

Sigman M, Howards SS. Male infertility. In: Walsh PC, Retik AB, Vaughan ED, Wein AJ, eds. *Campbell's Urology*, 7th ed. Philadelphia: WB Saunders, 1998.

 ## Kocher Maneuver

DESCRIPTION Reflection of the duodenum from right to left, exposing the right renal hilum and vessels

REFERENCE

Kabalin JN. Surgical anatomy of the retroperitoneum, kidneys, and ureter. In: Walsh PC, Retik AB, Vaughan ED, Wein AJ, eds. *Campbell's Urology*, 7th ed. Philadelphia: WB Saunders, 1998:61.

 ## Kock Pouch

DESCRIPTION A continent catheterizable urinary reservoir is created from 70 to 80 cm of small bowel. The mid 45-cm portion is folded into a U-shaped configuration and opened along its antimesenteric border, and the adjoining edges of the U are sutured together. The resulting U patch is folded again from top to bottom to form a reservoir. The 17-cm end limbs are intussuscepted and stapled to create nipple valves at each end. The ureters are anastomosed in the proximal afferent limb, where the nipple prevents reflux and the efferent limb is used to create a continent stoma, which is catheterized to empty the pouch.

REFERENCE

Benson MC, Olsson CA. Continent urinary diversion. In: Walsh PC, Retik AB, Vaughan ED, Wein AJ, eds. *Campbell's Urology*, 7th ed. Philadelphia: WB Saunders, 1998:3190–3245.

 ## Labial Adhesions and Fusion

DESCRIPTION Complete (fusion) or partial adherence of labia minora. Occurs in prepubescent girls and postmenopausal women. Not found at birth but is acquired. Fecal soiling as an infant, vulvovaginitis, eczema, dermatitis, and sexual abuse may be inciting factors. May cause voiding dysfunction in severe cases, with resulting hydroureteronephrosis

SYNONYMS

• Acquired postinflammatory cohesion of the labia minora
• Vulvar fusion
• Synechiae of the vulva

CAUSES

• Low estrogen levels contribute to a thin atrophic lining, which is easily denuded and later heals with adhesions.

TREATMENT

• Conjugated estrogen cream locally applied; surgical treatment for severe cases

REFERENCE

Berkowitz CD, Elvik SL, Logan MK. Labial fusion in prepubescent girls: A marker for sexual abuse? *Am J Obstet Gynecol* 1987;156(1):16–20.

 ## Lactate Dehydrogenase (LDH)—Urologic Considerations

DESCRIPTION LDH is a cellular enzyme useful in monitoring the treatment of germ cell tumors. It tends to have a low specificity (further impaired in smokers), and therefore must be correlated with other clinical findings and lab markers (i.e., alpha-fetoprotein and beta-hCG). There has been correlation with LDH and tumor "bulk."

REFERENCE

Weissbach L, Bussar-Maatz R, Mann K. The value of tumor markers in testicular seminomas. Results of a prospective multicenter study. *Eur Urol* 1997;32(1):16–22.

Lapides Classification of Voiding Dysfunction

 Lapides Classification of Voiding Dysfunction

DESCRIPTION   System for categorizing neurogenic voiding dysfunction into five areas:

• Sensory neurogenic bladder: Interrupted afferent bladder sensation can lead to chronic bladder distension and deterioration. Common processes include diabetes mellitus, tabes dorsalis, and pernicious anemia.
• Motor paralytic bladder: Destruction of parasympathetic motor innervation to the bladder results in painful overdistension initially and inability to initiate and maintain micturition. Common processes include pelvic surgery or trauma and possibly herpes zoster.
• Uninhibited neurogenic bladder: Injury to the corticoregulatory tract of the sacral spinal cord (micturition reflex center) leads to frequency, urgency, and urge incontinence. Common processes include cerebrovascular accident, brain or spinal cord tumor, Parkinson disease, and demyelinating disease.
• Reflex neurogenic bladder: Complete interruption of sensory and motor pathways between the sacral spinal cord and brain stem leads to lack of bladder sensation and inability to voluntarily micturate. Common processes include trauma and transverse myelitis.
• Autonomous neurogenic bladder: Complete motor and sensory separation from the sacral spinal cord leads to inability to voluntarily micturate and lack of reflex bladder activity and bladder sensation.

REFERENCE

Wein AJ. Pathophysiology and categorization of voiding dysfunction. In: Walsh PC, Retik AB, Vaughan ED, Wein AJ, eds. *Campbell's Urology*, 7th ed. Philadelphia: WB Saunders, 1998: 922–923.

 Laurence-Moon-Bardet-Biedl Syndrome

DESCRIPTION   This autosomal recessive disease was initially described in 1860 by Laurence-Moon and received a more exact description in 1920 by Bardet-Biedl. A wide variety of manifestations include retinal pigmentary dystrophy (previously termed *retinitis pigmentosa*), postaxial polydactyly, central obesity, mental retardation, and hypogenitalism. More recently, renal abnormalities have been described, including chronic glomerulonephritis, characteristic cystic tubular disease, lower urinary tract malformations, and defects of tubular concentrating ability. Renal failure is the major cause of morbidity and early mortality. Undescended or maldescended testes can be present neonatally in up to 25% of males.

SYNONYMS

• Bardet-Biedl syndrome: more general, including all of the above description
• Laurence-Moon syndrome: much rarer, differs with the above description, including progressive spastic paraparesis and distal muscle weakness but without polydactyly

REFERENCE

Beales PL, Warner AM, Hitman GA, Thakker R, Flinter FA. Bardet-Biedl syndrome: A molecular and phenotypic study of 18 families. *J Med Genet* 1997;34(2):92–98.

 Lazy Bladder Syndrome (Nurses Bladder)

DESCRIPTION   First described by Swenson in 1962, this condition occurs when children exhibit "holding" behavior and void very infrequently. It is more common in girls. Patients are prone to develop urinary tract infections due to urinary stasis and often have problems with constipation. Some patients have overflow or stress incontinence. The VCUG shows a large smooth-walled bladder, and ultrasound of the upper tract is usually normal. Urodynamic studies show large bladders with decreased sensation during bladder filling, low pressures, and large post-void residuals.

CAUSES

• Continuous voluntary suppression of the normal desire to void

SYNONYMS

• Nurses bladder
• Infrequent voiding syndrome

TREATMENT

• Timed voiding schedules, antibiotic suppression, biofeedback bladder training, intermittent catheterization

REFERENCE

Bauer SB, et al. The unstable bladder of childhood. *Urol Clin North Am* 1980;7:321.

 Leadbetter and Clarke Ureteral Anastomosis

DESCRIPTION   A nonrefluxing anastomosis is created by making a longitudinal incision through the taenia, just outside the mucosa. The ureter is laid over the mucosa and a small button hole is made through the mucosa to anastomose the spatulated end of the ureter. The taenia is closed over the ureter.

REFERENCE

Kay R. Reimplantation of the ureter. In: Novick AC, Streem SB, Pontes JE, eds. *Stewarts Operative Urology*. Baltimore: Williams & Wilkins, 1989:526–538.

 Leadbetter-Politano Ureteroneocystostomy

DESCRIPTION   Through a transvesical exposure, the ureter is mobilized from the bladder wall and surrounding peritoneum. A new ureteral hiatus is created 2 to 3 cm above the old hiatus. The ureter is then delivered behind the entire bladder, through the new hiatus and tunnel submucosally toward the old hiatus, where it is reimplanted.

REFERENCE

Kay R. Reimplantation of the ureter. In: Novick AC, Streem SB, Pontes JE, eds. *Stewarts Operative Urology*. Baltimore: Williams & Wilkins, 1989:526–538.

 Leak Point Pressure (LPP)

DESCRIPTION   The LPP is the pressure required to cause urinary leakage in the absence of a bladder contraction. An LPP of <60 cm H_2O suggests significant intrinsic sphincter deficiency. If the LPP is for 60 to 90, it suggests mild sphincter deficiency. Sphincter deficiency is minimal or absent with an LPP >90 cm H_2O. Performed during cystometric evaluation, the bladder is filled and the standing patient is asked to Valsalva until leakage occurs. The lowest pressure that results in leakage is the LPP.

SYNONYMS

• Valsalva leak point pressure

REFERENCE

Webster GD, Kreder KJ. Neurologic evaluation. In: Walsh PC, Retik AB, Vaughan ED, Wein AJ, eds. *Campbell's Urology*, 7th ed. Philadelphia: WB Saunders, 1998.

 LeBag Neobladder

DESCRIPTION   This is a modification of the Mainz I orthotopic neobladder, which uses only one ileal limb instead of two. The detubularized colon and a single segment of ileum can be joined using metal staplers to create a broad intestinal plate, which is then converted into a pouch with a ureterocolonic and urethral anastomosis.

REFERENCE

Benson MC, Olsson CA. Continent urinary diversion. In: Walsh PC, Retik AB, Vaughan ED, Wein AJ, eds. *Campbell's Urology*, 7th ed. Philadelphia: WB Saunders, 1998:3190–3245.

LeDuc Ureteral Anastomosis

DESCRIPTION   The end of the small bowel segment is opened 4 to 5 cm and a longitudinal incision is made in the mucosa, which is then raised. At the distal end of this incision, a hole is made through the wall. The ureter is pulled through this opening and laid in the mucosal incision. The mucosa is then sutured to the side of the ureter.

REFERENCE

McDougal WS. Use of intestinal segments and urinary diversion. In: Walsh PC, Retik AB, Vaughan ED, Wein AJ, eds. *Campbell's Urology*, 7th ed. Philadelphia: WB Saunders, 1998:3137–3144.

 ## LEOPARD Syndrome

DESCRIPTION   An autosomal dominant condition similar to Noonan syndrome, except for multiple lentigines (macule pigment accumulation of the dermis and epidermis). LEOPARD syndrome is the mnemonic for **l**entigines, **E**CG abnormalities, **o**cular hypertelorism/**o**bstructive cardiomyopathy, **p**ulmonary valve stenosis, **ab**normalities of genitalia in males, **r**etardation of growth, and **d**eafness. Cardiomyopathy is an important feature because it is associated with significant mortality. Genital hypoplasia in males, including a small penis and small, often undescended testicles, is the most common association. Hypospadias and delayed puberty may also be found.

SYNONYMS

- Multiple lentigines syndrome
- Progressive cardiomyopathic lentiginosis

TREATMENT

- Orchiopexy, repair of hypospadias

REFERENCE

Coppin BD, Temple IK. Multiple lentigines syndrome (LEOPARD syndrome or progressive cardiomyopathic lentiginosis). *J Med Genet* 1997; 34(7):582–586.

 ## Leriche Syndrome

DESCRIPTION   Described in 1923 as symptoms characteristic of thrombotic occlusion of the terminal aorta. It is caused by atherosclerosis of the arterial wall, with thrombus and gradual occlusion. Symptoms include fatigue of both lower limbs, symmetrical atrophy of lower extremities, pallor of legs/feet, and inability to maintain a stable erection due to inadequate arterial flow to the penis (hypogastric arterial obstruction). Gradual occlusion allows for collateral circulation; therefore, acute symptoms are unlikely.

SYNONYMS

- Gradual thrombotic obliteration of the abdominal aorta and iliac arteries

TREATMENT

- Bypass graft from aorta to iliac or common femoral arteries

REFERENCE

Krotovsky GS, Turpitko SA, Gerasimov VB, et al. Surgical treatment and prevention of vasculopathic impotence in conjunction with revascularization of the lower extremities in Leriche's syndrome. *J Cardiovasc Surg* 1991;32(3): 340–343.

 ## Lesch-Nyhan Syndrome

DESCRIPTION   First described in 1964 as an X-linked recessive disorder associated with failure to form hypoxanthine phosphoribosyltransferase. Caused by loss of function of the enzyme hypoxanthine–guanine phosphoribosyltransferase (HPRT). Manifestations are hyperuricemia and uric acid lithiasis, choreoathetosis, mental retardation, spastic cerebral palsy, and self-mutilation of fingers and lips by biting.

TREATMENT

- Allopurinol

REFERENCE

Nyhan WL, Wong DF. New approaches to understanding Lesch-Nyhan disease. *N Engl J Med* 1996;334(24):1602–1604.

 ## Leukemia—Urologic Considerations

DESCRIPTION   Leukemic infiltration of the testicle can be seen in children with acute lymphoblastic leukemia. The typical presentation is testicular enlargement, typically bilateral. Open testicular biopsy, bilaterally, should be performed along with bone marrow and CSF analysis for tumor recurrence. Orchiectomy is not indicated for leukemic infiltration. Testes were once a common site of relapse, but with current intensive chemotherapy regimens, the testicular relapse rate is <5%. No strong evidence to suggest increase in birth defects in children of leukemia survivors. Patients treated with cyclophosphamide-containing regimens are at risk for hemorrhagic cystitis and long-term urothelial tumors. See Section II, "Cystitis—Hemorrhagic (Infectious, Noninfectious)."

TREATMENT

- If the testicle is the isolated site of relapse, local irradiation (up to 20 Gy) to both testes and reinstitution of systemic chemotherapy can be curative.
- Therapy can cause irreversible damage to seminiferous tubules and Leydig cells. Patients can develop hypogonadotropic hypogonadism and low testosterone with azospermia.

REFERENCE

Pui CH, Rivera GK. Acute lymphoblastic leukemia. In: Rudolph AM, ed. *Rudolph's Pediatrics,* 19th ed. Norwalk, CT: Appleton & Lange, 1991

 ## Leukoplakia—Penis

DESCRIPTION   Solitary or whitish plaques with hyperkeratosis, parakeratosis, and hypertrophy of the squamous rete pegs, with edema and lymphocytic infiltration. Often involves the penile meatus and has been associated with in situ squamous cell carcinoma and verrucous carcinoma

TREATMENT

- Elimination of chronic irritation
- Circumcision
- Surgical excision with periodic biopsy of incompletely excised lesions

REFERENCE

Bissada NK. Conservative extirpative treatment of cancer of the penis. *Urol Clin North Am* 1992;19(2):283–290.

Lich-Gregoir Ureteral Reimplantation

 Lich-Gregoir Ureteral Reimplantation

DESCRIPTION   This extravesical, less invasive repair does not disrupt the ureteral trigonal continuity. A 4- to 5-cm trough is created by dissecting the detrusor of the mucosa, and the mobilized ureter is placed in the trough with the detrusor closed over it.

REFERENCE

Kay R. Reimplantation of the ureter. In: Novick AC, Streem SB, Pontes JE, eds. *Stewarts Operative Urology.* Baltimore: Williams & Wilkins, 1989:526–538.

 Lichen Nitidus—Penis

DESCRIPTION   Uncommon chronic inflammation appearing as skinflesh-colored papules with sharp demarcation and flat, shiny, and slightly elevated surfaces. Etiology is unknown, but it is believed to be a variant of lichen planus. Histologically, lymphocytes, histiocytes, and melanophages form a ball-like structure covered by epidermis with a characteristic "claw-like" projection of the rete ridges. Usually asymptomatic

TREATMENT

• Spontaneous healing is common.
• Oral histamines
• Topical antipruritics and topical corticosteroids may be helpful.

REFERENCE

Davis DA, Skidmore RA, Woosley JT. Lichen nitidus. *Urology* 1996;47(4):573.

 Lichen Planus—Penis

DESCRIPTION   Uncommon pruritic inflammation of the skin, which typically occurs on the penile glans. Benign and characterized by pruritic, violaceous, and flat-topped papules, and histologically by degeneration of basal cell–layer keratinocytes and dense infiltration of lymphocytes in the upper dermis "hugging" the epidermis. Multiple lesions occur and can ulcerate. Differential diagnoses include secondary syphilis, Bowen disease, psoriasis, Zoon's balanitis, and squamous cell carcinoma.

TREATMENT

• No specific treatment
• Symptomatic relief by antihistamines
• Ataractics, topical lotions

REFERENCE

Varghese M, Kindel S. Pigmentary disorders and inflammatory lesions of the external genitalia. *Urol Clin North Am* 1992;19(1):111–121.

 Lichen Sclerosis et Atrophicus

DESCRIPTION   Uncommon cutaneous disorder with a female predominance. Early lesions are characterized as either white macules, which may coalesce into patches, or flat, white, or pink depressed papules and plaques. Confluence of the papules and marked hyperkeratosis, and atrophy may develop. Extragenital areas (arms, shoulders, trunk, neck, and face) are less commonly affected in men. Dysuria, pruritus, and pain are associated with the disease process. Squamous cell carcinoma has been reported to occur.

SYNONYMS

• Lichen sclerosis
• The late stage evolves into balanitis xerotica obliterans.

TREATMENT

• Circumcision
• Topical treatments for nongenital areas

REFERENCE

Lipscombe TK, Wayte J, Wojnarowska F, Marren P, Luzzi G. A study of clinical and aetiological factors and possible associations of lichen sclerosus in males. *Australas J Dermatol* 1997;38(3):132–136.

 Lichen Simplex Chronicus

DESCRIPTION   Localized chronic pruritus with patches of dermatitis, resulting from chronic scratching/rubbing. Common sites are the perineum, thigh, scrotum, and vulva. Appear as multiple oval plaques that become thickened and scaly. Microscopically, resembles chronic dermatitis with hyperkeratosis and parakeratosis

SYNONYMS

• Circumscribed neurodermatitis

TREATMENT

• Breaking the scratch–itch cycle
• Systemic antipruritics
• Open wet compresses to affected areas

REFERENCE

Weyers W, Weyers I, Bonczkowitz M, Diaz-Cascajo C, Schill WB. Lichen amyloidosus: A consequence of scratching. *J Am Acad Dermatol* 1997;37(6):923–928.

 Lipoma—Bladder

DESCRIPTION   Bladder lipoma is a rare entity. It can be associated with a pelvic lipoma and has been reported to cause bladder outlet obstruction. A capsule circumscribes the homogenous, sharply marginated fat. It is benign and must be distinguished from liposarcoma, angiolipoma, and cystic teratoma, usually by CT scan.

TREATMENT

• Surveillance, unless symptomatic

REFERENCE

Berens BM, Azarvan A. Bladder outlet obstruction due to pelvic lipoma: Computerized tomography, magnetic resonance imaging and radiographic evaluation. *J Urol* 1991;145(1):138–139.

 Lipoma—Spermatic Cord

DESCRIPTION   Benign lobulated preperitoneal fat that can project down the cord. Accounts for up to 90% of spermatic cord tumors and is most commonly seen in adults. Histologic variants include angiolipoma, fibrolipoma, fibromyxolipoma, myxolipoma, and myxoid myolipoma. Can present as a mass and must be distinguished from adenomatoid tumor, leiomyoma, fibroma, liposarcoma, leiomyosarcoma, and fibrosarcoma. (See also Section I, "Spermatic Cord Mass.")

TREATMENT

• Complete excision at time of surgery

REFERENCE

Lioe TF, Biggart JD. Tumours of the spermatic cord and paratesticular tissue. A clinicopathological study. *Br J Urol* 1993;71(5):600–606.

Lipomatosis—Pelvic

DESCRIPTION   First described in 1959 as an overgrowth of fat in the perirectal and perivesical regions that can cause compression of the lower urinary tract and lead to uremia. Rare disease found primarily in men in the third to sixth decades of life. Approximately two-thirds of patients are African American, with an 18:1 male-to-female ratio. Lipomatous tissue is composed of mature adipose and may be associated with inflammation. Histopathologically, it is found to be dense, vascular, unencapsulated lipomatous tissue that commonly envelops the pelvic viscera. It differs from a simple lipoma by the fact that it does not arise from a single focus, is not encapsulated, and does not expand centrifugally. Clinical features vary from urinary frequency to constipation. On a plain abdominal x-ray, it presents with radiolucency of the perivesical areas. On cystography, a full bladder has an abnormal shape (banana shape) and position (superiorly as well as anteriorly). Pelvic lipomatosis has been associated with a higher incidence of hypertension. The cause, however, is not clear.

TREATMENT

• Surgical removal (difficult and feasible in select few patients)
• Supravesical urinary diversion

REFERENCE

Heyns CF. Pelvic lipomatosis: A review of its diagnosis and management. *J Urol* 1991;146(2):267–273.

 Lobar Nephronia

DESCRIPTION   Renal mass caused by acute focal infection without liquefaction. Clinical characteristics most frequently encountered are fever, flank pain, or back pain. Uroradiographic findings in this condition can mimic a renal abscess or neoplasm. Appropriate medical treatment will cause the infected mass to disappear, but scarring may occur. (See also Section II, "Pyelonephritis—Acute.")

SYNONYMS

• Acute lobar nephronia
• Acute focal bacterial nephritis

CAUSES

• Bacterial infection (*E. coli, Klebsiella, Aerobacter aerogenes, Proteus, Pseudomonas,* and *Candida albicans*)

TREATMENT

• Intravenous antibiotics
• Radiologic surveillance: CT scan or ultrasound

REFERENCE

Papanicolaou N, Pfister RC. Acute renal infections. *Radiol Clin North Am* 1996;34(5):965–995.

 Lord Procedure

DESCRIPTION   Described in 1964 as a bloodless operation for the treatment of hydroceles. Transscrotal incision, with the hydrocele being delivered from the scrotum. The testes are extruded and the tunica vaginalis is plicated with no resection of the hydrocele sac. Not suitable for thick-walled or multiloculated hydroceles due to the amount of bundled residual tissue. A Penrose drain is recommended.

REFERENCE

Oesterling JE. Scrotal surgery. In: Glenn JF, ed. *Urologic Surgery,* 4th ed. Philadelphia: JB Lippincott Co, 1991:924–926.

 Lowe Syndrome

DESCRIPTION   Described in 1952 as an X-linked recessive disorder manifested by congenital cataracts, hypotonia, developmental delay, poor growth, and renal tubular dysfunction. Proteinuria and aminoaciduria are present by 1 year, with gradual progression of Fanconi syndrome (typically failure to reabsorb water, electrolytes, bicarbonate, glucose, calcium, phosphorus, and small molecules). Polyuria, metabolic acidosis, hypophosphatemia with rickets, hypercalciuria, and sodium and potassium wasting can occur, and eventually end-stage renal disease. Nephrolithiasis has been reported due to the hypercalciuria.

SYNONYMS

• Oculocerebrorenal syndrome

TREATMENT

• Vitamin D supplements, with ultrasonographic surveillance for nephrolithiasis

REFERENCE

Sliman GA, Winters WD, Shaw DW, Avner ED. Hypercalciuria and nephrocalcinosis in the oculocerebrorenal syndrome. *J Urol* 1995;153(4):1244–1246.

 Lower Urinary Tract Symptoms (LUTS)

DESCRIPTION   Historically, urinary tract symptoms in older men were referred to as "prostatism." Since these symptoms may not be gender-specific, use of this term is no longer recommended. Prostatism also implies that the symptoms have a prostatic origin; however, even in men, the symptoms may not be caused by prostatic disease. Since voiding symptoms are neither pathognomonic for benign prostatic hyperplasia (BPH) nor specifically related to diseases of the prostate, a more accurate expression is the term *lower urinary tract symptoms* (LUTS). Historically, bladder outlet obstruction (BOO), LUTS, and hyperplasia of the prostate have been considered to be almost synonymous; however, an increasing number of studies now demonstrate that the correlations between these parameters are weak and symptoms may originate outside the lower urinary tract (i.e., polyuria as a cause of urinary frequency). Traditionally, LUTS has been divided into obstructive and irritative symptoms. Recently, it has been suggested that these effects are more appropriately termed *voiding symptoms* and *storage symptoms,* respectively.

• Voiding symptoms: weak stream, abdominal straining, hesitancy, intermittency, incomplete bladder emptying, dribbling, and dysuria
• Storage symptoms: frequency, nocturia, urgency, incontinence, and bladder pain

See also Section II, "Bladder Outlet Obstruction" and "Prostate—Benign Hyperplasia."

SYNONYMS

• Prostatism, bladder outlet obstruction

REFERENCE

Jepsen JV, Bruskewitz RC. Office evaluation of men with lower urinary tract symptoms. *Urol Clin North Am* 1998;25(4):545–554.

Lubb Syndrome

 Lubb Syndrome

DESCRIPTION   Very rare, incomplete androgen insensitivity of karyotype XY with testis but ambiguous genitalia. Nonfertile, with elevated testosterone and LH levels. Usually raised as female. (See Section I, "Ambiguous Genitalia.")

SYNONYMS

• Incomplete androgen insensitivity

TREATMENT

• Early gonadectomy and feminizing genitoplasty in infancy

REFERENCE

Snyder HM. Management of ambiguous genitalia in the neonate. In: Snyder NM, ed. *Urologic Surgery in Neonates and Young Infants,* 19th ed. Philadelphia: WB Saunders, 1988:346–348.

 Lymphangiogram—Pedal

DEFINITION   Contrast injection into lymphatic channels on the dorsum of foot to visualize retroperitoneal lymph nodes. Largely replaced by CT scan. Can be used to assess the retroperitoneal lymph nodes in patients with testicular cancer and prostatic cancer. Major advantage over CT scan is detection of architectural changes in nonenlarged lymph nodes. It is time consuming, invasive, does not opacify "sentinel" nodes, cannot differentiate between malignant and nonmalignant changes, and may cause fibrosis of lymph nodes due to reaction to the contrast medium.

REFERENCE

Pollack H. Tumors of the testis and testicular adnexa. In: Pollack H, ed. *Clinical Urography.* Philadelphia: WB Saunders, 1990:1424–1428.

 Lymphangioma—Bladder

DEFINITION   This is a rarely reported bladder lesion that presents with hematuria, and several cases are reported in children. Treatment is by partial cystectomy. This lesion is composed of multiple small cystic cavities filled with proteinaceous material typical of cavernous lymphangiomas.

REFERENCE

Bolkier M, Ginesin Y, Lichtig C, Levin DR. Lymphangioma of bladder *J Urol* 1983;129(5): 1049–1050.

 Lymphangioma—Renal

DESCRIPTION   Rare tumor, with one-third occurring in children and two-thirds in adults. Appears as a solitary encapsulated mass with multiple cysts. Microscopy reveals benign endothelial cells with septa, which may contain smooth muscle. If in the renal sinus, the mass may cause obstruction.

REFERENCE

Bostwick DG. Neoplasms of the kidney. In: Bostwick DG, Eble JN, eds. *Urological Surgical Pathology.* St Louis: Mosby, 1997:110.

 Lymphangioma—Scrotal

DESCRIPTION   Congenital malformations of the intrascrotal lymphatic system, which may form cystic masses. These lymphangiomas are benign tumors, occurring mostly in children. They are found relatively infrequently in the scrotum. Treatment consists of surgical excision. Unless completely removed, recurrences are common.

REFERENCE

MacMillan RW, MacDonald BR, Alpern HD. Scrotal lymphangioma. *Urology* 1984;23(1):79–80.

 Lymphoma—Urologic Considerations

DESCRIPTION   Lymphoma can involve any part of the urinary tract, but is more commonly seen in the testicle and kidney.

• Lymphoma represents a common cause of testicular cancer in older men. It may be a local tumor growth or a late manifestation of widespread disease. Over 50% of testicular tumors in men over 60 are lymphomas. Must be differentiated from seminoma. In adults, most are diffuse, large B-cell lymphomas; children can have Burkitt's lymphoma involving the testicle.
• Bladder involvement is usually secondary to systemic disease and is present in 13% of patients dying of non-Hodgkin's lymphoma. Primary bladder lymphoma occurs almost exclusively in females. Lesions may be sessile or polypoid. Should be differentiated from chronic inflammatory bladder involvement, small cell carcinoma, and a rare entity called lymphoma-like carcinoma
• Prostate lymphoma typically presents in older men, with symptoms of bladder outlet obstruction. PSA rarely elevated. Usually a manifestation of systemic disease, with primary prostate disease rare. Differential diagnosis includes chronic prostatitis with follicular hyperplasia, neuroendocrine prostate cancer, and granulomatous prostatitis.
• Adrenal involvement in up to 25% dying of systemic disease. Rare primary site of disease. Bilateral, clinical, adrenal involvement in 18% of non-Hodgkin's lymphoma and 9% of Hodgkin's lymphoma

TREATMENT

• Testicular lymphomas are usually managed by radical orchiectomy followed by systemic chemotherapy, depending on the extent of the disease. For stage I disease, 5-year survival is >60%; if advanced, survival at 5 years is <20%.
• Bladder lymphoma primary treated with radiation with reasonably good response rates. If bladder site is part of systemic manifestation, systemic therapy is used.
• Prostate lymphoma carries a poor prognosis, regardless of primary site; most die in less than 24 months. Systemic therapy with TUR for obstructive symptoms

REFERENCE

In: Bostwick DG, Eble JN, eds. *Urological Surgical Pathology.* St Louis: Mosby, 1997; 401, 403, 627–629.

 Macro-orchidism

DESCRIPTION   Macro-orchidism (MO) is the increase of the testicular volume, up to 25 mL in the adult male. It is frequently associated with mental retardation (MR) with fragile X-chromosome. MO has also been described in association with bilateral testicular tumors, idiopathic precocious puberty, juvenile hypothyroidism, and, more rarely, with congenital testicular cysts (cystic testicular dysplasia). Management of MO must be conservative in all cases, and testicular biopsy must only be performed to diagnose leukemic infiltration, carcinoma in situ (CIS), or as part of a fertility work-up. Macro-orchidism may be related pathogenically to some hormonal regulation mechanism or to a higher seminiferous tubule sensitivity to FSH.

REFERENCE

Martinez-Garcia F, Regadera-Gonzalez J, Cobo-Nunez P, Martin-Cordova C, Paniagua Gomez-Alvarez R, Nistal Martin de Serrano M. Macro-orchidism: New pathogenetic and histopathologic aspects. *Espanol Urol* 1994;47(1):59–65.

Madsen-Iversen Symptom Score

DESCRIPTION Self-administered questionnaires have been used as an investigational tool for the evaluation of bladder outlet obstruction. Generally replaced by the AUA and IPSS scoring systems. However, this system is still widely reported for ongoing clinical studies and has high correlation with other indices.

REFERENCES

Madsen PO, Iversen P. A point system for selecting operative candidates. In Hinman F Jr, ed. *Benign Prostatic Hypertrophy*. New York, Springer-Verlag, 1983:763.

Barry MJ, Fowler FJ Jr, O'Leary MP, et al. Correlation of the American Urological Association symptom index with self-administered versions of the Madsen-Iversen, Boyarsky, and Maine Medical Assessment Program symptom indexes. *J Urol* 1992;148:1558–1563.

 MAGPI Hypospadias Repair

DESCRIPTION The acronym MAGPI stands for meatal advancement and glanuloplasty procedure. After a circumferential subcoronal incision, the bridge of tissue immediately distal and dorsal to the meatus is split in a vertical fashion and closed in a horizontal orientation (Heineke-Mikulicz closure). The ventral edge of the new meatal opening is pulled up and the glans is reapproximated ventrally, which, in effect, advances the meatus.

REFERENCE

Duckett JW. Hypospadias. In: Walsh PC, Retik AB, Vaughan ED, Wein AJ, eds. *Campbell's Urology*, 7th ed. Philadelphia: WB Saunders, 1998:2093–2119.

 Mainz I Pouch Urinary Diversion

DESCRIPTION An orthotopic pouch is created by opening the cecum and two limbs of distal ileum, and the limbs are sutured to create a broad intestinal plate. After a tunneled ureterocolonic anastomosis is made, the cecal portion of the plate is anastomosed to the male urethral stump and the plate is closed into a sphere.

REFERENCE

Benson MC, Olsson CA. Continent urinary diversion. In: Walsh PC, Retik AB, Vaughan ED, Wein AJ, eds. *Campbell's Urology*, 7th ed. Philadelphia: WB Saunders, 1998:3190–3245.

 Mainz II Pouch Urinary Diversion

DESCRIPTION An augmented valved rectum is created by making a 10- to 12-cm rectosigmoid opening. The sigmoid colon is configured into a U shape, and the medial plate is closed. Ureters are implanted through submucosal tunnels. After securing the apex of the pouch to the sacral promontory, the remaining plate is closed.

REFERENCE

Benson MC, Olsson CA. Continent urinary diversion. In: Walsh PC, Retik AB, Vaughan ED, Wein AJ, eds. *Campbell's Urology*, 7th ed. Philadelphia: WB Saunders, 1998:3190–3245.

 Malacoplakia—Genitourinary

DESCRIPTION Malacoplakia, derived from the Greek term *soft plaque,* is a chronic inflammatory disease, the etiology of which remains obscure. It appears related to an underlying infectious process. It has a very low incidence and affects primarily the genitourinary tract. The diagnosis is made by biopsy. The pathologic specimens typical of malacoplakia consist of large histiocytes known as von Hansemann cells and intracytoplasmic inclusions known as Michaelis-Gutmann bodies. The goal of treatment is stabilizing the disease process by controlling urinary tract infection.

REFERENCE

Long JP Jr. Althausen AF. Malacoplakia: A 25-year experience with a review of the literature. *J Urol* 1989;141(6):1328–1331.

 Marshall-Marchetti-Krantz Cystourethropexy

DESCRIPTION Through a Pfannenstiel incision, the retropubic space is exposed and the urethra, vaginal wall, bladder neck, and bladder are identified. The original description reports placement of a three-paired No. 1 catgut suture to attach the paraurethral anterior vaginal wall to the back of the symphysis pubis, with the most proximal suture being at the bladder neck. Used for the treatment of stress incontinence in women. Now can be performed laparoscopically

REFERENCE

Raz S, Stothers L, Chopra A. Vaginal reconstructive surgery for incontinence and prolapse. In: Walsh PC, Retik AB, Vaughan ED, Wein AJ, eds. *Campbell's Urology*, 7th ed. Philadelphia: WB Saunders, 1998:1066–1094.

 Martius Flap

DESCRIPTION The advancement of the fibro-fatty labial tissue to the vaginal vault for the repair of vesicovaginal fistulas.

REFERENCE

Raz S. Vesicovaginal fistulas. In: *Atlas of Transvaginal Surgery*. Philadelphia: WB Saunders, 1992:1–155.

 Mathieu Hypospadias Repair

DESCRIPTION A ventral flap is mobilized based on the dartos blood supply, and it is transposed over the urethral plate to advance the meatus. The lateral wings of the glans are approximated over the repair.

REFERENCE

Duckett JW. Hypospadias. In: Walsh PC, Retik AB, Vaughan ED, Wein AJ, eds. *Campbell's Urology*, 7th ed. Philadelphia: WB Saunders, 1998:2093–2119.

 Maturation Arrest

DESCRIPTION The term *maturation arrest* has been used to describe testicular biopsies in cases of infertility. Two forms of maturation arrest have been described: spermatogenic arrest and spermatocytic (meiotic) arrest. The arrest is most frequently observed at primary spermatocyte level. Reversible arrest at that level can be due to heat, infections, and hormonal and nutritional factors. Irreversible arrest at primary spermatocyte or spermatid level has a genetic origin due to chromosomal anomalies. Occurs in somatic and germ cells

REFERENCE

Martin-du Pan RC, Campana A. Physiopathology of spermatogenic arrest. *Fertil Steril* 1993; 60(6):937–946.

Mayer-Rokitansky-Kuster-Hauser Syndrome

 Mayer-Rokitansky-Kuster-Hauser Syndrome

DESCRIPTION This eponym refers to congenital absence of the vagina, with some form of abnormal or absent uterus. The diagnosis is usually made when amenorrhea effects a normal pubertal female. Renal and skeletal anomalies are a common association. The defect involves mesodermal development and the mesonephric kidney, the latter resulting in abnormalities in the paramesonephros (uterus and vagina) and in the metanephric kidney.

REFERENCE

Griffin JE, Edwards C, Madden JD, Harrod MJ, Wilson JD. Congenital absence of the vagina. The Mayer-Rokitansky-Kuster-Hauser syndrome. [Review]. *Ann Intern Med* 1976;85(2):224–236.

 Mayo Clinic Grading System for Prostate Cancer

DESCRIPTION Not only does this grading system use assessment of glandular architecture similar to Gleason's, but also histologic criteria. Grading is done on a scale of 1 to 4, with 4 having the worst prognosis. Cellular features, such as cytoplasmic–nuclear–nucleolar morphology, mitotic activity, and tumor invasiveness, are all used to assign grade.

REFERENCE

Kozlowski JM, Grayhack JP. Carcinoma of the prostate. In: Gillenwater JY, Grayhack JT, Howards SS, Duckett JW, eds. *Adult and Pediatric Urology,* 2nd ed. St Louis: Mosby, 1991.

 McCune-Albright Syndrome

DESCRIPTION A syndrome characterized by a classic triad of fibrous dysplasia (cystic bone lesions), precocious puberty, and cutaneous pigmentation. Association with various endocrine abnormalities is common.

SYNONYMS

- Polyostotic fibrous dysplasia
- Osteitis fibroso cystica

TREATMENT

- Hyperthyrodism surgery
- Adrenalectomy

REFERENCE

Giovannelli G, Bernasconi S, Banchini G. McCune-Albright syndrome in a male child: A clinical and endocrinologic enigma. *J Pediatr* 1978;92:220.

 Meatal Stenosis—Urethral, Female

DESCRIPTION Distal urethral (meatal) stenosis is a recognized entity. Females with this condition present clinically with complaints ranging from urinary tract infection to enuresis. Distal urethral stenosis may be associated with the roentgenologic appearance of a prominent, collar-like vesical neck, which reflects generalized detrusor hypertrophy. When treatment is deemed necessary, the distal urethra is calibrated with bougies. (See also Section III, "Urethra—Meatus, Normal Caliber.")

REFERENCE

Perlmutter AD, Colodny A, Harris PD, Gross RE. Urethral meatal stenosis in female children simulating bladder-neck obstruction. *J Pediatr* 1966;69(5):739–743.

 Meatal Stenosis—Urethral, Male

DESCRIPTION Most commonly seen after neonatal circumcision. This acquired condition is theorized to follow a postsurgical inflammatory reaction at the glans, resulting in an extremely narrow meatus. Meatal stenosis is usually not apparent until the child is toilet trained. Strength and/or direction of stream can be effected. Dysuria, frequency, incontinence, and hematuria are symptoms that have been associated with this condition. Meatal stenosis rarely causes obstructive changes in the urinary tract. Meatoplasty is the corrective procedure for those requiring surgical correction. (See also Section III, "Urethra—Meatus, Normal Caliber.")

REFERENCE

Brem J, Jaffee SR. Hidden meatal stenosis in male infants and children. *Am Fam Physician* (GP) 1970;2(2):72–73.

 Meckel-Gruber Syndrome

DESCRIPTION Meckel-Gruber syndrome is a rare lethal autosomal recessive disorder with major characteristic features consisting of the triad occipital encephalocele, polydactyly, and bilateral polycystic kidneys. Prenatal sonographic examination has been demonstrated to be of reliable diagnostic accuracy. For this reason, appropriate prenatal counseling is advocated for those at high risk.

REFERENCE

Sepulveda W, Sebire NJ, Souka A, Snijders RJ, Nicolaides KH. Diagnosis of the Meckel-Gruber syndrome at eleven to fourteen weeks' gestation. *Am J Obstet Gynecol* 1997;176(2):316–319.

 Meckel Syndrome

DESCRIPTION Autosomal recessive syndrome that exhibits encephalocele, polydactyly, and microcephaly. Of urologic interest, renal cystic disease is common.

REFERENCE

Lippert M. Renal cystic disease. In: Gillenwater JY, Grayhack JT, Howards SS, Duckett JW, eds. *Adult and Pediatric Urology,* 3rd ed. St Louis: Mosby, 1996.

 Median Bar

DESCRIPTION *Median bar* refers to prostatic posterior commissural hyperplasia, which is acinar hyperplasia involving the posterior vesical lip, producing a wide bar. Patients suffering enlargement of the middle lobe or posterior commissure are more likely to develop obstructive symptoms, due to the tissue location, which easily obstruct the bladder neck. This explains the correlation between the size of the gland and the degree of obstruction.

REFERENCE

Randall A. *Surgical Pathology of Prostatic Obstruction.* Baltimore: Williams & Wilkins, 1931.

Medullary Cystic Kidney

DESCRIPTION A form of progressive renal disease with up to 75% of cases having medullary cysts, although it is primarily a tubulointerstitial disease. Juvenile nephronophthisis and medullary cystic disease are similar anatomically and clinically, but they have different modes of transmission and different clinical presentations. Juvenile nephronophthisis usually is inherited as an autosomal recessive trait (onset age: 6–20 years), and medullary cystic disease typically is inherited as an autosomal dominant trait and presents after the third decade. Patients present with polyuria and polydipsia due to salt wasting, a concentrating defect, anemia, and profound growth retardation. Juvenile nephronophthisis often is associated with disorders of the retina (i.e., retinitis pigmentosa), skeletal abnormalities, hepatic fibrosis, and Bardet-Biedl syndrome (obesity, mental retardation, polydactyly, retinitis pigmentosa, and hypogenitalism). On ultrasound or CT, the medullary cysts can be seen with parenchyma and may appear hyperechogenic due to tubulointerstitial fibrosis.

SYNONYMS

• Juvenile nephronophthisis, uremic medullary cystic disease, salt-losing enteropathy, and uremic sponge kidney

TREATMENT

• Sodium replacement initially, with dialysis and transplantation later. The graft appears to be resistant to the disease.

REFERENCE

Bernstein J, Gardner KD Jr. Familial juvenile nephronophthisis: Medullary cystic disease. In: Edelman CM Jr, ed. *Pediatric Kidney Disease.* Boston: Little, Brown, 1979:580.

 Megacalycosis

DESCRIPTION A nonobstructive enlargement of the calyces due to a congenital malformation of the renal papillae. There is no dilation of the renal pelvis, and there is no evidence of ureteropelvic junction obstruction. Found almost exclusively in males, it often presents in children due to a UTI work-up or in adults with hematuria and renal calculi. Must differentiate between hydronephrosis and UPV obstruction

TREATMENT

• None necessary. A diuretic renogram fails to demonstrate any obstruction.

REFERENCE

Gittes RF, Talner MB. Congenital magacalyces vs obstructive hydronephrosis. *J Urol* 1972; 108:833.

 Megacystis–Megaureter Syndrome

DESCRIPTION The term *megacystis-megaureter* describes the radiologic appearance of a large-capacity, thin-walled bladder and massive primary vesicoureteral reflux. The pathophysiology of these massively dilated ureters and the large-capacity bladder is the constant recycling of large volumes of refluxed urine. Bladder contractility is normal, even with a poorly developed trigone.

TREATMENT

• Correction of the reflux surgically should lead to a normal voiding pattern. (See also Section II, "Vesicoureteral Reflux—Pediatric.")

REFERENCE

Burbige KA, Lebowitz RL, Colodny AH, Bauer SB, Retik AB. The megacystis-megaureter syndrome. *J Urol* 1984;131(6):1133–1136.

 Melanoma—Adrenal

DESCRIPTION Primary malignant melanoma of the adrenal gland is an established entity. It originates in the adrenal medulla from cells derivative of the neural crest. Because of the high frequency of metastatic involvement of the adrenal by cutaneous and ocular melanomas, diagnosis can be difficult. Primary adrenal melanoma is a highly malignant tumor of middle age that often manifests as a painful flank mass. Distant lymph node metastases can be seen as a presenting sign. Treatment is not effective, with a mortality rate approaching 100% within 2 years.

REFERENCE

Dao AH, Page DL, Reynolds VH, Adkins RB Jr. Primary malignant melanoma of the adrenal gland. A report of two cases and review of the literature *Am Surgeon* 1990;56(4):199–203.

 Melanoma—Genitourinary

DESCRIPTION Malignant melanoma of the genitourinary tract is rarely a primary disease. However, lesions of the penis and urethra can present as primary sites of disease. Secondary melanoma of the GU tract is a common autopsy finding. The majority of patients whose secondary melanoma is discovered clinically die of metastatic disease within 2 years.

REFERENCE

Stein BS, Kendall AR. Malignant melanoma of the genitourinary tract. *J Urol* 1984;132(5): 859–868.

 Mesothelioma—Benign, Testicular Tunic

DESCRIPTION Both a benign papillary and nonpapillary (adenomatoid tumor) variety exists. The nonpapillary tumor is the most common tumor of the epididymis and cord. Both arise from the tunica vaginalis and are usually seen in young men between 20 and 50 years of age The most common clinical presentation is associated with a painless scrotal mass or hydrocele.

REFERENCE

Bostwick DG. Spermatic cord and testicular adnexa. In: Bostwick DG, Eble JN, eds. *Urological Surgical Pathology.* St Louis: Mosby, 1997.

 Mesothelioma—Malignant, Testicular Tunic

DESCRIPTION Mesothelioma is a rare tumor, affecting the serosal surface of pleura, pericardium, peritoneum, and tunica vaginalis (an extension of the peritoneum), which usually presents as an incidental finding at the time of hydrocele surgery. Less than 100 cases have been reported. It most commonly presents between the fifth and seventh decades, although it has been reported in a patient 10 years old. Patients typically present with a hydrocele, but the initial physical examination rarely suggests malignancy. Metastatic spread occurs early via the lymphatic system to the paraaortic, inguinal, and supraclavicular nodes. The tumor spreads less commonly via the bloodstream to the lungs and liver. In the absence of metastatic spread, aggressive local surgery seems to yield the best results. The role of adjuvant chemotherapy and radiotherapy is less clear.

REFERENCE

Eden CG, Bettochi C, Coker CB, Yates-Bell AJ, Pryor JP. Malignant mesothelioma of the tunica vaginalis. *J Urol* 1995;153[3 Pt 2]:1053–1054.

 Metapyrone

DESCRIPTION Cushing syndrome describes the symptom complex caused by excess circulating glucocorticoids. Metapyrone is a blocking agent used to reduce the secretion of functional steroids, thereby lessening the severity of symptoms. Metapyrone blocks the conversion of 11-deoxycortisol to cortisone. The usual dose is 250 to 500 mg three times daily, and does not usually result in salt wasting because of increased production of deoxycorticosterone, a potent mineralocorticoid.

REFERENCE

Scott HW Jr, Orth DN. Hypercortisolism. In: Surgery of the Adrenal Glands. Philadelphia: JB Lippincott Co, 1990.

Meyer-Weigert Law

DESCRIPTION In cases where separate ureteric buds on the same mesonephric duct form a completely duplicated collecting system, separate investigators (Weigert and then Meyer) noted that there exists a consistent relationship between the upper and lower pole orifices as they relate to one another on the trigone. The caudad, or distally placed, orifice actually drains the upper pole moiety; whereas the cranial, or superior, orifice drains the lower pole moiety. The distal orifice is more medial on the trigone, as opposed to the laterally placed cranial orifice. This is a reliable rule for cases of ureteral duplication.

REFERENCE

Schlussel RN, Retik AB. Anomalies of the Ureter. In: Walsh PC, Retik AB, Vaughan ED, Wein AJ, eds. *Campbell's Urology*, 7th ed. Philadelphia: WB Saunders, 1998:1817–1819.

 ## Michaelis-Gutmann Bodies

DESCRIPTION Michaelis-Gutmann bodies are the pathognomic finding in the benign inflammatory process known as malacoplakia. Light microscopy demonstrates a granulomatous inflammatory process, characterized by the accumulation of large mononuclear cells with abundant granular cytoplasm and PAS-positive calcific intracytoplasmic inclusions (so-called Michaelis-Gutmann bodies). On electron microscopy, such inclusions appear as concentric lamellated structures with a mineralized core.

REFERENCE

Lambird PA, Yardley JH. Urinary tract malakoplakia: Report of a fatal case with ultrastructural observations of Michaelis-Gutmann bodies. *Johns Hopkins Med J* 1970;126(1):1–14.

 ## Microlithiasis—Testis

DESCRIPTION Testicular microlithiasis is an uncommon condition characterized by the presence of calcifications within degenerating seminiferous tubules. A review of scrotal sonograms in adults revealed the incidence of bilateral testicular microlithiasis to be 0.6%. While the condition is considered to be benign, microlithiasis has been described in association with various testicular neoplasms. Testicular microlithiasis may be differentiated from tumorous calcifications by a combination of physical examination, tumor marker levels, and ultrasonographic examination. Currently, no particular etiologic relationship has been documented between testicular microlithiasis and testis tumor.

REFERENCE

Miller RL, Wissman R, White S, Ragosin R. Testicular microlithiasis: A benign condition with a malignant association [Review]. *J Clin Ultrasound* 1996;24(4):197–202.

 ## Milk–Alkali Syndrome

DESCRIPTION Hypercalcemia and alkalosis associated with the ingestion of large amounts of milk and antacids containing calcium and absorbable alkali. Patients can develop nephrocalcinosis and renal insufficiency but typically do not have hypercalciuria. The associated vomiting and dehydration can give further volume contraction and alkalosis.

TREATMENT

- Withdrawal of milk and alkali, with gentle hydration to lower serum calcium
- Vigorous hydration can result in rebound hypocalcemia due to the chronic suppression of the parathyroid glands.

REFERENCE

Smith SG. Milk-alkalai syndrome. In: Dambro M, ed. Griffith's 5-Minute Clinical Consult. Philadelphia: Lippincott Williams and Wilkins, 1999, 686.

 ## Mitrofanoff Principle

DESCRIPTION Originally, the author described excising the appendix with a button of cecum, reversing it, and tunneling it to create a catheterizable continent apparatus to be used in continent colonic urinary diversions.

REFERENCE

Benson MC, Olsson CA. Continent urinary diversion. In: Walsh PC, Retik AB, Vaughan ED, Wein AJ, eds. *Campbell's Urology*, 7th ed. Philadelphia: WB Saunders, 1998:3190–3245.

 ## Moskowitz's Vaginal Prolapse Repair

DESCRIPTION Through a transabdominal exposure, the procedure entails closing the cul-de-sac through placement of a series of pursestring sutures. The procedure was initially described to treat rectal prolapse by securing the rectum to the fixed vagina, and the same logic has been used to correct vaginal prolapse by fixing it to the rectum. Unfortunately, the rectum is not well anchored.

REFERENCE

Raz S, Stothers L, Chopra A. Vaginal reconstructive surgery for incontinence and prolapse. In: Walsh PC, Retik AB, Vaughan ED, Wein AJ, eds. *Campbell's Urology*, 7th ed. Philadelphia: WB Saunders, 1998:1066–1094.

 ## Mucormycosis—Genitourinary

DESCRIPTION Fungal infection that usually affects immunocompromised patients. A particular group at risk for disseminated disease is that of patients receiving hemodialysis and deferoxamine. The kidneys are the organs most often involved in the GU system. Penile involvement has also been reported. The course is usually fatal.

CAUSES

- The organism is one of the order Mucorales

TREATMENT

- Amphotericin B systemically; nephrectomy for involved kidney

REFERENCE

Wise GJ, Freyle J. Changing patterns in genitourinary fungal infections. AUA Update Series, Volume XVI, Lesson 1, 1997.

 ## Mulberry Stones

DESCRIPTION A term that refers to the surface appearance of irregular calcium oxalate stones often seen in the bladder

REFERENCE

Amis ES, Newhouse JH, eds. *Essentials of Uroradiology*, 1st ed. Boston: Little-Brown, 1991:224.

Müllerian Duct Remnants and Syndrome

DESCRIPTION Refers to the persistence of the müllerian duct structures (uterus, fallopian tubes) in the genotypically and phenotypically normal male that occurs due to the absence of Müllerian inhibiting substance. Patients present with cryptorchidism and hernia, with the persistent müllerian structures found within the hernia sac.

SYNONYMS

- Prostatic utricular cyst
- Müllerian duct cyst

REFERENCE

Buchloz NP, et al. Persistent Müllerian duct syndrome. *Eur Urol* 1998;34:230–232.

 ## Multilocular Cystic Kidney

DESCRIPTION Rare, less than 200 reported. Cystic tumor that compresses remainder of kidney. Children and adults equally affected. Defined by Boggs and Kimmelsteil in 1956. Criteria include multilocular mass, no communication between cysts or pelvis, epithelial lining, normal contralateral kidney, and absence of nephrons in cyst walls. Can present as abdominal or flank mass, hematuria, or abdominal pain. Can have sarcomas, adenocarcinoma, or Wilms' tumor in the walls of the cysts

SYNONYMS

- Partial or focal polycystic kidney
- Multicystic and cystic adenoma

TREATMENT

- Partial nephrectomy or radical nephrectomy is indicated.
- Follow-up is required because of local recurrence.

REFERENCE

Glassberg KI, Filmer RB. Renal dysplasia, renal hypoplasia, and cystic disease of the kidney. In: Kelalis PP, et al. *Clinical Pediatric Urology,* 3rd ed. Philadelphia: WB Saunders, 1992.

 ## Multiple Endocrine Neoplasia (MEN I, MEN II, and MEN III)

DESCRIPTION Refers to a group of inherited syndromes, with MEN types II and III of urologic interest because of the possibility of adrenal involvement, and type I MEN associated with hyperparathyroidism and renal stones

- MEN I: neuroendocrine parathyroid, pancreas, duodenal, and pituitary lesions
- MEN II: triad consisting of

—Pheochromocytoma
—Medullary carcinoma of the thyroid
—Parathyroid adenoma

SYNONYMS

- Sipple syndrome (MEN II)
- MEN III (IIb)

—Medullary carcinoma of the thyroid
—Pheochromocytoma
—Mucosal neuromas
—Thickened corneal nerves and alimentary tract
—Ganglioneuromatosis
—Marfanoid habitus

- Mucosal neuroma syndrome

REFERENCE

Rave F, Frank K, Meybeingtt P, Ziegler R. Pheochromocytoma in MEN. *Cardiology* 1985; 72[Suppl]:147.

 ## Multiple Myeloma—Urologic Considerations

DESCRIPTION A malignant proliferation of plasma cells derived from a single clone. The cause is unknown. The classic triad involves marrow plasmacytosis, lytic bone lesions, and a serum and/or urine M component. Renal failure occurs in 25% of patients. Hypercalcemia is the most common cause. There may be tubular precipitation of light-chain proteins (myeloma kidney), urinary obstruction due to uric acid or calcium-containing stones, or recurrent pyelonephritis. The development of a myeloma kidney can lead to the adult Fanconi syndrome, which is a type II proximal renal tubular acidosis.

REFERENCE

Alexanian R, Dimopoulos M. The treatment of multiple myeloma. *N Engl J Med* 1994;330:484.

 ## Mustarde Hypospadias Repair

DESCRIPTION A more extensive Mathieu technique in which the ventral flap is tubularized to form a neourethra and then transposed distally. The glans wings are again approximated over the neourethra.

REFERENCE

Duckett JW. Hypospadias. In: Walsh PC, Retik AB, Vaughan ED, Wein AJ, eds. *Campbell's Urology,* 7th ed. Philadelphia: WB Saunders, 1998:2093–2119.

 ## Myoglobin Nephrotoxicity

DESCRIPTION Renal failure associated with the excessive deposit of myoglobin into the serum following massive muscle necrosis. Renal failure is initiated by acute tubular obstruction and necrosis caused by free chelatable iron and ischemia. There are granular casts in the urine. Renal failure is initially manifested by oliguria and followed later by a polyuric state.

TREATMENT

- Should be prevented by maintaining fluid balance, with the use of diuretics, and hydration, with isotonic saline initially
- If renal failure develops, fluid retention should be avoided with limited infusion rates.
- In polyuric states, vigilant replacement of electrolytes is required.

REFERENCE

Abazzi ZA, et al. Acute renal failure complicating muscle crush injury. *Semin Nephrol* 1998;18:558–565.

Myoglobinuria

 Myoglobinuria

DESCRIPTION First described by Fleischer in 1881. *Myoglobinuria* refers to the presence of excessive amounts of myoglobin, a protein found in muscle, in the urine. Myoglobinuria occurs when the serum levels exceed the renal threshold. Myoglobin is released into the serum following massive muscle necrosis, known as rhabdomyolysis, and gives a cola-like color to the urine. Diagnosis is made by electrophoresis separation and radioimmunoassay. Serum creatinine kinase is elevated, and there is an absence of red cells in the urine.

CAUSES

- Ischemia
- Trauma
- Malignant hyperthermia
- Neuroleptic malignant syndrome
- Diabetic acidosis
- Infectious myositis
- Toxins
- Fluid/electrolyte imbalance

TREATMENT

- Remove the causative agent.
- Protect against renal failure by maintaining fluid balance with hydration and diuretics.

REFERENCE

Abazzi ZA, et al. Acute renal failure complicating muscle crush injury. *Semin Nephrol* 1998;18:558–565.

 Myolipoma—Renal

DESCRIPTION Renal angiomyolipoma (AML) is a benign tumor that may occur as an isolated phenomenon or as part of the syndrome associated with tuberous sclerosis. Renal AMLs are often bilateral and are prone to show profuse hemorrhage, large size, and multiplicity. The tumor is named for its three components: blood vessels, clusters of adipocytes, and sheets of smooth muscle. CT is the imaging of choice, and the presence of fat on CT is characteristic for AML. Presentation as incidental CT finding. Large tumors may cause local discomfort or GI symptoms, or patients may have sudden pain or hypotension due to massive hemorrhage within the tumor.

TREATMENT

- Asymptomatic lesions smaller than 4 cm may be observed.
- Growing lesions, large initial lesions, or symptomatic lesions should be treated. Initially, selective arterial embolization may be attempted. If embolization is unsuccessful, or there are multiple lesions that are not all characteristic of AML, or calcification is present, then the patient should undergo exploration and an attempt at conservative surgical excision.

REFERENCE

Steiner MS, Goldman SM, Fishman EK, et al. The natural history of renal angiomyolipoma. *J Urol* 1993;150:1782.

 Nagamatsu Incision

DESCRIPTION A dorsolumbar incision can be made over either the 11th or 12th rib. After rib removal, the diaphragm and pleura are retracted superiorly and the kidney and the adrenal may be exposed.

REFERENCE

Montague DK: Surgical incisions. In: Novick AC, Streem SB, Pontes JE, eds. *Stewarts Operative Urology*. Baltimore: Williams & Wilkins, 1989:15–40.

 Nelson Syndrome

DESCRIPTION Refers to the development of pituitary tumors (usually a chromophobe adenoma) seen in 10% to 20% of patients originally treated with bilateral adrenalectomy for Cushing disease. Felt to be caused by a lack of hypothalamic/pituitary feedback and resultant high levels of ACTH and related compounds. Patients must be followed with ACTH levels and imaging of the sella turcica.

TREATMENT

- Surgical excision
- Radiation therapy
- Prophylactic pituitary radiotherapy (shown to reduce the incidence of Nelson syndrome by 50%)

REFERENCES

Kasperlik-Zalusica AA. Early diagnosis of Nelson syndrome. *J Mol Neurosci* 1996;7(2):87–90.

 Nephritis—Radiation

DESCRIPTION Renal dysfunction occurs if 23 Gy or more of radiation therapy is administered to both kidneys during a period of 5 weeks or less. Histologic examination shows hyalinized glomeruli, atrophic tubules, interstitial fibrosis, and hyalinization of the media of renal arterioles. Radiation-induced renal ischemia causes tubulointerstitial damage, which may take months to manifest. Acute radiation nephritis presents with rapidly progressing azotemia, moderate-to-malignant hypertension, anemia, and proteinuria. More than 50% progress to chronic renal failure. Malignant hypertension may follow unilateral radiation and resolve with nephrectomy. This entity has essentially vanished, due to refinement in radiation therapy techniques.

REFERENCE

Kelly CJ, Neilson EG. Tubulointerstitial diseases. In: Brenner BM, ed. *The Kidney*, 5th ed. Philadelphia: WB Saunders, 1996:1655–1679.

 Nephrogenic Adenoma and Metaplasia

DESCRIPTION A rare lesion occurring in the bladder that histologically resembles primitive renal collecting tubules. It is a metaplastic response of urothelium to trauma, infection, radiation therapy, or chronic immunosuppression. Edema and inflammatory cell infiltration are common, but little nuclear atypia or mitotic activity is demonstrated. It is more common in men and is associated with symptoms of dysuria and urinary frequency.

TREATMENT

- Transurethral resection of the tumor, with extensive fulguration of the tumor base, with frequent follow-up cystoscopies and repeat resection, as needed, to control symptoms

REFERENCE

Navarre RJ Jr, Loening SA, et al. Nephrogenic adenoma: A report of nine cases and review of the literature. *J Urol* 1982;127:775.

Nephropathy—Analgesic

DESCRIPTION   Refers to a chronic interstitial nephritis seen in patients who consume large quantities of analgesics over many years. They usually suffer from chronic headaches or low back pain and have consumed a mixture of analgesics, including acetaminophen, aspirin, and NSAIDs. Their chronic use leads to recurrent papillary necrosis with impaired concentrating ability, sterile pyuria, and renal insufficiency. During periods of acute necrosis, they can have flank pain, pyuria, hematuria, and acute ureteral obstruction from passage of sloughed, necrotic papillary tissue. IVP shows the "ring sign," which refers to the contrast agent surrounding the sloughed papilla. Renal ultrasound shows small kidneys, with irregular thinning of the renal cortex. Renal biopsy shows interstitial infiltrates and fibrosis. The mechanism of injury is felt to be a combination of injury from the production of toxic metabolites and medullary ischemia. These patients have also been found to be at increased risk of developing transitional cell carcinoma of the urinary tract.

TREATMENT

• Cessation of drug use can lead to stabilization of renal function.

REFERENCE

Paller MS. Drug induced nephropathies. *Med Clin North Am* 1990;74:909–917.

 ## Nephropathy—Membranous

DESCRIPTION   Renal disease that manifests with nephrotic syndrome. Affects mainly middle-aged adults and can show either spontaneous remission or progression to end-stage renal disease. Microscopic hematuria is often present. Massive proteinuria, hypertension, and impaired renal function on presentation, and male gender, are all poor prognostic factors. Felt to be related to in situ formation of immune complexes. May be idiopathic or secondary to underlying disease process, such as malignancy, infection, drugs (gold, penicillamine), and systemic lupus erythematosus (SLE). Immunofluorescence often reveals deposits of IgG and complement. (See also Section II, "Nephrotic Syndrome.")

TREATMENT

• May respond to corticosteroids

REFERENCE

Glassock RJ, et al. Primary glomerular diseases. In: Brenner BM, ed. *The Kidney*, 5th ed. Philadelphia: WB Saunders, 1996:1392–1427.

 ## Nephropathy—Minimal Change

DESCRIPTION   Common cause of nephrotic syndrome, most often affecting children. Manifests as the nephrotic syndrome, with massive proteinuria and anasarca without hypertension. There is generally an absence of red or white blood cells in the urine. Histologic evaluation shows essentially no changes on light microscopy. Electron microscopy shows epithelial foot process fusion. The pathogenesis is unknown. (See also Section II, "Nephrotic Syndrome.")

TREATMENT

• Frequently undergoes spontaneous remission and is responsive to corticosteroid therapy; rarely progresses to chronic renal failure

REFERENCE

Glassock RJ, et al. Primary glomerular diseases. In: Brenner BM, ed. *The Kidney*, 5th ed. Philadelphia: WB Saunders, 1996:1392–1427.

 ## Nephropathy—Urate

DESCRIPTION   A disorder in which there is an abrupt deterioration in renal function, due to the renal tubular deposition of urate and uric acid crystals. This occurs almost exclusively in the setting of malignancies, such as leukemias and lymphomas, with rapid cell turnover, leading to increased purine metabolism and loss of nucleotides in the plasma. This is further enhanced by added acceleration of cell lysis, which occurs with chemotherapy and radiation used in these patients. Nucleotides are converted to urate by xanthine oxidase, resulting in hyperuricemia with levels between 25 and 90 mg/dL at the time of onset of renal dysfunction. (See also Section III, "Tumor Lysis Syndrome.") Diagnosis requires the appropriate clinical setting of increased cell lysis (usually with chemotherapy), oliguria, marked hyperuricemia, and hyperuricosuria. A urinary uric acid-to-creatinine ratio greater than 1 distinguishes this from other catabolic states with elevated serum urate levels and renal failure, such as trauma with rhabdomyolysis.

TREATMENT

• Prevention is the key, using xanthine oxidase inhibition with allopurinol and alkaline diuresis prior to initiation of chemotherapy.
• Occasionally, dialysis is required to correct azotemia and reduce urate levels.

REFERENCE

Conger JD. Acute uric acid nephropathy. *Med Clin North Am* 1990;74:859–871.

 ## Nesbit Chordee Repair

DESCRIPTION   One or more transverse ellipses are removed from the longer convex side, and the ellipses are closed transversely, which results in shortening of the longer side.

REFERENCE

Montague DK. Correction of chordee. In: Novick AC, Streem SB, Pontes JE, eds. *Stewarts Operative Urology*. Baltimore: Williams & Wilkins, 1989:822–825.

 ## Neuroendocrine Tumors— Genitourinary

DESCRIPTION   A group of tumors that share a characteristic morphology, often being composed of clusters and trabecular sheets of round "blue cells," granular chromatin, and an attenuated rim of poorly demarcated cytoplasm. Neuroendocrine tumors include carcinoids, small (oat) cell carcinomas, medullary carcinoma of the thyroid, Merkel cell tumor, cutaneous neuroendocrine carcinoma, pancreatic islet cell tumors, and pheochromocytoma. See also Section II, "Pheochromocytoma," and Section III, "Multiple Endocrine Neoplasia (MEN I, MEN II, and MEN III)" and "Prostate Cancer— Small Cell (Neuroendocrine)."

REFERENCE

Segen JC. *Dictionary of Modern Medicine*. Park Ridge, NJ: Parthenon Publishing Group, 1992.

 ## Neurofibromatosis—Urologic Considerations

DESCRIPTION   A hereditary disorder characterized by café-au-lait spots, cutaneous fibromas, and neurofibromas. Associated with renovascular lesions and pheochromocytomas. Vascular lesions are characterized by endothelial proliferation, with or without aneurysmal formation and cellular nodules in the vessel walls. The aorta is frequently involved, and the renal arteries may demonstrate long areas of stenosis that are generally best treated with revascularization rather than angioplasty. In addition, a thirty-fold increase in the incidence of neurofibromatosis in patients with Wilms' tumor has been reported.

REFERENCE

Saborio P, et al. Genetic renal disease. *Current Opinion Pediatrics* 1998;10:174–183.

NMP–22 Testing

 NMP–22 Testing

DESCRIPTION Nuclear matrix protein (NMP-22) has been found to serve as a urinary marker for transitional cell carcinoma. The NMP-22 test (Matritech, Inc., Newton, MA) is a quantitative immunoassay that measures nuclear matrix protein (NMP-22). In a multi-institutional trial, evaluating the role of NMP-22 as a predicator of the subsequent disease status of patients who had undergone TUR for bladder tumor, reports suggest a negative predictive value of 86% and a sensitivity of 100% in detecting invasive malignant tumor, with an overall sensitivity of 72%. The results of this study suggested that NMP-22 might be a helpful adjunct to cytology and cystoscopy in following up patients after TUR.

REFERENCES

Stampfer DS, et al. Evaluation of NMP22 in the detection of transitional cell carcinoma of the bladder. *J Urol* 1998;159:394–398.

Soloway MS, Briggman V, Carpinito GA, et al. Use of a new tumor marker, urinary NMP22, in the detection of occult or rapidly recurring transitional cell carcinoma of the urinary tract following surgical treatment. *J Urol* 1996;156: 363–367.

 Nocturnal Penile Tumescence Testing

DESCRIPTION *Nocturnal penile tumescence* refers to a recurring cycle of penile erections associated with rapid eye movement sleep. The primary goal of NPT testing is to distinguish between psychogenic and organic causes of impotence. Nocturnal monitoring devices measure the number of erectile episodes, maximal penile rigidity, tumescence, and duration of erections. This testing assumes that the mechanism for nocturnal erections is the same as that for erotically induced erections.

REFERENCE

Lue TF. Physiologe of penile erection. In: Walsh PC, Retik AB, Vaughan ED, Wein AJ, eds. *Campbell's Urology*, 7th ed. Philadelphia: WB Saunders, 1998:1186.

 Nonseminomatous Germ Cell Tumors

DESCRIPTION Nonseminomatous germ cell tumors include embryonal, teratoma, choriocarcinoma, and mixed tumors. Embryonal tumor (20% of germ cell tumors) has an adult variant and an infantile variant (yolk sac tumor), which is the most common testicular tumor in infants and children. The tumor marker alphafetoprotein is found in 70% of those tumors. Teratoma (5% of germ cell tumors) contains more than one germ cell layer in various stages of maturation. Pure choriocarcinoma is rare (less than 1% of germ cell tumors) and usually behaves in an aggressive fashion. The mixed-cell type accounts for 40% of germ cell tumors. Except for choriocarcinoma, which has early hematogenous spread, germ cell tumors spread in a stepwise lymphatic fashion. A classic presentation would be a painless enlargement of the testis. Approximately 10% of the patients would be asymptomatic, and 10% would present with symptoms of metastasis, back pain being the most common. hCG tumor marker should be found in 100% of choriocarcinoma cases, with a lesser incidence of the other types. Scrotal US is an essential part of the diagnostic work-up. If diagnosis is made, chest x-ray or CT should be used to rule out metastasis. Testicular cancers are misdiagnosed in approximately 25% of cases as epididymoorchitis, with hydrocele being the second most common misdiagnosis.

CAUSES

- None identified; suggestion of occasional familial clustering

TREATMENT

- See individual tumors in Section II.

REFERENCE

Mostofi FK. Testicular tumors: Epidemiologic, etiologic and pathologic features. *Cancer* 1973;32:1186.

 Noonan Syndrome

DESCRIPTION This syndrome consists of multiple congenital anomalies, including characteristic facial features, short stature, and chest deformity. Over half the males with Noonan syndrome have unilateral or bilateral cryptorchidism. Females can have delayed sexual maturation, but normal development is expected. Renal anomalies occur in 10% of children. Because congenital cardiac anomalies are found in half of the patients, all patients with this syndrome should have cardiac evaluation and close follow-up.

CAUSES

- Autosomal dominance

TREATMENT

- Growth hormone replacement may have value in treating short stature.

REFERENCE

Noonan JA. An update and review for the primary pediatrician. *Pediatrics* 1997;33:549

 Nutcracker Syndrome

DESCRIPTION This syndrome occurs secondary to compression of the left renal vein by the superior mesenteric artery and the aorta. Patients are usually young and previously healthy. Presentation classically is due to gross hematuria caused by left renal vein hypertension.

TREATMENT

- Various modalities, including nephrectomy, autotransplantation, renocaval reimplantation, venolysis
- Gore-Tex graft renal vein interposition and anterior nephropexy have been successful.

REFERENCE

Kim SH, Cho SW, Kim HD, Chung JW, Park JH, Han MC. Nutcracker syndrome: Diagnosis with Doppler US. R*adiology* 1996;198:93.

 Oligospermia

DESCRIPTION One of the components of a basic semen analysis is sperm count. Oligospermia occurs when sperm density is less than 20 million sperm per milliliter or a total count of less than 50 million sperm. Severe oligospermia occurs if counts are less than 10 million per milliliter, and may be due to hormone deficiency. Less than 20 million sperm per milliliter is associated with substantially decreased fertility rates. (See also Section I, "Infertility," and Section III, "Semen Analysis—Abnormal" and "Semen Analysis.")

REFERENCE

Sigman M, Howards SS. Male infertility. In: Walsh PC, Retik AB, Vaughan ED, Wein AJ, eds. *Campbell's Urology*, 7th ed. Philadelphia: WB Saunders, 1998:1299.

Omphalocele

DESCRIPTION This disorder is due to a defect in the umbilical ring, through which the peritoneum and an amnion-covered sac herniate. The incidence is 1 in 3200 to 10,000 live births. In more than half of the cases, multisystemic disorders are also present.

TREATMENT

• Small- to medium-sized defects can be closed primarily.
• Treatment options for difficult-to-treat giant omphaloceles include conservative therapy or Silastic chimneys.
• Conservative therapy allows epithelization of the omphalocele to occur, followed by repair of the residual ventral hernia.

REFERENCE

Nunchtern JG, Baxter R, Hatch El Jr. Non-operative initial management versus Silon chimney for treatment of giant omphalocele. *J Pediatr Surg* 1995;30:771.

 ## Opitz-Frias Syndrome

DESCRIPTION This condition is due to a defect of midline development, characterized by numerous congenital abnormalities, especially of the face. Many have hypertelorism and posterior rotated ears. Hypospadias is almost always present. Other manifestations include cleft lip and palate, high tracheal bifurcation, duodenal stricture, imperforate anus, lung hypoplasia, and cardiac abnormalities. Carriers show minimal abnormalities. It is more common in males. Perinatal mortality is around 30%.

SYNONYMS

• G syndrome (represents the family name of the original patients described.)

CAUSES

• Inheritance is autosomal dominant with incomplete penetrance.

REFERENCE

Conlon BJ, O'Dwyer TH. The G syndrome, Opitz oculo-genital-laryngeal syndrome, Opitz BBB/G syndrome, Opitz-Frias syndrome. *J Laryngol Otol* 1995;109(3):244–246.

 ## Orchitis—Granulomatous

DESCRIPTION This condition encompasses a group of disorders that have similar clinical and pathologic findings. It is usually of sudden clinical onset during the sixth or seventh decade of life. The patient may complain of a painful and swollen scrotum. Occasionally fever and/or skin changes may be present. Often, the diagnosis is rendered postoperatively after inguinal orchiectomy is performed for presumed malignancy and histology shows chronic inflammation with granuloma.

CAUSES

• The most common cause is from *Mycobacterium tuberculosis*.
• Brucellosis, actinomycosis, and sarcoidosis

TREATMENT

• If tuberculosis is suspected, antitubercular chemotherapy is warranted, with operative treatment for medical failures.
• For other causes, medical and/or surgical therapy can be utilized.

REFERENCE

Kahn IK, McAninch JW. Granulomatous diseases of the testis. *J Urol* 1980;123:868.

 ## Ormond Disease

DESCRIPTION Ormond disease is primary retroperitoneal fibrosis caused by a chronic inflammatory condition of unknown etiology. It may be unilateral or bilateral and is most common in men. It is primarily seen in adults, but children have been afflicted. Unilateral or bilateral ureteral obstruction can occur due to retroperitoneal fibrosis. (See also Section II, "Retroperitoneal Fibrosis.")

SYNONYMS

• Retroperitoneal fibrosis

TREATMENT

• Surgery is the main treatment. The ureters are mobilized away from the inflammatory process and intraperitonealized.
• Recently, laparoscopic treatment successes have been reported.

REFERENCE

Boeckmann W, Wolff JM, Adam G, Effert P, Jakse G. Laparoscopic bilateral ureterolysis in Ormond's disease. *Urol Int* 1996;56:133.

 ## Orofaciodigital Syndrome

DESCRIPTION These are a group of at least seven disorders characterized by oral, facial, and digital malformations. Abnormalities that may occur include median clefts of the upper lip, atypical cleft palates, epicanthal folds, forehead anomalies, and syndactyly. Many of these patients have mental retardation. Polycystic kidney disease is also associated with this syndrome. Hair and cutaneous anomalies suggest type I. Bilateral duplication of the great toes suggests type II.

CAUSES

• Type I is sporadic or X-linked. The remaining are autosomal recessive.

TREATMENT

• Surgical treatment of the individual facial and oral abnormalities, as needed
• Type I, because of its inheritance pattern, is usually lethal in males, and genetic counseling is warranted.
• If renal cysts are present, kidney function should be followed.

REFERENCE

Feather SA, Woolf AS, Donnai D, Malcolm S, Winter RM. The oral-facial-digital syndrome type 1 (OFD1), a cause of polycystic kidney disease and associated malformations, maps to Xp22.2-Xp22.3. *Hum Mol Genet* 1997;6:1163.

 ## Ossifying Renal Tumor of Infancy

DESCRIPTION Rare, calcified tumor in infancy, usually resembling a renal pelvis calculus. Occurs usually in first year of life. Gross hematuria is the most common presenting symptom. Anatomic and histologic origins are unclear but are thought to be of urothelial origin. Lesions are apparently benign, with no reported cases of recurrence or metastasis.

TREATMENT

• Surgical enucleation with renal-sparing procedure
• Careful follow-up with renal sonograms, as necessary

REFERENCE

Steffens J, et al. Ossifying renal tumor of infancy. *J Urol* 1993;149(5):1080–1081.

Ovarian Remnant Syndrome

 ## Ovarian Remnant Syndrome

DESCRIPTION This condition is a rare complication of bilateral oophorectomy and occurs when remnants of ovarian cortex are inadvertently left behind. The remaining ovarian tissue becomes functional and cystic. Typically, patients present with pelvic pain that can be chronic or intermittent. Symptoms may begin weeks to 5 years postoperatively.

TREATMENT

- Hormonal manipulation can be used as treatment.
- Excision of the ovarian remnant is the most widely accepted treatment method.
- Surgery is associated with an 8% to 10% recurrence rate.

REFERENCE

Lafferty HW, Angioli RA, Rudolph J, Penalver MA. Ovarian remnant syndrome: Experience at the Jackson Memorial Hospital, University of Miami, 1985 through 1993. *Am J Obstet Gynecol* 1996;174:641.

 ## Ovarian Vein Syndrome

DESCRIPTION Ureteral obstruction, usually right-sided, occurring secondary to occlusion by ovarian veins. The ovarian veins lie adjacent to the ureters, and dilation of these veins, especially during pregnancy, is thought to result in ureteral obstruction. The obstruction is usually seen around the third or fourth lumbar vertebrae. Symptoms include chronic flank pain, but colicky pain has also been found. The symptoms can also begin several days prior to menses and then regress. Diagnosis can be made by intravenous urogram, retrograde ureteropyelogram, and simultaneous angiography.

TREATMENT

- Ureteral stent placement or surgical mobilization of the ureter and ligation of the offending vein

REFERENCE

Resnick MI, Krush ED. In: Walsh PC, Retik AB, Vaughan ED, Wein AJ, eds. *Campbell's Urology*, 7th ed. Philadelphia: WB Saunders, 1998: 392–393.

 ## Oxylate-Associated Renal Disease

DESCRIPTION Hyperoxaluria is associated with calcium oxalate nephrolithiasis. An increased oxalate production, absorption, or idiopathic form might be responsible for the disease. In case of primary hyperoxaluria, stone formation usually starts during childhood, with eventual tubulointerstitial nephropathy and chronic renal failure. Oxalate deposition in heart, joints, and other tissues (oxalosis) may occur.

CAUSES

- Increased oxalate production
- Primary hyperoxaluria type I, due to defect of the enzyme alanine–glyoxylate amino transferase (AGT) in the liver
- Primary hyperoxaluria type II, due to deficiency of the hepatic enzymes D-glycerate dehydrogenase and glyoxylate reductase
- Increased hepatic conversion, due to pyridoxine deficiency, type I glycol ingestion, and methoxy flurane anesthesia
- Enteric hyperoxaluria
- Malabsorption from any cause
- Idiopathic

TREATMENT

- Pyridoxine supplements (200–400 mg/d) for primary hyperoxaluria
- Oral hydration; low-oxalate, low-fat diet for enteric hyperoxaluria
- Pyridoxine and thiazides for idiopathic hyperoxaluria

REFERENCES

Danpure CJ. Molecular and cell biology of primary hyperoxaluria type I. *Clin Invest Med* 1994;72:725.

Scheinman JI. Primary hyperoxaluria: Therapeutic strategies for the 90's. *Kidney Int* 1991;40: 389–399.

 ## *p53*—Urologic Considerations

DESCRIPTION The *p53* gene produces a nuclear phosphorylation protein, which has a tumor suppression function. Loss of wild-type *p53* is the most common genetic abnormality associated with transitional cell carcinoma. Its presence is associated with high grade, late stage, and relapse. Potentially, it may be useful in grading tumors. In prostate cancer, *p53* is associated with increased probability of biochemical relapse and is in a higher percentage of hormone refractory cancers.

REFERENCE

Minimo C, Tawfiek ER, Bagley D, McCue PA, Bibbo M. Grading of upper urinary tract transitional cell carcinoma by computed DNA content and p53 expression. *Urology* 1997;50:869.

 ## Pad Testing

DESCRIPTION Use as a clinical tool to assess the severity of urinary incontinence, often in association with micturition diary. The pad test provides a gross/semi-quantitative measurement of urine loss over a given period of time. Several types have been described, but none has met with widespread approval. One technique has a patient take Pyridium 200 mg tid and then change pads every 6 hours for a 24-hour period. The amount of staining is an estimate of incontinence. Another approach is to weigh the pads (1 g = 1 mL urine).

REFERENCE

Ryhammer AM, Djurhuus JC, Laurberg S. Pad testing in incontinent women: A review. *Int Urogynecol J Pelvic Floor Dysfunct* 1999; 10(2):111–115.

 ## Pagano Ureteral Anastomosis

DESCRIPTION A 4- to 5-cm linear incision is made through the taenia of the colon, and the mucosa is dissected from the submucosa to the level of the mesentery. The ureters are pulled through the lateral muscular wall and implanted distally into the mucosa. The serosa is reapproximated while incorporating mucosa in the midline.

REFERENCE

McDougal WS. Use of intestinal segments and urinary diversion. In: Walsh PC, Retik AB, Vaughan ED, Wein AJ, eds. *Campbell's Urology*, 7th ed. Philadelphia: WB Saunders, 1998:3137–3144.

Page Kidney

DESCRIPTION This condition was first described in 1939, after hypertension was created by wrapping cellophane around a canine kidney. Applied clinically, this term was given to hypertension that is secondary to subcapsular or perirenal compression resulting in renal ischemia. Elevated renin secretion from the compromised kidney and decreased renin production from the contralateral renal unit result. Diagnosis can be made with US, CT, or MRI, demonstrating a surrounding hematoma or fibrous capsule.

CAUSES

- Blunt trauma
- Closed renal biopsy
- Anticoagulation or tumor bleed

TREATMENT

- Observation
- ACE inhibitor therapy
- Open or percutaneous drainage or nephrectomy
- Spontaneous resolution can occur secondary to reabsorption of the hematoma.

REFERENCE

Vaughan ED, Sosa RE. Renovascular hypertension and other renal vascular disease. In: Walsh PC, Retik AB, Vaughan ED, Wein AJ, eds. *Campbell's Urology*, 7th ed. Philadelphia: WB Saunders, 1998:451–452.

 ## Paget Disease—Anogenital/Extramammary

DESCRIPTION Extramammary Paget disease is an adenocarcinoma of the epidermis that can exist in numerous areas, including the penis, scrotum, bladder, vulva, perianal area, umbilicus, axilla, and conjunctiva. An underlying adnexal neoplasm is associated half the time. An increased risk of other malignancies is present. Generally considered an adenocarcinoma that occurs in apocrine gland areas of the body. Mammary type originates from lactiferous ducts and extends into epidermis. Anogenital type usually slow growing and resembles dermatitis clinically and rarely involves the penile or scrotal skin. Often associated with underlying carcinoma such as bladder cancer, prostate cancer and urethral cancer. Typically presents in the 60s or 70s with lesions that are crusted, indurated, erythematous to whitish patches. Histologically, the intraepithelial neoplastic cells contain mucin and are PAS positive. Differential diagnosis includes squamous cell carcinoma in situ and malignant melanoma.

SYNONYMS

- Extramammary Paget disease
- Anogenital Paget disease

CAUSES

- Originates from pluripotent cells in epidermis that formed apocrine glands
- May also result from extracutaneous adenocarcinoma that spread into the epidermis

TREATMENT

- Excision of skin lesion and evaluation for underlying malignancy

REFERENCE

Balducci L, Crawford ED, Smith GF, Lambuth B, McGehee R, Hardy C. Extramammary Paget's disease: An annotated review. *Cancer Invest* 1988;6:293.

 ## Paget Disease—Bone

DESCRIPTION This condition affects up 10% of elderly individuals with a 3:1 male-to-female ratio. Bone pain is the most common presenting symptom. Paget disease of the spine may also be a cause of low back pain. The disorder is due to increased bone remodeling, bone hypertrophy, and bone deformity of uncertain origin. Paget disease is characterized by an initial phase of intense osteoclastic resorption, followed by an increase in bone formation, but the new skeletal tissues are deformed and prone to inducing pain and fracture. Approximately one-third of Paget disease cases have monostotic disease, with pelvic involvement in 72%. In these cases, the lumbar spine is involved in 58%, the thoracic spine in 45%, and the femur and skull in 55% and 42%, respectively. Patients' elevated alkaline phosphatase or bone pain may be due to Paget disease or other diseases, such as liver disease, renal disease, or metastatic prostate cancer. Radiographically, the localized enlargement of bone is a characteristic feature. Areas of lysis due to osteoclastic reabsorption can also be present. Can be confused with metastatic prostate cancer to bone. Suspect Paget disease over metastatic prostate cancer when there is widening of the bone, thickening of the cortex, and a prominent trabecular pattern.

SYNONYMS

- Osteitis deformans

TREATMENT

- Pain reduction and decreasing long-term complications are the main goals.
- Inhibitors of osteoclastic bone resorption, such as calcitonin (salmon calcitonin for nasal administration), plicamycin, and etidronate, as well as biphosphonates, are used to decrease the rate of bone remodeling.

REFERENCE

Delmas PD, Meunier PJ. The management of Paget's diseases of bone. *N Engl J Med* 1997;336:558.

 ## Paneth Cell–like Change—Prostate

DESCRIPTION Describes observation of prostatic glandular epithelium with distinct eosinophilic intracytoplasmic granules resembling Paneth cells, found in crypts of Lieberkühn in the small intestine. These cells are thought to represent a morphologic similarity to Paneth cells, rather than true Paneth cell metaplasia of the prostatic epithelium, due to presence of PSA and PAP on immunohistochemistry. Have been described in normal, hyperplastic, dysplastic, and malignant prostate tissue. Must be differentiated from other prostatic intracytoplasmic inclusions, including secretory vacuoles, melanin, CMV viral inclusions, or "virus-like" particles

REFERENCE

Weaver MG, et al. Paneth cell-like change of the prostate gland. *Am J Surg Pathol* 1992;16(1):62–68.

 ## Papillary Adenoma of the Prostatic Utricle

DESCRIPTION The prostatic utricle is a 6-mm-thin orifice found in the verumontanum. Its origin is as a müllerian remnant that projects back into the substance of the prostate. Papillary adenocarcinoma of the prostatic utricle is a rare malignancy with metastatic potential. Histologically, these tumors are composed of tall columnar cells with clear to eosinophilic cytoplasm with large nucleoli. The cells form glands with scant intervening stroma.

SYNONYMS

- Endometrial carcinoma of the prostate (because these tumors histologically resemble endometrial carcinoma)

TREATMENT

- Transurethral resection, radiotherapy, radical prostatectomy, or a combination of these has been utilized.
- Some advocate not using estrogen or castration, given the histologic resemblance to endometrial carcinoma.

REFERENCE

Merchant RF Jr, Graham AR, Bucher WC, Parker AC. Endometrial carcinoma of the prostatic utricle with osseous metastases. *Urology* 1976; 8:169.

Papillary Cystadenoma of the Epididymis

 Papillary Cystadenoma of the Epididymis

DESCRIPTION This is a rare, benign neoplasm that may be unilateral or bilateral. Patients often present with infertility. Histologically, they appear as papillary projections of clear cells that resemble clear cell renal carcinoma.

CAUSES

• Tumors are thought to arise from efferent duct epithelium.
• Because it is associated with von Hipple-Lindau (VHL) disease, evaluation for VHL should be performed in patients with this epididymal tumor.

TREATMENT

• No treatment is warranted, given its benign nature.

REFERENCE

Billesbolle P, Nielsen K. Papillary cystadenoma of the epididymis. *J Urol* 1988;139:1062.

 Papilloma—Bladder

DESCRIPTION A controversial diagnostic entity of the urinary bladder. The papillary lesion is small and unifocal, with a delicate fibrovascular stalk, and covered in cytologically and architecturally normal urothelium. Typically found in a younger age group than is bladder cancer. Recurrences are common, and future development of invasive urothelial tumors of the urinary tract occurs in <10%. Many consider the lesion to be a very low grade bladder cancer (grade I TCC) with limited potential to progress.

SYNONYMS

• WHO grade I papillary urothelial carcinoma
• Urothelial papilloma

TREATMENT

• Transurethral surgical resection is the main modality.
• These patients need to be followed closely, due to the increased risk of having a urothelial malignancy.
• No defined role for intravesical therapy

REFERENCE

Jordan, AM, et al. Transitional cell neoplasms of the urinary bladder: Can biologic potential be predicted based on histologic grading? *Cancer* 1987;60:2766–2774.

 Paquin Ureteral Reimplantation

DESCRIPTION Repair is done with a combined extravesical ureteral mobilization and intravesical implantation. A submucosal plane is developed towards the trigone with tenotomy succors, and the freshly spatulated ureter is reimplanted.

REFERENCE

Atala A, Keating MA. Vesicoureteral reflux and megaureter. In: Walsh PC, Retik AB, Vaughan ED, Wein AJ, eds. *Campbell's Urology*, 7th ed. Philadelphia: WB Saunders, 1998:1882–1896.

 Paraffinoma—Penile

DESCRIPTION Foreign-body reaction resulting from injection of paraffin, Vaseline, or other foreign-body material into penile shaft, in attempt to increase penile girth. Usually performed by patient or untrained person practicing medicine fraudulently. Complications usually occur, including penile deformity, skin necrosis, erectile dysfunction, and painful intercourse.

SYNONYMS

• Sclerosing lipogranuloma

TREATMENT

• Complete excision of affected skin and subcutaneous tissue
• Skin graft coverage (full-thickness or split-thickness skin graft)
• Flap coverage (usually scrotal) required if skin graft does not take

REFERENCE

Jeong JH, et al. A new repair for penile paraffinoma: Bilateral scrotal flaps. *Ann Plast Surg* 1996;37(4):386–393.

 Partin Tables

DESCRIPTION Nomograms for patients with biopsy-proven prostate cancer, developed by Alan Partin, incorporating PSA, TNM stage, and Gleason score, to predict rate of lymph node and distant spread. Used to predict whether patients have organ-confined cancer, and to allow more accurate treatment decisions. (See Partin Tables in the appendix.)

REFERENCE

Partin AW, et al. Combination of prostate-specific antigen, clinical stage, and Gleason score to predict pathologic stage of localized prostate cancer: A multi-institutional update. *JAMA* 1997;277(18):1445–1451.

 Patau Syndrome

DESCRIPTION This rare syndrome is associated with trisomy 13 and has a median survival of 3 months. The incidence is 1 in 6000 live births and is associated with multiple cardiac, neurologic, and renal abnormalities. Renal anomalies occur in about 80% of children. Unilateral renal agenesis, renal duplication, hydronephrosis, and polycystic kidneys have been associated with Patau syndrome.

REFERENCE

Martlew RA, Sharples A. Anesthesia in a child with Patau's syndrome. *Anesthesia* 1995;50:980.

 Pearly Papules of Penis

DESCRIPTION These are normal anatomic structures located on the proximal glans penis or corona. They appear as minute, dome-shaped, flesh-colored papules. The incidence is between 19% and 30%. These lesions are asymptomatic and can be confused with genital warts. Histologically, these papules are angiofibromas.

SYNONYMS

• Pearly penile papules

TREATMENT

• None needed

REFERENCE

Rehbein HM. Pearly penile papules: Incidence. *Cutis* 1977;19:54.

Pediculosis Pubis (Crab Lice)

DESCRIPTION Ectoparasitic infection, marked by severe pruritis and tending to have an incubation period of approximately 4 weeks. Signs include observation of the lice, 1- to 2-mm-long gray-brown organisms, on the skin or on the hair shafts.

CAUSES

- *Phthirus pubis*

TREATMENT

- Lindane 1% shampoo applied for 4 minutes and washed off (avoid during pregnancy or lactation and in children less than 2 years of age)
- Permethrin 1% cream rinse applied for 10 minutes and then washed off
- Piperonyl butoxide pyrethrin applied for 10 minutes and then washed off

REFERENCE

Buntin DM. The 1993 sexually transmitted disease treatment guidelines. *Semin Dermatol* 1994;13(4):269–274.

 ## Pelvis—Bifid

DESCRIPTION A normal variant seen in approximately 10% of patients where the pelvis divided into two major calyces just inside the kidney

REFERENCE

Bauer SB. Anomalies of the kidney and ureteropelvic junction. In: Walsh PC, Retik AB, Vaughan ED, Wein AJ, eds. *Campbell's Urology*, 7th ed. Philadelphia: WB Saunders, 1998.

 ## Pelvis—Extrarenal

DESCRIPTION Often a normal anatomic variant, can also be associated with conditions such as renal malrotation or ectopic kidney. Infrequently may cause urinary stasis and difficulties with infection and stones

REFERENCE

Bauer SB. Anomalies of the kidney and ureteropelvic junction. In: Walsh PC, Retik AB, Vaughan ED, Wein AJ, eds. *Campbell's Urology*, 7th ed. Philadelphia: WB Saunders, 1998.

 ## Penile Brachial Pressure Index

DESCRIPTION The penile brachial pressure index (PBI) can be defined as the penile systolic blood pressure divided by the brachial systolic blood pressure. A penile brachial index of 0.7 or less has been suggested to indicate arteriogenic impotence. However, due to several limitations, this test is considered an unreliable tool to exclude arteriogenic impotence.

REFERENCE

Metz P, Bengtsson J. Penile blood pressure. *Scand J Urol Nephrol* 1981;15:161.

 ## Penis—Agenesis (Aphallia)

DESCRIPTION Penile agenesis is a rare anomaly with an estimated incidence of about 1 in 10 million live births. Most of the cases have a 46,XY karyotype. The usual appearance is that of a well-developed scrotum with descended testes and an absent penile shaft. Associated anomalies are common. Associated urethral absence is usually accompanied by fatal anomalies. Immediate investigations for associated anomalies and karyotype are essential.

SYNONYMS

- Aphallia

CAUSES

- Failure of development of the genital tubercle

TREATMENT

- Surgical reconstruction/gender reassignment is recommended in the newborn.

REFERENCE

Oesch IL, Pinter A, Ransley PG. Penile agenesis: A report of six cases. *J Pediatr Surg* 1987;2:172–174.

 ## Penis—Angiosarcoma

DESCRIPTION Approximately 32 cases of penile angiosarcoma have been reported. No site of predilection is demonstrated. The tumor may be well circumscribed or diffuse. Death may occur 1 week to 5 years after presentation (mean: 13 months). The application of immunoperoxidase staining for factor VIII, present in normal endothelial cells, aids in diagnosis.

TREATMENT

- Local excision with lymph node dissection
- Local radiotherapy
- Systemic chemotherapy with more widespread tumor

REFERENCE

Kovacz J, Crouch RD. Sarcoma of the penis. *J Urol* 1958;80:43.

 ## Penis—Buried (Concealed/Hidden/Trapped)

DESCRIPTION Must be differentiated from an abnormally small penis. A *buried* or *concealed* penis refers to a normal-sized penis that is hidden because of the prepubic fat pad. Congenital causes or obesity can hide the penile shaft. The penis can usually be exposed by retracting skin lateral to the penile shaft. The iatrogenic hidden penis after circumcision is more properly called a "trapped penis." Children who undergo neonatal circumcision with testicular swelling or with a hernia or a webbed penis are at risk for excess penile shaft skin loss and a trapped penis. Theoretically, obese adults who undergo circumcision are also at risk for removal of excess shaft skin. Symptoms can sometimes be associated (balanitis, urinary tract infection, painful voiding, ballooning of the foreskin, and urinary retention).

SYNONYMS

- Inconspicious penis (general term for buried, trapped, or webbed penis)

TREATMENT

- Surgical correction is optional and controversial.
- Liposuction has been used in cases of extreme obesity.

REFERENCE

Donatucci CF, et al. Management of the buried penis in adults. *J Urol* 1998;159(2):420–424.

Penis—Cysts

 Penis—Cysts

DESCRIPTION   Epidermal cysts found on the ventral surfaces of the penis have been attributed to defective embryologic closure of the median raphe, anomalous developmental rests of the periurethral glands of Littre, development of apocrine cystadenomas ectopically, and anomalous budding and separation of urethral columnar epithelium from the urethra. Penile cysts are commonly found lying just beneath the median raphe and are most likely derived from urethral columnar epithelium. Patients are most often asymptomatic.

CAUSES

• Congenital anomaly

TREATMENT

• Surgical excision

REFERENCE

Paslin D. Urethroid cysts. *Arch Dermatol* 1983;119(1):89–90.

 Penis—Duplication (Diphallus)

DESCRIPTION   This is an extremely rare anomaly, with an incidence of 1 in 5 to 6 million births. According to Aleem's Classification, the condition may be true diphallia (complete or partial), or bifid phallus (complete or partial bifid glans or bifid penis). Usually, the penes are unequal in size and lie side by side. Associated anomalies are frequent. Ultrasound may help in differentiating true complete diphallia (two corpora cavernous in each penis) from complete bifid phallus (only one corpus cavernous in each penis).

SYNONYMS

• Diphallia

CAUSES

• Failure of fusion of paired mesodermal anlagen of the genital tubercle

TREATMENT

• Surgical reconstruction

REFERENCE

Aleem AA. Diphallia: Report of a case. *J Urol* 1972;108:357.

 Penis—Leiomyoma

DESCRIPTION   Penile leiomyoma is a rare benign tumor of smooth muscle, which commonly involves the shaft, with the glans penis involvement being next in frequency. These lesions tend to be small (1.0 cm in diameter), well circumscribed, rubbery in consistency, with light yellow to white cut surfaces. Electron microscopy and immunohistochemistry should be used to confirm diagnosis. Multiple recurrences are rare.

TREATMENT

• Primary excision of the tumor is the treatment of choice.

REFERENCE

Leoni S, Prandi S, Mora A. Leiomyoma of the prepuce. *Eur Urol* 1980;6(3):188–189.

 Penis—Leiomyosarcoma

DESCRIPTION   Penile leiomyosarcoma is a very rare malignant smooth muscle tumor that usually occurs in the fifth to seventh decades. Superficial lesions commonly arise from the dermis of the shaft or the smooth muscle of the glans penis and usually form subcutaneous nodules. Deep leiomyosarcoma is less common, arising from the smooth muscle of the corpora cavernosa, and tend to invade the urethra and metastasize early. These tumors are firm, gray-white, lobulated, and poorly circumscribed, and can range in size from 3 to 8 cm. Electron microscopy and immunohistochemistry should be used to confirm diagnosis.

TREATMENT

• Primary excision of the tumor is the treatment of choice in low-grade (superficial) tumors; however, the tumor tends to recur locally.
• In high-grade (deep) malignancies, the treatment is dependent on the age of the patient, size, location of the tumor, and the degree of invasiveness.

REFERENCE

Kathuria S, Jablokow VR, Molnar Z. Leiomyosarcoma of the penile prepuce with ultrastructural study. *Urology* 1986;27(6):556–557.

 Penis—Length

DESCRIPTION   Data on pediatric penile length considerations are discussed in Section II, "Microphallus (Micropenis)." At birth, dimensions of the normal term infant phallus are 3.5 ± 0.7 cm in stretched length and 1.1 ± 0.2 cm in diameter. In adults, concern over phallus size can direct some men to seek penile augmentation. There is no real cutoff between "normal" and "abnormal," since many variables (fat pad, erect vs. flaccid length) are present. For example, a large fat pad can cause a penis to become "buried" and give a shorter appearance (See Section III, "Penis—Buried"). One recent study provided the following data for their mean measurements in adults (length from penopubic skin to the meatus):

• Flaccid length: 8.85 cm; stretched length: 12.45 cm
• Erect length: 12.89 cm; flaccid girth: 9.71 cm; erect girth: 12.3 cm

REFERENCE

Wessels H, McAninich JW. Penis size: What is normal? *Contemp Urol* 1997;6671.

 Penis—Leukoplakia

DESCRIPTION   These lesions present as solitary or multiple white plaques, usually involving the penile meatus. Histologically, there is parakeratosis, hyperkeratosis, and hypertrophy of the rete pegs, with dermal edema and lymphocytic infiltration. Leukoplakia is commonly associated with in situ squamous cell carcinoma and verrucous carcinoma of the penis. Thus, close follow-up of the excision site with periodic biopsy of incompletely excised lesions is necessary to detect early malignant change.

TREATMENT

• Elimination of chronic irritation and circumcision may be indicated.
• Surgical excision and radiation have been used in the treatment of leukoplakia.

REFERENCE

Bain L, Geronemus R. The association of lichen planus of the penis with squamous cell carcinoma in situ and with verrucous squamous carcinoma. *J Dermatol Surg Oncol* 1989;15(4):413–417.

Penis—Metastasis

DESCRIPTION Metastatic disease to the penis is rare, with roughly 200 cases reported during the past 100 years. The bladder, prostate, rectum, and rectosigmoid are responsible for the greatest number of metastases. However, distal primaries (e.g., lung) have been reported. Several mechanisms might lead to this condition: direct extension, retrograde lymphatic spread, retrograde venous spread, direct arterial extension, secondary embolism, tertiary embolism, instrumental spread, and paradoxical spread. Patients may develop masses or "malignant priapism." Most patients die within 6 months of presentation. Penectomy may be indicated for pain or relief of urinary obstruction.

REFERENCE

Bachrach P, Dahlen CP. Metastatic tumors to the penis. *Urology* 1973;1(4):359–362

 ## Penis—Neurofibroma

DESCRIPTION Neurofibroma is a benign tumor of the neural sheath–forming cells (Schwann cells). It may occur as a solitary lesion or as part of systemic neurofibromatosis (von Recklinghausen disease). Solitary neurofibromas usually occur on the extremities as a discrete encapsulated mass, which rarely recurs after surgical removal and almost never undergoes malignant change. In contrast, systemic lesions are usually chronic and progressive, with a tendency for recurrence after surgical removal and malignant transformation. Diagnosis is made by open biopsy of the lesion, displaying sheets of spindle-shaped cells encapsulated by fibrous tissue under microscopy.

SYNONYMS

- Schwannoma

CAUSES

- Family history of neurofibromatosis

REFERENCE

Thompson PD, Harty JI, Koper D. Neurofibroma of penis. *Urology* 1992;40(6):555.

 ## Penis—Sclerosing Lipogranuloma

DESCRIPTION This inflammatory process is directed toward exogenous lipids and waxes that gain access to the dermis. It occurs most commonly among young men in the penis and scrotum secondary to attempts to enhance the size of the genitalia. The exogenous lipids prompt a foreign-body giant cell reaction, which is associated with variable fibrosis. In most instances, there is a history of trauma to the genital region. No specific treatment is available.

SYNONYMS

- Paraffinoma

CAUSES

- Trauma
- Injections of oil-based substances for either therapeutic or cosmetic purposes

REFERENCE

Matsuda T, Shichiri Y, Hida S, et al. Eosinophilic sclerosing lipogranuloma of the male genitalia not caused by exogenous lipids. *J Urol* 1988;140:1021.

 ## Penis—Sclerosing Lymphangitis

DESCRIPTION Firm and often asymptomatic subcutaneous cordlike swellings along the dorsal shaft of the penis or around the coronal sulcus. Can be confused with lymphangioma circumscriptum, a uncommon tumor of the lymphatic channels

SYNONYMS

- Mondor's phlebitis of the penis

CAUSES

- Thrombosis of the superficial venous plexus of the penis
- Probably secondary to trauma

TREATMENT

- None necessary; usually resolves in several weeks. Failure to resolve in a timely manner may require biopsy.

REFERENCE

Margolis DJ. Cutaneous diseases of the male external genitalia. In: Walsh PC, Retik AB, Vaughan ED, Wein AJ, eds. *Campbell's Urology*, 7th ed. Philadelphia: WB Saunders, 1998.

 ## Penis—Torsion

DESCRIPTION Congenital rotation of the penile shaft such that the median raphe spirals obliquely around the penile shaft. The external genitalia are otherwise normal, but may be associated with hypospadias or ventral hood penile deformity. The torsion tends to occur in a counterclockwise direction (i.e., the twist is to the left). Mainly a cosmetic issue, repair is usually not necessary if the rotation is <60 to 90 degrees.

TREATMENT

- Mild cases require only simply freeing the penile shaft of its investing tissue.

REFERENCE

Pomerantz P, et al. Isolated torsion of penis. Report of 6 cases. *Urology* 1978;11(1):37–39.

 ## Penis—Verrucous Carcinoma

DESCRIPTION Squamous cell carcinoma of the penis represents about 1% of cancers in men in the United States and 11% to 12% of all cancers in men in countries where circumcision is not routinely practiced. Verrucous carcinoma is an uncommon variant that accounts for only 5% to 16% of all penile squamous cell carcinomas. Diagnosis of verrucous carcinoma may be difficult because biopsies are usually performed on the superficial portion of the lesion. Therefore, it is crucial to have depth of the biopsy. Verrucous carcinoma exhibits an exophytic warty lesion of squamous cell carcinoma and endophytic growth where cellular atypia is noted. (See also Section II, "Penis Cancer—General.")

SYNONYMS

- Giant condyloma
- Buschke-Lowenstein tumor

CAUSES

- Lack of circumcision
- Prior trauma
- Previous disease
- Poor hygiene
- Phimosis
- Tight prepuce

TREATMENT

- Partial penectomy

REFERENCE

Kanik AB, Lee J, Wax F, Bhawan J. Penile verrucous carcinoma in a 37 yr old circumcised man. *J Am Acad Dermatol* 1997;37(2):329–331.

Penis—Webbed

 Penis—Webbed

DESCRIPTION A congenital condition in which the scrotal skin extends onto the ventral aspect of the penile shaft. While there are usually no associated abnormalities, there are a few reports of hypoplasia of the distal urethra. Occasionally, a webbed penis is the result of a circumcision in which there was excess removal of ventral penile shaft skin. Cosmetic repair is performed, as needed.

REFERENCE

Dilley AV, et al. Webbed penis. *Pediatr Surg Int* 1999;15(5–6):447–448.

 Penn Pouch

DESCRIPTION A continent urinary reservoir is created based on the Mitrofanoff principle, which uses the appendix as the catheterizable continent apparatus. The pouch is made from joining a detubularized colon and ileum.

REFERENCE

Benson MC, Olsson CA. Continent urinary diversion. In: Walsh PC, Retik AB, Vaughan ED, Wein AJ, eds. *Campbell's Urology*, 7th ed. Philadelphia: WB Saunders, 1998:3190–3245.

 Pereyra Urethropexy

DESCRIPTION Pereyra, in 1959, was the first to present a transvaginal approach to a urethropexy using a needle suture carrier, obviating the need for a transabdominal exposure. Through a T vaginal incision, the bladder neck and periurethral tissue are exposed. The suture carrier is passed through a suprapubic stab incision and, under digital guidance, delivered through the periurethral tissue, and the bladder neck is suspended with absorbable suture.

REFERENCE

Raz S, Stothers L, Chopra A. Vaginal reconstructive surgery for incontinence and prolapse. In: Walsh PC, Retik AB, Vaughan ED, Wein AJ, eds. *Campbell's Urology*, 7th ed. Philadelphia: WB Saunders, 1998:1066–1094.

 Pfannenstiel Incision

DESCRIPTION A transverse incision is centered approximately 2 fingerbreadths above the pubic symphysis. A transverse incision is made through the anterior rectus fascia, and entry into the retropubic space can be gained by separating the rectus muscle in the midline. Useful for bladder and other lower abdominal procedures.

REFERENCE

Montague DK. Surgical incisions. In: Novick AC, Streem SB, Pontes JE, eds. *Stewarts Operative Urology*. Baltimore: Williams & Wilkins, 1989:15–40.

 PLAP (Placental Alkaline Phosphatase)

DESCRIPTION PLAP is a fetal isoenzyme, which has a different structure than the adult alkaline phosphatase. It is one of many tumor markers used for diagnosis, staging, and monitoring of treatment response in patients with germ cell tumors. May be useful as a prognostic index. Although the individual sensitivity of PLAP is low, when combined with gamma-glutamyl transpeptidase (GGT), simultaneous determinations have shown elevation of one or both in 80% of patients with active disease.

REFERENCE

Javadpour N. Multiple biochemical tumor markers in testicular cancer. *Cancer* 1983;52:887.

 Plasmacytoma—Bladder

DESCRIPTION This tumor is characterized by a monotonous proliferation of plasma cells at variable stages of differentiation, with predominance of the immature variety. Five cases have been reported in the literature, with a mean age of 54 years, None of which had multiple myeloma at the time of diagnosis. Local suprapubic recurrences and regional lymph node metastasis may occur. Survival up to 12 years after diagnosis has been reported.

TREATMENT

- Subtotal cystectomy
- Radiation and chemotherapy.

REFERENCE

Yang C, Motteram R, Sandeman TF. Extramedullary plasmacytoma of the bladder: A case report and review of literature. *Cancer* 1982;50:146.

 Plasmacytoma—Testicular

DESCRIPTION Neoplastic collections of plasma cells occurring in the testicles. They are very rare tumors, with an incidence of approximately 1 in 1000 testicular tumors. They are most commonly associated with a previous or concurrent diagnosis of multiple myeloma and are generally not believed to occur as primary tumors.

TREATMENT

- Orchiectomy.

REFERENCE

Oppenheim PI, et al. Testicular plasmacytoma. *Arch Pathol Lab Med* 1991;115(6):629–632.

 Ploidy Analysis—Bladder Cancer

DESCRIPTION Ploidy is the chromosomal content of cells, which can be measured using flow cytometry. Ploidy analysis, when considered as an independent variable, is a fair predictor of clinical outcome. Tumor stage and grade are considered to be the most important predictors of survival. Although ploidy may be more significant in predicting survival than grade, the addition of ploidy to the known stage and grade of a bladder tumor usually does not drastically alter clinical management of a patient.

REFERENCE

Bittard H, et al. Clinical evaluation of cell deoxyribonucleic acid content measured by flow cytometry in bladder cancer. *J Urol* 1996; (155):1887–1891.

 Ploidy Analysis—Prostate Cancer

DESCRIPTION Ploidy is a variation in the number of chromosomes in a cell. Aneuploidy is a variation in the number of chromosomes in a cell that is other than a simple multiple of the number of chromosomes. In a prostate specimen, flow cytometry is used to measure the DNA content of the cells. DNA ploidy in addition to the histologic grading may improve the ability to predict the pathologic state and ultimately the prognosis. The frequency of aneuploidy increases with advancing stage of the tumor. Inherent problems with ploidy analysis include heterogeneity of DNA cell sampling, as well as whether it will change clinical management.

REFERENCE

Dejter SW, et al. Prognostic significance of DNA ploidy in carcinoma of prostate. *Urology* 1989;33:361–366.

Polyarteritis Nodosa—Urologic Considerations

DESCRIPTION   PAN is not well understood. It is believed to be caused by the deposition of immune complexes in the wall of primarily medium-sized arteries, causing deformative changes in the wall. This may lead to thickening and aneurysmal changes, causing acute renal hemorrhage and often leading to chronic renal failure.

TREATMENT

- Corticosteroids and azathioprine

REFERENCE

Litvak AS, et al. Urologic manifestation of polyarteritis nodosa. *J Urol* 1976;115(5):572–576, 1976.

 ## Polyembryoma

DESCRIPTION   Mixed germ cell tumor of the testis, containing embryonal carcinoma and yolk sac tumor. Histologic analysis reveals distinctive, well-organized pattern of embryoid bodies in a myxoid stroma, which resembles extraembryonic mesenchyme.

REFERENCE

Ulbright TM. Germ cell neoplasms of the testis. *Am J Surg Pathol* 1993;17(11):1075–1091.

 ## Polyorchidism

DESCRIPTION   This is a very rare condition characterized by multiple (more than two) testicles. It may be the result of transverse division of the urogenital ridge. It may be accompanied by inguinal hernias, torsion, or cryptorchidism. It is most often discovered as an asymptomatic swelling in the scrotum and usually occurs with its own separate epididymis and vas deferens. If a testicular tumor can be ruled out using ultrasound or MRI, and there are no other associated disorders, surgical exploration is not necessary.

TREATMENT

- Surveillance, exploration, and biopsy, if indicated

REFERENCE

Thum G. Polyorchidism. *J Urol* 1991;145(2): 370–372.

 ## Polypoid Cystitis

DESCRIPTION   Also known as papillary cystitis, it results from inflammation and edema in the bladder lamina propria, leading to papillary and polypoid mucosal lesions. Technically, *papillary cystitis* refers to long finger-like papillae, and *polypoid cystitis* is for the more broad-based lesions. The lesions are caused by edema and hypervascularity of the mucosa. Clinically, indwelling catheters or enterovesical fistulas are common causes, and it should be differentiated from papillary bladder cancer.

SYNONYMS

- Papillary cystitis

TREATMENT

- Usually resolves within 3 to 6 months after removal of the inflammatory stimulus; if necessary, the lesions can be resected. If the lesions persist, malignancy should be ruled out.

REFERENCE

Bostwick DG, Eble JN. *Urologic Surgical Pathology*. St Louis: Mosby, 1997:179–181.

 ## Polypoid Urethritis

DESCRIPTION   A urethral counterpart of polypoid cystitis, it occurs as single or multiple polypoid/papillary lesions. A nonneoplastic inflammatory lesion usually found in the prostatic urethra near the verumontanum. The lesions are edematous stroma with distended blood vessels and chronic inflammatory infiltrate.

TREATMENT

- Usually resolves after removal of the inflammatory stimulus; if necessary, resection of the lesions leads to cure. If the lesions persist, malignancy should be ruled out.

REFERENCE

Bostwick DG, Eble JN. *Urologic Surgical Pathology*. St Louis: Mosby, 1997:439.

 ## Polyuria

DESCRIPTION   Generally defined as greater than 3 L of urine output from a person without excessive fluid intake. It is useful to measure the urine osmolality to determine whether the polyuria is due to a water diuresis (urine osmolality <250 mOsmol/kg) or a solute diuresis (urine osmolality >300 mOsmol/kg). There are numerous causes of polyuria. A solute diuresis may be caused by excessive hypertonic saline infusion, high-protein feedings, uncontrolled diabetes, or postobstructive diuresis. A water diuresis can be caused by multiple conditions, including polydipsia, loop diuretics, diabetes insipidus, and infusion of hypotonic solutions.

TREATMENT

- Correct the underlying cause.

REFERENCE

Evaluation of the urologic patient. In: Walsh PC, Retik AB, Vaughan ED, Wein AJ, eds. *Campbell's Urology*, 7th ed. Philadelphia: WB Saunders, 1998:134.

 ## Postatrophic Hyperplasia of the Prostate

DESCRIPTION   Postatrophic hyperplasia is a histologic pattern showing atrophic and hyperplastic glands, sometimes with a small acinar configuration. Atrophy followed by hyperplasia results in acini with nuclear enlargement. Nucleoli are enlarged as well. The basal cell layer may be difficult to see, but its presence rules out prostate cancer. Immunohistochemistry with 34βE12 stain, which stains for basal cell cytokeratin, may be helpful. Can be confused with prostate cancer on needle biopsy and is a benign condition. See also Section III, "Atypical Small Acinar Proliferation—Prostate (ASAP)" and "Atypical Adenomatous Hyperplasia of the Prostate."

REFERENCE

Amin MB, et al. Postatrophic hyperplasia of the prostate gland: A detailed analysis of its morphology in needle biopsy specimens. *Am J Surg Pathol* 1999;23(8):925–931.

Postcoital Test

 Postcoital Test

DESCRIPTION This is a test that evaluates the interaction between sperm and cervical mucus. It determines the adequacy of sperm and the receptivity of cervical mucus. Testing consists of retrieving specimens from the posterior vaginal fornix, exocervix, and endocervical canal approximately 6 to 8 hours after intercourse. The test should be performed close to the time of ovulation, and couples are asked to abstain from sex 48 hours prior to the test. These specimens are examined to determine the number of motile sperm, with 10 sperm/HPF considered adequate and excluding the cervical mucosa as cause of infertility. When these test results are poor, the specimens may be repeated on another occasion, 1 to 3 hours after coitus.

SYNONYMS

• Sims-Huhner Test

REFERENCE

Moghissi KS. Postcoital test: Physiolgic basis, technique, and interpretation. *Fertil Steril* 1976;27(2)117–129.

 Postoperative Spindle Cell Nodule

DESCRIPTION These are benign lesions that appear 5 weeks to 3 months after surgical procedures in the lower urogenital tract. They grossly resemble a sarcoma and develop after damage to the bladder wall. Microscopically, they appear as intersecting spindle cells intermingle with inflammatory infiltrates. The main differential diagnosis is leiomyosarcoma. They have been reported most commonly in the bladder and prostate.

SYNONYMS

• Postoperative spindle cell nodule of Proppe
• Pseudosarcoma

TREATMENT

• Transurethral resection

REFERENCE

Young RH, Eble JN. Non-neoplastic disorders of the urinary bladder. In: Bostwick DG, ed. *Urologic Surgical Pathology*, 1st ed. St Louis: Mosby, 1997.

 Posttransplant Lymphoproliferative Disorder

DESCRIPTION There is an increased incidence of cancer with the use of immunosuppression in transplant patients. Posttransplant lymphoproliferative disorders, including lymphoma and Kaposi's sarcoma, have an incidence of 2.5% in cadaveric renal allografts. Epstein-Barr virus infection at the time of transplantation appears to be a significant risk factor. The lymphoproliferative disorder may be controlled by adjusting or stopping the immunosuppression.

REFERENCE

Cockfield SM, et al. Post-transplant lymphoproliferative disorder in renal allograft recipients. *Transplantation* 1993;56–60.

 Potter Syndrome/Potter Facies

DESCRIPTION A fetus with Potter syndrome may show signs of Potter facies (a flat nose, recessed chin, epicanthal folds, low-set ears) and limb abnormalities. These deformities are believed to be secondary to compression of the fetus due to severe oligohydramnios resulting from bilateral renal agenesis. Death usually results from respiratory insufficiency from lack of development of the alveolar sacs

SYNONYMS

• Oligohydramnios sequence

TREATMENT

• None; usually death immediately after birth

REFERENCE

Potter EL. Bilateral renal agenesis. *J Pediatr* 1946;29:68.

 Pouchitis

DESCRIPTION Pain in the region of a catheterizable stoma, along with an increase in pouch contractility. The increased contractility can cause temporary loss of the continence mechanism. The patient may complain of sudden, explosive loss of urine through the catheterizable stoma. Most caused by a bacterial infection that responds to a 10-day course of antibiotics based on sensitivity testing

REFERENCE

Benson MC, Olsson CA. Continent urinary diversion. In: Walsh PC, Retik AB, Vaughan ED, Wein AJ, eds. *Campbell's Urology*, 7th ed. Philadelphia: WB Saunders, 1998:3218.

 Prader-Willi Syndrome

DESCRIPTION This is secondary to a chromosomal abnormality consisting of partial deletion of the long-arm of chromosome 15. Children often present as obese, hypotonic, and retarded, with hypogonadism and cryptorchidism. Obesity and behavioral problems are the major cause of morbidity and mortality in affected individuals.

REFERENCE

Cassidy SB. Prader-Willi syndrome. *J Med Genet* 1997;34(11):917–923.

 Prehn's Sign

DESCRIPTION This is a test that may aid in the differentiation of epididymitis vs. testicular torsion. A positive test is indicated by relief of pain with elevation of the involved testicle, which suggests a diagnosis of epididymitis rather than testicular torsion. This is often not a reliable test.

REFERENCE

Gillenwater JY, Grayhack JT, Howards SS, Duckett JW, eds. *Adult and Pediatric Urology*, 3rd ed. St Louis: Mosby, 1996:68–69.

 Prentiss Maneuver

DESCRIPTION Additional cord length in an orchiopexy operation can be gained by incising the inguinal floor and ligating the inferior epigastric vessels. The internal ring and transversalis fascia are then closed lateral to the cord.

REFERENCE

Rozanski T, Bloom DA, Colodny A. Surgery of the scrotum and testis in children. In: Walsh PC, Retik AB, Vaughan ED, Wein AJ, eds. *Campbell's Urology*, 7th ed. Philadelphia: WB Saunders, 1998:2193–2198.

Preputial Stones

DESCRIPTION Preputial stones are rare occurrences. They generally occur in adults and are associated with poor genital hygiene, low socioeconomic status, and phimosis. Factors in preputial stone formation include obstruction, stasis, foreign body, nidus formation, and infection.

SYNONYMS

• Preputial calculi

TREATMENT

• Removal of stone and elimination of predisposing condition

REFERENCE

Ellis DJ, et al. Preputial calculus: A case report. *J Urol* 1986;136(2):464–465.

 ## Pressure–Flow Studies

DESCRIPTION The simultaneous measurement of bladder pressure and uroflow throughout the entire voiding cycle. Performed as part of urodynamic study, improves on some of the limitations of uroflowmetry alone. Measurements for this study can include the variables that affect the study: intravesical pressure, rectal pressure, intraurethral pressure, sphincter EMG, and urine flow rate. A small catheter is placed and used to fill the bladder and measure the flow. All variables are plotted and recorded simultaneously to compare the various readings at various points in the micturition study.

REFERENCE

Webster GD, Kreder KJ. Neurologic evaluation. In: Walsh PC, Retik AB, Vaughan ED, Wein AJ, eds. *Campbell's Urology,* 7th ed. Philadelphia: WB Saunders, 1998:939.

 ## Propantheline Stimulation Test

DESCRIPTION This test is used when involuntary detrusor contractions are demonstrated during cystometry to predict the outcome of pharmacologic treatment with anticholinergics. Propantheline bromide is an anticholinergic with side effects including dry mouth and blurred vision. Once involuntary detrusor contractions have been confirmed, 15 mg of propantheline bromide are administered parenterally. Once effects of the drug are noticed, cystometry is repeated. A positive response is defined as the complete abolition of involuntary detrusor contractions, or a 200% increase in the bladder volume at which they occur. If the parenteral dosage is effective, a favorable clinical response to the orally administered dose can be expected in most patients.

REFERENCE

Blaivis JG, et al. Urodynamic evaluation as a test of sacral cord function. *Urology* 1979;9:682.

 ## Prostate Calculi

DESCRIPTION These are more common in older males and are rarely found in children. They usually occur in clusters and are associated with other disease processes. They are generally asymptomatic but may cause symptoms such as decreased urinary stream, prostatism, and lower back pain. Rare a source of chronic bacterial prostatitis. Calculi may form secondary to calcification of corpora amylacea and simple precipitation of prostatic secretion.

TREATMENT

• Generally none
• Transurethral resection or total prostatectomy, if markedly symptomatic

REFERENCE

Klimas R, et al. Prostatic calculi: A review. *Prostate* 1985;7(1):91–96.

 ## Prostate Cancer—Gaeta Grading System

DESCRIPTION A system used to grade prostate cancer. Based on the histologic features of the least favorable-appearing cells seen in at least one-third of the sample. Both glands and cellular nuclei were graded separately on a scale from 1 to 4, the higher number being less differentiated. The system attempted to correlate grade with stage and survival.

• Grade 1: single, separate glands; small nuclei with inconspicuous nucleoli
• Grade 2: small or medium glands; pleomorphic nuclei with nucleomegaly
• Grade 3: small glands, including cribriform and scirrhous patterns; pleomorphic nuclei with nucleomegaly
• Grade 4: sheets of cells without glands; nuclei and nucleoli of any size; mitotic figures >3 per HPF

REFERENCE

Gaeta JF, Asirwatham JE, Miller G, et al. Histologic grading of primary prostatic cancer: A new approach to an old problem. *J Urol* 1980;123:689–693.

 ## Prostate Cancer—Gleason Grading System

DESCRIPTION The most commonly used system of grading adenocarcinoma of the prostate. It is based on data originally obtained in the VA Cooperative urologic research group. Based on architectural findings. Assigned by rating the predominant pattern a score of 1 to 5, and the second most predominant a similar score. The grades/patterns are added together to obtain a final Gleason score of 2 to 10. A lower score is more differentiated. Higher scores are less differentiated. (Note: An early version of the Gleason system included a clinical stage of 1 to 4 to create a Gleason "sum," but this is not currently used.)

• Pattern 1: lobular cluster of closely packed, single, separate, round uniform glands
• Pattern 2: same as pattern 1, except for less uniformity of gland spacing and shape, and tumor margin not well defined
• Pattern 3: single, separate, irregular glands, including cribriform and papillary patterns
• Pattern 4: coalescing and fused glands form cords, including solid and cribriform patterns; may have hypernephroid appearance (clear cells)
• Pattern 5: few or no glands; tumor in sheets or comedo pattern

REFERENCE

Gleason D. Histologic grading and clinical staging of carcinoma of the prostate. In: Tannenbaum M, ed. *Urologic Pathology: The Prostate.* Philadelphia: Lea & Febiger, 1997.

Prostate Cancer—Helpap Grading System

 Prostate Cancer—Helpap Grading System

DESCRIPTION Grading system reported in the literature that may be useful to differentiate low-risk (grade 1) from high-risk prostate cancer (grade 3)

- Grade 1a: well-differentiated glands
- Grade 1b: moderately differentiated glands
- Grade 2a: poorly differentiated, with moderate nuclear and nucleolar atypia, or mixed pattern with minor cribriform component
- Grade 2b: poorly differentiated, with marked nuclear and nucleolar atypia, or mixed pattern, with chiefly cribriform pattern
- Grade 3: solid trabecular pattern with marked atypia, with or without cribriform pattern

REFERENCE

Helpap B. Review of the morphology of prostatic carcinoma with special emphasis on subgrading and prognosis. *J Urol Pathol* 1993; 1:3–19.

 Prostate Cancer—Mayo Clinic Grading System

DESCRIPTION This grading system not only uses an assessment of glandular architecture similar to Gleason's, but also uses histologic criteria. Grading is done on a scale of 1 to 4, with 4 having the worst prognosis. Cellular features such as cytoplasmic-nuclear-nucleolar morphology, mitotic activity, and tumor invasiveness are all used to assign grade.

REFERENCE

Kozlowski JM, Grayhack JP. Carcinoma of the prostate. In: Gillenwater JY, Grayhack JT, Howards SS, Duckett JW, eds. *Adult and Pediatric Urology,* 2nd ed. St Louis: Mosby, 1991.

 Prostate Cancer—M.D. Anderson Grading System

DESCRIPTION Introduced as a new grading system for adenocarcinoma of the prostate in 1982, this grading system is based on the percentage of tumor that is differentiated (gland-forming) or undifferentiated (non–gland-forming). Grading is assigned by low-power ($\times 40$–$\times 100$) microscopic analysis. This system (MDAH) is rarely utilized today. Gleason and Mostofi grading systems remain the most popular classification schemes.

SYNONYMS

- Broders prostate cancer grading system
- Grade 1: 75% to 100% of tumor composed of glands
- Grade 2: 50% to 75% of tumor composed of glands
- Grade 3: 25% to 50% of tumor composed of glands
- Grade 4: 0% to 25% of tumor composed of glands

REFERENCES

Broders AC. Carcinoma grading and practical application. *Arch Pathol Lab Med* 1926;2: 376–381.

Brawn PN, Ayala AG, vonEschenbach AC. Histologic grading study of prostate adenocarcinoma: The development of a new system and comparison with other methods. *Cancer* 1982;49:525.

 Prostate Cancer—Mostofi (WHO) Grading System

DESCRIPTION Traditional grading system, generally replaced by the Gleason grading system

- Grade I: well differentiated, with slight nuclear anaplasia
- Grade II: moderately to poorly differentiated, with moderate nuclear anaplasia
- Grade III: poorly differentiated, with marked nuclear anaplasia, or undifferentiated carcinoma

SYNONYMS

- World Health Organization Grading System

REFERENCE

Mostofi FK. Grading of prostatic carcinoma. *Cancer Chemother Rep* 1975;59[Pt I]:111–117.

 Prostate Cancer—Mucinous Adenocarcinoma

DESCRIPTION These very rare tumors are histopathologically defined as having lakes of extracellular mucin, comprising at least 25% of the primary prostate tumor. It generally is considered to have a slightly worse prognosis than typical adenocarcinoma of the prostate. They appear to be hormonally refractory, and bone metastasis are common. Radiation and or surgery can be considered.

REFERENCE

Ro JY, Grignon DJ, Ayala AG, et al. Mucinous adenocarcinoma of the prostate: Histochemical and immunohistochemical studies. *Hum Pathol* 1990;21:593–600.

 Prostate Cancer—Risk Stratification

DESCRIPTION A challenge of prostate cancer is to choose the appropriate therapy based on the risk of disease progression. It is often useful to assign a relative "risk" to an individual. These risk groups were established from literature and based on known prognostic factors: PSA level, biopsy Gleason score, and 1992 AJCC T stage. One typical system is described here. Note that this is risk of PSA progression posttherapy and not overall or disease specific-survival.

- Low risk: stages T1c and T2a, PSA level of 10 ng/mL or less, and biopsy Gleason score of 6 or less (<25% PSA progression at 5 years post-therapy)
- Intermediate risk: PSA levels 10 to 20 ng/mL or lower, biopsy Gleason score of 7, or AJCC clinical stage T2b (25%–50% PSA progression at 5 years posttherapy)
- High risk: T2c disease or a PSA level >20 ng/mL or a biopsy Gleason score of 8 or more (>50% PSA progression at 5 years posttherapy)

REFERENCE

D'Amico AV, Whittington R, Malkowicz SB, et al. Biochemical outcome after radical prostatectomy, external beam radiation therapy, or interstitial radiation therapy for clinically localized prostate cancer. *JAMA* 1998;280(11):969–974.

Prostate Cancer—Small Cell (Neuroendocrine)

DESCRIPTION A rare subtype of malignancy of the prostate that has a rapidly fatal course. Considered to be a variant of Gleason 5 adenocarcinoma of the prostate, it is identical to small cell carcinomas of the lung and has neuroendocrine (small cell, oat cell) differentiation. In 50% of the cases, the tumors are mixed small cell carcinoma with adenocarcinoma. Neuroendocrine cells are identified by special staining (i.e., neuron-specific enolase [NSE] or other markers). It should be noted that the normal prostate does have some neuroendocrine positivity, but it is limited and can only be detected by staining. About 10% of acinar adenocarcinomas of the prostate can have Paneth-like cells (large eosinophilic cells) that are neuroendocrine, and today it is recognized that adenocarcinoma of the prostate that is not classified as neuroendocrine can have some patchy cells that stain as neuroendocrine cells. Large numbers of Gleason 5 cells in a prostate sample should prompt a neuroendocrine staining work-up of the sample. There can be a spectrum of differentiation of the tumors with a carcinoid-like pattern (low-grade neuroendocrine carcinoma) to the small cell undifferentiated type (oat cell), the highest grade of neuroendocrine tumor. Immunohistochemically, these cells can stain for serotonin, calcitonin, ACTH, hCG, and others. Most of these small cell tumors do not produce detectable levels of hormones but sometimes can produce detectable levels in the serum. They may also express and stain for PSA and acid phosphatase, but pure small cell carcinoma usually does not stain for PSA. At diagnosis, 70% of patients have metastatic disease, and visceral metastases are common (i.e., liver). The average survival is less than a year. Androgen receptor–positive tumors have a worse prognosis than tumors that do not express the receptor (median survival: 10 months vs. 30 months). Diagnosis is made by TRUS biopsy, symptoms associated with metastasis, and elevated LFTs and CEA.

SYNONYMS

- Small cell anaplastic carcinoma of the prostate (SCCP)
- Oat cell carcinoma of the prostate
- Neuroendocrine prostate cancer
- Carcinoid of the prostate

TREATMENT

- These tumors respond poorly to androgen ablation, but this should be attempted.
- Surgery and/or radiation therapy may provide local control.
- Chemotherapy with agents such as VP-16 and cisplatinum have some activity.

REFERENCE

Moore SR, Reinberg Y, Zhang G. Small cell carcinoma of prostate: Effectiveness of hormonal versus chemotherapy. *Urology* 1992;39(5):411–416.

 ## Prostate Cancer—Squamous and Adenosquamous

DESCRIPTION A rare lesion, it can arise in patients infected with *Schistosoma haematobium*. It can be confused with more common conditions, such as squamous metaplasia of the prostate due to infarction, radiation, and hormonal therapy. Pure primary squamous cell carcinoma of the prostate does not respond to estrogen therapy, and it does not develop elevated serum PSA or PAP levels with metastatic disease. Bone metastases are osteolytic instead of osteoblastic. Median survival is about 14 months.

REFERENCE

Bostwick DG. Neoplasms of the prostate. In: Bostwick DG, ed. *Urologic Surgical Pathology*, 1st ed. St Louis: Mosby, 1997.

 ## Prostate—Female

DESCRIPTION A coined radiologic expression that refers to an impression at the base of the female bladder seen on excretory urography or cystogram. The impression resembles an enlarged prostate in the male and can be caused by urethral diverticulum, benign and malignant tumors of the anterior vaginal wall, urethral neoplasm, and repair of stress urinary incontinence.

REFERENCE

Amis ES, Newhouse JH, eds. *Essentials of Uroradiology*, 1st ed. Boston: Little, Brown, 1991:289.

 ## Prostate Hyperplasia—Small Acinar Atypical

DESCRIPTION Histologic findings include nucleomegaly and prominent nucleoli. These lesions are found in ever-increasing numbers of prostate biopsies and are suspicious for but not diagnostic of malignancy. Subsequent biopsies have revealed adenocarcinoma in 45% of cases. Therefore, the histologic finding of atypical small acinar adenosis is highly predictive for malignancy.

TREATMENT

- Surveillance
- Repeat biopsy

REFERENCE

Iczkowski KA, et al. Atypical small acinar proliferation suspicious for malignancy in prostate needle biopsies. *Am J Surg Pathol* 1997;21(2):1489–1495.

 ## Prostate Infarction

DESCRIPTION The etiology of prostatic infarction is still unclear, although it has been linked to prostate hyperplasia. Histologic findings include infraction of prostatic epithelium, with hemorrhage and neutrophils in the intervening stroma. Recent infarcts generally do not have squamous metaplasia, whereas older ones do. Typically, the infarctions are multiple and located in the central and middle concentric zones of the middle third of the prostate. Prostatic infarction may elevate PSA levels.

REFERENCE

Brawn PN, et al. Characteristics of prostatic infarcts and their effect on serum prostate-specific antigen and prostatic acid phosphatase. *Urology* 1994;44(1):71–74.

 ## Prostate Massage

DESCRIPTION Repetitive prostatic massage is not a new tool in the urologists' armamentarium. It can be used to localize lower urinary tract infections or as a therapeutic modality. Once the most popular therapeutic maneuver used to treat prostatitis, it was abandoned as primary therapy almost 30 years ago. Based on experience reported outside North America and anecdotal experiences of some patients and their physicians, it may be making a comeback to treat certain forms of prostatitis, such as chronic abacterial prostatitis or chronic pelvic pain syndrome (see Section III). The prostate is massaged from the lateral border to the medial aspect on each side, from base to apex. Firm pressure is necessary to express prostatic fluid into the urethra. A sterile container should be held by the patient at the meatus to capture the expressed prostatic fluids (see also Section III, "Stamey Test"). The test is contraindicated in acute bacterial prostatitis.

REFERENCE

Nickel JC, Alexander R, Anderson R, et al. Prostatitis unplugged? Prostatic massage revisited. *Techniques Urol* 1999;5(1):1–7.

Prostatic Acid Phosphatase (PAP)

 Prostatic Acid Phosphatase (PAP)

DESCRIPTION Human PAP is a glycoprotein dimer of 102,000 MW. Its activity is much greater in the prostate than in any other tissue. PAP is not prostate-specific and can be found in other tissues. Historically, PAP was used a serum marker for the staging and detection of prostate cancer before the discovery of prostate-specific antigen. Although enzymatic elevation of PAP is associated with advanced prostate cancer, there are other causes of an elevated PAP, including liver, skeletal, and renal disease.

REFERENCES

Romas M, Kwan DJ. Prostatic acid phosphatase. *Urol Clin North Am* 1993;20:581–588.

Remynse LC, Begun FP, Jacobs SC, Lawson RK. Juxtaglomerular cell tumor with elevation of serum erythropoietin. *J Urol* 1989;142(6):1560–1562.

 Prostatic Urethral Polyps

DESCRIPTION Urethral polyps are rare abnormalities in male children, who present with hematuria or obstructive symptoms. Strangury may be seen, with large lesions on a long stalk. The diagnosis is by best confirmed by voiding cystourethrography. These polyps are nearly always in the prostatic fossa, although anterior urethral polyps have been reported. These are benign lesions and are not related to the polypoid masses of sarcoma botryoides.

TREATMENT

• Transurethral excision of the polyps

REFERENCE

Leibovitch I, Hanani J, et al. Hematuria and voiding disorders in children caused by congenital urethral polyps. Principles of diagnosis and management. *Eur Urol* 1993;23:382.

 Prostatitis—Mycotic

DESCRIPTION A type of granulomatous prostatitis caused by fungi and typically associated with systemic mycosis. Fungi can include blastomycosis, coccidiomycosis, cryptococcosis, histoplasmosis, and candida. Diagnosis is based on prostatic histology and culture results. For systemic therapy, see the specific agent.

REFERENCE

Schwartz J. Mycotic prostatitis. *Urology* 1982;19:1.

 Prostatitis—NIH Classification System

DESCRIPTION A new classification, proposed by an NIH working group, to more clearly define the different types of prostatitis, in order to improve the diagnosis and management of the disease. This system has not yet been validated in trials.

• Category I: acute bacterial prostatitis; acute infection of the prostate gland
• Category II: chronic bacterial prostatitis; recurrent infection of the prostate
• Category III: chronic abacterial prostatitis/chronic pelvic pain syndrome (CPPS); no demonstrable infection
• Category IIIA: inflammatory chronic pelvic pain syndrome; white cells in semen/EPS VB3
• Category IIIB: noninflammatory chronic pelvic pain syndrome; no white cells in semen/EPSNB3
• Category IV: asymptomatic inflammatory prostatitis; no symptoms

REFERENCE

Krieger JN, et al. NIH consensus definition and classification of prostatitis. *JAMA* 1999;282(3):236–237.

 Prostatitis—Stress

DESCRIPTION A subset of chronic abacterial noninflammatory prostatitis (prostatodynia), in which a pattern of excessive tension could be identified as a trigger of the syndrome. Symptoms usually respond to anxiolytic agents or behavorial modifications. See Section II, "Prostatitis—Nonbacterial, Noninflammatory (Prostatodynia)."

REFERENCE

Miller HC. Stress prostatitis. *Urology* 1988;32:507.

 Prostatodynia

DESCRIPTION Patients may present with multiple complaints, including pain in the perineum, lower back, or upon ejaculation; slow stream; and hesitancy. They exhibit no evidence of prostatic inflammation. Dysuria, frequency, and systemic signs are usually absent. Patients may suffer from associated personality disturbances. On physical examination, the prostate is normal, with no tenderness. Shows no evidence of inflammation on microscopic examination of expressed prostatic secretions and negative cultures. The cause of prostatodynia may be detrusor striated sphincter dyssynergia, tension myalgia of the pelvic floor, or overactivity of pelvic sympathetics.

SYNONYMS

• Prostatitis, chronic, nonbacterial, noninflammatory (stress) (see Section II)

TREATMENT

• Alpha-adrenergic blockade, others

REFERENCE

Orland SM, et al. Prostatitis, prostatosis, and prostatodynia. *Urology* 1985;25(5):439–459.

 Prosthesis—Infected Penile

DESCRIPTION A dreaded complication of penile prosthesis implantation. Rates of infection range from 1% to 8%; risk factors include spinal cord injury, diabetes mellitus (especially if poorly controlled with HgbA1C >11.5%), history of urinary tract infection, and multiple prosthesis operations. Usually occurs within 6 months after implantation, but delayed infection is also reported. Most common symptom is persistent pain; also present with erythema, drainage, or fever

CAUSES

• *Staphylococcus epidermidis* (most common)
• Gram-negative rods and yeast also common

TREATMENT

• Surgical removal
• Irrigation and antibiotic treatment
• Immediate salvage procedures with surgical removal
• Washout and immediate replacement have reported with good results: vigorous intraoperative irrigation with four different solutions, including vancomycin; immediate reimplantation of a new inflatable penile prosthesis; and postoperative outpatient antibiotics, with oral ciprofloxacin or IV vancomycin or cefazolin.

REFERENCE

Kaufman JM, et al. Immediate salvage procedure for infected penile prosthesis. *J Urol* 1998;159(3):816–818.

 Pruritus—External Genitalia, Male

DESCRIPTION Itching of the external genitalia can precede the appearance of a rash or other lesion. When the itching results in red, weeping skin with crusts, it is often called "eczematous dermatitis." The differential diagnosis of eczematous dermatitis includes eczema (atopic dermatitis), allergic dermatitis, seborrheic dermatitis, contact/irritant dermatitis, fixed drug reaction, balanitis candidal infection, or herpes. Other sexually transmitted diseases, such as scabies, can cause itching. (See specific lesion for further details.)

Some patients manifest itching with or without a demonstrable local factor. The skin may appear normal or demonstrate excoriation from

scratching or lichenification (skin thickening) from rubbing, or both. These patients tend to have diabetes, lymphoma, renal failure, end-stage liver disease, and depression with no pathogen identified. Tricyclic antidepressants and topical steroids are used with varying results.

REFERENCE

Lynch PJ, Edwards L. In: Cynch PJ, ed. Genital Dermatology. New York, Churchill Livingstone, pp 229–235.

 ## PSA—Age-Adjusted

DESCRIPTION An age-specific scale of normal PSA values has been proposed, based on the observation that PSA rises with age, in an effort to reduce unnecessary prostate biopsies. Patients with a benign digital rectal examination, with a PSA within the normal PSA range for age, would avoid prostate biopsy, even if PSA level is above the normal threshold of 4 ng/mL.

AGE (YEARS)	AGE-SPECIFIC REFERENCE RANGE
40–49	0.0–2.5 ng/mL
50–59	0.0–3.5 ng/mL
60–69	0.0–4.5 ng/mL
70–79	0.0–6.5 ng/mL

REFERENCE

Oesterling JE, et al. Serum prostate-specific antigen in a community based population of healthy men. *JAMA* 1993;270(7):860–864.

 ## PSA Density (PSAD)

DESCRIPTION Ratio of prostate-specific antigen (PSA) level to prostate size, as measured by transrectal ultrasound (TRUS). Proposed as a method to differentiate an elevated PSA between 4.0 and 10.0 ng/mL, without evidence of prostate cancer on digital rectal examination or TRUS, as due to benign prostatic hyperplasia or adenocarcinoma, to prevent unnecessary prostate biopsies. A PSAD of 0.15 or greater would warrant prostate biopsy. Use of PSA density remains controversial.

REFERENCE

Seaman E, et al. Prostate specific antigen density (PSAD): Role in patient evaluation and management. *Urol Clin North Am* 1993; 20:653–663.

 ## PSA—Free and Total

DESCRIPTION PSA is found either free in serum or bound to serum proteins. Patients with prostate cancer tend to have lower free PSA levels in proportion to total PSA. Measurement of the free PSA percentage can improve the specificity of PSA as a cancer screening test. Patients with mildly elevated PSA (4.0–10.0 ng/mL) would have prostate biopsy only if the free PSA percentage is low. The free PSA percentage threshold for biopsy is controversial, ranging from less than 15% to less than 25%, with a higher threshold having improved sensitivity and a lower threshold having improved specificity.

REFERENCE

Catalona WJ, et al. Use of the percentage of free prostate-specific antigen to enhance differentiation of prostate cancer from benign prostatic disease. *JAMA* 1998;279(19):1542–1547.

 ## PSA—Race-Adjusted

DESCRIPTION A separate proposed scale of normal PSA values, adjusted for race as well as age. Based on the observation that African-American males have higher average PSA values when adjusted for age, in the absence of prostate cancer. Developed to improve the sensitivity of PSA as a screening test in the African-American population, which has a significantly higher incidence and mortality from prostate cancer when compared with Caucasians. Use of these tables is controversial. (See also PSA—Walter Reed/CDPR Reference Ranges below.)

AGE (YEARS)	RACE-SPECIFIC REFERENCE RANGE	
	WHITES	BLACKS
40–49	0.0–2.5 ng/mL	0.0–2.0 ng/mL
50–59	0.0–3.5 ng/mL	0.0–4.0 ng/mL
60–69	0.0–3.5 ng/mL	0.0–4.5 ng/mL
70–79	0.0–3.5 ng/mL	0.0–5.5 ng/mL

REFERENCE

Morgan TO, Jacobsen SJ, McCarthy WF, Jacobson DG, Moul JW. Age-specific reference ranges for serum prostate-specific antigen in black men. *N Engl J Med* 1996;335:304–310.

 ## PSA RT-PCR

DESCRIPTION Use of reverse transcriptase–polymerase chain reaction (RT-PCR) to amplify mRNA transcripts of PSA. First clinical reports in 1992. These PSA mRNA species should theoretically only be present in prostate tissues. Tested in extraprostatic tissue of patients with biopsy-proven prostate cancer, including peripheral blood, lymph nodes, and bone marrow, to detect PSA mRNA transcripts and presumably prostate cells in extraprostatic sites. It is being investigated as an assay to detect micrometastasis of prostate cancer before clinical presentation or evidence of disease spread ("molecular staging"). Its clinical utility as a diagnostic assay remains uncertain.

REFERENCE

Gomella LG, Raj GV, Moreno JG. Reverse transcriptase polymerase chain reaction for prostate specific antigen in the management of prostate cancer. *J Urol* 1997;158:326–337.

 ## PSA Velocity

DESCRIPTION Measurement of change in serial measurements of PSA over time. A rate of rise in PSA of 0.75 ng/mL or greater per year is suspicious for prostate cancer, based on at least three separate assays 6 months apart. Measurement of PSA velocity has been advocated to improve the specificity of PSA as a prostate cancer screening test.

REFERENCE

Carter HB, et al. Longitudinal evaluation of prostate-specific antigen levels in men with and without prostate disease. *JAMA* 1992; 267:2215–2220.

PSA—Walter Reed/CDPR Reference Ranges

 PSA—Walter Reed/CDPR Reference Ranges

DESCRIPTION These are age-specific reference ranges for the PSA test, based on the 5th percentile of the distribution of PSA levels in the patients according to race. The reference range values are represented in the following table. (See also Section III, "PSA—Race-Adjusted.")

AGE	WHITE	BLACK
40–49	0.0–2.5	0.0–2.0
50–59	0.0–3.5	0.0–4.0
60–69	0.0–3.5	0.0–4.5
70–79	0.0–3.5	0.0–5.5

REFERENCE

Morgan TO, Jacobsen SJ, McCarthy WF, Jacobson DG, Moul JW. Age-specific reference ranges for serum prostate-specific antigen in black men. *N Engl J Med* 1996;335:304–310.

 Pseudodyssynergia (Hinman Syndrome)

DESCRIPTION Form of detrusor–external sphincter dyssynergia, in which there is voluntary contraction of external sphincter during detrusor contraction. Functional voiding dysfunction seen in children with intractable voiding symptoms, men with chronic prostatitis or prostatodynia, and women with urethral syndrome. May sometimes be a cause of urinary incontinence. Diagnosis based on urodynamic evidence of increased or vacillating external sphincter activity during detrusor contraction, usually with simultaneous elevation of intraabdominal pressure (indicating voluntary nature of contraction), without clinical evidence of neurologic deficit

SYNONYMS

- Nonneurogenic neurogenic bladder
- Hinman syndrome/Hinman-Allen syndrome (in children)
- Dysfunctional voiding syndrome

CAUSES

- Learned behavioral abnormality thought to be overcompensation of continence mechanism

TREATMENT

- Children need to be motivated to participate in the therapy.
- Need to teach how to void properly and how to defecate properly
- Timed voiding, voiding diary, double voiding, psychotherapy, and biofeedback may all be appropriate in select children.
- Anticholinergics may control instability; alpha-adrenergics may improve outlet resistance.
- Psychotherapy, with a change in parental attitude, can greatly improve the situation.

- Intermittent catheterization may be necessary in more difficult cases (e.g., with upper tract changes, failure to respond to less invasive measures).
- Biofeedback

REFERENCE

Kaplan SA, et al. Pseudodyssynergia (contraction of the external sphincter during voiding) misdiagnosed as chronic nonbacterial prostatitis and the role of biofeedback as a therapeutic option. *J Urol* 1997;157(6):2234–2237.

 PSMA (Prostate-Specific Membrane Antigen)

DESCRIPTION Membrane-bound protein found in prostatic epithelial cells. PSMA levels reported to be elevated in hormone refractory prostate cancer and with metastatic disease. Its use as a tumor marker, similar to PSA, is being investigated as a more accurate prognostic indicator.

REFERENCE

Murphy GP, et al. Evaluation and comparison of two new prostate carcinoma markers: Free-prostate specific antigen and prostate specific membrane antigen. *Cancer* 1996;78(4):809–818.

 Psoas Hitch Procedure

DESCRIPTION Used to replace short segments of distal ureteral loss or in combination with a ureteral reimplantation to provide a fixed posterior bladder wall. The bladder is mobilized and stretched superiorly along the axis of the ureteral deficit. The stretched bladder is then sutured to the fascia of the ilio-psoas muscle.

REFERENCE

Amis ES, Newhouse JH, eds. *Essentials of Uroradiology,* 1st ed. Boston: Little, Brown, 1991:370.

 Psoriasis—External Genitalia

DESCRIPTION Chronic papulosquamous skin disease frequently affecting external genitalia, more common in males. Genital involvement reported in 25% to 40% of patients with psoriasis. Lesions characteristically are sharply demarcated plaques with silvery, scaly patches. Most frequently involves penis in males and mons pubis, labia majora, and inguinal crease in females. Reported to increase risk of squamous cell carcinoma of genitalia

TREATMENT

- Topical steroids
- Tar preparations
- Good hygiene

REFERENCES

Farber EM, Nall L. Genital psoriasis. *Cutis* 1992;50(4):263–266.

Loughlin KR. Psoriasis: Association with 2 rare cutaneous urological malignancies. *J Urol* 1997;157(2):622–623.

 Pyelitis Cystica

DESCRIPTION Ingrowth of urothelial cells into lamina propria with subsequent liquefaction, giving cystlike appearance. Identical to cystitis cystica, occurring in the renal pelvis and calyces. Rare condition, usually associated with chronic infection. More common in females, and usually occurs above age 50 years. Presenting symptoms are related to chronic infections, including fever, dysuria, hematuria, and flank pain. Identified on radiographic studies as multiple small cysts up to 10 mm in diameter in renal pelvis and calyces, and confirmed by endoscopic biopsy. Not thought to be premalignant condition, but recommend urine cytology and biopsy to rule out other neoplastic conditions

REFERENCE

Gronlund A, Glenthoj A, Kvist E. Pyelitis cystica. *Scand J Urol Nephrol* 1997;31(5):509–511.

 Pyelitis Glandularis

DESCRIPTION In this condition, combined urothelial hyperplastic and metaplastic changes of the renal pelvis occur. Characteristic glandular structures haphazardly arranged within the lamina propria are seen. Those glands are lined by mucin-secreting columnar epithelial cells, which differentiate them from other forms of urothelial hyperplasia as Vonbrunn's nests and pyelitis cystica. It is not uncommon to see the later hyperplastic changes and pyelitis glandularis in a single specimen. Intracellular and luminal mucin can be demonstrated by mucicarmine stain. Most commonly, the overlying surface epithelium remains of the transitional cell type. However, metaplastic squamous epithelium or mucus-secreting columnar cells may be seen. Pyelitis glandularis is commonly focal. Extensive lesions with columnar cell metaplasia of the surface urothelium have high resemblance to colonic mucosa. However, the absence of muscularis mucosa helps distinguish these two entities.

REFERENCE

Krag DO, Alcott DL. Glandular metaplasia of the renal pelvis: Report of a case. *Am J Clin Pathol* 1957;29:672.

Pyonephrosis

DESCRIPTION   Infected, obstructed collecting system with grossly purulent drainage and suppurative necrosis of renal parenchyma. It can be a chronic, indolent infection, but it usually presents acutely with sepsis, flank pain, and ipsilateral loss of renal function. Immediate aspiration with retrograde or percutaneous catheter drainage is essential.

REFERENCE

Baumgarten DA, Baumgartner BR. Imaging and radiologic management of upper urinary tract infections. *Urol Clin North Am* 1997;24(3): 545–569.

 Q-tip Test

DESCRIPTION   The Q-tip test is also useful to evaluate the urethral axis and evidence of hypermobility in the evaluation of urinary incontinence in the female. A Q-tip is advanced transurethrally to the level of the bladder neck and observed for changes in angle during straining maneuvers. Hypermobility suggests that a bladder neck suspension may restore continence.

REFERENCE

Dupont MC, Albo ME, Raz S. Diagnosis of stress urinary incontinence. *Urol Clin North Am* 1996;23(3):407–415

 Quakel's Corporal Shunt

DESCRIPTION   Used for the treatment of priapism. Through a scrotal perineal approach, a longitudinal incision is made in the outer bulbar urethra (making sure not to completely traverse and injure the urethra), and a parallel incision is made in the corporal body. After irrigating stagnant corporal blood, these two incisions are anastomosed.

REFERENCE

Thomas AJ. Surgery for priapism. In: Novick AC, Streem SB, Pontes JE, eds. *Stewarts Operative Urology.* Baltimore: Williams & Wilkins, 1989:826–832.

 Raz Bladder Neck Suspension (Urethropexy)

DESCRIPTION   This one of many surgical bladder neck suspension techniques aiming to fix the vesicourethral junction in a physiologic position to correct genuine stress incontinence in females. A modification of the Pereyra needle suspension. Through an inverted U-shaped incision in the anterior vaginal wall, the operator performs (1) retropubic urethrolysis, (2) fingertip guidance of a double-pronged suture carrier placed through a suprapubic opening, and (3) placement of helical nonabsorbable sutures through the urethropelvic ligament, otherwise known as the endopelvic fascia. Cystoscopy is performed after the sutures are placed. Best suited for urethral and bladder neck hypermobility and no cystocele

REFERENCE

Raz S, Stothers L, Chopra A. Vaginal reconstructive surgery for incontinence and prolapse. In: Walsh PC, Retik AB, Vaughan ED, Wein AJ, eds. *Campbell's Urology,* 7th ed. Philadelphia: WB Saunders, 1998:1066–1094.

 Raz Vaginal Wall Sling

DESCRIPTION   Technique to treat urinary incontinence due to intrinsic sphincter dysfunction or anatomic incontinence. A modification of the original Raz bladder neck suspension, this technique provides support for both the bladder neck and mid-urethra. In addition to the principal maneuvers described in the Raz urethropexy, the author incorporates a patch of anterior vaginal wall with the suspension sutures at the level of the bladder neck, which, in effect, creates a hammock that serves as a backboard to the bladder neck and mid-urethra.

REFERENCE

Raz S, Stothers L, Chopra A. Vaginal reconstructive surgery for incontinence and prolapse. In: Walsh PC, Retik AB, Vaughan ED, Wein AJ, eds. *Campbell's Urology,* 7th ed. Philadelphia: WB Saunders, 1998:1066–1094.

 Reifenstein Syndrome

DESCRIPTION   Form of incomplete male pseudohermaphroditism, usually presenting with perineoscrotal hypospadias, and frequently cryptorchidism at birth, with azoospermia and incomplete virilization at puberty, and infertility and gynecomastia at or after puberty. Usually assigned to male sex at birth. Exhibit elevated levels of testosterone and luteinizing hormone

SYNONYMS

- Lubb syndrome
- Gilbert-Dreyfus syndrome
- Type 1 incomplete male pseudohermaphroditism

CAUSES

- Mutations in DNA-binding domain of androgen receptor, with varying degrees of androgen receptor dysfunction

TREATMENT

- Surgical repair of hypospadias and cryptorchidism
- Supplemental testosterone is *not* beneficial.

REFERENCES

Klocker H, et al. Point mutation in the DNA binding domain of the androgen receptor in two families with Reifenstein syndrome. *Am J Hum Genet* 1992;50(6):1318–1327.

Wilson JD, et al. *Harrison's Principle of Internal Medicine,* 12th ed. New York: McGraw-Hill, 1991:1808–1809.

 Reinke Crystals

DESCRIPTION   Cytoplasmic crystalloid inclusions found in human Leydig cells. Crystals are large, distinctive, and easily visible under light microscopy. Noted to increase in number with age. Their function or significance is unknown.

REFERENCE

Kerr JB. Ultrastructure of the seminiferous epithelium and intertubular tissue of the human testis. *J Electron Microsc Technique* 1991;19(2): 215–240.

Reiter Syndrome

 Reiter Syndrome

DESCRIPTION Classic triad of polyarthritis, conjunctivitis, and nongonococcal urethritis. Thought to be systematic inflammatory response triggered by microbial infection in genitourinary or gastrointestinal tracts. Arthritis usually asymmetric, with predominately lower extremity involvement. Joint aspiration typically sterile, but can exhibit bacterial fragments, DNA, RNA, and lipopolysaccharide indicative of latent infection. Association with HLA-B27 noted, and may confer susceptibility

SYNONYMS

- Reactive arthritis

CAUSES

- *Chlamydia trachomatis*
- *Salmonella* species
- *Shigella* species
- *Yersinia* species
- *Ureaplasma urealyticum*

TREATMENT

- Prolonged antibiotic treatment with tetracyclines
- Supportive care

REFERENCE

Hughes RA, Keat AC. Reiter's syndrome and reactive arthritis: A current view. *Semin Arthritis Rheum* 1994;24(3):190–210.

 Renal Agenesis

DESCRIPTION Congenital anomaly with absence of one or both kidneys. Bilateral agenesis, with associated renal failure, oligohydramnios, and hypoplastic lungs, incompatible with life (see Section III, "Potter Syndrome/Potter Facies"). Occurs in 1 in 3000 births. Unilateral renal agenesis is more common, occurring in 1 in 1000 births and more commonly in males. Associated with other anomalies, including single umbilical artery, absence of ipsilateral ureter and hemitrigone, vaginal atresia/agenesis (Mayer-Rokitansky syndrome), unilateral vas deferens agenesis/atresia, and seminal vesicle cysts. Other organ systems commonly affected: cardiovascular (30%) (valvular or septal cardiac anomalies); gastrointestinal (25%) (imperforate anus or atresia of anus or esophagus); and vertebral or pharyngeal anomalies. Patients are at risk for hypertension and renal failure, warranting yearly follow-up.

REFERENCE

Robson WLM, Leung AKC, Rogers RC. Unilateral renal agenesis. *Adv Pediatr* 1995;42:575–592.

 Renal Anatomy—Normal Radiographic Findings

DESCRIPTION In adults, a normal kidney is between three and four vertebral bodies in length. On ultrasonography, the normal right and left kidneys measure 10.7 cm and 11.1 cm, respectively; at autopsy, 11.2 cm and 11.8 cm, respectively; and on excretory urography, 12.6 cm and 13.8 cm, respectively. The majority of normal kidneys have 10 to 14 minor calyces.

REFERENCE

Amis ES, Newhouse JH, eds. *Essentials of Uroradiology*, 1st ed. Boston: Little, Brown, 1991:7.

 Renal Artery Aneurysm

DESCRIPTION Similar to arterial aneurysms in other locations, aneurysms can occur in renal arteries. Incidence ranges from 0.3% to 1.0% on radiographic studies, accounting for 1% of all arterial aneurysms and 10% of visceral aneurysms. Commonly bilateral or multiple (20% and 30%, respectively). Occur typically in the fifth or sixth decade of life, and slightly more common on the right. Classification includes saccular (most common), fusiform, dissecting, and intrarenal. Associated with hypertension, but a causal effect has not been shown. Spontaneous rupture is rare, but risk is increased during pregnancy. Presentation is usually secondary to hypertension, flank pain, hematuria, or an incidental finding on radiographic study.

CAUSES

- Atherosclerotic disease
- Fibromuscular dysplasia
- Congenital
- Trauma
- Intrarenal aneurysms: collagen vascular diseases (polyarteritis nodosa, Wegener's granulomatosis), infectious causes (syphilis or tuberculosis)

TREATMENT

- Surgical repair is indicated for symptomatic lesions, lesions >4.0 cm, spontaneous rupture, or asymptomatic lesions in high-risk patients (women of childbearing age or patients with functional or anatomic solitary kidney).

—Repair includes primary repair with excision of aneurysmal segment, or aortorenal bypass with vein.
—Extraanatomic bypass (hepatorenal, gastroduodenal–renal, or splenorenal) is useful for a severely calcified aorta or when aortic cross-clamping is undesirable.
—Autotransplantation is useful for complex repairs with long ischemic time.
—Percutaneous treatment with embolization or occlusion of aneurysmal segments is reserved for high-risk surgical candidates.

—Intraluminal vascular stent placement is being investigated.

REFERENCE

Cinat M, Yoon P, Wilson SE. Management of renal artery aneurysms. *Semin Vasc Surg* 1996;9(3):236–244.

 Renal Artery Fibromuscular Dysplasia

DESCRIPTION Fibromuscular diseases of the renal artery account for one-third of cases of renovascular hypertension. Four pathologic entities have been described. Intimal fibroplasia affects mainly children and young male adults. Angiographically, a smooth focal stenosis is typically seen at the midrenal artery or its branches. Prompt repair is advised because of the progressive nature of the disease. Fibromuscular hyperplasia of smooth muscle and fibrous tissue is rare, progressive, and affects mainly children and young adults. Medial fibroplasia is the most common (80%), affecting women in their 30s. On angiogram, it has the appearance of a string of beads. This lesion does not dissect, and complete occlusion has not been reported. Angioplasty is the treatment of choice. Perimedial fibroplasia is a tightly stenotic, progressive, lesion, affecting women 15 to 30 years of age. On angiography, extensive collateral vessels are commonly identified.

REFERENCE

Schreiber MJ, Pohl MA, Novick AC. The natural history of atherosclerotic and fibrous renal artery disease. *Urol Clin North Am* 1984;11:383.

 Renal Carcinoid Tumor

DESCRIPTION Rare tumor derived from enterochromaffin or amine precursor uptake and decarboxylation (APUD) cells, occurring most commonly in the gastrointestinal tract and lung, but also occurring in ovaries, testes, thymus, pancreas, and hepatobiliary system. Primary renal lesions are extremely rare, with only 32 cases reported. Thought to originate in renal collecting cells undergoing intestinal metaplasia or from teratomatous epithelial cells within the kidney. Horseshoe kidneys are shown to have a markedly elevated risk of carcinoid tumor, though still very rare, and may have a more benign course.

REFERENCE

Krishnan B, et al. Horseshoe kidney is associated with an increased relative risk of primary renal carcinoid tumor. *J Urol* 1997;157(6): 2059–2066.

Renal Cell Carcinoma—Papillary

DESCRIPTION   Uncommon variant of renal cell carcinomas, representing approximately 10% of renal cell carcinomas. Exhibit a tubulo-papillary growth pattern. Hereditary pattern demonstrated in a small number of families, and tending to be multifocal, bilateral, and associated with loss of short arm of chromosome 3

REFERENCE

Zbar B, et al. Hereditary papillary renal cell carcinoma: Clinical studies in 10 families. *J Urol* 1995;153(3):907–912.

 Renal Cell Carcinoma— Sarcomatoid

DESCRIPTION   Uncommon histologic variant of renal cell carcinoma, with an approximate incidence of 5% to 10% of all renal cell carcinomas. Histologically, composed of clear cells and pleomorphic spindle cells resembling sarcoma. Tends to have more malignant behavior and worse prognosis, with higher local recurrence, more frequent metastasis, and shorter survival

REFERENCE

Sella A, et al. Sarcomatoid renal cell carcinoma. A treatable entity. *Cancer* 1987;60(6): 1313–1318.

 Renal Cholesterol Microembolism Syndrome

DESCRIPTION   Cholesterol microembolism of the kidney is an uncommon cause of hypertensive urgency, affecting mainly elderly men with atherosclerotic vascular disease. Clinical findings include severe hypertension, digital gangrene, livedo reticularis, cerebrovascular accidents, gastrointestinal hemorrhage or infarction, bowel perforation, retinal emboli, and eosinophilia. Dialysis for renal insufficiency might be necessary. Diagnosis is made from clinical history, physical examination, lab findings, and selective renal angiogram, and is confirmed by renal biopsy. In the kidneys, intralobular and arcuate arteries are most frequently affected.

CAUSES

- Spontaneous
- Iatrogenic
- Angiographic manipulation
- Cardiovascular surgery
- Anticoagulant medications

TREATMENT

- Supportive
- Management of hypertension and renal insufficiency
- Control of the underlying pathology

REFERENCE

Lye WC, Cheah JS, Sinniah R. Renal cholesterol embolic disease. Case report and review of the literature. *Am J Nephrol* 1993;13:489.

 Renal Hemangioma

DESCRIPTION   These are benign vascular neoplasms, usually diagnosed in the third to fifth decade, with no sex predilection. The most common presenting symptom is intermittent hematuria. Angiographic appearance varies markedly. Hypervascular, hypovascular, and normal lesions have been reported. In the past, a clinical finding of unilateral hematuria and a suggestive angiographic pattern were the basis of preoperative diagnosis. Currently, hemangioma can be identified ureteroscopically, without the need for a biopsy, where they may appear as small, red, or bluish spots on the tip or base of a papilla, or they may be large, bulbous, erythematous lesions on the papillary tips. Pathologically, hemangiomas would have the gross appearance of a well-demarcated lesion that shows a cluster of blood-filled vascular channels. Microscopically, the majority of cases conform to the typical features of cavernous hemangioma, with variable large blood-filled vascular tributaries in a disorganized tangle. Variation in vascular wall thickness and structure indicates arterial and venous components. The benign cytologic feature of flat lining endothelial cells allows for differentiation of this lesion from angiosarcoma.

TREATMENT

- Ureteroscopic electrocauterization or laser ablation using holmium, ND:YAG, or a combination of both
- Surgical resection

REFERENCE

Waller JI, Throckmorton MA, Barbosa E. Renal hemangioma. *J Urol* 1995;74:186.

 Renal Hemangiopericytoma

DESCRIPTION   Rare primary sarcoma of the kidney, accounting for 1% to 3% of renal malignancies. Solid hypervascular mass with calcifications, originating from pericytes, located external to endothelial cells of capillaries, and enveloped by basement membrane. Can be metabolically active, secreting renin. Common presenting signs include flank pain, flank mass, hypertension, hypoglycemia, and hematuria. Can have malignant potential, and should be considered a surgical lesion.

TREATMENT

- Radical nephrectomy

REFERENCE

Bowers DL, et al. Renal hemangiopericytoma. Case report and review of the literature. *Urol Int* 1995;55(3):162–166.

 Renal Leiomyoma

DESCRIPTION   Rare benign renal tumor, with an incidence of 5% on autopsy series. Originates from smooth muscle, usually from renal capsule or vessels, and less commonly from renal pelvis. Radiographically, can appear as solid or cystic mass, difficult to differentiate from renal cell carcinoma, usually prompting radical nephrectomy

REFERENCE

Woo HH, Farnsworth RH. Renal leiomyoma. *Br J Urol* 1994;74(4):525–526.

 Renal Malrotation

DESCRIPTION   The abnormal orientation of the kidney, so that there is no medial position of the renal pelvis, with the calyces pointing laterally. May occur in cases of ectopia, fusion, and complete renal ascent. Incidence of 1 in 390. Three types:

- Nonrotation: The renal pelvis is anterior.
- Reverse rotation: The renal pelvis is lateral.
- Hyperrotation: The renal pelvis is posterior.

Symptoms are usually absent; occasionally, vague abdominal pain and/or vomiting due to renal obstruction. Patients may develop ureteral obstruction, infections, or calculi. Diagnosis is made typically on excretory urography with altered orientation of the calyces and pelves. Retrograde pyelography is often useful to define the anatomy. No treatment is necessary unless symptoms, stones, or obstruction become problematic. Follow-up ultrasound to evaluate for stones or hydronephrosis

REFERENCE

Kelalis P, King L, Belman B, eds. *Clinical Pediatric Urology*, 3rd ed, vol 1. 1992:505–507.

Renal Pseudotumors

 Renal Pseudotumors

DESCRIPTION   Benign condition of the kidney, mimicking renal neoplasm on radiographic studies. Most commonly is hypertrophied column of Bertin (sometimes referred to as an anomalous calyx), a prominent medullary column usually located between upper and middle pole calyceal infundibula, that can appear as a renal mass but is homogeneous with surrounding renal parenchyma, with normal appearing calyces. Other conditions giving appearance of renal tumor include fetal lobulation, lobar dysmorphism, dromedary hump, lobar nephronia, and renal sinus lipomatosis. (See also Section I, "Renal Masses—Benign and Malignant.")

REFERENCE

Bosniak MA. Problems in the radiologic diagnosis of renal parenchymal tumors. *Urol Clin North Am* 1993;20(2):217–230.

 Renal–Retinal Syndrome

DESCRIPTION   Actually a subtype of juvenile nephronophthisis. (See Section III, "Juvenile Nephronophthisis."). Occurs in about 1 out of 7 cases of JN. These patients have concomitant retinitis pigmentosa, which is slowly progressive and bilateral, with retinal degeneration. Rods are affected, leading to defective night vision that becomes symptomatic in early childhood. Midperipheral ring scotoma gradually widens. The retina becomes darkly pigmented, with a boney-spiculed appearance. The disk may look yellow and waxy.

SYNONYMS

• Juvenile nephronophthisis with retinal disease

CAUSES

• Autosomal recessive disease mapped to chromosome 2

TREATMENT

• Renal replacement therapy, as needed

REFERENCE

Lippert M. Renal cystic disease. In: Gillenwater JY, Grayhack JT, Howards SS, Duckett JW, eds. *Adult and Pediatric Urology*, 3rd ed. St Louis: Mosby, 1996.

 Renal Vein—Leiomyosarcoma of

DESCRIPTION   Rare tumor arising from smooth muscle element of renal vein, most commonly on left side. Striking female predominance (85% of the 27 reported cases), usually in sixth decade of life. Presenting symptoms include flank or abdominal pain, weight loss, and a palpable abdominal mass. Visualized with CT, revealing homogeneous, well-circumscribed mass at or near the renal hilum, commonly encasing renal vein. Mean survival is 28 months, with an aggressive malignant pattern to distant sites, including lung, liver, bone, skin and soft tissue, and brain.

TREATMENT

• Aggressive surgical resection with nephrectomy and en bloc resection
• Nonsurgical treatment with XRT and chemotherapy is ineffective.

REFERENCE

Brandes SB, et al. Leiomyosarcoma of the renal vein. *J Surg Oncol* 1996;63(3):195–200.

 Reninoma

DESCRIPTION   Rare tumor of the juxtaglomerular apparatus. Usual presentation is in a young female with severe, refractory, frequently paroxysmal, hypertension with hypokalemia, hyperaldosteronism, and elevated plasma renin levels. Tumors are typically small and not always visualized on CT scan. Selective renal vein sampling for renin may help localize the lesion. It is generally a benign tumor, although untreated hypertension can be fatal.

SYNONYMS

• Renin-secreting juxtaglomerular cell tumor

TREATMENT

• Radical nephrectomy

REFERENCE

Baert J, et al. Juxtaglomerular cell tumor: Importance of clinical suspicion. *Urol Int* 1995;54(3):171–174.

 Renoalimentary Fistula

DESCRIPTION   A broad group of nonanatomic communications between the upper urinary collecting system and the alimentary canal, with nephrocolic fistulas being the most common. Symptoms vary from gastrointestinal symptoms, such as nausea, vomiting, and diarrhea, to recurrent urinary tract infections with flank pain and fever. Retrograde ureterography is generally needed to illustrate the fistula. (See also Section I, "Fistula—Enterovesical.")

CAUSES

• Renal inflammatory disease (acute/chronic)
• Malignancy of either intestinal or renal origin
• Iatrogenic, e.g., percutaneous surgery
• Trauma

TREATMENT

• Conservative: stenting or nephrostomy tube
• Nephrectomy with removal of fistula tract and bowel resection

REFERENCE

Bissada NK, Cole AT, Fried FA. Reno-alimentary fistula: An unusual urological problem. *J Urol* 1973;110:273.

 Renobronchial Fistula

DESCRIPTION   Fistulous communication between pleural cavity and kidney, associated with pyelonephritis and perinephric abscess. Usually presents with flank or abdominal pain with ipsilateral pneumonia, and patients commonly have history of pyelonephritis or abdominal abscess. Can involve pleural space alone or erode into lung parenchyma and bronchial tree. Diagnosis is made with CT scan.

SYNONYMS

• Nephrobronchial fistula
• Renal—bronchopleural fistula

CAUSES

• Pyelonephritis with perinephric abscess
• Xanthogranulomatous pyelonephritis
• Most common pathogens: *E. coli* and *Proteus* species
• Tubercular infections also reported

TREATMENT

• Percutaneous or open drainage and antibiotic therapy acutely
• Often requires nephrectomy

REFERENCE

O'Brien JD, Ettinger NA. Nephrobronchial fistula and lung abscess resulting from nephrolithiasis and pyelonephritis. *Chest* 1995;108(4):1166–1168.

Renomedullary Interstitial Cell Tumor

DESCRIPTION Tumor of interstitial cells found within the juxtaglomerular apparatus, which are involved in prostaglandin metabolism and counterbalance the renin–angiotensin system. Small tumor nodules composed of interstitial cells common at autopsy, occurring in 44% of older individuals. Often incidentally discovered at nephrectomy for other causes. Do not appear to have any undue effect on arterial blood pressure

REFERENCE

Mai KT. Giant renomedullary interstitial cell tumor. *J Urol* 1994;151(4):986–988.

 ## Rete Testis—Adenocarcinoma

DESCRIPTION Rare, highly malignant tumor arising from rete testis. Usually occurs in older men, but reported in men as young as 17 years old. Commonly presents with painless scrotal mass or symptoms related to metastasis. Pathology reveals papillary adenocarcinoma in rete testis, commonly with local invasion. May be associated with maldescended testis or adenomatous hyperplasia of rete testis. Prognosis poor, with less than 50% survival at 1 year. Metastatic sites include retroperitoneal lymph nodes, lungs, bone, and liver. The diagnostic criteria include

- Tumor in mediastinum separate from body of testis
- Transition in rete testis from normal epithelium to neoplastic cells
- No evidence of teratoma
- No primary tumor elsewhere
- Intact parietal tunica

TREATMENT

- Radical orchiectomy is the mainstay of treatment.
- XRT and chemotherapy have limited efficacy for metastatic disease.
- Retroperitoneal lymph node dissection may have a role in the absence of metastasis.

REFERENCE

Gruber H, et al. Adenocarcinoma of the rete testis: Report of a case with surgical history of adenomatous hyperplasia of the rete testis. *J Urol* 1997;158(4):1525–1526.

 ## Retrocaval/Circumcaval Ureter

DESCRIPTION A rare congenital anomaly in which the infrarenal vena cava (IVC) is derived from right subcardinal or postcardinal vein, anterior to the ureter. The term *circumcaval ureter* refers to the ureter emerging medial to IVC after running behind it, where the term *retrocaval* applies for those ureters that only knuckle behind the IVC but reemerge laterally. Not all retrocaval/circumcaval ureters are obstructed. Males are affected 3 times more often than are females. Pain in the second, third, or fourth decade is the most common presentation. However, despite its congenital origin, symptoms are usually absent in childhood. Less commonly, patients present with hematuria or urinary tract infection.

REFERENCE

Bateson EM, Atkinson D. Circumcaval ureter: A new classification. *Clin Radiol* 1969;20:173.

 ## Retroperitoneal Lymphoma

DESCRIPTION Lymphoma involving retroperitoneal lymph nodes. Can be primary site of involvement or site of metastasis. Can cause extrinsic compression of ureters with obstructive uropathy. Positive diagnosis is made when a mass is visualized on CT scan or a ureteral obstruction is visualized with ultrasound or IVP. (See also Section I, "Retroperitoneal Mass.")

TREATMENT

- Systemic chemotherapy, with or without adjuvant radiotherapy
- Obstructive uropathy may require ureteral stenting or percutaneous decompression prior to chemotherapy.

REFERENCES

Klein EA, et al. Intraoperative consultation for the retroperitoneum and adrenal glands. *Urol Clin North Am* 1985;12(3):411–421.

Resnick MI, Kursh ED. Extrinsic obstruction of the ureter. In: Walsh PC, Retik AB, Vaughan ED, Wein AJ, eds. *Campbell's Urology*, 7th ed. Philadelphia: WB Saunders, 1998:411–414.

 ## Retroperitoneal Rheumatoid Nodules

DESCRIPTION Rheumatoid nodules (necrobiotic granulomas) are a common extraarticular manifestation of rheumatoid arthritis, usually found in subcutaneous tissue. They have been reported in numerous other locations, including blood vessels, larynx, pharynx, sclera, and extradural space. Genitourinary involvement is rare, including renal cortex and bladder. Retroperitoneal occurrence has been reported and can cause ureteral compression and obstruction, requiring ureterolysis and repair.

REFERENCE

Adelson GL, Saypol DC, Walker AN. Ureteral stenosis secondary to retroperitoneal rheumatoid nodules. *J Urol* 1982;127(1):124–125.

 ## Rhabdoid Tumor—Malignant

DESCRIPTION The most lethal renal neoplasm, formerly believed to be a form of Wilms' tumor. It comprises 2% of all renal tumors and affects children, with a median age of 1 year. The most common presentation is an abdominal mass detected in those young patients. Histologically, the cells are large, with large nuclei and very prominent nucleoli. In most cases, cytoplasmic eosinophilic inclusions (fibrils) can be demonstrated on electron microscopy. Although these large cells may suggest rhabdomyoblasts, actual presence of muscle could not be confirmed by light or electron microscopy. If striated muscle can be identified, as in conventional Wilms' tumor, the diagnosis of rhabdoid tumor can be excluded, and the outlook is better. Rhabdoid tumors tend to metastasize to the brain and have a high association with independent primary central nervous tumors. Extrarenal rhabdoid tumors also have been reported. The term *pseudomalignant rhabdoid tumors* refers to neoplasms lacking prominent nucleoli, exhibiting a serpentine growth pattern or containing malignant rhabdoid tumor-like cells in the background of a typical Wilms' tumor.

REFERENCE

Beckwith JB, Palmer NF. Histopathology and prognosis of Wilms' tumor: Results from the first National Wilms' Tumor Study. *Cancer* 1978;41:1937.

Rhabdomyolysis

 Rhabdomyolysis

DESCRIPTION Clinical syndrome of acute renal failure and myoglobinuria caused by damage or destruction of skeletal muscle. Mechanism of renal failure thought to be multifactorial, including hypovolemia from fluid sequestration in damaged muscle, direct tubular toxicity of myoglobin–metabolite hematin, or tubular obstruction due to myoglobin precipitation in acid environment. (See also Section III, "Myoglobinuria" and "Myoglobin Nephrotoxicity.")

CAUSES

- Burn injury
- Crush injury
- Compartment syndrome or ischemic injury to large muscle groups
- Seizures or malignant hyperthermia
- Prolonged coma
- Exaggerated lithotomy position during urologic, gynecologic, or orthopedic procedures

TREATMENT

- Aggressive fluid resuscitation with forced diuresis and urinary alkalinization
- Supportive care with intensive monitoring

REFERENCE

Biswas S, et al. Exaggerated lithotomy position-related rhabdomyolysis. *Am Surg* 1997;63(4):361–364.

 Rieger Syndrome

DESCRIPTION In the majority of cases, this is an autosomal dominant syndrome. It is manifested by ocular anomalies; maxillary hypoplasia; broad, flat nasal root; microdontia or anodontia; deafness; mental retardation; heart defects; and genitourinary anomalies in the form of hypospadias. An association with Down syndrome and Marfan syndrome has also been reported.

REFERENCE

Henkind P, Siegel IM, Carr RE. Mesodermal dysgenesis of the anterior segment: Rieger's anomaly. *Arch Ophthalmol* 1965;73:810.

 Rim Sign (Rim Nephrogram)

DESCRIPTION A radiographic appearance in which only a thin peripheral rind of renal tissue is visible. This condition occurs as a result of marked thinning of the parenchyma due to end-stage obstructive atrophy, and it usually denotes irretrievable renal function.

REFERENCE

Bedon WE, Levitt SB, Baker DH, et al. Hydronephrosis in infants and children: Value of high dosage excretory urography in predicting renal salvageability. *AJR* 1970;109:380.

 Robinow Syndrome

DESCRIPTION An autosomal dominant disease characterized by small genitalia, cryptorchidism, flat face, and short forearms

REFERENCE

Barkat AY, Seikaly MG, Perkaloustion VM. Urogenital abnormalities in genetic disease. *J Urol* 1986;136:778.

 Robson Staging System

DESCRIPTION Robson's modification of Flocks and Kadesky's staging system for renal cell carcinoma was the most commonly used in the United States. The fact that long-term evaluation of patients with stage IIIA without disease extension into perinephric fat and lymph nodes has shown survivals comparable to those of stages I and II, has currently led many investigators to prefer the TNM system prosed by IUAC. (See the appendix.) The Robson Staging system is as follows:

- Stage I: Tumor is confined within the kidney parenchyma (no involvement of perinephric fat, renal vein, or regional nodes).
- Stage II: Tumor involves the perinephric fat but is confined within Gerota's (including adrenal).
- Stage IIIA: Tumor involves the renal vein or inferior vena cava (IVC).
- Stage IIIB: Tumor involves regional lymph nodes.
- Stage IIIC: Tumor involves both local vessels and regional lymph nodes.
- Stage IVA: Tumor involves adjacent organs other than the adrenals (colon, pancreas, etc.).
- Stage IVB: distant metastasis

REFERENCE

Robson CJ, Churchill BM, Andreson W. The results of radical nephrectomy for renal cell carcinoma. *Trans Am Assoc Genitourin Surg* 1968; 60:122.

 Rokitansky-Kuster-Houser Syndrome

DESCRIPTION Absence of the vagina, with abnormal or absent uterus. Usually discovered during evaluation of a normal-appearing girl who presents with failure of menstruation at the time of expected puberty. Renal agenesis and skeletal anomalies are common. In some patients, cyclic abdominal pain suggestive of some functional endometrium is noted.

CAUSES

- Müllerian agenesis

TREATMENT

- Vaginal reconstruction with bowel or skin grafting

REFERENCE

Griffin JE, Edwards C, Madden JD, et al. Congenital absence of the vagina. The Mayer-Rokitansky-Kuster-Houser syndrome. *Ann Intern Med* 1976;85:224.

 Rosewater Syndrome

DESCRIPTION An infertility disorder associated with germ cell aplasia. On testicular biopsy, the seminiferous tubules would contain only Sertoli cells. This is considered irreversible and precludes germ cell restoration. Not infrequently, tubular and peritubular fibrosis would associate germ cell aplasia.

REFERENCE

Craig JM. The pathology of infertility. *Pathol Ann* 1975;10:299.

 Rovsing Syndrome

DESCRIPTION This is a symptom complex associated with horseshoe kidney, in which the patient experiences pain, nausea, and vomiting on hyperextension of the spine, due to compression of the isthmus of the fused kidney on the vena cava and aorta, accentuated by hypertension and accompanied by a sensation of fullness.

REFERENCE

Glenn JF. Analysis of 51 patients with horseshoe kidney. *N Engl J Med* 1959;261:684.

Rovsing's Polycystic Kidney Operation

DESCRIPTION Entails multiple unroofing of cysts, which do not prevent deterioration of renal function but may improve flank pain if the cysts cause obstruction of the collecting system.

REFERENCE

Novick AC, Streem AB. Surgery of the kidney. In: Walsh PC, Retik AB, Vaughan ED, Wein AJ, eds. *Campbell's Urology,* 7th ed. Philadelphia: WB Saunders, 1998:3055–3056.

 ## Sacral Agenesis—Urologic Considerations

DESCRIPTION The partial or complete absence of two or more lower vertebral bodies. Affected individuals may manifest a short gluteal crease, seen only inferiorly secondary to flattened buttocks. Other deformities, such as high-arched feet or claw or hammer toes, may be present. A standard anteroposterior or lateral film may be used to confirm the diagnosis. Symptoms of the disorder include upper or lower motor neuron lesions causing dysfunctional voiding.

CAUSES

- Maternal diabetes
- Genetic transmission
- Unknown teratogens

REFERENCE

Schranger-Stumpel C, Schrander J, Fryns JP, Hamers G. Caudal deficiency sequence in 7q terminal deletion. *Am J Med Genet* 1988;30(3):756–761.

 ## Sarcoidosis—Urologic Considerations

DESCRIPTION Sarcoidosis is a systemic granulomatous disease with unknown etiology. Most commonly affected sites include lungs, lymph nodes, central nervous system, skin, eyes, and liver, but genitourinary tract involvement has also been reported. Involvement of the bladder is most common, and exhibits gross hematuria and irritative voiding symptoms. Spinal cord involvement, with subsequent neurogenic lower urinary tract dysfunction, including detrusor hyperreflexia and detrusor–sphincter dyssynergia, has also been reported.

REFERENCES

Brownstein PK, et al. Sarcoidosis and malakoplakia. *Urology* 1975;6(2):249–251.

Fitzpatrick KJ, et al. Urologic manifestations of spinal cord sarcoidosis. *J Spinal Cord Med* 1996;19(3):201–203.

 ## Scabies

DESCRIPTION An intensely pruritic parasitic infection that affects simultaneous areas of the body, including the genitalia, anus, legs, hands, umbilicus, and axillae. Diagnosis can be made by identifying the mite expressed from the papular or linear burrow-like lesion. Transmission occurs from fomites or by direct contact with infected individuals, including sexual contact.

CAUSES

- *Sarcoptes scabiei*

TREATMENT

- Lindane 1% cream, washed off after 8 hours. Do not use in pregnant or lactating women or in children under 2 years.
- Permethrin 5% cream, washed off after 8 to 14 hours
- Crotamiton 10% cream for two consecutive nights; wash off 24 hours after the second application.
- Treat sex partners and close contacts.

REFERENCE

Peterson CM, Eichenfeld LF. Scabies. *Pediatr Ann* 1996;25(2):97–100.

 ## Scardino-Prince Pyeloplasty

DESCRIPTION An inverted J–configured incision is started on the anterior surface of the pelvis and brought down across the UPJ obstruction to a 1- to 2-cm point beyond the obstruction. The upper apex of the flap is then flipped down to the apex of the ureterotomy, where a 5-0 chromic stay suture is placed. The medial aspect of the flap is sutured to the lateral edge of the ureterotomy. The lateral edge of the flap is sutured to the lateral aspect of the ureterotomy, and the pelvis is closed. Used to treat UPJ obstruction

REFERENCE

Kay R. Procedures for ureteropelvic junction obstruction. In: Novick AC, Streem SB, Pontes JE, eds. *Stewarts Operative Urology.* Baltimore: Williams & Wilkins, 1989:220–233.

 ## Schiller-Duval Bodies

DESCRIPTION Perivascular papillary structures seen in histologic specimens of yolk sac tumors, similar to the endodermal sinuses of Duval in the placenta of the rat

REFERENCE

Moran CA, Suster S. Hepatoid yolk sac tumors of the mediastinum: A clinicopathologic and immunohistochemical study of four cases. *Am J Surg Pathol* 1997;21(10):1210–1214.

 ## Schistosomiasis—Urologic Considerations

DESCRIPTION Parasitic infection by the blood fluke *Schistosoma haematobium*. Has a broad spectrum of urologic manifestations, due to the parasite's life cycle: infection across the skin, hematogenous migration to perivesical venous plexus, transmural migration into bladder, shedding into urine. Typically, will exhibit polypoid urothelial mucosal lesions (active infection) or "sandy" patch flat, tan lesions (inactive infection). Can have significant upper urinary tract obstruction with chronic disease. Classic symptoms are hematuria and terminal dysuria. Linked to bladder cancer, occurring earlier in life (40–50 years old), and most commonly squamous cell carcinoma (60%–90%) and adenocarcinoma (5%–15%). Presence of fluke eggs in urinary sediment is diagnostic of schistosomiasis.

TREATMENT

- Medical management: metrifonate and praziquantel
- Surgical management: infection refractory to medical management; ureteral or bladder outlet obstruction; persistent or refractory hematuria; or malignancy

REFERENCES

Johansson SL, et al. Epidemiology and etiology of bladder cancer. *Semin Surg Oncol* 1997;13:291–298.

Smith JH, von Lichtenberg F. Parasitic diseases of the genitourinary system. In: Walsh PC, Retik AB, Vaughan ED, Wein AJ, eds. *Campbell's Urology,* 7th ed. Philadelphia: WB Saunders, 1998:733–757.

Schwannoma—Penile

 Schwannoma—Penile

DESCRIPTION A primary sarcoma arising from neural elements of the penis

SYNONYMS

- Penile neurofibrosarcoma

TREATMENT

- Surgical excision
- Radiation therapy
- Chemotherapy
- Observation

REFERENCE

Marsidi PJ, Winter CC. Schwannoma of the penis. *Urology* 1980;16:303.

 Schwannoma—Renal

DESCRIPTION A tumor arising from Schwann cell neural elements of the kidney

SYNONYMS

- Neurinoma
- Neurilemmoma

TREATMENT

- Surgical removal of the tumor
- Radiotherapy or chemotherapy is of unknown efficacy.

REFERENCE

Romics I, Bach D, Beutler W. Malignant schwannoma of the renal capsule. *Urology* 1992;40(5):453–455.

 Scleroderma—Urologic Considerations

DESCRIPTION Systemic, acquired disorder of connective tissue, including cutaneous sclerosis, visceral organ fibrosis, and vascular lesions. Commonly affects kidneys, with renal disease affecting 10% to 50% of patients. Lower urinary tract manifestations also reported, including bladder fibrosis, microscopic hematuria, urodynamic abnormalities, and poor compliance and obstructive uropathy. Lower urinary tract symptoms include urinary urgency, frequency, and incontinence.

SYNONYMS

- Systemic sclerosis

REFERENCE

Lally EV, et al. Pathologic involvement of the urinary bladder in progressive systemic sclerosis. *J Rheum* 1985;12:778–781.

 Sclerosing Adenosis of the Prostate

DESCRIPTION Part of histologic differential diagnosis of prostate cancer. Small glands with a proliferative stroma may be seen in needle biopsy or TUR specimens and have been misdiagnosed as cancer. Specimen will by immunoreactive with S-100 and smooth muscle actin, indicating a myoepithelial differentiation. Other features differentiating from cancer are that cells have bland nuclei and are sometimes surrounded by a hyaline-like sheath. (See also Section III, "Atypical Adenomatous Hyperplasia of the Prostate" and "Postatrophic Hyperplasia of the Prostate.")

SYNONYMS

- Pseudoadenomatoid tumor

REFERENCE

Epstein JI. Non-neoplastic diseases of the prostate. In: Bostwick D, et al. *Urologic Surgical Pathology*, 1st ed. St Louis: Mosby, 1997.

 Scrotum—Bifid

DESCRIPTION A disorder characterized by separation of the labioscrotal folds seen with midscrotal or perineal hypospadias and intersex disorders. Represents a spectrum of penoscrotal transposition abnormalities (see Section III, Scrotum—Engulfment")

CAUSES

- Failure of the genital swellings to fuse at the midline

TREATMENT

- Surgical realignment at the midline and hypospadias repair

REFERENCE

Sule JD, Skoog SJ, Tank ES. Perineal lipoma and the accessory labioscrotal fold: An etiological relationship. *J Urol* 1994;151(2):475–477.

 Scrotum—Engulfment

DESCRIPTION Most extreme form of penoscrotal transposition. Usually associated with hypospadias and chordee

SYNONYMS

- Penoscrotal transposition
- Scrotal engulfment

TREATMENT

- Hypospadias repair with scrotoplasty

REFERENCE

Parida SK, et al. Penoscrotal transposition and associated anomalies: Report of five new cases and review of the literature. *Am J Med Genet* 1995;59(1):68–75.

 Scrotum—Giant Neurilemmoma

DESCRIPTION Well-encapsulated tumors of neural elements within the scrotum. Most such tumors are benign, with malignant transformation as an extremely rare occurrence.

SYNONYMS

- Neurinoma
- Schwannoma

TREATMENT

- Surgical removal of lesion

REFERENCE

Fernandez MJ, Martino A, Khan H, Considine TJ, Burden J. Giant neurilemmoma: Unusual scrotal mass. *Urology* 1987;30(1):74–76.

Scrotum—Hemangioma

DESCRIPTION These lesions should be differentiated from angiokeratoma of Fordyce that appear in older men (see Section III). Scrotal hemangiomas are rare benign vascular lesions of the scrotum and can be seen in approximately 1% of newborns. Cutaneous hemangiomas (also called strawberry angiomas) may grow for up to 6 months and then undergo involution such that most do not need therapy. Subcutaneous hemangiomas are even more infrequent but tend to expand gradually and may clinically resemble a varicocele.

TREATMENT

• Large cutaneous lesions can be excised surgically or ablated with a laser.
• Most smaller lesions can be expected to involute over time.
• Subcutaneous lesions usually require surgical excision.

REFERENCE

Alter GJ, Trengove-Jones G, Horton CE Jr. Hemangioma of the penis and scrotum. *Urology* 1993;42(2):205–208.

 ## Scrotum—Hypoplasia

DESCRIPTION The unilateral or bilateral underdevelopment of the scrotum, which simulates labia majora, most commonly associated with cryptorchid testes and ambiguous genitalia

TREATMENT

• A testicular prosthesis can improve the cosmetic appearance of the scrotum.
• Testosterone cream can also be applied for an improved cosmetic result on the affected side.

REFERENCE

Maat-Kievit A, Brunner HG, Maaswinkel-Mooij P. Two additional cases of the Ohdo blepharophimosis syndrome. *Am J Med Genet* 1993;47(6):901–906.

 ## Scrotum—Idiopathic Calcinosis

DESCRIPTION Patients are typically young men and present with multiple hard nodules throughout the scrotal wall. Although the skin is usually intact, lesions may ulcerate. Thought to be caused by calcification of the scrotal dermal connective tissue (eccrine sweat glands) for unknown reasons. No therapy necessary unless there are recurrent episodes of infection; then surgical excision may help.

REFERENCE

Song DH, et al. Idiopathic calcinosis of the scrotum: Histopathologic observations of fifty-one nodules. *J Am Acad Dermatol* 1988;19: 1095–1101.

 ## Scrotum—Sebaceous Cyst

DESCRIPTION Benign cyst occurring on the scrotum and filled with a keratin-containing compound, often with a central pore

TREATMENT

• Excision, if symptomatic or infected

REFERENCE

Bennett RT, Palmer LS, Kreutzer ER. Massive scrotal epidermal inclusion cysts. *Urology* 1996;48(5):781–782.

 ## SEAPI Incontinence Classification System

DESCRIPTION SEAPI is an acronym for stress incontinence, emptying ability, anatomy, protection, and instability. Is useful as a reliable and uniform method of following the short- and long-term outcome of SUI surgery. This system is similar to the TNM tumor staging classification system in that each component is graded with a score from 0 (no symptoms) to 3 (severe symptoms). After completion of the evaluation of the incontinent patient, a preoperative subjective and objective SEAPI score is determined. These scores are then compared with postoperative SEAPI scores to access treatment outcome.

REFERENCE

Raz SR, Erickson DR. SEAPI QMM incontinence classification system. *Neurourol Urodyn* 1992;11:187.

 ## Seborrheic Dermatitis

DESCRIPTION Commonly referred to as "dandruff," it can be seen on the penis, anus, or pubic hair. Itching is the rule, with the lesions in hair-bearing areas having a red base and waxy yellow crust. While the organism *Pityrosporon orbiculare* is suspected, the exact agent is unknown.

TREATMENT

• Standard "anti-dandruff shampoos" are usually effective. Shampoo containing ketoconazole may be needed. Steroids should be used with caution, if at all, because this tends to be a lifelong problem.

REFERENCE

Margolis DJ. Cutaneous diseases of the male external genitalia. In: Walsh PC, Retik AB, Vaughan ED, Wein AJ, eds. *Campbell's Urology*, 7th ed. Philadelphia: WB Saunders, 1998.

 ## Semen Analysis—Abnormal

DESCRIPTION There is significant overlap between fertile, subfertile, and infertile populations; therefore, absolute parameters for infertility (except for aspermia or azoospermia) are difficult to measure precisely. In general, fertile populations demonstrate mean sperm densities between 70 and 80 million/mL. Assisted reproductive techniques are now able to overcome many of these abnormalities. (See also Section I, "Infertility," and Section III, "Semen Analysis, Technique and Normal Values)

SYNONYMS

• Oligozoospermia: sperm concentration $<20 \times 10^6$/mL
• Asthenospermia: $<50\%$ of spermatozoa with forward progression of 3 to 4
• Tetratozoospermia: $<50\%$ spermatozoa with normal morphology
• Oligoasthenoteratozoospermia: signifies disturbance of all three variables (combinations of two prefixes may also be used)
• Azoospermia: no sperm in the ejaculate
• Aspermia: no ejaculate
• Polyspermia: abnormally high sperm density ($>250 \times 10^6$/mL)
• Pyospermia: excess white cells ($>1 \times 10^6$/mL)

REFERENCE

Gilbert BR, Cooper GW, Goldstein M. Semen analysis in the evaluation of male factor subfertility. AUA Update Series, Volume XI, Lesson 32, 1992.

Semen Analysis—Technique and Normal Values

 Semen Analysis—Technique and Normal Values

DESCRIPTION The cornerstone of the male infertility work-up. (See also Section I, "Infertility," and Section III, "Semen Analysis—Abnormal.") After 48 to 72 hours of abstinence, a semen specimen is collected in a wide-mouth polypropylene container with a screw top. The sample is kept as close to body temperature as possible and delivered to the lab within 1.5 hours. Analysis includes (may vary slightly by laboratory) total seminal volume, sperm concentration, sperm motility, sperm morphology, fructose content, coagulation time, liquefaction time, viscosity, and leukocyte count. Newer computer-assisted systems can also evaluate curvilinear velocity, straight-line velocity, linearity, and amplitude of lateral head displacements. Antisperm antibodies may be considered a secondary test. Normal parameters are established by most labs. The following are general reference parameters and are typically determined on at least two specimens.

Volume	1.5–5.0 mL
Appearance	White, viscid, opaque
pH	7.2–7.8
Sperm density	$>20 \times 10^6$/mL
Total sperm count	$>40 \times 10^6$/mL
Motility	>60%
Forward progression	>50% or >2+ on a scale of 0–4 (0 no movement, 4 excellent forward progression)
Morphology	>60% normal
Viability	>50% (by dye exclusion)
Fructose, quantitative	>13 μmol per ejaculate
Liquefaction	10–20 minutes (measured on a scale of 0–4)
Agglutination	Minimal clumping (increased clumping suggests inflammatory/ immunologic process)

SYNONYMS

• Normozoospermia/normospermia

REFERENCE

Sheriff DS. Analysis of semen in a constantly changing social context of medicine. *Arch Androl* 1995;34(3):125–132.

 Seminal Vesicle Amyloidosis

DESCRIPTION A benign condition characterized by subepithelial deposition of amyloid in the seminal vesicles. Its incidence increases with increased age and can often be misinterpreted as regional spread of bladder or prostate cancer when those conditions are also present.

TREATMENT

• No treatment is necessary in asymptomatic cases.

REFERENCE

Coyne JD, Kealy WF. Seminal vesicle amyloidosis: Morphological, histochemical, and immunohistochemical observations. *Histopathology* 199322(2):173–176.

 Seminal Vesicle Cysts

DESCRIPTION Cysts, of either congenital or acquired origin, located in the seminal vesicles. Many studies in the past have linked such cysts to other genitourinary maladies, including renal agenesis, infertility, hematospermia, genitourinary infection, and adult polycystic kidney disease.

CAUSES

• Ejaculatory duct obstruction
• Basement membrane defect, especially in cysts associated with adult polycystic kidney disease

TREATMENT

• No treatment is necessary if asymptomatic.
• Aspiration, marsupialization, or excision, if symptomatic

REFERENCE

Beeby DI. Seminal vesicle cyst associated with ipsilateral renal agenesis: Case report and review of literature. *J Urol* 1974;112(1):120–122.

 Sertoli Only Syndrome

DESCRIPTION Patients usually have small-to-normal testes and azoospermic semen specimens. Phenotypically, these patients are normally virilized males. Histologically, Sertoli cells line the seminiferous tubules with a complete absence of germ cells and normal interstitium. Plasma FSH is usually elevated due to the absence of germ cells. Plasma testosterone and LH are normal. Diagnosis is based on an elevated FSH and fine-needle aspiration of the testis.

SYNONYMS

• Germinal cell aplasia

TREATMENT

• Testicular sperm extraction and intracytoplasmic sperm injection

REFERENCE

Odabas O, Ugras S, Aydin S, et al. Assessment of the testicular cytology by fine-needle aspiration and the imprint technique: Are they reliable diagnostic modalities? *Br J Urol* 1997; 79(3):445–448.

 Sex Reversal Syndrome

DESCRIPTION These patients demonstrate small, firm testes; frequent gynecomastia; small-to-normal penises; and azoospermia. Testicular biopsy may demonstrate seminiferous tubule sclerosis, causing elevated gonadotropins and decreased testosterone levels. Individuals are shorter than average height. There is no increase in the incidence of mental retardation, but there is an increase in hypospadias. While karyotyping demonstrates 46XX, molecular biologic mapping suggests that portions of the Y chromosome are present. It has been hypothesized that the portion of the Y chromosome containing the testes determining factor has been translocated. Diagnosis is based on karyotype, molecular biologic mapping, and PCR using Y-specific probes.

SYNONYMS

• XX male

TREATMENT

• If necessary, phenotypic gender assignment is done very early and appropriate surgical correction is performed.
• After puberty, management is more difficult because of andrologic problems such as hypogonadism, micropenis, undescended testes, lack of secondary sex characteristics, and impotence. Treatment plans would have to address these issues.

REFERENCE

Yamamoto M, Yokoi K, Katsuno S. A case of sex reversal syndrome with sex-determining region. *Nagoya J Med Sci* 1995;58(3-4):111–115.

 ## Sexual Function Survey

DESCRIPTION The IIEF is a 15-item, self-administered questionnaire scale for the assessment of erectile function that has been linguistically validated in ten languages (see Section VII). It addresses the relevant domains of male sexual function: erectile function (EF), orgasmic function (OF), sexual desire (SD), intercourse satisfaction (IS), and overall satisfaction. EF is represented in items 1, 2, 3, 4, 5, and 15 of the questionnaire, with a score range of 0 (or 1) to 5, a minimum score of 1, and a maximum score of 30. OF is represented in items 9 and 10, with a score range of 0 to 5, a minimum score of 0, and a maximum score of 10. SD is represented in items 11 and 12, with a score range of 1 to 5, a minimum score of 2, and a maximum score of 10. IS is covered in items 6, 7, and 8, with a score range of 0 to 5, a minimum score of 0, and a maximum score of 15. OS is covered in items 13 and 14, with a score range of 1 to 5, a minimum score of 2, and a maximum score of 10. In general, the lower the score, the worse the erectile function. (See Survey Instrument in the appendix.)

SYNONYMS

- International Index of Erectile Function (IIEF)

REFERENCE

Rosen RC, Riley A, Wagner G, Osterloh, Kirkpatrick J, Mishra A. I: The International Index of Erectile Function (IIEF): A multidimensional scale for assessment of erectile dysfunction. *Urology* 1997;49:822–830.

 ## Signet Ring Carcinoma— Prostate

DESCRIPTION A rare high-grade neoplasm that carries a poor prognosis. A gastrointestinal primary tumor should be considered with this pathology. This malignancy is more aggressive than other cell types. More than 50% of these patients die within a year of diagnosis.

TREATMENT

- Radiation
- Hormone therapy

REFERENCE

Smith C, Feddersen RM, Dressler L, et al. Signet ring cell adenocarcinoma of prostate. *Urology* 1994;43(3):397–400.

 ## Silber's Vasoepididymostomy

DESCRIPTION Silber in 1978 was the first to report the use of the microscope to perform a vasoepididymostomy. The distal epididymis is cut and, with the microscope, the tubule exuding semen is identified. The freshly cut mucosal lumen of the vas deferens is anastomosed to this tubule, and the adventitia of the vas is then anchored to the epididymal tunic. Used in selected cases of obstructive infertility

REFERENCE

Thomas AJ. Vasovasostomy. In: Novick AC, Streem SB, Pontes JE, eds. *Stewarts Operative Urology*. Baltimore: Williams & Wilkins, 1989:767–773.

 ## Smegma

DESCRIPTION Substance composed of desquamated cells that originate from the epithelium of the glans penis and on the inner surface of the foreskin. It is composed of 26% fat and 13% protein. It remains unclear whether smegma is only desquamated epithelial cells or whether secretions from preputial glands at the coronal sulcus contribute to smegma. The issue of smegma carcinogenicity is still controversial. Some believe that phimosis allows for retention of smegma, which is an irritant producing malignant transformation of the epithelium by direct contact.

TREATMENT

- Good hygiene

REFERENCE

Maden C, Sherman KJ, Beckmann AM, et al. History of circumcision, medical conditions, and sexual activity and risk of penile cancer. *J Natl Cancer Inst* 1993;85(1):19–24.

 ## Smith-Lemli-Opitz Syndrome

DESCRIPTION An autosomal recessive multisystemic disease found in newborns that present with hypospadias and cryptorchidism. Anomalies in other systems include pernicious anemia, mental retardation, syndactyly, renal abnormalities, and microcephaly. These patients have an inborn error of cholesterol biosynthesis, which results in deficiency of cholesterol and elevation of 7-dehydrocholesterol, a cholesterol precursor.

CAUSES

- Defect of the delta 5,7-sterol, delta 7-reductase

TREATMENT

- Patients can take cholesterol with or without bile acids.

REFERENCE

Jira P, Wevers R, de-Jong, et al. Treatment of Smith-Lemli-Opitz syndrome. *Am J Med Genet* 1997;68(3):311–314.

 ## Soap-Bubble Nephrogram

DESCRIPTION A radiographic appearance of the dilated pyelocalyceal system, due to end-stage obstruction atrophy, where overlapping curved, white densities several millimeters in thickness appear after intravenous or intraarterial injection of contrast material. Dilated calyces are represented by bubbles, and remnants of Bertin's columns appear as thin opacities between adjacent calyces.

REFERENCE

Ransley PG. Opacification of the renal parenchyma in obstruction and reflux. *Pediatr Radiol* 1976;4:226.

 ## Sperm Granuloma

DESCRIPTION Sperm granulomas form from the testicular end of the vas after vasectomy. Because sperm is highly antigenic, the inflammatory reaction creates a granuloma, which is usually asymptomatic. Some studies have shown that men who undergo vasectomy reversal have higher success rates if they have a sperm granuloma at the vasectomy site. A mass in the scrotum postvasectomy is diagnostic.

TREATMENT

- When chronic postvasectomy pain is localized to the sperm granuloma, the lesion should be excised and occluded with electrocautery.
- Postvasectomy congestive epididymitis may be relieved with open-ended vasectomy, which will produce a pressure-relieving sperm granuloma.

REFERENCE

Subhas T, Michaels T. The influence of scrotal heating prior to vasectomy on sperm granuloma formation and testicular activity. *Contraception* 1980;21(2):175–181.

Sperm Penetration Assay (SPA)

 Sperm Penetration Assay (SPA)

DESCRIPTION A test for infertility that assesses the ability of sperm to penetrate the ovum. The zona pellucida from hamster oocytes is removed, which allows capacitated human sperm to penetrate it. This assay requires the sperm to be able to undergo capacitation, the acrosome reaction, fusion with the oolemma, and incorporation into the ooplasm. If sperm penetration is between 10% and 30%, the sample is considered normal, but this bioassay is not standardized. Some studies have shown that IVF success is correlated with a positive SPA, while others have not. These inconsistencies require that the physician become familiar with the laboratory performing this test. Although there are controversies surrounding SPA, it is a test that should be performed for unexplained infertility.

SYNONYMS

- Humster test

REFERENCE

Anonymous. Consensus Workshop on Advanced Diagnostic Andrology Techniques. ESHRE (European Society of Human Reproduction and Embryology) Andrology Special Interest Group. *Hum Reprod* 1996;11(7):1463–1479.

 Spinal Cord Compression— Urologic Considerations

DESCRIPTION Spinal cord compression, if due to a urologic etiology, is most likely bone metastasis from prostate cancer. Other types of cancer must also be kept in mind. Symptoms include back pain, progressive weakness, sensory loss, and paralysis. Bowel and bladder dysfunction are late findings. Neurologic impairment can progress overnight, so patients must be followed carefully. Survival of patients with spinal cord compression due to metastasis is relatively poor. Forty-six percent of the patients survived less than 6 months, and 20% less than 2 months. (See also Section II, "Spinal Cord Injury—Urologic Considerations.") Diagnosis is based on findings of CT and MRI.

TREATMENT

- Radiation
- Glucocorticoids
- Flutamide
- Casodex
- DES
- Orchiectomy

REFERENCE

Kuban DA, el-Mahdi AM, Sigred SV, et al. Characteristics of spinal cord compression in adenocarcinoma of prostate. *Urology* 1986;28(5): 364–369.

 Splenogonadal Fusion

DESCRIPTION A rare congenital malformation in which there is an abnormal fusion between the spleen and the gonad or mesonephros derivatives. This fusion occurs in both sexes, but it is more common in males. Half of the cases are reported in children. The two types are continuous and discontinuous. In the continuous splenogonadal fusion, the main spleen is connected to the left gonad by a strand of tissue. This cord may be fibrous or splenic or contain beads of splenic tissue. The discontinuous type has no cord between the spleen and left gonad. One-third of all reported cases are associated with other congenital abnormalities, especially peromelia. The majority of cases present with scrotal mass or scrotal tenderness. Some are found incidentally during herniorrhaphy or orchidopexy. Although evaluation is usually done in the operating room, a technetium-99 colloid liver spleen scan can easily identify splenic tissue in the scrotum if splenogonadal fusion is suspected preoperatively. Scrotal ultrasound does not help diagnosis this entity.

TREATMENT

- Usually involves removing both the testis and adjoining mass
- If the diagnosis of discontinuous splenogonadal fusion is made before surgery, the splenic nodule can simply be excised.
- For the continuous variety, exploratory laparotomy is necessary to identify the anatomy involved and deal with the continuous cord.

REFERENCE

Gouw AS, Elema GD, Bink-Boelkens MT, de Jongh HJ, ten Kate LP. The spectrum of splenogonadal fusion. Case report and review of 84 reported cases. *Eur J Pediatr* 1985;144(4): 316–323.

 Squamous Metaplasia—Bladder

DESCRIPTION This term describes the replacement of normal urothelium by mature squamous epithelium. The nonkeratinizing form is thought to be a normal variant in premenopausal women, occurring under hormonal influence. This form is commonly found in the trigone. Cystoscopically, squamous metaplasia appears as a white patch. Keratinizing squamous metaplasia, also known as vesical leukoplakia, is a response to chronic irritation and infection. Some go on to develop squamous carcinoma. Keratinizing squamous metaplasia occurs often with long-term urinary catheters, a bladder stone, vesical schistosomiasis, and squamous carcinoma of the bladder.

SYNONYMS

- Pseudomembranous trigonitis
- Vesical leukoplakia

CAUSES

- Long-term indwelling urinary catheter
- Bladder stone
- Vesical schistosomiasis

TREATMENT

- Transurethral resection

REFERENCE

Adkas A, Turkeri L. The impact of squamous metaplasia in transitional cell carcinoma of the bladder. *Int Urol Nephrol* 1991;23(4):333–336.

 Stamey Procedure (Urethropexy)

DESCRIPTION Stamey was the first to report the use of the cystoscope to aid in the performance of a transvaginal urethropexy. In addition, the nonabsorbable sutures that are placed with a needle carrier incorporate a Dacron pledget to buttress the suture at the level of the bladder neck. Used to treat stress incontinence in women. Of the patients who have undergone this procedure, 82% of 192 were improved, and 65% of the 192 would be willing to undergo the procedure again. Another study showed that although the Stamey procedure has a high early success rate, the long-term results were poor. After 5 years, only 18% of 28 women remained dry. Concomitant abdominal hysterectomy, respiratory disease, and obesity were likely to point to a lower long-term cure rate. Possible complications include long-term erosion of suture into the urinary tract and long-term urinary retention if sutures are tied too tightly.

REFERENCE

O'Sullivan DC, Chilton CP, Munson KW. Should Stamey colposuspension be our primary surgery for stress incontinence? *Br J Urol* 1995;75(4): 457–460.

Stamey Test

DESCRIPTION The three-glass test described by Meares and Stamey is a method of collecting urine, which can provide information on the site of origin of red blood cells or bacteria. Though this method is effective in localizing the cause of hematuria, it is more commonly used in diagnosing prostatitis. A specimen is collected from the urethra, midstream urine, and prostatic secretions. The first-voided 10 mL of urine is the urethral specimen (VB1). The midstream urine of 10 mL (VB2) is collected after the patient has voided about 200 mL. The patient is then instructed to stop voiding, at which time the physician massages the prostate and collects the prostatic fluid. Afterward, the patient voids again, and a 10-mL specimen (VB3) is collected. Cultures are sent on the four specimens. When the bladder urine is sterile, urethral and prostatic infection can be differentiated by comparing the bacterial colony counts of VB1 and prostatic (EPS and VB3) counts. In urethral infections, the VB1 count is much higher than the EPS or VB3 count. The EPS and VB3 counts in prostatic infections significantly exceed the VB1 count. When interpreting bacterial colony counts, one must take into account that the VB3 specimen is a 100× dilution of prostatic fluid. When the bladder urine is infected, the infection cannot be localized, because all specimens will show heavy growth of organisms.

SYNONYMS

- Three-glass test

REFERENCE

Meares EM, Stamey TA. The diagnosis and management of bacterial prostatitis. *Br J Urol* 1972;44(2):175–179.

 Stauffer Syndrome

DESCRIPTION A syndrome associated with nonmetastatic hepatic dysfunction commonly seen in cases of renal cell carcinoma. Symptoms include fever, fatigue, and weight loss. The patient has unusual liver function tests, white blood cell loss, and areas of hepatic necrosis without hepatic metastasis. The presence of hepatic dysfunction should not be a contraindication to surgery. Hepatic function usually returns to normal after nephrectomy. If syndrome persists, it is a sign of recurrent tumor. Diagnostic indicators are elevation of alkaline phosphatase and bilirubin, hypoalbuminemia, prolonged PTT, and hypergammaglobulinemia.

CAUSES

- Associated with renal cell carcinoma

TREATMENT

- Nephrectomy

REFERENCE

Jacobi GH, Philipp T. Stauffer's syndrome—Diagnostic help in hypernephroma. *Clin Nephrol* 1975;4(3):113–115.

 Steinstrasse

DESCRIPTION A German expression for "street of stones." Multiple stone fragments in ureter after extracorporeal shock wave lithotripsy (ESWL). Characteristically find stone fragments in a line within ureter. Occasionally presents with renal colic, nausea, or vomiting

CAUSES

- Large stone or overfragmentation during ESWL

TREATMENT

- Observation only if symptoms tolerable or absent
- For severe colic or obstruction: ureteral stent placement, percutaneous nephrostomy, or ureteroscopic lithotripsy

REFERENCE

Weinerth JL, et al. Lessons learned in patients with large Steinstrasse. *J Urol* 1989;142:1425.

 Sting Procedure

DESCRIPTION Subureteric Teflon injection (Sting) is a procedure performed to correct vesicoureteral reflux. Pyrolyzed Teflon particles suspended in glycerin are injected deep into the ureter. Because migration of these Teflon particles to the pelvic lymph nodes, liver, lung, and brain has been demonstrated in laboratory models, other substances, such as collagen, may be used. The success rate is inferior to that of open surgery. About 70% have reflux resolution after one procedure. With repeat Sting procedures, the success rate increases to 90% to 95%.

REFERENCE

Aubert D, Zoupanos B, Destuynder O, Hurez F. Sting procedure in the treatment of secondary reflux in children. *Eur Urol* 1990;17(4):307–309.

 Stranguria

DESCRIPTION Sharp, stabbing, interrupted suprapubic and urethral pain at the end of urination. Micturition may occur in drops and is produced by spasmodic muscular contractions of the urethra and bladder.

SYNONYMS

- Strangury
- Terminal dysuria

CAUSES

- Inflammatory conditions of the bladder, prostate, or urethra
—Bacterial cystitis
—Idiopathic cystitis
—Granulomatous diseases
—Prostatitis
—Urethritis
- Malignancy
—Transitional cell carcinoma
—Carcinoma in situ
—Adenocarcinoma
—Squamous cell carcinoma
—Carcinosarcoma

TREATMENT

- Directed at specific etiology

REFERENCE

Brendler CB. Evaluation of the urologic patient. In: Walsh PC, Retik AB, Vaughan ED, Wein AJ, eds. *Campbell's Urology,* 7th ed. Philadelphia: WB Saunders, 1998.

 Streak Gonad

DESCRIPTION Patients with streak gonad usually present with female phenotype, primary amenorrhea, infantile breast status, sparse pubic and axillary hair, infantile external genitalia and vagina, atrophic vaginal smear, immature uterus, high serum FSH, low urinary estrogen, osteoporosis, and streak gonad. Diagnosis is made by measuring FSH, urinary estrogen, and karyotype. See Section II, "Gonadal Dysgenesis—(Mixed and Pure)."

TREATMENT

- Management includes laparotomy with excision of any intraabdominal testis or streak gonads. These masses then progress to develop malignancies, which may develop before puberty.
- Female sex assignment and reconstructive surgery are advised in cases with severely deficient virilization of the genitalia.

REFERENCE

Calabrese F, Valente M. Mixed gonadal dysgenesis: Histological and ultrastructural findings in two cases. *Int J Gynecol Pathol* 1996;15(3):270–275.

Strickler Ureteral Anastamosis

 ## Strickler Ureteral Anastamosis

DESCRIPTION   Through an extracolonic approach, a small linear incision is made in the taenia, and a small clamp is used to create a submucosal 3- to 4-cm tunnel exiting out of the colon laterally. The ureter is delivered through the tunnel, and the spatulated end is anastomosed to the mucosa and the taenia is closed while incorporating ureter adventitia.

REFERENCE

McDougal WS. Use of intestinal segments and urinary diversion. In: Walsh PC, Retik AB, Vaughan ED, Wein AJ, eds. *Campbell's Urology*, 7th ed. Philadelphia: WB Saunders, 1998:3137–3144.

 ## Struvite

DESCRIPTION   The mineral name for magnesium ammonium phosphate hexahydrate stones. See Section II, "Urolithiasis—Infectious (Struvite)."

 ## Studer Pouch

DESCRIPTION   An orthotopic neobladder is made, based on 60 cm of marsupialized ileum, which is configured and sutured into a W to create a broad intestinal plate. In addition, a nontubularized segment of ileum extends from a limb of the W, simulating a chimney. The ureters are implanted into the chimney. The intestinal plate is anastomosed to the urethra and then closed into a sphere.

REFERENCE

Benson MC, Olsson CA. Continent urinary diversion. In: Walsh PC, Retik AB, Vaughan ED, Wein AJ, eds. *Campbell's Urology*, 7th ed. Philadelphia: WB Saunders, 1998:3190–3245.

 ## Superficial Inguinal Pouch of Denis-Browne

DESCRIPTION   *Superficial inguinal pouch* is defined as the space distal to the internal inguinal ring, but above the inguinal canal between the external oblique fascia and Scarpa's fascia. Studies suggest that a testis in the superficial inguinal pouch is, in reality, a cryptorchid testis.

REFERENCE

Herzog B, Steigert M, Hadziselimovic F. Is a testis located at the superficial inguinal pouch (Denis-Browne pouch) comparable to a true cryptorchid testis? *J Urol* 1992;148(2 Pt 2): 622–623.

 ## Supernumerary Kidney

DESCRIPTION   Supernumerary kidney is a rare condition in which a free accessory renal organ exists as a distinct entity, with its own blood supply, and the presence of two normal kidneys. It is distinguished by its small size and/or abnormal position. The kidney is either a component of a bifid ureteral system or a completely duplicated system. When diagnosed, treatment for a supernumerary kidney should be based on pathologic processes affecting the kidney rather than its redundant appearance or abnormal position.

REFERENCE

N'Guessan G, Stephans FO. Supernumerary kidney. *J Urol* 1983;130:649.

 ## Swyer Syndrome

DESCRIPTION   A type of pure gonadal dysgenesis. Patients have bilateral streak gonads and often present as adolescent phenotypic females with delayed puberty. A 46XY genotype may develop rapid breast or clitoral enlargement due to hormonally active gonadoblastomas within the streak gonads. See Section II, "Gonadal Dysgenesis (Mixed and Pure)."

REFERENCE

Moreira-Filho CA, et al. H-Y antigen in Swyer syndrome and the genetics of XY gonadal dysgenesis. *Hum Genet* 1979;53(1):51–56.

 ## Systemic Lupus— Urologic Considerations

DESCRIPTION   The kidney is the organ most commonly affected by systemic lupus erythematosus (SLE). The renal manifestations of SLE vary from patient to patient. In mesangial lupus nephropathy, kidney function is normal, urinary abnormalities are minimal, and kidney biopsy findings are limited to expansion of the mesangium and immune complex deposition within the mesangium. However, for severe forms of lupus nephritis, patients will present with either diffuse proliferative or membranoproliferative nephritis. These forms of nephritis can cause impaired renal function, proteinuria, and an active urine sediment. Diagnosis of SLE is based on clinical and laboratory data. However, renal biopsy may be useful in assessing prognosis and determining therapy.

SYNONYMS

- Lupus nephritis

CAUSES

- Unknown etiology

TREATMENT

- Cytotoxic agents (pulse cyclophosphamide therapy) are superior to glucocorticoid therapy for the treatment of proliferative lupus nephritis.

REFERENCE

Boumpas, et al. SLE: Emerging concepts: Part I: Renal, neuropsychiatric, cardiovascular, pulmonary, and hematologic disease. *Ann Intern Med* 1995;122(12):940–950.

 ## Tabes Dorsalis

DESCRIPTION   Tertiary syphilis involving the dorsal spinal roots and posterior spinal column. Can present with voiding dysfunction, presumably due to loss of bladder sensation, with high residual volumes and urinary retention. Urodynamic evaluation reveals detrusor atony and detrusor areflexia.

SYNONYMS

- Neurosyphilis
- Tabetic bladder
- Tertiary syphilis

TREATMENT

- Penicillin for syphilis
- Clean intermittent catheterization for bladder atony

REFERENCE

Erturk E, et al. Voiding dysfunction in tertiary syphilis. *Urology* 1987;30(3):284–286.

Takayasu's Arteritis—Urologic Considerations

DESCRIPTION An inflammatory disease affecting the aorta and its main branches, causing stenosis or aneurysmal dilation of the affected vessels. Involvement of renal arteries might lead to renovascular hypertension. The disease is progressive and hard to manage.

CAUSES

- The etiology is unknown.

TREATMENT

- Angioplasty

REFERENCE

Kumar S, Mandalim R, Raovr K, et al. Percutaneous transluminal angioplasty in non-specific aortoarthritis (Takayasu's disease): Experience in 16 cases. *Cardiovasc Intervent Radiol* 1990;12:321.

 ## Teratoma, Sacrococcygeal—Urologic Considerations

DESCRIPTION Sacrococcygeal tumors are usually diagnosed in the neonate (1 in 40,000 births) and less frequently in infants or adults. Females are more affected than are males. Clinical presentation is usually in the form of palpable mass, skin discoloration, or hairy nevus. Frequently, the patient presents with bowel or urinary obstruction. Sacrococcygeal tumors of newborn and young adults are generally benign, whereas those discovered during infancy have a 50% chance of being malignant.

TREATMENT

- Wide, local excision of the tumor
- Adjunctive irradiation or chemotherapy is still uncertain.

REFERENCE

Richie JP. Neoplasms of the testis. In: Walsh PC, Retik AB, Vaughan ED, Wein AJ, eds. *Campbell's Urology*, 7th ed. Philadelphia: WB Saunders, 1998:2411–2452.

 ## Testis—Cysts

DESCRIPTION Nonneoplastic testicular cysts include hydatid, epidermoid, simple, and cystic dysplasia. These are very rare lesions and are generally clinically interpreted as neoplastic, until proven otherwise at the time of microscopic view. Hydatid cysts are rarely seen, except in the Middle East.

REFERENCE

Kumar PVN, Johanshahi SL. Hydatid cyst of testis: A case report. *J Urol* 1987;137:511.

 ## Testis—Dermoid Cyst

DESCRIPTION A primary non–germ cell tumor representing 1% of testis tumors, with half of the patients presenting in their 20s. Grossly, the lesions present as encapsuled intratesticular nodules, which are round and sharply circumscribed, with firm consistency. The cut surface reveals a grayish white, cheesy, amorphous mass. The microscopic picture is that of dense fibrous tissue lined by stratified squamous keratinized epithelium with degeneration and macrocalcification. The benign behavior of these tumors is the rule. Testicular ultrasound may aid in this tumor's differentiation from germ cell tumor. Most of the cases have been managed by radical orchiectomy. However, local excision has been equally successful in a small number of patients.

REFERENCE

Shah KH, Maxted WC, Chun B. Epidermoid cysts of the testis. *Cancer* 1981;47:577.

 ## Testis—Microlithiasis

DESCRIPTION Numerous and diffuse calcifications throughout the entire testicle seen on ultrasound. It is reported in undescended testicles (0.3% incidence), prepubertal Klinefelter syndrome, and male pseudohermaphroditism, and is slightly more common in prepubertal males. Infertility and malignancy have been reported to be associated with the condition, and some consider it possibly premalignant. Both seminomas and nonseminomatous germ cell tumors have been described in association with microlithiasis. Others suggest an association with carcinoma in situ of the testicle. Many advocate close surveillance of patients with testicular microlithiasis, such as yearly testicular ultrasound, physical examination, and judicious tumor marker determinations.

REFERENCE

Furness PD III, et al. Multi-institutional study of testicular microlithiasis in childhood: A benign or premalignant condition? *J Urol* 1998;160(3 Pt 2):1151–1154.

 ## Testis—Teratoma, Extragonadal

DESCRIPTION Primary tumors of extragonadal origin are rare. In a decreasing order of frequency, the most common sites are the mediastinum, retroperitoneum, sacrococcygeal region, and pineal gland. Histologically, all types of germ cell tumors are represented, with pure seminoma accounting for half of mediastinal and retroperitoneal tumors. Clinically, males are affected more than are females, with the exception of sacrococcygeal tumors, where females predominate. The majority of adults present with advanced local disease and distant metastasis. Patients with mediastinal extragonadal tumors are usually diagnosed in their 20s, with or without symptoms of chest pain, cough, or dyspnea. Patients with primary retroperitoneal tumors may present with abdominal or back pain, a palpable mass, or vascular obstruction. Tumors of the pineal gland usually present in children and young adults, with symptoms of increased intracranial pressure, oculomotor dysfunction, hearing loss, hypopituitarism, or hypothalamic disturbances.

CAUSES

- Displacement of primitive germ cell takes place during early embryonic migration from the yolk sac endoderm.
- Pluripotential cells persist in sequestered primitive rests during early somatic development.

TREATMENT

- Intensive chemotherapy regimens have shown some success in primary retroperitoneal seminoma.
- The nonseminomatous version has done poorly despite surgery, radiotherapy, and chemotherapy.
- Primary radiation therapy has been much favored for pineal tumors (a cerebrospinal fluid shunt may be required).

REFERENCE

Garnick MB, Canellos GP, Richie JP. Treatment and surgical staging of testicular and primary extragonadal germ cell cancer. *JAMA* 1983;250:1733.

Tethered Cord Syndrome

 Tethered Cord Syndrome

DESCRIPTION   Late sequelae of spinal dysraphism, in which fixation or scarring of the spinal cord and conus medullaris, due to prior spinal surgery, prevents normal cephalad migration of spinal cord with childhood growth, causing spinal cord ischemia. Usually manifests with change in voiding pattern, or with neurologic or musculoskeletal deficits. Urodynamic evaluation typically reveals detrusor hyperreflexia or detrusor areflexia. Detrusor–external sphincter dyssynergia or poor detrusor compliance with elevated bladder pressure can also be seen and warrant aggressive intervention. MRI is usually diagnostic. See also Section II, "Myelodysplasia (Myelomeningocele)—Urologic Considerations," and Section III, "Dysraphism—Spinal."

TREATMENT

• Surgery to untether spinal cord
• Urologic intervention, based on urodynamic findings

REFERENCE

Palmer LS, Richards I, Kaplan WE. Subclinical changes in bladder function in children presenting with nonurologic symptoms of the tethered cord syndrome. *J Urol* 1998;159(1): 231–234.

 Thiersch-Duplay Hypospadias Repair

DESCRIPTION   The distal urethral plate is tubularized to advance the meatus. The glans is reapproximated over the repair.

REFERENCE

Duckett JW. Hypospadias. In: Walsh PC, Retik AB, Vaughan ED, Wein AJ, eds. *Campbell's Urology*, 7th ed. Philadelphia: WB Saunders, 1998:2093–2119.

 Thompson Pyeloplasty

DESCRIPTION   It is used when insufficient renal pelvis is available to close, due to trauma or scarring. A triangular flap of renal capsule is sharply developed, and it is then flipped over onto the renal pelvic opening and closed with 5-0 chromic sutures.

REFERENCE

Kay R. Procedures for ureteropelvic junction obstruction. In: Novick AC, Streem SB, Pontes JE, eds. *Stewarts Operative Urology*. Baltimore: Williams & Wilkins, 1989:220–233.

 Thrombophlebitis—Superficial

DESCRIPTION   Local inflammatory process of superficial veins. Clinically, patients present with redness, tenderness, and swelling surrounding a palpable thrombosed superficial vein. In the upper limbs, it is usually caused by acidic fluid infusion or prolonged cannulation. In the lower limbs, it may be associated with varicose veins or DVT.

REFERENCE

Archer DS, Fowler PD. Comparison of oxyphenbutazone and placebo in the treatment of superficial thrombophlebitis: An object lesson in clinical trial design. *Practitioner* 1977;218:712.

 Tinea Cruris (Jock Itch)

DESCRIPTION   Dermatophytic infection of the crural areas of the genitalia. Clinically, reddish brown lesions with an elevated red border can be identified in the crural area, inner thigh, and scrotum. Penis involvement is rare. Postinflammatory hyperpigmentation may occur as a result of chronic or recurrent disease. Culture or KOH examination is necessary to confirm diagnosis. Scraping should be carried on the active border of the lesion, and reveals branching septate hyphae. Differential diagnosis includes erythrasma, psoriasis, and seborrheic dermatitis. Recurrent disease is not unusual, and treatment should be aimed toward active disease rather than postinflammatory hyperpigmentation. (See also Section III, "Pruritis—External Genitalia, Male.")

SYNONYMS

• Jock itch

CAUSES

• Dermatophytes: *Trichophyton rubrum, Trichophyton mentagrophytes, Epidermophyton floccosum*

TREATMENT

• Prevent skin maceration by keeping skin dry.
• Application of antifungal agents on overt lesions. Agents include Lotrimin, Mycelex, Loprox, Spectazole, Lamasil, and others for up to 14 days.
• Rarely, oral agents may be needed if topical agents fail. Ketoconazole (Nizoral) for 14 days (requires baseline laboratory monitoring CBC, LFTs)

REFERENCE

Geer DL. An overview of common dermatophytes. *J Am Acad Dermatol* 1994;31:S112.

 Torsion—Testicular Appendages

DESCRIPTION   Torsion of the appendix testis or appendix epididymis may be the most common cause of acute scrotal pain. The most common cause of acute scrotum in prepubertal boys (between 3 and 13 years); peak incidence between 9 and 13 years. Torsion of the appendix testis is the most common (>90% of torsed appendages). Torsion of a testicular appendage can be similar to testicular torsion; however, the pain of a torsed testicular appendage is less severe and has a crescendo pattern over a few days. Systemic symptoms (fever, nausea, and vomiting) are uncommon. If examined early in the course, a palpable, tender nodule may be appreciated in the superior portion of the testicle, as may be a blue discoloration in this same area, both of which are considered pathognomonic for this entity ("blue dot sign"). The torsed appendage may be visible through the scrotal wall when transilluminated early in the process. The testicle usually is not enlarged or indurated. As the inflammatory process progresses, edema and erythema develop and the swelling may become more severe, making the differentiation between a torsed appendix and a torsed testicle more difficult. Color Doppler ultrasonography and nuclear scintigraphy both demonstrate normal-to-increased testicular blood flow. (See also Section II, "Torsion—Testicular.")

CAUSES

• Possibly increased estrogen stimulation prior to the onset of puberty, which may cause the vestigial appendage to enlarge and strangulate
• May be precipitated by vigorous physical activity

TREATMENT

• Management is conservative (analgesics, scrotal support, and minimization of activity).
• Surgical exploration only if the diagnosis is not clear and testicular torsion is suspected
• If the pain becomes severe and refractory to analgesics and supportive care, surgical excision may be indicated, with minimal risk and prompt recovery.

REFERENCE

Burgher SW. Acute scrotal pain. *Emerg Med Clin North Am* 1988; 16(4):781–809.

Trichomoniasis

DESCRIPTION Sexually transmitted infection caused by the protozoan *Trichomonas vaginalis*. Rare cause of nongonococcal urethritis in men, common cause of vaginitis in women. Signs and symptoms include urethral discharge, dysuria, and the present of neutrophils in urethral secretions. A positive diagnosis is made by identification of the protozoan on wet mount.

TREATMENT

• Metronidazole 2 g orally for patient and sexual partners

REFERENCE

Krieger JN, et al. Clinical manifestations of trichomoniasis in men. *Ann Intern Med* 1993;118(11):844–849.

 Trigonitis

DESCRIPTION A commonly seen cause of microscopic hematuria in women. Nonkeratinized squamous epithelium is commonly seen on the trigone and bladder neck in up to 86% of women of reproductive age and in up to 75% after menopause. Considered a normal finding and is distinct from squamous metaplasia, which is considered a premalignant lesion. Cystoscopically, these are pale white-grey areas with irregular borders. This condition is not seen in men, except for some reports in men on estrogens for prostate cancer. Treatment is not necessary.

SYNONYMS

• Pseudomembranous trigonitis

REFERENCE

Stephenson TJ, et al. Pseudomembranous trigonitis of the bladder: Hormonal aetiology. *J Clin Pathol* 1989;42(9):922–926.

 Tri-Mix

DESCRIPTION A custom-compounded formulation for intracorporal injection therapy of erectile dysfunction. Typically consists of prostaglandin E1 (5.88 (g/mL), papaverine (18 mg/mL), and phentolamine (0.6 mg/mL)

 Trisomy 4 P

DESCRIPTION Hypertelorism and genitourinary anomalies in the form of hydronephrosis, hypospadias, and undescended testis

REFERENCE

Barakat AY, Seikaly MG, Derkaloustian VM. Urogenital abnormalities in genetic disease. *J Urol* 1986;136:778.

 Trisomy 8

DESCRIPTION This trisomy is associated with a large, square head; a prominent forehead; widely spaced eyes; a slender body; and genitourinary anomalies in the form of hydronephrosis, horse shoe kidney, reflux, hypospadias, and undescended testis.

REFERENCE

Mininberg, D. The genetic basis of urologic disease. AUA Update Series, 9:218, 1992.

 Trisomy 9

DESCRIPTION Small cranium and genitourinary anomalies in the form of renal hypoplasia and hypospadias

REFERENCE

Barakat AY, Seikaly MG, Derkaloustian VM. Urogenital abnormalities in genetic disease. *J Urol* 1986;136:778.

 Trisomy 9 P

DESCRIPTION Strabismus and genitourinary anomalies in the form of pancake kidney and undescended testis

REFERENCE

Barakat AY, Seikaly MG, Derkaloustian VM. Urogenital abnormalities in genetic disease. *J Urol* 1986;136:778.

 Trisomy 10 Q

DESCRIPTION Oval, flat face and genitourinary anomalies in the form of hydronephrosis and small penis

REFERENCE

Mininberg D. The genetic basis of urologic disease. AUA Update Series 9:218, 1992.

 Trisomy 11 Q

DESCRIPTION Flat nose, wide glabella, cleft lip/palate, and micropenis

REFERENCE

Mininberg D. The genetic basis of urologic disease. AUA Update Series 9:218, 1992.

 Trisomy 13

DESCRIPTION Polydactyly, congenital heart disease, and cystic kidney

REFERENCE

Barakat AY, Seikaly MG, Derkaloustian VM. Urogenital abnormalities in genetic disease. *J Urol* 1986;136:778.

 Trisomy 18 (Edwards Syndrome)

DESCRIPTION Hypertonia and genitourinary anomalies in the form of hydronephrosis and small penis. Hypoplasia of the labia majora may cause a false impression of a large clitoris.

REFERENCE

Barakat AY, Seikaly MG, Derkaloustian VM. Urogenital abnormalities in genetic disease. *J Urol* 1986;136:778.

Trisomy 20 P

 Trisomy 20 P

DESCRIPTION   Short nose, dental abnormalities, vertebral abnormalities, and polycystic kidney

REFERENCE

Mininberg D. The genetic basis of urologic disease. AUA Update Series 9:218, 1992.

 Trisomy 21

• See Section III, "Down Syndrome—Urologic Considerations."

 Trisomy 22

DESCRIPTION   Microcephaly, low-set ears, cleft palate, beaked nose, and microphallus

REFERENCE

Mininberg D. The genetic basis of urologic disease. AUA Update Series 9:218, 1992.

 Tubrous Sclerosis

DESCRIPTION   An autosomal dominant disease that clinically presents with a classic triad of epilepsy, mental retardation, and adenoma sebaceum. Named for the tubers or periventricular calcifications seen on CT scan. *Adenoma sebaceum* describes the facial angiofibromas around nasolabial regions and cheeks. The renal system may be free of anomalies or may display cysts (10%), angiomyolipomas (40%–80%), or both. AML can bleed, with increasing risk at 3.5 cm. Renal failure as a result of parenchymal compression by expanding cysts. Hypertension may also occur. Renal cell carcinoma in 2%

SYNONYMS

• Tuberous sclerosis complex
• Bourneville disease

CAUSES

• Autosomal dominant disease mapped to chromosome 16 or 9

TREATMENT

• Ultrasound is the method of choice for surveillance.
• Embolization is first-line treatment for hemorrhage from AML.

REFERENCE

Brenstein J, Robbins TO, Kissane JM. The renal lesion of tuberous sclerosis. *Semin Diagn Pathol* 1986;3:97–99.

 Tumor Lysis Syndrome (TLS)

DESCRIPTION   A syndrome associated with chemotherapy. Extensive metastatic tumor, pretreatment renal impairment, and markedly elevated LDH concentrations have been reported to be serious risk factors in developing TLS. Lab investigations would reveal hyperkalemia, hypocalcemia, hyperphosphatemia, and concurrent metabolic acidosis, as well as severe hyperuricemia with eventual renal failure. (See also Section III, "Nephropathy—Urate.")

REFERENCE

Ustundag Y, Boyacioglu S, Haznedaroglu IC, Baltali E. Acute tumor lysis syndrome associated with paclitaxel. *Ann Pharmacother* 1997;31:1548.

 Tumor Thrombus (Renal, Adrenal)

DESCRIPTION   Renal carcinoma may invade the main renal vein and extend into it as a tumor thrombus. The thrombus tends to grow into the vena cava only in a small number of cases. However, direct invasion of the vessel is uncommon. Preoperative assessment of the extent of venous involvement, using CT, MRI, or an inferior vena cavogram, is essential. Excision of renal carcinoma with caval extension is recommended and can be achieved safely, even with extension into the right atrium. However, this is seldom helpful for patients with regional and distant metastasis. The use of modern cardiac surgical techniques has facilitated tumor removal and improved survival rates.

REFERENCE

Calyman RV, Gonzalez R, Fraley EE. Renal cell carcinoma invading the inferior vena cava: Clinical review and anatomical approach. *J Urol* 1980;123:157.

 Tunica Albuginea Tumors and Cysts

DESCRIPTION   Tunica albuginea cysts usually present in the fifth and sixth decades of life. They may be unilocular or multilocular and are commonly found in the anterolateral aspect of the testis. Size varies from 2 to 4 mm. Cystic fluid is clear, with no spermatozoa. The epithelium lining the cysts may be either simple columnar or stratified cuboidal, supported by a thin layer of collagenized connective tissue. Those cystic malformations were considered very rare. However, with the current use of ultrasound, the incidence has been found to be much higher. See Section I, "Scrotum—Mass and/or Pain (Acute Scrotum)."

REFERENCE

Nistal M, Inguez L, Paniagua R. Cysts of the testicular parenchyma and tunica albuginea. *Arch Pathol Lab Med* 1989;113:902.

 Tunica Vaginalis Tumors

DESCRIPTION   Malignant mesothelioma of the tunica vaginalis is rare. However, increased frequency has been reported since 1980. Most of the patients are 40 to 79 years of age, with prior exposure to asbestos being reported in some. Microscopically, mesothelioma may be epithelial, fibrous, or a combination of both. The malignant nature of the disease is indicated by its frequent mitosis, nuclear atypia with prominent nucleoli, and invasion of adjacent structures or lymphatics. Positive staining with keratin and failure to stain with carcinoembryonic antigen indicate mesothelioma. In addition, an immunoperoxidase stain has been reported to be specific for the tumor. Computerized tomography and aspiration cytology may aid in preoperative diagnosis. See Section I, "Scrotum—Mass and/or Pain (Acute Scrotum)." Adjunct chemotherapy may be tried. However, its value has not been established.

REFERENCE

Chen KTK, Arhelger RB, Flam RS, et al. Malignant mesothelioma of tunica vaginalis testis. *Urology* 1982;20:316.

Turner Syndrome

DESCRIPTION   A sex chromosome abnormality with a 46,XO karyotype. It is characterized by primary amenorrhea, sexual infantilism, short stature, dysgenic ovaries, webbed neck, and a host of other congenital anomalies. The external genitalia are female but immature. Renal abnormalities are extremely common. Horseshoe kidney is the most common abnormality. Ultrasound is a good screening test to determine if any renal abnormalities are present.

REFERENCE

Jones KL. *Smith's Recognizable Patterns of Human Malformation,* 4th ed. Philadelphia: WB Saunders, 1998.

 Turner-Warwick Inlay Urethroplasty

DESCRIPTION   Through a midline scrotal incision, the urethral stricture is opened and scarred tissue is removed, leaving a strip of urethra in place. The edges of the scrotal incision are sutured to the urethral strip. In a second stage, the mature marsupialized urethra is tubularized with the surrounding scrotal skin and closed.

REFERENCE

Devine CJ, Devine PC. Operations for urethral stricture. In: Novick AC, Streem SB, Pontes JE, eds. *Stewarts Operative Urology.* Baltimore: Williams & Wilkins, 1989:650–680.

 Uninhibited Detrusor Contraction

DESCRIPTION   Uninhibited detrusor contraction leads to an overactive bladder. Bladder overactivity can result from damage to central inhibitory pathways, sensitization of peripheral afferent terminals in the bladder that unmask primitive voiding reflexes, or changes in bladder smooth muscle cells. In a majority of patients, hyperstimulation of the detrusor has a major impact on quality of life. Symptom assessment is diagnostically disappointing. Cystometry is essential if a definitive diagnosis is required.

SYNONYMS

• Overactive bladder
• Unstable bladder

TREATMENT

• Traditionally centers on the use of anticholinergic medications (oxybutynin, tolterodine, others)
• Estrogens may help in the postmenopausal woman.

REFERENCE

Anonymous. The overactive bladder: From basic science to clinical management consensus conference. *Urology* 1997;50[Suppl 6A]:1–114.

 Ureter—Agenesis/Atresia

DESCRIPTION   Bilateral ureteral agenesis can occur and is incompatible with life. Unilateral ureteral agenesis indicates failure of ureteral bud development and is often accompanied by ipsilateral renal agenesis or multicystic kidney. Ureteral atresia is caused by varying degrees of failure in ureteral bud development. When either atresia or agenesis is unilateral, it is usually asymptomatic and of no clinical significance. However, it can be associated with infection (UTI) on occasion.

REFERENCE

Morozumi M, Ogawa Y, Fujima M, Kitagawa R. Distal ureteral atresia associated with crossed renal ectopia with fusion: Recovery of renal function after release of a 10 yr ureteral obstruction. *Int J Urol* 1997;4(5):512–515.

 Ureter—Diverticulum

DESCRIPTION   Diverticula can be congenital or acquired, although most have been discovered in adults. Most diverticula are solitary outpouchings involving the distal ureters and upper portions of the pelvis. They are true diverticula composed of a muscular wall, which is lined by transitional cell epithelium. Renal pelvic diverticula tend to be larger than those found in the ureter. Diverticula may be associated with other pathology, such as Ask-Upmark kidney. The most common complications are infection and/or stone formation. Unlike diverticula found in the bladder and urethra, major complications and development of transitional cell carcinoma are rare.

REFERENCE

Murphy W. *Urological Pathology,* 2nd ed. Philadelphia: WB Saunders, 1997:127.

 Ureter—Duplication

DESCRIPTION   Duplication of ureters is a common anomaly. Duplication may be either complete or incomplete. Complete duplication is most often associated with vesicoureteral reflux, ectopic ureteral insertion, and ectopic ureterocele, all of which are more commonly found in females than in males. Incomplete duplication is most often associated with ureteropelvic junction obstruction of the lower pole of the kidney. Common clinical presentations include urinary tract infections (UTIs) and urinary incontinence. Diagnosis is made usually in childhood by ultrasound (US), excretory urography, and voiding cystourethrography.

SYNONYMS

• Bifid ureter (partial duplication)
• Double ureters (complete duplication)

CAUSES

• Congenital anomaly
• Environmental factors may also play a role.

TREATMENT

• In the presence of persistent reflux: ureteroneocystostomy
• If obstructed but in the absence of reflux: ureteropyelostomy

REFERENCE

Fernbach SK, Fernstein KA, Spencer K, Lindstrom CA. Ureteral duplication and its complications. *Radiographics* 1997;17(1):109–127.

 Ureter—Fibroepithelial Polyps

DESCRIPTION   Fibroepithelial polyps are rare benign neoplasms. The majority of these polyps are found at the ureteropelvic junction. Signs and symptoms are usually associated with ureteral obstruction (i.e., flank pain, hematuria). In addition, varying degrees of hydroureteronephrosis and ureteral intussusception have been described. Grossly, ureteral polyps are intraluminal lesions and most commonly covered with transitional epithelium. The bulk of the polyp is composed of vascularized collagenous fibrous tissue, with or without areas of chronic inflammation and edema. Ureteroscopy is often necessary to confirm the diagnosis.

SYNONYMS

• Fibromyxoma
• Myxoma
• Fibroma
• Vascular fibrous polyps

Ureter—"Fish Hook" (Reverse J)

TREATMENT

- Ureteroscopic resection
- Open ureterotomy with polypectomy or partial ureterectomy is a viable conservative treatment option if the diagnosis can be confirmed preoperatively.
- Many patients undergo nephroureterectomy for suspected malignancy.

REFERENCE

Bahnson RR, Blum MD, Carter MF. Fibroepithelial polyps of the ureter. *J Urol* 1984;132:343.

 Ureter—"Fish Hook" (Reverse J)

DESCRIPTION A radiographic appearance of the type I (low-loop) circumcaval ureter, in which the dilated proximal part of the ureter takes a characteristic "fish hook" or "reverse J" course. Ureteral dilation usually ends 1 to 2 cm lateral to the inferior vena cava (IVC), where the ureter turns upward at the border of the psoas muscle.

REFERENCE

Kenawi MM, Williams DI. Circumcaval ureter: A report of four cases in children with a review of the literature and a new classification. *Br J Urol* 1976;48:183.

 Ureter—Hemangioma

DESCRIPTION Hemangiomas are benign ureteral tumors. They may be the most common cause of chronic unilateral hematuria. Symptomatology may include hematuria, pain, hydronephrosis, bladder irritations, and palpable tumor. Varicoceles have also been found, but less frequently. Like other ureteral tumors, hemangiomas usually cause incomplete obstruction and may eventually cause complete obstruction with dilation of the urinary tract. As in a report by Hagen, "They present as red, slightly elevated structures, fairly diffusely demarcated from their surroundings." Urothelial malignancies must be excluded, especially in the elderly.

TREATMENT

- Flexible ureteropyeloscopy is considered a good diagnostic and therapeutic option in selected patients with unilateral hematuria of uncertain etiology.

REFERENCE

Kumon H, Masaya T, Yosuke M, Ohmori H. Endoscopic diagnosis and treatment of chronic unilateral hematuria of uncertain etiology. *J Urol* 1990;143(3):554–558.

 Ureter—J Hooking

DESCRIPTION With progressive benign prostatic hypertrophy, elevation of the trigone occurs, resulting in characteristic "J hooking" of the distal ureters. A reliable sign on IVP of significant prostatic hypertrophy

REFERENCE

Amis ES, Newhouse JH, eds. *Essentials of Uroradiology*, 1st ed. Boston: Little, Brown, 1991:320.

 Ureter—Leiomyoma

DESCRIPTION Leiomyomas of the urinary tract are rare (neoplasms of mesenchymal origin comprise less than 3% of all primary ureteral tumors). These benign tumors are seen predominantly between the fourth and fifth decades of life. The left ureter is more frequently affected. Diagnosis may be suggested by urinalysis, cytology, IVP, cytoscopy, and retrograde pyelogram. Immunohistochemical studies confirm the diagnosis.

TREATMENT

- These benign mesothelial tumors require conservative resection.
- Small lesions are potentially managed with endoscopic techniques.

REFERENCE

Zaiton, MM. Leiomyoma of ureter. *Urology* 1986;28(1):50–51.

 Ureter—Leiomyosarcoma

DESCRIPTION Leiomyosarcoma originating from the ureters is exceedingly rare. There have been 13 reported cases of primary leiomyosarcoma of the ureter. It is a disease that is very difficult to diagnose. Furthermore, it has a poor 5-year disease-specific survival. Patients present with flank pain, hematuria, and/or UTI. Radiographic examination includes IVP, retrograde pyelogram, and CT. Light microscopy immunohistochemical staining and electron microscopy should be used to confirm the diagnosis of leiomyosarcoma.

TREATMENT

- Tumor resection
- Possible nephroureterectomy, depending on tumor grade and stage
- Adjuvant radiation therapy may be helpful.

REFERENCE

Griffin JH, Waters WB. Primary leiomyosarcoma of the ureter. *J Surg Oncol* 1996;62(2): 148–152.

 Ureter—Metastasis

DESCRIPTION Carcinoma metastatic to the ureter is rare. According to a study by Richie, the sites of primary tumors that later involved the ureter, in order of frequency, were breast, colon/rectum, cervix, prostate, bladder, retroperitoneal lymphoma, and miscellaneous. There is a predilection for the lower third of the ureter. Furthermore, the longest time interval from primary tumor to diagnosis of ureteral obstruction ranged from 8 months to 9 years. Therapy of ureteral obstruction secondary to metastatic tumor must be considered carefully against the patient's prognosis.

REFERENCE

Richie JP, Withers G, Ehrlich RM. Ureteral obstruction secondary to metastatic tumors. *Surg Gynecol Obstet* 1979148:355–357.

Ureter—Nephrogenic Adenoma

DESCRIPTION Nephrogenic adenoma is rarely found in the ureter, but is more common in the bladder. It is a benign papillary and tubular proliferation in response to trauma, infection, or ionizing radiation.

TREATMENT

• Biopsy and fulguration (treated as a low-grade urothelial malignancy)

REFERENCE

Bostwick DG, ed. *Urologic Surgical Pathology,* 1st ed. St Louis: Mosby, 1997.

 Ureter—Neurofibroma

DESCRIPTION Grossly, neurofibromas may be single or multiple and comprise different-sized nodules. Histologically, they are composed of fascicles of elongated, spindle-shaped cells with thin, wavy nuclei in a collagenized background. Neurofibromas in the ureter are very rare. They do have an increased incidence in von Recklinghausen disease. Neurofibromas frequently recur and can cause death by urinary obstruction and renal failure.

CAUSES

• Von Recklinghausen disease

TREATMENT

• Endoscopic or open excision

REFERENCE

Bostwick DG, ed. *Urologic Surgical Pathology,* 1st ed. St Louis: Mosby, 1997.

 Ureter—Pipe Stem

DESCRIPTION A radiographic appearance seen in late stages of tuberculous involvement of the ureter. On IVP, the ureter appears straight with a narrow lumen, due to diffuse fibrotic changes of the wall.

CAUSES

• Tuberculous infection of the ureter

TREATMENT: *N/A*

REFERENCE

Murphy DM, Fallon B, Lane V, O'Flynn JD. Tuberculous stricture of ureter. *Urology* 1982;20:382.

 Ureter—Radiation Injury to

DESCRIPTION Clinically, radiation injury to the ureter will present as obstruction. Upper urinary tract obstruction secondary to the effects of radiation is generally reported to occur in about 5% of patients with ureteral encroachment, and in less than 1% of all treated patients. The ureters are relatively resistant to the effects of radiation, although there are some factors that are postulated to increase the chance of injury after radiation exposure: infection of the ureter, necrosis of the tumor invading the ureteral wall, and direct radiation injury to the ureteral wall.

CAUSES

• Radiation therapy of 8000 Gy or more results in a 40% urologic complication rate.
• A dose of 6000 Gy or less results in less than a 2% complication rate.

TREATMENT

• See Section II, "Ureter—Malignant Obstruction."

REFERENCE

Resnick MI, Kursh ED. Extrinsic obstruction of the ureter. In: Walsh PC, Retik AB, Vaughan ED, Wein AJ, eds. *Campbell's Urology,* 7th ed. Philadelphia: WB Saunders, 1998:409–410.

 Ureter—Retrocaval (Circumcaval, Postcaval)

DESCRIPTION A retrocaval ureter is a congenital anomaly in which the problem arises from the inferior vena cava rather than the ureter. Normally, the infrarenal vena cava derives from the supracardinal vein, which lies posterior to the ureter. If the infrarenal vena cava derives from either the persistent right subcardinal or postcardinal vein, both of which lie anterior to the ureter, a portion of the lumbar ureter becomes trapped behind the vena cava. Clinically, a retrocaval ureter may present as ureteral obstruction. Males are affected 3 times more often than are females. (See "Ureter—Shepherd's Crook," below.)

SYNONYMS

• Postcaval or circumcaval ureter

TREATMENT

• Surgery with transection of the ureter and re-anastomosis in front of the inferior vena cava

REFERENCE

Amis ES, Newhouse JH, eds. *Essentials of Uroradiology,* 1st ed. Boston: Little, Brown, 1991.

 Ureter—"Shepherd's Crook"

DESCRIPTION An S-shaped appearance of the circumcaval ureter on retrograde ureterography, where a normal-caliber ureter emerging at the medial aspect of the inferior vena cava (IVC) runs inferiorly between it and the aorta. On frontal projection, the ureter is medial to the lower lumbar pedicles, where it crosses anterior to the right iliac vessels to enter the pelvis. See "Ureter—Retrocaval (Circumcaval, Postcaval)" above.

REFERENCE

Kenawi MM, Williams DI. Circumcaval ureter: A report of four cases in children, with a review of the literature and a new classification. *Br J Urol* 1976;48:183.

 Ureter—Stricture

DESCRIPTION Strictures are one of the main causes for ureteral obstruction that might lead to hydronephrosis and renal function impairment. Ureteral strictures may present with an insidious onset of irreversibly damaged renal parenchymal due to slow development of silent hydronephrosis. Common signs of symptomatic stricture are flank pain, elevated creatinine level, or decreased urine output. Imaging studies with contrast are an essential part of the diagnostic work-up. The location and length of obstruction are important parameters for treatment planning.

CAUSES

• Iatrogenic (gynecologic or other pelvic surgeries)
• Instrumentation (ureteroscopy)
• Extrinsic trauma
• Postchemotherapy and radiation therapy
• Inflammatory and infectious factors (Crohn disease)
• Malignant (intrinsic or extrinsic)
• Congenital
• Sclerosing retroperitoneal fibrosis

TREATMENT

• Relieve the obstruction with concomitant antibiotic coverage, if needed.
• Surgical correction with endoscopic or open surgery

REFERENCE

Glenn SG. Ureteral stricture: In: Graham SD Jr, ed. *Glenn's Urologic Surgery.* Philadelphia: Lippincott-Raven, 1998:173–178.

Ureter—Valves

DESCRIPTION   Ureteral valves obstruct the forward flow of fluid, causing a proximal hydronephrosis. About 35% of ureteral valves occur at the ureteropelvic junction (UPJ); 60% occur near the ureterovesical junction, and 5% in the upper ureter. Valves are 3 times more common in males. They are usually unilateral, although they may be bilateral, and, if so, usually lead to renal failure. Seventy-five percent of valves occur on the left side.

TREATMENT

- Dependent on the location of the valve
- May include ureteral reimplantation (distal ureter), endoscopic ablation (midproximal ureter), or UPJ repair

REFERENCE

Amis ES, Newhouse JH, eds. *Essentials of Uroradiology,* 1st ed. Boston: Little, Brown, 1991:63.

 Urethra—Adenocarcinoma of Accessory Glands

DESCRIPTION   In males, the urethral accessory glands can develop rare, aggressive neoplasms that are difficult to diagnose because of the local destructive nature of the lesions (Cowper and Littre glands). Cowper's gland cancers are found in the bulbous urethra, while Littre's glands can arise along the entire urethra, but tend to arise distally. In females, Skene's glands can develop adenocarcinoma as well. Patients typically present with hematuria, dysuria, and progressive urinary obstruction. Management is similar to that for urethral adenocarcinoma.

SYNONYMS

- Adenocarcinoma of Cowper's gland
- Adenocarcinoma of Littre's glands
- Adenocarcinoma of Skene's (periurethral) glands

REFERENCE

Reuter V. Urethra. In: Bostwick DG, ed. *Urologic Surgical Pathology,* 1st ed. St Louis: Mosby, 1997.

 Urethra—Condyloma

DESCRIPTION   Condyloma is a common finding in the lower genital tract, but a rare finding in the urinary tract. In fact, condyloma of the urethra or bladder is often associated with immunosuppression. It is estimated that 0.5% to 5.0% of patients with condylomata of the genitalia may also have urethral involvement. Clinically, urethral involvement is suspected when pyuria or urethral discharge appears in a patient with genital verrucae.

SYNONYMS

- Condylomata acuminatum
- Venereal warts

CAUSES

- Human papillomavirus (HPV)

TREATMENT

- Cryotherapy
- Excision
- Laser ablation

REFERENCE

Huguet Perez J, et al. Urethral condyloma in the male: Experience with 48 cases. *Arch Esp Urol* 1996;49(7):675–680.

 Urethra—Diverticular Carcinoma

DESCRIPTION   Carcinoma of the urethral diverticulum is a rare pathologic entity commonly found in females. Average age at presentation is 52. Reported symptoms included urethral bleeding (most common), dysuria, vaginal mass, and urethral obstruction. Adenocarcinoma occurs more frequently than transitional and squamous cell cancers combined and carries a more favorable diagnosis. (See Section II, "Urethra Diverticula—Female" and "Urethra—Carcinoma, General.")

TREATMENT

- Surgical: Radical cystourethrectomy with pelvic node dissection is recommended by most authors.
- Diverticulectomy has been suggested for low-stage adenocarcinoma, if close follow-up is assured.

REFERENCE

Clayton M, Siami P, Guinan P. Urethral diverticular carcinoma. *Cancer* 1992;70:665.

 Urethra—Duplication

DESCRIPTION   Duplication of the urethra is rare and usually comes to the attention of pathologists at autopsy. Duplication of the urethra may be complete, extending from the bladder to the dorsum of the penis, or partial, extending from the dorsal surface or, less commonly, the ventral surface of the penis and ending blindly. In only 15% of cases of duplicated urethra, whether complete or partial, is there a connection with the functional urethra. Most cases are asymptomatic, but the most common complication is infection. Patients may have urinary obstruction caused by compression of the functional urethra by a mass of material in the blind, accessory urethra. In other cases, patients may complain of incontinence or double urinary stream.

TREATMENT

- Complete resection of the nonfunctioning urethra, if symptomatic

REFERENCE

Bostwick DG, ed. *Urologic Surgical Pathology,* 1st ed. St Louis: Mosby, 1997.

 Urethra—Hemangioma

DESCRIPTION   Urethral hemangiomas are extremely rare tumors. The lesion is believed to be congenital, arising from the embryonic rest of unipotent angioblastic cells that fail to develop into normal blood vessels. The clinical presentation is bloody urethral discharge or frank urethral bleeding. These lesions are benign in nature.

TREATMENT

- Local resection
- Electrocoagulation

REFERENCE

Hayashi, Igarashi, Sekine. Urethral hemangioma. *J Urol* 1997;158:539–540.

Urethra—Leiomyosarcoma

DESCRIPTION Leiomyosarcoma is a smooth muscle tumor that often exhibits necrosis, hemorrhage, and cystic degeneration. Leiomyosarcomas are extremely rare tumors that are more common in females than in males. Patients present with hematuria, pain, or mass. The prognosis is poor. (See Section I, "Urethral Mass.")

TREATMENT

- Radical excision of the tumor
- Radiation therapy may be considered.

REFERENCE

Bostwick DG, ed. *Urologic Surgical Pathology*, 1st ed. St Louis: Mosby, 1997.

 Urethra—Leukoplakia

DESCRIPTION The term *leukoplakia* refers to the presence of grossly discernible white patches commonly seen on the mucosal surfaces of areas of squamous metaplasia. There seems to be an increased incidence in diabetics as well as in those with chronic irritation or infection. Generally believed to be a premalignant lesion, it may progress to squamous cell carcinoma.

SYNONYMS

- Squamous metaplasia

CAUSES

- Chronic irritation
- Chronic infection

TREATMENT

- Biopsy and ablation

REFERENCE

Benson RC, et al. Relationship of urethral leukoplakia to urothelial malignancy. *J Urol* 1984;13:507–511.

 Urethra—Lymphoma

DESCRIPTION Primary malignant lymphoma rarely affects the lower urinary tract. When it does, it generally affects the bladder. Initial presentation within the urethra is extremely rare. Concurrent or subsequent regional or systemic lymphoma is generally the rule. Only 11 cases of lymphoma presenting in the urethra have been documented, and 10 were in women. (See Section III, "Lymphoma—Urologic Considerations.")

TREATMENT

- The high probability of regional or systemic extension is an argument against radiotherapy as a primary treatment.
- Chemotherapy is an excellent treatment, and the prognosis is good.

REFERENCE

Hatcher PA, et al. Primary lymphoma of the male urethra. *Urology* 1997;49(1):142–144.

 Urethra—Malacoplakia

DESCRIPTION This designation refers to a peculiar pattern of inflammatory reaction, characterized macroscopically by soft, yellow, slightly raised mucosal plaques. The disease shows a predilection for involving the bladder, ureter, renal pelvis, ureteropelvic junction, and urethra. The disease predominates in females in a 4:1 ratio, and the peak age is in the sixth decade. Apart from symptoms associated with urinary tract infections, the clinical manifestations are usually unremarkable. Most often, the bladder is involved, and symptoms of bladder irritability or hematuria may be present. Malacoplakia occurs with increased frequency in immunosuppressed transplant recipients.

CAUSES

- Pathogenesis is unknown, but an altered host response is suspected.
- There is an association with diabetes mellitus, alcoholic liver disease, sarcoidosis, and mycobacterial infection.

TREATMENT

- When the lower urinary tract is involved, long-term antibiotics are used successfully.

REFERENCE

Karaiossifidi H, et al. Malacoplakia of the urethra: A case of unique localization with followup [Review]. *J Urol* 1992;148(6):1903–1904.

 Urethra—Malignant Melanoma

DESCRIPTION Primary urethral malignant melanoma is rare, with less than 100 cases reported in the literature. Ninety percent of patients are diagnosed in the sixth or seventh decade. Eighty percent of cases were reported to be in the fossa navicularis and the meatus. The most common presentations are dysuria, hematuria, deviated urinary stream, or urinary obstruction. Endoscopically, a pigmented nodular mucosal mass or masses, which may be ulcerated, may be seen. Local recurrence is common. Metastasis is usually to inguinal and pelvic lymph nodes. Hematogenous spread to liver, lung, and brain is also common. Staging for urethral melanoma has not yet been standardized. Prognosis depends on the thickness of the lesion.

TREATMENT

- Surgical: urethrectomy or penectomy with regional lymph node dissection
- The role of radiotherapy, immunotherapy, or chemotherapy is yet to be defined.

REFERENCE

Kokatas NS, Kallis EG, Fokitis PJ. Primary malignant melanoma of male urethra. *Urology* 1982; 18:392.

 Urethra—Meatus, Normal Caliber

DESCRIPTION Normal limits of male urethral calibration are as follows:

- 6 weeks to 3 years: 15% <8Fr; 85% 10Fr
- 4 to 10 years: 8% "tight" 8Fr; 76% 12Fr
- 11 to 12 years: 5% <10Fr; 75% 14Fr

Normal limits for female urethra are as follows:

- 2 to 4 years: 14Fr
- 6 to 10 years: 16Fr
- 12 years: 20Fr
- >14 years: 24Fr

REFERENCE

Elder JS. Congenital abnormalities of the genitalia. In: Walsh PC, Retik AB, Vaughan ED, Wein AJ, eds. *Campbell's Urology*, 7th ed. Philadelphia: WB Saunders, 1998:2128, 2137; Table 69-3 (male), Table 69-4.

Urethra—Metastasis

 Urethra—Metastasis

DESCRIPTION Metastatic lesions to the urethra usually originate from the prostate, bladder, and rectum. However, origin from distant sites has been reported. In a patient with a known malignancy, pain, hematuria, and/or urethral obstruction may suggest the diagnosis.

REFERENCE

Roberets TW, Melicow MM. Pathology and natural history of urethral tumors in females. *Urology* 1977;10:583.

 Urethra—Nephrogenic Metaplasia (Adenoma)

DESCRIPTION Nephrogenic metaplasia is a rare metaplastic lesion of urethral epithelium, with a classic triad of tubular, cystic, and papillary–polypoid patterns microscopically. Occurs at all ages, with a 3:1 male predominance. 15% of nephrogenic metaplasia is found in the urethra. Presenting symptoms include irritative voiding symptoms and hematuria, or it may be asymptomatic. Diagnosed by cystoscopy and biopsy. Clinical course usually benign, although may persist or recur. Rarely, a metaplastic lesion can cause carcinoma.

SYNONYMS

- Adenomatoid metaplasia
- Adenomatoid tumor
- Adenomatous metaplasia
- Hamartoma
- Tubular metaplasia
- Nephrogenic adenoma

CAUSES

- Etiology unknown
- Associated with surgical trauma, calculi, indwelling catheter, chronic infections, and immunosuppression

TREATMENT

- Regular cytoscopic examination
- Removal of underlying cause
- Transurethral excision

REFERENCE

Duun S, Kirkeby L, Carstensen JM. Nephrogenic metaplasia of the bladder in renal transplant recipients. *Scand J Urol Nephrol* 1995;29:109–111.

 Urethra—Papilloma (Squamous and Transitional)

DESCRIPTION First described by Potts and Hirst in 1963, papillomas are rare benign, polypoid lesions occurring in transitional cell epithelium. Greater than 90% occur in the urinary bladder, predominantly in the trigone and bladder neck area. 3.5% of cases have been described in the prostatic urethra. 6:1 male predominance, with usual presentation in sixth to seventh decade. Etiology unknown; however, thought to represent a neoplasm. Usually presents with painless hematuria or obstruction. Potential for recurrence and association with transitional cell carcinoma requires consideration of papilloma as a premalignant condition. The patient should be followed with routine urine cytology and close urologic observation.

REFERENCE

Renfer LG, Kelley J, Belville WD. Inverted papilloma of the urinary tract: Histogenesis, recurrence, and associated malignancy. *J Urol* 1988;140:832–834.

 Urethra—Polyps (Fibroepithelial, Adenomatous, Inflammatory)

DESCRIPTION Uncommon benign polypoid of papillary lesions of the urethra. Usually limited to male patients and occur most often in children. Polyps vary in microscopic features, which results in classification into fibroepithelial, adenomatous, or inflammatory. Adenomatous polyps are thought to represent prostatic glandular material from a developmental error. Fibroepithelial and inflammatory polyps consist of stromal elements and an inflammatory infiltrate, respectively. Presenting symptoms can include hematuria, hematospermia, obstruction, or urinary tract infection. Cystourethroscopy with biopsy is the test of choice. Transurethral resection with fulguration is the treatment of choice. (See Section III, "Urethritis—Polypoid.")

REFERENCE

Walsh IP, Keane PF, Herron B. Benign urethral polyps. *Br J Urol* 1993;72:937–938.

 Urethra—Prolapse (Female)

DESCRIPTION Prolapse of the urethra is a rare condition, which has been described as complete eversion of urethral mucosa through the external urethral orifice. Etiology is unknown. Primarily a disease of African-American girls, vaginal bleeding is often the presenting symptom, followed by urinary complications such as dysuria. Associated factors involve increased abdominal pressure, such as coughing, constipation, and trauma or infections of the vagina or urinary tract. Management ranges from conservative medical treatment to a variety of surgical corrective procedures, such as excision and urethroplasty.

REFERENCE

Fernandes ET, Dekermacher S, Sabadin MA, Vaz F. Urethral prolapse in children. *Urology* 1993;41(3):240–242.

 Urethra—Villous Adenoma

DESCRIPTION An adenomatous lesion of the urethra, usually polypoid in nature, covered by mucinous material. Masses 2 to 4 cm in the urinary tract have been described. Onset possibly due to similar embryologic origin with rectosigmoid. Urinary obstruction and/or hematuria can be presenting symptoms. Best treated by complete removal, due to premalignant changes seen in some lesions and malignant potential seen in adenomas of the colon

REFERENCE

Ulgaba F, Matias-Guiu X, Badia F, Sole-Balcells F. Villous adenoma of the prostatic urethra. *Eur Urol* 1988;14:255–257.

Urethral Pressure Profile

DESCRIPTION The urethral pressure profile (UPP) is a graphic representation of the intraluminal pressure along the length of the urethra. This static study provides no assessment of physiologic urethral function during voiding. The micturitional urethral pressure profile, however, is a dynamic study that can be performed by withdrawing a catheter from the urethra during micturition. The study can define the site of urethral obstruction by demonstrating a drop in urethral pressure immediately distal to the obstructive lesion in the urethra.

REFERENCE

Sullivan MP, Comiter CV, Yalla SV. Micturitional urethral pressure profilometry. *Urol Clin North Am* 1996;23(2):263–278.

 Urethritis—Polypoid

DESCRIPTION An inflammatory reaction in the urethra, secondary to mechanical irritation, pressure, and/or cytotoxic effects, caused by indwelling catheters. The lesion is similar to that seen in polypoid cystitis, due to similar macroscopic and microscopic mucosal changes. Microscopically, the mucosa is usually polypoid in appearance, often with evidence of microabscesses and an inflammatory infiltrate. Its similarity to polypoid cystitis suggests that polypoid urethritis is reversible with removal of the indwelling catheter. [See Section III, "Urethra—Polyps (Fibroepithelial, Adenomatous, Inflammatory").]

REFERENCE

Norlen LJ, Ekelund P, Heddin H, Johansson SL. Effects of indwelling catheters on the urethral mucosa (polypoid urethritis). *Scand J Urol Nephrol* 1988;22:81–86.

 Urethrorrhagia—Idiopathic

DESCRIPTION Bleeding from the urethra or blood spotting on the undershorts in preadolescents. Benign lesion, self-limited in most cases. Etiology unknown, although some theories suggest infectious in nature. Intravenous pyelogram and voiding cystourethrogram can be used to rule out other problems in the differential diagnosis. Instrumentation via catheter or endoscope is not recommended, due to potential for urethral stricture and inadequacy of procedures to aid in diagnosis.

REFERENCE

Kaplan GW, Brock WA. Idiopathic urethrorrhagia in boys. *J Urol* 1982;158(5):1001–1003.

 Urinary Diversion Electrolyte Abnormalities

DESCRIPTION Fluid and electrolyte complications, which can arise from solute transfer from urine across a bowel segment used for urinary diversion. The specific segment of bowel used, the amount and time of contact of urine with bowel mucosa, the duration of the conduit, and renal function are all factors that can affect fluid and electrolyte balances.

- *Ileal and colonic conduits* can have hyperchloremic metabolic acidosis. The mechanism is the absorption of ammonium chloride (a weak acid) in exchange for carbonic acid (CO_2 and water). Treatment, if necessary, consists of urinary alkalinization (sodium bicarbonate, Bicitra, Polycitra) or blockade of chloride transport (chlorpromazine 25–50 mg tid or nicotinic acid 400 mg tid)
- *Jejunum* is least attractive for use in urinary diversions, due to its high absorptive capacity, and associated with hyponatremic, hyperkalemic metabolic acidosis with azotemia.
- *Stomach* segments cause a hypochloremic, hypokalemic metabolic alkalosis. Normally not a significant problem unless renal failure develops and the segment usually needs to be taken down
- *Distal ileum resection* may result in macrocytic anemia due to B12 deficiency over long periods and may require supplementation.

REFERENCE

Cruz DN, Huot SJ. Metabolic complications of urinary diversions: An overview. *Am J Med* 1997;102:477–484.

 Urinary Diversion— Risk of Malignancy

DESCRIPTON Segments of bowel used for urinary diversion have increased risk of malignant transformation. Some studies have shown an increase as high as 5% to 40% 10 to 20 years after a urinary diversion. Etiology is unknown. Adenocarcinomas, adenomatous polyps, sarcomas, transitional cell carcinomas, signet ring carcinomas, and squamous cell carcinomas have been identified. Routine urinary cytology and colonoscopy are recommended after 10 years following urinary diversion.

REFERENCE

Shokeir AA, Shamaa M, El-Mekresh MM, El-Baz M, Ghoneim MA. Late malignancy in bowel segments exposed to urine without fecal stream. *Urology* 1995;46(5):657–661.

 Urinary Flow Rate (Uroflowmetry)

DESCRIPTION Uroflowmetry is the study of urinary flow rate. *Urinary flow rate* is defined as the product of detrusor contractility against bladder outlet resistance. Deviations from normal urinary flow rate may represent abnormalities of either process. It should not be used alone, but in combination with a determination of bladder residual volume and symptoms to determine the presence of bladder outlet obstruction. To adequately interpret a uroflow, most investigators agree that a voided volume of <150 mL may not generate an adequate study. Normal values are as follows:

- Males: <40 years: >22 mL/s; 40 to 60 years: >18 mL/s; >60 years: >13 mL/s
- Female: <50 years: >25 mL/s; >50 years: >18 mL/s

Obstruction should be suspected at rates of 15 mL/s or less. The study consists of a graphical flow rate pattern, along with values for maximum flow rate, average flow rate, maximum flow time, and total flow time. Various nomograms have been published to aid in the interpretation of uroflow data (Siroky, Abrhams, and Griffiths). A normal graphical flow rate pattern represents a bell-shaped curve. (See also Section III, "Pressure—Flow Studies.")

REFERENCE

Webster G, Kreder KJ. The neurourologic evaluation. In: Walsh PC, Retik AB, Vaughan ED, Wein AJ, eds. *Campbell's Urology*, 7th ed. Philadelphia: WB Saunders, 1998.

 Urinary Residual Volume

DESCRIPTION Urinary residual volume is the amount of urine present in the urinary bladder immediately after a complete voiding. Also known as post-void residual, it can assist in differentiating between disorders of emptying and disorders of storage in urinary incontinence. Provides clinical quantitative information on the degree of obstruction in certain conditions, such as BPH, or efficiency of bladder emptying in neurogenic bladder. Chronic high urinary residual volumes can predispose to infection, bladder hypertrophy, ureterovesical reflux, increased intravesical pressure, incontinence, or loss of detrusor muscle tone. Residual volume is measured by ultrasound or catheterization. Usually interpreted in the context of uroflowmetry. Treatment of high urinary residual volumes is to treat the underlying cause.

SYNONYMS

- Residual
- Post-void residual

Urinoma (Perinephric Pseudocyst)

REFERENCE

Simforoosh N, Dadkhah F, Hosseini SY, Asgari MA, Nasseri A, Safarinejad MR. Accuracy of residual urine measurement in men: Comparison between real-time ultrasonography and catheterization. *J Urol* 1997;158:59–61.

 Urinoma (Perinephric Pseudocyst)

DESCRIPTION   A urinoma is a collection of urine into the perirenal space from chronically extravasated urine. The perirenal urine causes lipolysis of surrounding fat, creating a fibrous sac around the extravasated urine. Ureteral compromise can result, secondary to obstruction from the urinoma.

SYNONYMS

- Perinephric pseudocyst

CAUSES

- Ureteral obstruction secondary to stones, neoplasms, or bladder outlet obstruction
- Accidental or iatrogenic trauma of ureter or collecting system

TREATMENT

- Correction of underlying cause; may involve stent placement, percutaneous nephrostomy, and/or percutaneous drainage of urinoma

REFERENCE

Lang EK, Glorioso L. Management of urinomas by percutaneous drainage procedure. *Radiol Clin North Am* 1986;24(4):551–559.

 Urolithiasis—Indinavir

DESCRIPTION   Spectrum of asymptomatic crystalluria, renal colic secondary to urolithiasis with or without dysuria or urgency, seen in patients who are HIV infected and being treated with indinavir. (See Section II, "HIV Infection—Urologic Considerations.")

REFERENCE

Hermieu J, et al. Urolithiasis and the protease inhibitor indinavir. *Eur Urol* 1999;35:239–241.

 Urolithiasis—Matrix

DESCRIPTION   Rare renal calculus, which has been described as being composed of coagulated mucoids with little crystalline component. Found mostly in individuals with infection due to urease-producing organisms such as *Proteus*. Matrix calculi can be confused with uric acid calculi because they are radiolucent. Matrix calculi, however, are usually associated with alkaline urine from urinary tract infection, while uric acid calculi usually form in acidic sterile urine. (See also Section II, "Urolithiasis—Adult, General.")

SYNONYMS

- Matrix stone
- Matrix nephrolithiasis
- Matrix calculus

TREATMENT

- Lithotripsy, as indicated

REFERENCE

Kim SH, Lee SE, Park IA. CT and ultrasound features of renal matrix stones with calcified center. *J Comput Assist Tomogr* 1996;20(3):404–406.

 Urolithiasis—Triamterene

DESCRIPTION   Renal calculus consisting either completely or partially of triamterene, a potassium-sparing diuretic often used with hydrochlorothiazide in the treatment of hypertension. Promotion of nucleation and growth of renal calculi, especially calcium oxalate monohydrate, has been shown to occur from triamterene and its metabolites. They are usually radiopaque. Although rare, they usually occur in a patient with a history of urolithiasis. (See also Section II, "Urolithiasis—Adult, General.")

SYNONYMS

- Triamterene stone
- Triamterene nephrolithiasis
- Triamterene calculus

TREATMENT

- Avoid use of triamterene in patients with a history of urolithiasis.
- Discontinue use of triamterene in patients with triamterene urolithiasis.

REFERENCE

Carr MC, Prien EL Jr, Babayan RK. Triamterene nephrolithiasis: Renewed attention is warranted. *J Urol* 1990;144(6):1339–1440.

 Urolithiasis—Xanthine

DESCRIPTION   Renal calculus composed of xanthine. Usually associated with hereditary xanthinuria, an autosomal recessively inherited inborn error of metabolism characterized by a deficiency of xanthine oxidase. Other causes include allopurinol use in patients with Lesch-Nyhan syndrome, APRT deficiency, or endogenous uric acid overproduction. Xanthine calculi can be confused with uric acid calculi because they are both radiolucent. Xanthine calculi, however, are associated with low serum uric acid levels. (See also Section II, "Urolithiasis—Adult, General.")

SYNONYMS

- Xanthine stone
- Xanthine nephrolithiasis
- Xanthine calculus

TREATMENT

- High fluid intake
- Lithotripsy, if indicated

REFERENCES

Cameron JS, Moro F, Simmonds HA. Gout, uric acid, and purine metabolism in paediatric nephrology. *Pediatr Nephrol* 1993;7:105–118.

Jorgensen JB. Uroflowmetry. *Urol Clin North Am* 1996;23(2):237–242.

 VACTERL Association

DESCRIPTION   Congenital abnormality association involving defects in three or more of the following: vertebral defects, anal atresia, cardiac defects, esophageal atresia and/or tracheoesophageal fistula, renal dysplasia, and limb defects, especially radial limb defects. Also known as VATER syndrome

REFERENCE

Botto LD, et al. The spectrum of congenital anomalies of the VATER association: An international study. *Am J Med Genet* 1997;71:8–15.

Vaginal Agenesis

DESCRIPTION   Absence or failure of formation of the vagina. Occurs in 1 in 4000 to 1 in 5000 female births. 50% of the time, vaginal agenesis is associated with renal abnormalities, such agenesis or ectopia. Uterine abnormalities are commonly associated as well. Etiology has been theorized to be a defect in the embryologic development of a single mesonephric duct. Patient usually comes to attention due to primary amenorrhea. Surgical reconstruction with the use of grafts or flaps is the treatment of choice.

REFERENCE

Marshall FF. Vaginal abnormalities. *Urol Clin North Am* 1978;5(1):155–159.

 Vaginal Duplication

DESCRIPTION   Rare abnormality in embryologic development, which results in duplication of the vagina. Caused by failure of a primitive septum in the uterovaginal canal to regress or abnormalities in the fusion of paramesonephric ducts during weeks 8 and 9 of embryologic development of the upper vagina. The lower vagina develops from the urogenital sinus when the sinovaginal bulbs fuse. Abnormalities in the fusion can result in different vaginal abnormalities, including duplication. Presenting symptoms can include dysmenorrhea at menarche or a lower abdominal mass. Surgical correction of the septum is the treatment of choice for vaginal duplication.

REFERENCE

Burbige KA, Hensle TW. Uterus didelphys and vaginal duplication with unilateral obstruction presenting as a newborn abdominal mass. *J Urol* 1984;132(6):1195–1198.

 Valsalva Maneuver

DESCRIPTION   A maneuver effected by a forced expiratory effort against a voluntarily closed airway, which causes increased intrathoracic and intraabdominal pressure and impedes venous return to the right atrium. The maneuver may increase the degree of varicocele dilatation, aiding in diagnosis. It can also be used to measure the pressure required to cause leakage in the absence of a bladder contraction, which correlates with the degree of urinary incontinence. The Valsalva maneuver can also be used to aid in micturition in those with hypotonic bladders by increasing intravesical pressure. (See also Section III, "Leak Point Pressure.")

REFERENCE

Desautel MG, Kapoor R, Badlani GH. Sphincteric incontinence: The primary cause of post-prostatectomy incontinence in patients with prostate cancer. *Neurourol Urodyn* 1997;16(3):153–160.

 Vanishing Testis Syndrome

DESCRIPTION   A condition in which a normal genotypic 46XY male has absent or rudimentary testes with otherwise normal differentiation of internal and external structures. Infertility is inevitable, despite aggressive testosterone replacement therapy.

SYNONYMS

- Bilateral anorchia
- Gonadal agenesis
- Testicular regression syndrome
- XY agonadism

CAUSES

- Vascular compromise in utero, infection in utero, testicular torsion in utero

TREATMENT

- Testosterone replacement therapy to induce virilization

REFERENCE

Gong M, Geary ES, Shortliffe LM. Testicular torsion with contralateral vanishing testis. *Urology* 1996;48(2):306–307.

 Vas Deferens—Calcification

DESCRIPTION   Calcification of the vas deferens (CVD) is a rare finding that is primarily detected in radiologic examinations. It usually presents asymptomatically. A majority of the patients with calcification of the vas deferens are diabetics in their fifth or sixth decade of life. For these diabetic patients, CVD has a bilateral and symmetrical presentation. In addition, a minority of patients will present with postinflammatory CVD, which usually has a unilateral and segmental presentation.

REFERENCE

Grunebaum M. The calcified vas deferens. *Isr J Med Sci* 1971;7:311.

 Vasculitis—Urologic Considerations

DESCRIPTION   Vasculitis is a common reaction to injury caused by a multitude of different processes, including autoimmunity, infection, and hypersensitivity. There is a very strong correlation between the presence of antineutrophil cytoplasmic antibodies (ANCA) and the various types of systemic vasculitis that cause crescentic glomerulonephritis and/or focal necrotizing glomerulonephritis. Depending on the type of vasculitis, patients present with different signs and symptoms. Furthermore, some types can progress to chronic renal failure. However, upon renal biopsy, similar pathologic presentations are demonstrated.

SYNONYMS

- Various types
  - Henoch-Schönlein purpura
  - Polyarteritis nodosa (PAN)
  - Hypersensitivity angitis
  - Wegener's granulomatosis
  - Lymphomatoid granulomatosis

TREATMENT

- ANCA titers have proved to be extremely useful in the management of patients. They are a help in diagnosis, and even more important as a guide to maintenance immunosuppressive therapy.
- Cytotoxic agents and corticosteroids are effective, depending on the type of vasculitis.

REFERENCE

Rees AJ. Vasculitis and the kidney. *Curr Opin Nephrol Hypertens* 1996;5(3):273–281.

Venous Leak Syndrome

 Venous Leak Syndrome

DESCRIPTION Venous leakage is a common cause of vascular impotence due to veno-occlusive dysfunction. Possible leak sites are the superficial and deep dorsal veins, cavernosal venous system, and glans or corpus spongiosum. The majority of patients would have more than one leak site. Diagnosis can be demonstrated by pharmacocavernosography.

CAUSES

- Congenital
- Iatrogenic
- Neovascularity associated with inflammatory reactions secondary to stricture disease or Peyronie disease.

TREATMENT

- Surgical correction
- Combination of pharmacologic injection therapy with a venous constriction system or a vacuum device

REFERENCE

Shabsigh R., Fishman IJ, Toombs BD, Skolkin M. Venous leaks: Anatomical and physiological observations. *J Urol* 1991;146:1260.

 Videourodynamics

DESCRIPTION A technique in which urodynamic studies are performed at the same time as fluoroscopy of the lower urinary tract. The cystometry and pressure–flow studies are conducted in the same manner as regular urodynamics. The only difference is the addition of contrast and fluoroscopy. Radiation exposure is usually limited to less than 20 seconds. Adding simultaneous video enhances the evaluation of all patients, especially for more complex urodynamic problems. Videourodynamics is helpful when results from simple urodynamics do not agree with the clinical scenario. In complex bladder outlet obstruction, this technique can identify whether it occurs at the bladder neck, the prostatic urethra, or the distal sphincter. It is also helpful in the identification of bladder neck dysfunction in young men with voiding problems and in neurogenic patients with dyssynergia of the distal sphincter. In incontinence evaluation, videourodynamics can help identify the presence and degree of vesical neck hypermobility, the degree of proximal urethral weakness, and the degree and type of cystocele present. In neurogenic bladders, simultaneous video screening aids in diagnosing proximal and distal sphincter dyssynergia and demonstrates the presence of reflux and bladder diverticula. The presence of reflux, bladder and urethral diverticula, fistula, and stones can be identified and characterized.

REFERENCE

McGuire EJ, Cespedes RD, Cross CA, et al. Videourodynamic studies. *Urol Clin North Am* 1996; 23(2):309–321.

 Villous Adenoma—Bladder/Urethra

DESCRIPTION Villous adenomas of the bladder and urethra are rare and histologically identical to those found in the colon. These tumors are more frequently found in the urachus at the dome of the bladder. On cystoscopy, these villous adenomas appear as exophytic papillary masses. Histologically, villous adenomas are complex branching papillary structures lined by a pseudostratified epithelium containing goblet cells. Often, this tumor is associated with cystitis glandularis. Villous adenoma of the urethra has been reported in both males and females. In males, villous adenoma may be associated with urinary retention, hematuria, and difficulty in micturition. In females, it may be less symptomatic and present with a slowly growing mass in the urethra. When villous adenomas are found, primary intestinal tumor must be ruled out. After resection of the adenoma, the patient must be followed for recurrence or malignancy because their behavior is unpredictable. Diagnosis is made with urine cytology, cystogram, cystoscopy, or biopsy.

TREATMENT

- Transurethral resection
- Cystectomy

REFERENCE

Channer JL, Williams JL, Henry L. Villous adenoma of the bladder. *J Clin Pathol* 1993;46(5):450–452.

 Vimentin—Staining

DESCRIPTION Monoclonal antibodies can be used to identify cell products or surface markers by directing antibodies against intermediate filaments. This facilitates the classification of otherwise poorly differentiated tumors. Vimentin is the predominant intermediate filament in mesenchymal cells, and it is found in all fibroblasts. Vimentin is less specific than the other intermediate filaments in immunocytochemistry because certain epithelial tumors (e.g., renal cell carcinoma) may co-express keratin and vimentin.

REFERENCE

Cotran R, Kumar V, Robbins S. *Pathologic Basis of Disease,* 5th ed. 1995:299.

 Vitiligo—Urological Considerations

DESCRIPTION A depigmentation of the skin, in which sharply bordered patches of skin become white. This is distinct from postinflammatory skin depigmentation in that there is no preceding inflammatory process. The etiology is probably autoimmune, and it is estimated to involve the external genitalia only in 0.3% of the adult male population. Treatment is optional and can include steroids, uv light, skin grafting, and cosmetic covering.

REFERENCE

Margolis DJ. Cutaneous diseases of the male external genitalia. In: Walsh PC, Retik AB, Vaughan ED, Wein AJ, eds. *Campbell's Urology,* 7th ed. Philadelphia: WB Saunders, 1998.

 Voiding Diary

DESCRIPTION A tool often used in association with pad testing to document the nature and severity of incontinence. A data sheet, maintained by the patient over a representative 24-hour period, typically documents the following:

- Time of urge to void
- Strength of urge or pain
- Time of actual void
- Voided volume
- Incontinence (stress, urge, unaware)
- Amount of leakage (small, medium, large)

REFERENCE

Blaivas JG, et al. Urinary incontinence. In: Walsh PC, Retik AB, Vaughan ED, Wein AJ, eds. *Campbell's Urology,* 7th ed. Philadelphia: WB Saunders, 1998:1021.

VURD Syndrome

DESCRIPTION VURD stands for vesicoureteral reflux associated with renal dysplasia. This term applies to children with posterior urethral valves in which there is massive reflux into a dysplastic nonfunctioning kidney. Approximately 15% of the patients with posterior urethral valves have this syndrome. Some believe that severe unilateral vesicoureteral reflux is protective of the contralateral nonrefluxing kidney. Diagnosis is made using kidney ultrasound, voiding cystourethrogram, nuclear imaging of kidneys, and serum creatinine levels.

CAUSES

- Posterior urethral valves

TREATMENT

- The patient should be observed first to see if kidney function returns. If function does not return, then nephrectomy is considered.

REFERENCE

Donnelly LF, Gylys-Morin VM, Wacksman J, et al. Unilateral vesicoureteral reflux: Association with protected renal function in patients with posterior urethral valves. *AJR* 1997;168(3): 823–826.

 WAGR Syndrome (Wilms' Tumor, Aniridia, Genital Anomaly, Retardation Syndrome)

DESCRIPTION This is one of the Wilms' tumor–associated syndromes, presenting in children less than 3 years of age. It causes mental retardation and genitourinary manifestations in the form of renal hypoplasia, ectopia, fusions, duplications, cystic disease, hypospadias, cryptorchidism, pseudohermaphroditism. Physical examination may also reveal ear deformities, umbilical/inguinal hernias, and aniridia.

REFERENCE

Kirsch AJ, Snyder HM III. What's new and important in pediatric urologic oncology. AUA Update Series, 17:83, 1998.

 Wallace Ureteral Anastomosis

DESCRIPTION The spatulated ureters are laid adjacent and the apex of each is sutured. The medial and lateral walls are then sutured together in either an interrupted or running fashion. The Y configured ureters are then anastomosed to the end of the small bowel segment.

REFERENCE

McDougal WS. Use of intestinal segments and urinary diversion. In: Walsh PC, Retik AB, Vaughan ED, Wein AJ, eds. *Campbell's Urology*, 7th ed. Philadelphia: WB Saunders, 1998:3137–3144.

 Walter Reed Staging System—Testis Cancer

DESCRIPTION These are lymphangiographic criteria used to evaluate the presence and location of testicular neoplasm metastases. The following lymphangiographic patterns were found to be useful in assessing metastatic disease: filling defects, lymph node enlargement and masses, lymphatic obstruction and collateral vessel formation, and an increase or decrease in the number of lymph nodes.

REFERENCE

Maier JG, Schamter DT. The role of lymphangiography in the diagnosis and treatment of malignant testicular tumors. *AJR* 1972;114:482.

 Waterhouse Friederichsen Syndrome

DESCRIPTION Acute adrenocortical insufficiency in children suffering from septicemia with *Pseudomonas* or meningococcemia, leading to acute hemorrhagic destruction of both adrenal glands

REFERENCE

Rao RH, et al. Bilateral massive adrenal hemorrhage: Early recognition and treatment. *Ann Intern Med* 1989;116:227.

 Waterhouse Urethral Stricture Repair

DESCRIPTION Through a combined abdominal and perineal approach, a wedge of pubis is resected with a Gigli saw. The membranous stricture is identified and excised. The distal urethra is mobilized off the corporal bodies, and the spatulated urethral edges are reanastomosed.

REFERENCE

Devine CJ, Devine PC. Operations for urethral stricture. In: Novick AC, Streem SB, Pontes JE, eds. *Stewarts Operative Urology*. Baltimore: Williams & Wilkins, 1989:650–680.

 Weddellite

DESCRIPTION Mineral name for calcium oxylate dihydrate stones. (See Section II, "Urolithiasis—Calcium Oxylate/Phosphate.")

 Wegener's Granulomatosis

DESCRIPTION Systemic granulomatous vasculitis, most commonly affecting the upper and lower respiratory tracts and the kidneys, affecting small arteries and venules. Respiratory infiltrates or sinusitis are commonly the presenting symptoms, as well as constitutional symptoms (weight loss, fever, etc.). Renal involvement is usually vasculitis-induced chronic renal failure, but can have acute fulminant glomerulonephritis. Other urologic manifestations include granulomatous necrotizing prostatitis, urethritis, or epididymo-orchitis. Hemorrhagic cystitis is common, but usually iatrogenic secondary to cyclophosphamide treatment. Diagnosis is made by

- Granulomatous necrotizing vasculitis (lung biopsy)
- Focal necrotizing glomerulonephritis (renal biopsy)
- Red cell casts in voided urine (glomerulonephritis)
- Antineutrophil cytoplasmic antibodies (ANCA) (useful for follow-up)

TREATMENT

- Cyclophosphamide
- Corticosteroids
- Other cytotoxic and immunosuppressive agents: methotrexate, cyclosporine, FK-506
- Surveillance cystoscopy when cyclophosphamide used

REFERENCE

Duna GF, et al. Wegener's granulomatosis. *Rheum Dis Clin North Am* 1995;21(4):949–986.

Whewellite

 Whewellite

DESCRIPTION Mineral name for calcium oxylate monohydrate stones. (See Section II, "Urolithiasis—Calcium Oxylate/Phosphate.")

 Whitaker Test

DESCRIPTION Antegrade pressure–flow study to assess for renal obstruction. Used to determine if pelvocaliectasis or hydronephroureterosis seen radiographically represents functional obstruction or anatomic dilation. Technically difficult, invasive test, requiring placement of percutaneous antegrade catheter into renal pelvis, with simultaneous monitoring of bladder and renal pelvic pressures during set flow rate of 10 mL/min. Elevation of renal pelvic pressure over bladder pressure indicates degree of renal obstruction. A Foley catheter must be in the bladder.

RENAL PELVIS—BLADDER PRESSURE DIFFERENTIAL	DEGREE OF OBSTRUCTION
<13 cm H_2O	Normal
14–20 cm H_2O	Mild obstruction
21–34 cm H_2O	Moderate obstruction
>35 cm H_2O	Severe obstruction

SYNONYMS

- Urodynamic antegrade pyelogram
- Ureteral perfusion test
- Pressure–flow Whitaker examination

REFERENCE

Whitaker RH. The Whitaker Test. *Urol Clin North Am* 1979;6(3):529–539.

 Whitlockite

DESCRIPTION Mineral name for tricalcium phosphate stones. (See Section II, "Urolithiasis—Calcium Oxylate/Phosphate.")

 WHO Classification of Bladder Tumors

DESCRIPTION The WHO histologic classification of urinary bladder tumors is as follows. A pathology working group is currently preparing a modification of this classification.

- Epithelial tumors

—Transitional cell papilloma
—Transitional cell papilloma, inverted type
—Squamous cell papilloma

- Transitional cell carcinoma

—Variants of transitional cell carcinoma
   —With squamous metaplasia
   —With glandular metaplasia
   —With squamous and glandular metaplasia
—Squamous cell carcinoma
—Adenocarcinoma
—Undifferentiated carcinoma

- Nonepithelial tumors

—Benign
—Malignant
—Rhabdomyosarcoma
—Others

- Miscellaneous tumors

—Pheochromocytoma
—Lymphomas
—Carcinosarcoma
—Malignant melanoma
—Others

- Metastatic tumors and secondary extensions, unclassified tumors, epithelial abnormalities

—Papillary (polypoid) "cystitis"
—Von Brunn's nests
—"Cystitis" cystica
—Glandular metaplasia
—"Nephrogenic adenoma"
—Squamous metaplasia

- Tumor-like lesions

—Follicular cystitis
—Malakoplakia
—Amyloidosis
—Fibrous (fibroepithelial) polyp
—Endometriosis
—Hamartomas
—Cysts

REFERENCE

Mostofi FK, Sobin IH, Torloni H, et al. Histological typing of urinary bladder tumors. *WHO* 1973;10:21.

 Wilms' Tumor Staging System (National)

DESCRIPTION A unified system developed to aid in the conduct of clinical trials now widely used for clinical staging treatment decisions. (See Section II, "Wilms' Tumor.")

- Stage I: Tumor is limited to kidney and is completely excised.
- Stage II: Tumor extends beyond the kidney (regional extension) but is completely removed. There is no residual tumor at or beyond the surgical margins.
- Stage III: Residual nonhematogenous tumor is confined to the abdomen. This may occur as positive lymph nodes, peritoneal contamination by tumor, positive surgical margins, or locally unresectable tumor.
- Stage IV: hematogenous metastases; involves distant organs, e.g., lung, liver, bone, brain
- Stage V: bilateral renal involvement

REFERENCE

D'Angio GJ, Breslow W, Beckwith JB, et al. Treatment of Wilms' Tumor: Results of the Third National Wilms' Tumor Study. *Cancer* 1989;64: 349–360.

 Winter Corporal Shunt

DESCRIPTION A shunt between the corpora and glans penis. A Tru-Cut biopsy needle is inserted through the tip of the glans and into the corpora, and a core of tissue is removed. Through the same glans puncture site, the Tru-Cut can be reinserted in order to create two fistulas at the end of both corpora. Used in the treatment of priapism

REFERENCE

Thomas AJ. Surgery for priapism. In: Novick AC, Streem SB, Pontes JE, eds. *Stewarts Operative Urology*. Baltimore: Williams & Wilkins, 1989: 826–832.

Wolffian Duct Remnants

DESCRIPTION Normally, an embryo develops two sets of paired Müllerian and Wolffian (mesonephric) ducts. In females, virilization of the Wolffian system fails to occur, and Wolffian vestiges may persist as the epoophoron, Gartner's duct, or the appendix vesiculosa, commonly forming paraovarian cysts. In males, virilization of the Wolffian duct gives rise to epididymis, vas deferens, ejaculatory duct and seminal vesicles. The rostral end of the Wolffian duct occasionally persists as a vestigial remnant, the appendix epididymis. Remnants of the mesonephric tubules may persist as a cystic structure, the paradidymis.

SYNONYMS

- Paradidymis
- Appendix epididymis

REFERENCE

Wilson JD, Griffin JE, George FW, et al. The role of gonadal steroids in sexual differentiation. *Recent Prog Horm Res* 1981;37:1.

 ## Xanthoma—Bladder

DESCRIPTION Collection of foamy histocytes found in the lamina propria in patients with disorders of lipid metabolism

REFERENCE

Nishimura K, Nozawa M, Hara T, et al. Xanthoma of the bladder. *J Urol* 1995;153:1912.

 ## XO Syndrome

DESCRIPTION A sex chromosome syndrome with an incidence of 1 in 10,000 newborn females. Clinically, patients present with short stature, primary amenorrhea, webbed neck, shieldlike chest, and coarctation of the aorta. Genitourinary anomalies include horseshoe kidney and infantile genitalia. Due to the increased incidence of aortic aneurysm formation and rupture associated with the disease, a routine echocardiogram should be performed, and a routine intravenous pyelography or ultrasound to rule out a surgically correctable renal abnormality is indicated.

SYNONYMS

- Turner syndrome

TREATMENT

- Hormonal therapy in the form of growth hormone, estrogen, and medroxy progesterone, aimed toward maximizing final height, induction of secondary sexual characteristics, and menarche

REFERENCE

Mininberg D. The genetic basis of urologic disease. AUA Update Series, 9:218, 1992.

 ## XX Male Reversal Syndrome

DESCRIPTION A rare disorder of phenotypic males who have a 46XX karyotype. Physical examination may reveal short stature; small, firm testes; a small- to normal-sized penis; hypospadias; and gynecomastia. Azoospermia is typical. Seminiferous tubule sclerosis can be shown on testicular biopsy. Lab investigations would reveal high gonadotropin levels and decreased testosterone levels. In most cases, DNA fragments from the short arm of the Y chromosome can be detected in the distal end of the short arm of the X chromosome.

REFERENCE

Petit C, Chapelle A, Levilliers J, et al. An abnormal terminal X-Y interchange accounts for most but not all cases of human XX maleness. *Cell* 1987;49:595.

 ## XXX Syndrome

DESCRIPTION Triple X chromosome abnormality accrues in approximately 1.2 in 1000 liveborn females. There are no specific diagnostic features. Menstrual irregularities and mental retardation have been reported. Fertility is usually preserved, and many XXX females give normal offspring.

REFERENCE

Sills JA, Brown JK, Grace E, Wood SM, Barclay GR, Urbaniak SJ. XXX syndrome associated with immunoglobulin deficiency and epilepsy. *J Pediatr* 1978;93:469.

 ## XXXY Syndrome

DESCRIPTION Rare variant of Klinefelter syndrome (47XXY), with additional X chromosome (48XXXY). Phenotype similar to 47XXY, with more pronounced features. Frequently exhibit microphallus, hypoplastic testicles, cryptorchidism, hypospadias, and gynecomastia. Infertile, with azoospermia. Usually are mentally retarded, and have characteristic faces

TREATMENT

- Supplemental testosterone may be beneficial for virilization at puberty.

REFERENCE

Linden MG, et al. Sex chromosome tetrasomy and pentasomy. *Pediatrics* 1995;96(4 Pt 1): 672–682.

 ## XXY Syndrome (Klinefelter Syndrome)

DESCRIPTION A syndrome characterized by the presence of an extra X chromosome, resulting in a hypogonadal male. Affected individuals are tall, with a eunuchoid habitus, small firm testes, and gynecomastia. Mental retardation and psychiatric disturbances have also been identified. Elevated gonadotropins and azoospermia are typically present. Seminiferous tubular sclerosis is a common finding on testicular biopsy. The diagnosis may be made with a chromatin-positive buccal smear, indicating the presence of an extra X chromosome. Karyotypes usually demonstrate 47XXY or the milder mosaic pattern, 46XY, 47XXY.

CAUSES

- Nondysjunction of the meiotic chromosomes of the gametes from either parent

TREATMENT

- No therapy to improve spermatogenesis in Klinefelter syndrome
- In mosaic Klinefelter syndrome with severe oligospermia, intracytoplasmic injection with IVF is technically possible.

REFERENCE

Klinefelter HG Jr, Reifenstein EC Jr, Albright F. Syndrome characterized by gynecomastia, aspermatogenesis without aleydigism and increased secretion of follicle stimulating hormone. *J Clin Endocrinol* 1942;2:615.

 ## Yolk Sac Tumor—Bladder

DESCRIPTION Yolk sac tumor of the bladder is very rare. It has the same pathologic characteristics as its counterparts in any other part of the body, and it is managed in the same way. (See Section III, "Yolk Sack Tumor—Prostate.")

REFERENCE

Messing EM, Catalona W. Urothelial tumors of the urinary tract. In: Walsh PC, Retik AB, Vaughan ED, Wein AJ, eds. *Campbell's Urology*, 7th ed. Philadelphia: WB Saunders, 1998:2327–2410.

Yolk Sac Tumor—Prostate

 Yolk Sac Tumor—Prostate

DESCRIPTION Extragonadal germ cell tumor located in the prostate, similar to yolk sac tumor found in the testis. Primary site of presentation in the prostate is extremely rare, with only a few reported cases. Increased incidence of extragonadal germ cell tumor reported with Klinefelter syndrome. Fetoprotein commonly elevated, and used as tumor marker; human chorionic gonadotropin not elevated. Schiller-Duval bodies evident on histology

SYNONYMS

• Endodermal sinus tumor

TREATMENT

• Multimodal: cisplatinum-based combination chemotherapy and radical surgery

REFERENCE

Tay HP, et al. Primary yolk sac tumor of the prostate in a patient with Klinefelter's syndrome. *J Urol* 1995;153(3):1066–1069.

 Young–Dees–Leadbetter Bladder Reconstruction

DESCRIPTION This procedure is used to achieve a functional bladder neck closure (i.e., establish continence) in children with exstrophy; also for urinary incontinence in nonexstrophy conditions, although generally no longer widely used. Through an anterior cystotomy a rectangular area between the distal urethra and trigone is demarcated. Flaps lateral to this are developed and used to tubularize a neourethra over a 10Fr catheter.

REFERENCE

Duckett JW, Caldamone AA. Bladder and urachus. In: Kelalis P, King L, Belman B, eds. *Clinical Pediatric Urology,* 2nd ed., Philadelphia: WB Saunders, 1985:735.

 Young's Classification of Posterior Urethral Valves

DESCRIPTION Young described three general types of posterior urethral valves:

• Type I: The valves are continuous with the verumontanum and take an anterior course, dividing into two forklike processes in the region of the bulbomembranous junction. Usually, anterior fusion of the valves is not complete; however, some cases exhibit complete anterior fusion and cleft between the folds posteriorly. A subdivision of type I consists of a single instead of double valve. Type I valves are the most common.
• Type II: Same as type I, but the valves, rather than taking an anterior course, would tend to pass from the upper aspect of the verumontanum towards the internal sphincter, where it divides into two forklike processes. (Note: Type II valves are now thought to be nonexistent.)
• Type III: The valves have no relation to the verumontanum; instead, they are attached to the entire circumference of the urethra at any level, with a small opening in the center, and they have been called "iris valves" due to their resemblance to the iris of the eye. Incomplete varieties of this type (crescentic or semilunar) have been described. Type III valves are a more distal diaphragmatic obstruction, similar to a urethral membrane.

REFERENCE

Young HH, Frantz WA, Baldwin JC. Congenital obstruction of the posterior urethra. *J Urol* 1919;3:289.

 Young Syndrome

DESCRIPTION Obstructive azoospermia in patients with frequent respiratory infections or bronchiectasis. Motile sperm, with normal cilia and vas deferens

CAUSES

• Inspissated secretions, causing epididymal obstruction

TREATMENT

• Vasoepididymostomy, but fertility rates remain poor

REFERENCE

Hughes TM III, et al. Young's syndrome: An often unrecognized correctable cause of obstructive azoospermia. *J Urol* 1987;137(6):1238–1240.

 Zellweger Syndrome

DESCRIPTION Family of diseases of inborn errors of metabolism. Causes agenesis or disruption of peroxisomes. Autosomal recessive inheritance pattern, with an incidence of 1 in 25,000 to 1 in 50,000 live births. Characteristics include severe developmental delay, sensorineural deafness, renal cysts, retinal dysfunction, hepatomegaly, and characteristic facies. Usually lethal in childhood, with rare patients surviving into adolescence and adulthood. Positive diagnosis is made by serum assay of very long chain fatty acids (VLCFA) and dihydroxyacetone phosphate acyl transferase (DHAP-AT). Related disorders include

• Neonatal adrenoleukodystrophy (NALD)
• Infantile Refsum disease (IRD)
• Hyperpipecolic acidemia (HPA)
• Pseudo-Zellweger syndrome

TREATMENT

• No known treatment

REFERENCE

Fitzpatrick, D. Zellweger syndrome and associated phenotypes. *J Med Genet* 1996;33:863.

 Zona Pellucida Binding Assay

DESCRIPTION An assay used to counsel patients about their chances of success with IVF. Being species-specific, the human sperm-ZP binding requires human oocytes. Different sources of oocytes can be used, such as postmortem, IVF surplus, or surgical specimens. Oocytes are bisected, and half of the zona acts as the control. Different preservation methods are available, such as salt storage, dimethyl sulfoxide freezing, or ultra-low-temperature freezing. The assay is essentially composed of two steps: initial attachment, followed by irreversible binding. After repeated rinsing, the number of tightly bound spermatozoa to ZP is counted using phase contrast microscopy. This can be expressed as the hemizona index, which is the number of the patient's bound spermatozoa divided by the bound spermatozoa from the fertile control donor multiplied by 1003. Using a cut off of 35%, the hemizona index has been used by some to predict IVF success rate.

REFERENCE

Oehninger S, et al. Hemizona assay and its impact on the identification and treatment of human sperm dysfunctions. *Andrologia* 1992; 24:307.

Section IV
Urine Studies

Urine Studies

 ## Normal Urinalysis Values

- Appearance: "yellow, clear," or "straw colored, clear"
- Specific gravity

—Neonate: 1.012
—Infant: 1.002 to 1.006
—Child and adult: 1.001 to 1.035 (with normal fluid intake 1.016–1.022)

- pH

—Newborn/neonate: 5 to 7
—Child and adult: 4.6 to 8.0

- Negative for bilirubin, blood, acetone, glucose, protein, nitrite, leukocyte esterase, reducing substances
- Trace: urobilinogen
- RBC: male: 0 to 3/HPF; female: 0 to 5/HPF
- WBC: 0 to 4/HPF
- Epithelial cells: occasional
- Hyaline casts: occasional
- Bacteria: none
- Crystals: some limited crystals, based on urine pH (see below)

 ## Differential Diagnosis for Routine Urinalysis

- Appearance

—Colorless: diabetes insipidus, diuretics, excess fluid intake
—Dark: acute intermittent porphyria, malignant melanoma
—Cloudy: urinary tract infection (pyuria), amorphous phosphate salts (phosphaturia is normal in alkaline urine), blood, mucus, bilirubin
—Pink/red
  —Heme positive: blood, hemoglobin, sepsis, dialysis, myoglobin
  —Heme negative: food coloring, beets, sulfa drugs, nitrofurantoin, salicylates
—Orange/yellow: dehydration, phenazopyridine (Pyridium), rifampin, bile pigments
—Brown/black: Myoglobin, bile pigments, melanin, cascara, iron, nitrofurantoin, metronidazole, alkaptonuria
—Green: urinary bile pigments, indigo carmine, methylene blue
—Foamy: proteinuria, bile salts

- pH

—Acidic: High-protein (meat) diet, ammonium chloride, mandelic acid and other medications, acidosis (due to ketoacidosis [starvation, diabetic], chronic obstructive pulmonary disease [COPD])
—Basic: urinary tract infections (UTIs), renal tubular acidosis, diet (high-vegetable, milk, immediately after meals), sodium bicarbonate therapy, vomiting, metabolic alkalosis, diuretic therapy

- Specific gravity

—Usually corresponds with osmolarity, except with osmotic diuresis. A value >1.023 indicates normal renal concentrating ability.
  —Increased: volume depletion, congestive heart failure (CHF), adrenal insufficiency, diabetes mellitus, inappropriate antidiuretic hormone (ADH), increased proteins (nephrosis); if markedly increased (1.040–1.050), suspect artifact or excretion of radiographic contrast media.
  —Decreased: diabetes insipidus, pyelonephritis, glomerulonephritis, water load with normal renal function

- Bilirubin

—Positive: obstructive jaundice (intrahepatic and extrahepatic), hepatitis (note: false positive with stool contamination)

- Blood

—Positive: See Section I, "Hematuria."
—Note: If the dipstick is positive for blood, but no red cells are seen, there may be free hemoglobin from trauma, from a transfusion reaction, or from lysis of RBCs (RBCs will lyse if the pH is <5 or >8), or there may be myoglobin present because of a crush injury, burn, or tissue ischemia.

- Glucose

—Positive: diabetes mellitus, pancreatitis, pancreatic carcinoma, pheochromocytoma, Cushing disease, shock, burns, pain, steroids, hyperthyroidism, renal tubular disease, iatrogenic causes.
(Note: The glucose oxidase technique in many kits is specific for glucose and will not react with lactose, fructose, or galactose.)

- Ketones

—Detects primarily acetone and acetoacetic acid and not β-hydroxybutyric acid
  —Positive: Starvation, high-fat diet, diabetic ketoacidosis, vomiting, diarrhea, hyperthyroidism, pregnancy, febrile states (especially in children)

- Nitrite

—Many bacteria will convert nitrates to nitrite. (See also the section on Leukocyte Esterase, below.)
  —Positive: infection (A negative test does not rule out infection, because some organisms, such as *Streptococcus faecalis* and other gram-positive cocci, will not produce nitrite, and the urine must also be retained in the bladder for several hours to allow the reaction to take place.)

- Protein

—Indication by dipstick of persistent proteinuria should be quantified by 24-hour urine studies.
  —Positive: pyelonephritis, glomerulonephritis, Kimmelstiel-Wilson syndrome (diabetes), nephrotic syndrome, myeloma, postural causes, preeclampsia, inflammation and malignancies of the lower tract, functional causes (fever, stress, heavy exercise), malignant hypertension, CHF

- Leukocyte esterase

—This test detects 5 or greater WBCs/HPF or lysed WBCs. When combined with the nitrite test, it has a predictive value for urinary tract infection of 74% if both tests are positive, and >97% if both tests are negative.
  —Positive: infection (false-positive with vaginal contamination)

- Reducing substance

—Positive: glucose, fructose, galactose, false-positives (vitamin C, salicylates, antibiotics, etc.)

- Urobilinogen

—Positive: cirrhosis, CHF with hepatic congestion, hepatitis, hyperthyroidism, suppression of gut flora with antibiotics (Note: With obstructive jaundice, urobilinogen is usually normal, but bilirubin is elevated.)

Urine Sediment

Many labs no longer do microscopic examinations unless specifically requested or if there is evidence of an abnormal finding on the dipstick test (such as positive leukocyte esterase).

- Red blood cells (RBCs): trauma, pyelonephritis, genitourinary TB, cystitis, prostatitis, stones, tumors (malignant and benign), coagulopathy, and any cause of blood on dipstick test (see above on hemoglobin)
- White blood cells (WBCs): infection anywhere in the urinary tract, TB, renal tumors, acute glomerulonephritis, radiation, interstitial nephritis (analgesic abuse)
- Epithelial cells: acute tubular necrosis (ATN), necrotizing papillitis (most epithelial cells are from an otherwise unremarkable urethra)
- Parasites: *Trichomonas vaginalis, Schistosoma haematobium* infections
- Yeast: *Candida albicans* infection (especially in diabetics, immunosuppressed patients, or if a vaginal yeast infection is present)
- Spermatozoa: normal in males immediately after intercourse or nocturnal emission
- Crystals: Note that urine should be examined fresh and warm because crystalluria may be observed when urine cools.

—Abnormal: cystine, sulfonamide, leucine, tyrosine, cholesterol
—Normal in acid urine: oxalate (small square crystals with a central cross), uric acid.
—Normal in alkaline urine: calcium carbonate, triple phosphate (resemble coffin lids)

- Contaminants: cotton threads, hair, wood fibers, amorphous substances (all usually unimportant).
- Mucus: Large amounts suggest urethral disease (normal from ileal conduit or other forms of urinary diversion).
- Glitter cells: WBCs are lysed in hypotonic solution.
- Casts: The presence of casts in a urine sample localizes some or all of the disease process to the kidney itself.

—Hyaline casts (occasionally acceptable, unless they are "numerous"), benign hypertension, nephrotic syndrome, after exercise
—RBC casts: acute glomerulonephritis, lupus nephritis, subacute bacterial endocarditis (SBE), Goodpasture disease, after a streptococcal infection, vasculitis, malignant hypertension
—WBC casts: pyelonephritis
—Epithelial (tubular) casts: tubular damage, nephrotoxin, virus
—Granular casts: breakdown of cellular casts, leads to waxy casts; "dirty brown granular casts" typical for ATN
—Waxy casts (end stage of granular casts): severe, chronic renal disease; amyloidosis
—Fatty casts: nephrotic syndrome, diabetes mellitus, damaged renal tubular epithelial cells
—Broad casts: chronic renal disease

 Spot or Random Urine Studies

The so-called spot urine is often ordered to aid in diagnosing various conditions. It relies on only a small sample (10–20 mL) of urine.

- Spot urine for β_2-microglobulin (<0.3 mg/L)

—A marker for renal tubular injury
—Increased: diseases of the proximal tubule (ATN, interstitial nephritis, pyelonephritis), drug-induced nephropathy (aminoglycosides), diabetes, trauma, sepsis

- Spot urine for electrolytes

—The usefulness of this assay is limited because of large variations in daily fluid and salt intake, and the results are usually indeterminate if a diuretic has been given. (See also Section I, "Anuria and Oliguria.")
—Sodium <10 mEq/L (mmol/L): volume depletion, hyponatremic states, prerenal azotemia (CHF, shock, etc.), hepatorenal syndrome, glucocorticoid excess
—Sodium >20 mEq/L (mmol/L): syndrome of inappropriate antidiuretic hormone (SIADH), acute tubular necrosis (usually >40 mEq/L), postobstructive diuresis, high salt intake, Addison disease, hypothyroidism, interstitial nephritis
—Chloride <10 mEq/L (mmol/L): chloride-sensitive metabolic alkalosis (vomiting, excessive diuretic use), volume depletion
—Potassium <10 mEq/L (mmol/L): hypokalemia, potassium depletion, extrarenal loss
—Spot urine for protein (normal: <10 mg/dL [0.1 g/L] or <20 mg/dL [0.2 g/L] for a sample taken in the early morning)
—See Section I, "Proteinuria," for the differential diagnosis of protein in the urine.

- Spot urine for erythrocyte morphology

—The morphology of RBCs in a sample of urine that tests positive for blood may give some indication of the nature of the hematuria. Eumorphic red cells are typically seen in cases of postrenal, nonglomerular bleeding. Dysmorphic red cells are more likely associated with glomerular causes of bleeding. Each reference lab has standards, but as a general rule, the presence of >90% dysmorphic erythrocytes in patients with asymptomatic hematuria indicates a renal glomerular source of bleeding, especially if associated with proteinuria and/or casts (i.e., IgA nephropathy, poststreptococcal GN, sickle cell disease or trait, etc.). If (90% eumorphic erythrocytes or even "mixed" results (10%–90% eumorphic erythrocytes), this indicates a postrenal cause of hematuria, requiring a complete urologic evaluation (i.e., hypercalcuria, urolithiasis, cystitis, trauma, tumors, hemangioma, exercise-induced, BPH, etc.).

- Spot urine for osmolality (75–300 mOsmol/kg [mmol/kg]; varies with water intake)

—Patients with normal renal function should concentrate >800 mOsmol/kg (mmol/kg) after a 14-hour fluid restriction; <400 mOsmol/kg (mmol/kg) is a sign of renal impairment.
—Increased: dehydration, SIADH, adrenal insufficiency, glycosuria, high-protein diet
—Decreased: excessive fluid intake, diabetes insipidus, acute renal failure, medications (acetohexamide, glyburide, lithium)

- Spot urine for myoglobin (qualitative negative)

—Positive: skeletal muscle conditions (crush injury, electrical burns, carbon monoxide poisoning, delirium tremens, surgical procedures, malignant hyperthermia), polymyositis

Urine Studies

 24-Hour Urine Studies

- Calcium, urine

—Normal: calcium-free diet <150 mg/24 h (3.7 mmol/d); average calcium diet (600–800 mg/24 h) 100 to 250 mg/24 h (2.5–6.2 mmol/d).
—Increased: hyperparathyroidism, hyperthyroidism, hypervitaminosis D, distal renal tubular acidosis (type I), sarcoidosis, immobilization, osteolytic lesions (bony metastasis, multiple myeloma), Paget disease, glucocorticoid excess, immobilization
—Decreased: medications (thiazide diuretics, estrogens, oral contraceptives), hypothyroidism, renal failure, steatorrhea, rickets, osteomalacia

- Catecholamines, fractionated

—Used to evaluate neuroendocrine tumors, including pheochromocytoma and neuroblastoma. Avoid caffeine and methyldopa (Aldomet) prior to the test.
  —Normal: Values are variable and dependent on the assay method used. Norepinephrine 15 to 80 mg/24 h [SI: 89–473 nmol/24 h], epinephrine 0 to 20 mg/24 h [SI: 0–118 nmol/24 h], dopamine 65 to 400 mg/24 h [SI: 384–2364 nmol/24 h]
  —Increased: pheochromocytoma, neuroblastoma, epinephrine administration, presence of drugs (methyldopa, tetracyclines cause false increases)

- Cortisol, free

—Used to evaluate adrenal cortical hyperfunction; screening test of choice for Cushing syndrome
  —Normal: 10 to 110 mg/24 h [SI: 30–300 nmol]
  —Increased: Cushing syndrome (adrenal hyperfunction), stress during collection, oral contraceptives, pregnancy

- Creatinine clearance

—Normal
  —Adult male: total creatinine 1 to 2 g/24 h (8.8–17.7 mmol/d); clearance 85 to 125 mL/min/1.73 m^2
  —Adult female: total creatinine 0.8 to 1.8 g/24 h (7.1–15.9 mmol/d); clearance 75 to 115 mL/min 1.73 m^2 (1.25–1.92 mL/s/1.73 m^2)
  —Child: total creatinine (>3 years) 12 to 30 mg/kg/24 h; clearance 70 to 140 mL/min/1.73 m^2 (1.17–2.33 mL/s/1.73 m^2)
—Decreased: A decreased creatinine clearance results in an increase in serum creatinine, usually secondary to renal insufficiency. See Section I, "Renal Failure—Acute" and "Renal Failure—Chronic" for the differential diagnosis of increased serum creatinine.
—Increased: early diabetes mellitus, pregnancy

- Creatinine clearance determination

—Creatinine clearance is one of the most sensitive indicators of early renal insufficiency. Clearances are ordered on patients with suspected renal disease and are useful for following patients who are taking nephrotoxic medications, such as gentamicin. Clearance normally decreases with age. A creatinine clearance of 10 to 20 mL/min indicates severe renal failure, and a clearance of less than 10 mL/min usually indicates the need for dialysis.

To determine a creatinine clearance, order a concurrent serum creatinine and a 24-hour urine creatinine. A shorter time interval can be used (e.g., 12 hours), but remember that the formula must be corrected for this change and that a 24-hour sample is less prone to collection error.

Creatinine clearance (mL/min)
$$= \frac{\text{urine volume} \times \text{urine creatinine}}{\text{time}}$$

where time = 1440 minutes if 24-hour collection.

Some clinicians advocate a preliminary determination to see if the urine sample is valid, by determining first if the sample contains at least 18 to 25 mg/kg/24 h of creatinine for adult males or 12 to 20 mg/kg/24 h for adult females. This preliminary test is not a requirement but can confirm if a 24-hour sample was collected or if some of the sample was lost.

If the patient is an adult (150 lb = body surface area of 1.73 m^2), adjustment of the clearance for body size is not routinely done. Adjustment for pediatric patients, however, is a necessity. If the values in the previous example were for a 10-year-old boy who weighed 70 lb (1.1 m^2), the clearance would be

- Cysteine

—Used to detect cystinuria, homocystinuria
  —Normal: 40 to 60 mg/g creatinine
  —Increased: heterozygotes <300 mg/g creatinine/d; homozygotes >250 mg/g creatinine

- 5-Hydroxyindoleacetic acid (5-HIAA)

—5-HIAA is a serotonin metabolite and is useful in diagnosing carcinoid syndrome.
  —Normal: 2 to 8 mg [SI: 10.4–41.6 mmol]/24-h urine collection
  —Increased: carcinoid tumors (except rectal), certain foods (banana, pineapple, tomato, walnuts, avocado), phenothiazine derivatives

- Metanephrines

—These are metabolic products of epinephrine and norepinephrine, a primary screening test for pheochromocytoma.
  —Normal: <1.3 mg/24 h (7.1 mmol/L) for adults, but variable in children
  —Increased: pheochromocytoma, neuroblastoma (neural crest tumors), false-positive with drugs (phenobarbital, guanethidine, hydrocortisone, monoamine oxidase [MAO] inhibitors)

- Protein (see Section I, "Proteinuria")

—Normal: <150 mg/24 h (<0.15 g/d)
—Increased: Nephrotic syndrome is usually associated with >4 g/24 h.

- 17-Ketogenic steroids (17-KGS, corticosteroids)

—Overall adrenal function test, largely replaced by serum or urine cortisol levels
  —Normal: males: 5 to 24 mg/24 h (17–83 mmol/24 h); females: 4 to 15 mg/24 h (14–52 mmol/24 h)
  —Increased: adrenal hyperplasia (Cushing syndrome), adrenogenital syndrome
  —Decreased: panhypopituitarism, Addison disease, acute steroid withdrawal

- 17-Ketosteroids, total (17-KS)

—Measures dehydroepiandrosterone (DHEA), androstenedione (adrenal androgens); largely replaced by assay of individual elements
  —Normal: adult males: 8 to 20 mg/24 h (28–69 mmol/L); adult females: 6 to 15 mg/dL (21–52 mmol/L). Note: low values in prepubertal children
  —Increased: adrenal cortex abnormalities (hyperplasia [Cushing disease], adenoma, carcinoma, adrenogenital syndrome), severe stress, adrenocorticotropic hormone (ACTH) or pituitary tumor, testicular interstitial tumor and arrhenoblastoma (both produce testosterone)
  —Decreased: panhypopituitarism, Addison disease, castration in men

- Vanillylmandelic acid (VMA)

—VMA is the urinary product of both epinephrine and norepinephrine; good screening test for pheochromocytoma; also used to diagnose and follow up neuroblastoma and ganglioneuroma
  —Normal: <7 to 9 mg/24 h (35–45 mmol/L)
  —Increased: pheochromocytoma, other neural crest tumors (ganglioneuroma, neuroblastoma), factitious (chocolate, coffee, tea, methyldopa)

Commonly Used Medications in Urology

Acetaminophen (Tylenol, Others)

This section is designed to be a quick reference of commonly used medications in urology. You should be familiar with all the indications, contraindications, adverse effects, and drug interactions of any medication that you prescribe. Such detailed information is beyond the scope of this book and can be found in the package insert, *Physicians' Desk Reference* (*PDR*), or the American Hospital Formulary Service.

Medications are listed in alphabetical order by generic name. Some of the more common trade names are listed for each medication. Common uses of the medication in urology are listed rather than the official "labeled indications" (FDA-approved) because many available medications are used to treat various conditions based on the medical literature and are not listed in the package insert. This information is based on the author's review of the literature and is representative of urology practice patterns in the United States. Where no pediatric dosage is provided, the implication is that the use of the agent is not well established in this age group. Please note that the medications that fall in the categories of cephalosporins, nonsteroidal antiinflammatory drugs (NSAIDs), and systemic steroids are listed separately under these headings. Controlled substances are indicated by the symbol [C].

This chapter is modified and reproduced with permission from *Clinicians' Pocket Drug Reference, Urology Edition*, Gomella LG, Das A, 1999. Philadelphia: Palm Medical.

 ### Acetaminophen (Tylenol, Others)

COMMON USES   Treatment of mild pain, headache, and fever

ACTIONS   Nonnarcotic analgesic; inhibits the synthesis of prostaglandins and inhibits the hypothalamic heat-regulating center

DOSAGE   Adult: 650 mg po or pr q4–6h or 1000 mg po q6h; do not exceed 4 g per 24 hours; peds <12 years: 10 to 15 mg/kg/dose po or pr q4–6h; do not exceed 26 g per 24 hours

SUPPLIED   Tablets 160, 325, 500, or 650 mg; tablets, chewable, 80 or 160 mg; liquid 100 or 120 mg/25 mL, or 120, 160, 167, 325, or 500 mg/5 mL; drops 48 mg/mL, 60 mg/06 mL; suppositories 120, 125, 300, 325, or 650 mg

NOTES   Has no antiinflammatory or platelet-inhibiting action; decrease dose with alcohol use; overdose causes hepatotoxicity, which is treated with *N*-acetylcysteine; charcoal is not usually recommended.

 ### Acetaminophen with Butalbital and Caffeine (Fioricet) [C]

COMMON USES   Mild pain, headache, especially associated with stress

ACTIONS   Nonnarcotic analgesic

DOSAGE   1 to 2 tablets or capsules po q4–6h prn

SUPPLIED   Each tablet or capsule contains 325 mg acetaminophen, 40 mg caffeine, and 50 mg butalbital.

NOTES   May be habit forming

 ### Acetaminophen with Codeine (Tylenol #1, #2, #3, #4) [C]

COMMON USES   #1, #2, #3 for relief of mild-to-moderate pain; #4 for relief of moderate-to-severe pain

ACTIONS   Combined effects of acetaminophen and a narcotic analgesic

DOSAGE   Adult: 12 tablets q3–4h prn; peds: acetaminophen 10 to 15 mg/kg/dose; codeine 05- to 10-mg/kg dose q4–6h (useful dosing guide: 3–6 years, 5 mL per dose; 7–12 years, 10 mL per dose)

SUPPLIED   Tablets 300 mg APAP and codeine; capsules 325 mg APAP and codeine; liquids acetaminophen 120 mg, and codeine 12 mg per 5 mL

NOTES   Codeine in #1: 75 mg; #2: 15 mg; #3: 30 mg; #4: 60 mg

 ### Acetazolamide (Diamox)

COMMON USES   Diuresis and alkalinization of urine

ACTIONS   Carbonic anhydrase inhibitor; decreases renal excretion of hydrogen and increases renal excretion of sodium, potassium, bicarbonate, and water

DOSAGE   Adult: Diuretic: 250 to 375 mg IV or po q24h; peds: diuretic: 5 mg/kg/24 h po or IV; alkalinization of urine: 5 mg/kg/dose po bid-tid

SUPPLIED   Tablets 125 mg, 250 mg; capsule SR 500 mg, injection 500 mg/vial

NOTES   May increase risk of calcium phosphate stones. Contraindicated in renal failure, sulfa hypersensitivity; follow Na+ and K+; watch for metabolic acidosis; sustained release dosage forms are *not* recommended for use in epilepsy.

 ### Acetohydroxamic Acid (Lithostat)

COMMON USES   Used in conjunction with antibiotics in patients with infection stones

ACTIONS   Irreversible inhibitor of urease

DOSAGE   250 mg q8h

SUPPLIED   250-mg tablets

NOTES   Used in patients with infection stones when surgical intervention is contraindicated. Can cause headache, nausea, anemia

Acyclovir (Zovirax)

COMMON USES Treatment of herpes simplex and herpes zoster viral infections

ACTIONS Interferes with viral DNA synthesis

DOSAGE Adults:

- Oral: initial genital herpes: 200 mg po q4h while awake, for a total of 5 capsules/d for 10 days
- Chronic suppression: 400 mg po bid-tid
- Intermittent therapy: as for initial treatment, except treat for 5 days initiated at the earliest prodrome
- Herpes zoster: 800 mg po 5 times per day
- Intravenous: 5 to 10 mg/kg/dose IV q8h
- Peds: 5 to 10 mg/kg/dose IV or po q8h or 750 mg/m^2/24 h divided q8h

SUPPLIED Capsules 200 mg; tablets 400 mg, 800 mg; suspension 200 mg/5 mL; injection 500 mg/vial

NOTES Adjust the dose in renal insufficiency.

 Allopurinol (Zyloprim, Lopurin, Others)

COMMON USES Treatment of hyperuricemia of malignancy, gout, and uric acid urolithiasis

ACTIONS Xanthine oxidase inhibitor, which decreases the production of uric acid

DOSAGE Adult: initial 100 mg po qd; usual 300 mg po qd, maximum dose 800 mg/d; peds: Use only for treating hyperuricemia of malignancy in children: 10 mg/kg/24 h divided q6–8h (maximum: 600 mg/24 h)

SUPPLIED Tablets 100 mg, 300 mg

NOTES Aggravates acute gouty attack; do *not* begin until acute attack resolves; should be taken after meals

 Alprostadil (Caverject, Edex)

COMMON USES Treatment of erectile dysfunction due to neurogenic, vasculogenic, or mixed etiology

ACTIONS Relaxes smooth muscles, dilates cavernosal arteries, increases lacunar spaces and entrapment of blood by compressing venules against tunica albuginea

DOSAGE 0.2 to 6.0 μg intracavernosal; adjusted to individual needs

SUPPLIED Caverject: 6.15, 11.9, 23.2, or 46.2 μg vials with or without diluent syringes; Edex: 5-, 10-, 20-, 40-μg vials with syringes

NOTES Penile pain is the most common side effect. Dosage must be titrated at the physician's office. Patients should be informed of other side effects, including priapism, penile fibrosis, and hematoma.

 Alprostadil Urethral Suppository (Muse)

COMMON USES Treatment of erectile dysfunction

ACTIONS Alprostadil (PGE1) is absorbed through urethral mucosa. A portion of the administered dose is transported to the corpus cavernosa, where it acts as a vasodilator and smooth muscle relaxant.

DOSAGE 125- to 1000-μg system 5 to 10 minutes prior to sexual activity

SUPPLIED 125, 250, 500, 1000 μg with a transurethral delivery system

NOTES Hypotension, dizziness, syncope, penile pain, and priapism have been reported. Dose titration should be administered under the supervision of a physician.

 Amikacin (Amikin)

COMMON USES Treatment of serious infections caused by gram-negative bacteria and mycobacterial infections

ACTIONS Aminoglycoside antibiotic; inhibits protein synthesis

DOSAGE

- Adults and peds: 5 to 7.5 mg/kg/dose divided q8–24h based on renal function
- Neonates (<1200 g, 0 to 4 weeks): 7.5 mg/kg/dose q12h
- Postnatal age <7 days, 1200 to 2000 g: 7.5 mg/kg/dose q12h; >2000 g: 10 mg/kg/dose q12h
- Postnatal age >7 days, 1200 to 2000 g: 7 mg/kg/dose q8h; >2000 g: 7.5 to 10.0 mg/kg/dose q8h

SUPPLIED Injection 100 mg/2 mL, 500 mg/2 mL

NOTES May be effective against gram-negative bacteria resistant to gentamicin and tobramycin; monitor renal function carefully for dosage adjustments; monitor serum levels.

 Aminobenzoate Potassium (Potaba)

COMMON USES Oral therapy for Peyronie disease

ACTIONS Possible increase in oxygen uptake at the tissue level

DOSAGE 12 g/d in 4 to 6 divided doses

SUPPLIED 0.5-, 2-g tablets or capsules

NOTES Contraindicated in patient taking sulfonamides

Aminocaproic Acid (Amicar)

 Aminocaproic Acid (Amicar)

COMMON USES Treatment of excessive bleeding resulting from systemic hyperfibrinolysis and urinary fibrinolysis

ACTIONS Inhibits fibrinolysis via inhibition of plasminogen activator substances

DOSAGE Adults: 5 g IV or po, followed by 1 to 125 g/h IV or po; peds: 100 mg/kg IV, then 1 g/m²/h to maximum of 18 g/m²/d

SUPPLIED Tablets 500 mg; syrup 250 mg/mL; injection 250 mg/mL

NOTES Administer for 8 hours or until bleeding is controlled; contraindicated in disseminated intravascular coagulation; *not for upper urinary tract bleeding*

 Amino-Cerv pH 5.5 Cream

COMMON USES Mild cervicitis, postpartum cervicitis/cervical tears, postcauterization, postcryosurgery, and postconization

ACTIONS N/A

DOSAGE 1 applicatorful intravaginally qHS for 2 to 4 weeks

SUPPLIED Vaginal cream

NOTES Contains 8.34% urea, 0.5% sodium propionate, 0.83% methionine, 0.35% cystine, 0.83% inositol, benzalkonium chloride

 Aminoglutethimide (Cytadren, Elipten, Orimeten)

COMMON USES Adrenal cortex carcinoma, Cushing syndrome, and prostate cancer

ACTIONS Inhibits adrenal steroidogenesis and adrenal conversion of androgens to estrogens

DOSAGE 750 to 1500 mg/d in divided doses, plus dexamethasone 2 to 5 mg/d or hydrocortisone 20 to 40 mg/d

SUPPLIED Tablets 250 mg

NOTES Toxicity includes adrenal insufficiency ("medical adrenalectomy"), hypothyroidism, masculinization, hypotension, vomiting, rare hepatotoxicity, rash, myalgia, and fever.

 Amitriptyline (Elavil, Others)

COMMON USES Treatment for interstitial cystitis and chronic pain

ACTIONS Tricyclic antidepressant; inhibits reuptake of serotonin and norepinephrine by the presynaptic neuronal membrane

DOSAGE Adults: Initially 30 to 50 mg po qHS, may increase to 300 mg qHS; peds: *not recommended* for children < 12 years, unless for chronic pain: 01 mg/kg PO qHS initially, then advance over 2 to 3 weeks to 0.5 to 2.0 mg/kg po qHS

SUPPLIED Tablets 10, 25, 50, 75, 100, 150 mg; injection 10 mg/mL

NOTES Strong anticholinergic side effects; may cause urine retention and sedation; overdose may be fatal.

 Ammonium Aluminum Sulfate (Alum)

COMMON USES Hemorrhagic cystitis

ACTIONS Protein precipitation over the bleeding surface

DOSAGE 1% to 2% solution used with constant bladder irrigation with NSS

SUPPLIED Available in a powder form; prepared solutions, which can be stored up to 8 weeks

NOTES Can be used safely without anesthesia and in the presence of vesicoureteral reflux. Encephalopathy has been reported; thus, it is recommended to obtain aluminum levels, especially in patients with renal insufficiency.

 Amoxicillin (Amoxil, Larotid, Polymox, Others)

COMMON USES Treatment of infections due to susceptible gram-positive bacteria (streptococci), and gram-negative bacteria (*Haemophilus influenzae, E. coli, Proteus mirabilis*)

ACTIONS Beta-lactam antibiotic; inhibits cell wall synthesis

DOSAGE Adults: 250 to 500 mg po tid; peds: 25 to 100 mg/kg/24 h po divided q8h

SUPPLIED Capsules 250 mg, 500 mg; chewable tablets 125 mg, 250 mg; suspension 50 mg/5 mL, 125 mg/5 mL, 250 mg/5 mL

NOTES Cross-hypersensitivity with penicillin; may cause diarrhea; skin rash is common; many hospital strains of *E. coli* are resistant. Can be given to neonates and during pregnancy.

 Amoxicillin and Clavulanic Acid (Augmentin)

COMMON USES Treatment of infections caused by beta-lactamase–producing strains of *H. influenzae, Staphylococcus aureus,* and *E. coli*

ACTIONS Combination of a beta-lactam antibiotic and a beta-lactamase inhibitor

DOSAGE Adult: 250 to 500 mg as amoxicillin po q8h; peds: 20 to 40 mg/kg/d as amoxicillin po divided q8h

SUPPLIED (amoxicillin/clavulanic acid) Tablets 250/125 mg, 500/125 mg; chewable tablets 125/3125 mg, 250/625 mg; suspension 125/3125 mg per 5 mL, 250/625 mg per 5 mL

NOTES Do not substitute two 250-mg tablets for one 500-mg tablet, or an overdose of clavulanic acid will occur; may cause diarrhea and GI intolerance

Amphotericin B (Fungizone)

COMMON USES Treatment of severe systemic fungal infections. Intravesical amphotericin can be used for fungal infections of the urinary tract.

ACTIONS Binds to ergosterol in the fungal membrane, altering membrane permeability

DOSAGE

• Adults and peds: test dose of 1 mg in adults or 0.1 mg/kg to 1.0 mg in children, then 0.25 to 15.0 mg/kg/24 h IV over 4 to 6 hours. Doses often range from 25 to 50 mg qd or every other day. Total dose varies with indication.
• Intravesical therapy: 50 mg in 1000 mL of water or 5% dextrose at 42 mL/h. For outpatient therapy, use 100 mg in 500 mL of water.
• Renal collecting system: 10 to 24 mg/d for up to 15 days. Scheduling similar to intravesical therapy. Use only after obstructive uropathy is corrected.

SUPPLIED Powder for injection 50 mg/vial

NOTES Monitor renal function; hypokalemia and hypomagnesemia may be seen from renal wasting; pretreatment with acetaminophen and antihistamines (Benadryl) help minimize adverse effects associated with IV infusion.

 Amphotericin B Lipid Complex (Abelcet)

COMMON USES Treatment of aspergillosis in patients refractory or intolerant to conventional amphotericin B

ACTIONS Binds to sterols in the cell membrane, resulting in changes in membrane permeability

DOSAGE 5 mg/kg/d IV administered as a single daily dose. Infuse at a rate of 25 mg/kg/h.

SUPPLIED Injection 100 mg

NOTES Filter solution with a 5-μ micron filter needle; *do not* mix in electrolyte-containing solutions; if infusion exceeds 2 hours, mix content of the bag

 Ampicillin (Amcill, Omnipen, Others)

COMMON USES Treatment of susceptible gram-negative (*Shigella, Salmonella, E. coli, H. influenzae, P. mirabilis*) and gram-positive (streptococci) bacteria

ACTIONS Beta-lactam antibiotic; inhibits cell wall synthesis

DOSAGE

• Adults: 500 mg —2 g IM or IV q6h or 250 to 500 mg po q6h
• Peds

—Neonates <7 days: 50 to 100 mg/kg/24 h IV divided q8h
—Term infants: 75 to 150 mg/kg/24 h divided q6–8h IV or po
—>1 Month and children: 100 to 200 mg/kg/24 h divided q4–6h IM or IV; 50 to 100 mg/kg/24 h divided q6h po up to 250 mg/dose

SUPPLIED Capsules 250 mg, 500 mg; suspension 100 mg/mL, 125 mg/5 mL, 250 mg/5 mL, 500 mg/5 mL; powder for injection 125-mg, 250-mg, 500-mg, 1-g, 2-g, 10-g vials

NOTES Cross-hypersensitivity with penicillin; can cause diarrhea and skin rash; many hospital strains of *E. coli* are now resistant. Can be given to neonates and during pregnancy

 Ampicillin/Sulbactam (Unasyn)

COMMON USES Treatment of infections caused by beta-lactamase–producing strains of *Staphylococcus aureus, Enterococcus, H. influenzae, Proteus mirabilis,* and *Bacteroides* species

ACTIONS Combination of a beta-lactam antibiotic and a beta-lactamase inhibitor

DOSAGE Adult: 15 to 30 g IM or IV q6h; peds: dosed by ampicillin content (see Ampicillin)

SUPPLIED Powder for injection 15-g, 30-g vials

NOTES 2:1 ratio of ampicillin to sulbactam; adjust dosage in renal failure; observe for hypersensitivity reactions.

 Antithymocyte Globulin [ATG] (Atgam)

COMMON USES Management of allograft rejection in transplant patients

ACTIONS Reduces the number of circulating, thymus-dependent lymphocytes

DOSAGE Adults and peds: 10 to 15 mg/kg/d

SUPPLIED Injection 50 mg/mL

NOTES Do not administer to a patient with a history of severe systemic reaction to any other equine gamma globulin preparation; discontinue treatment if severe unremitting thrombocytopenia or leukopenia occurs.

 Aspirin (Bayer, St Joseph, Others)

COMMON USES Mild pain, headache, fever, inflammation, prevention of emboli, and prevention of myocardial infarction

ACTIONS Prostaglandin inhibitor

DOSAGE

• Adults: pain, fever: 325 to 650 mg q4–6h po or pr
• Peds: *Caution:* Use is linked to Reye syndrome; avoid use with viral illness in children.
• Antipyretic: 10 to 15 mg/kg/dose po or pr q4h up to 80 mg/kg/24 h

SUPPLIED Tablets 325 mg, 500 mg; chewable tablets 81 mg; enteric-coated tablets 165, 325, 500, 650, 975 mg; tablets SR 650 mg, 800 mg; tablets, effervescent, 325 mg, 500 mg, suppositories 120, 200, 300, 600 mg

NOTES GI upset and erosion are common adverse reactions; discontinue use 1 week prior

to surgery to avoid postoperative bleeding complications.

Aspirin with Butalbital and Caffeine (Fiorinal) [C]

COMMON USES Mild pain, headache, especially when associated with stress

ACTIONS Nonnarcotic analgesic

DOSAGE 1–2 tablets (capsules) po q4–6h prn

SUPPLIED Each capsule or tablet contains 325 mg aspirin, 40 mg caffeine, 50 mg butalbital

NOTES Also available with codeine: #1: 75 mg; #2: 15 mg; #3: 30 mg; significant drowsiness associated with use

Aspirin with Codeine (Empirin #1, #2, #3, #4) [C]

COMMON USES Relief of mild-to-moderate pain

ACTIONS Combined effects of aspirin and codeine

DOSAGE Adults: 1–2 tablets po q4–6h prn; peds: aspirin 10 mg/kg/dose; codeine 0.5–10 mg/kg/dose q4h

SUPPLIED Tablets 325 mg and codeine, as below

NOTES Codeine in #1: 75 mg; #2: 15 mg; #3: 30 mg; #4: 60 mg

 ## Azathioprine (Imuran)

COMMON USES Adjunct for the prevention of rejection following organ transplantation; rheumatoid arthritis; systemic lupus erythematosus

ACTIONS Immunosuppressive agent; antagonizes purine metabolism

DOSAGE Adults and peds: 1 to 3 mg/kg IV or po daily

SUPPLIED Tablets 50 mg; injection 100 mg/20 mL

NOTES May cause GI intolerance; do not administer vaccines while patient is taking azathioprine; injection should be handled with cytotoxic precautions.

 ## Azithromycin (Zithromax)

COMMON USES Treatment of skin structure infections and nongonococcal urethritis

ACTIONS Macrolide antibiotic; inhibits protein synthesis

DOSAGE Adults: nongonococcal urethritis: 1 g as a single dose; peds: 12 mg/kg/d for 5 days

SUPPLIED Capsules 250 mg, suspension 1-g single-dose packet; suspension 100 mg/5 mL, 200 mg/5 mL

NOTES Should be taken on an empty stomach

 ## Aztreonam (Azactam)

COMMON USES Treatment of infections caused by aerobic gram-negative bacteria, including *Pseudomonas aeruginosa*

ACTIONS Monobactam antibiotic; inhibits cell wall synthesis

DOSAGE

- Adults: 1–2 g IV/IM q6–12h
- Peds

—Premature infants: 30 mg/kg/dose IV q12h
—Term infants, children: 30 mg/kg/dose q6–8h

SUPPLIED Injection 500 mg, 1 g, 2 g

NOTES Not effective against gram-positive or anaerobic bacteria; may be given to penicillin-allergic patients; can be given to patients with renal insufficiency

 ## Bacillus Calmette-Guérin (TheraCys, Tice BCG)

COMMON USES Intravesical treatment of superficial bladder carcinoma (CIS and for prophylaxis of recurrent papillary tumors)

ACTIONS Immunomodulator

DOSAGE Bladder cancer three 27 mg (TheraCys) or 1 to 8 × 10⁸ CFU (Tice BCG) 7 to 14 days after biopsy weekly for 6 weeks. Repeat cycle ×1 if no response. Various maintenance schedules described after 6-week treatment and include monthly for 6 to 12 months or three weekly doses at 3 months, then every 6 months thereafter.

SUPPLIED Injection 27 mg (34 ± 3 × 10⁸ CFU) per vial (TheraCys), 1 to 8 × 10⁸ CFU per vial (Tice BCG)

NOTES Dilute in 50 mL preservative-free saline, instill by gravity catheter, and retain for 2 hours; change position every 15 minutes. Intravesical toxicity includes hematuria, urinary frequency, dysuria, bacterial urinary tract infection. Rare BCG-osis or BCG sepsis (see Section II, "BCG Sepsis"). *Do not administer in less than 7 days after TURBT or biopsy, or with traumatic catheterization.*

 ## Baclofen (Lioresal)

COMMON USES Management of spasticity secondary to severe chronic disorders, such as multiple sclerosis or spinal cord lesions

ACTIONS Centrally acting skeletal muscle relaxant; inhibits transmission of both monosynaptic and polysynaptic reflexes at the spinal cord

DOSAGE

- Adults: initially, 5 mg po tid; increase every 3 days to maximum effect; maximum 80 mg/d
- Peds: 2 to 7 years: 10 to 15 mg/d divided q8h; titrate to effect or a maximum of 40 mg/d; >8 years: maximum of 60 mg/d

SUPPLIED Tablets 10, 20 mg

NOTES Use caution in epileptics and neuropsychiatric disturbances

Basiliximab (Stimulect)

COMMON USES Treatment of acute renal transplantation in combination with cyclosporine

ACTIONS Monoclonal antibody that blocks IL-2 receptor on T cells

DOSAGE 2 doses, 20 mg each IV over 15 minutes, 2 hours before transplant and the other 4 days after; peds: 12 mg/m^2 (maximum, 20 mg) administered as above

SUPPLIED Injectable

NOTES Combination human–mouse antibody; no significant side effects reported

 Belladonna and Opium Suppositories (B & O Supprettes) [C]

COMMON USES Treatment of bladder spasms, moderate-to-severe pain

ACTIONS Antispasmodic

DOSAGE Insert one suppository rectally q6h prn

- 15A = 30 mg powdered opium; 162 mg belladonna extract
- 16A = 60 mg powdered opium; 162 mg belladonna extract
- Peds: 3 to 7 years one-half 15A suppository q6h prn

SUPPLIED Suppositories 15A, 16A

NOTES Anticholinergic side effects; caution subjects about sedation, urinary retention, and constipation.

 Benzquinamide (Emete-Con)

COMMON USES Nausea and vomiting

ACTIONS Antiemetic; acts on the chemoreceptor trigger zone

DOSAGE 50 mg IM q3–4h prn

SUPPLIED Powder for injection 50 mg/vial. Note: Alternative antiemetic when phenothiazine or antihistamine is contraindicated

 Betamethasone (Calestone). See Systemic Steroids

 Bethanechol (Urecholine, Duvoid, Various)

COMMON USES Neurogenic atony of the bladder with urinary retention, acute postoperative and postpartum functional (nonobstructive) urinary retention

ACTIONS Stimulates cholinergic receptors in the smooth muscle of the bladder and GI tract

DOSAGE
- Adults: 10 to 50 mg po tid-qid or 2.5 to 5.0 mg SQ tid-qid and prn
- Peds: 0.6 mg/kg/24 h po divided tid-qid or 0.15 to 2.0 mg/kg/d SQ divided 3 to 4 times

SUPPLIED Tablets 5 mg, 10 mg, 25 mg, 50 mg; injection 5 mg/mL

NOTES Contraindicated in bladder outlet obstruction, asthma, coronary artery disease; *do not* administer IM or IV.

 Bicalutamide (Casodex)

COMMON USES Advanced prostate cancer (in combination with gonadotropin-releasing hormone agonists such as leuprolide or goserelin)

ACTIONS Nonsteroidal antiandrogen

DOSAGE 50 mg daily

SUPPLIED Capsules 50 mg

NOTES Toxicity includes hot flashes, loss of libido, impotence, diarrhea, nausea, vomiting, gynecomastia, and LFT elevation. Follow LFTs. Under research at 150 mg/day.

 Bisacodyl (Dulcolax)

COMMON USES Constipation, bowel prep

ACTIONS Stimulates peristalsis

DOSAGE
- Adults: 5 to 15 mg po or 10 mg rectally prn
- Peds
—<2 years: 5 mg rectally prn
—>2 years: 5 mg po or 10 mg rectally prn

SUPPLIED Enteric-coated tablets 5 mg; suppository 5 mg, 10 mg

NOTES *Do not* use with an acute abdomen or bowel obstruction. *Do not* chew tablets. *Do not* give within 1 hour of antacids or milk.

 Bleomycin Sulfate (Blenoxane)

COMMON USES Testicular carcinomas and squamous cell carcinoma of the penis

ACTIONS Induces breakage (scission) of single- and double-stranded DNA

DOSAGE 10 to 20 mg (U)/m^2 once or twice weekly

SUPPLIED Injection 15 mg (15 U)

NOTES Toxicity includes hyperpigmentation (skin staining), hypersensitivity (rash to anaphylaxis). Test dose of 1 mg (U) recommended, especially in lymphoma patients; fever in 50%; lung toxicity (idiosyncratic and dose-related) pneumonitis may progress to fibrosis. Note: Serious lung toxicity is most likely when total dose exceeds 400 mg (U).

Bumetanide (Bumex)

 Bumetanide (Bumex)

COMMON USES Diuresis

ACTIONS Loop diuretic; inhibits reabsorption of sodium and chlorine in the ascending loop of Henle and distal renal tubule

DOSAGE

• Adults: 05 to 20 mg po daily; 05 to 10 mg IV every 8 to 24 hours
• Peds: 0.015 to 0.1 mg/kg/d po, IV, IM divided q6–24h

SUPPLIED Tablets 0.5 mg, 1 mg; injection 0.25 mg/mL

NOTES Monitor fluid and electrolyte status during treatment.

 Bupivacaine (Marcaine)

COMMON USES Peripheral nerve block

ACTIONS Local anesthetic

DOSAGE Adults and peds: Dose is dependent on the procedure, vascularity of the tissues, depth of anesthesia, and degree of muscle relaxation required. Max dose in 70 kg adult is 70 mL of 0.25% solution.

SUPPLIED Injection 0.25%, 0.5%, 0.75%

NOTES Should *only* be used by an experienced physician

 Buprenorphine (Buprenex) [C]

COMMON USES Relief of moderate-to-severe pain

ACTIONS Opiate agonist–antagonist

DOSAGE 0.3 to 0.6 mg IM or slow IV push q6h prn

SUPPLIED Injection 0.324 mg/mL (equal to 0.3 mg of buprenorphine)

NOTES May induce withdrawal syndrome in opioid-dependent patients

 Butorphanol (Stadol)

COMMON USES Treatment of moderate-to-severe pain

ACTIONS Opiate agonist–antagonist with central analgesic actions

DOSAGE 1 to 4 mg IM or IV every 3 to 4 hours prn; *headaches:* 1 spray in 1 nostril, may be repeated one time

SUPPLIED Injection 1 mg/mL, 2 mg/mL; nasal spray 10 mg/mL

NOTES May induce withdrawal syndrome in opioid-dependent patients

 Captopril (Capoten)

COMMON USES Treatment of hypertension, CHF, left ventricular dysfunction (LVD), and diabetic nephropathy

ACTIONS Angiotensin converting enzyme inhibitor

DOSAGE

• Adults

—Hypertension: initially, 25 mg po bid–tid; titrate to a maintenance dose every 1 to 2 weeks by 25-mg increments per dose (maximum 450 mg/d) to desired effect.
—CHF: initially, 6.25 to 12.5 mg po tid; titrate to desired effect
—LVD: 50 mg po tid
—Diabetic nephropathy: 25 mg po tid

• Peds

—Infants <2 months: 005 to 05 mg/kg/dose po q8–24h
—Children: Initially, 015 mg/kg/dose po; titrate to a maximum of 6 mg/kg/d

SUPPLIED Tablets 125, 25, 50, 100 mg

NOTES Use with caution in renal failure. Give 1 hour before meals; can cause rash, proteinuria, and cough

 Carbenicillin (Geocillin)

COMMON USES Urinary tract infections due to susceptible strains of *E. coli, Proteus, Morganella, Pseudomonas, Providencia, Enterobacter, Enterococci*

ACTIONS Inhibits cell wall synthesis

DOSAGE 1 to 2 tablets q6h

SUPPLIED 382-mg tablets

NOTES Hypersensitivity reactions, dosage adjustment in patients with renal impairment. Useful in prostatitis

 Carboplatin (Paraplatin)

COMMON USES Testicular cancer and autologous transplantation in high doses

ACTIONS DNA cross-linker; forms DNA-platinum adducts

DOSAGE 360 mg/m² (ovarian carcinoma), area under the curve (AUC) dosing 4 to 7 mg/mL (using Calvert formula: mg = AUC × [25 + calculated GFR]); also may be adjusted based on pretreatment platelet count, creatinine clearance, and BSA (Egorin's formula); up to 1500 mg/m² used in autologous bone marrow transplantation setting

SUPPLIED Injection 50 mg, 150 mg, 450 mg

NOTES Toxicity includes myelosuppression, nausea and vomiting, diarrhea, nephrotoxicity, hematuria, neurotoxicity, hepatic enzyme elevations. Physiologic dosing based on either Calvert's or Egorin's formula allows larger doses to be given with reduced toxicity.

 Cefaclor (Ceclor). See Cephalosporins, First Generation

 Cefadroxil (Duricef, Ultracef). See Cephalosporins, First Generation

 Cefamandole (Mandol). See Cephalosporins, Second Generation

 Cefazolin (Ancef, Kefzol). See Cephalosporins, First Generation

Cephalosporins—Second Generation

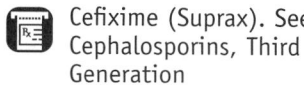 Cefixime (Suprax). See Cephalosporins, Third Generation

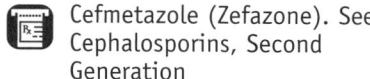 Cefmetazole (Zefazone). See Cephalosporins, Second Generation

Cefonicid (Monocid). See Cephalosporins, Second Generation

Cefoperazone (Cefobid). See Cephalosporins, Third Generation

Cefotaxime (Claforan). See Cephalosporins, Third Generation

Cefotetan (Cefotan). See Cephalosporins, Second Generation

Cefoxitin (Mefoxin). See Cephalosporins, Second Generation

Cefpodoxime (Vantin). See Cephalosporins, Third Generation

Cefprozil (Cefzil). See Cephalosporins, Second Generation

Ceftazidime (Fortaz, Ceptaz, Tazidime, Tazicef). See Cephalosporins, Third Generation

Ceftibuten (Cedax). See Cephalosporins, Third Generation

Ceftizoxime (Cefizox). See Cephalosporins, Third Generation

Ceftriaxone (Rocephin). See Cephalosporins, Third Generation

Cefuroxime (Ceftin, Zinacef). See Cephalosporins, Second Generation

Cephalexin (Keflex, Keftab). See Cephalosporins, First Generation

Cephalothin (Keflin). See Cephalosporins, First Generation

Cephapirin (Cefadyl). See Cephalosporins, First Generation

Cephradine (Velosef, Anspor). See Cephalosporins, First Generation

Cephalosporins—First Generation

COMMON USES   Treatment of infections caused by susceptible strains of *Staphylococcus, E. coli, Proteus,* and *Klebsiella,* involving the skin and urinary tract

ACTIONS   Bactericidal; inhibits cell wall synthesis

DOSAGE   See below, under specific agents.

SUPPLIED   See below, under specific agents.

NOTES   Cefazolin is the most widely used for surgical prophylaxis.

• Cefadroxil (Duricef, Ultracef)

—Adult dosage: 500 to 1000 mg q12–24h
—Peds dosage (divided doses): 30 mg/kg/d (bid)
—Supplied: 500-, 1000-mg tablets; 125, 250, 500 mg/5 mL

• Cefazolin (Ancef, Kefzol)

—Adult dosage: 1 to 2 g IV q8h
—Peds dosage (divided doses): 50 to 100 mg/kg/d (q8h)
—Supplied: 500-, 1000-mg vial for IV mixture

• Cephalexin (Keflex)

—Adult dosage: 250 to 500 mg qid
—Peds dosage (divided dosage): 25 to 100 mg/kg/d (q6h)
—Supplied: 250-, 500-mg caps, tabs; 125, 250 mg/5 mL

• Cephalothin (Keflin)

—Adult dosage: 1 to 2 g q6h
—Peds dosage (divided doses): 75 to 125 mg/kg/d (q6h)
—Supplied: 250-, 500-mg vial for IV mixture

• Cephapirin (Cefadyl)

—Adult dosage: 1 to 2 g q6h
—Peds (divided doses): 40 to 80 mg/kg/d (q6h)
—Supplied: vials for IV mixture

• Cephradine (Velosef)

—Adult dosages: 250 to 500 mg qid
—Peds (divided doses): 25 to 50 mg/kg/d (q6h)
—Supplied: 250-, 500-mg caps

 Cephalosporins—Second Generation

COMMON USES   Treatment of infections caused by susceptible bacteria, involving the skin, urinary tract, abdomen, and gynecologic system

ACTIONS   Bactericidal; inhibits cell wall synthesis

DOSAGE   See below, under specific agents.

SUPPLIED   See below, under specific agents.

NOTES   Has more gram-negative activity than first-generation cephalosporins. Cefaclor has good activity against *H. influenzae.* Cefmetazole and cefotetan have activity against anaerobes. Cefoxitin has the best activity against anaerobes. Cefuroxime crosses the blood-brain barrier.

• Cefaclor (Ceclor)

—Adult dosages: 250 to 500 mg po q8h
—Peds dosages (divided doses): 20 to 40 mg/kg/d (q8h)
—Supplied: 250-, 500-mg caps; 125, 250, 375 mg/5 mL

• Cefamandole (Mandol)

—Adult dosages: 1 to 2 g IV q4–6h
—Peds dosages (divided doses): 100 to 150 mg/kg/d (q4–6h)
—Supplied: 1-, 2-g vials for IV

• Cefmetazole (Zefazone)

—Adult dosages: 1 to 2 g IV q8h
—Peds dosages: N/A
—Supplied: vials for IV mixture

• Cefonicid (Monocid)

—Adult dosages: 1 to 2 g IV q24h
—Peds dosages: N/A
—Supplied: 1-g vials for IV

• Cefotetan (Cefotan)

—Adult dosages: 1 to 2 g IV q6h
—Peds dosages (divided doses): 40 to 80 mg/kg/d (q12h)
—Supplied 1-, 2-g vials for IV

Cephalosporins—Third Generation

- Cefoxitin (Mefoxin)
—Adult dosages: 1 to 2 g IV q6h
—Peds dosages (divided doses): 80 to 160 mg/kg/d (q6h)
—Supplied: 1-, 2-g vials for IV
- Cefprozil (Cefzil)
—Adult dosages: 250 to 500 mg po bid
—Peds dosages (divided doses): 75 to 15 mg/kg/d (q6h)
—Supplied: 250-, 500-mg tabs
- Cefuroxime (Zinacef, Ceftin)
—Adult dosages: 750 to 1500 mg IV q8h; 250 to 500 mg po bid
—Peds dosages (divided doses): 100 to 150 mg/kg/d (q8h)
—Supplied: 750-, 1500-mg vials; 125-, 250-, 500-mg tablets

 Cephalosporins—Third Generation

COMMON USES Treatment of infections caused by susceptible bacteria, involving the skin, urinary tract, febrile neutropenia, and septicemia

ACTIONS Bactericidal; inhibits cell wall synthesis

DOSAGE See below, under specific agents.

SUPPLIED See below, under specific agents.

NOTES Has more gram-negative activity and less gram-positive activity than the first- or second-generation cephalosporins. These may be used in combination with aminoglycosides. Cefpodoxime has drug interactions with agents increasing gastric pH. Ceftazidime has the best activity against *Pseudomonas*. Cefoperazone should be administered with vitamin K. Ceftibuten should be taken on an empty stomach.

- Cefixime (Suprax)
—Adult dosages: 200 to 400 mg po q12–24h
—Peds dosages (divided doses): 8 mg/kg/d (q12–24h)
—Supplied: 200-, 400-mg tabs; 100 mg/5 mL
- Cefoperazone (Cefobid)
—Adult dosages: 1 to 2 g IV q12h
—Peds dosages (divided doses): 100 to 150 mg/kg/d (q4–6h)
—Supplied: 1-, 2-g solutions IV
- Cefotaxime (Claforan)
—Adult dosages: 1 to 2 g IV q4–8h
—Peds dosages (divided doses): 100 to 200 mg/kg/d (q6–8h)
—Supplied: 500 mg; 1, 2 g for IV
- Cefpodoxime (Vantin)
—Adult dosages: 200 to 400 mg q12
—Peds dosages (divided doses): 10 mg/kg/d (q12h)
—Supplied: 100-, 200-mg tabs

- Ceftazidime (Fortaz, Ceptaz, Tazidime, Tazicef)
—Adult dosages: 1 to 2 g q8h
—Peds dosages (divided doses): 30 to 50 mg/kg/d (q8h)
—Supplied: 500 mg; 1-, 2-g vials
- Ceftibuten (Cedax)
—Adult dosages: 400 mg qd
—Peds dosages (divided doses): 9 mg/kg/d (qd)
—Supplied: 400-mg tabs; 90 mg/5 mL
- Ceftizoxime (Cefizox)
—Adult dosages: 1 to 2 g q8–12h
—Peds dosages (divided doses): 150 to 200 mg/kg/d (q6–8h)
—Supplied: 1-, 2-g solutions IV
- Ceftriaxone (Rocephin)
—Adult dosages: 1 to 2 g q8–12
—Peds dosages (divided doses): 50 to 100 mg/kg/d (q8h)
—Supplied: 250-, 500-mg; 1-g vials

 Charcoal, Activated (Superchar, Actidose, Liqui-Char)

COMMON USES To help identify urinary–intestinal fistulas

ACTIONS Adsorbent detoxicant

DOSAGE One bottle po

SUPPLIED 25-, 50-g unit-dose bottles

NOTES Some liquid-dosage forms are in a sorbitol base. Check urine for charcoal paper stone (urine strainer useful) to see if enterovesical fistulas exists.

 Chlorothiazide (Diuril)

COMMON USES Diuresis and urinary lithiasis

ACTIONS Thiazide diuretic

DOSAGE
- Adults: 500 mg to 10 g po or IV qd-bid
- Peds: 20 to 30 mg/kg/24 h po divided bid

SUPPLIED Tablets 250 mg, 500 mg; suspension 250 mg/5 mL; injection 500 mg/vial

NOTES Contraindicated in anuria

 Chlorthalidone (Hygroton, Others)

COMMON USES Diuresis and urinary lithiasis

ACTIONS Thiazide diuretic; decreases hypercalcuria

DOSAGE Adults: 50 to 100 mg po qd; peds: 2 mg/kg/dose po 3 times weekly or 1 to 2 mg/kg po daily

SUPPLIED Tablets 25 mg, 50 mg, 100 mg

NOTES Contraindicated in anuric patients

 Cholestyramine (Questran)

COMMON USES Used in patients with persistent diarrhea due to the loss of the terminal ileum that has been used as a reconstructive part of a urinary diversion or reservoir

ACTIONS Binds bile acids in the intestine to form insoluble complexes

DOSAGE
- Adults: individualize dose to 4 g 1 to 6 times a day
- Peds: 240 mg/kg/d in 3 divided doses

SUPPLIED 4 g cholestyramine resin/9 g of powder

NOTES Mix 4 g cholestyramine in 2 to 6 oz of noncarbonated beverages

Cimetidine (Tagamet)

COMMON USES Duodenal ulcer, ulcer prophylaxis in hypersecretory states such as trauma, burns, and surgery

ACTIONS Histamine-2 receptor antagonist

DOSAGE

• Adults

—Active ulcer: 2400 mg/d IV continuous infusion, or 300 mg IV q6–4h; 400 mg po bid, or 800 mg qHS
—Maintenance therapy: 400 mg po qHS

• Peds

—Neonates: 10 to 20 mg/kg/24 h or IV divided q4–6h
—Children: 20 to 40 mg/kg/24 h po or IV divided q4–6h

SUPPLIED Tablets 200 mg, 300 mg, 400 mg, 800 mg; liquid 300 mg/5 mL; injection 300 mg/2 mL

NOTES Extend the dosing interval with renal insufficiency; decrease the dose in the elderly.

 ## Ciprofloxacin (Cipro)

COMMON USES Broad-spectrum activity against a variety of gram-positive and gram-negative aerobic bacteria

ACTIONS Quinolone antibiotic; inhibits DNA gyrase

DOSAGE

• Adults: 250 to 750 mg po q12h, or 200 to 400 mg IV q12h
• Peds: *not recommended for use in children <18 years old*

SUPPLIED Tablets 250 mg, 500 mg, 750 mg; injection 200 mg, 400 mg

NOTES Little activity against streptococci; drug interactions with theophylline, caffeine, sucralfate, and antacids; nausea, vomiting, and abdominal discomfort are common side effects; *contraindicated in pregnancy and nursing mothers*

 ## Cisplatin (Platinol)

COMMON USES Testicular cancers, bladder cancer, and penile cancer

ACTIONS DNA binding, intrastrand cross-linking, formation of DNA adducts

DOSAGE 20 mg/m^2/d $\times$ 5 days every 3 weeks, 120 mg/m^2 every 3 to 4 weeks, 100 mg/m^2 on days 1 and 8 every 20 days, IV

SUPPLIED Injection 10 mg, 50 mg

NOTES Toxicity includes allergic reactions, nausea and vomiting, nephrotoxicity (exacerbated by concurrent administration of other nephrotoxic drugs and minimized by saline infusion and mannitol diuresis), high-frequency hearing loss in approximately 30%, peripheral "stocking glove" type neuropathy, cardiotoxicity (ST-T wave changes), hypomagnesemia, mild myelosuppression, hepatotoxicity. Renal impairment is dose-related and cumulative.

 ## Clarithromycin (Biaxin)

COMMON USES Treatment of skin and skin structure infections and infections caused by nontuberculous *Mycobacterium*

ACTIONS Macrolide antibiotic

DOSAGE

• Adults: 250 to 500 mg po bid
• *Mycobacterium*: 500 to 1000 mg po bid
• Peds: 75 mg/kg/dose po bid

SUPPLIED Tablets 250 mg, 500 mg; suspension 125 mg/5 mL, 250 mg/5 mL

NOTES Increases theophylline and carbamazepine levels; avoid concurrent use with astemizole, and terfenadine and cisapride.

 ## Clindamycin (Cleocin)

COMMON USES Susceptible strains of streptococci, pneumococci, staphylococci, and gram-positive and gram-negative anaerobes; no activity against gram-negative aerobes and bacterial vaginosis

ACTIONS Bacteriostatic, interferes with protein synthesis

DOSAGE

• Adults: 150 to 450 mg po qid; 300 to 600 mg IV q6h or 900 mg IV q8h
• Vaginal: One applicatorful qHS for 7 days
• Peds

—Neonates: 1 to 15 mg/kg/24 h divided q6–8h
—Children >1 month old: 10 to 30 mg/kg/24 h divided q6–8h, to a maximum of 4 g/d

SUPPLIED Capsules 75 mg, 150 mg; suspension 75 mg/5 mL; injection 300 mg/2 mL; vaginal cream 2%

NOTES Beware of diarrhea that may represent pseudomembranous colitis caused by *C. difficile* if used orally.

 ## Clomiphene Citrate (Clomid, Serophene)

COMMON USES Idiopathic oligospermia

ACTIONS Stimulate the release of pituitary gonadotropins

DOSAGE 25 to 50 mg/d

SUPPLIED 50-mg tablets

NOTES Pregnancy rates are less than 30%. Hypersensitivity reactions have been reported.

Clonidine, Oral (Catapres)

 Clonidine, Oral (Catapres)

COMMON USES Hypertension; opioid and tobacco withdrawal

ACTIONS Centrally acting alpha-adrenergic stimulant

DOSAGE Adults: 0.10 mg po bid adjusted daily by 0.1- to 0.2-mg increments (maximum 24 mg/d); peds: 5 to 25 mg/kg/24 h divided q6h

SUPPLIED Tablets 0.1, 0.2, 0.3 mg

NOTES Dry mouth, drowsiness, and sedation occur frequently; more effective for hypertension when combined with diuretics; rebound hypertension can occur with abrupt cessation of doses >0.2 mg bid (See transdermal dose below.)

 Clonidine, Transdermal (Catapres TTS)

COMMON USES Hypertension, management of hot flushes associated with treatment of prostate cancer

ACTIONS Centrally acting alpha-adrenergic stimulant

DOSAGE Apply 1 patch every 7 days to a hairless area on the upper arm or torso; titrate according to individual therapeutic requirements.

SUPPLIED TTS-1, TTS-2, TTS-3 (programmed to deliver 0.1, 0.2, 0.3 mg, respectively, of clonidine per day for 1 week)

NOTES Doses above two TTS-3 are usually not associated with increased efficacy. (See side effects for Clonidine, Oral, above.)

 Clotrimazole (Lotrimin, Mycelex)

COMMON USES Treatment of candidiasis and tinea infections

ACTIONS Antifungal agent; alters cell wall permeability

DOSAGE

- Oral: one troche dissolved slowly in mouth 5 times a day for 14 days
- Vaginal: cream: one applicatorful qHS for 7 to 14 days
- Tablets: 100 mg vaginally qHS for 7 days or 200 mg (2 tabs) vaginally qHS for 3 days or 500 mg tab vaginally HS $\times$ 1
- Topical: Apply 3 to 4 times daily for 10 to 14 days

SUPPLIED 1% cream, solution, lotion; troche 10 mg; vaginal tablets 100, 500 mg; vaginal cream 1%. Note: Oral prophylaxis commonly used in immunosuppressed patients.

 Clotrimazole and Betamethasone (Lotrisone)

COMMON USES Fungal skin infections

ACTIONS Imidazole antifungal and anti-inflammatory

DOSAGE Apply and gently massage into the area twice a day for 2 to 4 weeks.

SUPPLIED Cream 15 g and 45 g

NOTES Contraindicated in children and varicella

 Cloxacillin (Tegopen)

COMMON USES Treatment of infections caused by susceptible strains of *Staphylococcus* and *Streptococcus*

ACTIONS Bactericidal; inhibits cell wall synthesis

DOSAGE

- Adults: 250 to 500 mg q6h
- Peds: 50 to 100 mg/kg/d divided q6h

SUPPLIED 250-, 500-mg capsules; 125 mg/5 mL oral solution

NOTES Administer on an empty stomach.

 Codeine [C]

COMMON USES Mild-to-moderate pain

ACTIONS Narcotic analgesic

DOSAGE

- Adults: 15 to 60 mg po or IM qid prn
- Peds: 05 to 10 mg/kg/dose po or IM q4–6h prn

SUPPLIED Tablets 15 mg, 30 mg, 60 mg; solution 15 mg/5 mL; injection 30 mg/mL, 60 mg/mL

NOTES Most often used in combination with acetaminophen for pain; 120 mg IM equivalent to 10 mg morphine IM

 Colchicine

COMMON USES Acute gout, Peyronie disease

ACTIONS Inhibits migration of leukocytes and reduces production of lactic acid by leukocytes

DOSAGE P. uronie disease: Initially 0.6 mg po bid for 2 to 3 weeks, then check for bone marrow suppression. If no bone marrow suppression, then continue for 3 to 4 months

SUPPLIED

- Tablets 0.5 mg, 0.6 mg; injection 1 mg/2 mL

NOTES Caution in elderly and patients with renal impairment. Side effects include bone marrow suppression, GI upset, and decreased sperm count.

 Cortisone (Cortone). See Systemic Steroids

Cyclophosphamide (Cytoxan, Endoxan, Neosar)

COMMON USES Neuroblastoma, transitional cell carcinomas, and prostate cancer

ACTIONS Converted to acrolein and phosphoramide mustard, the active alkylating moieties

DOSAGE 500 to 1500 mg/m² as single dose at 2- to 4-week intervals, 18 g/m² to 160 mg/kg (or approximately 12 g/m² in a 75-kg individual) in bone marrow transplantation setting

SUPPLIED Tablets 25 mg, 50 mg; injection 100 mg, 200 mg, 500 mg

NOTES Toxicity includes myelosuppression (leukopenia and thrombocytopenia), sterile hemorrhagic cystitis, SIADH, alopecia, anorexia, nausea and vomiting; common. Hepatotoxicity and, rarely, interstitial pneumonitis may occur. Irreversible testicular atrophy (with oligospermia) may occur. Cardiotoxicity rarely occurs (high-dose therapy). Second malignancies (bladder cancer and acute leukemias) reported; cumulative risk of 35% at 8 years, 107% at 12 years. Preventive measures to avoid hemorrhagic cystitis are often applied in high-dose regimens and may include continuous bladder irrigation and Mesna uroprotection.

 ## Cyclosporine (Sandimmune, Neoral)

COMMON USES Prophylaxis of organ rejection in kidney transplants in conjunction with adrenal corticosteroids

ACTIONS Immunosuppressant; reversible inhibition of immunocompetent lymphocytes

DOSAGE Adults and Peds
• Oral: 15 mg/kg/d beginning 12 hours prior to transplant; after 2 weeks, taper dose by 5 mg per week to 5 to 10 mg/kg/d
• IV: If the patient is unable to take orally, give one-third oral dose IV.

SUPPLIED Capsules 25 mg, 100 mg; oral solution 100 mg/mL; injection 50 mg/mL

NOTES May elevate BUN and creatinine, which may be confused with renal transplant rejection; should be administered in glass containers; has many drug interactions; Neoral and Sandimmune are not interchangeable. Renal transplant levels: 50 to 250 mg/mL (RIA).

 ## Dactinomycin (Actinomycin D, Cosmegen)

COMMON USES Choriocarcinoma, Wilms' tumor, rhabdomyosarcoma, and testicular cancer

ACTIONS DNA intercalating agent

DOSAGE 0.5 mg/d × 5 days, 2 mg/week for 3 consecutive weeks, 15 μg/kg or 0.45 mg/m²/d (maximum of 0.5 mg) × 5 days every 3 to 8 weeks in pediatric sarcoma

SUPPLIED Injection 05 mg

NOTES Toxicity includes myelosuppression, immunosuppression, nausea and vomiting, alopecia, acne from skin changes and hyperpigmentation, radiation recall phenomenon, phlebitis and tissue damage with extravascular extravasation, hepatotoxicity

 ## Dacilizumab (Zenapax)

COMMON USES Treatment of acute renal transplantation in combination with cyclosporine

ACTIONS Monoclonal antibody that blocks IL-2 receptor on T cells

DOSAGE 1 mg/kg IV in 50 mL over 15 minutes; first dose before transplant and then 4 more doses at 14-day intervals

SUPPLIED Injectable

NOTES Combination human–mouse antibody; no significant side effects reported

 ## Dantrolene (Dantrium)

COMMON USES Treatment of clinical spasticity resulting from upper motor neuron disorders such as spinal cord injuries, strokes, cerebral palsy, or multiple sclerosis; treatment of malignant hyperthermic crisis

ACTIONS Skeletal muscle relaxant

DOSAGE
• Adults: spasticity: initially, 25 mg po qd; titrate to effect by 25 mg up to a maximum dose of 100 mg po qid prn.
• Peds: initially, 0.5 mg/kg/dose bid; titrate by 0.5 mg/kg to effectiveness up to a maximum dose of 3 mg/kg/dose qid prn.
• Adults and peds: malignant hyperthermia: treatment: continuous rapid IV push beginning at 1 mg/kg until symptoms subside or 10 mg/kg is reached
• Postcrisis follow-up: 4 to 8 mg/kg/d in 3 to 4 divided doses for 1 to 3 days to prevent recurrence

SUPPLIED Capsules 25, 50, 100 mg; powder for injection, 20 mg/vial

NOTES Monitor ALT and AST closely

 ## Demeclocycline (Declomycin)

COMMON USES Treatment of SIADH

ACTIONS Antagonizes action of ADH on renal tubules

DOSAGE 300 to 600 mg po q12h

SUPPLIED Capsules 150 mg; tablets 150 mg, 300 mg

NOTES Reduce the dose in renal failure. May cause diabetes insipidus

Desmopressin (DDAVP, Stimate)

 Desmopressin (DDAVP, Stimate)

COMMON USES Enuresis

ACTIONS Synthetic analog of vasopressin, a naturally occurring human antidiuretic hormone; increases factor VIII

DOSAGE Peds >6 years: 20 μg intranasally at bedtime, escalate as needed to 40 μg; oral, 0.05 to 0.4 mg bid-tid. Start at 0.05 mg bid; titrate dose.

SUPPLIED Nasal solution 01 mg/mL, 15 mg/mL; 0.1- and 0.2-mg tablets

NOTES In very young and old patients, adjust fluid intake to avoid water intoxication and hyponatremia. No adverse side effects noted, even when used for more than 12 months. Used with caution in patients at risk for electrolyte changes or fluid retention (congestive heart failure, renal insufficiency, and cystic fibrosis), as this can cause electrolyte abnormalities (hyponatremia).

 Dexamethasone (Decadron). See Systemic Steroids

 Dextran 40 (Rheomacrodex)

COMMON USES Plasma expander for adjunctive therapy in shock; prophylaxis of DVT and thromboembolism

ACTIONS Expands plasma volume; decreases blood viscosity

DOSAGE
• Shock: 10 mL/kg infused rapidly, with maximum dose of 20 mL/kg in the first 24 hours; total daily dosage beyond 24 hours should not exceed 10 mL/kg and should be discontinued after 5 days.
• Prophylaxis of DVT and thromboembolism: 10 mL/kg IV on day of surgery, followed by 500 mL IV daily for 23 days; then 500 mL IV every 23, days based on patient's risk factors, for up to 2 weeks

SUPPLIED 10% dextran 40 in 0.9% sodium chloride or 5% dextrose

NOTES Observe for hypersensitivity reactions; monitor renal function and electrolytes.

 Dezocine (Dalgan)

COMMON USES Relief of moderate-to-severe pain

ACTIONS Narcotic agonist–antagonist

DOSAGE 5 to 20 mg IM or 25 to 10 mg IV q2–4h prn

SUPPLIED Injection 5 mg/mL, 10 mg/mL, 15 mg/mL

NOTES May cause withdrawal in patients dependent on narcotics

 Diclofenac (Cataflam, Voltaren). See Nonsteroidal Antiinflammatory Drugs

 Dicloxacillin (Dynapen)

COMMON USES Treatment of infections caused by susceptible strains of *Staphylococcus* and *Streptococcus*

ACTIONS Bactericidal; inhibits cell wall synthesis

DOSAGE
• Adults: 250 to 500 mg q6h
• Peds: 125 to 250 mg/kg/d divided q6h

SUPPLIED 250-, 500-mg capsules

NOTES Administer to patient with an empty stomach.

 Dicyclomine (Bentyl)

COMMON USES Treatment of hyperreflexive bladders

ACTIONS Smooth muscle relaxant

DOSAGE
• Adults: 20 mg po tid
• Peds

—Infants >6 months: 5 mg/dose tid-qid
—Children: 10 mg/dose tid-qid

SUPPLIED Capsules 10 mg, 20 mg; tablets 20 mg; syrup 10 mg/5 mL; injection 10 mg/mL

NOTES Anticholinergic side effects may limit the dose.

 Diethylstilbestrol (DES)

COMMON USES Advanced prostate cancer

ACTIONS Synthetic estrogen; suppression of testosterone production, possibly direct suppression of prostate cancer cells

DOSAGE 1 to 3 mg qd

SUPPLIED 1-, 5-mg tablets

NOTES Thromboembolic disease, breast tenderness, and changes in libido

 Diflunisal (Dolobid)

COMMON USES Mild-to-moderate pain

ACTIONS Nonsteroidal antiinflammatory agents

DOSAGE Pain: 500 mg po bid

SUPPLIED Tablets 250 mg, 500 mg

NOTES May prolong prothrombin time

 Dimethyl Sulfoxide (DMSO) (RIMSO-50)

COMMON USES Intravesical therapy for interstitial cystitis

ACTIONS Membrane penetrant; anti-inflammatory, local analgesic, and cholinesterase inhibitor

DOSAGE 50 mL of 50% solution given intravesically

SUPPLIED 50-mL bottles

NOTES Garlic-like taste and odor

Diphenhydramine (Benadryl, Others)

COMMON USES Allergic reactions; potentiate narcotics, sedation, and treatment of extrapyramidal reactions

ACTIONS Antihistamine, antiemetic

DOSAGE Adults: 25 to 50 mg po IV or IM bid-tid; peds: 5 mg/kg/24 h po or IM divided q6h (maximum of 300 mg/d)

SUPPLIED Tablets and capsules 25 mg, 50 mg; elixir 125 mg/5 mL; syrup 125 mg/5 mL; injection 10 mg/mL, 50 mg/mL

NOTES Anticholinergic side effects, including dry mouth, urinary retention; causes sedation; increase the dosing interval in moderate-to-severe renal failure.

 ### Docusate Calcium (Surfak, Others). See Docuset Sodium

 ### Docusate Potassium (Dialose). See Docuset Sodium

 ### Docusate Sodium (DOSS, Colace, Others)

COMMON USES Constipation-prone patient; adjunct to painful anorectal conditions (hemorrhoids). Used often in postprostatectomy patients

ACTIONS Stool softener

DOSAGE

- Adults: 50 to 500 mg po qd
- Peds

—Infants to 3 years: 10 to 40 mg/24 h divided qd-qid
—3 to 6 years: 20 to 60 mg/24 h divided qd-qid
—6 to 12 years: 40 to 120 mg/24 h divided qd-qid

SUPPLIED

- Calcium: capsules 50 mg, 240 mg
- Potassium: capsules 100 mg, 240 mg
- Sodium: capsules 100 mg, 240 mg, 250 mg, 300 mg; syrup 50 mg/15 mL, 60 mg/15 mL; liquid 150 mg /15 mL; solution 50 mg/mL

NOTES No significant side effects, no laxative action

 ### Doxazosin (Cardura)

COMMON USES Treatment of symptomatic benign prostatic hyperplasia and nonbacterial prostatitis

ACTIONS Alpha-1-adrenergic blocker; relaxation of bladder neck smooth muscle fibers

DOSAGE Initially 1 mg po qd; may be increased to 16 mg po qd

SUPPLIED Tablets 1 mg, 2 mg, 4 mg, 8 mg

NOTES Doses greater than 4 mg increase the likelihood of excessive postural hypotension.

 ### Doxepin (Sinequan, Adapin)

COMMON USES Treatment of urge incontinence and chronic pain

ACTIONS Tricyclic antidepressant; increases the synaptic concentrations of serotonin or norepinephrine in the CNS

DOSAGE 25 to 150 mg po qd usually qHS but can be in divided doses

SUPPLIED Capsules 10 mg, 25 mg, 50 mg, 75 mg, 100 mg, 150 mg; oral concentrate 10 mg/mL

NOTES Anticholinergic, CNS and cardiovascular side effects

 ### Doxorubicin (Adriamycin, Doxil, Rubex)

COMMON USES Soft-tissue sarcomas, Wilms' tumor, neuroblastoma, bladder cancer (intravesical)

ACTIONS Anthracene antibiotic; DNA intercalating agent, inhibitor of DNA topoisomerase I and II

DOSAGE 60 to 75 mg/m^2 every 3 weeks, reduced cardiotoxicity with weekly (20 mg/m^2/wk) or continuous infusion (60–90 mg/m^2 over 96 hours) schedules. Intravesically, 50 mg in 50 mL water, instilled weekly for 4 to 8 weeks; a single dose can be given immediately after TUR to prevent recurrence.

SUPPLIED Injection 10 mg, 20 mg, 50 mg, 100 mg, 200 mg

NOTES Toxicity includes myelosuppression; extravasation leads to tissue damage (do not administer IM or subcutaneously); venous streaking and phlebitis may occur; nausea, vomiting and diarrhea, mucositis, radiation recall phenomenon. Cardiomyopathy rare but dose-related; limit of 550 mg/m^2 cumulative dose (400 mg/m^2 if history of mediastinal irradiation). Chemical cystitis and bladder contracture can occur when used intravesically. No formal labeling for intravesical use

 ### Doxycycline (Vibramycin)

COMMON USES Broad-spectrum antibiotic, including activity against *Rickettsiae, Chlamydia,* and *Mycoplasma pneumoniae*

ACTIONS Tetracycline; interferes with protein synthesis

DOSAGE Adults: 100 mg po q12h first day, then 100 mg po qd or bid or 100 mg IV q12h; peds >8 years: 5 mg/kg/24 h po, up to a maximum of 200 mg/d, divided qd or bid

SUPPLIED Tablets 50 mg, 100 mg; capsules 50 mg, 100 mg; syrup 50 mg/5 mL; powder for oral suspension 25 mg/5 mL; powder for injection 100 mg, 200 mg per vial

NOTES Tetracycline of choice for patients with renal impairment

Dronabinol (Marinol) [C]

COMMON USES Nausea and vomiting associated with cancer chemotherapy; appetite stimulation

ACTIONS Antiemetic; inhibits the vomiting center in the medulla

DOSAGE

• Adults and peds: *antiemetic:* 5 to 15 mg/m²/dose q4–6h prn
• Adults: *appetite:* 2.5 mg po before lunch and supper

SUPPLIED Capsules 2.5 mg, 5 mg, 10 mg

NOTES Principle psychoactive substance present in marijuana; many CNS side effects

 Droperidol (Inapsine)

COMMON USES Nausea and vomiting, premedication for anesthesia

ACTIONS Tranquilization, sedation, and antiemetic

DOSAGE

• Adults

—Nausea: 1.25-2.5 mg IV prn
—Premedication: 2.5 to 1.0 mg IV

• Peds: 0.1 to 0.15 mg/kg/dose

SUPPLIED Injection 2.5 mg/mL

NOTES May cause drowsiness, moderate hypotension, and occasionally tachycardia

 Econazole (Spectazole)

COMMON USES Treatment of most tinea, cutaneous *Candida,* and tinea versicolor infections

ACTIONS Topical antifungal

DOSAGE Apply to affected areas bid (qd for tinea versicolor) for 2 to 4 weeks.

SUPPLIED Topical cream 1%

NOTES Relief of symptoms and clinical improvement may be seen early in treatment, but the course of therapy should be carried out to avoid recurrence.

 Enoxacin (Penetrex)

COMMON USES Treatment of UTIs and gonorrhea

ACTIONS Quinolone antibiotic; inhibits DNA gyrase

DOSAGE 200 to 400 mg po bid; *gonorrhea:* 400 mg as a single dose

SUPPLIED Tablets 200 mg, 400 mg

NOTES Significant drug interaction with theophylline and caffeine

 Enoxaparin (Lovenox)

COMMON USES Prevention of DVT

ACTIONS Low-molecular-weight heparin

DOSAGE 30 mg SC twice daily

SUPPLIED Injection 30 mg/0.3 mL

NOTES Does not significantly affect bleeding time, platelet function, PT, or APTT

 Ephedrine

COMMON USES Retrograde ejaculation and enuresis

ACTIONS Sympathomimetic that stimulates both alpha and beta receptors

DOSAGE

• Adults: 25 to 50 mg qid
• Peds: 0.2 to 0.3 mg/kg/dose q4–6h prn

SUPPLIED Capsules 25 mg, 50 mg; syrup 11 mg/5 mL, 20 mg/5 mL

 Epinephrine (Adrenalin, Sus-Phrine, Others)

COMMON USES Priapism, anaphylactic reactions, and can be used with local anesthetics

ACTIONS Beta-adrenergic agonist with some alpha effects

DOSAGE

• Adults

—Anaphylaxis: 0.3 to 0.5 mL of 1:1000 dilution SQ; may repeat q10–15min to maximum of 1 mg/dose and 5 mg/d
—Priapism: 03 mL of 1:1000 dilution mixed with NSS. The solution is then injected into the corpora cavernosum at 5- to 10-minute intervals.

SUPPLIED Injection 1:1000, 1:10,000, 1:100,000; suspension for injection 1:200

NOTES Only to be used for low-flow priapism. Corpora must be evacuated and irrigated.

Epoetin alfa (Epogen, Procrit)

COMMON USES Treatment of anemia associated with chronic renal failure and patients receiving cancer chemotherapy. Treatment for anemic patients scheduled to undergo elective surgery. This reduces the need for allogenic blood transfusions.

ACTIONS Erythropoietin supplementation

DOSAGE Adults and peds: 50 to 150 U/kg 3 times weekly; adjust dose every 4 to 6 weeks as needed. Preoperatively, 300 U/kg/d for 10 days before surgery, the day of surgery, and for 4 days after surgery

SUPPLIED Injection 2000 U, 3000 U, 4000 U, 10,000 U

NOTES May cause hypertension, headache, tachycardia, nausea, and vomiting

 Erythromycin (E-Mycin, Ilosone, Erythrocin, ERYC, Others)

COMMON USES Infections caused by Group A streptococci (*S. pyrogenes*), alpha-hemolytic streptococci, and *N. gonorrhoeae* infections in penicillin-allergic patients; *S. pneumoniae, Mycoplasma pneumoniae,* and Legionnaire disease, bowel preparation

ACTIONS Bacteriostatic, interferes with protein synthesis

DOSAGE Adults: 250 to 500 mg po qid or 500 mg-1 g IV qid 1 g of erythromycin base at staggered time intervals for bowel prep; peds: 30 to 50 mg/kg/24 h PO or IV divided q6h, to a maximum of 2 g/d

SUPPLIED
• Powder for injection as lactobionate and gluceptate salts: 250 mg, 500 mg, 1 g; base: tablets 250 mg, 333 mg, 500 mg; and capsules 125 mg, 250 mg
• Estolate: chewable tablets 125 mg, 250 mg; capsules 125 mg, 250 mg; drops 100 mg/mL; suspension 125 mg/5 mL, 250 mg/5 mL
• Stearate: tablets 250 mg, 500 mg
• Ethylsuccinate: chewable tablets 200 mg; tablets 400 mg; suspension 200 mg/5 mL, 400 mg/5 mL

NOTES Frequent, mild GI disturbances; estolate salt is associated with cholestatic jaundice; erythromycin base not well absorbed from the GI tract; some forms, such as ERYC, are better tolerated with respect to GI irritation. Lactobionate salt contains benzyl alcohol; therefore, use with caution in neonates; used as part of the "Condon bowel prep."

 Esterified Estrogens (Estratab, Menest)

COMMON USES Atrophic vaginitis and female hypogonadism

ACTIONS Estrogen supplementation

DOSAGE Hypogonadism: 2.5 mg po qd-tid

SUPPLIED Tablets 0.3 mg, 0.625 mg, 1.25 mg, 2.5 mg

 Estradiol Topical (Estrace)

COMMON USES Atrophic vaginitis

ACTIONS Estrogen supplementation

DOSAGE 2 to 4 g daily × 2 weeks, then 1 g 1 to 3 times a week, applied topically

SUPPLIED Vaginal cream

 Estradiol Transdermal (Estraderm)

COMMON USES Female hypogonadism

ACTIONS Hormonal replacement

DOSAGE 0.05-mg patch twice weekly; adjust dose as necessary to control symptoms.

SUPPLIED Transdermal Patches 0.05 mg, 0.1 mg (delivers 0.05 mg or 0.1 mg per 24 hours)

 Estramustine Phosphate (Estracyte, Emcyt)

COMMON USES Advanced prostate cancer

ACTIONS Antimicrotubule agent, weak estrogenic and antiandrogenic activity

DOSAGE 140 to 1400 mg/d in divided doses

SUPPLIED Capsules 140 mg

NOTES Toxicity includes nausea and vomiting, exacerbation of preexisting congestive heart failure, gynecomastia in 20% to 100%

 Estrogen, Conjugated (Premarin)

COMMON USES Atrophic vaginitis and palliative therapy of advanced prostatic carcinoma

ACTIONS Hormonal replacement

DOSAGE 0.3 to 1.25 mg/d po cyclically; prostatic carcinoma requires 125 to 25 mg po tid

SUPPLIED Tablets 0.3 mg, 0.625 mg, 0.9 mg, 1.25 mg, 2.5 mg; injection 2.5 mg/mL

NOTES Do not use in pregnancy; associated with an increased risk of endometrial carcinoma, gallbladder disease, and thromboembolism and possibly breast cancer. Generic products are *not* equivalent.

 Ethacrynic Acid (Edecrin)

COMMON USES Rapid diuresis

ACTIONS Loop diuretic; inhibits reabsorption of sodium and chlorine in the ascending loop of Henle and distal renal tubule

DOSAGE
• Adults: 50 to 200 mg po qd or 50 mg IV prn
• Peds: 1 mg/kg/dose IV. Repeated doses are not recommended.

SUPPLIED Tablets 25 mg, 50 mg; powder for injection 50 mg

NOTES Contraindicated in anuria; many severe side effects

 Ethambutol (Myambutol)

COMMON USES Tuberculosis (TB), other mycobacterial infections, and BCG-induced TB

ACTIONS Inhibits cellular metabolism

DOSAGE Adults and peds >12 years: 15 to 25 mg/kg po daily as single dose

SUPPLIED Tablet 100 mg, 400 mg

NOTES May cause vision changes and GI upset

Ethinyl Estradiol (Estinyl, Feminone)

 Ethinyl Estradiol (Estinyl, Feminone)

COMMON USES Female hypogonadism

ACTIONS Estrogen supplementation

DOSAGE 0.02 to 1.5 mg/d divided qd tid

SUPPLIED Tablets 0.02 mg, 0.05 mg, 0.5 mg

 Etodolac (Lodine). See Nonsteroidal Antiinflammatory Drugs

 Etoposide (VePesid) [VP-16]

COMMON USES Testicular cancer

ACTIONS Topoisomerase II inhibitor

DOSAGE 50 mg/m^2/d IV × 3 to 5 days, 50 mg/m^2/d po × 21 days (bioavailability of oral formulation approximately 50% of IV form)

SUPPLIED Capsules 100 mg; oral solution 100 mg/5 mL; injection 100 mg

NOTES Toxicity includes myelosuppression, nausea and vomiting, alopecia; hypotension may occur if infused too rapidly; anaphylaxis or lesser hypersensitivity reactions (wheezing) rarely occur; potential for secondary leukemias

 Famotidine (Pepcid)

COMMON USES Duodenal ulcer, ulcer prophylaxis in hypersecretory states such as trauma, burns, and surgery

ACTIONS H2-antagonist; inhibits gastric acid secretion

DOSAGE

• Adults

—Ulcer: 20 to 40 mg po HS or 20 mg IV q12h
—Hypersecretory: 20 to 160 mg po q6h

• Peds: 1 to 2 mg/kg/d

SUPPLIED Tablets 10 mg, 20 mg, 40 mg; suspension 40 mg/5 mL; injection 10 mg/mL

NOTES Decrease the dose in severe renal failure.

 Famciclovir (Famvir)

COMMON USES Management of acute herpes zoster (shingles) and genital herpes infections

ACTIONS Oral form of penciclovir, a novel nucleoside analog that inhibits viral DNA synthesis

DOSAGE

• Zoster: 500 mg po q8h
• Simplex: 125 to 250 mg po bid

SUPPLIED Tablets 125 mg, 250 mg, 500 mg

 Fenoprofen (Nalfon). See Nonsteroidal Antiinflammatory Drugs

 Fentanyl Transdermal System (Duragesic)

COMMON USES Management of chronic pain

ACTIONS Narcotic

DOSAGE Apply patch to upper torso every 72 hours. Dose is calculated from the narcotic requirements for the previous 24 hours.

SUPPLIED Transdermal patches that deliver 25 μg/h, 50 μg/h, 75 μg/h, 100 μg/h

NOTES 0.1 mg of fentanyl is equivalent to 10 mg of morphine IM

 Finasteride (Proscar)

COMMON USES Treatment of symptomatic benign prostatic hyperplasia; reduces the risk of retention and need for surgery such as TURP. Prostate bleeding control.

ACTIONS Inhibits 5-alpha-reductase

DOSAGE 5 mg po qd

SUPPLIED Tablets 5 mg

NOTES May take 3 to 6 months to see effect on urinary symptoms. Appears to work better on larger glands(>40 cc^3). Decreases serum PSA levels to approximately 50% of baseline at 6 months. Use the "multiply by 2" rule to maintain the usefulness of PSA as a screening tool for prostate cancer (Guess et al. *J Urol* 1996; 158:3–9.)

 Flavoxate (Urispas)

COMMON USES Symptomatic relief of dysuria, urgency, nocturia, suprapubic pain, urinary frequency and incontinence

ACTIONS Counteracts smooth muscle spasm of the urinary tract

DOSAGE 100 to 200 mg po tid-qid

SUPPLIED Tablets 100 mg

NOTES May cause drowsiness, blurred vision, and dry mouth

Fluconazole (Diflucan)

COMMON USES *Candida* infections of the peritoneum and urinary tract; prevention of candidiasis in patient receiving chemotherapy or radiation; and candidal vaginitis

ACTIONS Antifungal; inhibits fungal cytochrome P-450 sterol demethylation

DOSAGE
- Adults: 100 to 400 mg po or IV qd
—Vaginitis: 150 mg po as single dose
- Peds: 3 to 6 mg/kg po or IV qd

SUPPLIED Tablets 50 mg, 100 mg, 150 mg, 200 mg; suspension 10 mg/mL, 40 mg/mL; injection 2 mg/mL

NOTES Adjust the dose in renal insufficiency; oral dosing produces the same blood levels as IV; therefore, the oral route should be used whenever possible.

 Flucytosine (Ancobon)

COMMON USES Treatment of serious fungal infections caused by susceptible strains of *Candida* or *Cryptococcus*

ACTIONS It disrupts fungal protein and DNA synthesis.

DOSAGE 100 to 150 mg/kg/d given in divided doses at 6-hour intervals

SUPPLIED 250-, 500-mg tablets are available

NOTES It is readily absorbed by the gastrointestinal tract and widely distributed. Doses must be adjusted in patients with renal insufficiency. Bone marrow suppression can occur, but resolves when the drug is stopped.

 Fludrocortisone Acetate (Florinef)

COMMON USES Partial treatment for adrenocortical insufficiency

ACTIONS Mineralocorticoid replacement

DOSAGE
- Adults: 0.05 to 0.2 mg po qd
- Peds: 0.05 to 0.1 mg po qd

SUPPLIED Tablets 0.1 mg

NOTES For adrenal insufficiency, must be used in conjunction with a glucocorticoid supplement; dosage changes based on plasma renin activity

 Flurbiprofen (Ansaid). See Nonsteroidal Antiinflammatory Drugs

 Fluorouracil [5-FU] (Adrucil)

COMMON USES Bladder and prostate cancer

ACTIONS Inhibitor of thymidylate synthase (interferes with DNA synthesis, S-phase specific)

DOSAGE 370 to 1000 mg/m²/d × 1 to 5 days, intravenously as IV push to 24-hour continuous infusions, protracted venous infusion of 200 to 300 mg/m²/d

SUPPLIED Injection 500 mg

NOTES Toxicity includes stomatitis, esophagopharyngitis, diarrhea, anorexia, nausea and vomiting. Myelosuppression (leukocytopenia, thrombocytopenia, and anemia); rash, dry skin, and photosensitivity occur frequently. Tingling in the hands and feet, followed by pain (palmar–plantar erythrodysesthesia), may occur; phlebitis and discoloration may occur at injection sites.

 Flutamide (Eulexin)

COMMON USES Advanced prostate cancer (in combination with gonadotropin-releasing hormone agonists such as leuprolide or goserelin); in combination with radiation therapy for localized prostate cancer in combination with LH-RH analogue

ACTIONS Nonsteroidal antiandrogen

DOSAGE 250 mg orally three times daily (750 mg total)

SUPPLIED Capsule 125 mg

NOTES Must monitor LFT's before treatment and during therapy. Hepatic toxicity can be seen. Other toxicity includes hot flashes (60%), loss of libido, impotence (33%), diarrhea, nausea and vomiting, and gynecomastia (9%). These have been noted in patients receiving flutamide plus a GnRH agonist; therefore, it is difficult to discern the contribution of flutamide.

 Formalin (Lazerformalyde)

COMMON USES Hemorrhagic cystitis

ACTIONS It acts by hydrolyzing proteins and coagulating the tissue on a superficial level.

DOSAGE 1% to 10 % solution given only with general or regional anesthesia

SUPPLIED Available in 3-oz plastic bottle instillation only.

NOTES Before formalin is administered, vesicoureteral reflux must be identified and prevented, if found. Higher concentrations may cause fibrosis of the bladder.

Foscarnet (Foscavir)

COMMON USES Treatment of acyclovir-resistant herpes infections

ACTIONS Inhibits viral DNA polymerase and reverse transcriptase

DOSAGE Induction: 60 mg/kg IV q8h for 14 to 21 days; maintenance: 90 to 120 mg/kg IV qd (Monday–Friday)

SUPPLIED Injection 24 mg/mL

NOTES Dosage must be adjusted for renal function; nephrotoxic; monitor ionized calcium closely (causes electrolyte abnormalities); administer through a central line.

 Fosfomycin Tromethamine (Monurol)

COMMON USES Uncomplicated urinary tract infections from *E. coli* and *Enterococcus*

ACTIONS Bactericidal; inhibits cell wall synthesis

DOSAGE One sachet dissolved in 3 to 4 oz of water

SUPPLIED Single-dose sachet containing 3 g of fosfomycin

NOTES Used to treat uncomplicated urinary tract infections with a single dose. Drug interactions with metoclopramide and cimetidine. Use cautiously in pregnant patients.

 Furosemide (Lasix)

COMMON USES Rapid diuresis

ACTIONS Loop diuretic; inhibits sodium and chlorine reabsorption in the ascending loop of Henle and distal renal tubule

DOSAGE
• Adults: 20 to 80 mg po or IV qd or bid
• Peds: 1 mg/kg/dose IV q6–12h; 2 mg/kg/dose po q12–24h

SUPPLIED Tablets 20 mg, 40 mg, 80 mg; solution 10 mg/mL, 40 mg/5 mL; injection 10 mg/mL

NOTES Monitor for hypokalemia; use with caution in hepatic disease; high doses of the IV form may cause ototoxicity.

 Gallium Nitrate (Ganite)

COMMON USES Treatment of hypercalcemia of malignancy; bladder cancer

ACTIONS Inhibits resorption of calcium from the bones

DOSAGE Hypercalcemia: 100 to 200 mg/m^2/d for 5 days; cancer: 350 mg/m^2 continuous infusion × 5 days to 700 mg/m^2 rapid intravenous infusion every 2 weeks in antineoplastic settings

SUPPLIED Injection 25 mg/mL

NOTES Can cause renal insufficiency; may cause hypocalcemia, hypophosphatemia, and decreased bicarbonate; <1 % of patients developed acute optic neuritis; for bladder cancer use in combination with vinblastine and ifosfamide

 Ganciclovir (Cytovene)

COMMON USES Prevention of CMV disease in transplant recipients

ACTIONS Inhibits viral DNA synthesis

DOSAGE
• Adults and peds
—IV: 5 mg/kg IV q12h for 14 to 21 days, then maintenance of 5 mg/kg IV qd for 7 days/week or 6 mg/kg IV qd for 5 days/week
• Adults
—PO: following induction, 1000 mg po tid

SUPPLIED Capsules 250 mg; injection 500 mg

NOTES This is *not* a cure for CMV; granulocytopenia and thrombocytopenia are the major toxicities; injection should be handled with cytotoxic precautions, and capsules should be taken with food.

 Gentamicin (Garamycin)

COMMON USES Serious infections caused by susceptible *Pseudomonas, Proteus, E. coli, Klebsiella, Enterobacter,* and *Serratia,* and for initial treatment of gram-negative sepsis

ACTIONS Bactericidal, inhibits protein synthesis

DOSAGE
• Adults: 3 to 5 mg/kg/24 h IV divided q8–24h
• Peds
—Infants <7 days
—<1200 g: 25 mg/kg/dose q18–24h
—>1200 g: 25 mg/kg/dose q12–18h
—Infants >7 days: 25 mg/kg/dose IV q8–12h
—Children: 25 mg/kg/dose IV q8h

SUPPLIED Injection 10 mg/mL, 40 mg/mL

NOTES Nephrotoxic and ototoxic; decrease dose with renal insufficiency; monitor creatinine clearance and serum concentration for dosage adjustments. Drug levels: 4 to 10 µg/mL, through <2 µg/mL

 Gonadorelin (Lutrepulse)

COMMON USES Primary hypothalamic amenorrhea

ACTIONS Stimulates the pituitary to release the gonadotropins LH and FSH

DOSAGE 5 to 20 µg IV q 90 minutes for 21 days, using a reservoir and pump

SUPPLIED Injection 800 µg, 32 mg

NOTES Risk of multiple pregnancies

Ibuprofen (Advil, Motrin). See Nonsteroidal Antiinflammatory Drugs

 Goserelin Acetate (Zoladex)

COMMON USES Advanced prostate cancer; stage B₂/C prostate cancer in combination with flutamide for external beam radiation

ACTIONS Slow release form of LH-RH agonist, thereby inhibiting the release of gonadotropin, decreasing testosterone levels

DOSAGE 3.6 mg SQ (implant) every 28 days, or 10.8 mg every 3 months

SUPPLIED Subcutaneous implant (3.6 mg and 10.8 mg)

NOTES Toxicity includes hot flashes in 50%, decreased libido and gynecomastia each in 9%, transient exacerbation of cancer-related bone pain in 17%, ("flare reaction"); edema, anorexia, and nausea all occur in less than 10%.

 Granisetron (Kytril)

COMMON USES Prevention of nausea and vomiting associated with emetogenic cancer therapy

ACTIONS Serotonin receptor antagonist

DOSAGE

• Adults and peds: 10 μg/kg IV 30 minutes prior to initiation of chemotherapy
• Adults: 1 mg po 1 hour prior to chemotherapy, then 12 hours after

SUPPLIED Tablets 1 mg; injection 1 mg/mL

 Heparin Sodium

COMMON USES Treatment and prevention of venous thrombosis and pulmonary emboli

ACTIONS Acts with antithrombin III to inactivate thrombin and to inhibit thromboplastin formation

DOSAGE

• Adult

—Prophylaxis: 3000 to 5000 U SQ q8–12h
—Treatment of thrombosis: loading dose of 50 to 75 U/kg IV, then 10 to 20 U/kg IV qh (adjust based on PTT)

• Peds

—Infants: Load 50 U/kg IV bolus, then 20 U/kg/h IV by continuous infusion.
—Children: Load 50 U/kg IV, then 15 to 25 U/kg continuous infusion or 100 U/kg/dose q4h IV intermittent bolus

SUPPLIED Injection 10 U/mL, 100 U/mL, 1000 U/mL, 5000 U /mL, 10,000 U/mL, 20,000 U/mL, 40,000 U/mL

NOTES Follow PTT, thrombin time, or activated clotting time to assess effectiveness; heparin has little effect on prothrombin time; with proper dose, PTT is about 1.5 to 2.0 times the control; can cause thrombocytopenia; follow platelet counts.

 Hydrochlorothiazide (HydroDIURIL, Esidrix, Others)

COMMON USES Diuresis and urinary lithiasis

ACTIONS Thiazide diuretic; inhibits sodium reabsorption in the distal tubule, causes calcium resorption

DOSAGE Adults: 25 to 100 mg po qd in single or divided doses; peds: 2 to 3 mg/kg/24 h po divided bid

SUPPLIED Tablets 25 mg, 50 mg, 100 mg; oral solution 50 mg/5 mL, 100 mg/mL

NOTES Hypokalemia is frequent; hyperglycemia, hyperuricemia, hyperlipidemia, and hyponatremia are common side effects.

 Hydrocortisone (Cortef). See Systemic Steroids

 Hydromorphone (Dilaudid) [C]

COMMON USES Management of moderate-to-severe pain

ACTIONS Narcotic analgesic

DOSAGE 1 to 4 mg po, IM, IV, or pr q4–6h prn

SUPPLIED Tablets 1 mg, 2 mg, 3 mg, 4 mg; injection 1 mg/mL, 2 mg/mL, 3 mg/mL, 4 mg/mL, 10 mg/mL; suppositories 3 mg

NOTES 15 mg IM equivalent to 10 mg morphine IM

 Hyoscyamine (Anaspaz, Levsin, Levsinex, Cystospaz)

COMMON USES Control of bladder spasms

ACTIONS Anticholinergic, antispasmodic

DOSAGE

• Oral: 0.125 to 0.25 mg po tid-qid (Levsin SL sublingual)
• IV: 0.25 to 0.5 mg SC, IM, or IV 2 to 4 times daily, as needed

SUPPLIED Tablets 0.125 mg, 0.15 mg; capsules, time-released, 0.375 mg; solution 0.125 mg/mL; elixir 0.125 mg/5 mL; injection 0.5 mg/mL

NOTES May cause dizziness, blurred vision, dry mouth, difficulty in urination

 Ibuprofen (Advil, Motrin). See Nonsteroidal Antiinflammatory Drugs

Ifosfamide (IFEX, Holoxan)

 Ifosfamide (IFEX, Holoxan)

COMMON USES Soft-tissue sarcoma and testicular cancer

ACTIONS Alkylating agent

DOSAGE 12 g/m^2/d $\times$ 5 days by bolus or continuous infusion; 24 g/m^2/d $\times$ 3 days; with mesna uroprotection (see Mesna)

SUPPLIED Injection 1g, 3 g

NOTES Toxicity includes hemorrhagic cystitis, nephrotoxicity, nausea and vomiting, mild-to-moderate leukopenia, lethargy and confusion, alopecia, hepatic enzyme elevations

 Imipenem/Cilastatin (Primaxin)

COMMON USES Treatment of serious infections caused by a wide variety of susceptible bacteria; inactive against *Staphylococcus aureus*, group A and B streptococci, and others

ACTIONS Bactericidal; interferes with cell wall synthesis

DOSAGE Adults: 250 to 500 mg (imipenem) IV q6h; peds: 60 to 100 mg/kg/24h IV divided q6h

SUPPLIED Injection (imipenem/cilastatin) 250 mg/250 mg, 500 mg/500 mg

NOTES Seizures may occur if the drug accumulates; adjust the dosage for renal insufficiency, to avoid drug accumulation if calculated creatinine clearance is <70 mL/min.

 Imipramine (Tofranil)

COMMON USES Treatment of enuresis, incontinence, retrograde ejaculation, and chronic pain

ACTIONS Tricyclic antidepressant; increases synaptic concentration of serotonin and/or norepinephrine in the CNS

DOSAGE
• Adults: 50 to 150 mg po qHS, not to exceed 200 mg/24 h
• Peds
—Enuresis >6 years: 10 to 25 mg po qHS; increase by 10 to 25 mg at 1- to 2-week intervals; treat for 2 to 3 months, then taper.

SUPPLIED Tablets 10 mg, 25 mg, 50 mg; capsules 75 mg, 100 mg, 125 mg, 150 mg; injection 125 mg/mL

NOTES Do not use with MAO inhibitors; less sedation than amitriptyline

 Imiquimod Cream, 5% (Aldara)

COMMON USES Treatment of external genital warts

ACTIONS Exact mechanism unknown. It is suggested that it may induce cytokines.

DOSAGE Applied 3 times a week and should be left on the skin for 6 to 10 hours for a maximum of 16 weeks

SUPPLIED Single-dose packets that contain 250 mg of the cream

NOTES Local skin reactions are common.

 Indapamide (Lozol)

COMMON USES Diuresis and urinary lithiasis

ACTIONS Thiazide diuretic; enhances sodium, chloride, and water excretion in the proximal segment of the distal tubule

DOSAGE 25 to 50 mg po qd

SUPPLIED Tablets 25 mg

NOTES Doses greater than 5 mg do not have additional effects on lowering blood pressure.

 Indomethacin (Indocin). See Nonsteroidal Antiinflammatory Drugs

 Interferon-Alpha (Roferon-A, Intron A)

COMMON USES Renal cell carcinoma, bladder cancer, condyloma acuminata

ACTIONS Direct antiproliferative action against tumor cells and modulation of the host immune response

DOSAGE
• Alpha-2A (Roferon): 3 million IU daily for 16 to 24 weeks SQ or IM
• Alpha-2B (Intron): 2 million IU/m^2 IM or SC 3 times a week for 2 to 6 months; intravesically 50 to 100 millions weekly in 30 to 50 mL distilled water weekly for 6 to 8 weeks

SUPPLIED Injection

NOTES May cause flu-like symptoms; fatigue is common; anorexia occurs in 20% to 30% of patients; neurotoxicity may occur at high doses; neutralizing antibodies can occur in up to 40% of patients receiving prolonged therapy; bladder administration only associated with low-grade fever and malaise. Combination BCG and interferon under study as intravesical therapy.

Interferon-Gamma-1b (Actimmune)

COMMON USES   Management of chronic granulomatous disease

ACTIONS   Biologic response modifier

DOSAGE   50 μg/m² SC 3 times weekly

SUPPLIED   Injection 100 μg

NOTES   100 μg = 3 million units; may cause flu-like syndrome

 Interleukin-2 (Aldesleukin, Proleukin, Teceleukin)

COMMON USES   Renal cell carcinoma

ACTIONS   Acts via IL-2 receptor; numerous immunomodulatory effects

DOSAGE   600,000 IU/kg q8h $\times$ 14 doses (FDA-approved dose/schedule for RCC). Multiple continuous infusion and SQ dosing schedules (including "high-dose" therapy with 24 $\times$ 106 IU/m² IV q8h on days 1 to 5, 12 to 16)

SUPPLIED   Injection 12 mg (22 $\times$ 106 U), 100 μg

NOTES   Toxicity includes flu-like syndrome (malaise, fever, chills), nausea, vomiting, diarrhea, increased serum bilirubin. Capillary leak syndrome may develop with hypotension, pulmonary edema, fluid retention, and weight gain. Renal toxicity and mild hematologic toxicity (anemia, thrombocytopenia, leukopenia) and secondary eosinophilia may be seen. Cardiac toxicity (myocardial ischemia and atrial arrhythmias) may occur. Neurologic toxicity (CNS depression, somnolence, rarely coma, delirium). Pruritic skin rashes, urticaria, and erythroderma are common. Continuous infusion schedules are less likely to result in severe hypotension and fluid retention.

 Isoniazid (INH)

COMMON USES   Treatment and prophylaxis of *Mycobacterium* spp infections

ACTIONS   Bactericidal; interferes with mycolic acid synthesis, thus disrupting the bacterial cell wall

DOSAGE

- Adults

—Active TB: 5 mg/kg/24 h po or IM qd (usually 300 mg/d)
—Prophylaxis: 300 mg po qd for 6 to 12 months

- Peds

—Active TB: 10 to 20 mg/kg/24 h po or IM qd to a maximum of 300 mg/d
—Prophylaxis: 10 mg/kg/24 h po qd

SUPPLIED   Tablets 50 mg, 100 mg, 300 mg; syrup 50 mg/5 mL; injection 100 mg/mL

NOTES   Can cause severe hepatitis; given with other antituberculous drugs for active tuberculosis; consult the *MMWR* for the latest recommendations on the treatment and prophylaxis of tuberculosis; IM route rarely used; to prevent peripheral neuropathy, can give pyridoxine 50 to 100 mg/d. See also Section II, "BCG Sepsis."

 Itraconazole (Sporanox)

COMMON USES   Treatment of systemic fungal infections caused by *Aspergillus, Blastomycosis,* and *Histoplasma*

ACTIONS   Inhibits synthesis of ergosterol

DOSAGE   200 mg po qd-bid

SUPPLIED   Capsules 100 mg

NOTES   Administer with meals or cola; should not be used concurrently with H2 antagonist, omeprazole, antacids, terfenadine, astemizole, or cisapride

 Ketoconazole (Nizoral)

COMMON USES   Treatment of systemic fungal infections; topical cream for localized fungal infections due to dermatophytes and yeast, advanced prostate carcinoma

ACTIONS   Inhibits fungal cell wall synthesis; surpasses androgen production and enhances clearance at androgens

DOSAGE

- Adults

—Prostate cancer: 1200 mg po daily with hydrocortisone replacement
—Oral: 200 mg po qd; increase to 400 mg po qd for very serious infections
—Topical: Apply to the affected area once daily.

- Peds >2 years: 5 to 10 mg/kg/24 h po divided q12–24h

SUPPLIED   Tablets 200 mg; suspension 100 mg/5 mL; topical cream 2%; shampoo 2%

NOTES   Associated with severe hepatotoxicity; monitor LFTs closely throughout the course of therapy; drug interaction with any agent increasing gastric pH, preventing absorption of ketoconazole; avoid concurrent use with astemizole, terfenadine or cisapride; may enhance oral anticoagulants; may react with alcohol to produce disulfiram-like reaction

 Ketoprofen (Orudis). See Nonsteroidal Antiinflammatory Drugs

 Ketorolac (Toradol). See Nonsteroidal Antiinflammatory Drugs

 Lactobacillus (Lactinex Granules)

COMMON USES   Control of diarrhea, especially after antibiotic therapy

ACTIONS   Replaces normal intestinal flora

DOSAGE   Adult and peds > 3 years: 1 packet, 2 capsules, or 4 tablets with meals or liquids tid-qid

SUPPLIED   Tablets; capsules; enteric-coated capsules; powder in packets 1 g

Lansoprazole (Prevacid)

 Lansoprazole (Prevacid)

COMMON USES Treatment of duodenal ulcers, erosive esophagitis, and hypersecretory conditions

ACTIONS Proton pump inhibitor

DOSAGE 15 to 30 mg po once daily

SUPPLIED Capsules 15 mg, 30 mg

 Leuprolide (Lupron and Lupron Depot)

COMMON USES Treatment of prostate cancer and central precocious puberty (CPP); endometriosis and uterine fibroids

ACTIONS LH-RH agonist; paradoxically inhibits release of gonadotropin, resulting in decreased LH and testosterone levels

DOSAGE

• Adults

—Prostate: 7.5 mg IM q28d or 22.5 mg IM q3mo or 30 mg IM q4mo

• Peds: CPP: 50 μg/kg/d as a daily SQ injection; may titrate upward by 10 mg/kg/d until total downregulation is achieved

—Depot
  —<25 kg: 75 mg IM every 4 weeks
  —>25 to 37.5 kg: 11.25 mg IM every 4 weeks
  —>37.5 kg: 15 mg IM every 4 weeks

SUPPLIED Injection 5 mg/mL; depot 7.5, 22.5, and 30 mg; Depot-Ped 7.5 mg, 11.25 mg, 15 mg

NOTES Toxicity includes hot flashes, gynecomastia, nausea and vomiting, constipation, anorexia, dizziness, headache, insomnia, paresthesias, peripheral edema, bone pain ("flare reaction" 7–10 days after first dose due to transient testosterone increase)

 Levofloxacin (Levaquin)

COMMON USES Broad-spectrum activity against a variety of gram-positive and gram-negative aerobic bacteria

ACTIONS Quinolone antibiotic; inhibits DNA gyrase

DOSAGE 500 mg q24h

SUPPLIED 250-, 500-mg tablets; injection in 20 mL of concentrated solution containing 500 mg or 250 mg

NOTES Drug interactions with theophylline, caffeine, sucralfate, and antacids; nausea, vomiting, and abdominal discomfort are common. Contraindicated in pregnancy

 Levorphanol (Levo-Dromoran) [C]

COMMON USES Moderate-to-severe pain

ACTIONS Narcotic analgesic

DOSAGE 2 mg po or SC prn

SUPPLIED Tablets 2 mg; injection 2 mg/mL

 Lidocaine (Xylocaine)

COMMON USES Local anesthetic

ACTIONS Anesthetic

DOSAGE 1 to 28 mL of 1% solution for 70-kg adult

SUPPLIED Injection 0.5%, 1%, 2%, 4%, 10%, 20%, topical gel

NOTES Epinephrine may be added for local anesthesia, to prolong the effect and help decrease bleeding. Do *not* use lidocaine with epinephrine on digits, ears, or nose, because vasoconstriction may cause necrosis. Intraurethral administration of viscous gel for minor procedures such as cystoscopy

 Lindane (Kwell)

COMMON USES Crab lice and scabies

ACTIONS An ectoparasiticide and ovicide

DOSAGE

• Adults and Peds

—Cream or lotion: Apply a thin layer after bathing and leave in place for 24 hours; pour on laundry.
—Shampoo: Apply 30 mL and develop a lather with warm water for 4 minutes; comb out nits.

SUPPLIED Cream 1%, lotion 1%, shampoo 1%

NOTES Caution with overuse; may be absorbed into blood

 Lomefloxacin (Maxaquin)

COMMON USES Treatment of UTI caused by gram-negative bacteria; prophylaxis in transurethral procedures

ACTIONS Quinolone antibiotic; inhibits DNA gyrase

DOSAGE 400 mg po qd

SUPPLIED Tablets 400 mg

NOTES May cause photosensitivity

 Loracarbef (Lorabid)

COMMON USES Broad-spectrum antibiotic for urinary tract infections and pyelonephritis

ACTIONS Inhibits cell wall synthesis

DOSAGE

• Adults: 200 to 400 mg once daily
• Peds: 15 mg/kg/d in divided doses twice a day

SUPPLIED 200-, 400-mg tablets; oral suspension 100 mg/5 mL or 200 mg/5 mL

NOTES Hypersensitivity reactions; gastrointestinal disturbances; dosage adjustment for renal impairment

Magnesium Citrate

COMMON USES Vigorous bowel prep; constipation

ACTIONS Saline cathartic

DOSAGE
- Adult: 120 to 240 mL po prn
- Peds: 0.5 mL/kg/dose, up to maximum 200 mL po

SUPPLIED Effervescent solution

NOTES Do not use in renal insufficiency or intestinal obstruction.

 Magnesium Hydroxide (Milk of Magnesia)

COMMON USES Constipation, light bowel prep

ACTIONS Saline laxative

DOSAGE
- Adult: 15 to 30 mL po prn
- Peds: 0.5 mL/kg/dose po prn

SUPPLIED Suspension 8%, tablets 325 mg

NOTES Do not use in renal insufficiency or intestinal obstruction.

 Magnesium Oxide (Beelith, Uro-Mag, Mag-Ox 400, Maox)

COMMON USES Replacement for low plasma levels, treatment of urinary lithiasis

ACTIONS Increases urinary magnesium levels

DOSAGE 400 to 800 mg/d divided qd-qid; Beelith 362 mg tablets qd

SUPPLIED Capsules 140 mg; tablets 400 mg, 420 mg; Beelith 362-mg tablets

NOTES GI side effects are most common.

 Mannitol

COMMON USES Osmotic diuresis (oliguria, anuria, renal transplantation, TUR syndrome)

ACTIONS Osmotic diuretic

DOSAGE
- Adult: diuresis: 0.2 g/kg/dose IV over 35 minutes; if no diuresis within 2 hours, discontinue
- Peds: diuresis: 0.75 g/kg/dose IV over 3 to 5 minutes; if no diuresis within 2 hours, discontinue
- Adult and peds: cerebral edema: 0.25 g/kg/dose IV push repeated at 5-minute intervals prn; increase incrementally to 1 g/kg/dose prn intracranial hypertension

SUPPLIED Injection 5%, 10%, 15%, 20%, 25%

NOTES Caution with CHF or volume overload

 Megestrol Acetate (Megace)

COMMON USES Treatment of "hot flushes" from hormonal therapy for prostate cancer

ACTIONS Hormone; progesterone analogue

DOSAGE 10 to 20 mg bid

SUPPLIED Tablets 20 mg, 40 mg; solution 40 mg/mL

NOTES May induce DVT; do not abruptly discontinue therapy.

 Meperidine (Demerol) [C]

COMMON USES Relief of moderate-to-severe pain

ACTIONS Narcotic analgesic

DOSAGE Adult: 50 to 150 mg po or IM q3–4h prn; peds: 115 mg/kg/dose po or IM q3–4h prn

SUPPLIED Tablets 50 mg, 100 mg; syrup 50 mg/mL; injection 10 mg/mL, 25 mg/mL, 50 mg/mL, 75 mg/mL, 100 mg/mL

NOTES 75 mg IM equivalent to 10 mg morphine IM; beware of respiratory depression; should *not* be used in renal failure

 Mesna (Mesnex)

COMMON USES Reduces the incidence of ifosfamide- and cyclophosphamide-induced hemorrhagic cystitis

ACTIONS Antidote; binds urotoxic metabolites

DOSAGE 20% of the ifosfamide dose (w/w) or cyclophosphamide dose IV at 15 minutes prior to and 4 and 8 hours after chemotherapy

SUPPLIED Injection 100 mg/mL

 Metyrapone (Metopirone)

COMMON USES Diagnostic test for hypothalamic–pituitary adrenocorticotropic hormone (ACTH) function

ACTIONS Inhibits adrenocortical synthesis by blocking 11b-hydroxylase

DOSAGE Metapyrone test
- Day 1: control period—Collect 24 h urine to measure 17-hydroxycorticosteroids (17-OHCS) or 17-ketogenic steroids (17-KSG).
- Day 2: ACTH test—Administer 50 U of ACTH infused over 8 hours and measure 24-hour urinary steroids.
- Days 3 to 4: rest period
- Day 5: Administer metyrapone with milk or a snack.
- Adults: 750 mg po q4h for 6 doses
- Peds: 15 mg/kg q4h for 6 doses (minimum 250-mg dose). Day 6: Determine 24-hour urinary steroids.

SUPPLIED Tablets 250 mg

NOTES Normal 24-hour urine 17-OHCS is 3 to 12 mg; following ACTH, it increases to 15 to 45 mg/24 h; normal response to metyrapone is a twofold to fourfold increase in 17-OHCS excretion; drug interactions with phenytoin, cyproheptadine, and estrogens may lead to a subnormal response.

Methadone (Dolophine) [C]

 Methadone (Dolophine) [C]

COMMON USES Severe pain; detoxification and maintenance of narcotic addiction

ACTIONS Narcotic analgesic

DOSAGE

- Adult: 25 to 10 mg IM q8h or 5 to 15 mg po q8h (titrate as needed)
- Peds: 0.7 mg/kg/24 h po or IM divided q8h

SUPPLIED Tablets 5 mg, 10 mg; oral solution 5 mg/5 mL, 10 mg/5 mL; injection 10 mg/mL

NOTES Equianalgesic with parenteral morphine; long half-life; increase the dose slowly to avoid respiratory depression.

 Methenamine Mandelate (Uroquid)

COMMON USES Suppression or elimination of bacteriuria associated with chronic and recurrent infections of the urinary tract

ACTIONS Releases formaldehyde in acidic urine, which is nonspecifically bactericidal

DOSAGE Initially, 2 tablets 4 times a day. Maintenance: 2 to 4 tablets daily in divided doses

SUPPLIED Each tablet contains 500 mg of methenamine mandelate.

NOTES Contraindicated in patients with renal insufficiency, severe hepatic disease, and severe dehydration

 Methotrexate (Folex, Rheumatrex)

COMMON USES Treatment of trophoblastic tumors (chorioepithelioma, choriocarcinoma, chorioadenoma destruens, and hydatidiform mole), penile cancer, bladder cancer, and advanced prostate cancer

ACTIONS Inhibits dihydrofolate reductase–mediated generation of tetrahydrofolate

DOSAGE

- Cancer

—"Conventional dose": 15 to 30 mg po or IV 1 to 2 times/week every 1 to 3 weeks
—"Intermediate dose": 50 to 240 mg or 0.5 to 1 g/m^2 IV $\times$ 1 every 4 days to 3 weeks
—"High dose": 1 to 12 g/m^2 IV $\times$ 1 every 1 to 3 weeks; 12 mg/ m^2 (maximum of 15 mg) intrathecally, weekly until CSF cell count returns to normal

SUPPLIED Tablets 25 mg; injection 25 mg/mL, 25 mg/mL; preservative-free injection 25 mg/mL

NOTES Toxicity includes myelosuppression, nausea, vomiting, anorexia, mucositis, diarrhea, hepatotoxicity (transient and reversible; may progress to atrophy, necrosis, fibrosis, cirrhosis), rashes, dizziness, malaise, blurred vision, renal failure, pneumonitis, and rarely, pulmonary fibrosis. Chemical arachnoiditis and headache may occur with intrathecal delivery. "High-dose" therapy requires "leucovorin rescue" in order to prevent severe hematologic and mucosal toxicity; monitor blood counts and methotrexate levels carefully.

 Methylprednisolone (Medrol). See Systemic Steroids

 Methyltestosterone Capsules (Testred)

COMMON USES Testosterone replacement, hypogonadism, selected cases of delayed puberty

ACTIONS Increase circulating testosterone level

DOSAGE 10 to 50 mg daily

SUPPLIED 10-mg capsules

NOTES Gynecomastia, acne, breast tenderness, male-pattern baldness

 Metoclopramide (Reglan, Clopra, Others)

COMMON USES Relief of diabetic gastroparesis; symptomatic gastroesophageal reflux; relief of cancer chemotherapy–induced nausea and vomiting

ACTIONS Stimulates motility of the upper GI tract and blocks dopamine in the chemoreceptor trigger zone

DOSAGE

- Adult

—Reflux: 1.0 to 15 mg po 30 minutes AC and HS
—Antiemetic: 13 mg/kg/dose IV 30 minutes prior to antineoplastic agent, then q2h for 2 doses, then q3h for 3 doses

- Peds

—Reflux: 0.1 mg/kg/dose po qid
—Antiemetic: 1 to 2 mg/kg/dose IV on same schedule as adults

SUPPLIED Tablets 5 mg, 10 mg; syrup 5 mg/5 mL; solution 10 mg/mL; injection 5 mg/mL

NOTES Dystonic reactions common with high doses that can be treated with IV Benadryl; can also be used to facilitate small bowel intubation and radiologic evaluation of the upper GI tract

Metronidazole (Flagyl, MetroGel)

COMMON USES Amebiasis, trichomoniasis, *C. difficile,* anaerobic infections, and bacterial vaginosis

ACTIONS Interferes with DNA synthesis

DOSAGE

• Adult

—Anaerobic infections: 500 mg IV q6–8h
—Trichomoniasis: 250 mg po tid for 7 days or 2 g po in 1 dose
—*C. difficile:* 500 mg po or IV q8h for 7 to 10 days
—Vaginosis: 1 applicatorful intravaginally bid or 500 mg po bid for 7 days

• Peds

—Anaerobic infections: 30 mg/kg/24 h po or IV divided q6h

SUPPLIED Tablets 250 mg, 500 mg; topical gel 0.75%; injection 500 mg

NOTES For *Trichomonas* infections, also treat the partner; reduce the dose in hepatic failure; no activity against aerobic bacteria; use in combination in serious mixed infections; may cause disulfiram-like reaction

 Mezlocillin (Mezlin)

COMMON USES Treatment of infections caused by susceptible gram-negative bacteria (including *Klebsiella, E. coli, Proteus, Enterobacter, P. aeruginosa,* and *Serratia*) involving the skin, urinary tract, abdomen, and septicemia

ACTIONS Bactericidal; inhibits cell wall synthesis

DOSAGE Adults: 3 g q4–6h; peds: 200 to 300 mg/kg/d divided q4–6h

SUPPLIED In a powder form: 1-, 2-, 3-, 4-, and 20-g vials. These must be prepared just prior to infusion with NSS, sterile water, or 5% dextrose injection

NOTES Dose must be adjusted in patients with renal impairment

 Miconazole (Monistat)

COMMON USES Severe systemic fungal infections, including coccidioidomycosis, candidiasis, *Cryptococcus,* and others; various tinea forms; cutaneous candidiasis; vulvovaginal candidiasis; tinea versicolor

ACTIONS Fungicidal; alters permeability of the fungal cell membrane

DOSAGE

• Adult

—Systemic: Dosage ranges from 200 to 3600 mg/24 h IV, based on diagnosis, divided into 3 doses
—Topical: Apply to the affected area twice daily for 24 weeks.
—Intravaginally: Insert 1 full applicator or suppository at bedtime for 7 days.

• Peds: 20 to 40 mg/kg/24 h IV divided q8h

SUPPLIED Injection 10 mg/mL; topical cream 2%, lotion 2%, powder 2%, spray 2%, vaginal suppositories 200 mg; vaginal cream 2%

NOTES Antagonistic to amphotericin B in vivo; rapid IV infusion may cause tachycardia or arrhythmias; may potentiate warfarin drug activity

 Mineral Oil

COMMON USES Constipation

ACTIONS Emollient laxative

DOSAGE

• Adult: 15 to 45 mL po prn
• Peds >6 years: 10 to 20 mL po bid

SUPPLIED Liquid

 Minocycline Hydrochloride (Minocin)

COMMON USES Broad-spectrum antibiotic against *Staphylococcus, Streptococcus, Chlamydia, Rickettsia,* and *Neisseria*

ACTIONS Bacteriostatic; inhibits protein synthesis

DOSAGE

• Adults: 200 mg initially, followed by 100 mg q12h
• Peds: For children above 8 years old, the loading dose is 4 mg/kg, followed by 2 mg/kg q12h.

SUPPLIED 50-, 100-mg tablets

NOTES Nausea, vomiting, and diarrhea are common. Can stain tooth enamel in children less than 8 years of age. Use cautiously in pregnancy. Do not use in patients with impaired renal function.

 Misoprostol (Cytotec)

COMMON USES Prevention of NSAID-induced gastric ulcers. Used for patients who are on long-term management with NSAIDs

ACTIONS Synthetic prostaglandin with both antisecretory and mucosal protective properties

DOSAGE 200 μg po qid

SUPPLIED Tablets 100 to 200 μg

NOTES *Do not* take if pregnant; can cause miscarriage, with potentially dangerous bleeding; GI side effects are common.

Mitomycin-C (Mutamycin)

 Mitomycin-C (Mutamycin)

COMMON USES Combination with other agents for metastatic stomach and pancreatic cancer; bladder cancer (intravesically)

ACTIONS Alkylating agent; may also generate oxygen-free radicals, which induce DNA strand breaks

DOSAGE 20 to 40 mg in 40 mL of NSS via a urethral catheter once a week for 8 weeks, which is followed by monthly treatments for 1 year; single dose after TUR may prevent recurrence

SUPPLIED Injection 5 mg, 20 mg

NOTES Follow CBC; can cause myelosuppression. Common side effects when used intravesically are irritative symptoms, bladder contracture, chemical cystitis, and palmar and facial skin rashes. No formal labeling for bladder cancer

 Mitotane (Lysodren)

COMMON USES Palliative treatment of inoperable adrenal cortex carcinoma

ACTIONS Exact action unclear; induces mitochondrial injury in adrenocortical cells

DOSAGE 8 to 10 g daily in 3 to 4 divided doses (begin at 2 g daily with full glucocorticoid replacement therapy)

SUPPLIED Tablets 500 mg

NOTES Toxicity includes anorexia, nausea, vomiting, diarrhea. Acute adrenal insufficiency may be precipitated by physical stresses (shock, trauma, infection); corticosteroid replacement is necessary. Allergic reactions (rarely), visual disturbance, hemorrhagic cystitis, albuminuria, hematuria, hypertension or hypotension, minor aches, and fever

 Mitoxantrone Hydrochloride (Novantrone)

COMMON USES Advanced hormone-refractory prostate cancer

ACTIONS DNA intercalating agent, inhibitor of DNA topoisomerase II

DOSAGE 12 to 14 mg/m² every 3 weeks with prednisone 5 mg po BID

SUPPLIED Injection 20 mg, 25 mg, 30 mg

NOTES Toxicity includes myelosuppression, nausea, vomiting, stomatitis, alopecia (infrequent), cardiotoxicity; cumulative dose should not exceed 160 mg/m² in patients having received mediastinal radiation therapy, or 120 mg/m² in patients who have received prior anthracycline therapy

 Morphine (Roxanol, Duramorph, MS Contin)[C]

COMMON USES Relief of severe pain

ACTIONS Narcotic analgesic

DOSAGE
- Adults
—Oral: 10 to 30 mg q4h prn; sustained-release tablets 30 to 60 mg q8–12h
—IV/IM: 25 to 15 mg q4h prn
- Peds: 01 to 02 mg/kg/dose IM/IV q24h prn up to maximum 15 mg/dose

SUPPLIED Tablets 10, 15, 30 mg; SR tablets 15, 30, 60 mg; solution 10, 20, 100 mg; suppositories 5, 10, 20 mg; injection 2, 4, 5, 8, 10, 15 mg/mL; preservative-free injection 0.5, 1 mg/mL

NOTES Large number of narcotic side effects; may require scheduled dosing to relieve severe chronic pain

 Muromonab-CD3 (Orthoclone OKT3)

COMMON USES Treatment of acute rejection following organ transplantation

ACTIONS Murine monoclonal antibody; binds to CD3 protein on T-lymphocytes, blocks antigen recognition and clears CD3- positive T cells from circulation

DOSAGE Adults: 5 mg IV qd for 10 to 14 days; peds: 01 mg/kg/d for 10 to 14 days

SUPPLIED Injection 5 mg/5 mL

NOTES Is a murine antibody; may cause significant fever and chills after the first dose

 Mycophenolate Mofetil (CellCept)

COMMON USES Prevention of organ rejection following transplantation

ACTIONS Inhibits immunologically mediated inflammatory responses

DOSAGE 1 g po bid

SUPPLIED Capsules 250 mg

NOTES Used in conjunction with corticosteroids and cyclosporin

 Nabumetone (Relafen). See Nonsteroidal Antiinflammatory Drugs

 Nafcillin (Unipen)

COMMON USES Treatment of infections caused by susceptible strains of *Staphylococcus* and *Streptococcus*

ACTIONS Bactericidal; inhibits cell wall synthesis

DOSAGE
- Adults: 1 to 2 g q4–6h
- Peds: 50 to 200 mg/kg/d divided q4–6h

SUPPLIED 250-mg capsules

NOTES No dosage adjustments for renal function

Nalbuphine (Nubain)

COMMON USES Moderate-to-severe pain

ACTIONS Narcotic agonist–antagonist; inhibits ascending pain pathways

DOSAGE

- Adults: 10 to 20 mg IM/IV q4–6h prn
- Peds: 0.2 mg/kg IV/IM to maximum dose of 20 mg

SUPPLIED Injection 10 mg/mL, 20 mg/mL

NOTES Causes CNS depression and drowsiness; use with caution in patients receiving opiate drugs.

 Nalidixic Acid (NegGram)

COMMON USES Urinary tract infections caused by susceptible strains *of Proteus, Klebsiella, Enterobacter,* and *E. coli,* but not *Pseudomonas*

ACTIONS Inhibits bacterial RNA and DNA synthesis

DOSAGE Adult: 1 g po qid for 7 to 14 days; peds: 55 mg/kg/24 h in 4 divided doses

SUPPLIED Tablets 250 mg, 500 mg, 1 g; suspension 250 mg/5 mL

NOTES Resistance emerged within 48 hours in a significant percentage of trials; may enhance effect of oral anticoagulants; may cause CNS adverse effects, which reverse on discontinuation of the drug

 Naloxone (Narcan)

COMMON USES Reversal of narcotic effect

ACTIONS Competitive narcotic antagonist

DOSAGE

- Adult: 0.4 to 2.0 mg IV, IM, or SQ q5min; maximum total dose of 10 mg
- Peds: 0.01 to 1.0 mg/kg/dose IV, IM, or SQ; may repeat IV q3min for 3 doses prn

SUPPLIED Injection 0.4 mg/mL, 10 mg/mL; neonatal injection 0.02 mg/mL

NOTES May precipitate acute withdrawal in addicts; if no response after 10 mg, suspect a nonnarcotic cause

 Naproxen (Naprosyn). See Nonsteroidal Antiinflammatory Drugs

 Naproxen Sodium (Anaprox, Alleve). See Nonsteroidal Antiinflammatory Drugs

 Neomycin–Polymyxin Bladder Irrigant Solution

COMMON USES Continuous irrigant for prophylaxis against bacteriuria and gram-negative bacteremia associated with indwelling catheter use

ACTIONS Bactericidal antibiotic

DOSAGE 1 mL irrigant added to 1 L 0.9% NaCl; continuous irrigation of the bladder with 12 L of solution per 24 hours

SUPPLIED Ampules 1 mL, 20 mL

NOTES Potential for bacterial or fungal superinfection; possibility for neomycin-induced ototoxicity or nephrotoxicity

 Neomycin Sulfate

COMMON USES Preoperative bowel prep

ACTIONS Aminoglycoside; suppresses GI bacterial flora

DOSAGE

- Adult: 3 to 2 g/24 h po in 3 to 4 divided doses
- Peds: 50 to 100 mg/kg/24 h po in 3 to 4 divided doses

SUPPLIED Tablets 500 mg; oral solution 125 mg/5 mL

NOTES Part of Condon bowel prep

 Nilutamide (Nilandron)

COMMON USES Used in combination with surgical castration for the treatment of metastatic prostate cancer

ACTIONS Blocks the effects of testosterone at the androgen receptor level

DOSAGE 300 mg/d in divided doses for the first 30 days, then 150 mg/d

SUPPLIED 50-mg tablets

NOTES Toxicity can include hot flashes, loss of libido, impotence, diarrhea, nausea, vom

iting, gynecomastia, hepatic dysfunction (follow LFTs), and interstitial pneumonitis.

 Nifedipine (Procardia, Procardia XL, Adalat, Adalat CC)

COMMON USES Management of autonomic hyperreflexia

ACTIONS Calcium channel blocking agent

DOSAGE 10 to 20 mg 30 minutes prior to catheterization

SUPPLIED Capsules 10, 20 mg

NOTES Headaches are common on initial treatment; reflex tachycardia may occur with regular-release dosage forms; Adalat CC and Procardia XL are not interchangeable dosage forms.

Nitrofurantoin (Macrodantin, Furadantin, Macrobid)

 Nitrofurantoin (Macrodantin, Furadantin, Macrobid)

COMMON USES Prevention and treatment of urinary tract infections

ACTIONS Bacteriostatic; interferes with carbohydrate metabolism

DOSAGE

- Adult

—Suppression: 50 to 100 mg po qd
—Treatment: 50 to 100 mg po qid; Macrobid: 100-mg tablets bid

- Peds: 5 to 7 mg/kg/24 h in 4 divided doses

SUPPLIED Capsules and tablets 50 mg, 100 mg; SR capsule 100 mg; suspension 25 mg/5 mL. Macrobid is available in 100-mg tablets

NOTES GI side effects common; should be taken with food, milk, or antacid; macrocrystals (Macrodantin) cause less nausea than other forms of the drug.

 Nizatidine (Axid)

COMMON USES Duodenal ulcer, ulcer prophylaxis in hypersecretory states such as trauma, burns, and surgery

ACTIONS H2 receptor antagonist

DOSAGE 150 mg po bid or 300 mg po qHS; maintenance: 150 mg po qHS

SUPPLIED Capsules 150 mg, 300 mg

 Nonsteroidal Antiinflammatory Drugs (NSAIDs)

COMMON USES Analgesic, antipyretic, prostatitis, and other inflammatory processes

ACTIONS Nonsteroid antiinflammatory agents; mechanism of action is not completely understood. It may be related to prostaglandin synthetase inhibition.

DOSAGE See below

SUPPLIED See below

NOTES May cause peptic ulcers, GI bleeding, papillary necrosis, interstitial nephritis, and liver enzyme elevation. Hypersensitivity reactions have been reported.

Acetic Acids

- Diclofenac (Cataflam, Voltaren)

—Dosage: 50 to 75 mg bid-tid
—Supplied: 25-, 50-, 75-mg tabs

- Etodolac (Lodine)

—Dosage: 200 to 400 mg bid-tid
—Supplied: 200-, 300-mg caps; 400-, 500-mg tabs

- Indomethacin (Indocin)

—Dosage: 25 to 50 mg bid-tid
—Supplied: 25-, 50-, 75-mg caps

- Ketorolac (Toradol)

—Dosage: IV/IM 15 to 30 mg q6h/10 mg q6h po
—Supplied: 10 mg tabs; 15 or 30 mg/mL for injection

- Nabumetone (Relafen)

—Dosage: 1000 to 2000 mg/d divided qd-bid
—Supplied: 500-, 750-mg tabs

- Sulindac (Clinoril)

—Dosage: 150 to 200 mg bid
—Supplied: 150-, 200-mg tabs

- Tolmetin (Tolectin)

—Dosage: 200 to 600 mg tid
—Supplied: 200-, 600-mg tabs; 400-mg caps

Oxicams

- Piroxicam (Feldene)

—Dosage: 10 to 20 mg qd
—Supplied: 10-, 20-mg caps

Propionic Acids

- Fenoprofen (Nalfon)

—Dosage: 300 to 600 mg tid-qid
—Supplied: 200-, 300-, 600-mg tabs

- Flurbiprofen (Ansaid)

—Dosage: 50 to 100 mg bid-qid
—Supplied: 50-, 100-mg tabs

- Ibuprofen (Advil, Motrin)

—Dosage: 300 to 800 mg tid-qid
—Supplied: 50-, 100-, 200-, 400-, 600-mg tabs

- Ibuprofen (Pediprophen)

—Dosage (Peds): 10 to 15 mg/kg/dose tid-qid
—Supplied: 100 mg/5 mL suspension; 40 mg/mL drops

- Ketoprofen (Orudis)

—Dosage: 50 to 75 mg tid-qid
—Supplied: 25-, 50-, 75-mg caps

- Naproxen (Naprosyn)

—Dosage: 250 to 500 mg bid
—Supplied: 375-, 500-mg tabs

- Naproxen sodium (Anaprox, Alleve)

—Dosage: 275 to 550 mg bid
—Supplied: 275-, 550-mg tabs

- Oxaprozin (Daypro)

—Dosage: 600 to 1200 mg qd
—Supplied: 600-mg tabs

 Norfloxacin (Noroxin)

COMMON USES Treatment of complicated and uncomplicated urinary tract infections due to a wide variety of gram-negative bacteria, prostatitis, and infectious diarrhea

ACTIONS Inhibits DNA gyrase

DOSAGE Adult: 400 mg po bid; peds: *not recommended for use in patients <18 years of age*

SUPPLIED Tablets 400 mg

NOTES *Not* for use in pregnancy; drug interactions with antacids, theophylline, and caffeine; good concentrations in the kidney and urine, poor blood levels. *Do not* use for urosepsis.

Nystatin (Mycostatin, Nilstat)

COMMON USES   Treatment of mucocutaneous *Candida* infections (thrush, vaginitis)

ACTIONS   Alters membrane permeability

DOSAGE

• Adult

—Oral: 400,000 to 600,000 U po "swish and swallow" qid
—Vaginal: 1 tab per vagina qHS
—Topical: Apply 2 to 3 times daily to the affected area.

• Peds

—Infants: 200,000 U po q6h
—Children: See Adult dosage.

SUPPLIED   Oral suspension 100,000 U/mL; oral tablets 500,000 U; troches 200,000 U; vaginal tablets 100,000 U; topical cream and ointment 100,000 U/g

NOTES   Not absorbed orally; therefore, not effective for systemic infections

 Ofloxacin (Floxin)

COMMON USES   Treatment of infections of the lower respiratory tract. skin and skin structure, and urinary tract; prostatitis; uncomplicated gonorrhea; and *Chlamydia* infections

ACTIONS   Bactericidal; inhibits DNA gyrase

DOSAGE

• Adult: 200 to 400 mg po bid or IV q12h
• Peds: should *not* be used in children <18 years of age

SUPPLIED   Tablets 200 mg, 300 mg, 400 mg; injection 20 mg/mL, 40 mg/mL

NOTES   May cause nausea, vomiting, diarrhea, insomnia, and headache; drug interactions with antacids, sucralfate, and aluminum-, calcium-, magnesium-, iron-, or zinc-containing products, which decrease the absorption of ofloxacin; may increase theophylline levels

 Omeprazole (Prilosec)

COMMON USES   Treatment of duodenal ulcers. Metabolic alkalosis associated with using stomach as a urinary reservoir.

ACTIONS   Proton-pump inhibitor

DOSAGE   20 to 40 mg po bid-qd

SUPPLIED   Capsules 20 mg

 Ondansetron (Zofran)

COMMON USES   Prevention of nausea and vomiting associated with cancer chemotherapy and postoperative nausea and vomiting

ACTIONS   Serotonin receptor antagonist

DOSAGE

• Adult and peds

—Chemotherapy: 0.15 mg/kg/dose IV prior to chemotherapy, then repeated 4 and 8 hours after the first dose or 4 to 8 mg po tid; administer the first dose 30 minutes prior to chemotherapy.

• Adults

—Postoperative: 4 mg IV immediately before induction of anesthesia or postoperatively

SUPPLIED   Tablets 4 mg, 8 mg; injection 2 mg/mL

NOTES   May cause diarrhea and headache

 Oxacillin (Bactocill)

COMMON USES   Treatment of infections caused by susceptible strains of *Staphylococcus* and *Streptococcus*

ACTIONS   Bactericidal; inhibits cell wall synthesis

DOSAGE   Adults: 1 to 2 g q4–6h; peds: 150 to 200 mg/kg/d divided q6h

SUPPLIED   250-, 500-mg capsules

 Oxaprozin (Daypro). See Nonsteroidal Antiinflammatory Drugs

 Oxybutynin (Ditropan, Ditropan XL)

COMMON USES   Symptomatic relief of urgency, nocturia, and incontinence associated with neurogenic or reflex neurogenic bladder

ACTIONS   Direct antispasmodic effect on smooth muscle, mild local anesthetic effects

DOSAGE

• Adult and peds >5 years: 5 mg po tid-qid
• Adult: extended-release 5 mg po qd; can titrate up to 30 mg po qd
• Peds 1 to 5 years: 0.2 mg/kg/dose 2 to 4 times a day

SUPPLIED   Tablets 5 mg; syrup 5 mg/5 mL; extended-release tablets 5 and 10 mg (Ditropan XL)

NOTES   Anticholinergic side effects (dry mouth, constipation, dry eyes, somnolence, others). Suggestion of efficacy when liquid formulation directly instilled in augmented bladder or neobladder

 Oxycodone and Acetaminophen (Percocet, Tylox) [C]

COMMON USES   Management of moderate-to-severe pain

ACTIONS   Narcotic analgesic

DOSAGE

• Adults: 12 tablets/capsules po q4–6h prn
• Peds: oxycodone 0.05 to 0.15 mg/kg/dose

q4–6h prn

SUPPLIED

• Percocet tab: 5 mg oxycodone, 325 mg acetaminophen
• Tylox capsule: 5 mg oxycodone, 500 mg acetaminophen
• Solution: 5 mg oxycodone and 325 mg acetaminophen per 5 mL

Paclitaxel (Taxol)

 Paclitaxel (Taxol)

COMMON USES Treatment of bladder and prostate cancer

ACTIONS Mitotic spindle poison promotes microtubule assembly and stabilization against depolymerization

DOSAGE 135 to 250 mg/m^2 as a 3- to 24-hour intravenous infusion

SUPPLIED Injection 300 mg

NOTES Toxicity includes hypersensitivity reactions (dyspnea, hypotension, urticaria, rash) usually within 10 minutes of starting infusion; can be minimized by corticosteroid and antihistamine pretreatment. Myelosuppression, peripheral neuropathy, transient ileus, myalgia, bradycardia, hypotension, mucositis, diarrhea, nausea and vomiting, fever, rash, headache, phlebitis. Hematologic toxicity is schedule dependent; leukopenia is dose-limiting by 24-hour infusion; neurotoxicity is dose-limiting by short (1- to 3-hour) infusion. This agent must be infused in glass or polyolefin containers using polyethylene-lined nitroglycerin tubing sets. Use of polyvinyl chloride infusion sets will result in leaching of plasticizer.

 Pamidronate (Aredia)

COMMON USES Treatment of hypercalcemia of malignancy; palliation of symptomatic bone metastases

ACTIONS Inhibition of normal and abnormal bone resorption

DOSAGE Hypercalcemia: 60 mg IV over 4 hours or 90 mg IV over 24 hours

SUPPLIED Powder for injection 30 mg, 60 mg, 90 mg

NOTES Toxicity includes fever, tissue irritation at the site of injection, uveitis, fluid overload, hypertension, abdominal pain, nausea and vomiting, constipation, urinary tract infection, bone pain, hypokalemia, hypocalcemia, hypomagnesemia, and hypophosphatemia.

 Papaverine Hydrochloride

COMMON USES Treatment of erectile dysfunction due to neurogenic, vasculogenic, or mixed etiology

ACTIONS Relaxes smooth muscle, dilates cavernosal arteries, increases lacunar spaces and entrapment of blood by compressing venules against tunica albuginea

DOSAGE Start at 6 to 12 mg, intracorporeally; titrate to the optimum dosage.

SUPPLIED Multi-dose vials, 30 mg/mL, 10 mL

NOTES Dosage must be titrated at the physician's office.

 Penicillamine (Cuprimine)

COMMON USES Treatment of cystine calculi or cystinuria

ACTIONS Reduces cystine levels in urine

DOSAGE
- Adults: 1 to 4 g/d
- Peds: 30 mg/kg/d

SUPPLIED 125-, 250-mg tablets

NOTES D-penicillamine side effects: gastrointestinal (nausea, vomiting, diarrhea, anorexia), impaired sense of smell and taste, pharyngitis, rash, ecchymoses, hypersensitivity reactions, hematologic abnormalities (leukopenia, thrombocytopenia, anemia), proteinuria, nephrotic syndrome. Must administer supplemental vitamin B6 (0.7 mg/kg/d). For each 250-mg increment in dose, expect a decrease of 75 to 100 mg cystine/d. Should be given on an empty stomach

 Penicillin G Aqueous (Potassium or Sodium) (Pfizerpen, Pentids)

COMMON USES Most gram-positive infections (except penicillin-resistant staphylococci), including streptococci, *N. meningitidis*, syphilis, clostridia, corynebacteria, and some coliforms

ACTIONS Bactericidal; inhibits cell wall synthesis

DOSAGE
- Adult: 400,000 to 800,000 U po qid; IV doses vary greatly; depending on indications, range from 12 to 24 million units/d
- Peds

—Newborns <1 week: 25,000 to 50,000 U/kg/dose IV q12h
—Infants 1 week to 1 month: 25,000 to 50,000 U/kg/dose IV q8h
—Children: 100,000 to 300,000 U/kg/24h IV divided q4h

SUPPLIED Tablets 200,000 U, 250,000 U, 400,000 U, 800,000 U; suspension 200,000 U/5 mL, 400,000 U/5 mL; powder for injection

NOTES Beware of hypersensitivity reactions.

 Penicillin G Benzathine (Bicillin)

COMMON USES Useful as a single-dose treatment regimen for glomerulonephritis prophylaxis and syphilis

ACTIONS Bactericidal; inhibits cell wall synthesis

DOSAGE
- Adult: 12 to 24 million U deep IM injection q2–4 weeks
- Peds: 50,000 U/kg/dose to a maximum of 24 million U/dose deep IM injection q2–4 weeks

SUPPLIED Injection 300,000 U/mL, 600,000 U/mL

NOTES Sustained action with detectable levels up to 4 weeks; considered drug of choice for treatment of noncongenital syphilis; Bicillin LA contains the benzathine salt only; Bicillin CR contains a combination of the benzathine and procaine (300,000 U procaine with 300,000 U benzathine/mL, or 900,000 U benzathine with 300,000 U procaine/2 mL)

Penicillin G Procaine (Wycillin, Others)

COMMON USES Moderately severe infections caused by penicillin G–sensitive organisms that respond to low, persistent serum levels

ACTIONS Bactericidal; inhibits cell wall synthesis

DOSAGE
- Adult: 300,000 to 12 million U/d IM divided qd-bid
- Peds: 25,000 to 50,000 U/kg/d IM divided qd-bid

SUPPLIED Injection 300,000 U/mL, 500,000 U/mL, 600,000 U/mL

NOTES A long-acting parenteral penicillin; blood levels up to 15 hours; give probenecid at least 30 minutes prior to administration of penicillin to prolong action.

 ### Penicillin V (Pen-Vee K, Veetids, Others)

COMMON USES Most gram-positive infections, including streptococci, *N. meningitidis*, syphilis, clostridia, corynebacteria, and some coliforms

ACTIONS Bactericidal; inhibits cell wall synthesis

DOSAGE
- Adult: 250 to 500 mg po q6h
- Peds: 25 to 50 mg/kg/24 h po in 4 divided doses

SUPPLIED Tablets 125 mg, 250 mg, 500 mg; suspension 125 mg/5 mL, 250 mg/5 mL

NOTES A well-tolerated oral penicillin; 250 mg = 400,000 U Pen G

 ### Pentosan Polysulfate Sodium (Elmiron)

COMMON USES For bladder pain and discomfort associated with interstitial cystitis

ACTIONS Heparin-like compound. It has anticoagulant and fibrinolytic effects. The mechanism in interstitial cystitis is unknown.

DOSAGE 100 mg po tid

SUPPLIED 100-mg capsules

NOTES Alopecia, diarrhea, nausea, and headaches have been reported.

 ### Pentazocine (Talwin) [C]

COMMON USES Management of moderate-to-severe pain

ACTIONS Partial narcotic agonist–antagonist

DOSAGE
- Adults: 30 mg IM or IV; 50 to 100 mg po q3–4h prn
- Peds

—5 to 8 years: 15 mg IM q4h prn
—8 to 14 years: 30 mg IM q4h prn

SUPPLIED Tablets 50 mg (with naloxone 0.5 mg); injection 30 mg/mL

NOTES 30 to 60 mg IM equianalgesic to 10 mg morphine IM; associated with considerable dysphoria

 ### Permethrin (Nix, Elimite)

COMMON USES Treatment of lice and scabies

ACTIONS Pediculicide

DOSAGE Adult and peds: Saturate the hair and scalp; allow it to remain in the hair for 10 minutes before it rinsing out.

SUPPLIED Topical liquid 1%; cream 5%

 ### Phenazopyridine (Pyridium, Others)

COMMON USES Symptomatic relief of discomfort from lower urinary tract irritation

ACTIONS Local anesthetic on urinary tract mucosa

DOSAGE Adult: 100 to 200 mg po tid; peds 6 to 12 years: 12 mg/kg/24 h po in 3 divided doses

SUPPLIED Tablets 100 mg, 200 mg

NOTES GI disturbances; causes red-orange urine color, which can stain clothing

 ### Phenylephrine (Neo-Synephrine)

COMMON USES Intracavernosal treatment for priapism

ACTIONS Alpha-adrenergic agonist

DOSAGE 10 mg/mL mixed with 19 mL of NSS. Given every 5 to 10 minutes intercavernously until detumescence is obtained

SUPPLIED Injection 10 mg/mL

NOTES The corpora cavernosa must be irrigated and evacuated, as needed.

 ### Phenylpropanolamine (Dexatrim, Acutrim, Ornade, Entex LA, Others)

COMMON USES Treatment of stress urinary incontinence in women

ACTIONS Stimulates alpha-1-adrenergic receptors in the bladder neck and proximal urethra

DOSAGE 25 to 75 mg tid, 75-mg SR capsule bid; ornade BID

SUPPLIED 25-, 50-mg tablets; 75-mg sustained-release capsules; Ornade: 75 mg phenylpropanolamine/12 mg chlorpheniramine 1 tab bid

Piperacillin (Pipracil)

 Piperacillin (Pipracil)

COMMON USES Treatment of infections caused by susceptible gram-negative bacteria (including *Klebsiella, E. coli, Proteus, Enterobacter, P. aeruginosa,* and *Serratia*) involving the skin, urinary tract, abdomen, and septicemia

ACTIONS Bactericidal; inhibits cell wall synthesis

DOSAGE Adults: 3g q4–6h; peds: 200 to 300 mg/kg/d divided q4–6h

SUPPLIED In a powder form: 2-, 3-, 4-, and 40-g vials. These must be prepared just prior to infusion with NSS, sterile water, or 5% dextrose injection.

NOTES Must be adjusted in patients with renal impairment. Best activity against *Pseudomonas*

 Piperacillin-Tazobactam (Zosyn)

COMMON USES Treatment of infections caused by susceptible gram-negative bacteria (including *Klebsiella, E. coli, Proteus, Enterobacter, P. aeruginosa,* and *Serratia*) involving the skin, urinary tract, abdomen, and septicemia

ACTIONS Bactericidal; inhibits cell wall synthesis

DOSAGE 3.375 g q6h

SUPPLIED In a powder form: 225-, 3375-, 45-, and 405-g vials. These must be prepared just prior to infusion with NSS, sterile water, or 5% dextrose injection.

NOTES Must be adjusted in patients with renal impairment. Tazobactam is a beta-lactamase inhibitor

 Piroxicam (Feldene). See Nonsteroidal Antiinflammatory Drugs

 Plicamycin (Mithracin)

COMMON USES Treatment of hypercalcemia of malignancy; disseminated embryonal cell carcinoma or germ cell tumors of the testis

ACTIONS Antibiotic; binding to outside of DNA molecule, interrupting DNA-directed RNA synthesis, DNA intercalation

DOSAGE
- Hypercalcemia: 25 μg/kg/d IV on alternate days for 3 to 8 doses
- Cancer: 25 to 30 μg/kg/d for 8 to 10 days

SUPPLIED Injection 2500 μg

NOTES Toxicity includes thrombocytopenia and drug-induced deficiency of clotting factors II, V, VII, and X, resulting in bleeding and bruising.

 Podophyllin (Podocon-25, Condylox Gel 0.5%, Condylox)

COMMON USES Topical treatment of genital warts

ACTIONS Direct antimitotic effect. The exact mechanism is unknown.

DOSAGE Condylox gel is applied 3 consecutive days per week for 4 weeks. Podocon-25 is used sparingly on the lesion and left on for 1 to 4 hours, then thoroughly washed off.

SUPPLIED Podocon-25 is supplied in 15-mL bottles. Condylox gel is available in 35 g of a clear gel, and Condylox topical solution is also available in 35 g of clear solution in a bottle.

NOTES Podocon-25 is to be applied only by the physician, not dispensed to the patient. Avoid using these agents on pregnant patients.

 Polyethylene Glycol–Electrolyte Solution (Go-Lytely, GoLyte)

COMMON USES Bowel cleansing prior to examination or surgery

ACTIONS Osmotic cathartic

DOSAGE Adults: Following a 3- to 4-hour fast, drink 240 mL of solution every 10 minutes until 4 L are consumed. peds: 25 to 40 mL/kg/h for 4 to 10 hours

SUPPLIED Powder for reconstitution to 4 L in container

NOTES First bowel movement should occur in approximately 1 hour; may cause some cramping or nausea

 Potassium Acid Phosphatase (K-Phos)

COMMON USES Use in patients with an elevated urinary pH. By acidifying the urine, it increases the antibacterial effect of methenamine mandelate.

ACTIONS Urine acidifier

DOSAGE Two tablets dissolved in 6 to 8 ounces of water 4 times daily with meals and at bedtime

SUPPLIED Each tablet contains 500 mg of potassium acid phosphate, 114 mg of phosphorus, and 144 mg (37 mEq) of potassium.

NOTES Contraindicated in patients with infected phosphate stones and severely impaired renal function. Patients should be advised to avoid the use of antacids containing aluminum, calcium, or magnesium, which may prevent the absorption of phosphate.

Potassium Citrate (Urocit-K)

COMMON USES Management of recurrent nephrolithiasis; RTA with calcium stones, hypocitraturic calcium oxalate nephrolithiasis of any etiology; uric acid lithiasis with or without calcium stones

ACTIONS Increases urinary citrate levels and increases urinary pH to 6 to 7 to decrease stone formation

DOSAGE 20 to 30 mEq/d divided tid or qid with meals

SUPPLIED Wax matrix tablets 5 and 10 mEq

NOTES Contraindicated in hyperkalemia and/or renal insufficiency; monitor serum potassium and acid-base status; encourage adequate hydration (>2 L urine/d). Monitor 24-hour urine citrate levels and/or urine pH to monitor effect

 Potassium Supplements (Kaon, Kaochlor, K-Lor, Slow-K, Micro-K, Klorvess, Others)

COMMON USES Prevention or treatment of hypokalemia (often related to diuretic use). Use in patients with hypokalemia from treatment with thiazides for urinary lithiasis

ACTIONS Supplementation of potassium

DOSAGE Adult: 8 to 24 mEq/d po divided qd-bid; peds: Calculate the potassium deficit.

SUPPLIED
- Potassium chloride
  —Liquid: 20, 30, 40 mEq/15 mL
  —Powder packets: 15, 20, 25 mEq
  —Tablets CSR: 6.7, 8, 10, 20 mEq
  —Capsules CSR: 10 mEq
- Potassium bicarbonate
  —Effervescent tablets: 20, 25, 50 mEq

NOTES Can cause GI irritation; powder and liquids must be mixed with beverage (unsalted tomato juice very palatable); use cautiously in renal insufficiency, and along with NSAIDs and ACE inhibitors

 Praziquantel (Biltricide)

COMMON USES Treatment of urinary schistosomiasis

ACTIONS Interferes with the ion transport mechanism of the schistosome tegument, which results in a sudden contraction of the parasite's musculature

DOSAGE Single dose of 40 mg/kg

SUPPLIED 600-mg tablets

NOTES Hypersensitivity reactions have been reported. Otherwise, it is well tolerated.

 Prazosin (Minipress)

COMMON USES Treatment of symptomatic benign prostatic hyperplasia

ACTIONS Peripherally acting alpha-adrenergic blocker (alpha-1 antagonist)

DOSAGE Adult: 1 mg po tid; can increase to a total daily dose of 20 mg/d

SUPPLIED Capsules 1 mg, 2 mg, 5 mg

NOTES Can cause orthostatic hypotension; therefore, patient should take first dose at bedtime; tolerance develops to this effect; tachyphylaxis may result.

 Prednisolone (Delta-Cortef). See Systemic Steroids

 Prednisone (Deltasone). See Systemic Steroids

 Probenecid (Benemid, Others)

COMMON USES Prevention of gout and hyperuricemia; prolongs serum levels of penicillins or cephalosporins

ACTIONS Renal tubular blocking agent

DOSAGE Adult (antibiotic effect): 1 to 2 g po 30 minutes prior to dose of antibiotic; peds >2 years: 25 mg/kg, then 40 mg/kg/d po divided qid

SUPPLIED Tablets 500 mg

 Prochlorperazine (Compazine)

COMMON USES Treatment of nausea and vomiting

ACTIONS Phenothiazine; blocks postsynaptic mesolimbic dopaminergic receptors in the brain

DOSAGE
- Adult: 5 to 10 mg po tid-qid, or 25 mg pr bid, or 5 to 10 mg deep IM q4–6h
- Peds: 0.1 to 0.15 mg/kg/dose IM q4–6h or 0.4 mg/kg/24 h po divided tid-qid

SUPPLIED Tablets 5 mg, 10 mg, 25 mg; SR capsules 10 mg, 15 mg, 30 mg; syrup 5 mg/5 mL; suppositories 2.5 mg, 5 mg, 25 mg; injection 5 mg/mL

NOTES Extrapyramidal side effects common; treat acute extrapyramidal reactions with diphenhydramine.

 Propantheline (Pro-Banthine)

COMMON USES Symptomatic treatment of ureteral and bladder spasm

ACTIONS Antimuscarinic agent

DOSAGE Adult: 15 mg po ac and 30 mg po HS; peds: 1 to 3 mg/kg/24 h po divided tid-qid

SUPPLIED Tablets 7.5 mg, 15 mg

NOTES Anticholinergic side effects such as dry mouth and blurred vision are common.

 Propoxyphene (Darvon, Darvocet) [C]

COMMON USES Treatment of mild-to-moderate pain

ACTIONS Narcotic analgesic

DOSAGE 65 to 100 mg po q4h prn

SUPPLIED
- Darvon (Propoxyphene HCl) 32 mg, 65 mg
- Darvon-N (propoxyphene napsylate) 100 mg = 65 mg of propoxyphene HCl
- Darvocet-N: propoxyphene napsylate/acetaminophen
- Darvon compound: propoxyphene HCl/aspirin/caffeine

NOTES An intentional overdose can be lethal.

Pseudoephedrine (Sudafed, Novafed, Afrinol, Others)

 Pseudoephedrine (Sudafed, Novafed, Afrinol, Others)

COMMON USES Oral therapy for stress urinary incontinence, retrograde ejaculation, and priapism

ACTIONS Stimulates alpha-adrenergic receptors, resulting in vasoconstriction

DOSAGE
- Adult: 30 to 60 mg po q6–8h; SR capsules 120 mg po q12h
- Peds: 4 mg/kg/24 h po divided qid

SUPPLIED Tablets 30, 60 mg; capsules 60 mg; SR tablets 120, 240 mg; SR capsules 120 mg; liquid 75 mg/8 mL, and 15, 30 mg/5 mL

NOTES Contraindicated in patients with poorly controlled hypertension or coronary artery disease, and patients taking MAO inhibitors; an ingredient in many cough and cold preparations

 Pyrazinamide

COMMON USES Treatment of active tuberculosis

ACTIONS Bacteriostatic; mechanism unknown

DOSAGE
- Adult: 15 to 30 mg/kg/24 h po divided tid-qid, maximum dose is 3 g/d
- Peds: 15 to 30 mg/kg/d po divided bid or qd

SUPPLIED Tablets 500 mg

NOTES May cause hepatotoxicity; use in combination with other antituberculosis drugs; Consult the *MMWR* for the latest recommendations on the treatment of tuberculosis. See Section II, "BCG Sepsis."

 Ranitidine (Zantac)

COMMON USES Duodenal ulcer, ulcer prophylaxis in hypersecretory states such as trauma, burns, and surgery

ACTIONS H2 receptor antagonist

DOSAGE
- Adult: 150 mg po bid, 300 mg po qHS, or 50 mg IV q6–8h; or 400 mg IV/d continuous infusion, then maintenance of 150 mg po qHS
- Peds: 0.75 to 1.5 mg/kg/dose IV q6–8h or 1.25 to 2.50 mg/kg/dose po q12h

SUPPLIED Tablets 75 mg, 150 mg, 300 mg; syrup 15 mg/mL; injection 25 mg/mL

NOTES Reduce dose with renal failure; note that oral and parenteral doses are different.

 Renacidin (Contains Citric acid, Glucono-delta-lactone, and Magnesium Carbonate)

COMMON USES Irrigation is used for prevention and dissolution of urinary calculi.

ACTIONS Dissolves urinary calculi, specifically stones composed of calcium phosphate, ammonium phosphate, or magnesium phosphate

DOSAGE Initially, the renal pelvis must be irrigated with NSS at 120 mL/h for 24 to 48 hours. Renacidin irrigation is then continued at 120 mL/h for 24 to 48 hours.

SUPPLIED 500-mL containers

NOTES Hypermagnesemia; only to be given if there is no urine infection, no leakage, and no flank pain

 Rifampin (Rifadin)

COMMON USES Tuberculosis, treatment and prophylaxis of *N. meningitidis*, *H. influenzae*, or *S. aureus* carriers

ACTIONS Inhibits DNA-dependent RNA polymerase activity

DOSAGE
- Adult

—*N. meningitidis* and *H. influenzae* carrier: 600 mg po qd × 4 days
—Tuberculosis: 600 mg po or IV qd, or twice weekly with combination-therapy regimen
—Peds: 10 to 20 mg/kg/dose po or IV qd-bid

SUPPLIED Capsules 150 mg, 300 mg; injection 600 mg

NOTES Multiple side effects; causes orange-red discoloration of bodily secretions, including tears; never used as a single agent to treat active tuberculosis infections

 Rofecoxib (Vioxx)

COMMON USES Osteoarthritis and pain such as dysmenorrhea

ACTIONS COX-2 inhibitor. The antiinflammatory effect of NSAIDs is due mainly to inhibition of the enzyme cyclooxygenase (COX), which is required for synthesis of prostaglandins and thromboxanes. Two COX isoforms have been identified. COX-1 is expressed constitutively in most tissues; it is thought to protect the gastric mucosa. COX-2 is mainly induced at sites of inflammation. Older NSAIDs block both COX isoforms; rofecoxib inhibits COX-2, but not COX-1.

DOSAGE Pain: 50 mg once daily; osteoarthritis: 12.5 to 25.0 mg once daily

SUPPLIED 12.5-mg and 25-mg tablets; oral suspension 12.5 mg/5 mL, 25 mg/5 mL

NOTES Preliminary data suggest that it may have activity in chronic prostatitis

Samarium (Sm 153) Lexidronam (Quadramet)

COMMON USES Relief of pain in patients with confirmed osteoblastic bone lesions

ACTIONS Radioactive agent that has affinity for bone and concentrates in areas of bone turnover

DOSAGE 1 mCi/kg IV

SUPPLIED 2-mL fill size, with total activity of 100 mCi, or 3-mL fill size, with total activity of 150 mCi

NOTES Side effects include flare-up reaction, bone marrow suppression, and hypersensitivity reactions. Patients should be hydrated prior to receiving Quadramet.

 ## Sertraline Hydrochloride (Zoloft)

COMMON USES Treatment of premature ejaculation

ACTIONS Inhibitor of neuronal serotonin reuptake

DOSAGE 50 mg qd

SUPPLIED 25-, 50-, 100-mg tablets

 ## Sildenafil Citrate (Viagra)

COMMON USES Oral therapy for erectile dysfunction

ACTIONS Potentiates normal physiologic response, causing penile erection after sexual arousal. Nitric oxide (NO) released from nerve endings binds to smooth muscle of corporal bodies, causing formation of cGMP, which relaxes smooth muscle and engorges corporal bodies. Detumescence occurs by conversion of cGMP to Gme by phosphodiesterase type 5. Sildenafil inhibits this phosphodiesterase responsible for cGMP breakdown, resulting in increased cGMP activity.

DOSAGE 25 to 100 mg 1 hour prior to sexual activity

SUPPLIED 25-, 50-, 100-mg tablets

NOTES Contraindicated in patients on nitroglycerines. Headache, flushing, visual disturbances ("blue haze"), and dyspepsia have been reported. For effect, must have sexual stimulation approximately 1 hour after dose

 ## Silver Sulfadiazine (Silvadene)

COMMON USES Prevention of sepsis in second-degree and third-degree burns

ACTIONS Bactericidal

DOSAGE Adult and peds: Aseptically cover the affected area with 1/16-inch coating bid.

SUPPLIED Cream 1%

NOTES Can have systemic absorption with extensive application

 ## Sodium Bicarbonate

COMMON USES Alkalinization of urine (i.e., uric acid stones) and treatment of metabolic acidosis secondary to urinary reservoir reconstruction

ACTION Alkalinization of urine

DOSAGE Adult and peds: Titrate to effect, based on blood gases or urine pH. Typical dose for uric acid calculi: 650 mg PO Q6-8h.

SUPPLIED Injection 0.5 mEq/mL, 1 mEq/mL; tablets 325 mg, 650 mg

NOTES 1 g neutralizes 12 mEq of acid.

 ## Sodium Polystyrene Sulfonate (Kayexalate)

COMMON USES Treatment of hyperkalemia

ACTIONS Sodium and potassium ion exchange resin

DOSAGE
• Adults: 15 to 60 g po, or 30 to 60 g pr q6h, based on serum K+
• Peds: 1 g/kg/dose po or pr q6h, based on serum K+

SUPPLIED Powder; suspension 15 g/60 mL sorbitol

NOTES Can cause hypernatremia; given with an agent such as sorbitol to promote movement through the bowel

 ## Sodium Citrate (Bicitra)

COMMON USES Alkalinization of urine

ACTIONS Absorbed and metabolized as sodium bicarbonate

DOSAGE
• Adults: 2 to 6 teaspoonfuls (10–30 mL) diluted in 1 to 3 oz of water after meals and at bedtime
• Peds: 1 to 3 teaspoonfuls (5–15 mL) diluted in 1 to 3 oz of water after meals and at bedtime

SUPPLIED 15-, 30-mL unit dose; 16 (473 mL) or 4 (118 mL) fluid ounces

NOTES Should not be given to patients on aluminum-based antacids. Contraindicated in patients with severe renal impairment on sodium-restricted diets.

 ## Sodium Oxychlorosene (Clorpactin WCS-90)

COMMON USES Intravesical treatment of interstitial cystitis

ACTIONS Complete-spectrum antimicrobial

DOSAGE 0.1% to 0.4% solution in sterile water or isotonic saline given only with general or regional anesthesia

SUPPLIED 2-g bottles

 ## Spironolactone (Aldactone)

COMMON USES Treatment of hyperaldosteronism

ACTIONS Aldosterone antagonist, potassium-sparing diuretic

DOSAGE
• Adult: 25 to 100 mg po qid
• Peds: 1 to 33 mg/kg/24 h po divided bid-qid

—Neonates: 0.5 to 1.0 mg/kg/dose q8h

SUPPLIED Tablets 25, 50, 100 mg

NOTES Can cause hyperkalemia and gynecomastia; avoid prolonged use; diuretic of choice for cirrhotic edema and ascites

Steroids: Systemic

 Steroids: Systemic

The following relates only to the commonly used systemic glucocorticoids.

COMMON USES Endocrine disorders (adrenal insufficiency), allergic states, edematous states (cerebral, nephrotic syndrome), immunosuppression for transplantation, hypercalcemia, malignancies (breast, lymphomas), preoperatively (in any patient who has been on steroids in the previous year, known hypoadrenalism, preoperatively for adrenalectomy)

ACTIONS N/A

DOSAGE Varies with indications and institutional protocols. Some commonly used dosages are listed below:

• Acute adrenal insufficiency (addisonian crisis): hydrocortisone 100 mg IV q8h
• Chronic adrenal insufficiency: hydrocortisone 20 mg po qam, 10 mg po qpm
• Perioperative steroid coverage: hydrocortisone 100 mg IV night prior to surgery, 1 hour preoperatively, intraoperatively, and 4, 8, and 12 hours postoperatively; POD#1 100 mg IV q6h; POD#2 100 mg IV q8h; POD#3 100 mg IV q12h; POD#4 50 mg IV q12h; POD#5 25 mg IV q12h; then, resume prior oral dosing if chronic use, or discontinue if only perioperative coverage required

SUPPLIED See below.

NOTES All can cause hyperglycemia, adrenal suppression; never acutely stop steroids, especially if chronic treatment; taper dose; equivalent dose for all agents; potency related to other agents

SHORT-ACTING STEROIDS
• Cortisone (Cortone)

—Equivalent dose: 25 mg
—Antiinflammatory potency: 8
—Supplied: 50 mg/10 mL injection; 25-mg tab

• Hydrocortisone (Cortef)

—Equivalent dose: 20 mg
—Antiinflammatory potency: 10
—Supplied: 50 mg/5 mL injection

INTERMEDIATE-ACTING STEROIDS
• Methylprednisolone (Medrol)

—Equivalent dose: 4 mg
—Antiinflammatory potency: 5
—Supplied: 4-mg tabs

• Prednisolone (Delta-Cortef)

—Equivalent dose: 5 mg
—Antiinflammatory potency: 4
—Supplied: 20 mg/1 mL suspension

• Prednisone (Deltasone)

—Equivalent dose: 5 mg
—Antiinflammatory potency: 4
—Supplied: 5 mg/5 mL suspension; 1-, 2.5-, 5-, 10-, 20-, 50-mg tabs

LONG-ACTING STEROIDS
• Betamethasone (Calestone)

—Equivalent dose: 06 to 075 mg
—Antiinflammatory potency: 20 to 30
—Supplied: 30 mg/5 mL injection

• Dexamethasone (Decadron)

—Equivalent dose: 0.75 mg
—Antiinflammatory potency: 20 to 30
—Supplied: 4 mg/mL available in 1-, 5-, 25-mL vials for injection; 0.75-, 4-mg tabs

 Streptomycin

COMMON USES Treatment of tuberculosis or serious *Enterococcus* infections

ACTIONS Aminoglycoside; interferes with protein synthesis

DOSAGE 1 to 4 gm per day IM in 1 to 2 divided doses

SUPPLIED Injection 400 mg/mL

NOTES Increased incidence of vestibular toxicity

 Strontium-89 Chloride (Metastron)

COMMON USES Management of bone pain in patients with osseous metastasis

ACTIONS A calcium analogue taken up by bone in areas of active osteogenesis with selective radiation of metastasis

DOSAGE 148 MBq (4 mCi) IV slowly, or 15 to 22 MBq/kg

SUPPLIED Injectable

NOTES Administered by radiation oncology; caution with platelet counts <60,000 or WBC of <2400

 Sulfamethoxazole (Gantanol)

COMMON USES Acute, recurrent, or chronic urinary tract infections due to susceptible organisms (*E. coli, Klebsiella, Enterobacter, Staphylococcus,* and *Proteus*)

ACTIONS Inhibits bacterial synthesis of dihydrofolic acid; bacteriostatic

DOSAGE
• Adults: 1 to 2 g daily in divided doses
• Peds

—Initial dose: 50 to 60 mg/kg, followed by 25 to 30 mg/kg twice daily.
—Maximum dose: should not exceed 75 mg/kg/d

SUPPLIED 500-g tablets

NOTES Should not be used in infants less than 2 months old. Hypersensitivity reactions. Dosage adjustment for impaired renal function

 Sulindac (Clinoril). See Nonsteroidal Antiinflammatory Drugs

 Tacrolimus (Prograf) [FK-506]

COMMON USES Prophylaxis of organ rejection

ACTIONS Macrolide immunosuppressant

DOSAGE
• IV: 0.05 to 0.1 mg/kg/d as continuous infusion
• PO: 0.15 to 0.3 mg/kg/d divided into 2 doses

SUPPLIED Capsules 1 mg, 5 mg; injection 5 mg/mL

NOTES May cause neurotoxicity and nephrotoxicity

Tamoxifen (Nolvadex)

COMMON USES Idiopathic oligospermia

ACTIONS Nonsteroidal antiestrogen, mixed agonist–antagonist effect

DOSAGE 10 to 20 mg/d

SUPPLIED Tablets 10, 20 mg

NOTES Skin rash, dizziness, headache, and peripheral edema may occur. Acute flare of bone metastasis pain and hypercalcemia may occur. With high doses, retinopathy reported

 Tamsulosin Hydrochloride (Flomax)

COMMON USES Treatment of symptomatic benign prostatic hyperplasia

ACTIONS Alpha-1-adrenergic blocker (highly selective for alpha-1a and alpha-1d subtypes); relaxation of bladder neck smooth muscle fibers

DOSAGE 0.4 or 0.8 mg po qd

SUPPLIED 0.4- to 0.8-mg capsules

NOTES May have fewer side effects than other alpha-blockers

 Terazosin (Hytrin)

COMMON USES Benign prostatic hyperplasia and autonomic hyperreflexia

ACTIONS Alpha-1 blocker (blood vessel and bladder neck/prostate)

DOSAGE Initially, 1 mg po HS; titrate up to maximum of 20 mg po qHS

SUPPLIED Tablets 1 mg, 2 mg, 5 mg, 10 mg

NOTES Hypotension and syncope following first dose; dizziness, weakness, nasal congestion, peripheral edema common; must be used with thiazide diuretic

 Terbutaline (Brethine, Bricanyl)

COMMON USES Treatment of low-flow priapism

ACTIONS Sympathomimetic

DOSAGE 5 to 10 mg SQ or po

SUPPLIED Tablets 2.5 mg, 5 mg; injection 1 mg/mL

NOTES Exercise caution with diabetes, hypertension, and hyperthyroidism; high doses may precipitate beta-1-adrenergic effects.

 Terconazole (Terazol 7)

COMMON USES Vaginal fungal infections

ACTIONS Topical antifungal

DOSAGE 1 applicatorful intravaginally qHS for 7 days

SUPPLIED Vaginal cream 0.4%

 Testosterone Injection (Delatestryl, Virilon)

COMMON USES Testosterone replacement, hypogonadism, enhancement of genital growth in children undergoing genital reconstruction (hypospadias, epispadias)

ACTIONS Increases circulating testosterone level

DOSAGE

- Adult: 200 mg/mL given IM
- Peds: in reconstruction, 25 mg/m weekly 3 to 4 weeks prior to surgery

SUPPLIED Virilon is available in 10-mL vials of 200 mg/mL. Delatestryl is available in 1-mL vials of 200 mg/mL.

NOTES Gynecomastia, breast tenderness, and acne are reported. Avoid in patients with prostate cancer.

 Testosterone Transdermal System (Testoderm, Androderm)

COMMON USES Testosterone replacement, hypogonadism

ACTIONS Increases circulating testosterone level

DOSAGE Testoderm is applied on the scrotal area with the 4 mg or 6 mg/d system for 6 to 8 weeks. Androderm is applied on the back, abdomen, or thighs with the 2.5 mg or 5 mg/d system for 6 to 8 weeks.

SUPPLIED Androderm is available in a 25 mg/d system in a carton of 60, or in a 5 mg/d system in a carton of 30. Testoderm is available in cartons of 30 for both the 4 and 6 mg/d systems.

NOTES Local irritation, including itching and discomfort. Gynecomastia, acne, and breast tenderness have been reported.

 Tetracycline (Achromycin V, Sumycin)

COMMON USES Broad-spectrum antibiotic treatment against *Staphylococcus, Streptococcus, Chlamydia, Rickettsia,* and *Mycoplasma*

ACTIONS Bacteriostatic; inhibits protein synthesis

DOSAGE

- Adult: 250 to 500 mg po bid-qid
- Peds >8 years: 25 to 50 mg/kg/24 h po q6–12h. *Do not* use in children <8 years old.

SUPPLIED Capsules 100 mg, 250 mg, 500 mg; tablets 250 mg, 500 mg; oral suspension 250 mg/5 mL

NOTES Can stain tooth enamel and depress bone formation in children; caution with use in pregnancy. *Do not* use in the presence of impaired renal function (see Doxycycline).

Ticarcillin (Ticar)

 Ticarcillin (Ticar)

COMMON USES Treatment of infections caused by susceptible gram-negative bacteria (including *Klebsiella, E. coli, Proteus, Enterobacter, P. aeruginosa,* and *Serratia*) involving the skin, urinary tract, abdomen, and septicemia

ACTIONS Bactericidal; inhibits cell wall synthesis

DOSAGE Adults: 3 g q4–6h; peds: 200 to 300 mg/kg/d divided q4–6h

SUPPLIED In powder form: 1-, 3-, and 6-g vials. These must be prepared just prior to infusion with NSS, sterile water, or 5% dextrose injection.

NOTES Must be adjusted in patients with renal impairment. May cause hypokalemia

 Ticarcillin-Clavulanate (Timentin)

COMMON USES Treatment of infections caused by susceptible gram-negative bacteria (including *Klebsiella, E. coli, Proteus, Enterobacter, P. aeruginosa,* and *Serratia*) involving the skin, urinary tract, abdomen, and septicemia

ACTIONS Bactericidal; inhibits cell wall synthesis

DOSAGE Adults: 3.1 g q4–6h IV; peds: 200 to 300 mg/kg/d divided q4–6h IV

SUPPLIED In powder form: 31-g vials. These must be prepared just prior to infusion with NSS, sterile water, or 5% dextrose injection.

NOTES Must be adjusted in patients with renal impairment. May cause hypokalemia

 Tioconazole (Vagistat)

COMMON USES Vaginal fungal infections

ACTIONS Topical antifungal

DOSAGE 1 applicatorful intravaginally at bedtime (single dose)

SUPPLIED Vaginal ointment 65%

 Tobramycin (Nebcin)

COMMON USES Serious gram-negative infections, especially *Pseudomonas*

ACTIONS Aminoglycoside; inhibits protein synthesis

DOSAGE Adults: 1 to 25 mg/kg/dose IV q8–24h; peds: 25 mg/kg/dose IV q8h

SUPPLIED Injection 10 mg/mL, 40 mg/mL

NOTES Nephrotoxic and ototoxic; decrease dose with renal insufficiency; monitor creatinine clearance and serum concentrations for dosage adjustments.

 Tolmetin (Tolectin). See Nonsteroidal Antiinflammatory Drugs

 Tolterodine Tartrate (Detrol)

COMMON USES Overactive bladder with symptoms of urinary frequency, urgency, or urge incontinence

ACTIONS Competitive muscarinic receptor antagonist

DOSAGE 1 to 2 mg po bid

SUPPLIED 1-, 2-mg tablets

NOTES Contraindicated in patients with urinary or gastric retention, and narrow-angle glaucoma. Has drug interactions with cytochrome P450 3A4 inhibitors (e.g., erythromycin, ketoconazole). Anticholinergic side effects: dry mouth, dyspepsia, constipation, and xerophthalmia

 Tramadol (Ultram)

COMMON USES Management of moderate-to-severe pain

ACTIONS Centrally acting analgesic

DOSAGE 50 to 100 mg po q4–6h prn, not to exceed 400 mg/d

SUPPLIED Tablets 50 mg

 Triamcinole Acetonide and Nystatin (Mycolog-II)

COMMON USES Cutaneous candidiasis

ACTIONS Antifungal and antiinflammatory

DOSAGE Apply lightly to area 2 times a day; maximum 25 days

SUPPLIED Cream and ointment 15, 30, 60, 120 mg

NOTES Contraindicated in varicella

 Tricitrates Oral Solution (Polycitra, Polycitra LC, Polycitra K)

COMMON USES Alkalinization of urine

ACTIONS Absorbed and metabolized as potassium bicarbonate and sodium bicarbonate

DOSAGE
• Adults: 3 to 6 teaspoonfuls (15–30 mL) diluted in water 4 times a day
• Peds: 1 to 3 teaspoonfuls (5–15 mL) diluted in water 4 times a day

SUPPLIED 16 fluid ounces

NOTES Contraindicated in severe renal impairment with oliguria or azotemia, untreated Addison disease, or severe myocardial infarction

Thiotepa/Triethylene-thiophosphoramide (Thio-TEPA, TESPA, TSPA, Thioplex)

COMMON USES Breast, ovarian cancer; intracavitary for serosal malignant implants; intravesical for superficial papillary bladder cancer

ACTIONS Polyfunctional alkylating agent; nitrogen mustard–like action

DOSAGE Intravesical: 60 mg in 30 to 60 mL saline, and held for 2 hours, if possible; treat weekly for 4 weeks. An additional 4-week course can be given, with caution because myelosuppression can occur.

SUPPLIED Injection 15 mg

NOTES Toxicity includes myelosuppression, nausea, vomiting, dizziness, headache, allergy, and paresthesias. When given intravesically, it can cause irritative voiding symptoms, cystitis, nausea, vomiting, leukopenia, and thrombocytopenia. This drug has a low molecular weight and may be absorbed by the bladder urothelium and may cause myelosuppression. Check CBC when on therapy. If WBC <4500 μL or platelets <100,000 μL, hold therapy until counts normalize.

 Trimethobenzamide (Tigan)

COMMON USES Treatment of nausea and vomiting

ACTIONS Inhibits medullary chemoreceptor trigger zone

DOSAGE
• Adult: 250 mg po, or 200 mg pr or IM tid-qid prn
• Peds: 20 mg/kg/24 h po, or 15 mg/kg/24 h pr or IM in 3 to 4 divided doses (not recommended for infants)

SUPPLIED Capsules 100 mg, 250 mg; suppositories 100 mg, 200 mg; injection 100 mg/mL

NOTES In the presence of viral infections, it may contribute to Reye syndrome; may cause parkinsonian-like syndrome

 Trimethoprim (Trimpex, Proloprim)

COMMON USES Urinary tract infections due to susceptible gram-positive and gram-negative organisms; often used for suppression of UTIs

ACTIONS Inhibits dihydrofolate reductase

DOSAGE
• Adults: 100 mg po bid, or 200 mg po qd
• Peds: 4 mg/kg/d in 2 divided doses

SUPPLIED Tablets 100 mg, 200 mg

NOTES Reduce the dose in renal failure.

 Trimethoprim-Sulfamethoxazole (Co-trimoxazole, Bactrim, Septra)

COMMON USES Urinary tract infections, otitis media, sinusitis, bronchitis, *Shigella*, *Pneumocystis carinii*, *Nocardia*

ACTIONS Dual effect of sulfamethoxazole-inhibiting synthesis of dihydrofolic acid and trimethoprim-inhibiting dihydrofolate reductase to cause impaired protein synthesis

DOSAGE
• Adult

—1 double-strength (DS) tablet po bid, or 5 to 10 mg/kg/24 h (based on trimethoprim component) IV in 3 to 4 divided doses
—*Pneumocystis carinii*: 15 to 20 mg/kg/d IV or po (trimethoprim component) in 4 divided doses
—*Nocardia*: 10 to 15 mg/kg/d IV or po (trimethoprim component) in 4 divided doses

• Peds: 8 to 10 mg/kg/24 h (trimethoprim) po divided into 2 doses or 3 to 4 doses IV; *do not* use in a newborn.

SUPPLIED Tablets, regular, 80 mg TMP and 400 mg SMX; tablets, DS, 160 mg TMP and 800 mg SMX; oral suspension 40 mg TMP and 200 mg SMX per 5 mL; injection 80 mg TMP and 400 mg SMX per 5 mL

NOTES Synergistic combination; reduce the dosage in renal failure.

 Trovafloxacin (Trovan)

COMMON USES Intraabdominal infections, skin and skin structure infections, urinary tract infections, and chronic bacterial prostatitis; current recommendations are that the use of Trovan be limited to serious limb or life threatening infections.

ACTIONS Quinolone antibiotic; inhibits DNA gyrase

DOSAGE 200-mg PO bid or 300-mg IV BID in hospital setting, with monitoring of liver function testing

SUPPLIED 100-, 200-mg tablets; injectable

NOTES Liver toxicity a significant problem especially with treatments over 2 weeks; hypersensitivity reactions reported; may have interactions with theophylline and warfarin

 Valacyclovir (Valtrex)

COMMON USES Treatment of herpes zoster

ACTIONS Prodrug of acyclovir, inhibits viral DNA replication

DOSAGE
• Zoster 1 g po tid for 7 days
• Simplex: 500 mg po BID for 5 days

SUPPLIED Caplets 500 mg

 Valrubicin (Valstar)

COMMON USES Intravesical treatment of BCG-refractory CIS when immediate cystectomy would be associated with unacceptable morbidity or mortality

ACTIONS Semisynthetic doxorubicin analogue; cytotoxic

DOSAGE 800 mg intravesically weekly for 6 weeks

SUPPLIED Liquid 200 mg/5 mL

NOTES Dilute 800 mg in approximately 75 mL normal saline; minimal systemic absorption with intact bladder; do not use within 1 to 2 weeks of biopsy because systemic absorption can cause myelosuppression; can cause local bladder symptoms; contraindicated with bladder capacity of <75 mL or active UTI

Vancomycin (Vancocin, Vancoled)

 Vancomycin (Vancocin, Vancoled)

COMMON USES Serious infections due to methicillin-resistant staphylococci and in enterococcal endocarditis in combination with aminoglycosides in penicillin-allergic patients; oral treatment of *C. difficile* pseudomembranous colitis

ACTIONS Inhibits cell wall synthesis

DOSAGE
• Adults: 1 g IV q12h; for colitis 125 to 500 mg po q6h
• Peds (*not* neonates): 40 mg/kg/24 h IV in divided doses q12–6h

SUPPLIED Capsules 125 mg, 250 mg; powder for oral solution; powder for injection 500 mg, 1000 mg, 10 g per vial

NOTES Ototoxic and nephrotoxic; not absorbed orally; provides local effect in gut only; IV dose must be given slowly over 1 hour to prevent "red-man syndrome"; adjust the dose in renal failure.

 Vinblastine (Velban, Velbe)

COMMON USES Testicular cancer, choriocarcinoma, bladder cancer, and renal cell carcinoma

ACTIONS Inhibits microtubule assembly through binding to tubulin

DOSAGE 0.1 to 0.5 mg/kg/wk (4–20 mg/m^2)

SUPPLIED Injection 10 mg

NOTES Toxicity includes myelosuppression (especially leukopenia), nausea and vomiting (rarely), constipation, neurotoxicity (similar to that listed for vincristine but less frequent), alopecia, and rash. Myalgia and tumor pain are common.

 Vincristine (Oncovin)

COMMON USES Rhabdomyosarcoma, Wilms' tumor, neuroblastoma, and penile cancer

ACTIONS Promotes disassembly of mitotic spindle, causing metaphase arrest

DOSAGE 0.4 to 1.4 mg/m^2 (single doses do not usually exceed 2 mg)

SUPPLIED Injection 1 mg, 5 mg

NOTES Toxicity includes neurotoxicity (commonly dose-limiting), jaw pain (trigeminal neuralgia), fever, fatigue, anorexia, constipation, and paralytic ileus; bladder atony reported; no significant myelosuppression is observed with standard doses. Soft-tissue necrosis may occur with extravasation.

 Vitamin E (Unique E, Others)

COMMON USES Oral treatment of Peyronie disease

ACTIONS Antioxidant

DOSAGE 2 capsules daily

SUPPLIED 400-IU capsules

 Warfarin Sodium (Coumadin)

COMMON USES Prophylaxis and treatment of pulmonary embolism and venous thrombosis, atrial fibrillation with embolization, other postoperative indications

ACTIONS Inhibits vitamin K–dependent production of clotting factors in the order of VII, IX, X, and II

DOSAGE
• Adult: Need to individualize dosage to keep international normalized ratio (INR) 2.0 to 3.0 for most indications. For mechanical heart valves, the desired INR is 25 to 35. Initially, 10 to 15 mg po, IM, or IV qd for 13 days; then maintenance, 2 to 10 mg po, IV, or IM qd; follow daily PT/INR during the initial phase to guide dosage.
• Peds: 0.05 to 0.34 mg/kg/24 h po, IM, or IV qd. Follow PT closely to adjust dosage.

SUPPLIED Tablets 2 mg, 25 mg, 5 mg, 75 mg, 10 mg; powder for injection 50 mg/vial

NOTES INR is the preferred laboratory test, rather than the ratio of the patient's prothrombin time (PT) to control; INR needs to be checked periodically while on maintenance dose; beware of bleeding caused by overanticoagulation (PT > 3 times control or INR > 50–60). Caution the patient on the effects of taking Coumadin with other medications, especially aspirin. To rapidly correct over-Coumadinization, use vitamin K or fresh-frozen plasma, or both. It is highly teratogenic; *do not* use in pregnancy.

 Yohimbine (Yocon, Yohimex)

COMMON USES May have activity as an aphrodisiac. Tried experimentally for erectile dysfunction

ACTIONS Blocks presynaptic alpha-2-adrenergic receptors; increases parasympathetic activity and decreases sympathetic activity

DOSAGE 1 tablet tid

SUPPLIED 5.4-mg tablets

NOTES Contraindications include hypersensitivity and renal diseases; may cause tachycardia

Section VI

Alternate Therapies in Urology

African Plum (*Pygeum africanum*)

These are common agents that are not FDA approved but are available to patients through health food stores and other commercial outlets. Phytotherapies and other supplements are under study, but none has undergone extensive placebo-controlled trials in the United States. Many of these alternative therapies are included as part of other combination therapies and may be sold under a variety of trade names.

 ## African Plum (*Pygeum africanum*)

DESCRIPTION The extract, Tadenan®, is derived from the bark of the African plum tree and is taken for the treatment of BPH and LUTS. Multiple formulations are available. The mode of action is thought to be via inhibition of fibroblast growth and antiinflammatory, as well as antiestrogenic, effects. Much inconclusive data exist showing decreases in symptom score and an increase in flow rate. A double-blind, placebo-controlled trial (IPSS-Tadenan) recently commenced, with data anticipated in the near future. No side effects have been noted.

REFERENCES

Lowe FC, et al. Phytotherapy in the treatment of benign prostatic hyperplasia: An update. *Urology* 1999;53(4):671–678.

Breza J, et al. Efficacy and acceptability of Tandenam® (*Pygeum africanum* extract) in the treatment of benign prostatic hyperplasia (BPH): A multi-culture trial in Central Europe. *Curr Med Res Opin* 1998;14:127–139.

 ## Bazoton (*Radix urticae*)

DESCRIPTION This plant extract is used in the treatment of BPH. The active ingredients are thought to include its steroid–glycoside composition. This has been reported to be an inhibitor of the sex-steroid binding globulin. There are few studies, some of which report a marginal decrease in PVR and an increase in maximal urine flow. There are no reported side effects.

REFERENCE

Romics I. Observations with Bazoton in the management of prostatic hyperplasia. *Int Urol Nephrol* 1987;19:293–297.

 ## Capsaicin (*Capsicum*)

DESCRIPTION This is the main pungent ingredient of the hot peppers in the genus *Capsicum*. It is used in a diluted form as an intravesical treatment for overactive bladders. The mode of action is by the selective activation of sensory nerve fibers and by a specific neurotoxin effect on C afferent fibers. Multiple studies have documented symptomatic and urodynamic improvement in patients treated with capsaicin. Adverse events include suprapubic pain, gross hematuria, and incontinence, all of which resolved.

REFERENCE

Chancellor MB, et al. Intravesical capsaicin and resiniferatoxin therapy: Spicing up the ways to treat the overactive bladder. *J Urol* 1999;162:3–11.

 ## Cranberries (*Vaccinium macrocarpon*)

DESCRIPTION The juice or extract of the berry is used for the treatment or prevention of urinary tract infections. It contains a unique blend of organic acids, being quinic, malic, and citric acid. Furthermore, it contains fructose and a nondialyzable polymeric compound, both of which inhibit bacterial adherence. A double-blind, placebo-controlled trial showed an approximate 50% decrease in both bacteruria and pyuria in women in the treatment arm after 2 months. Further studies are necessary.

REFERENCES

Avorn J, et al. Reduction of bacteruria and pyuria after ingestion of cranberry juice. *JAMA* 1994;271:751–754.

Sobota AE, et al. Inhibition of bacterial adherence by cranberry juice: Potential use for the treatment of urinary tract infections. *J Urol* 1984;131:1013–1016.

 ## Heather (*Calluna vulgaris*)

DESCRIPTION The medicinal portion consists of the entire herb (leaves, flowers, roots) ground and boiled to create a decoction that is taken for its diuretic properties and treatment of the kidneys, LUTS, and BPH. Active compounds include flavanoid and sitosterols. The claimed efficacy has not been documented in studies.

REFERENCE: N/A

 ## PC-SPES

DESCRIPTION Commercially available combination herbal therapy used by some patients with prostate cancer. Consists of eight herbs: chrysanthemum, isatis, licorice, *Ganoderma lucidium*, *Panax pseudo-ginseng*, *Rabdosia rubescens*, saw palmetto, and scutellaria (skullcap). It has potent estrogenic activity. Its use is associated with breast tenderness, loss of libido, and decreased PSA and testosterone, and it may confound the results of standard and experimental studies.

REFERENCE

DiPaola RS, et al. Clinical and biologic activity of an estrogenic herbal combination (PC-SPES) in prostate cancer. *N Engl J Med* 1998;339(12):785–791.

 ## Permixon® (*Serenoa repens*)

DESCRIPTION This is the branded version of the saw palmetto, an extract of the dried, ripe fruit from a dwarf palm tree of the family Arecaceae. It is the most widely studied agent in its category for use in treatment of BPH or lower urinary tract symptoms (LUTS). Consists mainly of sitosterols and flavonoids with varied mechanisms. It has an antiandrogenic and antiprostaglandin effect. It does not decrease the size of the prostate. There are no known health hazards or adverse effects. PSA effect not clear.

REFERENCES

Plosker Gl, et al. *Serenoa repens* (Permixon®): A review of its pharmacological and therapeutic efficacy in benign prostatic hyperplasia. *Drugs Aging* 1996;9(5):379–395.

Lowe FC, et al. Meta-analysis of clinical trials of Permixon. *J Urol* 1998;159(2):257.

 ## Pumpkin Seed (*Cucurbita pepo*)

DESCRIPTION Fresh and dried seeds are taken whole or ground for the treatment of BPH or irritable bladder symptoms. Active compounds are thought to be phytosterols. As there are no documented clinical studies, evidence establishing efficacy is empirical. There are no known side effects.

REFERENCE

Carbin BE, et al. Treatment of benign prostatic hyperplasia with phytosterols. *Br J Urol* 1990;66:639–641.

Rye Pollen (*Secale cereale*)

DESCRIPTION   A pollen extract obtained by the microbial digestion and extraction by water or organic solvents. The branded version is Cernilton. Active ingredients are thought to include β-sitosterols. It is taken for the treatment of BPH, prostatitis, and prostatodynia. The water-soluble portion was found to inhibit immortal prostate cancer cell line growth as well as the growth of epithelial and stromal BPH cells in vitro. The exact mode of action is unknown. No conclusive long-term studies exist; however one study has shown a decrease in PVR and an improvement in the IPSS score.

REFERENCES

Habib FK, et al. The identification of a prostate inhibitory substance in a pollen extract. *Prostate* 1995;26:133–139.

Buck AC, et al. Treatment of outflow tract obstruction due to benign prostatic hyperplasia with pollen extract Cernilton. A double-blind, placebo-controlled study. *Br J Urol* 1990;66:398–404.

 ## Saw Palmetto (*Sabal serrulata, Serona repens*). See Permixon

 ## Selenium

DESCRIPTION   A trace mineral taken that may prevent the development of prostate cancer. Epidemiologic studies have shown that it may, in fact, have a protective effect in the chemoprevention of various cancers, including prostate. One randomized study looking at selenium and skin cancer incidentally displayed a decrease in the incidence of prostate cancer in those patients receiving supplemental selenium.

REFERENCES

Clark LC, et al. Effects of selenium supplementation for cancer prevention in patients with carcinoma of the skin. A randomized controlled trial. *JAMA* 1997;276:1957.

Fair WR, et al. Cancer of the prostate: A nutritional disease? *Urology* 1997;50(6):840–848.

 ## South African Star Grass (*Hypoxis rooperi*)

DESCRIPTION   An extract taken mainly for BPH symptoms. Active compounds are thought to include sitosterols as well as other sterols. The mode of action is thought to be via induction of apoptosis by TGF-beta1. However, this has never been proven in vivo. Recent data suggest that IPSS, urinary flow rate, and post-void residual all improve with the use of sitosterols. Adverse effects were not reported. Further confirmatory studies are needed.

REFERENCES

Klippel KF, et al. The German BPH-Phytotherapy Study Group: A multicentric, placebo-controlled, double-blind clinical trial of beta-sitosterol (phytosterol) for the treatment of benign prostatic hyperplasia. *Br J Urol* 1997;80:427–432.

Burges RL, et al. Randomized placebo-controlled, double-blind clinical trial of beta-sitosterols in patients with benign prostatic hyperplasia. *Lancet* 1995;345:1529–1532.

 ## Stinging Nettle (*Urtica dioica*)

DESCRIPTION   The herb consists of fresh and dried ground portions of the flower and stem, taken either orally as a powder or tea for the treatment of BPH as well as kidney infections or stones. It acts as a diuretic. Active compounds include histamine, serotonin, acetylcholine, formic acid, flavonoids, and sterols, among others. Effects are thought to include an increase in the maximum urinary flow rate and a reduction in the post-void residual. One study showed an increase in IPSS scores vs. placebo. No significant health hazards or side effects are known.

REFERENCE

Engelmann U, et al. Therapie der benignen Prostathyperplasie mit Bazoton Liquidum. *Urologe B* 1996;36:287–291.

 ## Yohimbine

DESCRIPTION   An extract of the bark of the Yohim tree, taken for erectile dysfunction. The mode of action is as an alpha-adrenergic antagonist. Conflicting studies show no significant difference from placebo, while others show positive response rates of up to 62% in psychogenic impotence. Regardless, it continues to be widely prescribed, as well as purchased, in over-the-counter forms.

REFERENCES

Morales A, et al. Non-hormonal pharmacological treatment of organic impotence. *J Urol* 1982;128:45.

Reid K, et al. Double-blind trial of yohimbine in the treatment of psychogenic impotence. *Lancet* 1987;2:421–423.

Appendix:
Reference Tables

Appendix: Reference Tables

Table 1. TNM Classification

TNM stands for "tumor, nodes, metastasis" and is a universally accepted classification system for malignancy staging. The UICC (Union Internationale Contre le Cancer) and the AJCC (American Joint Committee on Cancer) have adopted this system, and the complete listing for all tumor sites appears in the Fifth Edition of the *AJCC Cancer Staging Manual* (1997). The following is a highly selected listing of commonly encountered solid tumors in urologic practice (adrenal, bladder, cervix, colon and rectum, kidney, ovary, uterus, prostate, penis, testes, renal pelvis/ureter, and urethra). Where appropriate, other common staging systems are noted (e.g., Duke's classification of colon cancer).

ADRENAL

TNM	DEFINITION
T1	Tumor <5 cm, no capsule invasion
T2	Tumor >5 cm, no capsule invasion
T3	Invasion into periadrenal fat
T4	Tumor invading adjacent organs
N0	Negative lymph nodes
N1	Positive regional lymph nodes
M0	No metastases
M1	Distant metastases

BLADDER

TNM	DEFINITION

Primary Tumor (T)

TX	Primary tumor cannot be assessed
T0	No evidence of primary tumor
Tis	Carcinoma in situ: "flat tumor"
Ta	Noninvasive papillary carcinoma
T1	Tumor invades subepithelial connective tissue
T2	Tumor invades superficial muscle (inner half)
T3	Tumor invades deep muscle or perivesical fat
T3a	Tumor invades deep muscle (outer half)
T3b	Tumor invades perivesical fat
T4	Tumor invades any of the following: prostate, uterus, vagina, pelvic wall, abdominal wall

Lymph Node (N)

NX	Regional lymph nodes cannot be assessed
N0	No regional lymph node metastasis
N1	Metastasis in a single lymph node, 2 cm or less in greatest dimension
N2	Metastasis in a single lymph node, more than 2 cm but not more than 5 cm in greatest dimension, or multiple lymph nodes, none more than 5 cm in greatest dimension
N3	Metastasis in a lymph node more than 5 cm in greatest dimension

Distant Metastasis (M)

MX	Presence of distant metastasis cannot be assessed
M0	No distant metastasis
M1	Distant metastasis

CERVIX

TNM	DEFINITION

Primary Tumor (T)

TX	Primary tumor cannot be assessed
T0	No evidence of primary tumor
Tis	Carcinoma in situ
T1	Cervical carcinoma confined to uterus
T1a	Preclinical invasive carcinoma diagnosed by microscopy only
T1a1	Minimal microscopic stromal invasion
T1a2	Tumor with invasive component 5 mm or less in depth taken from the base of the epithelium and 7 mm or less in horizontal spread
T1b	Tumor larger than T1a2
T2	Cervical carcinoma invades beyond uterus but not to pelvic wall or to the lower third of vagina
T2a	Tumor without parametrial invasion
T2b	Tumor with parametrial invasion
T3	Cervical carcinoma extends to pelvic wall or involves lower third of vagina or causes hydronephrosis or nonfunctioning kidney
T3a	Tumor involves lower third of the vagina, no extension to pelvic wall
T3b	Tumor extends to pelvic wall or causes hydronephrosis or nonfunctioning kidney
T4	Tumor invades mucosa of bladder or rectum or extends beyond the true pelvis

Lymph Node (N)

NX	Regional lymph nodes cannot be assessed
N0	No regional lymph node metastasis
N1	Regional lymph node metastasis

Distant Metastasis (M)

MX	Presence of distant metastasis cannot be assessed
M0	No distant metastasis
M1	Distant metastasis

COLON AND RECTUM

TNM	DEFINITION

Primary Tumor (T)

TX	Primary tumor cannot be assessed
T0	No evidence of primary tumor
Tis	Carcinoma in situ
T1	Tumor invades submucosa
T2	Tumor invades muscularis propria
T3	Tumor invades through muscularis propria into subserosa, or into nonperitonealized pericolic or perirectal tissues
T4	Tumor perforates visceral peritoneum, or directly invades other organs or structures

Lymph Node (N)

NX	Regional lymph nodes cannot be assessed
N0	No regional lymph node metastasis
N1	Metastasis in one to three pericolic or perirectal lymph nodes
N2	Metastasis in four or more pericolic or perirectal lymph nodes
N3	Metastasis in any lymph node along course of a major named vascular trunk

Distant Metastasis (M)

MX	Presence of distant metastasis cannot be assessed
M0	No distant metastasis
M1	Distant metastasis

Dukes' Classification (Aster-Coller Modification) of Colon Cancer

Stage A:	Limited to the mucosa
Stage B1:	Into muscularis propria, nodes negative
Stage B2:	Extends through entire wall, nodes negative
Stage C1:	Extends into muscularis propria, nodes positive
Stage C2:	Extends through entire wall, nodes positive
Stage D:	Metastatic disease

KIDNEY

TNM	DEFINITION

Primary Tumor (T)

TX	Primary tumor cannot be assessed
T0	No evidence of primary tumor
T1	Tumor 7 cm or less in greatest dimension limited to the kidney
T2	Tumor more than 7 cm in greatest dimension limited to the kidney
T3	Tumor extends into major veins or invades adrenal gland or perinephric tissues but not beyond Gerota's fascia
T3a	Tumor invades adrenal gland or perinephric tissues but not beyond Gerota's fascia
T3b	Tumor grossly extends into renal vein(s) or vena cava below diaphragm
T4	Tumor invades beyond Gerota's fascia

Lymph Node (N)

NX	Regional lymph nodes cannot be assessed
N0	No regional lymph node metastasis
N1	Metastasis in a single lymph node
N2	Metastasis in more than 1 lymph node

KIDNEY

TNM	DEFINITION

Distant Metastasis (M)

MX	Presence of distant metastasis cannot be assessed
M0	No distant metastasis
M1	Distant metastasis

OVARY

TNM	FIGO[a]	DEFINITION

Primary Tumor (T)

TNM	FIGO	DEFINITION
TX		Primary tumor cannot be assessed
T0	I	No evidence of primary tumor
T1		Tumor limited to ovaries
T1a	Ia	Tumor limited to one ovary; capsule intact, no tumor on ovarian surface
T1b	Ib	Tumor limited to both ovaries; capsules intact, no tumor on ovarian surface
T1c	Ic	Tumor limited to one or both ovaries with any of the following: capsule ruptured, tumor on ovarian surface, malignant cells in ascites, or peritoneal washings
T2	II	Tumor involves one or both ovaries with pelvic extension
T2a	IIa	Extension or implants on uterus or tubes
T2b	IIb	Extension to other pelvic tissues
T2c	IIc	Pelvic extension (2a or 2b) with malignant cells in ascites or peritoneal washing
T3	III[b]	Tumor involves one or both ovaries with microscopically confirmed or N1 peritoneal metastasis outside the pelvis or regional lymph node metastasis
T3a	IIIa	Microscope peritoneal metastasis beyond pelvis
T3b	IIIb	Macroscopic peritoneal metastasis beyond pelvis 2 cm or less in greatest dimension
T3c	IIIc	Peritoneal metastasis beyond pelvis more than 2 cm in greatest or N1 dimension or regional lymph node metastasis

Lymph Node (N)

NX	Regional lymph nodes cannot be assessed
N0	No regional lymph node metastasis
N1	Regional lymph node metastasis

Distant Metastasis (M)

TNM	FIGO	DEFINITION
MX		Presence of distant metastasis cannot be assessed
M0		No distant metastasis
M1	IV	Distant metastasis (excludes peritoneal metastasis)

[a]FIGO, Fédération Internationale de Gynécologie et d'Obstétrique.

[b]Note: Liver capsule metastasis is T3/stage III, liver parenchymal metastasis M1/stage IV. Pleural effusion must have positive cytology for M1/stage IV.

Appendix: Reference Tables

Table 1. TNM Classification (continued)

UTERUS

TNM	FIGO[a]	DEFINITION
Primary Tumor (T)		
TX		Primary tumor cannot be assessed
T0		No evidence of primary tumor
Tis	0	Carcinoma in situ
T1	I	Tumor confined to corpus
T1a	Ia	Uterine cavity 8 cm or less in length
T1b	Ib	Uterine cavity more than 8 cm in length
T2	II	Tumor invades cervix but does not extend beyond uterus
T3	III	Tumor extends beyond uterus but not outside true pelvis
T4[b]	IVa	Tumor invades mucosa of bladder or rectum or extends beyond the true pelvis
Lymph Node (N)		
NX		Regional lymph nodes cannot be assessed
N0		No regional lymph node metastasis
N1		Regional lymph node metastasis
Distant Metastasis (M)		
MX		Presence of distant metastasis cannot be assessed
M0		No distant metastasis
M1	IVb	Distant metastasis

[a]FIGO, Fédération Internationale de Gynécologie et d'Obstétrique.

[b]Note: The presence of bullous edema is not sufficient evidence to classify a tumor as T4.

PROSTATE

TNM		AMERICAN UROLOGICAL ASSOCIATION (A-D)	
T0	No evidence of primary tumor	Stage A	No palpable lesion
T1a	Three or fewer microscopic foci of carcinoma	A1	Focal
T1b	More than three microscopic foci of carcinoma	A2	Diffuse
T1c	No palpable tumor, diagnosed by elevated PSA		
T2	Tumor present clinically or grossly, limited to the gland	Stage B	Confined to prostate
T2a	Tumor 1.5 cm or less in greatest dimension, with normal tissue on two sides	B1	Small, discrete nodule
T2b	Tumor more than 1.5 cm in greatest dimension or in more than one lobe	B2	Large or multiple nodules or areas
T3	Tumor invades the prostatic apex, or into or beyond the prostatic capsule, bladder neck, or seminal vesicle, but is not fixed	Stage C	Localized to periprostatic area
		C1	No involvement of seminal vesicle, <70 g
T4	Tumor is fixed or invades adjacent structures other than those listed in T3	C2	Involvement of seminal vesicles, >70 g
N1	Metastasis in a single lymph node, 2 cm or less in greatest dimension	Stage D[a]	Metastatic disease
N2	Metastasis in a single lymph node, more than 2 cm but not more than 5 cm in greatest dimension, or multiple lymph nodes, none more than 5 cm in greatest dimension	D1	Pelvic lymph node metastases or ureteral obstruction causing hydronephrosis
N3	Metastasis in a lymph node more than 5 cm in greatest dimension	D2	Bone or distant lymph node or organ or soft-tissue metastases
M1	Distant metastasis		

[a]"Informal" Definitions: D0, only increased markers (no radiographic evidence of metastasis); D1.5, rising PSA after failed local therapy; D2.5, increasing PSA after nadir; D3, hormone refractory disease; D3.5, normally sensitive; D4, normally insensitive.

PENIS

TNM	DEFINITION

Primary Tumor (T)

TX Primary tumor cannot be assessed
T0 No evidence of primary tumor
Tis Carcinoma in situ
Ta Noninvasive verrucous carcinoma
T1 Tumor invades subepithelial connective tissue
T2 Tumor invades corpus spongiosum or cavernosum
T3 Tumor invades urethra or prostate
T4 Tumor invades other adjacent structures

Lymph Node (N)

NX Regional lymph nodes cannot be assessed
N0 No regional lymph node metastasis
N1 Metastasis in a single superficial inguinal lymph node
N2 Metastasis in multiple or bilateral superficial inguinal lymph nodes
N3 Metastasis in deep inguinal or pelvic lymph node(s), unilateral or bilateral

Distant Metastasis (M)

MX Distant metastasis cannot be assessed
M0 No distant metastasis
M1 Distant metastasis

TESTES

TNM	DEFINITION

Primary Tumor (T)

TX Primary tumor cannot be assessed (if no radical orchiectomy has been performed, TX is used)
T0 No evidence of primary tumor
Tis Intratubular germ cell neoplasia (carcinoma in situ)
T1 Tumor limited to testis and epididymis without vascular/lymphatic invasion; tumor may invade tunica albuginea, but not tunica vaginalis
T2 Tumor limited to testis and epididymis with vascular/lymphatic invasion, or tumor extending through tunica albuginea with involvement of tunica vaginalis
T3 Tumor invades spermatic cord with or without vascular/lymphatic invasion
T4 Tumor invades scrotum with or without vascular/lymphatic invasion

Lymph Node (N)

NX Regional lymph nodes cannot be assessed
N0 No regional lymph node metastasis
N1 Metastasis with a lymph node mass 2 cm or less in greatest dimension or multiple lymph nodes, none more than 2 cm in greatest dimension
N2 Metastasis with a lymph node mass more than 2 cm but not more than 5 cm in greatest dimension, or multiple lymph nodes, any one mass more than 2 cm but not more than 5 cm in greatest dimension
N3 Metastasis with a lymph node mass more than 5 cm in greatest dimension

Distant Metastasis (M)

MX Distant metastasis cannot be assessed
M0 No distant metastasis
M1 Distant metastasis
M1a Nonregional lymph node or pulmonary metastasis
M1b Distant metastasis other than to nonregional lymph nodes and lungs
*Note: Regional lymph nodes are considered the periaortic, preaortic, interaortocaval, paracaval, precaval, retrocaval, and retroaortic nodes.

Serum Tumor Markers (S)

SX Serum marker studies not available or not performed
S0 Serum marker study levels within normal limits

	LDH		hCG (mIU/mL)		AFP (ng/mL)
S1	$<1.5 \times N$	and	<5000	and	<1000
S2	$1.5–10.0 \times N$	or	$5000–50,000$	or	$1000–10,000$
S3	$>10 \times N$	or	$>50,000$	or	$>10,000$

Where N designates the upper limit of normal for the LDH assay

Appendix: Reference Tables

Table 1. TNM Classification (continued)

RENAL PELVIS AND URETER

TNM	DEFINITION

Primary Tumor (T)

TX	Primary tumor cannot be assessed
T0	No evidence of primary tumor
Ta	Noninvasive papillary carcinoma
Tis	Carcinoma in situ
T1	Tumor invades subepithelial connective tissue
T2	Tumor invades muscularis
T3	(Renal pelvis) Tumor invades beyond muscularis into peripelvic fat or renal parenchyma
	(Ureter) Tumor invades beyond muscularis into periureteric fat
T4	Tumor invades adjacent organs or through the kidney into perinephric fat

Lymph Node (N)

NX	Regional lymph nodes cannot be assessed
N0	No regional lymph node metastasis
N1	Metastasis in a single lymph node 2 cm or less in greatest dimension
N2	Metastasis in a single lymph node more than 2 cm but not more than 5 cm in greatest dimension, or multiple lymph nodes, none more than 5 cm in greatest dimension
N3	Metastasis in a lymph node more than 5 cm in greatest dimension

Distant Metastasis (M)

MX	Distant metastasis cannot be assessed
M0	No distant metastasis
M1	Distant metastasis

URETHRA

TNM	DEFINITION

Primary Tumor (T)

TX	Primary tumor cannot be assessed
T0	No evidence of primary tumor

Urethra (male and female)

Ta	Noninvasive papillary, polypoid, or verrucous carcinoma
Tis	Carcinoma in situ
T1	Tumor invades subepithelial connective tissue
T2	Tumor invades any of the following: corpus spongiosum, prostate, periurethral muscle
T3	Tumor invades any of the following: corpus cavernosum, beyond the prostatic capsule, anterior vagina, bladder neck
T4	Tumor invades other adjacent organs

Transitional Cell Carcinoma of Prostate (prostatic urethra)

Tis pu	Carcinoma in situ, involvement of the prostatic urethra
Tis pd	Carcinoma in situ, involvement of the prostatic ducts
T1	Tumor invades subepithelial connective tissue
T2	Tumor invades any of the following: prostatic stroma, corpus spongiosum, periurethral muscle
T3	Tumor invades any of the following: corpus cavernosum, beyond the prostatic capsule, bladder neck (extraprostatic extension)
T4	Tumor invades other adjacent organs (invasion of the bladder)

Lymph Nodes (N)

NX	Regional lymph nodes cannot be assessed
N0	No regional lymph node metastasis
N1	Metastasis in a single lymph node 2 cm or less in greatest dimension
N2	Metastasis in a single lymph node more than 2 cm in greatest dimension, or multiple lymph nodes

Distant Metastasis (M)

MX	Distant metastasis cannot be assessed
M0	No distant metastasis
M1	Distant metastasis

Fleming ID, Cooper JS, Henson DE, et al., eds. *AJCC Cancer Staging Manual.* Philadelphia: Lippincott, 1997.

Table 2. AUA Symptoms Score (See Section III, page 625, for Additional Information)

	NOT AT ALL	LESS THAN 1 TIME IN 5	LESS THAN HALF THE TIME	ABOUT HALF THE TIME	MORE THAN HALF THE TIME	ALMOST ALWAYS	YOUR SCORE
1. Incomplete emptying Over the past month, how often have you had a sensation of not emptying your bladder completely after you finished urinating?	0	1	2	3	4	5	
2. Frequency Over the past month, how often have you had to urinate again less than two hours after you finished urinating?	0	1	2	3	4	5	
3. Intermittency Over the past month, how often have you found you stopped and started again several times when you urinated?	0	1	2	3	4	5	
4. Urgency Over the past month, how often have you found it difficult to postpone urination?	0	1	2	3	4	5	
5. Weak Stream Over the past month, how often have you had a weak urinary stream?	0	1	2	3	4	5	
6. Straining Over the past month, how often have you had to push or strain to begin urination?	0	1	2	3	4	5	

	NONE	1 TIME	2 TIMES	3 TIMES	4 TIMES	5 TIMES OR MORE	
7. Nocturia Over the past month, how many times did you most typically get up to urinate from the time you went to bed at night until the time you got up in the morning?	0	1	2	3	4	5	

Total I-PSS Score

QUALITY OF LIFE DUE TO URINARY SYMPTOMS	DELIGHTED	PLEASED	MOSTLY SATISFIED	MIXED—ABOUT EQUALLY SATISFIED AND DISSATISFIED	MOST DISSATISFIED	UNHAPPY	TERRIBLE
If you were to spend the rest of your life with your urinary condition just the way it is now, how would you feel about that?	0	1	2	3	4	5	6

The International Prostate Symptom Score (I-PSS) is based on the answers to seven questions concerning urinary symptoms. Each question allows the patient to choose one of five answers indicating increasing severity of the particular symptom. The answers are assigned points from 0 to 5. The total score can therefore range from 0 to 35 (asymptomatic to very symptomatic). Furthermore, the International Scientific Committee (SCI) recommends the use of only a single question to assess the quality of life. The answers to this question range from "delighted" to "terrible" or 0 to 6. Although this single question may or may not capture the global impact of benign prostatic hyperplasia (BPH) symptoms or quality of life, it may serve as a valuable starting point for a doctor-patient conversation.

The SCI strongly recommends that all physicians who counsel patients suffering from symptoms of prostatism utilize these measures not only during the initial interview but also during and after treatment in order to monitor treatment response.

The SCI, under the patronage of the World Health Organization (WHO) and the International Union Against Cancer (UICC), has agreed to use the symptom index for BPH, which has been developed by the American Urological Association (AUA) Measurement Committee, as the official worldwide symptoms assessment tool for patients suffering from prostatism.

(With permission from Merck Pharmaceuticals, "International Prostate Symptom Score, 983703(1)-07-PRO.)

Table 3. Partin Tables (See Section III, page 678, for Additional Information)

Nomogram for Prediction of Final Pathological Stage[1]

GLEASON SCORE	PSA 0.0-4.0 ng/mL CLINICAL STAGE							PSA 4.1-10.0 ng/mL CLINICAL STAGE							PSA 10.1-20.0 ng/mL CLINICAL STAGE							PSA >20.0 ng/mL CLINICAL STAGE						
	T1a	T1b	T1c	T2a	T2b	T2c	T3a	T1a	T1b	T1c	T2a	T2b	T2c	T3a	T1a	T1b	T1c	T2a	T2b	T2c	T3a	T1a	T1b	T1c	T2a	T2b	T2c	T3a
Organ-Confined Disease																												
2-4	90	80	89	81	72	77	—	84	70	83	71	61	66	43	76	58	75	60	48	53	—	—	38	58	41	29	—	—
5	82	66	81	68	57	62	40	72	53	71	55	43	49	27	61	40	60	43	32	36	18	—	23	40	26	17	19	8
6	78	61	78	64	52	57	35	67	47	67	51	38	43	23	—	33	55	38	26	31	14	—	17	35	22	13	15	6
7	—	43	63	47	34	38	19	49	29	49	33	22	25	11	33	17	35	22	13	15	6	—	—	18	10	5	6	2
8-10	—	31	52	36	24	27	—	35	18	37	23	14	15	6	—	9	23	14	7	8	3	—	3	10	5	3	3	1
Established Capsular Penetration																												
2-4	9	19	10	18	25	21	—	14	27	15	26	35	29	44	20	36	22	35	43	37	—	—	47	34	48	52	—	—
5	17	32	18	30	40	34	51	25	42	27	41	50	43	57	33	50	35	50	57	51	59	—	57	48	60	61	55	54
6	19	35	21	34	43	37	53	27	44	30	44	52	46	57	—	49	38	52	57	50	54	—	51	49	60	57	51	46
7	—	44	31	45	51	45	52	36	48	40	52	54	48	48	38	46	45	55	51	45	40	—	—	46	51	43	37	2
8-10	—	43	34	47	48	42	—	34	42	40	49	46	40	34	—	33	40	46	38	33	26	—	24	34	37	28	23	17
Seminal Vesicle Involvement																												
2-4	0	1	1	1	2	2	—	1	2	1	2	4	5	10	2	4	2	4	7	8	—	—	9	7	10	14	—	—
5	1	2	1	2	3	3	7	2	3	2	3	5	6	12	3	5	3	5	8	9	15	—	10	9	11	15	19	26
6	1	2	1	2	3	4	7	2	3	2	3	5	6	11	—	4	4	5	7	9	14	—	8	8	10	13	17	21
7	—	6	4	6	10	12	19	6	9	8	10	15	18	26	8	11	12	14	18	22	28	—	—	22	24	27	32	36
8-10	—	11	9	12	17	21	—	10	15	15	19	24	28	35	—	15	20	22	25	30	34	—	20	31	33	33	38	40
Lymph Node Involvement																												
2-4	0	0	0	0	0	0	—	0	1	0	0	1	1	1	0	2	0	1	1	1	—	—	4	1	1	3	—	—
5	0	1	0	0	1	1	2	1	2	0	1	2	2	3	3	5	1	2	4	4	7	—	10	3	3	7	7	11
6	1	2	0	1	2	2	5	3	5	1	2	4	4	9	—	13	3	4	10	10	18	—	23	7	8	16	17	26
7	—	6	1	2	5	5	9	8	12	3	4	9	9	15	18	24	8	9	17	18	26	—	—	14	14	25	25	32
8-10	—	14	4	5	10	10	—	18	23	8	9	16	17	24	—	40	16	17	29	29	37	—	51	24	24	36	35	42

[1]Numbers represent the percent predictive probability (95% confidence interval) of the patient having a given final pathological stage based on a multinomial log-linear regression of all 3 variables combined.

How to Use the Nomogram

1. Select a clinical stage by the TNM classification system

TNM STAGE	DESCRIPTION	WHITMORE-JEWETT STAGE	DESCRIPTION
T1a	Nonpalpable, with 5% or less of resected tissue with cancer, low grade	A1	Same as TNM
T1b	Nonpalable, with greater than 5% of resected tissue with cancer and/or high grade	A2	Same as TNM
T1c	Nonpalpable, but serum PSA elevated	B0	Same as TNM
T2a	Palpable, half of 1 lobe or less	B1N	Palpable, less than 1 lobe, surrounded by normal tissue
T2b	Palpable, greater than half of 1 lobe but not both lobes	B1	Palpable, less than 1 lobe
T2c	Palpable, involves both lobes	B2	Palpable, 1 entire lobe or mroe
T3a	Palpable, unilateral, capsular penetration	C1	Palpable, outside capsule, not into seminal vesicles

2. Select a serum PSA level, using a monoclonal assay

3. Select a Gleason score

The nomogram will predict the final pathological stage based on a multinomial log-linear regression of all three variables combined.

For example:
With a stage T2a, PSA 14, Gleason score 6, the nomogram calculates:

Percent probability of organ-confined disease:	38%
Percent probability of capsular penetration:	52%
Percent probability of seminal vesicle involvement:	5%
Percent probability of lymph node involvement:	4%

(With permission from TAP Pharmaceuticals, "Nomogram for Prediction of Final Pathological Stage.")

Table 4. Catheter Sizing Guide

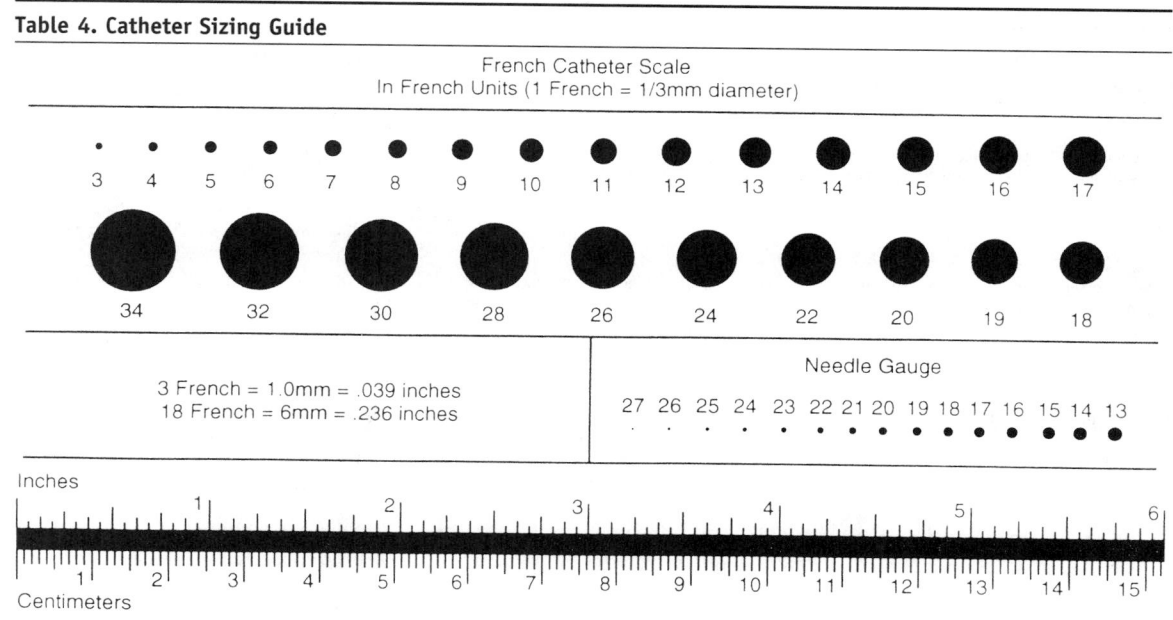

French Catheter Scale
In French Units (1 French = 1/3mm diameter)

3 4 5 6 7 8 9 10 11 12 13 14 15 16 17

34   32   30   28   26   24   22   20   19   18

3 French = 1.0mm = .039 inches
18 French = 6mm = .236 inches

Needle Gauge

27 26 25 24 23 22 21 20 19 18 17 16 15 14 13

Inches

Centimeters

Appendix: Reference Tables

Table 5. Sex Function Survey

Individual items of International Index of Erectile Function Questionnaire and response options (US version). For additional information, see Section III, "Sex Function Survey."

QUESTION*	_RESPONSE OPTIONS_
Q1: How often were you able to get an erection during sexual activity? **Q2:** When you had erections with sexual stimulation, how often were your erections hard enough for penetration?	0 = No sexual activity 1 = Almost never/never 2 = A few times (much less than half the time) 3 = Sometimes (about half the time) 4 = Most times (much more than half the time) 5 = Almost always/always
Q3: When you attempted sexual intercourse, how often were you able to penetrate (enter) your partner? **Q4:** During sexual intercourse, _how often_ were you able to maintain your erection after you had penetrated (entered) your partner?	0 = Did not attempt intercourse 1 = Almost never/never 2 = A few times (much less than half the time) 3 = Sometimes (about half the time) 4 = Most times (much more than half the time) 5 = Almost always/always
Q5: During sexual intercourse, _how difficult_ was it to maintain your erection to completion of intercourse?	0 = Did not attempt intercourse 1 = Extremely difficult 2 = Very difficult 3 = Difficult 4 = Slightly difficult 5 = Not difficult
Q6: How many times have you attempted sexual intercourse?	0 = No attempts 1 = One to two attempts 2 = Three to four attempts 3 = Five to six attempts 4 = Seven to ten attempts 5 = Eleven+ attempts
Q7: When you attempted sexual intercourse, how often was it satisfactory for you?	0 = Did not attempt intercourse 1 = Almost never/never 2 = A few times (much less than half the time) 3 = Sometimes (about half the time) 4 = Most times (much more than half the time) 5 = Almost always/always
Q8: How much have you enjoyed sexual intercourse?	0 = No intercourse 1 = No enjoyment 2 = Not very enjoyable 3 = Fairly enjoyable 4 = Highly enjoyable 5 = Very highly enjoyable
Q9: When you had sexual stimulation _or_ intercourse, how often did you ejaculate? **Q10:** When you had sexual stimulation _or_ intercourse, how often did you have the feeling of orgasm or climax?	0 = No sexual stimulation/intercourse 1 = Almost never/never 2 = A few times (much less than half the time) 3 = Sometimes (about half the time) 4 = Most times (much more than half the time) 5 = Almost always/always
Q11: How often have you felt sexual desire?	1 = Almost never/never 2 = A few times (much less than half the time) 3 = Sometimes (about half the time) 4 = Most times (much more than half the time) 5 = Almost always/always
Q12: How would you rate your level of sexual desire?	1 = Very low/none at all 2 = Low 3 = Moderate 4 = High 5 = Very high
Q13: How satisfied have you been with your overall _sex life_? **Q14:** How satisfied have you been with your _sexual relationship_ with your partner?	1 = Very dissatisfied 2 = Moderately dissatisfied 3 = About equally satisfied and dissatisfied 4 = Moderately satisfied 5 = Very satisfied
Q15: How do you rate your _confidence_ that you could get and keep an erection?	1 = Very low 2 = Low 3 = Moderate 4 = High 5 = Very high

*All questions are preceded by the phrase "Over the past 4 weeks."

Reproduced with permission from Rosen RC, Riley A, Wagner G, Osterloh J, Kirkpatrick J, Mishra A. I: The international index of erectile function (IIEF): A multidimensional scale for assessment of erectile dysfunction. _Urology_ 1997;49:822–830.

Index

Page numbers in boldface indicate major discussion.

Index

Index

Index

Index

Index

Index